D1688092

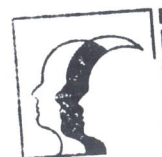

DIAGNOSTIC IMAGING
NUCLEAR MEDICINE

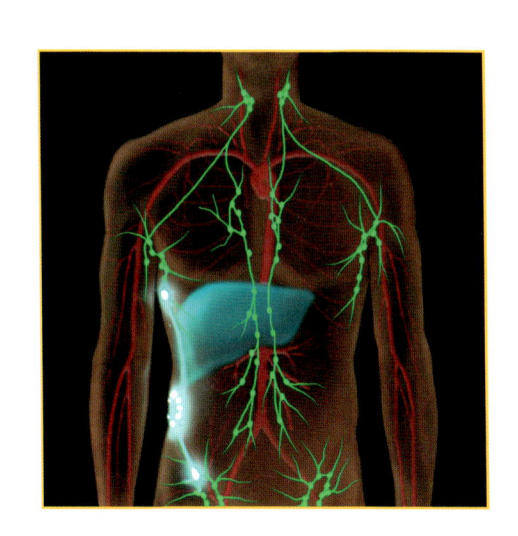

DIAGNOSTIC IMAGING
NUCLEAR MEDICINE

Kathryn A. Morton, MD
Professor of Radiology
University of Utah School of Medicine
Salt Lake City, Utah

Paige B. Clark, MD
Assistant Professor of Nuclear Medicine
Department of Radiology
Wake Forest University Health Sciences
Winston-Salem, North Carolina

Todd M. Blodgett, MD
Chief of Cancer Imaging
Department of Radiology
University of Pittsburgh Medical Center
Pittsburgh, Pennsylvania

Carl R. Christensen, MD
Assistant Professor of Radiology
University of Utah School of Medicine
Salt Lake City, Utah

Janis P. O'Malley, MD
Associate Professor of Radiology
Director of Nuclear Medicine and Clinical PET
University of Alabama
Birmingham, Alabama

Jeffrey S. Stevens, MD
Associate Professor of Radiology
Director of Nuclear Medicine
Oregon Health and Science University
Portland, Oregon

Crispin A. Chinn, MD
Director of Nuclear Medicine
Providence St. Vincent Hospital
Portland, Oregon

Alan D. Waxman, MD
Director of Nuclear Medicine
Co-Chair, Department of Imaging
Cedars-Sinai Medical Center
S. Mark Taper Imaging Center

Clinical Professor of Radiology
University of Southern California School of Medicine
Los Angeles, CA

Robert W. Nance, Jr., MD
Assistant Professor Radiology/Nuclear Medicine
Oregon Health and ScienceUniversity
Portland, Oregon

Anita J. Thomas, MD
Assistant Professor of Nuclear Medicine
Department of Radiology
Wake Forest University Health Sciences
Winston-Salem, North Carolina

Ralph Drosten, MD
Assistant Professor of Radiology
University of Utah School of Medicine
Salt Lake City, Utah

Thomas F. Heston, MD
Medical Director
Northwest Molecular
Kellogg, Idaho

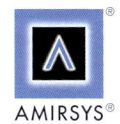

AMIRSYS®
Names you know, content you trust®

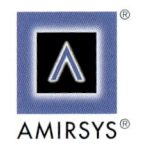

AMIRSYS®
Names you know, content you trust®

First Edition

Text and Radiologic Images - Copyright © 2007 Todd M. Blodgett, MD, Crispin A. Chinn, MD, Carl R. Christensen, MD, Paige B. Clark, MD, Ralph Drosten, MD, Thomas F. Heston, MD, Kathryn A. Morton, MD, Robert W. Nance, Jr., MD, Janis P. O'Malley, MD, Jeffrey S. Stevens, MD, Anita J. Thomas, MD, Alan D. Waxman, MD

Drawings - Copyright © 2007 Amirsys Inc.

Compilation - Copyright © 2007 Amirsys Inc.

All rights reserved. No part of this publication may be reproduced, stored in a retrieval system, or transmitted, in any form or media or by any means, electronic, mechanical, photocopying, recording, or otherwise, without prior written permission from Amirsys Inc.

Composition by Amirsys Inc, Salt Lake City, Utah

Printed in Canada by Friesens, Altona, Manitoba, Canada

ISBN-13: 978-1-4160-3339-4
ISBN-10: 1-4160-3339-4
ISBN-13: 978-0-8089-2382-4 (International English Edition)
ISBN-10: 0-8089-2382-X (International English Edition)

Notice and Disclaimer

The information in this product ("Product") is provided as a reference for use by licensed medical professionals and no others. It does not and should not be construed as any form of medical diagnosis or professional medical advice on any matter. Receipt or use of this Product, in whole or in part, does not constitute or create a doctor-patient, therapist-patient, or other healthcare professional relationship between Amirsys Inc. ("Amirsys") and any recipient. This Product may not reflect the most current medical developments, and Amirsys makes no claims, promises, or guarantees about accuracy, completeness, or adequacy of the information contained in or linked to the Product. The Product is not a substitute for or replacement of professional medical judgment. Amirsys and its affiliates, authors, contributors, partners, and sponsors disclaim all liability or responsibility for any injury and/or damage to persons or property in respect to actions taken or not taken based on any and all Product information.

In the cases where drugs or other chemicals are prescribed, readers are advised to check the Product information currently provided by the manufacturer of each drug to be administered to verify the recommended dose, the method and duration of administration, and contraindications. It is the responsibility of the treating physician relying on experience and knowledge of the patient to determine dosages and the best treatment for the patient.

To the maximum extent permitted by applicable law, Amirsys provides the Product AS IS AND WITH ALL FAULTS, AND HEREBY DISCLAIMS ALL WARRANTIES AND CONDITIONS, WHETHER EXPRESS, IMPLIED OR STATUTORY, INCLUDING BUT NOT LIMITED TO, ANY (IF ANY) IMPLIED WARRANTIES OR CONDITIONS OF MERCHANTABILITY, OF FITNESS FOR A PARTICULAR PURPOSE, OF LACK OF VIRUSES, OR ACCURACY OR COMPLETENESS OF RESPONSES, OR RESULTS, AND OF LACK OF NEGLIGENCE OR LACK OF WORKMANLIKE EFFORT. ALSO, THERE IS NO WARRANTY OR CONDITION OF TITLE, QUIET ENJOYMENT, QUIET POSSESSION, CORRESPONDENCE TO DESCRIPTION OR NON-INFRINGEMENT, WITH REGARD TO THE PRODUCT. THE ENTIRE RISK AS TO THE QUALITY OF OR ARISING OUT OF USE OR PERFORMANCE OF THE PRODUCT REMAINS WITH THE READER.

Amirsys disclaims all warranties of any kind if the Product was customized, repackaged or altered in any way by any third party.

Library of Congress Cataloging-in-Publication Data

Diagnostic imaging nuclear medicine / [edited by] Kathryn A. Morton, Paige B. Clark. — 1st ed.
  p. ; cm.
 Includes bibliographical references.
 ISBN-13: 978-1-4160-3339-4
 ISBN-10: 1-4160-3339-4
 ISBN-13: 978-0-8089-2382-4 (international English ed.)
 ISBN-10: 0-8089-2382-X (international English ed.)
 1. Diagnostic imaging—Handbooks, manuals, etc. 2. Nuclear medicine—Handbooks, manuals, etc. I. Morton, Kathryn A. II. Clark, Paige B.
  [DNLM: 1. Diagnostic Imaging—methods—Handbooks. 2. Nuclear Medicine—methods—Handbooks. 3. Radiopharmaceuticals—Handbooks. WN 39 D5359 2007]
 RC78.7.D53D5282 2007
 616.07'57—dc22

2007035165

To my husband, Mike Poler. His unfailing support and
encouragement made this book possible.
KAM

For my family.
PBC

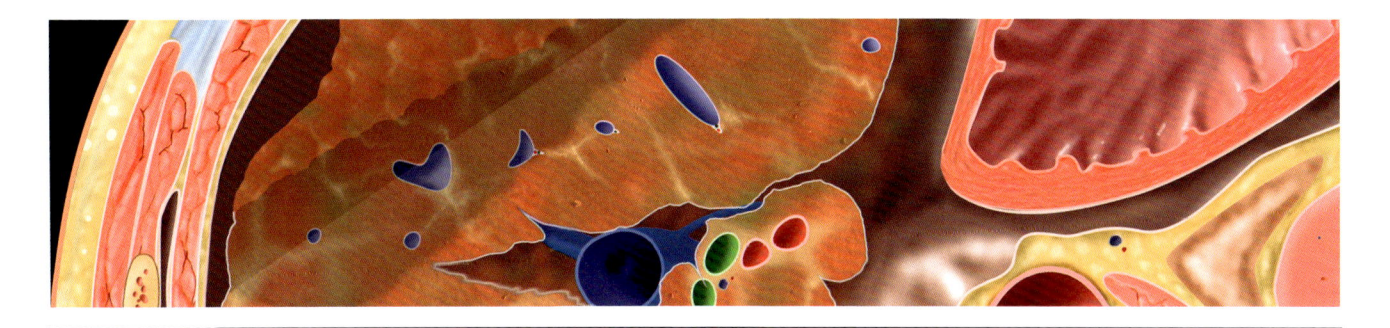

DIAGNOSTIC IMAGING: NUCLEAR MEDICINE

We at Amirsys and Elsevier are proud to present **Diagnostic Imaging: Nuclear Medicine**, the thirteenth volume in our acclaimed Diagnostic Imaging (DI) series. We began this precedent-setting, image- and graphic-rich series with David Stoller's Diagnostic Imaging: Orthopaedics. The next volumes, DI: Brain, DI: Head and Neck, DI: Abdomen, DI: Spine, DI: Pediatrics, DI: Obstetrics, DI: Chest, DI: Breast, DI: Ultrasound, DI: Pediatric Neuroradiology and DI: Emergency are now joined by Kathryn Morton and Paige Clark's fabulous new textbook, DI: Nuclear Medicine.

Nuclear medicine is an integral part of diagnostic imaging, yet it is relatively unfamiliar territory to many general and subspecialty radiologists. The application of exciting new techniques such as PET/CT have brought nuclear medicine squarely to the forefront in cancer imaging. We are thrilled to have Morton and Clark's DI: Nuclear Medicine join the Amirsys "family" of imaging textbooks. They have done a superb job in bringing together standard imaging techniques such as high-resolution CT, MR and ultrasound and correlating them with the most-up-to-date nuclear medicine scans available. Because the DI series is printed with glorious full four-color illustrations throughout each book, studies such as SPECT and fused FDG PET/CT can be shown in all their magnificence. DI: Nuclear Medicine is a feast for the eye as well as the intellect! Just look at the superb chapter on seizure evaluation as an example.

As always, the unique bulleted format of the DI series allows our authors to present approximately twice the information and four times the images per diagnosis compared to the old-fashioned traditional prose textbook. All DI books follow the same format, which means that our many readers find the same information in the same place—every time! And in every body part! Our innovative visual differential diagnosis "thumbnail" provides you with an at-a-glance look at entities that can mimic the diagnosis in question and has been highly popular (and much imitated). For example, the chapter on Metastases to the Lungs and Mediastinum shows beautiful images of sarcoidosis, reactivated tuberculosis, and normal thymus in its differential diagnosis image gallery. The DDx gallery for Alzheimer Disease shows FDG PET in normal pressure hydrocephalus, Lewy body disease, and stroke. How great is that??!!

In summary, **Diagnostic Imaging: Nuclear Medicine** is a product designed with you, the reader, in mind. The old, worn-out joke about "unclear medicine" should be retired. **Diagnostic Imaging: Nuclear Medicine** makes this fascinating, burgeoning field clear and vibrant to both subspecialty experts and general radiologists alike. We think you'll find this new volume a highly efficient and wonderfully rich resource that will significantly enhance your practice—and find a welcome place on your bookshelf. Enjoy!

Anne G. Osborn, MD
Executive Vice President & Editor-in-Chief, Amirsys, Inc.

H. Ric Harnsberger, MD
CEO & Chairman, Amirsys, Inc.

Paula J. Woodward, MD
Senior Vice President & Medical Director, Amirsys, Inc.

B.J. Manaster, MD
Vice President & Associate Medical Director, Amirsys, Inc.

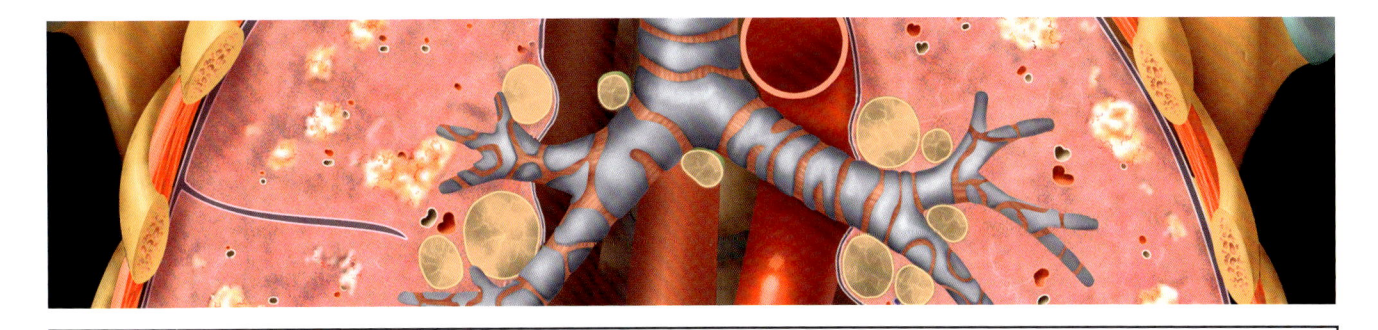

FOREWORD

Diagnostic Imaging: Nuclear Medicine is organized and edited in the popular format used for other books in this series. The lead author, Dr. Morton is unusual in that she is both an excellent radiologist and an outstanding clinical nuclear medicine physician. She is also well recognized and respected in the nuclear medicine research community. Dr. Clark is a vibrant rising star in the nuclear medicine field, both in clinical expertise as well as research. The contributing authors represent a well-balanced cadre of some of the most experienced and respected names in nuclear medicine today, as well as experts with strong multi-modality perspectives in diagnostic imaging. Together, they are an unbeatable team.

The authors have succeeded in presenting a well-balanced and fair appraisal of the best imaging approach to a vast array of common and not-so-common clinical problems that face diagnostic imagers in nuclear medicine. The book defines the appropriate role of nuclear medicine in the context of other powerful imaging modalities today. This includes important protocol information to allow optimization of a "best practice" imaging approach to specific problems. Hundreds of superb well-reproduced images and graphic illustrations are included, a hallmark of the Diagnostic Imaging series. Important clinical information regarding the diseases addressed is also included. The general organization is spare and direct in its bulleted format, with key points highlighted, making this a quick and easy reference for the practicing radiologist, nuclear medicine practitioner, as well as clinicians. Diagnostic Imaging: Nuclear Medicine should withstand the test of time as well-worn addition to any radiology reading room.

Edward V. Staab, MD
Professor of Nuclear Medicine
Department of Radiology
Wake Forest University Health Sciences
Winston-Salem, North Carolina

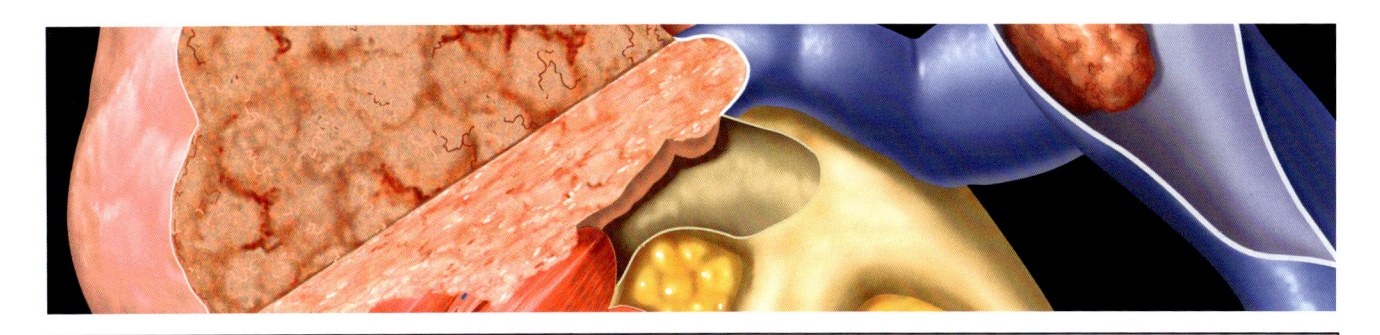

PREFACE

There are many outstanding radiology text books available today, addressing both general radiology as well as specific imaging subspecialties. In the face of literally hundreds of available text books, the Amirsys Diagnostic Imaging series has risen rapidly in popularity as one of the best selling imaging text book series of all time. Diagnostic Imaging: Nuclear Medicine rounds out this series, focusing on conventional nuclear medicine imaging, PET and PET/CT, radionuclide therapy, and the more commonly used in-vitro diagnostic determinations. We have strived to fill an un-met need in providing a quick and practical guide for radiologists and nuclear medicine physicians "in the trenches". The bulleted format is easy to digest and conveys clinically relevant information concisely and rapidly, providing a real-time reference for the reading room. The hundreds of images included are clear and convey typical and atypical examples of specific diagnoses, as well as "mimics" and potential pitfalls that complicate diagnostic accuracy.

This book is comprehensive in that it addresses the most common nuclear medicine diagnoses encountered in daily practice, as well those with which most imagers have less experience. The book provides thorough and concise information regarding nuclear medicine diagnostic and therapeutic procedures, including appropriate study selection, protocol advice and interpretive guidance. It also summarizes the key findings shown by CT, MR, ultrasound and other radiographic modalities for each diagnosis. Most importantly, it addresses the most appropriate role for nuclear medicine within the framework of all imaging modalities and options available to answer a specific clinical question, without hype or subspecialty bias. In short, this nuclear medicine book is practical, accessible and in-touch with the realities of multimodality diagnostic imaging.

Kathryn A. Morton, MD
Professor of Radiology
University of Utah School of Medicine
Salt Lake City, Utah

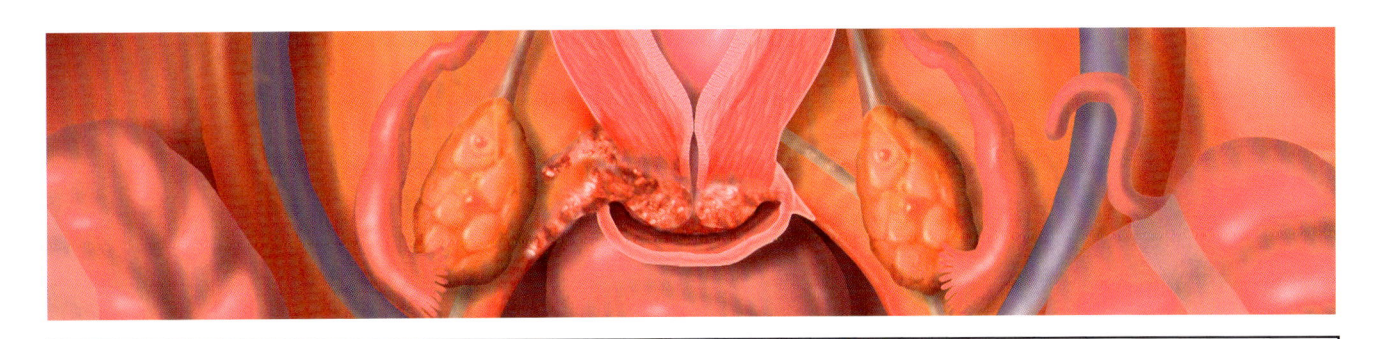

ACKNOWLEDGMENTS

Illustrations
Richard Coombs, MS
James A. Cooper, MD
Lane R. Bennion, MS

Image/Text Editing
Douglas Grant Jackson
Amanda Hurtado
Christopher Odekirk

Medical Text Editing
Edward V. Staab, MD

Associate Editor
Kaerli Main

Production Lead
Melissa A. Hoopes

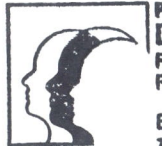

PRAXIS
DR. MED. BORIS KIRSCHSIEPER
FACHARZT FÜR NUKLEARMEDIZIN
FACHARZT FÜR DIAGNOSTISCHE RADIOLOGIE

BALGER STRASSE 50   TEL: (07221) 91 27 94
79532 BADEN-BADEN   FAX: (07221) 91 27 98

WEB: WWW.PRAXIS-KIRSCHSIEPER.DE
E-MAIL: INFO@PRAXIS-KIRSCHSIEPER.DE

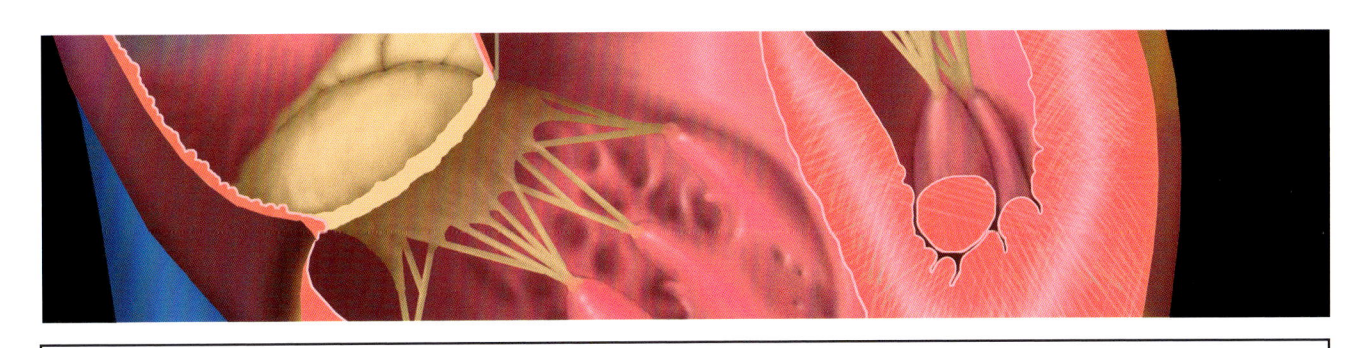

SECTIONS

Musculoskeletal 1

Vascular and Lymphatics 2

Cardiovascular 3

Chest and Mediastinum 4

CNS 5

Head and Neck 6

Thyroid/Parathyroid 7

Gastrointestinal 8

Genitourinary 9

HemeOnc Procedures & Therapies 10

Oncology, Other 11

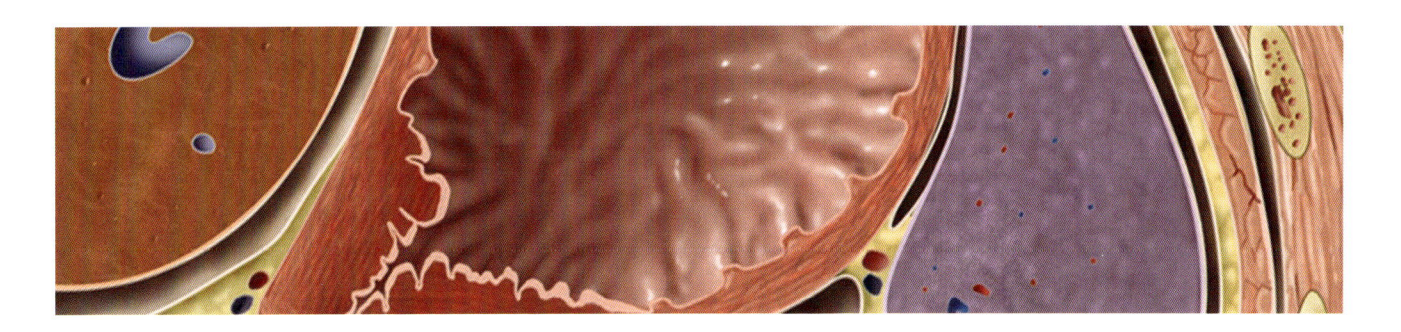

TABLE OF CONTENTS

SECTION 1
Musculoskeletal

Benign Bone Tumors

Osteoid Osteoma *Anita J. Thomas, MD*	1-2
Enchondroma *Robert W. Nance, Jr., MD*	1-6
Fibrous Cortical Defect *Robert W. Nance, Jr., MD*	1-8
Bone Cyst, Aneurysmal *Robert W. Nance, Jr., MD*	1-10
Bone Cyst, Solitary (Unicameral) *Paige B. Clark, MD*	1-12
Giant Cell Tumor *Jeffrey S. Stevens, MD & Kevin J. Limbaugh, MD*	1-16

Malignant Bone Tumors

Skeletal Metastases *Carl R. Christensen, MD*	1-18
Superscan *Carl R. Christensen, MD*	1-24
Osteosarcoma *Alan D. Waxman, MD*	1-28
Ewing Sarcoma *Crispin A. Chinn, MD*	1-34
Chondrosarcoma *Alan D. Waxman, MD & Kathryn A. Morton, MD*	1-38
Prostate Cancer, Bone Metastases *Crispin A. Chinn, MD*	1-42

Therapy

Palliation of Metastatic Bone Pain *Jeffrey S. Stevens, MD & Kevin J. Limbaugh, MD*	1-44

Infection

Cellulitis *Crispin A. Chinn, MD*	1-48
Osteomyelitis, Appendicular *Carl R. Christensen, MD*	1-52
Osteomyelitis, Axial *Paige B. Clark, MD*	1-58
Osteomyelitis, Temporal Bone *Kathryn A. Morton, MD*	1-60
Osteomyelitis, Feet *Anita J. Thomas, MD*	1-62
Osteomyelitis, Pediatric *Carl R. Christensen, MD*	1-66

Metabolic Bone Disease

Hyperparathyroidism *Carl R. Christensen, MD*	1-72
Osteomalacia *Kathryn A. Morton, MD*	1-76
Hypertrophic Osteoarthropathy *Carl R. Christensen, MD*	1-80

Dysplasias

Paget Disease *Janis P. O'Malley, MD*	1-86
Fibrous Dysplasia *Carl R. Christensen, MD*	1-90
Melorheostosis *Janis P. O'Malley, MD*	1-92
Multiple Enchondromatoses *Anita J. Thomas, MD*	1-96
Multiple Hereditary Exostoses *Anita J. Thomas, MD*	1-100

Avascular Necrosis

Osseous Necrosis *Anita J. Thomas, MD*	1-104
Legg-Calve Perthes Disease *Anita J. Thomas, MD*	1-108

Surgical Assessment

Joint Prostheses, Painful *Paige B. Clark, MD*	1-110
Failed Back Surgery Syndrome *Kathryn A. Morton, MD & Eryn Caamano, MD*	1-112

Skeletal Trauma

Insufficiency Fracture *Kathryn A. Morton, MD*	1-118
Fracture *Kathryn A. Morton, MD & Carl R. Christensen, MD*	1-124
Trauma, Non-Accidental *Robert W. Nance, Jr., MD*	1-126
Stress Fracture *Carl R. Christensen, MD*	1-128

Regional Pain Evaluation

Arthritis, Non-Infectious *Carl R. Christensen, MD*	1-132
Complex Regional Pain Syndrome *Paige B. Clark, MD*	1-136
Hip Pain *Anita J. Thomas, MD*	1-140
Wrist Pain *Anita J. Thomas, MD*	1-144
Calcaneal Pain *Paige B. Clark, MD & Laura Noelle Shashy*	1-150
Knee Pain *Paige B. Clark, MD & Andrea M. Davis*	1-154

Skeletal Muscle & Soft Tissues

Heterotopic Ossification *Carl R. Christensen, MD*	1-158
Skeletal Muscle Disorders *Christopher Hanrahan, MD & Kathryn A. Morton, MD*	1-164
Amyloidosis *Carl R. Christensen, MD*	1-168

Bone Marrow Disorders

Hematoproliferative Disorders *Kathryn A. Morton, MD*	1-170
Sickle Cell Disease, Bone Pain *Paige B. Clark, MD & Matthew Mattern, MD*	1-176
Multiple Myeloma *Alan D. Waxman, MD*	1-180

SECTION 2
Vascular and Lymphatics

Lymphatic

Lymphedema *Marte Wasserman, MD*	2-2
Sentinel Lymph Node Mapping *Robert W. Nance, Jr., MD*	2-4

Vascular

Large Vessel Vasculitis *Kathryn A. Morton, MD*	2-8
Atherosclerosis *Kathryn A. Morton, MD*	2-10
Vascular Thrombosis *Kathryn A. Morton, MD*	2-14
Vascular Graft Infection *Kathryn A. Morton, MD*	2-16

SECTION 3
Cardiovascular

Introduction and Overview

Cardiovascular Overview *Paige B. Clark, MD*	3-2

Cardiac

Cardiomyopathy *Thomas F. Heston, MD*	3-6
Valvular Heart Disease *Thomas F. Heston, MD & Carter Newton, MD*	3-12
Myocardial Ischemia *Keiichiro Yoshinaga, MD* *Rob Beanlands, MD & Thomas F. Heston, MD*	3-16
Myocardial Viability *Keiichiro Yoshinaga, MD* *Rob Beanlands, MD & Thomas F. Heston, MD*	3-22
Myocardial Infarction *Keiichiro Yoshinaga, MD* *Rob Beanlands, MD & Thomas F. Heston, MD*	3-26
Cardiac Transplant *Thomas F. Heston, MD*	3-32
Left-to-Right Intracardiac Shunts *Jeffrey S. Stevens, MD & Kevin J. Limbaugh, MD*	3-36
Right-to-Left Intracardiac Shunts *Jeffrey S. Stevens, MD & Kevin J. Limbaugh, MD*	3-38

SECTION 4
Chest and Mediastinum

Introduction and Overview

V/Q Scan Overview *Kathryn A. Morton, MD*	4-2

Lung Ventilation & Perfusion Abnormalities

V/Q, Pulmonary Embolism *Daniel Worsley, MD*	4-6
V/Q, Quantitative *Robert W. Nance, Jr., MD*	4-10

Lung Infection & Inflammation

Pneumocystis Carinii Pneumonia *Alan D. Waxman, MD*	4-16
Interstitial Lung Disease *Kathryn A. Morton, MD*	4-20
Granulomatous Disease *Kathryn A. Morton, MD*	4-24

Lung Cancer

Solitary Pulmonary Nodule 4-28
Ralph Drosten, MD & Alan D. Waxman, MD

Non-Small Cell Lung Cancer 4-32
Ralph Drosten, MD

Metastases, Lungs & Mediastinum 4-38
Ralph Drosten, MD

Pleura

Pleural Disease, Malignant & Inflammatory 4-42
Ralph Drosten, MD

Mediastinum

Thymic Evaluation 4-46
Ralph Drosten, MD

Pericardial Disease, Malignant & Inflammatory 4-50
Ralph Drosten, MD

SECTION 5
CNS

Introduction and Overview

Brain Imaging Overview 5-2
Kathryn A. Morton, MD

Vascular Assessment

Brain Death 5-4
Robert W. Nance, Jr., MD

Cerebral Vascular Occlusion 5-10
Kathryn A. Morton, MD

Blood Brain Barrier Disruption 5-14
Robert W. Nance, Jr., MD

Seizure Assessment

Seizure Evaluation 5-16
Alan D. Waxman, MD

Dementia & Neurodegenerative

Alzheimer Disease 5-22
Alan D. Waxman, MD

Dementia & Neurodegenerative, Other 5-26
Alan D. Waxman, MD & Doug Liou

Neurooncology

Gliomas & Astrocytomas 5-32
Todd M. Blodgett, MD & Alex Ryan, MD

Primary CNS Lymphoma 5-36
Marte Wasserman, MD

Metastases, Brain 5-40
Paige B. Clark, MD

Radiation Necrosis vs. Recurrent Tumor 5-44
Kathryn A. Morton, MD

CSF Imaging

CSF Leak 5-50
Jeffrey S. Stevens, MD & Kevin J. Limbaugh, MD

Ventricular Shunt Dysfunction 5-54
Kathryn A. Morton, MD

Normal Pressure Hydrocephalus 5-58
Kathryn A. Morton, MD

Miscellaneous

Heterotopic Gray Matter 5-64
Kathryn A. Morton, MD

Brain Infection & Inflammation 5-70
Kathryn A. Morton, MD

Psychiatry, Drug Addiction & Forensics 5-74
Jeffrey S. Stevens, MD & Kevin J. Limbaugh, MD

SECTION 6
Head and Neck

Squamous Cell Carcinoma of the Head and Neck

SCCHN, Staging 6-2
Todd M. Blodgett, MD & Alex Ryan, MD

SCCHN, Primary Unknown 6-6
Todd M. Blodgett, MD & Alex Ryan, MD

SCCHN, Therapeutic Assessment/Restaging 6-8
Todd M. Blodgett, MD & Alex Ryan, MD

Miscellaneous Primary Head and Neck Tumors

Parotid and Salivary Tumors 6-12
Todd M. Blodgett, MD & Alex Ryan, MD

Neuroendocrine Tumors, Head & Neck 6-14
Todd M. Blodgett, MD & Alex Ryan, MD

Miscellaneous

Lacrimal Complex Dysfunction 6-18
Paige B. Clark, MD

SECTION 7
Thyroid/Parathyroid

Introduction and Overview

Thyroid Overview 7-2
Kathryn A. Morton, MD & Paige B. Clark, MD

Parathyroid

Parathyroid Adenoma, Typical 7-6
Paige B. Clark, MD

Parathyroid Adenoma, Ectopic 7-10
Paige B. Clark, MD

xix

Hyperthyroidism

Graves Disease 7-12
Janis P. O'Malley, MD

Hashimoto Thyroiditis 7-16
Janis P. O'Malley, MD

Multinodular Goiter 7-20
Janis P. O'Malley, MD

Thyroid Adenoma, Hyperfunctioning 7-24
Janis P. O'Malley, MD

Subacute Thyroiditis 7-28
Janis P. O'Malley, MD

I-131 Hyperthyroid Therapy 7-32
Janis P. O'Malley, MD

Thyroid, Benign Miscellaneous

Ectopic Thyroid 7-36
Janis P. O'Malley, MD

Congenital Hypothyroidism 7-40
Janis P. O'Malley, MD

Benign Thyroid Conditions, PET 7-44
Crispin A. Chinn, MD

Thyroid Cancer

Well-Differentiated Thyroid Cancer 7-48
Crispin A. Chinn, MD & Kathryn A. Morton, MD

I-131 Thyroid Cancer Therapy 7-54
Crispin A. Chinn, MD

Well-Differentiated Thyroid Cancer, PET 7-58
Crispin A. Chinn, MD

Medullary Thyroid Cancer 7-62
Kathryn A. Morton, MD

SECTION 8
Gastrointestinal

Introduction and Overview

GI Anatomy & Imaging Issues 8-2
Kathryn A. Morton, MD

Biliary

Acute Calculous Cholecystitis 8-4
Carl R. Christensen, MD

Acute Acalculous Cholecystitis 8-10
Carl R. Christensen, MD

Chronic Cholecystitis 8-16
Carl R. Christensen, MD

Biliary Leak 8-20
Carl R. Christensen, MD

Common Bile Duct Obstruction 8-22
Carl R. Christensen, MD

Choledochal Cyst 8-24
Carl R. Christensen, MD

Biliary Bypass Obstruction 8-28
Carl R. Christensen, MD

Biliary Atresia 8-30
Jeffrey S. Stevens, MD & Kevin J. Limbaugh, MD

Cholangiocarcinoma 8-34
Todd M. Blodgett, MD & Alex Ryan, MD

Gallbladder Cancer 8-38
Janis P. O'Malley, MD

Hepatic

Focal Nodular Hyperplasia 8-42
Carl R. Christensen, MD

Hepatic Cirrhosis 8-46
Kathryn A. Morton, MD

Hypersplenism 8-52
Kathryn A. Morton, MD

Hepatic Metastases 8-56
Todd M. Blodgett, MD & Alex Ryan, MD

Hepatoblastoma 8-60
Kathryn A. Morton, MD

Hepatocellular Carcinoma 8-64
Kathryn A. Morton, MD & Marte Wasserman, MD

Cavernous Hemangiomas 8-70
Carl R. Christensen, MD

Adrenal

Adrenal Malignancy 8-74
Kathryn A. Morton, MD

Pheochromocytoma 8-80
Kathryn A. Morton, MD & Janis P. O'Malley, MD

Neuroblastoma 8-84
Jeffrey S. Stevens, MD & Kevin J. Limbaugh, MD

Spleen

Asplenia/Polysplenia Syndromes 8-90
Paige B. Clark, MD

Accessory & Ectopic Splenic Tissue 8-94
Jeffrey S. Stevens, MD & Kevin J. Limbaugh, MD

Oropharynx & Esophagus

Esophageal Cancer 8-98
Marte Wasserman, MD

Esophageal Dysmotility 8-102
Paige B. Clark, MD & Heather M.N. Clark, BA

Stomach

Gastritis 8-106
Todd M. Blodgett, MD & Alex Ryan, MD

Gastric Emptying Disorders 8-108
Paige B. Clark, MD & Heather M.N. Clark, BA

Gastric Carcinoma 8-112
Todd M. Blodgett, MD & Alex Ryan, MD

Intestine

Intestinal Cancer, Primary and Staging 8-116
Todd M. Blodgett, MD & Alex Ryan, MD

Intestinal Cancer, Therapy Eval./Restaging 8-120
Todd M. Blodgett, MD & Alex Ryan, MD

Meckel Diverticulum 8-122
Jeffrey S. Stevens, MD & Kevin J. Limbaugh, MD

GI Bleeding Localization 8-126
Alan D. Waxman, MD

Inflammatory Bowel Disease 8-130
Paige B. Clark, MD & Matthew Mattern, MD

Pancreas

Pancreatitis 8-134
Todd M. Blodgett, MD & Alex Ryan, MD

Pancreatic Adenocarcinoma 8-136
Janis P. O'Malley, MD

Islet Cell Tumors 8-140
Kathryn A. Morton, MD & Janis P. O'Malley, MD

Miscellaneous

Intraabdominal Infection 8-144
Kathryn A. Morton, MD

Carcinoid Tumor 8-150
Robert W. Nance, Jr., MD

GI Stromal Tumors 8-154
Crispin A. Chinn, MD

Peritoneal Systemic Shunt Evaluation 8-158
Crispin A. Chinn, MD

Diaphragmatic Patency Determination 8-162
Jeffrey S. Stevens, MD & Kevin J. Limbaugh, MD

Intraarterial Hepatic Pump Evaluation 8-164
Paige B. Clark, MD

SECTION 9
Genitourinary

Kidney

Renal Cortical Scar 9-2
Kathryn A. Morton, MD

Renal Ectopy 9-6
Jeffrey S. Stevens, MD & Kevin J. Limbaugh, MD

Renovascular Hypertension 9-10
Janis P. O'Malley, MD

Acute Renal Failure 9-14
Janis P. O'Malley, MD

Renal Masses 9-20
Kathryn A. Morton, MD

Renal Cell Carcinoma 9-22
Todd M. Blodgett, MD & Alex Ryan, MD

Pyelonephritis 9-26
Paige B. Clark, MD

Renal Transplant 9-30
Janis P. O'Malley, MD

Renal Function Quantification 9-36
Janis P. O'Malley, MD

Collecting System

Obstructive Uropathy 9-40
Kathryn A. Morton, MD

Reflux Uropathy 9-44
Anita J. Thomas, MD

Urinary Bladder & Epithelial Cancer 9-48
Todd M. Blodgett, MD
Alex Ryan, MD & Paige B. Clark, MD

Testes

Testicular Torsion 9-52
Anita J. Thomas, MD

Testicular Cancer 9-56
Kathryn A. Morton, MD

Ovaries

Ovaries, Normal & Benign Pathology 9-60
Todd M. Blodgett, MD

Ovarian Cancer 9-62
Todd M. Blodgett, MD

Uterus

Uterus, Normal & Benign Pathology 9-66
Todd M. Blodgett, MD

Cervical Cancer 9-68
Todd M. Blodgett, MD & Alex Ryan, MD

Endometrial Cancer 9-72
Todd M. Blodgett, MD & Alex Ryan, MD

Prostate

Prostate Cancer, Antibody Scan 9-76
Robert W. Nance, Jr., MD

SECTION 10
HemeOnc Procedures & Therapies

Therapy - Oncology

Phosphorus-32 Therapies 10-2
Kathryn A. Morton, MD

Hepatic Arterial Y-90 Microspheres 10-4
Kathryn A. Morton, MD

Radiolabeled Antibody Therapy 10-8
Jeffrey S. Stevens, MD & Kevin J. Limbaugh, MD

Hematologic Procedures

RBC Survival & Splenic Sequestration 10-12
Kathryn A. Morton, MD

Red Cell Mass and Plasma Volume 10-14
Kathryn A. Morton, MD

Schilling Test 10-16
Jeffrey S. Stevens, MD & Kevin J. Limbaugh, MD

SECTION 11
Oncology, Other

Lymphoma

Lymphoma, Benign Mimics 11-2
Ralph Drosten, MD

Hodgkin Lymphoma Staging 11-6
Ralph Drosten, MD

Lymphoma Post-Therapy Evaluation 11-10
Kathryn A. Morton, MD & Ralph Drosten, MD

Non-Hodgkin Lymphomas, Low Grade 11-16
Kathryn A. Morton, MD & Ralph Drosten, MD

Non-Hodgkin Lymphoma Staging 11-20
Ralph Drosten, MD & Kathryn A. Morton, MD

Melanoma

Melanoma Staging 11-24
Crispin A. Chinn, MD

Melanoma Therapy Eval./Restaging 11-28
Crispin A. Chinn, MD

Breast Cancer

Breast, Benign Disease 11-32
Kathryn A. Morton, MD

Breast Cancer, Primary 11-34
Alan D. Waxman, MD

Breast Cancer, Staging/Restaging 11-40
Alan D. Waxman, MD

Miscellaneous

Adenocarcinoma of Unknown Primary 11-46
Todd M. Blodgett, MD

Paraneoplastic Disorders 11-48
Kathryn A. Morton, MD

DIAGNOSTIC IMAGING
NUCLEAR MEDICINE

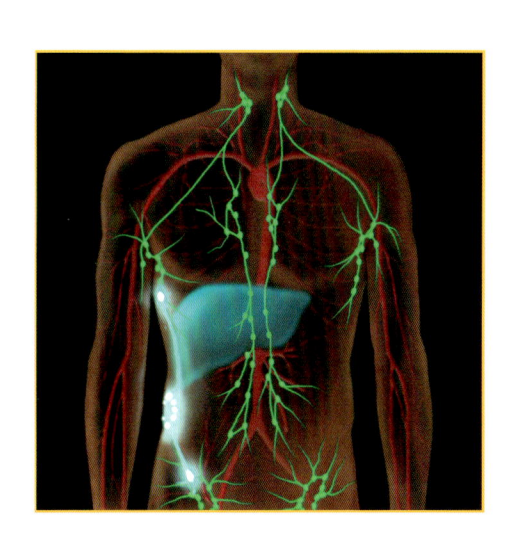

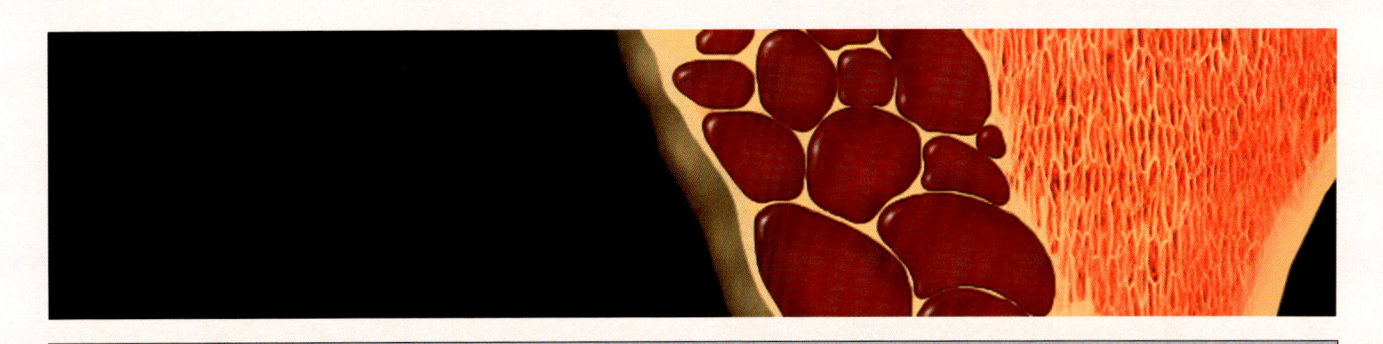

SECTION 1: Musculoskeletal

Benign Bone Tumors
Osteoid Osteoma	1-2
Enchondroma	1-6
Fibrous Cortical Defect	1-8
Bone Cyst, Aneurysmal	1-10
Bone Cyst, Solitary (Unicameral)	1-12
Giant Cell Tumor	1-16

Malignant Bone Tumors
Skeletal Metastases	1-18
Superscan	1-24
Osteosarcoma	1-28
Ewing Sarcoma	1-34
Chondrosarcoma	1-38
Prostate Cancer, Bone Metastases	1-42

Therapy
Palliation of Metastatic Bone Pain	1-44

Infection
Cellulitis	1-48
Osteomyelitis, Appendicular	1-52
Osteomyelitis, Axial	1-58
Osteomyelitis, Temporal Bone	1-60
Osteomyelitis, Feet	1-62
Osteomyelitis, Pediatric	1-66

Metabolic Bone Disease
Hyperparathyroidism	1-72
Osteomalacia	1-76
Hypertrophic Osteoarthropathy	1-80

Dysplasias
Paget Disease	1-86
Fibrous Dysplasia	1-90
Melorheostosis	1-92
Multiple Enchondromatoses	1-96
Multiple Hereditary Exostoses	1-100

Avascular Necrosis
Osseous Necrosis	1-104
Legg-Calve Perthes Disease	1-108

Surgical Assessment
Joint Prostheses, Painful	1-110
Failed Back Surgery Syndrome	1-112

Skeletal Trauma
Insufficiency Fracture	1-118
Fracture	1-124
Trauma, Non-Accidental	1-126
Stress Fracture	1-128

Regional Pain Evaluation
Arthritis, Non-Infectious	1-132
Complex Regional Pain Syndrome	1-136
Hip Pain	1-140
Wrist Pain	1-144
Calcaneal Pain	1-150
Knee Pain	1-154

Skeletal Muscle & Soft Tissues
Heterotopic Ossification	1-158
Skeletal Muscle Disorders	1-164
Amyloidosis	1-168

Bone Marrow Disorders
Hematoproliferative Disorders	1-170
Sickle Cell Disease, Bone Pain	1-176
Multiple Myeloma	1-180

OSTEOID OSTEOMA

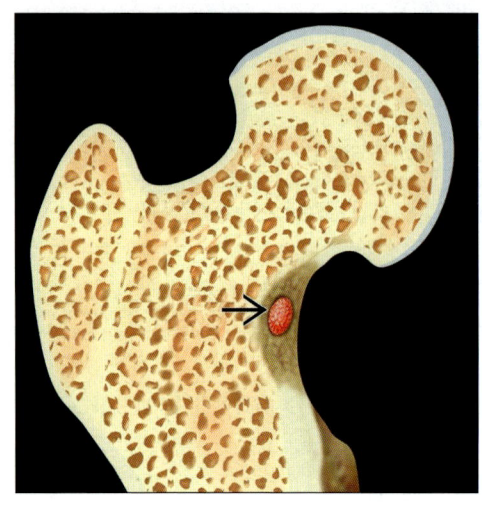

Coronal graphic shows intracortical osteoid osteoma in the femoral neck. The nidus is red →.

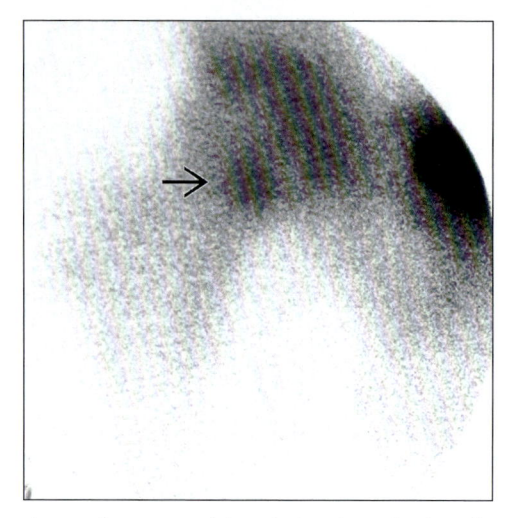

Anterior bone scan of the right hip shows focal uptake in the right femoral head/neck → in a patient with a surgically proven osteoid osteoma. (Courtesy B. Manaster, MD).

TERMINOLOGY

Definitions
- Benign skeletal neoplasm
  - Composed centrally of osteoid and woven bone in highly vascular connective tissue
  - Surrounded by dense sclerotic bone
  - Painful

IMAGING FINDINGS

General Features
- Best diagnostic clue
  - Three-phase bone scan: Highly vascular lesion with intense uptake on angiographic, blood pool and delayed images
  - Plain film: Lytic lesion, well-defined central nidus, ranging from lucent to dense depending on amount of calcification, surrounded by sclerotic bone
- Location
  - Cortical: Most common (80-90%)
    - Femur and tibia: Most frequent sites (> 50%)
    - Diaphyseal or metaphyseal
    - Cortical lesions associated with large amount of sclerosis
  - Medullary/cancellous
    - Predilection for femoral neck, small bones of hands and foot, vertebral posterior elements
    - Usually juxtaarticular
    - Less associated sclerosis
  - Subperiosteal
    - Arises as soft tissue mass adjacent to bone
    - Typically along medial aspect of femoral neck
    - May also be in hands and feet; neck of talus
    - Usually juxtaarticular or paraarticular
    - May be associated with a large amount of periostitis
  - Uncommon: Skull/facial bones
  - Rarely polyostotic
- Size
  - Usually < 1.5 cm
  - Range: 0.5-2.0 cm
- Morphology: Lucent nidus with marked surrounding sclerotic reaction

Nuclear Medicine Findings
- Three-phase bone scan

DDx: Mimics of Osteoid Osteoma

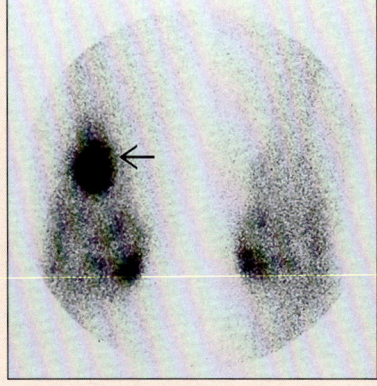

Enchondroma 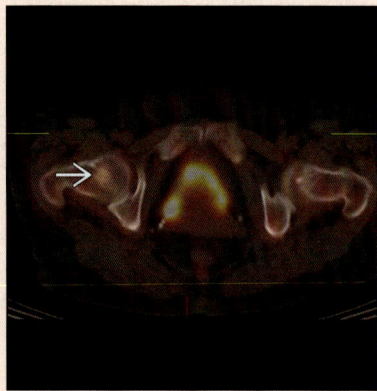 | *Sclerotic Metastasis* 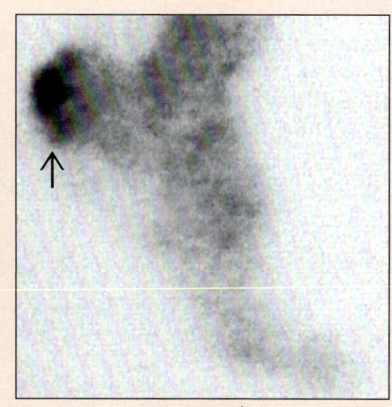 | *Osteomyelitis*

OSTEOID OSTEOMA

Key Facts

Imaging Findings
- Three-phase bone scan: Highly vascular lesion with intense uptake on angiographic, blood pool and delayed images
- Double density sign: Focal increased activity in nidus with surrounding focus of increased activity in sclerosis
- Bone scan useful for localizing lesion (e.g., in young patient with back pain)
- Negative bone scan excludes the diagnosis
- Bone scan to evaluate for polyostotic lesions (rare)
- Bone scan helpful in identifying residual nidus in symptomatic patients post treatment
- SPECT images useful when attempting to localize lesion and planar images negative

Top Differential Diagnoses
- Osteomyelitis, Chronic
- Stress Fracture
- Osteoma
- Osteoblastoma
- Metastasis
- Eosinophilic Granuloma

Clinical Issues
- Classic presentation: Pain, worse at night, relieved by aspirin
- Young population
- May spontaneously regress
- Initial treatment: Conservative
- Surgical treatment: Complete nidus removal curative

  - Hypervascular on flow and immediate static bone scan images
  - Increased activity on delayed bone scan images
  - Double density sign: Focal increased activity in nidus with surrounding focus of increased activity in sclerosis
- Whole body bone scan
  - Increased activity in lesion(s)

Radiographic Findings
- Lytic bone lesion with well-defined central nidus
- Lesion ranges from lucent to dense depending on amount of calcification
- Lesion surrounded by sclerotic bone
- Well-delineated from adjacent bone

CT Findings
- Lytic bone lesion with well-defined central nidus, ranging from lucent to dense depending on amount of calcification, surrounded by sclerotic bone
- Well-delineated from adjacent bone
- Best seen with thin sections

MR Findings
- Variable, nonspecific findings
- Nidus: Low-intermediate signal on T1WI; high signal on T2WI
- Calcification: Low signal intensity

Imaging Recommendations
- Best imaging tool
  - Plain film, CT
    - Lesion best delineated on these modalities
  - Three-phase and whole body bone scan
    - Bone scan useful for localizing lesion (e.g., in young patient with back pain)
    - Negative bone scan excludes the diagnosis
    - Bone scan to evaluate for polyostotic lesions (rare)
    - Bone scan helpful in identifying residual nidus in symptomatic patients post treatment
    - Intraoperative scintigraphy may aid in identifying nidus
- Protocol advice
  - Tc-99m MDP: 20-30 mCi (740 MBq to 1.11 GBq) IV
    - Children: 250-300 µCi/kg (9-10 MBq/kg) Tc-99m MDP IV
  - Three phase bone scan
    - Spot images over clinically painful region
    - Angiographic phase: Dynamic 1-3 second images for one minute
    - Blood pool phase: Static image for 3-5 minutes
    - Delayed phase: Spot images over chest and axial skeleton with 500K to 1 million counts, 150-250K counts in extremities
    - Often perform whole body scan as well, as primary lesion already characterized by plain film, CT
  - Whole body bone scan
    - Image anteriorly and posteriorly
    - Spot views as necessary
    - Pinhole collimator useful for small lesions
    - SPECT images useful when attempting to localize lesion and planar images negative

DIFFERENTIAL DIAGNOSIS

Osteomyelitis, Chronic
- Three phase bone scan
  - Angiographic phase: Increased activity
  - Blood pool phase: Increased activity
  - Delayed phase: Increased activity; no double density sign
- Linear tract extends away from lesion on anatomic images

Stress Fracture
- Three phase bone scan: Positive three phase bone scan
  - Angiographic phase: Increased activity
  - Blood pool phase: Increased activity
  - Delayed phase: Oval or fusiform increased activity with long axis parallel to axis of bone
- Anatomic imaging: Linear tract perpendicular to bone, adjacent new bone formation

OSTEOID OSTEOMA

Osteoma
- Bone scan: No increased activity in latent lesions, no nidus
  - May have some uptake in active lesions
- Anatomic imaging: Well-defined, round, dense sclerotic lesion attached to underlying bone
- Size: 1-5 cm

Osteoblastoma
- Bone scan: Intense uptake of radiotracer
- Anatomic imaging: Expansile, circumscribed lytic lesion involving extremities and posterior elements of spine
  - May also have some reactive sclerosis
- Larger nidus
- Tends to progress

Metastasis
- Whole body bone scan: Increased activity in (usually) multiple, scattered sites
- Anatomic imaging: Irregular areas of lytic, mixed or sclerotic bone destruction
- Less likely to be solitary
- Axial skeleton predominance

Eosinophilic Granuloma
- Well-defined lytic lesion without sclerotic rim
- Bone scan usually shows increased uptake, but may have normal uptake or decreased uptake with surrounding halo

PATHOLOGY

General Features
- Etiology
  - Controversial
  - Post-traumatic, developmental, inflammatory etiologies postulated
- Epidemiology: 10-12% of benign bone tumors
- Associated abnormalities
  - Scoliosis if located in vertebral posterior elements
  - Limb overgrowth if located near growth plate

Gross Pathologic & Surgical Features
- Granular bone, round or oval
- Sharp margins with adjacent bone

Microscopic Features
- Composed of osteoid and woven bone
- Tissue between the osteoid is fibrovascular
- Osteoblasts common at the edge of the osteoid

CLINICAL ISSUES

Presentation
- Most common signs/symptoms
  - Classic presentation: Pain, worse at night, relieved by aspirin
  - Systemic symptoms absent
  - Pain may be referred to adjacent joint
- Other signs/symptoms
  - Swelling may be associated with superficial lesions
  - Joint effusions and synovitis can occur if intraarticular

Demographics
- Age
  - Young population
    - Usually 10-20 years
    - Rarely < 2 or > 50 years
  - Almost always occurs in Caucasians
- Gender: Male predominance: 1.6-4.0:1

Natural History & Prognosis
- May spontaneously regress
- Complete surgical removal curative
- Symptoms recur if nidus not completely removed
- No growth progression

Treatment
- Initial treatment: Conservative
  - May treat with NSAIDs
  - Spontaneous regression possible
- Surgical treatment: Complete nidus removal curative
  - Curretage
  - En bloc resection
- Percutaneous
  - CT-guided removal
  - CT-guided radio-frequency ablation
  - CT-guided drilling followed by ethanol injection
  - CT-guided thermocoagulation

DIAGNOSTIC CHECKLIST

Consider
- Vascular lesion in young patient
- Consider medical management initially as lesions can regress

Image Interpretation Pearls
- Characteristic anatomic imaging findings of central nidus surrounded by sclerotic bone
- Markedly vascular on flow studies, increased uptake on delayed images
  - May appreciate double density sign on bone scan
- Precise anatomic localization needed prior to treatment as entire nidus should be completely removed

SELECTED REFERENCES

1. Vanderschueren GM et al: Osteoid osteoma: clinical results with thermocoagulation. Radiology. 224(1):82-6, 2002
2. Gangi A et al: Interstitial laser photocoagulation of osteoid osteomas with use of CT guidance. Radiology. 203(3):843-8, 1997
3. Goldman AB et al: Osteoid osteomas of the femoral neck: report of four cases evaluated with isotopic bone scanning, CT, and MR imaging. Radiology. 186(1):227-32, 1993
4. Kransdorf MJ et al: Osteoid osteoma. Radiographics. 11(4):671-96, 1991
5. Helms CA et al: Osteoid osteoma: radionuclide diagnosis. Radiology. 151(3):779-84, 1984

OSTEOID OSTEOMA

IMAGE GALLERY

Typical

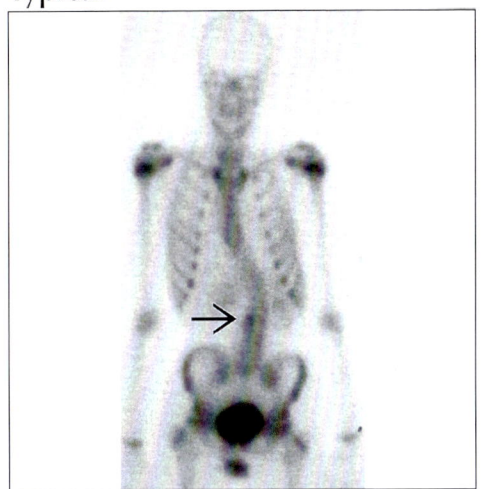

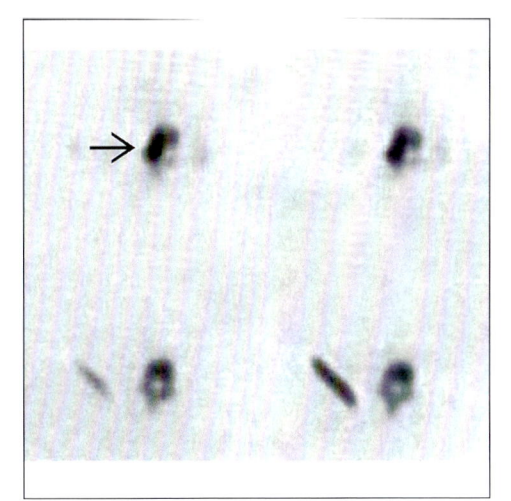

(Left) Anterior bone scan shows a focal area of increased uptake ➔ in a patient with new onset of painful scoliosis. See next image. *(Right)* Axial bone scan SPECT in same patient as left shows localization of uptake in vertebral posterior elements ➔. See next image.

Typical

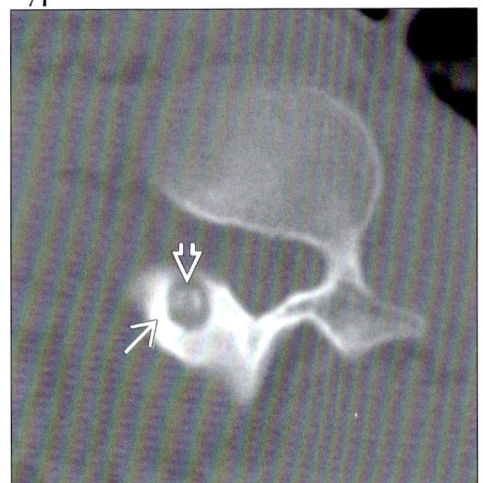

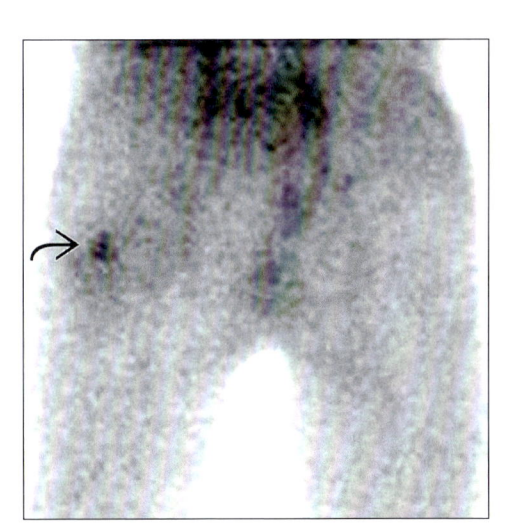

(Left) Axial NECT in same patient as previous image shows central partially calcified nidus ➔ surrounded by sclerotic rim ➔. *(Right)* Anterior bone scan immediate static image shows hyperemia in right hip ➔ in a patient with hip pain. See next image.

Typical

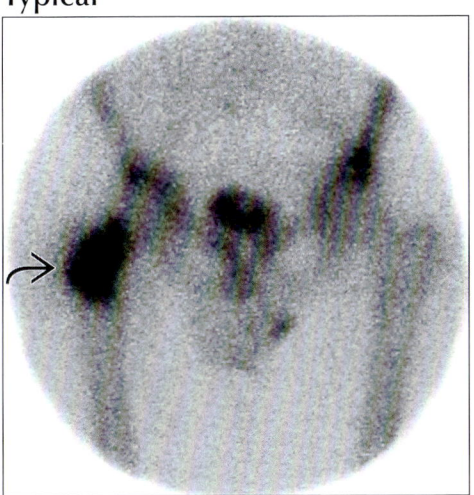

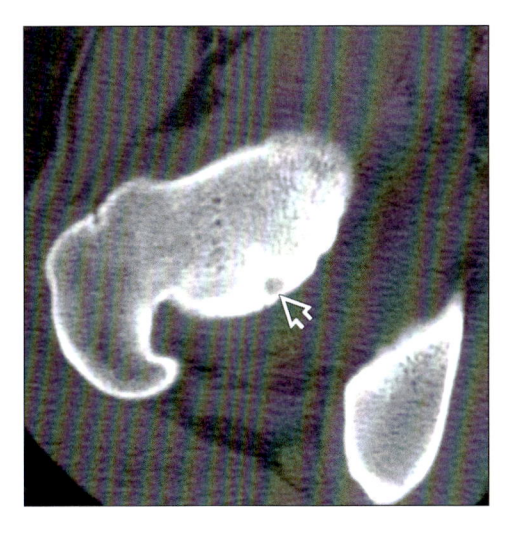

(Left) Anterior bone scan delayed image in same patient as previous image shows marked uptake in right femoral neck and proximal femur ➔. See next image. *(Right)* Axial CECT in same patient as left shows small lucent focus in femoral neck surrounded by sclerotic bone ➔, signifying osteoid osteoma.

ENCHONDROMA

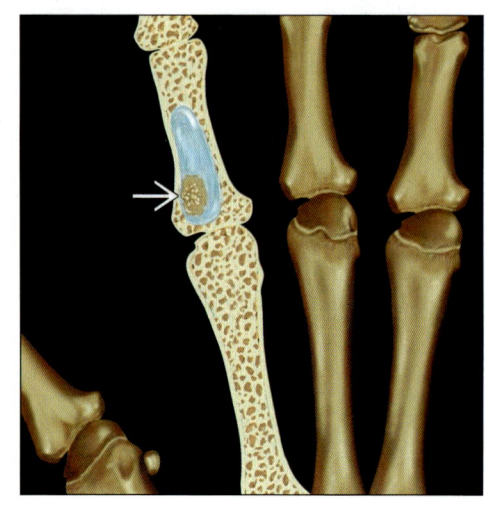

Graphic shows cartilaginous, partially calcified enchondroma in medullary space of proximal phalanx ➡.

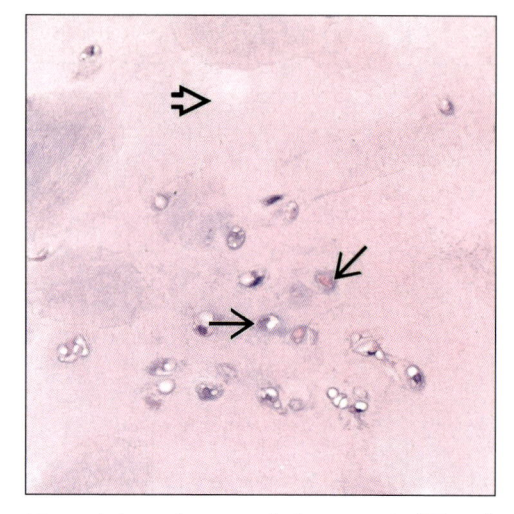

Histopathology shows cartilaginous matrix ➢ with several chondrocytes ➡ in place of normal marrow and trabeculae. (Courtesy A. Mansoor, MD).

TERMINOLOGY

Definitions
- Benign cartilaginous neoplasm in bone
  - 12-14% of benign bone neoplasms
  - 3-8% of all osseous neoplasms

IMAGING FINDINGS

General Features
- Location
  - Often in small bones of feet or hands
  - Diaphyseal regions of short tubular bones, metaphyseal regions of long bones
- Morphology
  - Usually solitary
  - If multiple, consider Ollier disease, Mafucci syndrome

Nuclear Medicine Findings
- Tc-99m MDP bone scan
  - Usually mildly ↑ or normal activity on bone scan
  - Fracture, sarcomatous degeneration: Tend to have ↑ bone scan activity, hyperemia on vascular phase
    - However, magnitude of uptake on bone scan not reliable in distinguishing from enchondroma
  - Assess for multiple lesions on whole body scan
    - Ollier disease, Mafucci syndrome

Imaging Recommendations
- Best imaging tool
  - Plain film and CT
    - Chondroid matrix in medullary-centered lytic regions
    - Pathologic fractures
    - Aggressive characteristics worrisome for sarcoma
    - Lytic-appearing areas in medullary space, +/- chondroid calcifications
- Additional nuclear medicine imaging options
  - FDG PET: Focal hypermetabolic activity worrisome for sarcomatous degeneration if fracture excluded
    - However, benign enchondroma can show ↑ FDG
- MR
  - Lobulated borders
  - May have ↑ T2 signal due to water in hyaline cartilage

DDx: Mimics of Solitary Enchondromas

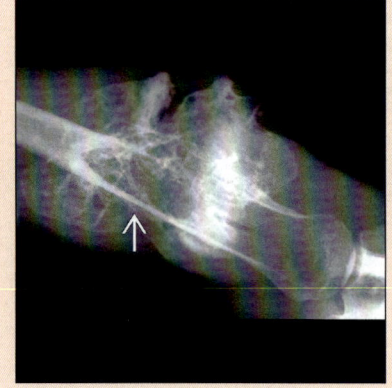

Chondrosarcoma

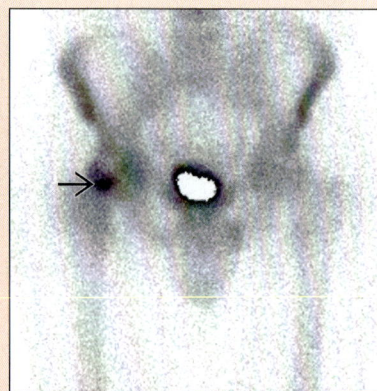

Bone Infarction

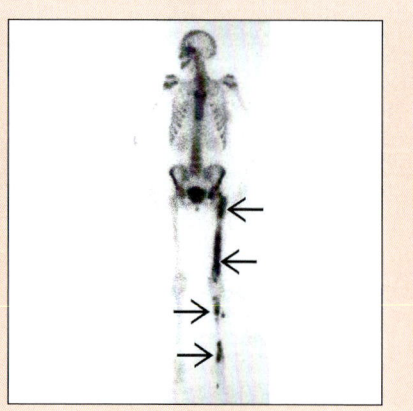

Multiple Enchondromatosis

ENCHONDROMA

Terminology
- Benign cartilaginous neoplasm in bone

Imaging Findings
- Often in small bones of feet or hands
- Diaphyseal regions of short tubular bones, metaphyseal regions of long bones
- Usually mildly ↑ or normal activity on bone scan
- Fracture, sarcomatous degeneration: Tend to have ↑ bone scan activity, hyperemia on vascular phase

Key Facts
- Assess for multiple lesions on whole body scan

Top Differential Diagnoses
- Multiple enchondromatosis
- Bone infarction
- Chondrosarcoma (typically ↑ on vascular phase)
- Nonossifying fibroma
- Simple bone cyst
- Fibrous dysplasia
- Eosinophilic granuloma

DIFFERENTIAL DIAGNOSIS

With Calcification
- Multiple enchondromatosis
- Bone infarction
- Chondrosarcoma (typically ↑ on vascular phase)

Without Calcification
- Nonossifying fibroma
- Simple bone cyst
- Fibrous dysplasia
- Eosinophilic granuloma

PATHOLOGY

General Features
- Associated abnormalities
  - Risk of sarcomatous degeneration
  - Pathologic fracture

Gross Pathologic & Surgical Features
- Ectopic hyaline cartilage rests in intramedullary bone
- Replaced trabeculae with mineralized, unmineralized cartilage

CLINICAL ISSUES

Presentation
- Most common signs/symptoms
  - Pain (with or without pathologic fracture)
  - Often asymptomatic
- Other signs/symptoms: Growth through cortex + soft tissue mass highly suggestive of sarcomatous transformation

Demographics
- Age: Pediatric to young adult, can be found later

DIAGNOSTIC CHECKLIST

Consider
- Bone scan useful to rule out multiple enchondromatosis
- Highly increased activity on bone scan: May be due to sarcomatous degeneration, pathologic fracture

SELECTED REFERENCES
1. Wang K et al: Bone scintigraphy in common tumors with osteolytic components. Clin Nucl Med. 30(10):655-71, 2005
2. Woertler K: Benign bone tumors and tumor-like lesions: value of cross-sectional imaging. Eur Radiol. 13(8):1820-35, 2003
3. Flemming DJ et al: Enchondroma and chondrosarcoma. Semin Musculoskelet Radiol. 4(1):59-71, 2000
4. Brien EW et al: Benign and malignant cartilage tumors of bone and joint: their anatomic and theoretical basis with an emphasis on radiology, pathology and clinical biology. I. Intramedullary cartilage tumors. Skeletal Radiol. 26(6):325-353, 1997

IMAGE GALLERY

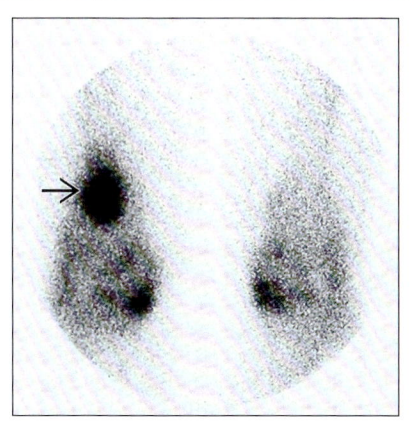

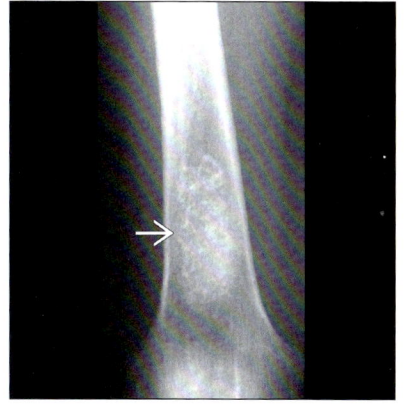

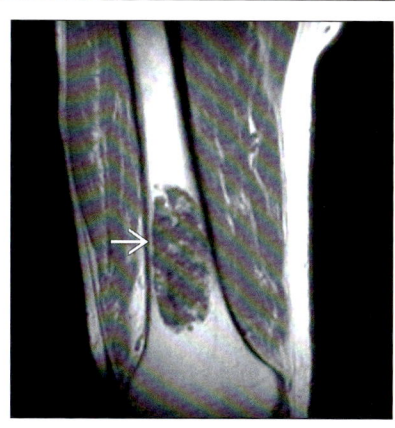

(Left) Anterior bone scan of knees shows lesion ➡ in patient with painful distal femur. Magnitude of uptake cannot reliably differentiate between enchondroma and chondrosarcoma. (Courtesy D. Sauser, MD). *(Center)* Plain film in same patient as previous image shows medullary chondroid matrix ➡, indicative of enchondroma. *(Right)* Coronal T1WI MR in same patient as previous image shows chondroid matrix ➡ against fat-replaced normal marrow.

FIBROUS CORTICAL DEFECT

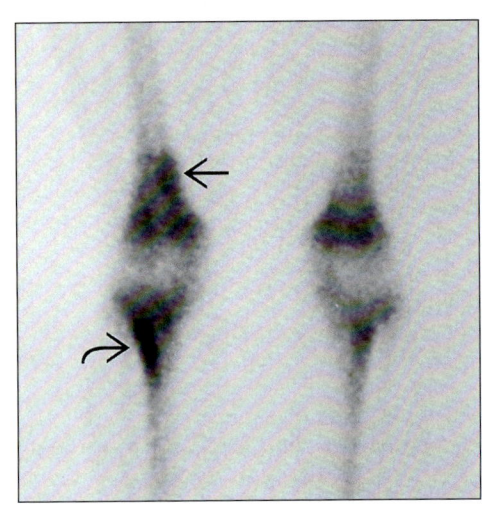

Anterior bone scan shows mildly increased uptake in the distal right femur ➡ and proximal tibia ➡. See next image.

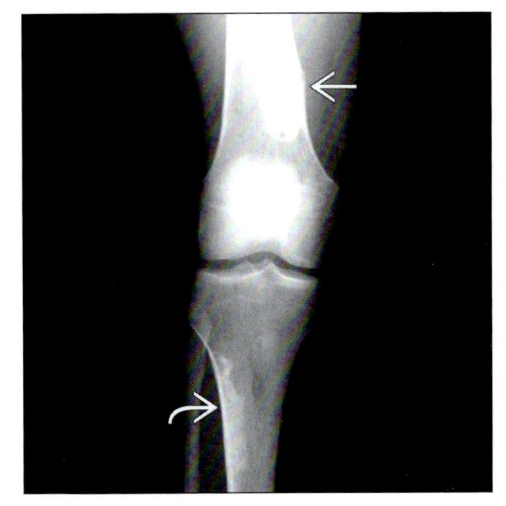

Plain film in the same patient as previous image shows FCDs corresponding to abnormal bone scan activity in the distal right femur ➡ and proximal tibia ➡.

TERMINOLOGY

Abbreviations and Synonyms
- Metaphyseal fibrous defect: Fibrous cortical defect if small, non-ossifying fibroma if large

Definitions
- Fibrous cortical defect (FCD)
  - FCD: Small, metaphyseal cortical fibrous bone lesion with sclerotic margin
  - Nonaggressive
  - Size < 3 cm
- Non-ossifying fibroma (NOF)
  - NOF: Larger, intramedullary bone lesion with sclerotic, scalloped margin
  - Also called fibroxanthoma
  - May be symptomatic, risk of pathologic fracture
  - Size > 3 cm

IMAGING FINDINGS

General Features
- Best diagnostic clue
  - Plain film: Metadiaphyseal, eccentric, ovoid bone lesion with sclerotic margin; may be multiloculated
  - Bone scan: Normal or mildly increased activity compared with normal bone; significantly increased activity suggests pathologic fracture, other lesion
    - Can be masked by normal epiphyseal activity in immature bone
- Location
  - Metaphyseal distal femur and tibia (80%)
    - Less common: Mandible (often ossifying), proximal femur
    - Unusual sites: Pelvis, ribs, vertebrae
  - Commonly monostotic; may be polyostotic

Imaging Recommendations
- Best imaging tool
  - Plain film usually diagnostic
  - MR usually low on T1, T2, or enhanced imaging

DIFFERENTIAL DIAGNOSIS

Primary Bone Malignancy
- Osteosarcoma, chondrosarcoma, fibrosarcoma
- Increased activity on bone scan

DDx: Mimic of Fibrous Cortical Defects in the Forearms

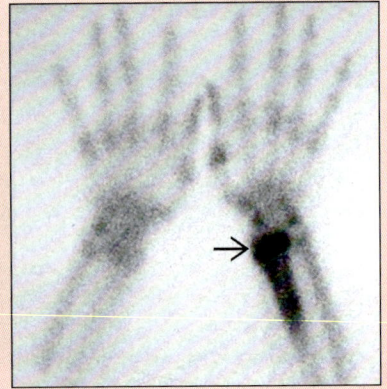

Pathologic Fracture

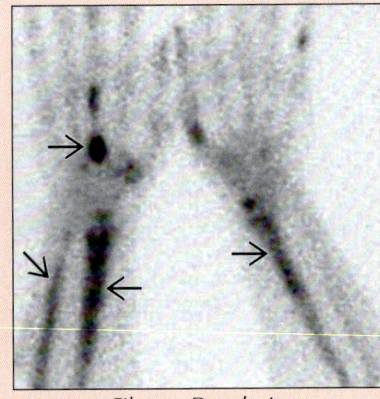

Fibrous Dysplasia

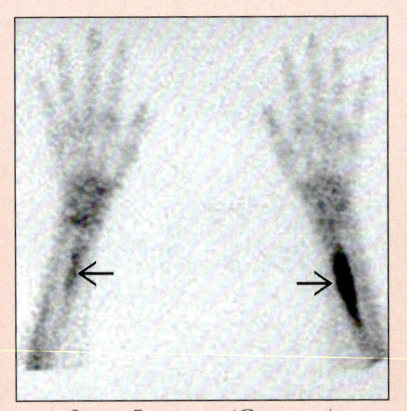

Stress Fractures (Gymnast)

FIBROUS CORTICAL DEFECT

Key Facts

Terminology
- FCD: Small, metaphyseal cortical fibrous bone lesion with sclerotic margin
- NOF: Larger, intramedullary bone lesion with sclerotic, scalloped margin

Imaging Findings
- Bone scan: Normal or mildly increased activity compared with normal bone; significantly increased activity suggests pathologic fracture, other lesion

Top Differential Diagnoses
- Primary Bone Malignancy
- Fibrous Dysplasia
- Osteoid Osteoma
- Trauma

Clinical Issues
- Smaller lesions may spontaneously resolve
- Pathologic fracture rare

Fibrous Dysplasia
- Ground-glass on plain film
- More likely polyostotic than FCD

Osteoid Osteoma
- Central nidus
- Increased activity peripherally
- Pain

Trauma
- Cortical avulsion has similar location on bone scan
- More increased activity on bone scan than FCD

PATHOLOGY

Gross Pathologic & Surgical Features
- Cortically centered, white fibrous lesions

Microscopic Features
- Whorls of fibrous tissue
- Fibroblasts, giant cells, foam cells
- Collagen
- Absent osteoclasts, osteoblasts

CLINICAL ISSUES

Presentation
- Most common signs/symptoms: Asymptomatic, incidental finding
- Other signs/symptoms
  - Pain from pathologic fracture
  - Cutaneous cafe au lait spots with multiple NOF (Jaffe Campanacci syndrome)

Demographics
- Age: Usually presentation at 5-20 yrs
- Gender: Possible male predominance

Natural History & Prognosis
- Smaller lesions may spontaneously resolve
- Pathologic fracture rare
  - Most occur where lesion extends > 50% in anteroposterior and transverse plane
- Progression in size, pathologic fracture in small lesion raises question of initial diagnosis

Treatment
- If symptomatic, curettage and packing

DIAGNOSTIC CHECKLIST

Image Interpretation Pearls
- Bone scan: Monostotic focus of normal to mildly increased activity in metadiaphyseal location suggests diagnosis; plain film correlation diagnostic

SELECTED REFERENCES

1. Biermann JS: Common benign lesions of bone in children and adolescents. J Pediatr Orthop. 22(2):268-73, 2002

IMAGE GALLERY

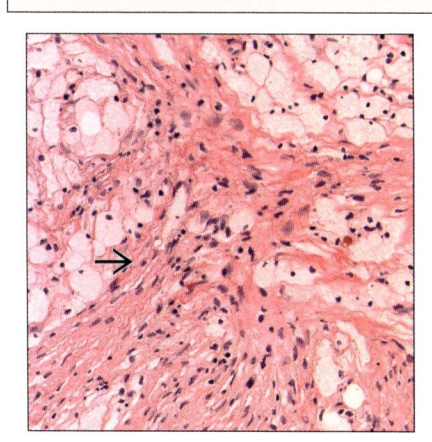

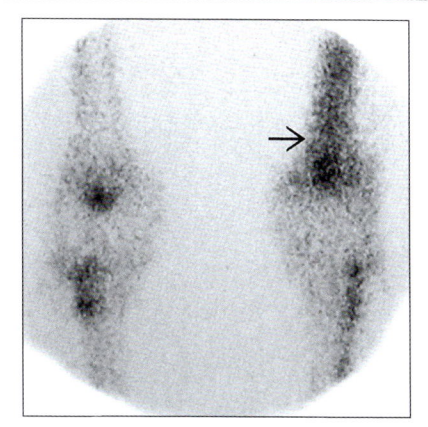

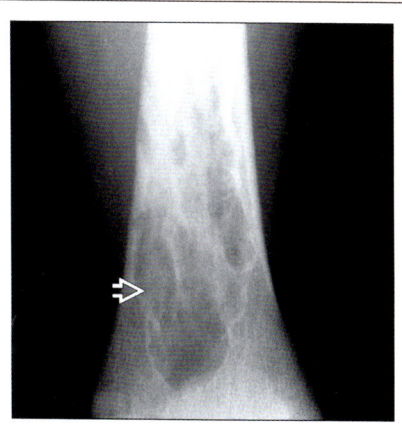

(Left) Histopathology slide of fibrous cortical defect shows whorls of fibrous tissue ➔ in this section of cortical bone, with absence of osteocytes and osteoblasts. (Center) Anterior bone scan in a patient with left knee pain shows mildly increased activity in the left distal femur ➔. See next image. (Right) Radiograph in the same patient as previous image shows a large lucent lesion with sclerotic margin ➔ consistent with NOF. This lesion is at risk for pathologic fracture.

BONE CYST, ANEURYSMAL

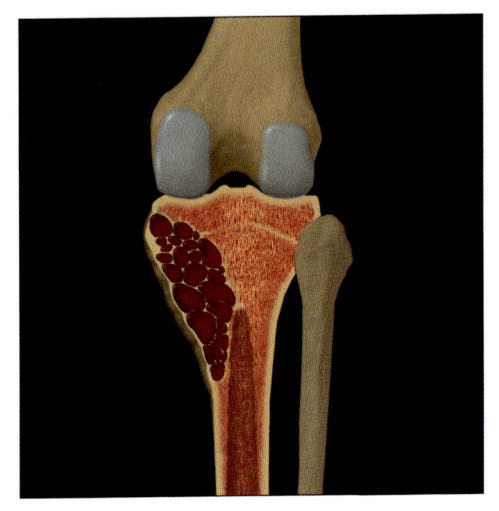

Graphic of ABC shows the expanded vascular spaces, few coarsened thickened trabecula remaining, and expanded thinned cortex.

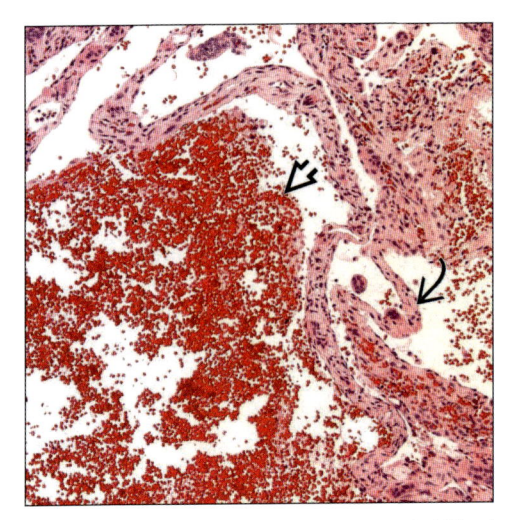

Tissue pathology slide of ABC shows expanded blood spaces and vessels full of erythrocytes ⇨ and remaining displaced trabeculae and bone tissue ➔. (Courtesy A. Mansoor, MD).

TERMINOLOGY

Abbreviations and Synonyms
- Aneurysmal bone cyst (ABC)

Definitions
- Benign bone tumor (~ 1% of primary bone lesions)
- Expansile lytic lesion, thin wall, blood-filled, cystic
  - 70% primary; 30% secondary (in preexisting bone lesion)
- Staging
  - Stage 1: Latent, stable, or heals spontaneously
  - Stage 2: Active, progressive, no cortical destruction
  - Stage 3: Locally aggressive, cortical destruction
- Can regress, recur post-treatment, become aggressive
  - Recurrence higher in young children, stage 3

IMAGING FINDINGS

General Features
- Best diagnostic clue
  - Plain film findings depend on phase
    - Phase 1: Small, lytic, thinned cortex, ↓ trabeculae
    - Phase 2: Rapid enlargement, "blown-out"
    - Phase 3: Slow, no growth
    - Phase 4: Healing, dense irregular remodeled bone, cavity ossification/calcification
  - Nuclear medicine: Tc-99m MDP bone scan
    - Evaluate skeleton for multiple ABCs: ~ 8% of patients with ABC have > 1
- Location: Lower leg 24%, femur 13%, upper extremity 21%, spine 16%, pelvis & sacrum 12%

Nuclear Medicine Findings
- Tc-99m MDP bone scan
  - Moderate to intense activity with central photopenia = doughnut sign (~ 65% of ABC)
    - Also seen with giant cell tumors (check radiograph), chondrosarcoma (> 40 y, metaphyseal/diaphyseal), telangiectatic osteosarcoma
  - Whole body bone scan to detect multiple lesions, fracture or aggressive portion of lesion
  - Three-phase bone scan for degree of remodeling, stage
    - Phase 1: ↑ Blood flow; phase 2: ↑ Blood pool; phase 3: Peripheral activity 2° to remodeling

DDx: Mimics of Aneurysmal Bone Cyst

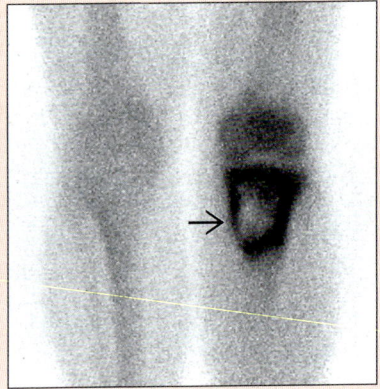

Giant Cell Tumor

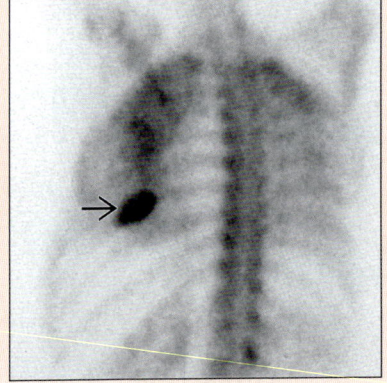

Brown Tumor

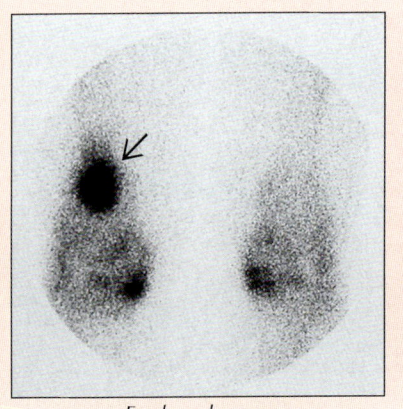

Enchondroma

BONE CYST, ANEURYSMAL

Key Facts

Terminology
- Benign bone tumor (~ 1% of primary bone lesions)
- Expansile lytic lesion, thin wall, blood-filled, cystic
- Stage 1: Latent, stable, or heals spontaneously
- Stage 2: Active, progressive, no cortical destruction
- Stage 3: Locally aggressive, cortical destruction

Imaging Findings
- Tc-99m MDP bone scan
- Moderate to intense activity with central photopenia = doughnut sign (~ 65% of ABC)
- Whole body bone scan to detect multiple lesions, fracture or aggressive portion of lesion
- Three-phase bone scan for degree of remodeling, stage

Clinical Issues
- Age: 10-30 y, peak ~ 16 y
- Surgery cures 70-90%

DIFFERENTIAL DIAGNOSIS

Enchondroma
- Radiographic findings usually help distinguish

Giant Cell Tumor
- Histopathologic evaluation often necessary

Hyperparathyroidism, Primary or Secondary
- Brown tumors

Osteoblastoma
- Histopathologic evaluation often needed

Osteosarcoma
- Telangiectatic osteosarcoma can mimic ABC

PATHOLOGY

General Features
- Etiology: Benign neoplasm, chromosomal abnormalities

CLINICAL ISSUES

Presentation
- Most common signs/symptoms
  - Pain
  - Pathologic fracture

Demographics
- Age: 10-30 y, peak ~ 16 y
- Gender: M:F = 1:2

Treatment
- Surgery cures 70-90%
  - Curettage + bone graft/cementation; excision for recurrent/aggressive
- Embolization
  - Vertebral, pelvic, extensive disease
- Radiation therapy
  - Incomplete resection, aggressive/recurrent

DIAGNOSTIC CHECKLIST

Image Interpretation Pearls
- Doughnut sign: ABC, giant cell tumor, chondrosarcoma, telangiectatic osteosarcoma
- ~ 8% of patients with ABC will have > 1 lesion
- Most recurrences within 2 y of treatment

SELECTED REFERENCES
1. Wang K et al: Bone scintigraphy in common tumors with osteolytic components. Clin Nucl Med. 30(10):655-71, 2005
2. Kransdorf MJ et al: Aneurysmal bone cyst: concept, controversy, clinical presentation, and imaging. AJR Am J Roentgenol. 164(3):573-80, 1995

IMAGE GALLERY

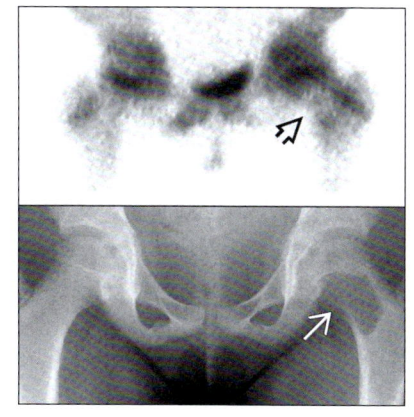

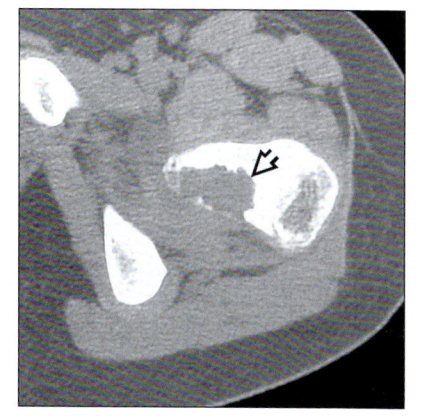

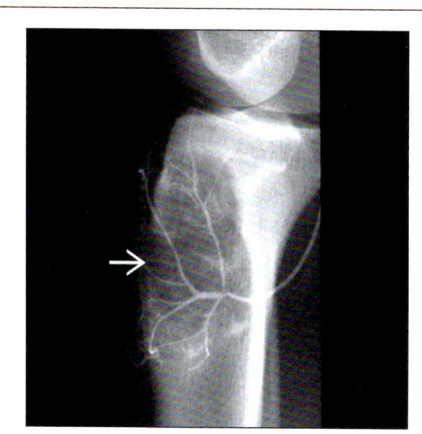

(Left) Anterior planar Tc-99m MDP bone scan (upper panel) shows photopenic lesion in left femoral neck ⇨, corresponding to the expansile, lytic ABC ⇨ on plain film (lower panel). (Center) Axial NECT of left femoral neck in same patient as previous image shows markedly thinned cortex posteriorly ⇨ in the ABC. (Right) Medial angiogram shows tibial ABC ⇨ during embolization treatment.

BONE CYST, SOLITARY (UNICAMERAL)

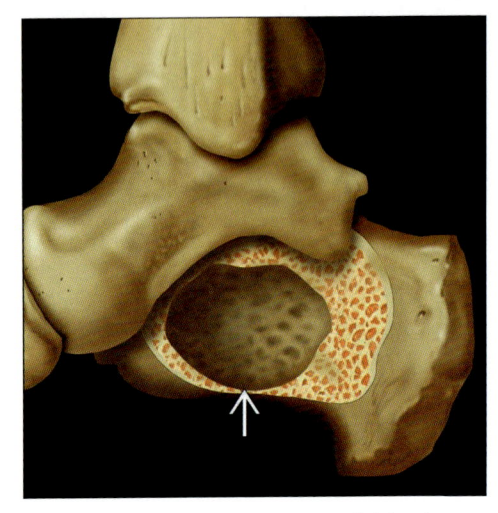

Graphic of posterior foot shows a well-defined, cystic lesion ➡ representing SBC. The calcaneus is a favored location of SBC in adults.

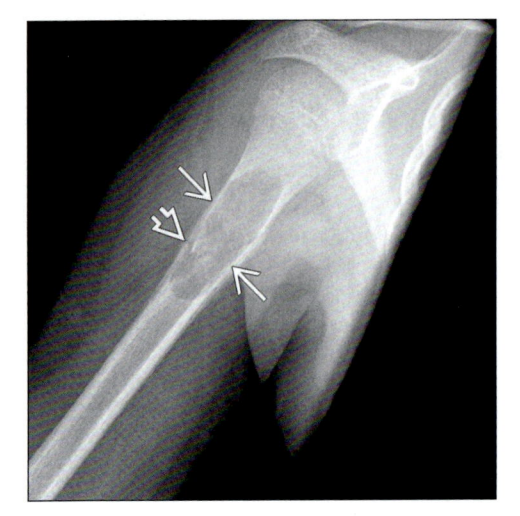

Anterior radiograph of the right arm shows a well-defined lucent lesion ➡ with an associated fracture ⇨ an in young patient with arm pain due to SBC.

TERMINOLOGY

Abbreviations and Synonyms
- Solitary or simple bone cyst (SBC)
- Unicameral bone cyst

Definitions
- Tumor-like lesion of unknown etiology, attributed to local disturbance of bone growth

IMAGING FINDINGS

General Features
- Best diagnostic clue
  - Well-defined, central, lytic lesion on plain film, CT
  - Bone scan: Mild increased activity peripherally with central photopenia; may be relatively normal
- Location
  - Active phase: Proximal metaphysis, adjacent to epiphyseal cartilage
  - Latent phase: Migration into diaphysis with growth
  - Does not cross growth plate
  - Bones
    - Humerus and femur: 60-80%
    - Calcaneus, talus, ilium: 50% (older patients)
    - Spine, sacrum, craniofacial bones: Rare
- Size: 2-15 cm (average 6-8 cm)
- Morphology: Well-defined, lytic lesion

Nuclear Medicine Findings
- Bone Scan
  - Vascular phase is usually negative
  - Peripheral: Mild increased radiotracer activity
  - Central: Decreased radiotracer activity
  - May show no increased activity
  - Focal significant uptake often indicates associated fracture
  - Use of SPECT/CT evolving, may optimize characterization of primary bone lesions on bone scan

Radiographic Findings
- Radiography
  - Centrally located, well-defined, expansile, lucent lesion
  - Long axis parallel to long axis of host bone
  - Sclerotic margin
  - Scalloping of underlying cortex

DDx: Mimics of Solitary Bone Cyst

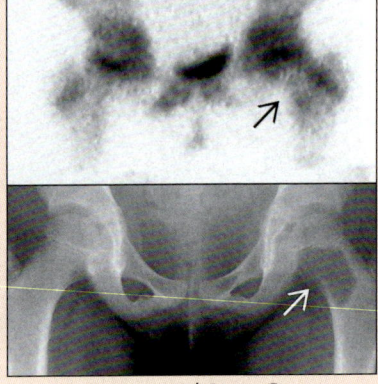

Aneurysmal Bone Cyst 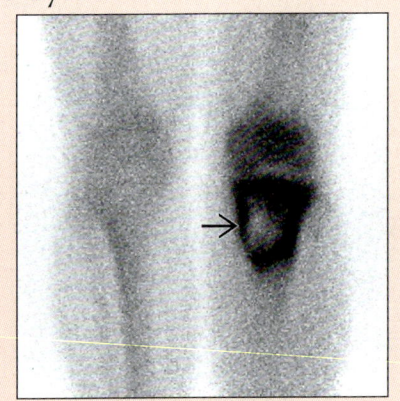 *Giant Cell Tumor* 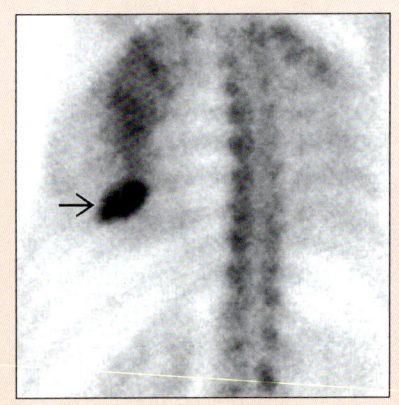 *Brown Tumor*

BONE CYST, SOLITARY (UNICAMERAL)

Key Facts

Imaging Findings
- Well-defined, central, lytic lesion on plain film, CT
- Bone scan: Mild increased activity peripherally with central photopenia; may be relatively normal
- Fallen fragment sign secondary to pathologic fracture on plain film = pathognomonic for SBC

Top Differential Diagnoses
- Aneurysmal Bone Cyst (ABC)
- Fibrous Dysplasia
- Fibroxanthoma
- Bone Abscess
- Enchondroma
- Langerhans Cell Histiocytosis
- Brown Tumors

Clinical Issues
- Most lesions asymptomatic
- 66% of cysts present with pathologic fractures
- Spontaneous regression in majority of cases
- Recurrence rate after injection, curettage: 20-45%

Diagnostic Checklist
- SBC on bone scan: Peripherally increased activity with central photopenia; may have minimal activity
- Very intense increased activity on bone scan with acute pain may represent pathologic fracture
- Postsurgical bone scan: Increased activity after instrumentation, with bone healing; should decrease over time
- Bone scan with SPECT/CT may be used for optimal characterization

---

  - Cortex never completely disrupted
  - Fluid-filled cavity (fluid/fluid levels)
  - No periosteal reaction unless fractured
  - No extension into soft tissues
  - Fallen fragment sign secondary to pathologic fracture on plain film = pathognomonic for SBC
    - Fragment migrates to dependent portions of cyst
  - Increased density/sclerosis after steroid injection

CT Findings
- NECT
  - Fluid-filled cavity
    - HU: 15-20
    - Can have fluid-fluid levels
  - Helpful in evaluating anatomically complex areas (pelvis, spine)
  - Determine extent of lesion
- CECT
  - No enhancement
  - Helpful in differentiating cyst from solid lesion

MR Findings
- T1WI: Low to intermediate signal intensity
- T2WI
  - High signal intensity
  - Heterogeneous signal in case of fracture (blood products)
- T1 C+
  - No enhancement
  - Differentiate cystic from solid lesions
- Fluid-fluid levels
- Septations

Imaging Recommendations
- Best imaging tool
  - Radiographs diagnostic
  - CT for anatomically complex areas (spine, pelvis)
- Protocol advice
  - Tc-99m MDP bone scan: 20-30 mCi (740 MBq-1.11 GBq) MDP IV adults; (age +1/age +7) x adult dose for children
  - Anterior and posterior whole body images to determine if lesion monostotic
  - Static planar views over area of interest to evaluate primary lesion, pathologic fracture
  - Three-phase bone scan may be useful to help characterize primary bone lesion (e.g., vascularity, soft tissue involvement)

DIFFERENTIAL DIAGNOSIS

Aneurysmal Bone Cyst (ABC)
- Eccentric, expansile lesion
- Periosteal reaction
- Geographic type of bone destruction
- Surrounding edema
- Prominent fluid-fluid levels

Fibrous Dysplasia
- No trabeculation
- Ground glass, smoky appearance
- No "fallen-fragment sign" in case of fracture

Fibroxanthoma
- Eccentric lesion
- Thin or scalloped sclerotic margins

Bone Abscess
- Periosteal reaction
- Cortical destruction
- Sinus tract, sequestration

Enchondroma
- Calcified matrix
- Lytic in hands

Langerhans Cell Histiocytosis
- Destructive lesion
- Surrounding bone marrow edema

Brown Tumors
- Hyperparathyroidism (HPT)
- Associated with other features of HPT
  - Subperiosteal resorption, osteopenia

BONE CYST, SOLITARY (UNICAMERAL)

PATHOLOGY

General Features
- General path comments
  - Fluid containing lesion lined by mesenchymal cells
  - Only primary true cyst of bone that conforms to pathologic definition of cyst
- Genetics: Case report of translocation (16;20)(p11.2;q13)
- Etiology
  - Unknown
  - Appears to be reactive, developmental rather than neoplastic
  - Possibly due to lymphatic or venous obstruction or synovial rests that produce joint fluid
  - Venous obstruction in area of rapidly growing and remodeling bone
- Epidemiology: 3% of primary bone lesions

Gross Pathologic & Surgical Features
- Intact specimens rarely seen
- Intramedullary cavity filled with clear or yellow fluid with low viscosity
- Fluid under pressure
- Septation with multiple cavities occasionally seen
- Spongy component composed of multiple smaller cysts can be present
- Wall composed of paper thin (1 mm), tan-yellow fibrous tissue with bony ridges
- Intact periosteum

Microscopic Features
- No epithelial lining in wall of lesion
  - Fibrous and granulation tissue, hemosiderin deposits, small lymphocytes within cyst wall
  - Giant cells of osteoclastic type in cyst wall
  - Fibrinous debris may undergo calcification simulating cementum
- Fluid usually shows elevated alkaline phosphatase
- Fluid contains prostaglandins and interleukins (can cause bone resorption)
- Blood products in cyst fluid in case of prior fracture

CLINICAL ISSUES

Presentation
- Most common signs/symptoms
  - Most lesions asymptomatic
  - Pain
  - Swelling
  - Stiffness at closest joint
- Clinical Profile
  - 66% of cysts present with pathologic fractures
    - Sudden onset of pain
    - Often occurs during exercise
  - Growth arrest in 10% of patients
    - Due to pathologic fracture (± surgical curettage), extension to physeal plate
  - Older patients with involvement of atypical sites usually asymptomatic
    - Calcaneus, talus, ilium

Demographics
- Age: 10-20 years, 3-14 years: 80%
- Gender: M:F = 2-3:1

Natural History & Prognosis
- Benign lesion, no malignant transformation
- Enlarge during skeletal growth
- Inactive, latent after skeletal maturity
- Spontaneous regression in majority of cases
- Recurrence rate after injection, curettage: 20-45%

Treatment
- Trephination: Multiple holes drilled into lesion ± irrigation
  - Performed under general anesthesia
- Dual needle aspiration and percutaneous injection of corticosteroids (80-200 mg methylprednisolone)
  - 1-3 injections at 2 month intervals
- Percutaneous injection of demineralized bone matrix and autogenous bone marrow
- Open curettage with bone graft in weight bearing bones
  - Recurrence 40-45%
  - Damage to growth plate may result in growth arrest
- Subtotal resection, allografting, packing with synthetic materials

DIAGNOSTIC CHECKLIST

Image Interpretation Pearls
- SBC on bone scan: Peripherally increased activity with central photopenia; may have minimal activity
- Very intense increased activity on bone scan with acute pain may represent pathologic fracture
- Postsurgical bone scan: Increased activity after instrumentation, with bone healing; should decrease over time
- Bone scan with SPECT/CT may be used for optimal characterization

SELECTED REFERENCES

1. Horger M et al: The role of single-photon emission computed tomography/computed tomography in benign and malignant bone disease. Semin Nucl Med. 36(4):286-94, 2006
2. Wilkins RM: Unicameral bone cysts. J Am Acad Orthop Surg. 8(4):217-24, 2000
3. Lokiec F et al: Simple bone cyst: etiology, classification, pathology, and treatment modalities. J Pediatr Orthop B. 7(4):262-73, 1998
4. Abdel-Dayem HM: The role of nuclear medicine in primary bone and soft tissue tumors. Semin Nucl Med. 27(4):355-63, 1997
5. Capanna R et al: Unicameral and aneurysmal bone cysts. Orthop Clin North Am. 27(3):605-14, 1996
6. Conway WF et al: Miscellaneous lesions of bone. Radiol Clin North Am. 31(2):339-58, 1993
7. Struhl S et al: Solitary (unicameral) bone cyst. The fallen fragment sign revisited. Skeletal Radiol. 18(4):261-5, 1989
8. McGlynn FJ et al: The fallen fragment sign in unicameral bone cyst. Clin Orthop Relat Res. (156):157-9, 1981
9. Gilday DL et al: Benign bone tumors. Semin Nucl Med. 6(1):33-46, 1976

BONE CYST, SOLITARY (UNICAMERAL)

IMAGE GALLERY

Typical

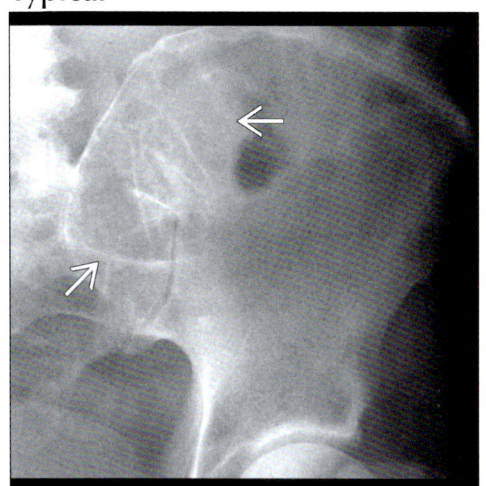

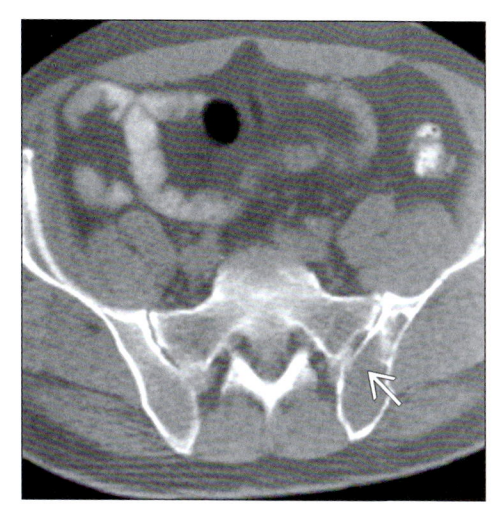

(Left) Anteroposterior radiograph shows a large, expansile, lytic lesion with pseudotrabeculations ➡ located in the posterior left iliac wing of an adult. See next 2 images. *(Right)* Axial NECT in same patient as previous image, shows the expansile, lytic lesion in left ilium ➡. No aggressive features are present, consistent with SBC. See next image.

Typical

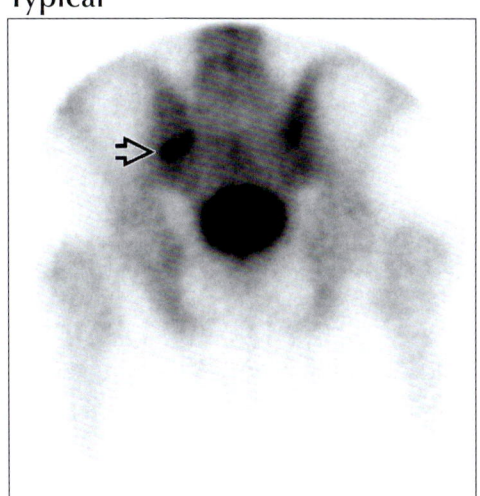

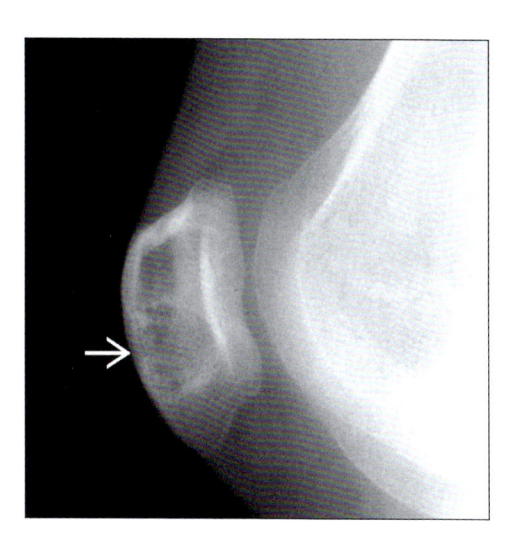

(Left) Posterior bone scan in the same patient as previous 2 images, shows minimally increased ➡ activity in SBC in left ilium. Focal activity associated with a SBC is often due to fracture. (Courtesy B. Manaster, MD, PhD). *(Right)* Lateral radiograph of a 34 year old male with painful thigh, shows lytic lesion with pseudotrabeculations occupying much of the patella ➡, an unusual location for SBC. Biopsy confirmed. (Courtesy B. Manaster, MD PhD).

Typical

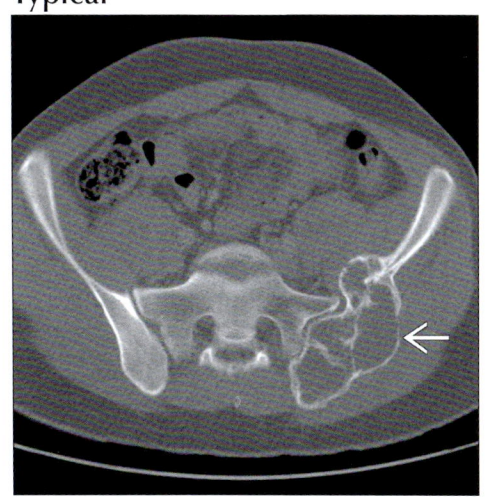

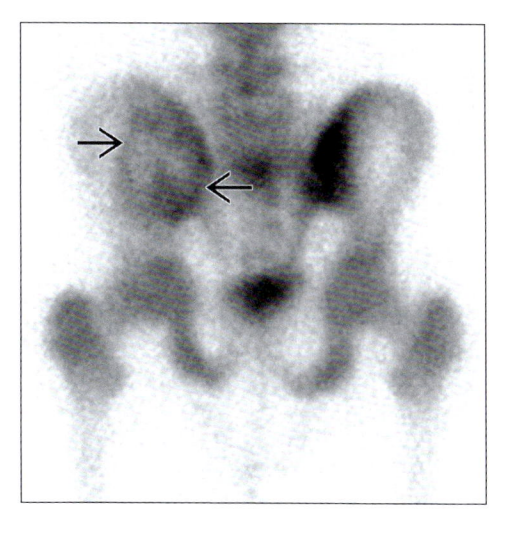

(Left) Axial NECT shows a well-defined, expansile, lytic lesion in left ilium ➡ consistent with SBC. See next image. *(Right)* Posterior bone scan shows a lesion with peripherally mild increased activity ➡ and central photopenia in left ilium, typical in appearance for SBC.

GIANT CELL TUMOR

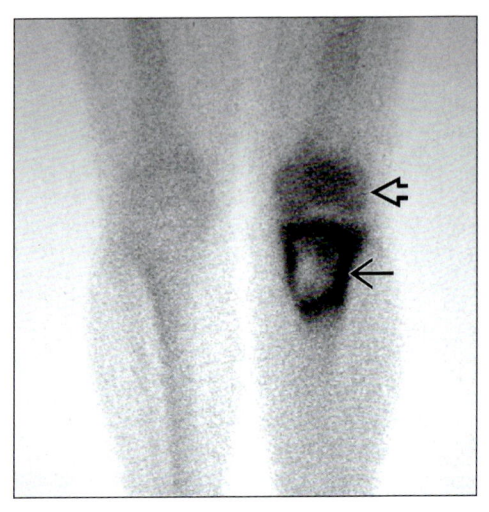

Anterior bone scan shows increased activity with a commonly seen central area of photopenia in proximal tibia ⇨. Activity in distal femur is secondary to reactive hyperemia ⇨. (All images courtesy D. Sauser, MD).

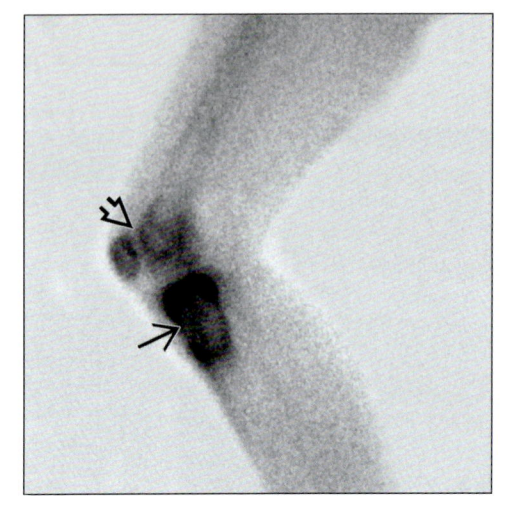

Left lateral bone scan shows (same patient as previous image) the proximal tibial lesion with central photopenia ⇨ and reactive hyperemia in the distal femur and patella ⇨.

TERMINOLOGY

Abbreviations and Synonyms
- Giant cell tumor (GCT), osteoclastoma

Definitions
- Locally aggressive tumor composed of osteoclastic giant cells involving the epiphysis

IMAGING FINDINGS

General Features
- Best diagnostic clue: Lytic epiphyseal lesion on plain radiograph extending to subchondral bone without surrounding sclerosis
- Location: Metaphyseal side of growth plate, usually long bones, knee most common
- Size: Range 2-20 cm, mean 5-7 cm
- Morphology: Lytic lesion without bone or cartilage matrix extending to subchondral bone

Nuclear Medicine Findings
- PET: Hypermetabolism (reported SUVs 1.8-9.4)

- Bone Scan
  - Radionuclide angiogram, capillary phase, and delayed images will likely all be positive
  - A central photopenic region is frequently present
  - Additional sites of uptake may indicate metastatic GCT

Radiographic Findings
- Radiography: Well-marginated lytic lesion without marginal sclerosis with septations and no bone or cartilage matrix

CT Findings
- Soft tissue attenuation with foci of lower attenuation from hemorrhage or necrosis

Imaging Recommendations
- Best imaging tool
  - Plain radiograms and MRI preferred
  - Bone scan is sensitive but not specific
- Protocol advice: Whole body bone scan should always be obtained to detect additional lesions (GCT may be metastatic in 3-5%)

DDx: Example of Giant Cell Tumor of Entire Sacrum

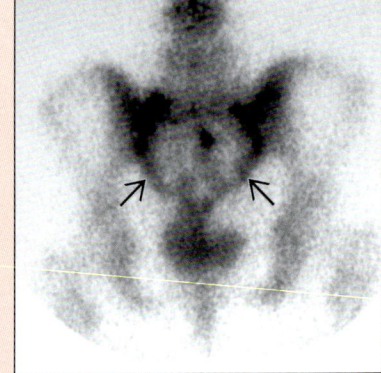

Posterior Bone Scan

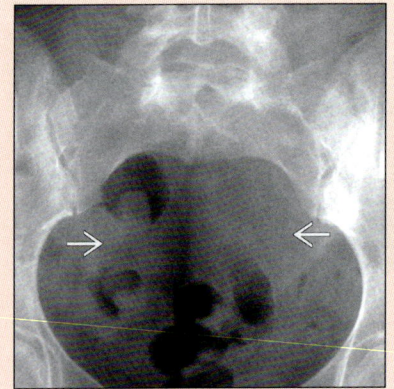

Plain Radiograph

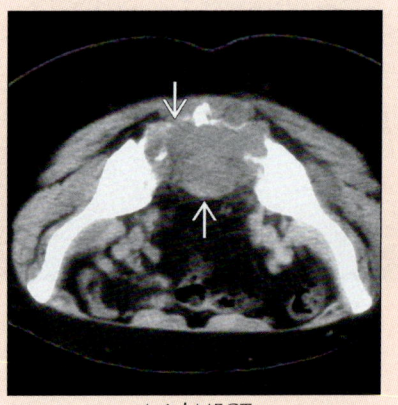

Axial NECT

GIANT CELL TUMOR

Key Facts

Terminology
- Locally aggressive tumor composed of osteoclastic giant cells involving the epiphysis

Imaging Findings
- Best diagnostic clue: Lytic epiphyseal lesion on plain radiograph extending to subchondral bone without surrounding sclerosis
- Location: Metaphyseal side of growth plate, usually long bones, knee most common
- Radionuclide angiogram, capillary phase, and delayed images will likely all be positive
- Plain radiograms and MRI preferred
- Bone scan is sensitive but not specific
- Protocol advice: Whole body bone scan should always be obtained to detect additional lesions (GCT may be metastatic in 3-5%)

DIFFERENTIAL DIAGNOSIS

Tumors, Recent Fractures, Osteomyelitis
- This is the typical spectrum of diagnoses for positivity on all three bone scan phases

PATHOLOGY

General Features
- Epidemiology: Accounts for 20% of all benign bone tumors and 5% of all bone tumors

Gross Pathologic & Surgical Features
- Well-demarcated, well-delineated peripherally, expansion of surrounding bone

Microscopic Features
- Multinucleated osteoclastic giant cells with no bone or cartilage matrix

CLINICAL ISSUES

Presentation
- Most common signs/symptoms: Pain and swelling in the affected area
- Other signs/symptoms: 12% present with pathologic fracture

Demographics
- Age: After skeleton is mature (typically age 20-40)
- Gender: Slight female predominance

Natural History & Prognosis
- 25-50% local recurrence rate
- Can rarely undergo sarcomatous degeneration
- Lung metastases from histologically benign GCT occurs in an estimated 3% of patients

Treatment
- Surgical resection and/or radiotherapy

DIAGNOSTIC CHECKLIST

Image Interpretation Pearls
- Bone scans are sensitive but nonspecific
- Value of bone scan is to exclude additional lesions

SELECTED REFERENCES

1. Turcotte RE: Giant cell tumor of bone. Orthop Clin North Am. 37(1):35-51, 2006
2. James SL et al: Giant-cell tumours of bone of the hand and wrist: a review of imaging findings and differential diagnoses. Eur Radiol. 15(9):1855-66, 2005
3. Strauss LG et al: 18F-FDG kinetics and gene expression in giant cell tumors. J Nucl Med. 45(9):1528-35, 2004
4. Yasko AW: Giant cell tumor of bone. Curr Oncol Rep. 4(6):520-6, 2002
5. Goodgold HM et al: Scintigraphic features of giant cell tumor. Clin Nucl Med. 9(9):526-30, 1984
6. Levine E et al: Scintigraphic evaluation of giant cell tumor of bone. AJR Am J Roentgenol. 143(2):343-8, 1984

IMAGE GALLERY

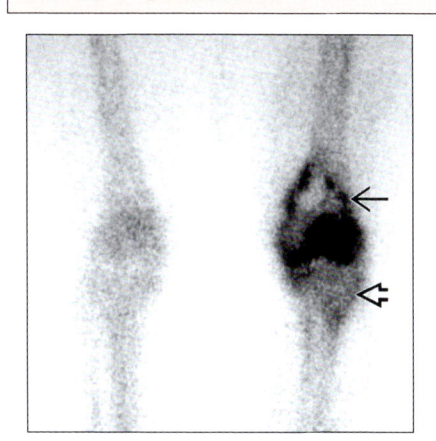

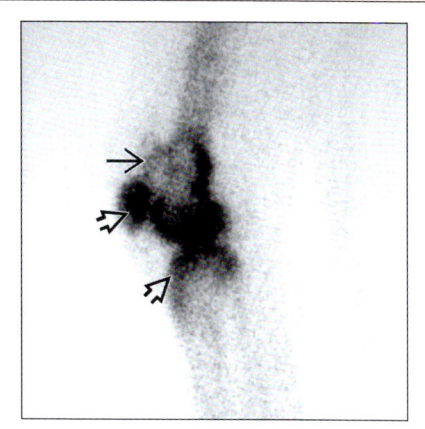

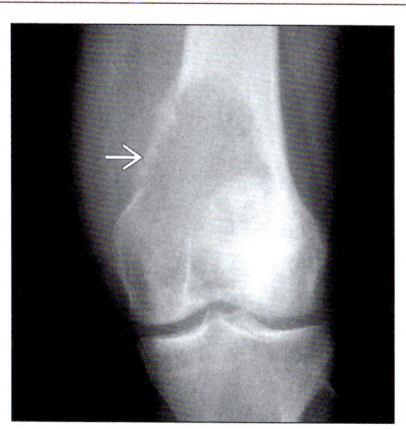

(Left) Anterior bone scan shows a distal femoral GCT with central necrosis ➔ and reactive hyperemia on the opposite side of the knee joint ➔. See next image. (Center) Left lateral bone scan shows the distal femoral lesion ➔ with reactive change due to hyperemia in the patella and proximal tibia ➔. (Right) Anterior radiograph shows the lytic lesion without sclerotic margin with septations and no bone or cartilage matrix in the distal femur ➔.

SKELETAL METASTASES

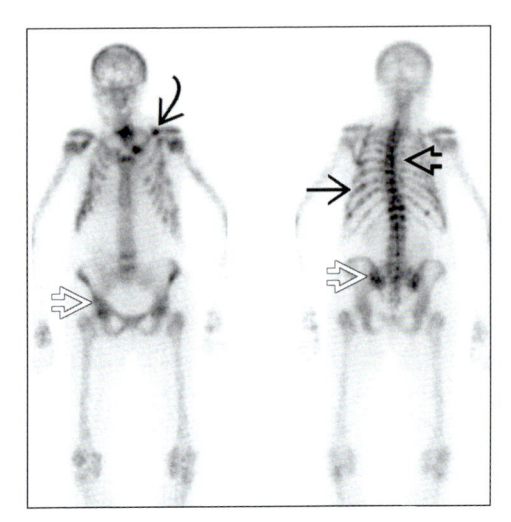

Anterior and posterior bone scan shows increased activity in extensive diffuse bony metastases: Ribs ➔, spine ⮞, clavicle ➔, and pelvis ➔.

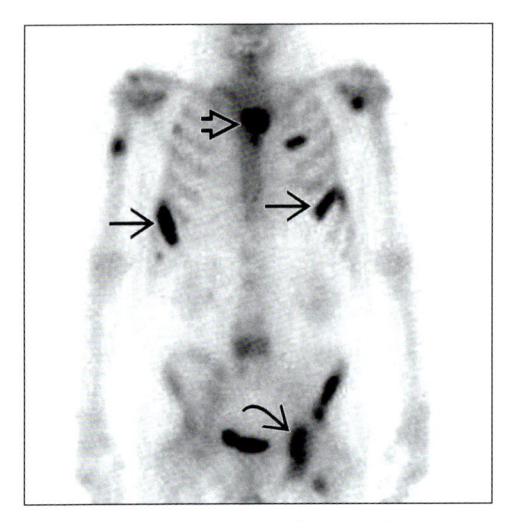

Anterior bone scan shows typical elongated appearance of multiple scattered bone metastases: Ribs ➔, manubrium ⮞, left acetabulum ➔.

TERMINOLOGY

Abbreviations and Synonyms
- Bone metastases, metastatic lesions to bone, secondary bone tumors

Definitions
- Rests of ectopic, viable, replicating neoplastic cells

IMAGING FINDINGS

General Features
- Best diagnostic clue
  - Scattered multiple sites typical, mapping areas of accelerated osteoblastic remodeling
    - Most lesions demonstrate increased tracer activity
- Location
  - Ribs, spine, pelvis, appendicular bones (esp. proximal femurs and humeri), sternum, calvarium
    - Randomly distributed (versus patterns of trauma, systemic disease or other benign process)
    - Especially areas of red marrow
    - May involve all or almost all of marrow space
    - Less common distally in long bones
- Morphology
  - Infiltrative, elongated appearance, may be expansile
    - Focal activity or regional patterns may represent fracture/arthropathy, not metastatic disease

Nuclear Medicine Findings
- Typical appearance: Scattered bone lesions with predilection for red marrow (axial, proximal appendicular)
  - Single lesions less commonly neoplastic, however metastatic disease not excluded
  - Ribs: Linear uptake
  - Vertebrae: Asymmetrical, not confined to endplate
  - Distal long bones: Less common pattern, more common in renal cell, lung, thyroid cancer
- Most metastases show focal ↑ tracer accumulation on bone scan, indicating cortical remodeling
- Some tumors may be photopenic (usually aggressive, overwhelmingly osteolytic/osteoclastic)
  - Renal cell carcinoma, thyroid carcinoma, poorly differentiated anaplastic tumors
    - Occasionally lung, breast, neuroblastoma, myeloma

DDx: Abnormal Skeletal Tracer Uptake in Cancer Patients

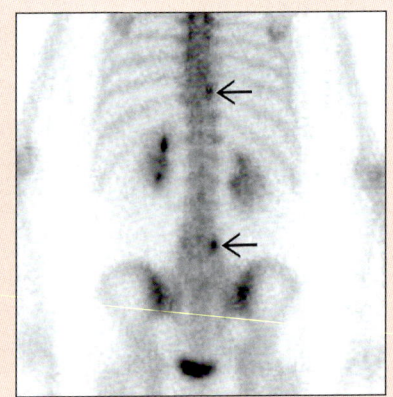

Degenerative Changes

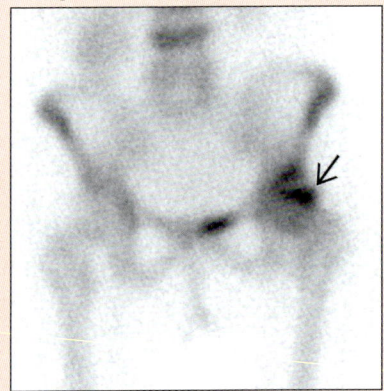

Avascular Necrosis

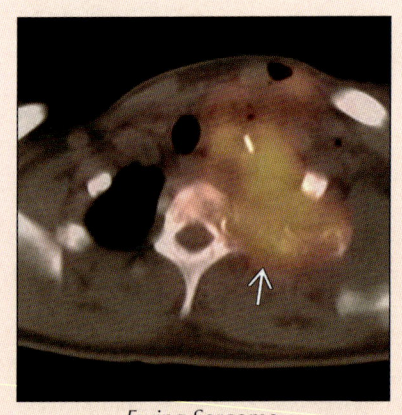

Ewing Sarcoma

SKELETAL METASTASES

Key Facts

Imaging Findings
- Typical appearance: Scattered bone lesions with predilection for red marrow (axial, proximal appendicular)
- Most metastases show focal ↑ tracer accumulation on bone scan, indicating cortical remodeling
- Some tumors may be photopenic (usually aggressive, overwhelmingly osteolytic/osteoclastic)
- "Flare" phenomenon: Increased conspicuity and number of lesions can occur with healing and osteoblastic remodeling by 4-6 weeks post therapy
- Disseminated bone lesions may yield diffusely increased activity: "Superscan"
- F-18 FDG PET: More sensitive/specific than bone scan, includes whole-body soft tissue evaluation
- F-18 NaF PET: Excellent PET bone agent, currently not reimbursed
- Plain film and CT: Sclerotic, lytic or mixed lesions
- MR: Decreased T1, intermediate or increased T2 and gadolinium-enhanced signal in lytic metastases

Top Differential Diagnoses
- Degenerative Processes, Arthropathies
- Healing Fracture or Bone Injury
- Primary Bone Tumors
- Avascular Necrosis, Osteonecrosis, Infarct
- Metabolic Disease, Infection, or Inflammation

Diagnostic Checklist
- Single lesions may be difficult to categorize, necessitating additional imaging

---

- Lesions may be photopenic following radiotherapy
- Often surrounded by reactive rim of activity
- Tumors typically confined to marrow space may have no significant cortical remodeling; therefore, may not be visualized on bone scan
  - Multiple myeloma, lymphoma, leukemia
- "Flare" phenomenon: Increased conspicuity and number of lesions can occur with healing and osteoblastic remodeling by 4-6 weeks post therapy
  - Do not confuse for disease progression, bone pain may also increase during flare
  - Exercise caution in interpretation for ~ 3-6 months, activity declines and tends to resolve thereafter
  - F-18 FDG PET can help distinguish treatment induced flare and tumor response from progression
  - Consider with "mixed" bone scan post-therapy: Some lesions resolved, some stable, some new
- Disseminated bone lesions may yield diffusely increased activity: "Superscan"
  - Diffuse increased skeletal activity with relative absence of normal renal, soft tissue activity
    - Breast, prostate cancer most common cancers with superscan

Imaging Recommendations
- Best imaging tool
  - Tc-99m whole body bone scan
    - Tc-99m methylene diphosphonate (MDP) or Tc-99m hydroxymethylene diphosphonate (HDP)
    - Diagnosis, staging, restaging, response to therapy
    - Most efficient imaging modality: Allows whole body evaluation with single study
    - Widely available, well tolerated
    - Sensitivity 80-90%, better than plain radiograph or CT but somewhat nonspecific
    - Plain film correlation for further characterization/ambiguity; additional evaluation with CT or MR as necessary
  - FDG PET and whole body MR have been utilized, not standard of care (↑ cost, limited availability)
- Protocol advice
  - Whole body bone scan
    - Adult dose: 20-25 mCi (740-925 MBq) Tc-99m MDP or HDP IV
    - Pediatric dose: As low as 2 mCi (74 MBq) according to dose algorithms; e.g., ages < 12 y use Webster rule: (Age+1/age+7) x adult dose
    - Hydrate patient prior to procedure to promote soft tissue washout, improves target:background activity
    - Inject in extremity away from sites of interest to prevent false (+) due to endovascular pooling, venous valvular adherence
    - Image at 3-4 hours, 2-3 hours longer with poor cardiac output, renal failure; up to 24 h in difficult cases
    - Best target:background at 6-12 h
    - Image after patient voids; catheterization may be useful, "sit on detector" view to distinguish bladder from bone activity
    - Whole body scan: 1 million count anterior/posterior planar image
    - Spot images: Static 500k count images of lateral skull, pelvis, lumbar spine, any areas of concern
    - SPECT regions of clinical concern if planar image unrevealing; fusion to CT or MR useful
- Additional nuclear medicine imaging options
  - F-18 FDG PET: More sensitive/specific than bone scan, includes whole-body soft tissue evaluation
    - Reveals marrow lesions in FDG-avid disease prior to cortical effects (often before bone scan becomes positive)
    - Ineffective for tumors that are not FDG-avid: Prostate cancer, highly mucinous tumors, occasionally renal cell carcinoma
    - Also limited in some sclerotic metastases
    - Detects 75% more breast and lung bone metastases than conventional bone scan
  - F-18 NaF PET: Excellent PET bone agent, currently not reimbursed
- Correlative imaging features
  - Evaluation of specific lesions or focal regions of concern, generally not whole body surveys
  - Plain film and CT: Sclerotic, lytic or mixed lesions

SKELETAL METASTASES

- Plain radiographs relatively insensitive, requiring loss of 40-60% of mineralization to be apparent
  - MR: Decreased T1, intermediate or increased T2 and gadolinium-enhanced signal in lytic metastases
    - Decreased T1 and T2 in sclerotic lesions
    - No enhancement in necrotic lesions

DIFFERENTIAL DIAGNOSIS

Degenerative Processes, Arthropathies
- Common at acromioclavicular/sternoclavicular joints, disc spaces, facets, esp. cervical and lower lumbar spines
  - Also at first carpal metacarpal joints, knees, feet

Healing Fracture or Bone Injury
- Usually focal rather than infiltrative or elongated
- Correlate with patient history
- Exclude pathologic fracture

Physiologic Activity
- Sacroiliac joints, kidneys, bladder, nasopharynx, calvarium (skull may be patchy)
- Growth plates in skeletally immature patient
  - May obscure underlying metastatic disease such as neuroblastoma; look for asymmetry

Primary Bone Tumors
- Lymphoma, myeloma, enchondroma, osteoma, fibrous dysplasia
  - Activity in enchondroma may be benign, suspect if changes occur

Avascular Necrosis, Osteonecrosis, Infarct
- Especially at femoral heads, humeral heads, knees
- Steroids, trauma, pancreatitis, sickle cell disease, radiation necrosis, alcohol use, collagen vascular disease

Metabolic Disease, Infection, or Inflammation
- Brown tumor of hyperparathyroidism
- Cushing disease, steroids
- Orthopedic hardware complication
  - Failure, loosening, infection, particle/cement disease
- Periodontal disease
- Paget disease

PATHOLOGY

General Features
- Etiology
  - Vascular spread by both arterial and venous routes of dissemination
    - Direct extension from adjacent tumor and lymphangitic spread can also occur
  - Adults: Breast cancer, prostate cancer, renal cell carcinoma, bronchogenic cancer, colon cancer, carcinoid = common primary tumors
  - Children: Neuroblastoma, Ewing sarcoma, rhabdosarcoma, retinoblastoma, medulloblastoma
- Associated abnormalities: Pathologic fractures

CLINICAL ISSUES

Presentation
- Most common signs/symptoms
  - Bone pain in absence of (or with trivial) corresponding insult
  - Lesion noted incidentally on conventional imaging
- Other signs/symptoms
  - Abnormal alkaline phosphatase elevation
    - May be absent in 50% of patients

Demographics
- Age: Most often adults corresponding to overall ↑ cancer incidence with age

Natural History & Prognosis
- Metastatic disease to bone indicates distant disease, advanced stage, portends a generally worsened prognosis
  - May lead to pathologic fracture secondary to compromised structural integrity, disorganized reparative response, demineralization
  - Contributes to pain and decreased quality of life

Treatment
- Systemic chemotherapy, targeted external beam radiotherapy, occasionally radiotherapy mediated by beta-emitting radioisotopes, e.g., Sr-89
  - Sr-89 chloride internal radiotherapy as palliation for pain efficacious in ≤ 80%
    - Decreases pain, analgesic therapy, delays opioid treatment; improves quality of life
    - May result in leukothrombopenia
    - Does not treat metastases
- Vertebroplasty with polymethylmethacrylate

DIAGNOSTIC CHECKLIST

Image Interpretation Pearls
- Suspicious for metastases: Increased tracer localization in lesions not attributable to trauma, degenerative changes or physiologic activity
- Photopenic lesions are suspicious for highly aggressive lesions, marrow fibrosis (often post-radiation) or marrow replacement (hemangioma)
- Single lesions may be difficult to categorize, necessitating additional imaging
  - Solitary skull lesions often benign (can be seen in ~ 10% of patients without metastatic disease)

SELECTED REFERENCES

1. Fujimoto R et al: Diagnostic accuracy of bone metastases detection in cancer patients: comparison between bone scintigraphy and whole-body FDG-PET. Ann Nucl Med. 20(6):399-408, 2006
2. Schmidt GP et al: Screening for bone metastases: whole-body MRI using a 32-channel system versus dual-modality PET-CT. Eur Radiol. 2006
3. Schneider JA et al: Flare on bone scintigraphy following Taxol chemotherapy for metastatic breast cancer. J Nucl Med. 35(11):1748-52, 1994

SKELETAL METASTASES

IMAGE GALLERY

Typical

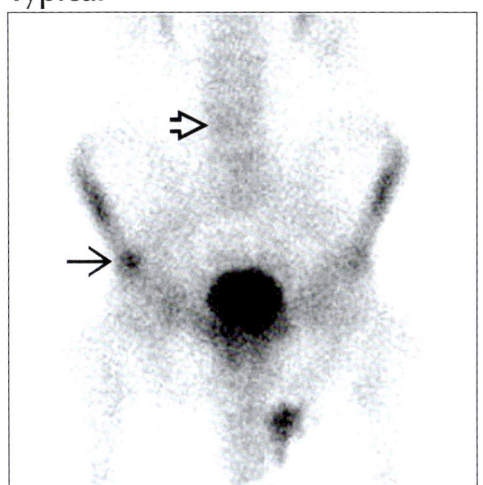

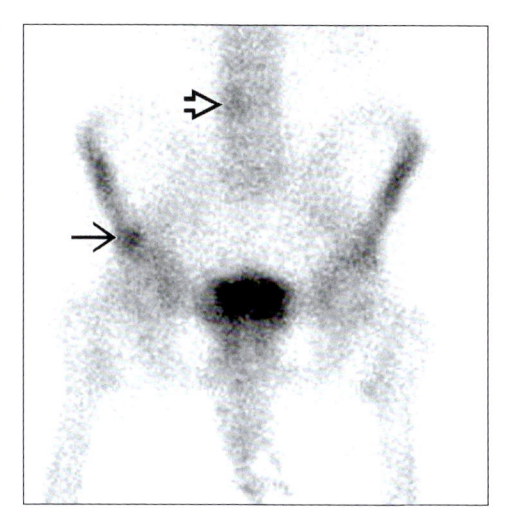

(**Left**) Anterior bone scan shows increased activity in a right acetabular lesion ➔ confirmed as metastases on CT, and a subtle right L4 vertebral lesion ⇨ with no corresponding CT abnormality. See next image. (**Right**) Anterior bone scan in same patient three months later, shows right acetabular metastases ➔ and increased conspicuity of L4 vertebral metastasis ⇨, confirmed on MR.

Typical

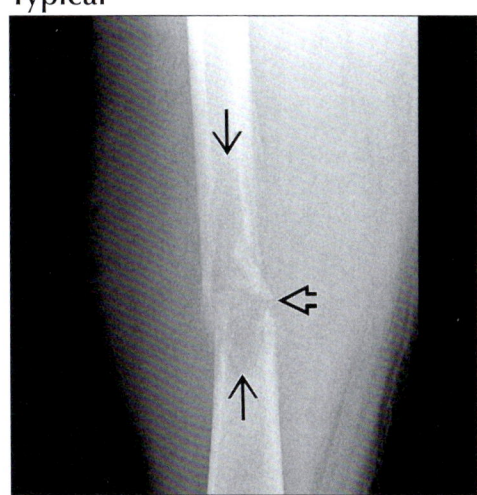

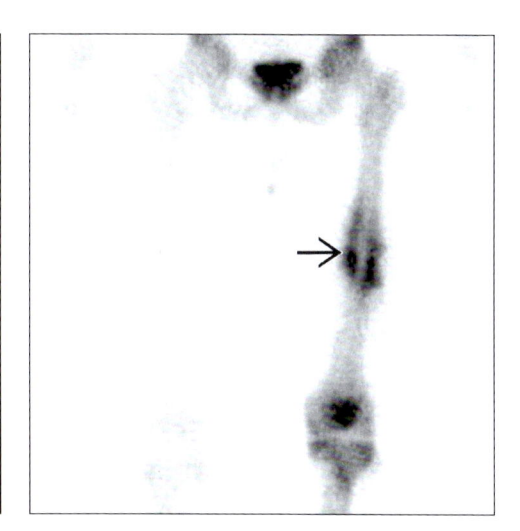

(**Left**) Posterior plain film shows lytic demineralization ➔ with pathologic fracture through lesion ⇨, demonstrating typical infiltrative appearance of lytic metastases. See next image. (**Right**) Anterior bone scan shows increased activity in the mid-left femoral metastatic lesion ➔ following open reduction internal fixation.

Variant

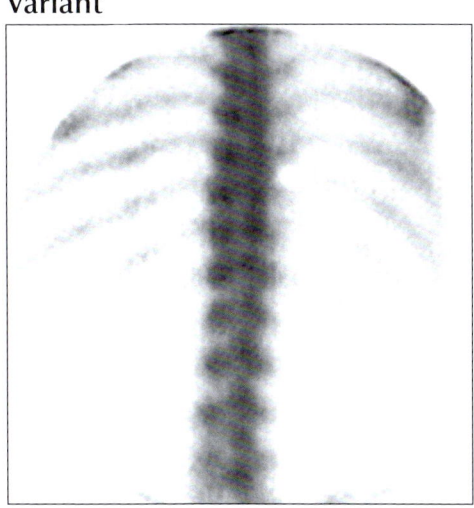

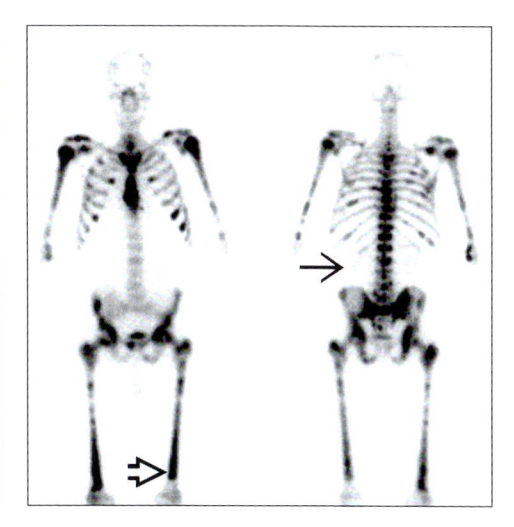

(**Left**) Posterior bone scan shows diffuse, uniform tracer uptake in bony structures without apparent renal or soft tissue activity, consistent with superscan. Typically, metastatic pattern is more patchy. (**Right**) Anterior and posterior typical superscan due to metastatic disease shows patchy diffuse increased skeletal activity ending in distal femurs ⇨, minimal renal activity ➔.

SKELETAL METASTASES

(Left) Left lateral bone scan contiguous increased activity in cervical spine ➔ with absence of calvarial activity ➔, consistent with headless-type superscan. (Right) Posterior bone scan in blood pool phase shows renal excretion of tracer ➔, early deposition in thoracic vertebra ➔ and ribs ➔. Photopenic L-spine and pelvis ➔ is consistent with previous radiation.

Variant

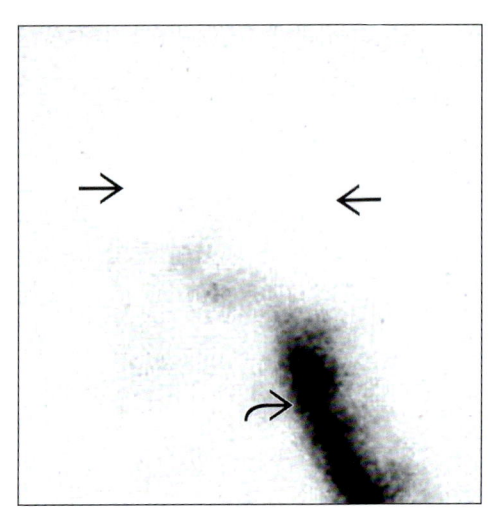

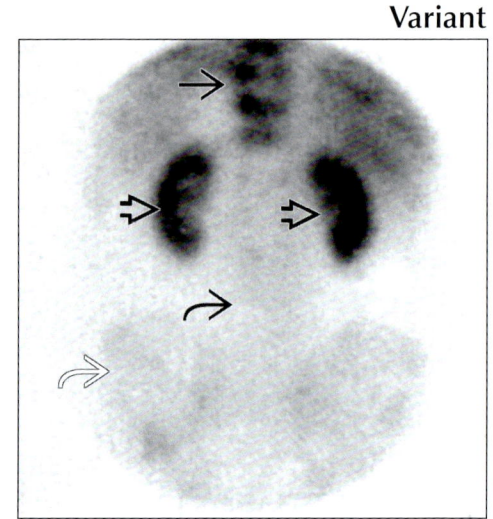

Variant

(Left) Anterior bone scan shows photopenic lesion in left margin of sternum ➔ in patient with breast cancer. This lesion was not evident on CT. Note additional metastasis in manubrium ➔. See next image. (Right) Anterior bone scan in same patient at left shows photopenic abnormality of the right ileum with subtle rim of activity ➔, indicating another lytic metastasis.

Variant

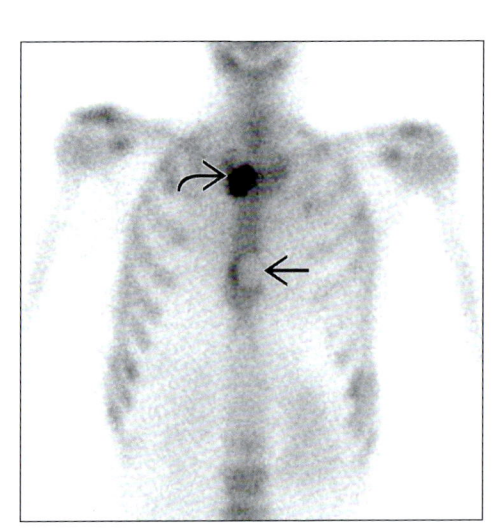

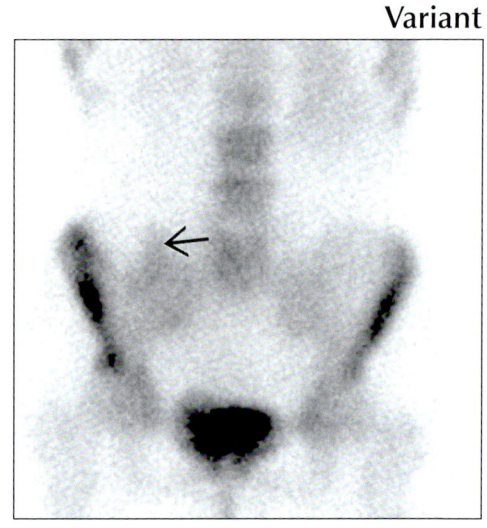

(Left) Anterior and posterior bone scan shows multiple, scattered foci of increased activity in osteoblastic lesions ➔ with coexistent photopenic right anterior rib lesion ➔. See next image. (Right) Axial CECT in same patient at left shows expansile lytic metastatic lesion of the rib ➔ corresponding to the photopenic lesion on bone scan.

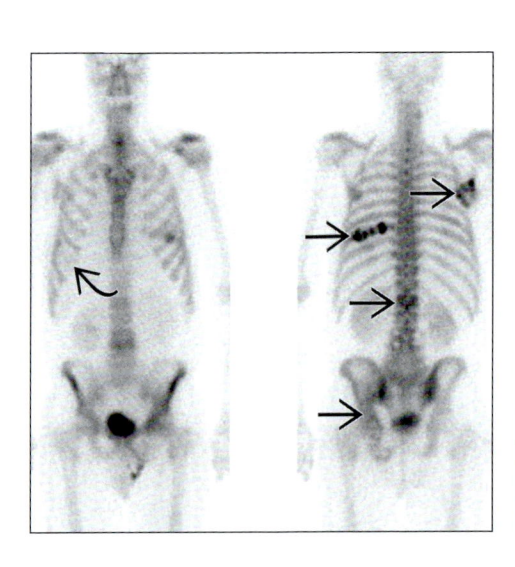

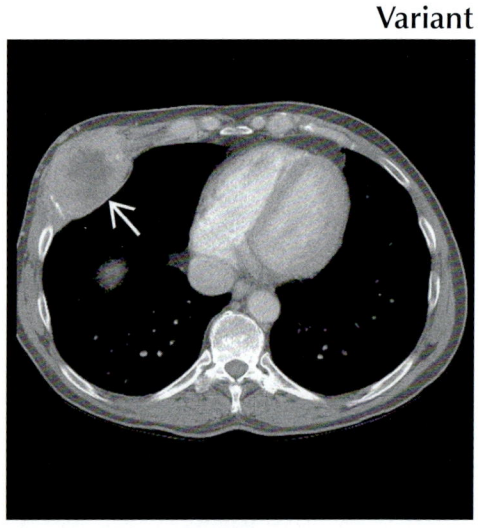

SKELETAL METASTASES

Typical

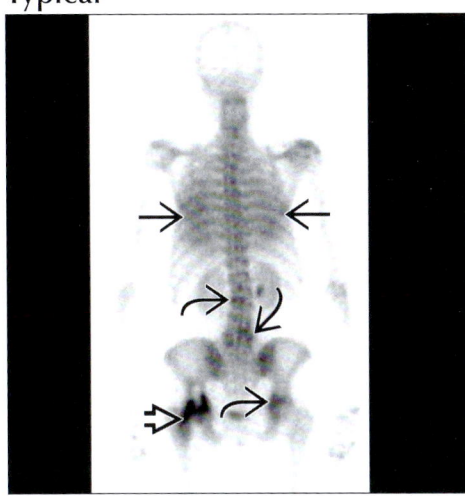

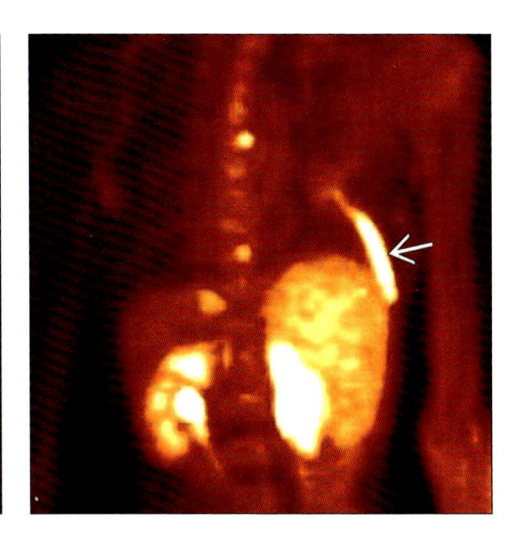

(Left) Posterior bone scan shows bone metastasis ➡ and hazy activity overlying lungs ➡, indicating malignant pleural effusions. Also note areas of degenerative change ➡. (Right) MIP F-18 FDG PET shows typical elongated, infiltrative appearance of FDG-avid right rib metastases ➡.

Typical

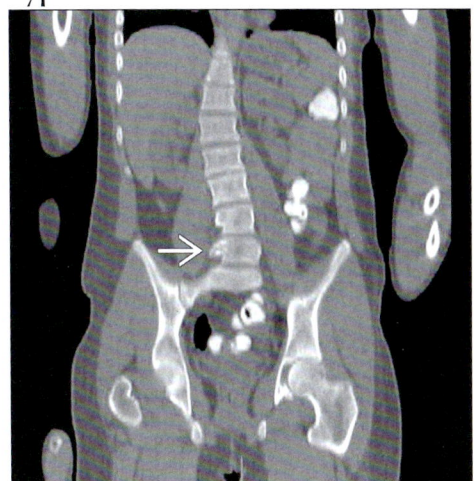

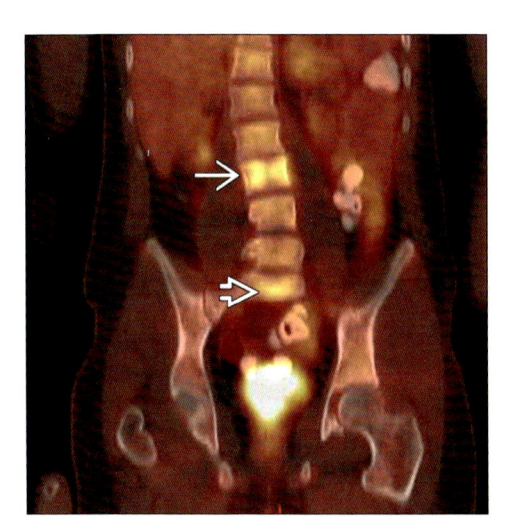

(Left) Coronal NECT shows scoliotic curvature with mild degenerative changes ➡ laterally, but no definite lytic or blastic metastases. See next image. (Right) Coronal FDG PET/CT in same patient at left shows hypermetabolic metastases at L3 ➡ and S1 ➡, occult by CT, illustrating the sensitivity of PET for bone lesions.

Typical

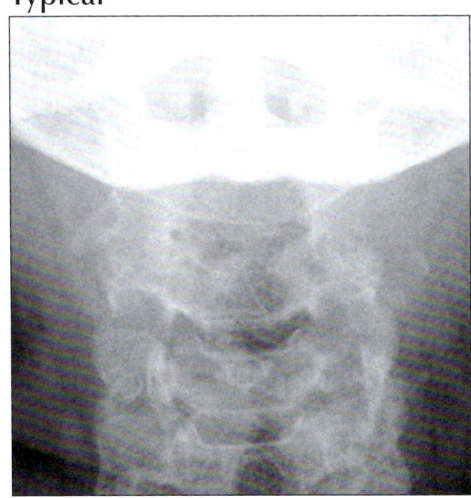

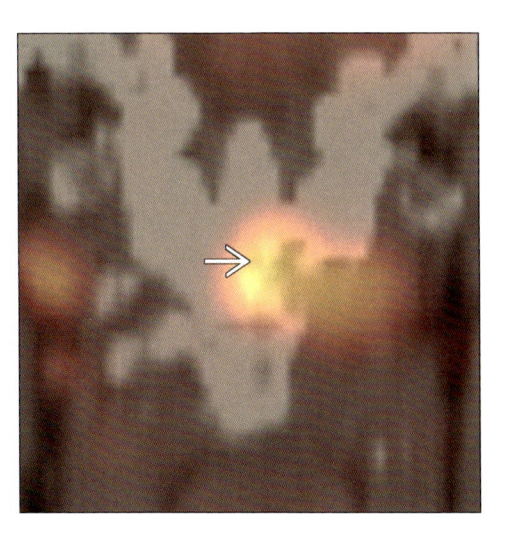

(Left) Anterior-posterior plain film of upper cervical spine shows no focal lytic or sclerotic lesions in patient with neck pain. (Right) Coronal fused FDG PET/CT in same patient at left shows FDG-avid lytic metastases ➡ of left C2 vertebral body with destructive changes extending to midline.

SUPERSCAN

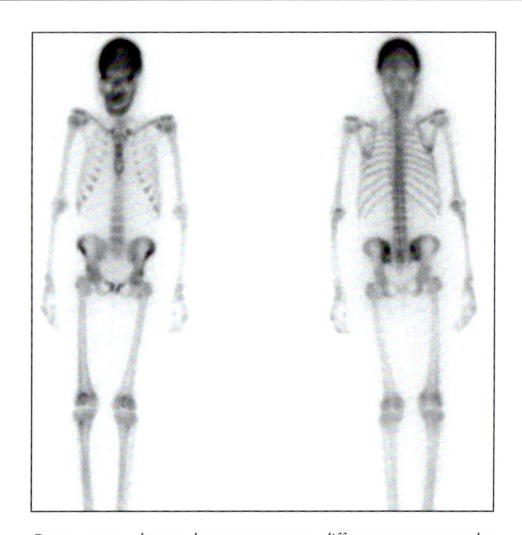

Bone scan shows homogeneous diffuse tracer uptake throughout entire skeleton, intense in calvarium, with absence of renal and soft tissue uptake (metabolic superscan pattern).

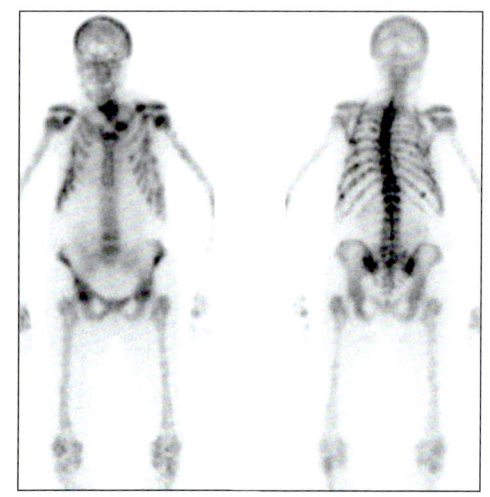

Anterior and posterior mineral phase planar imaging shows a heterogeneous superscan pattern, (diffuse metastatic disease). Note the near complete absence of the kidneys.

TERMINOLOGY

Abbreviations and Synonyms
- Super bone scan
- Beautiful bone scan
- Supernormal bone scan

Definitions
- Diffusely increased bony visualization usually with absent or near complete absence of soft tissue, renal, and bladder tracer activity

IMAGING FINDINGS

General Features
- Best diagnostic clue
  - Elevated widespread skeletal uptake of Tc-99m diphosphonate tracer
    - Early diffuse uptake of tracer in bones on vascular phase images
    - Relative absence of renal cortical activity on delayed images
    - Relative decrease in soft tissue activity
    - Activity typically present in bladder unless renal failure
    - Activity may be seen in collecting system if obstructed
- Location
  - Metastatic disease
    - Metastatic pattern follows red marrow distribution: Axial and proximal appendicular skeleton
    - Expansion of central bone marrow into periphery: Extension into more distal long bones
    - Metastatic pattern: Often spares the calvarium, resulting in the so called "headless" bone scan pattern
  - Metabolic disease and excessively delayed imaging in normal patient: Diffuse pattern
    - Diffuse pattern: Involves entire skeleton, including peripheral skeleton (hands, feet)
- Morphology
  - Metastatic pattern
    - Metastatic: Usually heterogeneous or patchy
    - In rare cases, extensive metastatic involvement can be near-confluent on bone scan
  - Metabolic pattern

DDx: Atypical Homogeneous Superscan Due to Mets (Medulloblastoma)

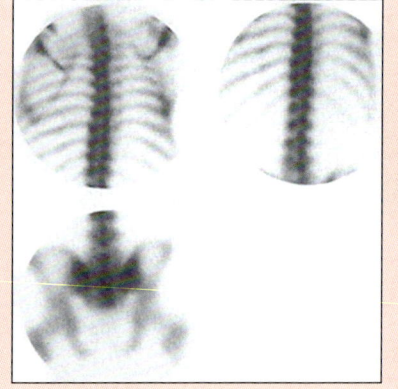

Kidneys Not Visible   *Distal Femur Cutoff*   *Forearms Not Visible*

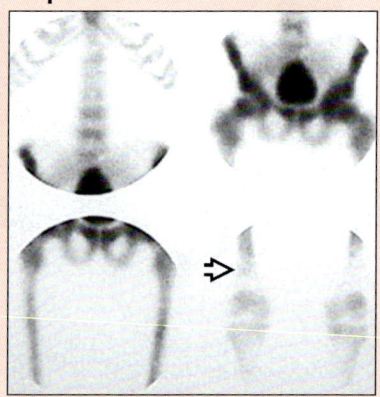

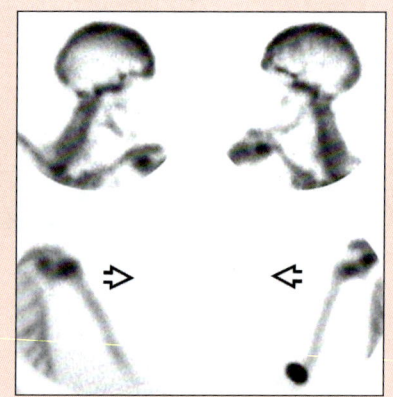

SUPERSCAN

Key Facts

Terminology
- Super bone scan
- Beautiful bone scan
- Supernormal bone scan

Imaging Findings
- Elevated widespread skeletal uptake of Tc-99m diphosphonate tracer
- Early diffuse uptake of tracer in bones on vascular phase images
- Relative absence of renal cortical activity on delayed images
- Relative decrease in soft tissue activity
- Activity typically present in bladder unless renal failure
- Activity may be seen in collecting system if obstructed

- Metastatic pattern follows red marrow distribution: Axial and proximal appendicular skeleton
- Metastatic pattern: Often spares the calvarium, resulting in the so called "headless" bone scan pattern
- Diffuse pattern: Involves entire skeleton, including peripheral skeleton (hands, feet)
- Metastatic: Usually heterogeneous or patchy
- In rare cases, extensive metastatic involvement can be near-confluent on bone scan
- Metabolic: Homogeneous, or confluent tracer uptake
- Metabolic: Transverse sternal and sternomanubrial activity ("striped tie" or "necktie" sign)
- Metabolic: Often intense calvarial activity
- Anterior rib ends may be hot (costochondral junctions) in osteomalacia

---

- Metabolic: Homogeneous, or confluent tracer uptake
- Metabolic: Transverse sternal and sternomanubrial activity ("striped tie" or "necktie" sign)
- Metabolic: Often intense calvarial activity
- Anterior rib ends may be hot (costochondral junctions) in osteomalacia

Nuclear Medicine Findings
- Bone Scan
  - Early localization in bones on vascular phase images - particularly vertebral and pelvic
  - Increased skeletal activity on mineral phase images
  - Skeletal tracer activity is so intense that renal and soft tissue activity appear absent in comparison
  - Tc-99m-diphosphonates (MDP, HDP): Conventional tracers for radionuclide bone scanning
    - Tc-99m-dimercaptosuccinate [Tc-99 (V) DMSA]: Rarely used as a confirmatory imaging tracer in equivocal cases; a tumor labeling agent
    - Areas of specific concern can be evaluated with spot films or correlated with other imaging modalities
  - "Headless bone scan" is an uncommon manifestation of metastatic superscan inferring a probable diagnosis of prostate cancer
    - Prostate cancer rarely metastasizes to the cranial vault, (approximately 7%), thus prostate cancer patients with superscans often demonstrate a headless appearance
    - Mechanism of headless bone scan: Markedly low calvarial tracer activity relative to diffusely increased activity in the remainder of the bony structures
  - Comparison with conventional plain film radiography, CT, or MR is useful in patients with initial or equivocal findings
  - Reduced sensitivity of Tc-99m diphosphate scan for metastatic disease
    - Multiple myeloma, neuroblastoma, and purely lytic disease (some lung cancer, breast cancer, renal cell cancer)

Imaging Recommendations
- Best imaging tool: Delayed Tc-99 MDP imaging, (standard mineral phase)
- Protocol advice
  - Mineral phase imaging should be performed 3-4 hours after injection as standard protocol
    - Earlier imaging results in residual soft tissue tracer activity and insufficient chemisorption to skeletal bone
    - Avoid abnormally long uptake times (> 4 h) as they may result in false positive superscan patterns, clearance of soft tissue and renal activity
  - More delayed imaging may be necessary in patients with poor cardiac function or renal insufficiency
    - Allows sufficient clearance of soft tissue background and blood pool tracer
- Other imaging modalities
  - PET and PET/CT
    - Poorly sensitive in prostate cancer and renal cell carcinoma
    - Not CMS approved for many types of tumors
    - Role in many types of tumors not yet established
    - F-18-NaF may ultimately replace conventional bone scan
    - FDG PET detects 75% more sites of bone mets than conventional bone scan for breast and lung cancer bony mets
  - MR
    - Indicated as first line in acute back pain in presence of cancer (with or without bone scan findings) to exclude epidural tumor
    - Confirmation of metastatic disease when homogeneous superscan in cancer patient
  - CT
    - Assessment of painful lytic bone lesions and subtle pathologic fractures
    - More sensitive than plain film in identifying lytic lesions in the spine
  - Plain radiography
    - Best when reserved for confirmation of suspected degenerative changes as cause of bone scan abnormalities

SUPERSCAN

DIFFERENTIAL DIAGNOSIS

Diffuse Metastases
- Prostate cancer, breast cancer, lung, renal cell carcinoma, bladder, lymphoma

Metabolic Disease
- Hyperparathyroidism
  - Secondary hyperparathyroidism more likely to present with abnormal bone scan findings than primary hyperparathyroidism
- Osteomalacia
- Secondary hypertrophic osteoarthropathy (HPOA)

Paget Disease
- Often patchy but usually involves entire bone - both lytic and sclerotic components are "hot"
- Suspected with both anterior and posterior element uptake on bone scan
- Common, and may therefore co-exist with metastatic disease
- MRI: Typically with normal marrow signal with Paget disease
- Plain film, CT: Coarsened trabeculae, thickened cortex, reduced size of marrow cavity

Delayed Imaging of a Normal Patient
- Imaging later than the normal 3-4 hours may result in sufficient soft tissue and renal clearance to result in false diagnosis of "superscan"
- As little as 5-6 hours may be enough delay to result in soft tissue and renal clearance mimicking a superscan pattern

PATHOLOGY

General Features
- Etiology
  - From rapid and increased deposition of calcium pyrophosphate as the result of abnormal osteoblastic activity
  - Tc-99m diphosphonate is an analog of calcium pyrophosphate (hydroxyapatite)
  - Reduced radionuclide activity in soft tissues and excretion by the kidneys is both relative and absolute (less available for soft tissue uptake or renal clearance)
- Associated abnormalities: Bone pain, elevated alkaline phosphatase and serum calcium levels, pathological insufficiency fractures, spinal cord compression

CLINICAL ISSUES

Presentation
- Most common signs/symptoms: Diffuse bone pain
- Other signs/symptoms
  - Elevated alkaline phosphatase
  - Elevated acid phosphatase
  - Abnormal titer of serological markers IgG-VCA and IgA-VCA

Treatment
- Sr-89 and Sm-153 for palliation of bone pain due to metastatic disease
- Biochemical modulation, pamidronate, cisplatin, futraful, uracil, diethylstilbestrol diphosphate, dexamethasone, and endocrine therapy
- Tc-99 (V) DMSA concentration in skeletal metastases can reveal potential therapeutic potential for Re-188 and Re-186 (V) DMSA regimens
- Radiation therapy can target specific regions when clinically appropriate (focal pain, risk of spinal cord compression or pathologic fracture)

DIAGNOSTIC CHECKLIST

Consider
- Increased skeletal activity relative to soft tissues including decreased or absent renal visualization
- Delayed imaging in a normal patient

Image Interpretation Pearls
- Look for decreased soft tissue and kidney activity during examination of every bone scan
  - If there are functioning kidneys, there should be some bladder activity
- Superscan can be difficult to diagnose when uptake is uniform
- Diffuse activity, down to small bones of hands and feet suspicious for metabolic disease
- Patchy activity, relative sparing of distal axial skeleton, calvarium more consistent with metastatic disease

SELECTED REFERENCES

1. Basu S et al: 99Tc(m)(V)DMSA scintigraphy in skeletal metastases and superscans arising from various malignancies: diagnosis, treatment monitoring and therapeutic implications. Br J Radiol. 77(916):347-61, 2004
2. Pour MC et al: Diffuse increased uptake on bone scan: super scan. Semin Nucl Med. 34(2):154-6, 2004
3. Hoshi S et al: Complete regression of bone metastases on super bone scan, by low-dose cisplatin, UFT, diethylstilbestrol diphosphate, and dexamethasone in a patient with hormone-refractory prostate cancer. Int J Clin Oncol. 8(2):118-20, 2003
4. Kim S et al: "Superscan" in an autosomal-dominant benign form of osteopetrosis. Clin Nucl Med. 26(7):636-7, 2001
5. Evans JC et al: Extensive soft tissue uptake of 99Tcm methylene diphosphonate in a patient with multiple myeloma. Br J Radiol. 73(873):1018-20, 2000
6. Yuksel D et al: The role of Tc-99m (V) DMSA scintigraphy in the evaluation of superscan on bone scintigraphy. Clin Nucl Med. 25(3):193-6, 2000
7. Liu RS et al: Superscan in patients with nasopharyngeal carcinoma. Clin Nucl Med. 21(4):302-6, 1996
8. Massie JD et al: The headless bone scan: an uncommon manifestation of metastatic superscan in carcinoma of the prostate. Skeletal Radiol. 17(2):111-3, 1988
9. Datz FL: Beautiful Bone Scan. In: Gamuts in Nuclear Medicine. 2nd ed. Norwalk, CT: Appleton & Lange. 88-89, 1987

SUPERSCAN

IMAGE GALLERY

Typical

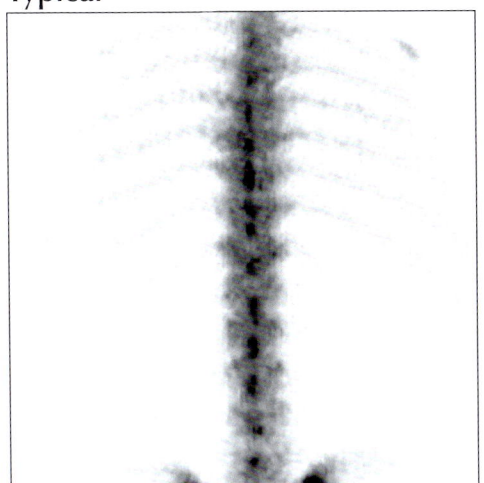

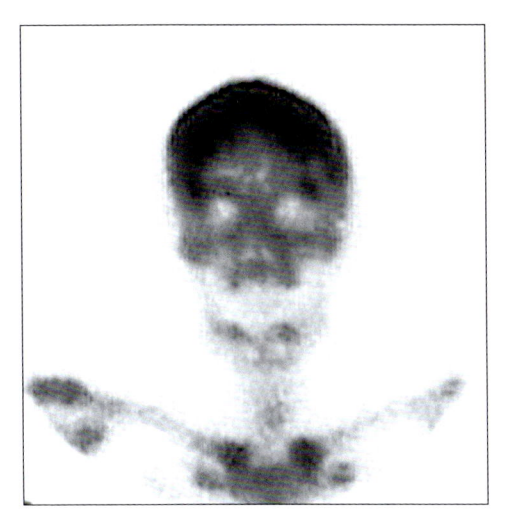

(Left) Posterior bone scan shows nonvisualization of kidneys, homogeneous diffuse skeletal uptake in patient with metabolic superscan pattern. See next image. *(Right)* Bone scan of skull shows diffuse intense calvarial uptake due to metabolic superscan (secondary hyperparathyroidism).

Variant

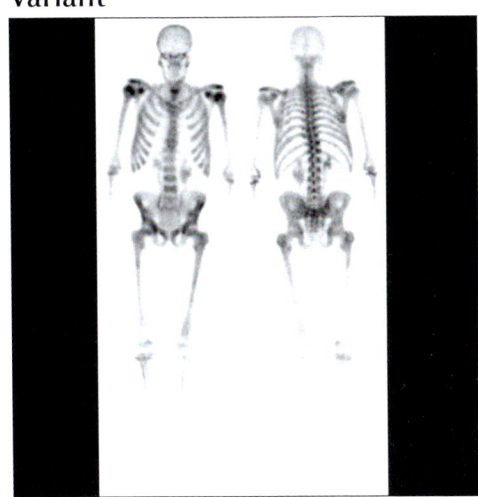

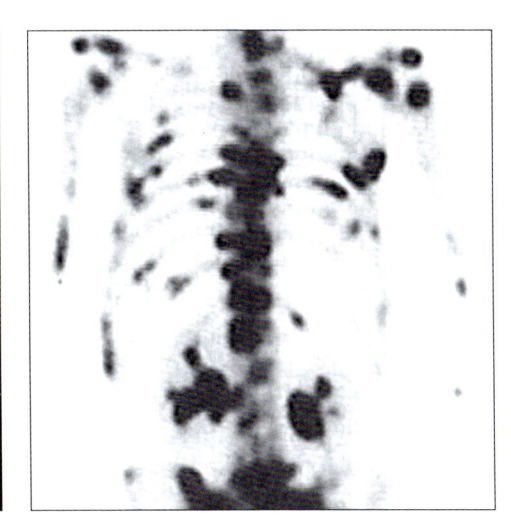

(Left) Bone scan shows slightly inhomogeneous, intense, near confluent uptake throughout axial and proximal appendicular skeleton and absence of soft tissue uptake (superscan). Bilateral renal collecting system uptake is due to obstruction. *(Right)* Posterior bone scan shows a heterogeneous superscan pattern of tracer accumulation with absence of renal parenchyma. The renal pelvises are prominent secondary to distal obstruction.

Typical

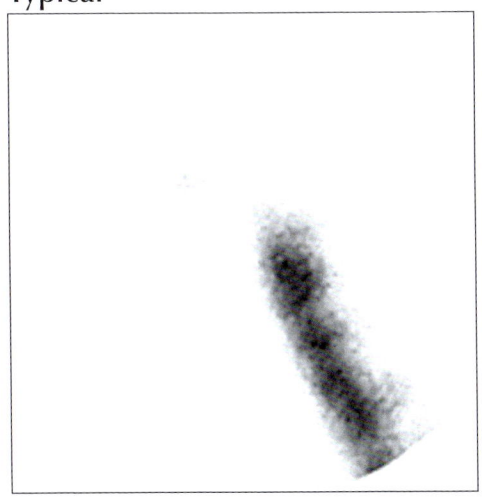

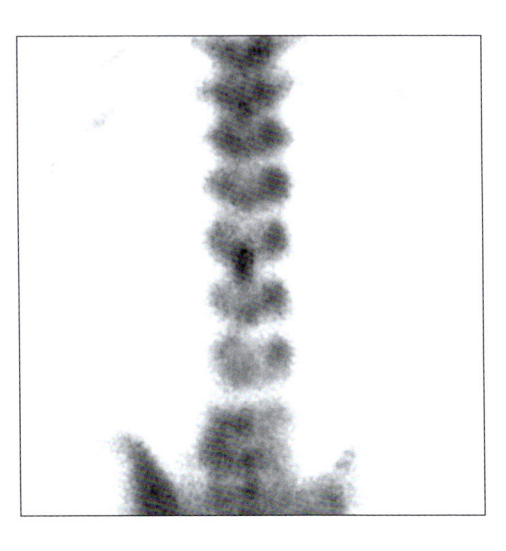

(Left) Left lateral bone scan of the head and neck shows diffuse activity within the cervical spine, but almost no activity in the bones of the face and calvarium ("headless" superscan pattern). See next image. *(Right)* Posterior bone scan shows heterogeneous, intense uptake, absence of renal visualization (metastatic superscan patterns).

OSTEOSARCOMA

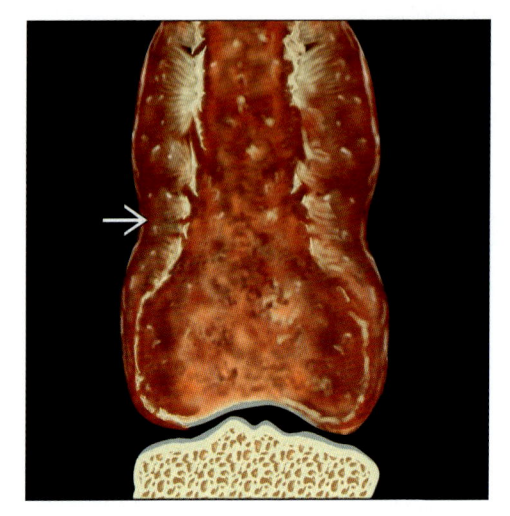

Graphic shows bone mass with cortical expansion and bone destruction in metaphyseal region distal femur, the most common location for primary osteosarcoma.

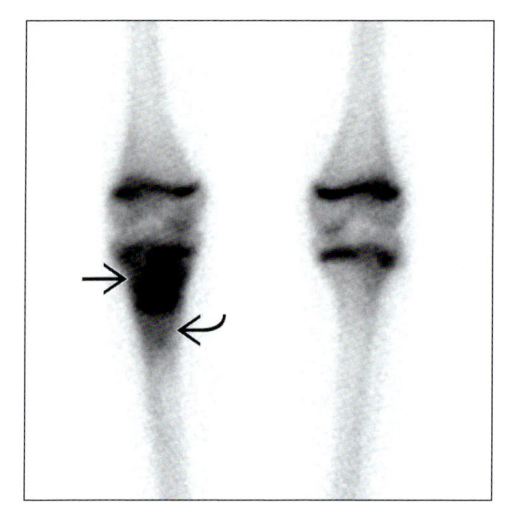

Anterior bone scan shows characteristic increased activity in osteosarcoma of proximal tibia. Smaller focus distally is suggestive of skip metastasis.

TERMINOLOGY

Abbreviations and Synonyms
- Osteogenic sarcoma; osteosarcoma; primary bone sarcoma

Definitions
- Primary malignant tumor of bone whose cells produce osteoid and have osteoblastic differentiation

IMAGING FINDINGS

General Features
- Best diagnostic clue
  - Radiograph, CT or MR: Heterogeneous metaphyseal mass
  - Tc-99m MDP bone scan: Increased activity in primary tumor, metastases (bone, lung)
  - FDG PET, Tl-201, Tc-99m Sestamibi (MIBI), Ga-67: Increased activity with ring appearance (indicates high grade osteosarcoma) in primary tumor
- Location
  - Regions of rapid bone growth, i.e., metaphyseal long bone
    - Femur: 42% (75% distal)
    - Tibia: 19% (80% proximal)
    - Humerus: 10% (90% proximal)
    - Pelvis: 8%
    - Jaw: 8%
- Morphology: Bone mass with cortical expansion, destruction of bone elements and lack of sclerotic rim

Nuclear Medicine Findings
- Bone Scan
  - Increased activity in primary tumor and metastases to bone, lung
  - SPECT images may show ring appearance
- FDG PET, Tl-201, Tc-99m MIBI, Ga-67
  - Tl-201, MIBI, FDG PET: High grade tumors = intense activity around photopenic region (less obvious with lower grade tumor)
  - FDG PET: Most reliable to follow therapeutic response
  - Ga-67: Increased activity in primary tumor, metastases; not helpful in following response to therapy

DDx: Common Lesions Simulating Osteosarcoma

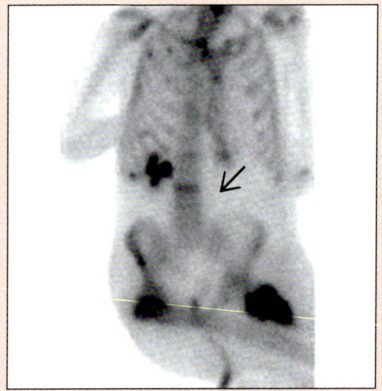

Heterotopic Bone

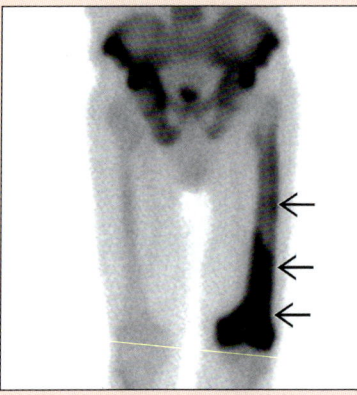

Paget Disease

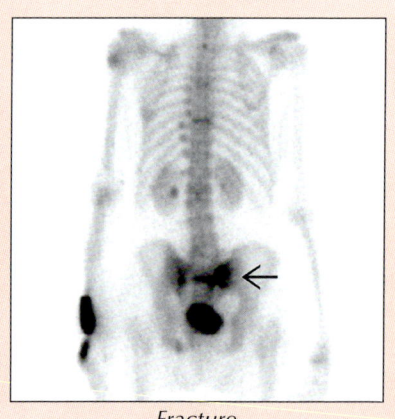

Fracture

OSTEOSARCOMA

Key Facts

Terminology
- Primary malignant tumor of bone whose cells produce osteoid and have osteoblastic differentiation

Imaging Findings
- Radiograph, CT or MR: Heterogeneous metaphyseal mass
- Tc-99m MDP bone scan: Increased activity in primary tumor, metastases (bone, lung)
- Tl-201, MIBI, FDG PET: High grade tumors = intense activity around photopenic region (less obvious with lower grade tumor)
- Ga-67: Increased activity in primary tumor, metastases; not helpful in following response to therapy
- FDG PET/CT: Assess heterogeneous lesions for optimal biopsy site, whole body staging, evaluate response to therapy, restage

Top Differential Diagnoses
- Trauma
- Infection
- Paget Disease
- Other Primary Bone Tumor
- Benign Bone Lesions
- Bone Metastases

Clinical Issues
- Pain localized to a palpable mass
- 10-20% of patients have metastatic disease at presentation
- Metastasis commonly involve lung and bone

Imaging Recommendations
- Best imaging tool
  - Radiography: Plain film first-line for initial presentation
  - Bone scan: Evaluate for multifocal disease, distant metastases
  - MR: Extent of intramedullary disease, soft tissue involvement, skip lesions
  - CT: Tumor extent, pulmonary metastases
  - FDG PET/CT: Assess heterogeneous lesions for optimal biopsy site, whole body staging, evaluate response to therapy, restage
  - Tl-201, Tc-99m MIBI, FDG PET: Better than CT/MR for tumor grading, estimating percentage of tumor necrosis
  - FDG PET: Standardized uptake value (SUV) shows good correlation with histopathologic grade, tumor cellularity, Ki-67 labeling, mitotic activity, overexpression of p53
  - FDG PET: Superior to MR/CT in detection/localization of recurrent tumor in patients with metallic prosthetic devices or hardware
  - FDG PET: Differentiation of benign residual masses from tumor best assessed with PET/CT (vs. CT or MR)
- Protocol advice
  - Bone scan
    - 20-30 mCi (740-1110 MBq) Tc99m-MDP IV
    - Planar whole body scan
    - SPECT for spine or chest lesions
  - Whole body scans
    - 3 mCi (111MBq) Tl-201 IV
    - 20-30 mCi (740-1110 MBq) Tc-99m MIBI IV
    - 10-20 mCi (370-740 MBq) FDG IV
    - 10 mCi (370 MBq) Ga-67 IV
- Correlative imaging features
  - CT and MR: May not indicate disease activity accurately (important in following tumor response to therapy)
  - MR: May overestimate residual disease following therapy due to Gadolinium enhancement in non-malignant reactive tissue and inflammation
  - Whole body PET/CT with MR = best methods to define disease extent, therapeutic response

DIFFERENTIAL DIAGNOSIS

Trauma
- Positive on Tl-201, Tc-99m MIBI, bone scan and FDG PET
  - Especially with fracture, hematoma
- Findings most evident in acute, early subacute phases

Infection
- Especially with abscess or extensive erosion

Paget Disease
- Bone scan may be strongly positive while Tl-201, Tc-99m MIBI and FDG PET most often demonstrate mild to moderate activity

Other Primary Bone Tumor
- Primary bone tumors other than osteosarcoma

Benign Bone Lesions
- Osteochondroma, enchondroma, chronic osteomyelitis, fibrous dysplasia, hereditary exostoses, bone infarct
  - Associated with increased risk of osteosarcoma
- Aneurysmal bone cyst, eosinophilic granuloma, osteoid osteoma

Bone Metastases
- Characteristic multifocal pattern of increased activity in skeleton
- Patient history of primary malignancy

PATHOLOGY

General Features
- Genetics
  - Germline mutation of retinoblastoma gene: Increased risk of osteosarcoma

OSTEOSARCOMA

- Li-Fraumeni syndrome: Germline mutation of p53 tumor suppressor gene, slight increased risk
- Rothmund-Thompson syndrome: Autosomal recessive, high risk of osteosarcoma (~ 30%); truncating mutation of RECQLA gene frequent
- Pagetoid osteosarcoma: Associated with loss of heterozygosity of chromosome 18
- Epidemiology
  - Ranks second in overall frequency in primary bone tumors behind multiple myeloma
  - Represents 5% of childhood cancers
  - Incidence in US: 4.8 cases/million/year in people < 20 years
  - Increased incidence with prior irradiation or chemotherapy
    - Radiation-induced osteosarcoma peak occurrence ~ 12-16 yrs
- Associated abnormalities
  - Benign bone disorders
    - Paget disease, osteochondroma, chronic osteomyelitis, multiple hereditary exostosis, fibrous dysplasia, bone infarcts

Gross Pathologic & Surgical Features
- Gross appearance often hemorrhagic, large destructive fleshy mass arising in metaphysis
- 90% of osteosarcomas are high grade intramedullary

Microscopic Features
- Malignant sarcomatous stroma with osteoid and bone
- Subclassification dependent on the differentiation of primitive mesenchymal cells toward bone, cartilage or fibrous tissue

Staging, Grading or Classification Criteria
- Enneking system staging
  - IA: Low grade tumor, intracompartmental
  - IB: Low grade tumor, extracompartmental
  - IIA: High grade tumor, intracompartmental
  - IIB: High grade tumor, extracompartmental
  - III: Any grade tumor with metastasis
- Staging system for spinal tumors: Complex, based on anatomic location of a spinal segment about a clock face and location

CLINICAL ISSUES

Presentation
- Most common signs/symptoms
  - Pain localized to a palpable mass
    - Frequently begins after injury, may be intermittent and worse with activity
  - Lymphadenopathy usually absent
  - 10-20% of patients have metastatic disease at presentation
  - Metastasis commonly involve lung and bone

Demographics
- Age
  - Bimodal distribution
    - 75% < 20 years, 15-20% > 65 years
    - Males slightly higher incidence than females
    - African American higher incidence than Caucasian

Natural History & Prognosis
- Untreated tumors progress at variable rates depending on tumor grade and host factors
- High grade tumors metastasize rapidly with lung and bone frequent sites
- Long term survival ~ 60-70%
- Long term prognosis dependent on response to neoadjuvant therapy, complete tumor resection

Treatment
- Neoadjuvant chemotherapy with complete resection followed by additional chemotherapy: Best opportunity for cure
- Surgery alone: Low 5 year survival in high grade tumors (approximately 10-20%)
- Surgical resection with limb sparing performed unless amputation required for completeness
- Radiation therapy: Not commonly used; however, wide surgical margins + radiation may improve survival in selected locations (e.g., pelvis)
- 3 or fewer pulmonary metastases: Resection + chemotherapy improves survival

DIAGNOSTIC CHECKLIST

Consider
- FDG PET/CT to optimize biopsy site: Highest grade areas (most active) best determine tumor grade, prognosis
- FDG PET/CT for staging and monitoring therapy
- Tl-201 acceptable alternative to PET in grading osteosarcoma, monitoring therapeutic response

Image Interpretation Pearls
- Rim of increased activity surrounding a photopenic center in untreated osteosarcoma with Tl-201, Tc-99m MIBI and FDG PET suggests a high grade tumor
- FDG PET/CT: High SUV associated with high grade osteosarcoma; also seem in giant cell tumors, fibrous dysplasia, sarcoidosis, lymphoma, Langerhans histiocytosis
- FDG PET/CT: Increasing FDG activity in region of previously treated tumor accurately predicts recurrence

SELECTED REFERENCES

1. Hicks RJ: Functional imaging techniques for evaluation of sarcomas. Cancer Imaging. 5(1):58-65, 2005
2. Brenner W et al: PET imaging of osteosarcoma. J Nucl Med. 44(6):930-42, 2003
3. Garcia R et al: Comparison of fluorine-18-FDG PET and technetium-99m-MIBI SPECT in evaluation of musculoskeletal sarcomas. J Nucl Med. 37(9):1476-9, 1996
4. Caner B et al: Technetium-99m-MIBI uptake in benign and malignant bone lesions: a comparative study with technetium-99m-MDP. J Nucl Med. 33(3):319-24, 1992
5. Ramanna L et al: Thallium-201 scintigraphy in bone sarcoma: comparison with gallium-67 and technetium-MDP in the evaluation of chemotherapeutic response. J Nucl Med. 31(5):567-72, 1990

OSTEOSARCOMA

IMAGE GALLERY

Typical

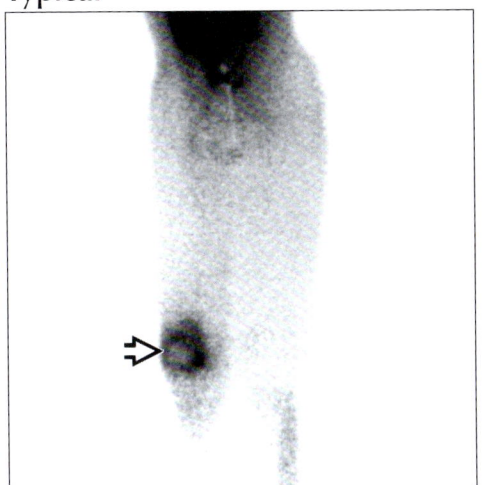

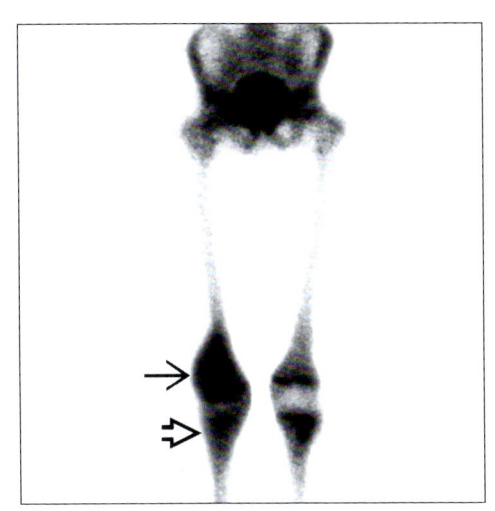

(Left) Anterior Tl-201 scintigraphy in a patient with high grade osteosarcoma of distal right femur ⇒. The ring appearance is due to outward tumor growth and central necrosis. See next image. *(Right)* Anterior Tc-99m MDP bone scan in the same patient as previous image, shows intense cortical bone activity →. Note lack of ring appearance on bone scan. Associated uptake in tibia ⇒ may be due to reactive hyperemia.

Typical

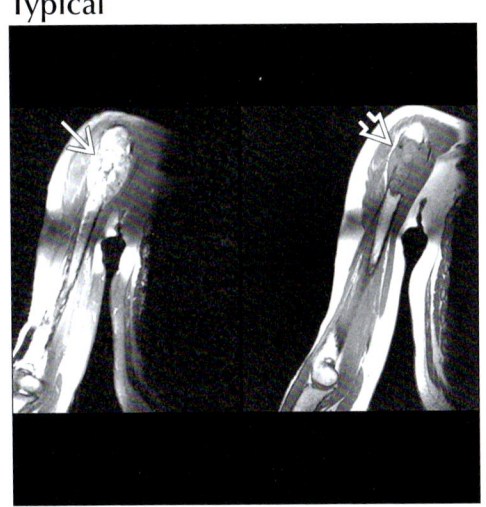

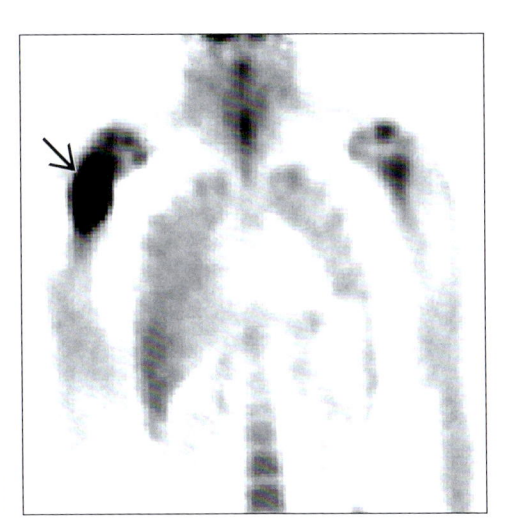

(Left) MR of right shoulder shows bright signal on T2WI ⇒ and low signal on T1WI ⇒ in osteosarcoma of the right proximal humerus. See next image. *(Right)* FDG PET in the same patient as previous image shows intense FDG activity → in the right humerus osteosarcoma, correlated with high tumor grade.

Typical

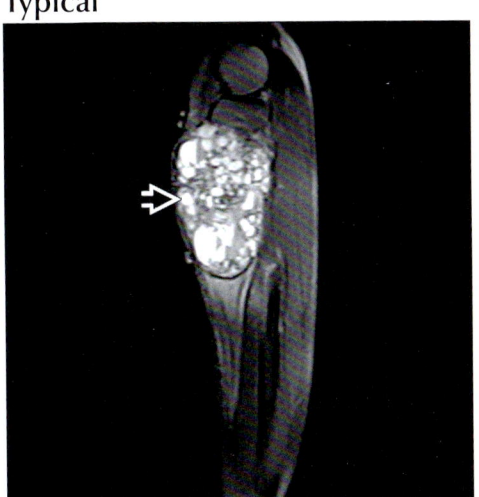

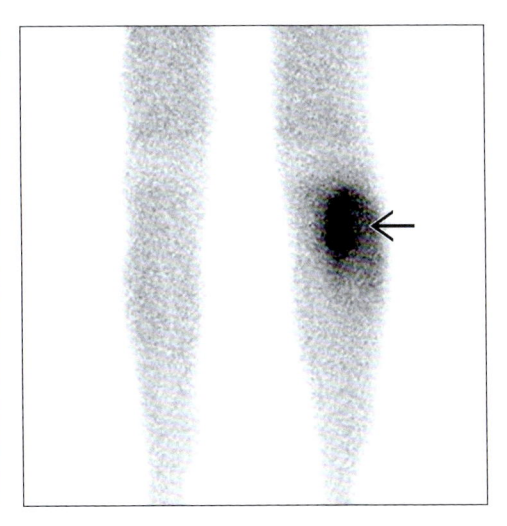

(Left) T2WI MR of the left proximal tibia shows the heterogeneous appearance of intermediate grade osteosarcoma ⇒. See next image. *(Right)* Anterior Tl-201 scintigraphy in the same patient as previous image shows moderate activity without a high grade ring pattern →.

OSTEOSARCOMA

(Left) Coronal FDG PET shows intensely increased activity in the left tibial osteosarcoma ➔ prior to neoadjuvant chemotherapy. See next image. (Right) FDG PET in the same patient as previous image after chemotherapy shows markedly decreased activity ➔, correlated with 95% tumor necrosis at surgery.

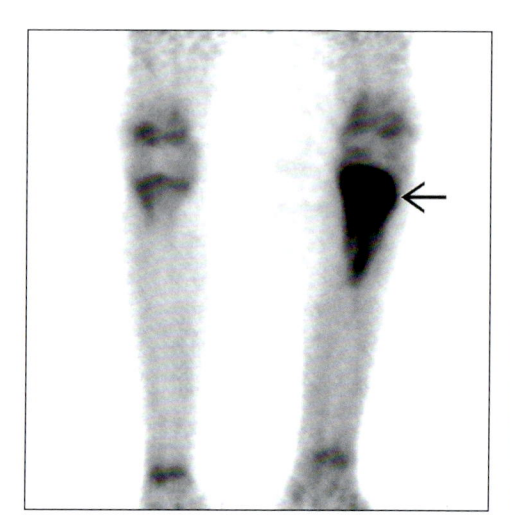

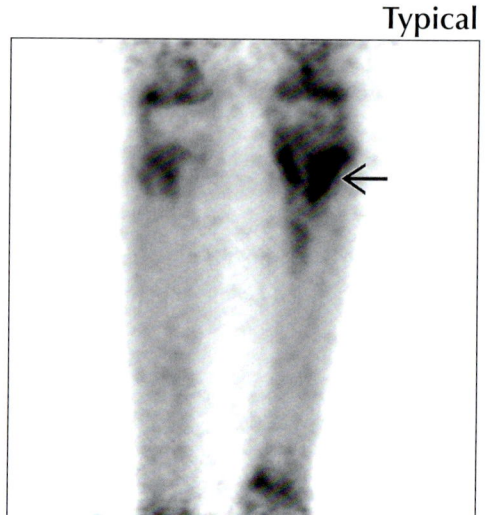

(Left) Axial CT in a patient with osteosarcoma of the right maxillary sinus wall prior to treatment ➔. See next image. (Right) Axial FDG PET in the same patient as previous image shows intensely increased activity in osteosarcoma ➔. See next image.

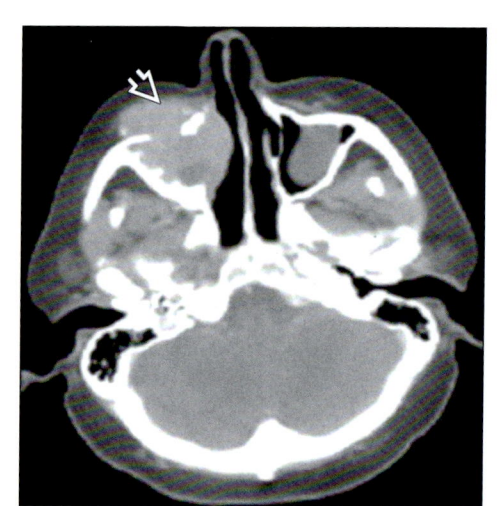

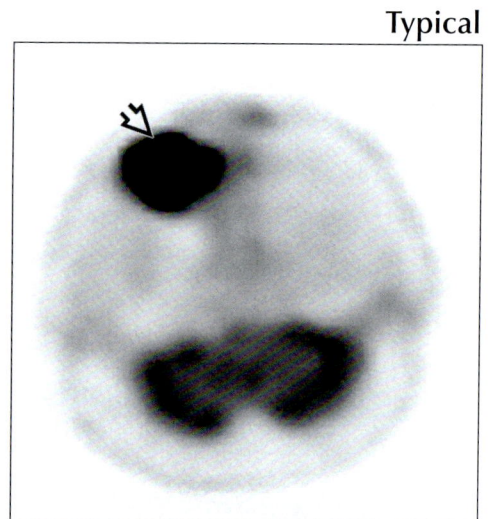

(Left) Axial CT in the same patient as previous image following surgery and chemotherapy shows interval decrease in the size of the soft tissue mass ➔. See next image. (Right) Axial FDG PET in the same patient as previous image shows no increased activity in the region of the tumor ➔, signifying response to therapy.

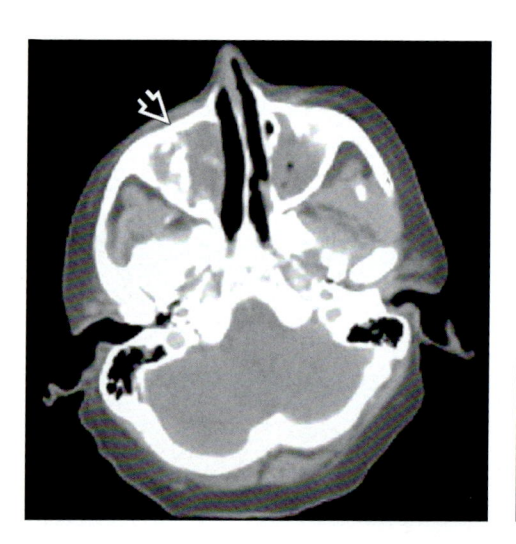

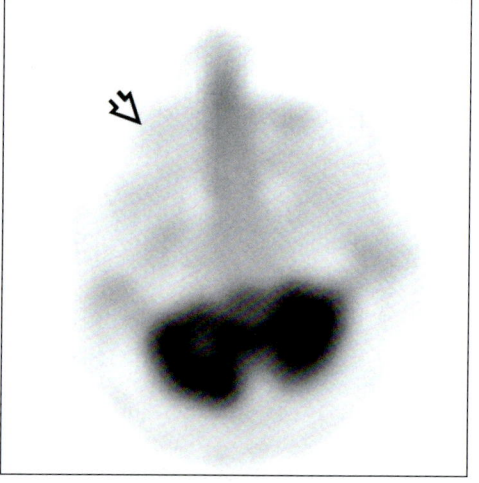

OSTEOSARCOMA

Typical

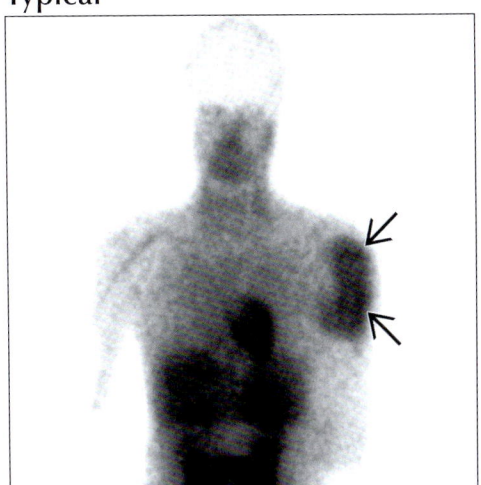

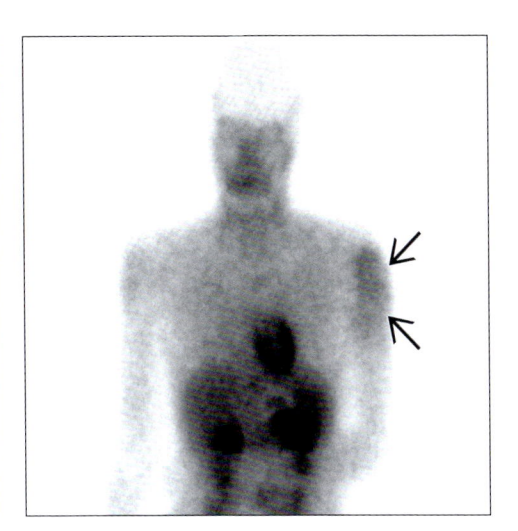

(Left) Anterior Tl-201 scintigraphy in a patient with osteosarcoma of the left proximal humerus shows increased activity ➡ prior to neoadjuvant chemotherapy. See next 5 images. *(Right)* Anterior Tl-201 scintigraphy in the same patient as previous image, after chemotherapy, shows moderately decreased activity ➡, consistent with response to therapy.

Typical

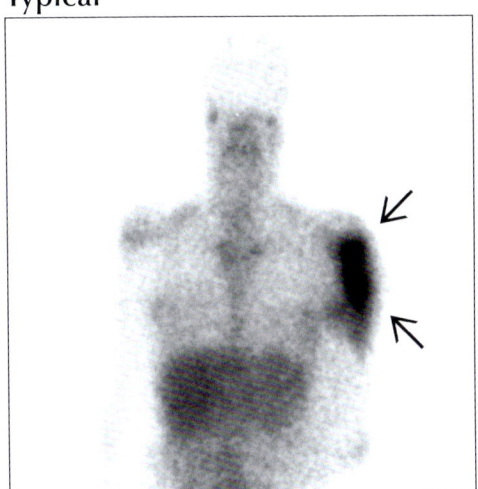

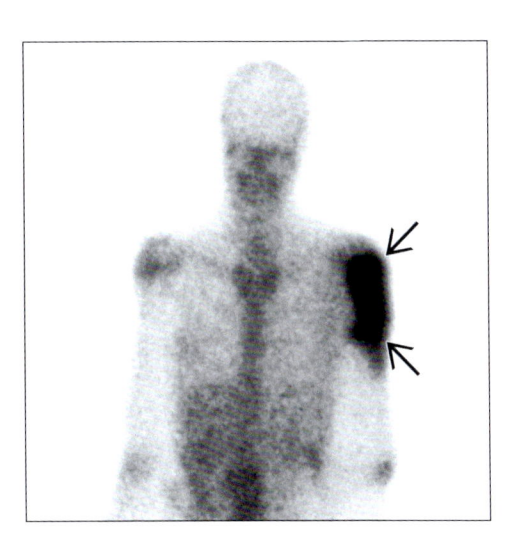

(Left) Anterior pretreatment Ga-67 scintigraphy in the same patient as previous shows intense uptake in the left proximal humerus osteosarcoma ➡. *(Right)* Anterior Ga-67 scintigraphy in the same patient as previous image, after chemotherapy, shows increased Ga-67 activity in the lesion ➡ despite good clinical response. See next image.

Typical

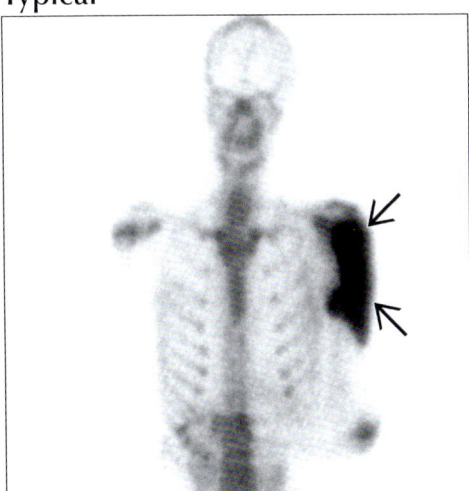

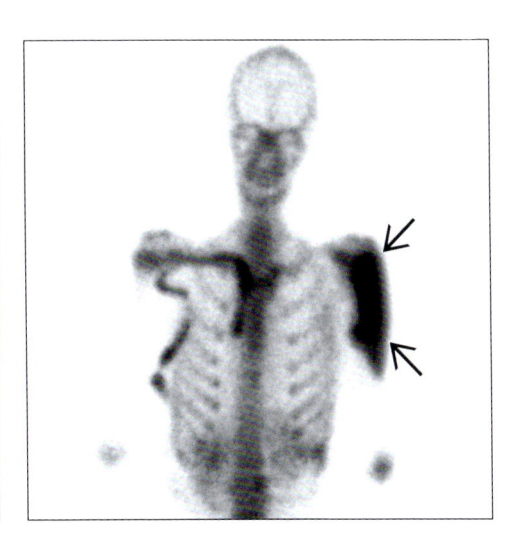

(Left) Pretreatment anterior bone scan in the same patient as previous image shows intense tumor uptake ➡. See next image. *(Right)* Anterior bone scan in the same patient as previous image, after chemotherapy, shows similar activity in the treated lesion ➡. Ga-67 scintigraphy and bone scan tend to reflect bone healing and thus show increased/similar activity to pretreatment scans.

EWING SARCOMA

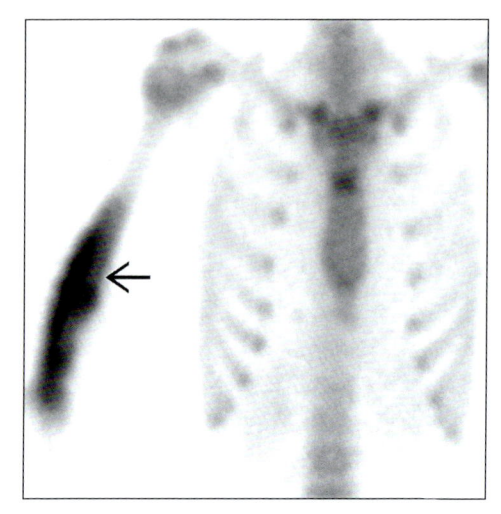

Anterior bone scan shows increased uptake in an expanded right distal humeral diaphysis ➔ compatible with a Ewing sarcoma in a 10 year old female with arm pain.

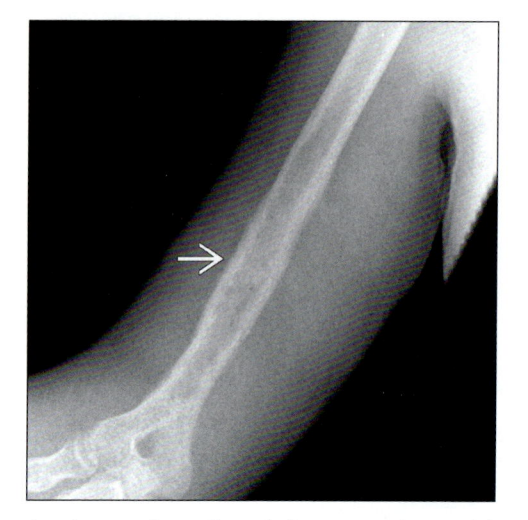

Anterior-posterior radiograph in same patient at left shows expansile permeative lytic lesion in humeral diaphysis. Note irregular amorphous periosteum ➔.

TERMINOLOGY

Abbreviations and Synonyms
- Ewing sarcoma (ES)

Definitions
- Malignant primary bone tumor
  - One of two most common primary bone tumors in children
  - Composed of small round cells
- Named after James Ewing in 1920
  - Co-founder of American Cancer Society in 1913

IMAGING FINDINGS

General Features
- Best diagnostic clue
  - Permeative appearance on radiographs
    - "Moth-eaten"
  - Adjacent extraosseous large soft tissue component on radiographs, CT
  - Bone scan: Increased activity in primary and metastatic lesions; rare photopenic lesions if tumor aggressive
- Location
  - Primary
    - May develop in any bone
    - Majority in pelvis or lower extremities
    - Not uncommon to occur in ribs
    - If in long bones, most commonly metadiaphyseal or diaphyseal
    - Usually medullary cavity instead of cortex
  - Metastases
    - Reported ≤ 30%
    - Lungs
    - Pleural space
    - Other bones
    - Lymph nodes
    - Brain (unusual)
- Size
  - Varies
  - Small bone metastases can be missed
- Morphology
  - Commonly poorly marginated
  - Aggressive periosteal margins

DDx: Mimics of Ewing Sarcoma on Bone Scan

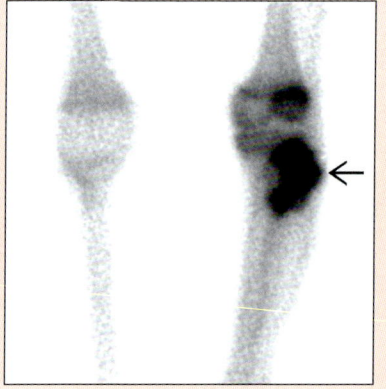

Osteosarcoma

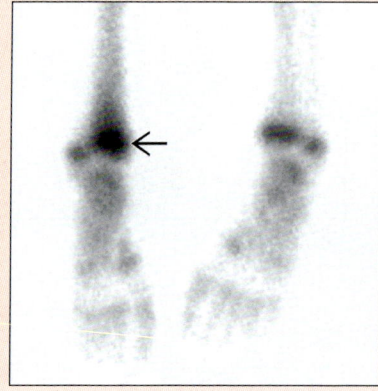

Osteomyelitis

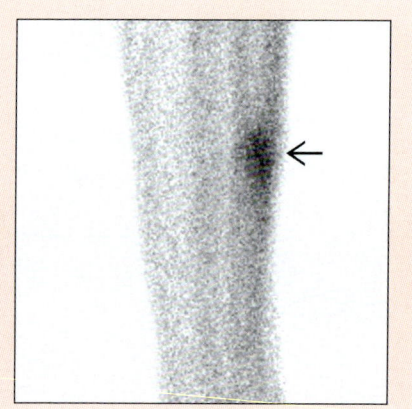

Stress Fracture

EWING SARCOMA

Key Facts

Terminology
- Malignant primary bone tumor
- One of two most common primary bone tumors in children

Imaging Findings
- Primary: Increased uptake on angiographic, blood pool and delayed images on three-phase bone scan
- Metastases: Scattered foci of increased uptake, axial > appendicular skeleton
- Photopenic lesions reported with aggressive tumors
- Equivocal bone scan lesions can be correlated with MR, radiographs
- As with any imaging examination, very small metastases can be missed on bone scan
- Bone scan not sensitive for local extent of disease (e.g., "skip lesions")
- ES demonstrates moderate to high uptake of FDG
- Ga-67 historically used for monitoring therapy
- If successful treatment, greater decrease in Ga-67 uptake compared with bone scan

Top Differential Diagnoses
- Malignant bone tumors
- Benign bone tumors
- Osteomyelitis
- Fracture

Clinical Issues
- Age: Typically 5-20 yrs
- Presence of metastases = key prognostic indicator
- Treatment often consists of combination of chemotherapy, surgical resection, radiotherapy

Nuclear Medicine Findings
- Tc-99m MDP bone scan
  - Primary: Increased uptake on angiographic, blood pool and delayed images on three-phase bone scan
  - Metastases: Scattered foci of increased uptake, axial > appendicular skeleton
  - Skeletal metastases seen in 10-40% of patients with Ewing sarcoma
  - Photopenic lesions reported with aggressive tumors

Imaging Recommendations
- Best imaging tool
  - Tc-99m MDP bone scan
    - Three-phase bone scan: Angiographic and blood pool phases can give additional information regarding soft tissue extent (however, better delineated with MR)
    - Whole body scan: Initial staging for bone metastases; sensitivity ~ 71%
    - Equivocal bone scan lesions can be correlated with MR, radiographs
    - As with any imaging examination, very small metastases can be missed on bone scan
    - Bone scan not sensitive for local extent of disease (e.g., "skip lesions")
    - May be useful to evaluate response to therapy
  - Radiograph
    - First step in work-up of suspected bone lesion
    - ES may resemble osteomyelitis
  - MR
    - Most specific imaging test for ES
    - Accurately defines local/soft tissue extent
    - Identifies noncontiguous medullary lesions in same bone as primary ("skip lesions")
    - Helps further characterize lesion, differentiate from osteomyelitis
    - Useful to assess for local recurrence
    - Whole body MR for metastases usually not practical; sensitivity reported at 82%
  - CT
    - Especially useful for staging chest
- Additional nuclear medicine imaging options
  - FDG PET
    - Superior to bone scan for detection of osseous metastases
    - Useful to assess response to induction chemotherapy
    - Small case series of 10 patients reported 96% sensitivity, 78% specificity on examination-based analysis
    - Differentiation between primary benign and malignant bone tumors with FDG PET scan of uncertain clinical utility
    - ES demonstrates moderate to high uptake of FDG
  - Ga-67
    - Ga-67 historically used for monitoring therapy
    - If successful treatment, greater decrease in Ga-67 uptake compared with bone scan
    - Large amount of residual uptake = relapse

DIFFERENTIAL DIAGNOSIS

Other Bone Tumors
- Malignant bone tumors
  - Osteosarcoma high on differential diagnosis of ES
    - Can occur in same age range
    - Also may have large soft tissue component
    - Bone metastases unusual without lung metastases
  - Primary bone lymphoma
  - Malignant fibrous histiocytoma
  - Acute leukemia
  - Metastases (e.g., neuroblastoma)
- Benign bone tumors
  - Eosinophilic granuloma
  - Giant cell tumor

Osteomyelitis
- ES can also cause fever, increased erythrocyte sedimentation rate
- Sequestration on radiograph favors osteomyelitis
- If aspiration yields bacteria = osteomyelitis
- If aspiration cultures negative (even with purulent material present) = tumor

EWING SARCOMA

Fracture
- Can usually be diagnosed by clinical history, radiographs
- If necessary, follow-up radiograph or MR
- Pathologic fracture occasionally occurs with ES

PATHOLOGY

General Features
- Genetics: Limited evidence of increased cancer risk in other family members
- Epidemiology
  - 2 cases per 1,000,000 children worldwide
  - Reported increased incidence if parents work on farms
    - Possibly fertilizer or pesticide exposure
  - More common in Caucasians
  - Rare in African-Americans

Gross Pathologic & Surgical Features
- Soft
- Grayish white
- ± Necrosis

Microscopic Features
- Small round blue-cell tumor

CLINICAL ISSUES

Presentation
- Most common signs/symptoms: Pain, swelling at tumor site
- Other signs/symptoms
  - Fever
  - Fatigue
  - Weight loss

Demographics
- Age: Typically 5-20 yrs
- Gender: Male to female ratio 1.5:1

Natural History & Prognosis
- Presence of metastases = key prognostic indicator
  - Overall survival ~ 75% for localized disease
  - Overall survival ≤ 30% for metastatic disease
  - If isolated pulmonary metastases, prognosis slightly better than extrapulmonary metastases
- Reported worse prognosis in adolescents
  - Children: 62% five-year survival
  - Adolescents: 30% five-year survival
- Also associated with worse prognosis
  - Large tumor size
  - Pelvic location

Treatment
- Treatment often consists of combination of chemotherapy, surgical resection, radiotherapy
  - Considered a "systemic disease" as most patients have subclinical metastases at time of presentation
- Local disease
  - Chemotherapy
    - Primary induction therapy prior to surgery
  - Surgery
    - Limb salvage often attempted
  - Radiotherapy
    - ES fairly radiosensitive
    - Definitive radiotherapy sometimes indicated when resection not possible
- Metastatic disease
  - Radiotherapy to primary site, bone metastases
  - Chemotherapy
- Recurrent disease
  - If localized, consider repeating surgery, radiation

DIAGNOSTIC CHECKLIST

Consider
- MR for primary characterization, local extent of disease
- Whole body bone scan for osseous metastatic survey

Image Interpretation Pearls
- Consider ES in the differential diagnosis in a young patient clinically suspected of having osteomyelitis on three-phase bone scan
  - Obtaining whole body scan at time of three-phase bone scan can be useful
- Correlate equivocal bone scan findings with plain film, MR
- Post-surgical change can show increased bone uptake on bone scan
  - MR best to distinguish local recurrence
  - Image entire bone with MR to increase sensitivity for "skip lesions"

SELECTED REFERENCES

1. Bernstein M et al: Ewing's sarcoma family of tumors: current management. Oncologist. 11(5):503-19, 2006
2. Gyorke T et al: Impact of FDG PET for staging of Ewing sarcomas and primitive neuroectodermal tumours. Nucl Med Commun. 27(1):17-24, 2006
3. Stiller CA et al: Bone tumours in European children and adolescents, 1978-1997. Report from the Automated Childhood Cancer Information System project. Eur J Cancer. 42(13):2124-35, 2006
4. Alfeeli MA et al: Ewing sarcoma of the rib with normal blood flow and blood pool imagings on a 3-phase bone scan. Clin Nucl Med. 30(9):610-1, 2005
5. Khoury JD: Ewing sarcoma family of tumors. Adv Anat Pathol. 12(4):212-20, 2005
6. Kutluk MT et al: Treatment results and prognostic factors in Ewing sarcoma. Pediatr Hematol Oncol. 21(7):597-610, 2004
7. Aoki J et al: FDG PET of primary benign and malignant bone tumors: standardized uptake value in 52 lesions. Radiology. 219(3):774-7, 2001
8. Daldrup-Link HE et al: Whole-body MR imaging for detection of bone metastases in children and young adults: comparison with skeletal scintigraphy and FDG PET. AJR Am J Roentgenol. 177(1):229-36, 2001
9. Estes DN et al: Primary Ewing sarcoma: follow-up with Ga-67 scintigraphy. Radiology. 177(2):449-53, 1990
10. Reinus WR et al: Radiology of Ewing's sarcoma: Intergroup Ewing's Sarcoma Study (IESS). Radiographics. 4(6):929-44, 1984

EWING SARCOMA

IMAGE GALLERY

Typical

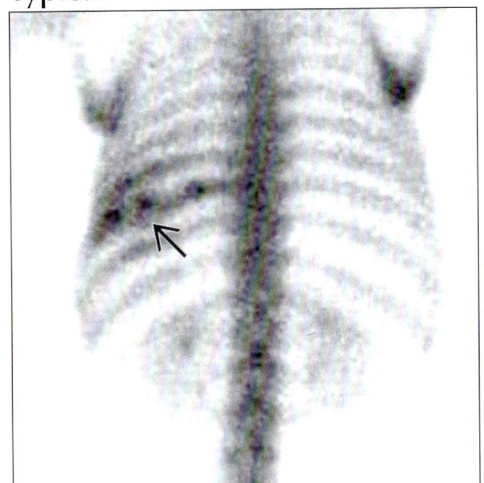

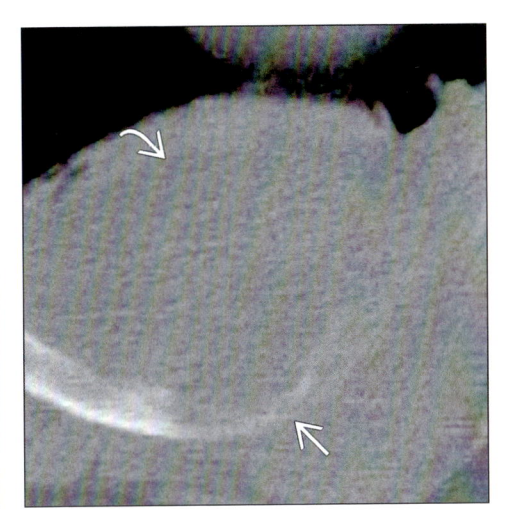

(Left) Posterior bone scan shows segmental uptake in left 8th and 9th posterior ribs ➔ in an adolescent patient with back pain and fever. *(Right)* Axial NECT in same patient at left shows rib destruction ➔ and a large soft tissue mass ➔, biopsy-proven Ewing sarcoma.

Typical

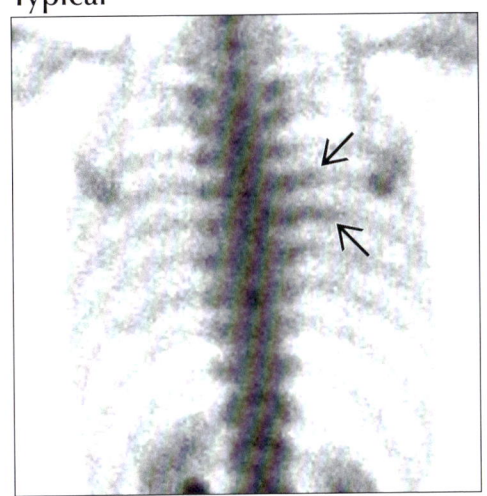

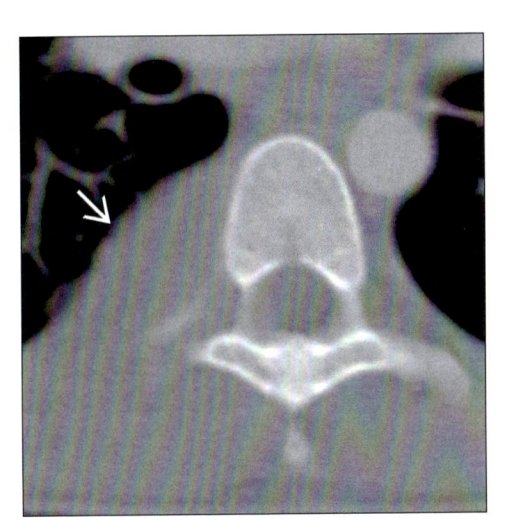

(Left) Posterior bone scan shows subtle increased right paraspinal rib uptake ➔ at multiple levels in patient presenting with leg and back pain. *(Right)* Axial NECT in same patient at left shows right paraspinal soft tissue mass ➔ compatible with Ewing sarcoma. This was treated with surgical resection and external beam radiation.

Typical

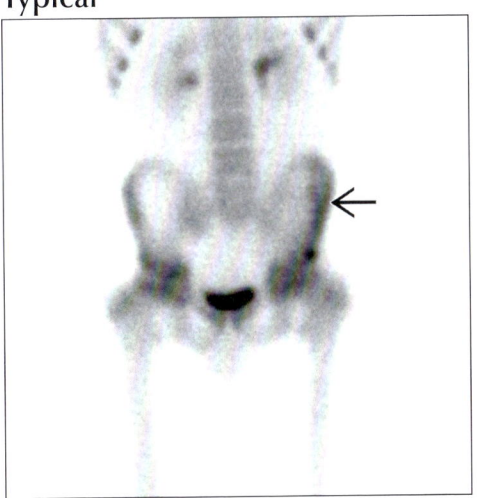

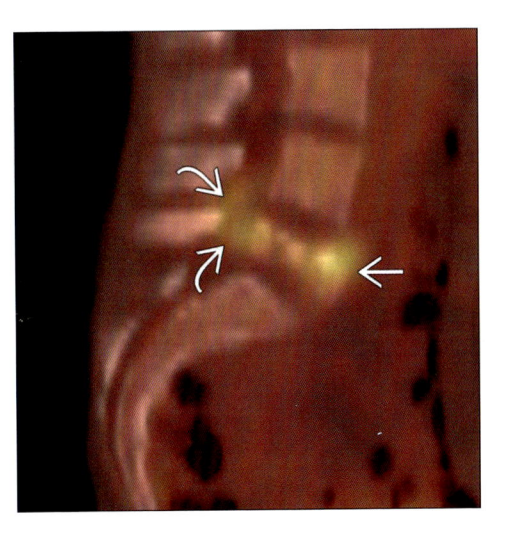

(Left) Anterior bone scan shows increased uptake in left pelvis ➔ in a 5 year old boy with Ewing sarcoma. Bone scan performed for staging showed no additional bony metastases. *(Right)* Sagittal FDG PET/CT in patient with L5 Ewing sarcoma shows moderate hypermetabolism in collapsed L5 vertebral body ➔, extending posteriorly into spinal canal ➔.

CHONDROSARCOMA

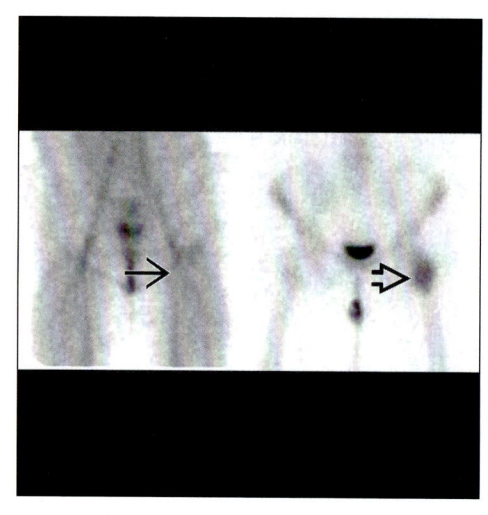

Angiographic phase bone scan shows no hyperemia ➡ and delayed phase bone scan shows increased uptake ⊳ in patient with pain and known enchondroma of proximal left femur. See next image.

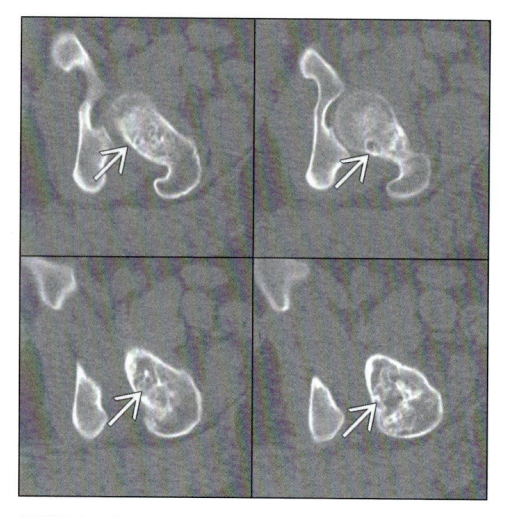

NECT in the same patient as previous image shows dense calcification ➡ without cortical disruption or soft tissue mass. Curettage revealed low grade chondrosarcoma.

TERMINOLOGY

Definitions
- Chondrosarcoma: Primary malignant tumor of bone whose cells produce hyaline cartilage resulting in abnormal cartilage and/or bone

IMAGING FINDINGS

General Features
- Best diagnostic clue
  - Lytic mass, ± chondroid matrix, cortical disruption, soft tissue extension
  - FDG PET activity proportional to tumor grade
- Location
  - Classified as central (within intramedullary canal), periosteal or peripheral
  - Predominantly axial; most common in pelvis, femur, humerus, rib, scapula
  - Occasionally found in sternum, skull, spine
  - In long bones, proximal metaphysis most common
  - Unusual de novo in hands and feet

Nuclear Medicine Findings
- FDG PET
  - FDG uptake depends on tumor grade: Grade III > grade II > grade I
  - PET cannot differentiate benign cartilaginous tumor vs. grade I chondrosarcoma
  - High pretreatment SUV predictive of higher grade chondrosarcoma
  - High SUV associated with high GLUT-1 expression, mitotic scoring and p53 overexpression
  - PET highly sensitive for detecting high grade chondrosarcoma metastases
  - PET insensitive for detecting low grade chondrosarcoma metastases
- Tc-99m MDP bone scan
  - Bone scan differentiation of benign (osteochondroma, enchondroma) vs. malignant lesions unreliable
  - High negative predictive value: Absence of activity in suspicious finding on X-ray, CT or MR makes malignancy unlikely

Imaging Recommendations
- Best imaging tool

DDx: Mimics of Chondrosarcoma

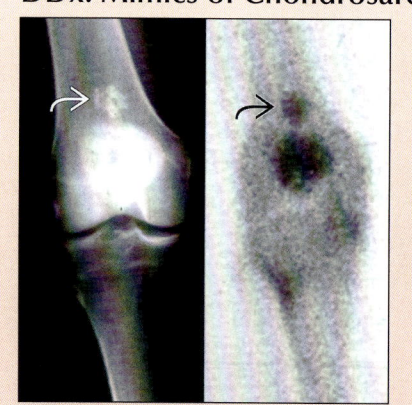

Enchondroma

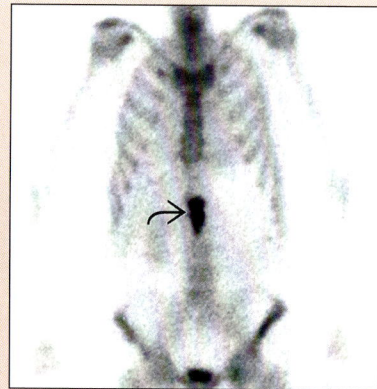

Cartilage Injury (Surgical)

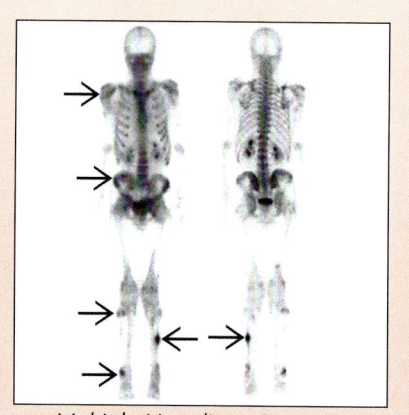

Multiple Hereditary Exostoses

CHONDROSARCOMA

Key Facts

Imaging Findings
- FDG uptake depends on tumor grade: Grade III > grade II > grade I
- PET cannot differentiate benign cartilaginous tumor vs. grade I chondrosarcoma

Top Differential Diagnoses
- Neoplasm
- Trauma
- Infection
- Bone Infarction

Clinical Issues
- Pain and regional swelling (≥ 60%)
- Pathologic fracture may be first sign
- Metastatic spread more common with high grade tumors: Regional lymph nodes, lungs
- Low grade chondrosarcoma: Adequate surgical resection with limb salvage when possible
- High grade chondrosarcoma: Surgical resection with chemotherapy or radiation

Diagnostic Checklist
- FDG PET/CT to evaluate primary chondrosarcoma: Low vs. high grade
- FDG PET/CT for optimizing biopsy approach; biopsy region of highest SUV
- FDG PET/CT for staging and therapeutic assessment
- Absence of FDG activity: Benign etiology
- Low level FDG activity: Indeterminate for benign vs. malignant etiology
- Increasing FDG activity following chemotherapy = treatment failure, recurrence

---

- Plain film for initial screen
  - Lucent lesion with matrix calcification
  - Cortical destruction and/or soft tissue extension suggests highly malignant lesion
  - Tumor size poorly assessed
- MR best for evaluating extent of tumor
  - T1WI: Low to intermediate signal intensity
  - T2WI: ↑ Signal (hyaline cartilage), ↓ signal in areas of mineralization
  - MR useful to evaluate thickness of cartilage cap of osteochondromas, identify malignant transformation
  - T1 C+: Enhancement of septa, capsule; nonenhancing hyaline cartilage, cystic mucoid tissue, necrosis
- NECT: Chondroid matrix mineralization of "rings and arcs" characteristic; nonmineralized portions hypodense to muscle
  - CT: Assess distant metastases
- FDG PET/CT: Assess tumor activity, establish optimal biopsy site, detect distant metastases, monitor therapy
- Protocol advice
  - PET/CT: 10-20 mCi (370-740 MBq) F-18 FDG IV; no carbohydrate for minimum of 6 hours prior to study, no exercise for 24 hours
  - Bone scan: 20-30 mCi (740-1110 MBq) Tc99m MDP IV; whole body anterior and posterior scan; SPECT spine, chest lesions
- Correlative imaging features
  - Tumor grading best with FDG PET/CT; bone scan X-ray, CT and MR useful for grading but not as accurate
  - FDG PET/CT superior to CT and MR when metallic hardware present
  - Disease extent and response to therapy best assessed with MR and FDG PET/CT
  - Ultrasonography: Limited utility, may establish biopsy site in extramedullary extension

DIFFERENTIAL DIAGNOSIS

Neoplasm
- Multiple benign tumors: Enchondroma, osteochondroma, fibrous dysplasia, hereditary multiple exostosis
- Other primary bone tumors: Chondroblastic osteosarcoma, fibrosarcoma

Trauma
- Especially in subacute phase with callous formation
- Acute phase non pathologic fracture vs. pathologic

Infection
- Abscess, extensive destructive osteomyelitis

Bone Infarction
- Decreased or increase activity on bone scan, depending on early or reparative phase

PATHOLOGY

General Features
- Genetics
  - No consistent, well-defined genetic risk; however, gene alterations are present
  - Some hereditary conditions predispose subjects to chondrosarcoma formation
    - Ollier disease (multiple enchondromatosis): Slight ↑ risk of chondrosarcoma
    - Multiple hereditary exostosis (osteochondromatoses): ↑ Risk of osteosarcoma 0.6-2.8%
    - Maffucci syndrome (enchondromas, hemangiomas and bone deformities): ~ 25% risk of developing chondrosarcoma
    - Wilms tumor: Rare association with chondrosarcoma
- Etiology
  - Unclear in most cases
  - Higher risk in patients with Paget disease, prior radiation treatments, chemotherapy

CHONDROSARCOMA

- Epidemiology
  - Third most common primary bone tumor behind osteosarcoma and multiple myeloma
  - Represents ~ 25% of primary malignant bone tumors (500 new cases/yr)
- Associated abnormalities: Benign bone disorders (e.g., enchondroma, osteochondroma, Paget disease)

Gross Pathologic & Surgical Features

- General: Primary chondrosarcoma
  - Pelvis most common site
    - Size variable, may exceed 6 cm if untreated
    - Cut surface demonstrates hyaline cartilage with blue and white color
    - Central tumors may have extensive intramedullary spread
- Juxtacortical chondrosarcoma: < 2% of chondrosarcomas
  - Femur most common site (metaphysis > diaphysis)
- Mesenchymal chondrosarcoma: 2% of chondrosarcomas
  - Maxilla, mandible common sites
- Clear cell chondrosarcoma: 2% of chondrosarcomas
  - Epiphyses of long bones most common site
- Dedifferentiated chondrosarcoma: 11% of all chondrosarcomas
  - Common in pelvis, proximal femur/humerus, distal femur, ribs
  - May be intraosseous or extraosseous mass

Microscopic Features

- General: Primary chondrosarcoma
  - Irregular lobules of cartilage separated by narrow fibrous bands
  - Mitotic forms: Widespread in grade III tumors, scattered in grade II, not seen in grade I
  - Matrix varies from mature hyaline to myxoid stroma
  - Spindle cells in grade III
- Juxtacortical chondrosarcoma
  - Well-differentiated hyaline cartilaginous lobules
  - Grade III tumors uncommon
- Mesenchymal chondrosarcoma
  - Variable-shaped tumor cells with irregular chromatin; mitotic rate varies
  - Sparse cartilaginous areas
- Clear cell chondrosarcomas
  - Lobular cartilaginous nests with clear cells
  - Rare mitoses, sparse matrix formation

Staging, Grading or Classification Criteria

- Musculoskeletal Tumor Society stage
  - IA: Low grade, within bone, no metastasis
  - IB: Low grade, outside bone, no metastasis
  - IIA: High grade, within bone, no metastasis
  - IIB: High grade, outside bone no metastasis
  - IIIA: Any grade, inside bone, with metastasis
  - IIIB: Any grade, outside bone, with metastasis
- Grade
  - I: Low grade, closely resembling normal cartilage but may surround lamellar bone and contain atypical cells
  - II: Intermediate grade, with more cells, nuclear atypia, hyperchromatic nuclei, larger nuclear size than grade I
  - III: High grade, with marked pleomorphism, large cells, marked hyperchromatic nuclei, occasional giant cells, frequent mitosis, necrosis

CLINICAL ISSUES

Presentation

- Most common signs/symptoms
  - Pain and regional swelling (≥ 60%)
    - Pathologic fracture may be first sign
    - Metastatic spread more common with high grade tumors: Regional lymph nodes, lungs

Demographics

- Age
  - Low incidence in children
  - Central: Peak 5th-7th, secondary 4th-5th decade
  - Juxtacortical: 80% > 20 yrs
  - Mesenchymal: 80% between 10-40 yrs
  - Clear cell: 3rd-4th decade
  - Dedifferentiated: Most > 50 years
- Gender: Male:female = 1.5-2.1

Natural History & Prognosis

- Untreated tumors progress at variable rates depending on tumor histology, host factors
- Metastatic potential, five-year survival and recurrence rate depend on grade
  - Grade I: 0%, 90%, low
  - Grade II: 10-15%, 81%, fair
  - Grade III: > 50%, 29%, high
  - Dedifferentiated: > 95%, < 10% (1 yr), high

Treatment

- Low grade chondrosarcoma: Adequate surgical resection with limb salvage when possible
- High grade chondrosarcoma: Surgical resection with chemotherapy or radiation

DIAGNOSTIC CHECKLIST

Consider

- FDG PET/CT to evaluate primary chondrosarcoma: Low vs. high grade
- FDG PET/CT for optimizing biopsy approach; biopsy region of highest SUV
- FDG PET/CT for staging and therapeutic assessment

Image Interpretation Pearls

- Absence of FDG activity: Benign etiology
- Low level FDG activity: Indeterminate for benign vs. malignant etiology
- Increasing FDG activity following chemotherapy = treatment failure, recurrence

SELECTED REFERENCES

1. Brenner W et al: FDG PET imaging for grading and prediction of outcome in chondrosarcoma patients. Eur J Nucl Med Mol Imaging. 31(2):189-5, 2004
2. Aoki J et al: FDG-PET in differential diagnosis and grading of chondrosarcomas. J Comput Assist Tomogr. 23:603-8, 1999

CHONDROSARCOMA

IMAGE GALLERY

Typical

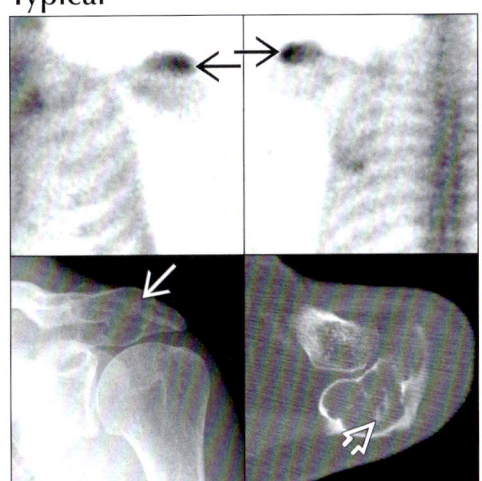

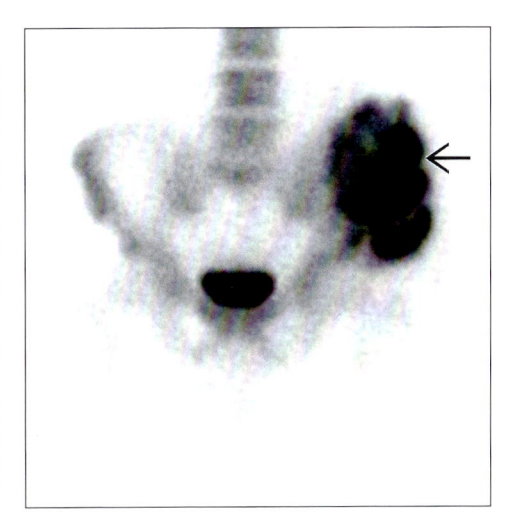

(Left) Bone scan shows ↑ uptake in left acromion ➡. Radiograph shows expansile lesion ➡. NECT shows low attenuating hyaline cartilage matrix with "ring and arc" mineralization ➡, typical of chondrosarcoma. *(Right)* Anterior bone scan of pelvis shows expansile lesion of left iliac wing ➡ with intense uptake, typical of high grade chondrosarcoma. See next 4 images.

Typical

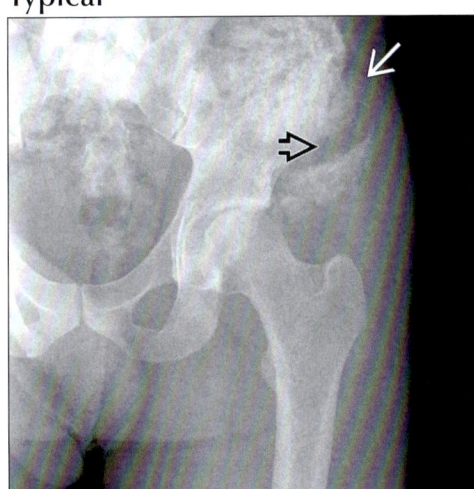

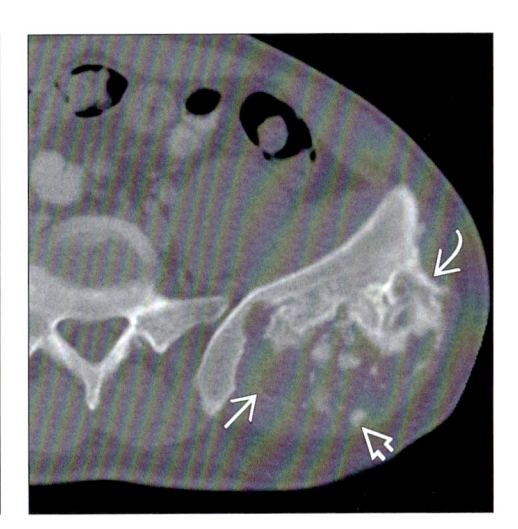

(Left) Radiograph in same patient as previous shows irregular calcified mass ➡ of left iliac wing extending into soft tissue. Regions of low density ➡ suggest chondroid matrix. See next image. *(Right)* NECT in the same patient as previous image shows mass with low attenuation (hyaline cartilage) ➡, calcified matrix ➡, and rings and arcs ➡, typical of high grade chondrosarcoma. See next image.

Typical

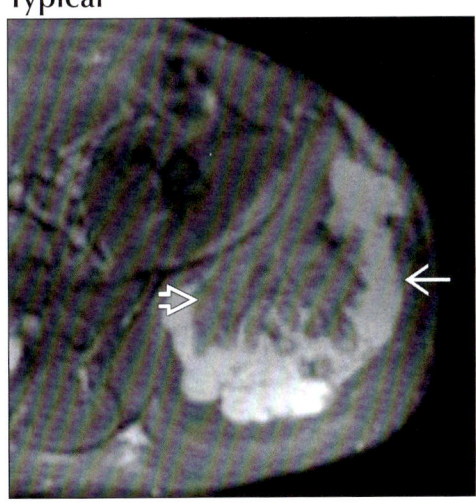

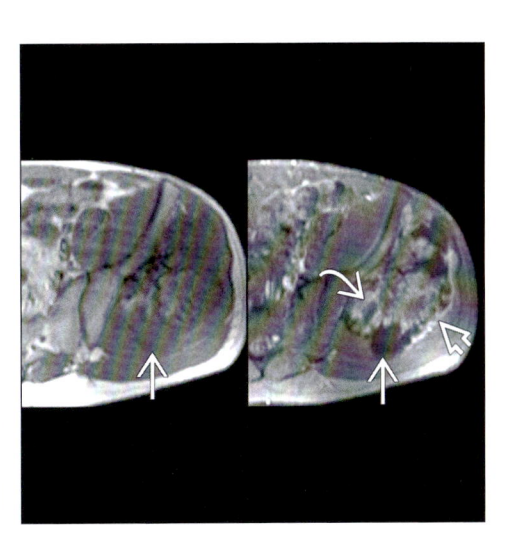

(Left) T2WI MR in same patient as previous shows high signal in hyaline cartilage ➡ due to high water content. Regions of lobulated low signal represent mineralized matrix ➡. *(Right)* T1WI shows nonenhancing areas of hyaline cartilage ➡. T1 C+ shows enhancing septa ➡ and enhancing capsule ➡, typical of chondrosarcoma.

PROSTATE CANCER, BONE METASTASES

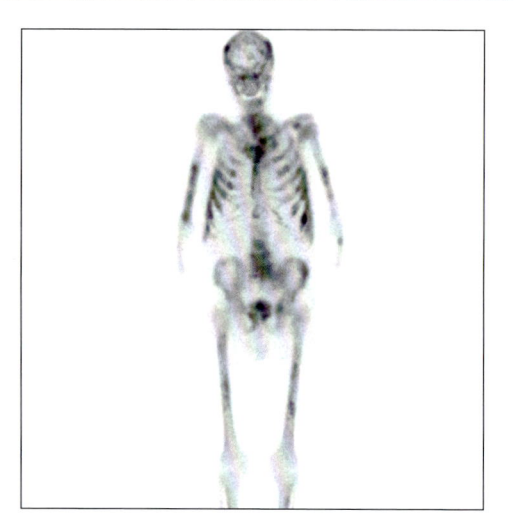

Anterior bone scan shows multiple bony metastases, including to the calvarium, bilateral humeri, multiple ribs, sternum, lumbar spine, pelvis, and both femurs. See next image.

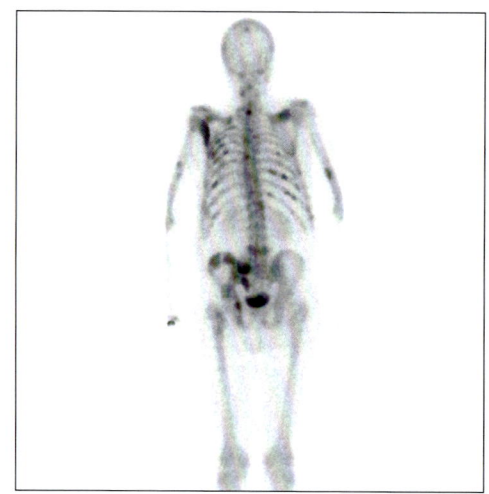

Posterior bone scan shows additional lesions including the scapulae and thoracic spine.

TERMINOLOGY

Definitions
- Malignant tumor of glandular origin from the prostate gland

IMAGING FINDINGS

General Features
- Best diagnostic clue: Multiple areas of uptake on bone scan with sclerotic lesions on CT, plain radiograph
- Location
  ○ Axial skeleton, proximal appendicular skeleton
  ○ Calvarium, distal appendicular skeleton often spared ("legless and headless" appearance on bone scan)
- Size: Different sizes, from small focal to confluent

Nuclear Medicine Findings
- Bone Scan
  ○ Fairly intense bony uptake in multiple areas, mostly in axial, proximal appendicular skeleton
  ○ Solitary hot spots are more likely benign, even if known extraosseous malignancy
  ○ Secondary/complicated findings
    ▪ Flare response rarely occurs later than 6 months after treatment; can result in transient worsening of bone scan with chemo or hormone therapy; typically regresses in 2-3 months

Imaging Recommendations
- Best imaging tool
  ○ Whole body bone scan
    ▪ Consider for bone scan: PSA 20 ng/ml or greater, locally advanced disease, or Gleason score ≥ 8
    ▪ Value of bone scan with PSA < 20 ng/ml is not established
  ○ Plain radiograph, CT: Sclerotic mets, lytic with more poorly differentiated tumor
- Protocol advice: If patient has back pain, SPECT or MR indicated even with normal planar images

DIFFERENTIAL DIAGNOSIS

Occult Fracture in the Elderly
- Vertebral compression spine fractures are especially common in the elderly

DDx: Mimics of Prostate Cancer Bone Metastases

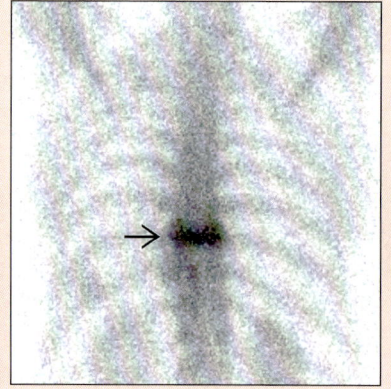

T9 Fracture

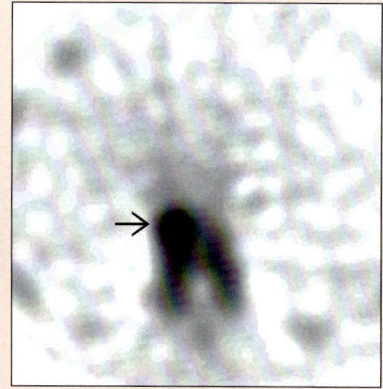

Osteophyte

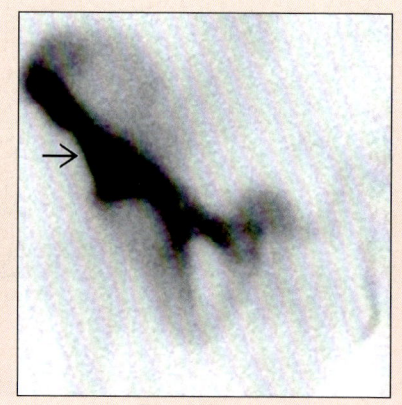

Paget Disease

PROSTATE CANCER, BONE METASTASES

Key Facts

Imaging Findings
- Axial skeleton, proximal appendicular skeleton
- Calvarium, distal appendicular skeleton often spared ("legless and headless" appearance on bone scan)
- Solitary hot spots are more likely benign, even if known extraosseous malignancy

- Flare response rarely occurs later than 6 months after treatment; can result in transient worsening of bone scan with chemo or hormone therapy; typically regresses in 2-3 months
- Consider for bone scan: PSA 20 ng/ml or greater, locally advanced disease, or Gleason score ≥ 8
- Value of bone scan with PSA < 20 ng/ml is not established
- Plain radiograph, CT: Sclerotic mets, lytic with more poorly differentiated tumor

Osteoarthritis
- Contour of osteophytes will project beyond expected location of vertebral body
- Benign facet disease is at the level of the disc space, compared to pedicle disease at the level of the vertebral body

Paget Disease
- Correlation with plain films is important to demonstrate thick coarsened trabeculae along with cortical thickening

PATHOLOGY

General Features
- Genetics: Men with an affected brother or father 2x as likely to develop prostate cancer
- Epidemiology
  - Incidence
    - Accounts for 33% (232,090) of new cancer cases in men (2005)
    - African-American men 58% higher incidence than Caucasians
  - Mortality: 30,350 deaths in US in 2005

Microscopic Features
- Primarily osteoblastic activity, although also osteoclastic activity

CLINICAL ISSUES

Demographics
- Age: More than 70% of patients diagnosed with prostate cancer are > 65 years

DIAGNOSTIC CHECKLIST

Image Interpretation Pearls
- Correlate uptake in weight bearing areas with plain films to evaluate for an impending pathologic fracture

SELECTED REFERENCES
1. Jemal A et al: Cancer statistics, 2005. CA Cancer J Clin. 55(1):10-30, 2005
2. Routh JC et al: Adenocarcinoma of the prostate: epidemiological trends, screening, diagnosis, and surgical management of localized disease. Mayo Clin Proc. 80(7):899-907, 2005
3. Abuzallouf S et al: Baseline staging of newly diagnosed prostate cancer: a summary of the literature. J Urol. 171(6 Pt 1):2122-7, 2004
4. Wu PS et al: Clinical significance of solitary rib hot spots on bone scans in patients with extraskeletal cancer: correlation with other clinical manifestations. Clin Nucl Med. 27(8):567-71, 2002
5. Han LJ et al: Comparison of bone single-photon emission tomography and planar imaging in the detection of vertebral metastases in patients with back pain. Eur J Nucl Med. 25(6):635-8, 1998

IMAGE GALLERY

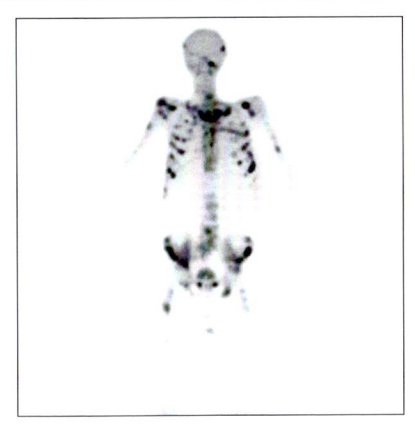

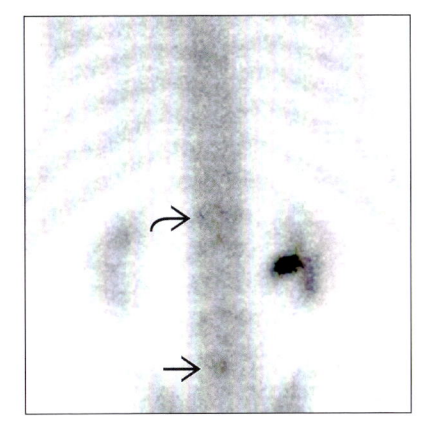

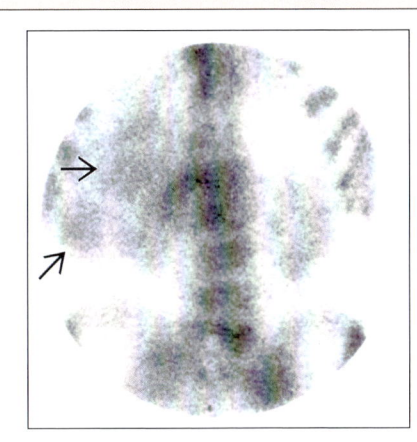

(Left) Anterior bone scan shows multiple bony metastases with relative sparing of distal appendicular skeleton. Almost no soft tissue or renal activity is consistent with a superscan. (Center) Posterior bone scan shows subtle uptake at T12 ➔ and L4 ➔. Confirmed to be metastatic disease on MR. The L4 lesion causes severe spinal stenosis and canal compromise. (Right) Anterior bone scan shows patchy liver uptake ➔ from extensive liver metastases due to poorly differentiated prostate cancer.

PALLIATION OF METASTATIC BONE PAIN

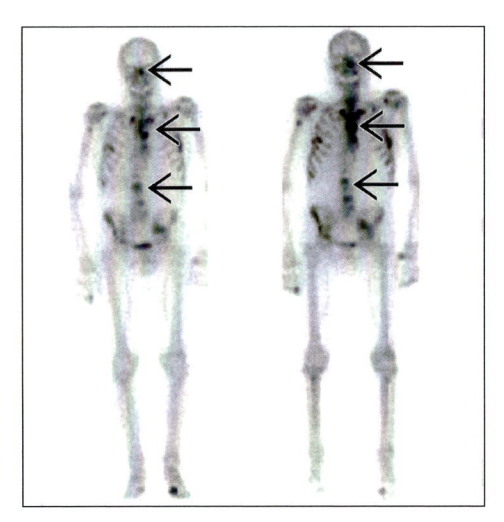

Anterior bone scan with Tc-99m MDP (left) and Sm-153 (right) shows matching increased activity ➔ in patient with diffuse bone pain from metastatic prostate cancer (Courtesy Cytogen Corp).

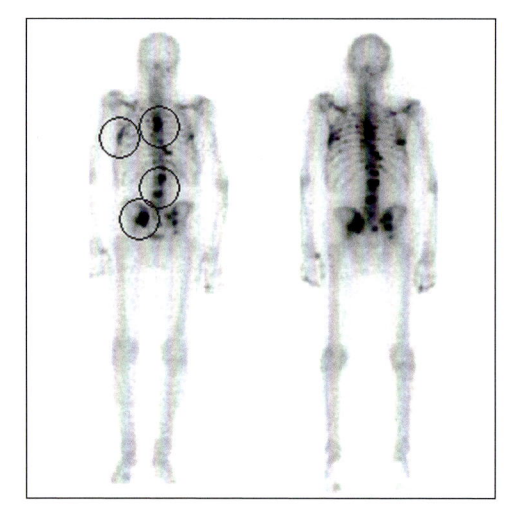

A pain map (same patient as previous) on posterior Tc-99m MDP image (left). Tracer localization in same regions on Sm-153 image (right) predicts good response (Courtesy Cytogen Corp).

TERMINOLOGY

Abbreviations
- Samarium 153 (Sm-153)
- Strontium 89 (Sr-89)
- Phosphorus 32 (P-32)

Definitions
- Bone pain
  - Common symptom of advanced bony metastases, major impact on quality of life
  - Initially, pain intermittent, variable intensity
  - Progresses to chronic pain, breakthrough episodes
    - Mechanical allodynia: Normal usually nonpainful activity (e.g., coughing) painful
  - Most common indications
    - Metastatic prostate, breast cancer
    - 85% of men who die of prostate cancer have bone metastases
  - Less frequent indication
    - Lung, kidney, thyroid cancer
- Palliative radiopharmaceutical treatment of metastatic bone pain refractory to analgesics
  - Does not affect survival
    - However, may ↓ tumor load
    - Some patients with prostate cancer show ↓ PSA post treatment
  - Mechanism not well understood
    - Beta-emitting radiopharmaceutical delivers localized radiation to metastatic sites
    - May ↓ tumor volume
    - Likely ↓ in circulating cytokine, humoral factors that sensitize and stimulate nerve endings
  - Sm-153
    - Weight-based dosing: 1 mCi (37 MBq)/kg maximum
    - T½ 1.9 days
    - Mixed beta and gamma emitter
    - 640, 710, and 810 keV beta emissions
    - Can image 103 keV gamma emissions
    - Labeled to bisphosphonate ethylenediaminetetramethylene phospate (EDTMP) (↑ bone-seeking properties)
    - Urinary excretion: Complete ~ 6 hrs after administration
  - Sr-89
    - Usual therapeutic dose 4 mCi (148 MBq)
    - T½ 50.3 days
    - Pure beta emitter (1.49 MeV maximum energy)
    - Bremsstrahlung imaging possible, but not practical
    - Physiologic distribution mimics calcium
    - Used in patients with moderate pain, reasonable life expectancy due to long response duration
  - P-32
    - T½ 14.3 days
    - Pure beta emitter
    - Bremsstrahlung imaging possible, but not practical
    - Major drawback: Normal marrow receives high radiation dose relative to metastatic deposits (⇒ myelosuppression)
    - Not widely used for bone pain palliation since 1980s
    - Also used to treat hematologic disease, primarily polycythemia vera
  - Rhenium 186 (Re-186)
    - Widely used in Europe, not approved in United States
    - Labeled to a bisphosphonate
    - Gamma emission suitable for imaging
  - Rhenium 188 (Re-188), Tin 117m (Sn-117m), Radium 223 (Ra-223), Lutetium 177 (Lu-177)
    - Primarily investigational
    - Not currently in clinical use

PALLIATION OF METASTATIC BONE PAIN

Key Facts

Terminology
- Samarium 153 (Sm-153)
- Strontium 89 (Sr-89)
- Palliative radiopharmaceutical treatment of metastatic bone pain refractory to analgesics
- Does not affect survival
- Beta-emitting radiopharmaceutical delivers localized radiation to metastatic sites
- May ↓ tumor volume
- Likely ↓ in circulating cytokine, humoral factors that sensitize and stimulate nerve endings

Pre-procedure
- Recent Tc-99m MDP bone scan showing metastases
- Complete blood count
- Creatinine
- Other contraindications not present

Procedure
- Outpatient treatment after informed consent and discussion of radiation safety precautions
- Adequate IV access essential as dose infiltration can ⇒ soft tissue necrosis
- Slow IV injection of radiopharmaceutical followed by saline flush
- Although not essential, imaging can verify uptake in painful lesions

Problems & Complications
- Myelotoxicity
- Dose infiltration
- Transient ↑ in pain
- Nausea/vomiting
- Musculoskeletal complaints
- Bleeding

PRE-PROCEDURE

Indications
- Palliative treatment of diffuse metastatic bone pain refractory to conventional analgesics
- Treatment can be repeated
  - Same treatment guidelines as for initial therapy
    - Duration of response may ↓
    - Risk of myelotoxicity generally ↑

Contraindications
- Acute or chronic renal failure (glomerular filtration rate < 30 ml/min)
  - Excretion primarily renal for most agents
  - Poor renal function delays tracer clearance
- Patient at high risk for pathologic fracture/cord compression (surgical, radiotherapy emergencies)
- Hemoglobin < 90 g/L
- White blood cells < 4,000 cells/mm³
- Platelets < 100,000/mm³
- Pregnancy
- Life expectancy < 3 months (especially for long T½ agents)
- Urinary incontinence/obstruction not absolute contraindication
  - Consider catheterization, stenting prior to treatment

Getting Started
- Things to Check
  - Recent Tc-99m MDP bone scan showing metastases
    - Most predictable response to treatment in bone scan + lesions
    - Symptoms can be mapped to bone scan to confirm pain caused by lesions
    - Superscan or diffuse proximal long bone activity = extensive marrow involvement; may predict myelotoxicity
  - Complete blood count
  - Creatinine
  - Other contraindications not present
- Equipment List: As with all beta emitters, a plastic syringe shield decreases bremsstrahlung radiation

PROCEDURE

Patient Position/Location
- Best procedure approach: Outpatient treatment after informed consent and discussion of radiation safety precautions

Equipment Preparation
- Adequate IV access essential as dose infiltration can ⇒ soft tissue necrosis

Procedure Steps
- Slow IV injection of radiopharmaceutical followed by saline flush
- If Sm-153 used, can perform whole body imaging

Findings and Reporting
- Although not essential, imaging can verify uptake in painful lesions

Alternative Procedures/Therapies
- Radiologic
  - External beam radiation
    - Radionuclide therapy and external beam radiation can be given concurrently
    - Preferred modality for localized pain, impending pathologic fracture
    - Pain may ↓ within 48 hours of treatment
    - For diffuse pain, hemibody and whole body radiotherapy effective for pain control (↑ bone marrow, pulmonary, gastrointestinal toxicity)
    - Typically a quicker symptomatic response than treatment with radiopharmaceutical; response duration often shorter
- Surgical: Treatment of lesions at risk for pathologic fracture
- Other
  - Bisphosphonates
    - ↓ Osteoclast-mediated bone resorption
    - ↓ Complication rates associated with osteolytic metastases
    - Promote repair by ↑ osteoblast differentiation, bone formation

PALLIATION OF METASTATIC BONE PAIN

- Better established for breast cancer, multiple myeloma; less clear for prostate cancer
- Chemotherapy
  - Variable evidence that chemotherapy alone effective in pain control
  - Has been used as a radiosensitizer for Sr-89 with some success

POST-PROCEDURE

Expected Outcome
- Overall response rates
  - Sm-153: 65-80%
  - Sr-89: 60-84%
  - P-32: 77-84%
- Time to onset of palliation
  - Sm-153: 2-7 days
  - Sr-89: 7-21 days
  - P-32: ≤ 14 days
- Duration of response
  - Sm-153: Mean 8 weeks (4-35 weeks range)
  - Sr-89: Mean 6 months (≤ 14 months)
  - P-32: Mean 2-4 months
- Transient increased pain may occur 2-3 days after treatment
  - Usually self-limited
  - Most prominent with Sr-89 treatment, rare with Sm-153
  - May suggest a good therapeutic response

Things To Do
- CBC every 1-2 weeks until evidence of hematopoietic recovery

PROBLEMS & COMPLICATIONS

Problems
- Most common reason for treatment failure = poor patient selection
  - Positive bone scan mapped to bone pain = highest likelihood of response
- Response less predictable in patients with primarily osteolytic lesions

Complications
- Most feared complication(s)
  - Myelotoxicity
    - Critical organ: Bone marrow
    - Most patients typically develop transient myelosuppression 4-8 weeks after therapy
    - Duration and severity variable depending on radionuclide, dose, and bone marrow reserve
    - Myelotoxicity may be cumulative for repeat treatments
    - Toxicity can be more severe in patients with subclinical disseminated intravascular coagulation (10-20% of patients with advanced prostate cancer)
    - Myelotoxicity especially prominent with P-32 treatment
  - Dose infiltration
    - Beta-emitting radiopharmaceutical delivered to skin/tissues around IV site
    - Can ⇒ skin, muscle necrosis requiring surgical intervention
    - Ensure properly working IV before administration
- Other complications
  - Transient ↑ in pain
    - Increase dose of breakthrough analgesics often required
  - Nausea/vomiting
  - Musculoskeletal complaints
  - Bleeding
  - Case reports of leukemia following treatment with Sr-89 (causal relationship not established)

SELECTED REFERENCES

1. Bauman G et al: Radiopharmaceuticals for the palliation of painful bone metastasis-a systemic review. Radiother Oncol. 75(3):258-70, 2005
2. Damerla V et al: Recent developments in nuclear medicine in the management of bone metastases: a review and perspective. Am J Clin Oncol. 28(5):513-20, 2005
3. Lewington VJ: Bone-seeking radionuclides for therapy. J Nucl Med. 46 Suppl 1:38S-47S, 2005
4. Liepe K et al: Systemic radionuclide therapy in pain palliation. Am J Hosp Palliat Care. 22(6):457-64, 2005
5. Liepe K et al: The benefit of bone-seeking radiopharmaceuticals in the treatment of metastatic bone pain. J Cancer Res Clin Oncol. 131(1):60-6, 2005
6. Pinski J et al: Prostate cancer metastases to bone: pathophysiology, pain management, and the promise of targeted therapy. Eur J Cancer. 41(6):932-40, 2005
7. Reisfield GM et al: Radiopharmaceuticals for the palliation of painful bone metastases. Am J Hosp Palliat Care. 22(1):41-6, 2005
8. Lam MG et al: 186Re-HEDP for metastatic bone pain in breast cancer patients. Eur J Nucl Med Mol Imaging. 31 Suppl 1:S162-70, 2004
9. Maini CL et al: 153Sm-EDTMP for bone pain palliation in skeletal metastases. Eur J Nucl Med Mol Imaging. 31 Suppl 1:S171-8, 2004
10. Pandit-Taskar N et al: Radiopharmaceutical therapy for palliation of bone pain from osseous metastases. J Nucl Med. 45(8):1358-65, 2004
11. Sapienza MT et al: Retrospective evaluation of bone pain palliation after samarium-153-EDTMP therapy. Rev Hosp Clin Fac Med Sao Paulo. 59(6):321-8, 2004
12. Sartor O et al: Samarium-153-Lexidronam complex for treatment of painful bone metastases in hormone-refractory prostate cancer. Urology. 63(5):940-5, 2004
13. Ashayeri E et al: Strontium 89 in the treatment of pain due to diffuse osseous metastases: a university hospital experience. J Natl Med Assoc. 94(8):706-11, 2002
14. Lewington VJ: A practical guide to targeted therapy for bone pain palliation. Nucl Med Commun. 23(9):833-6, 2002
15. Giammarile F et al: Bone pain palliation with strontium-89 in cancer patients with bone metastases. Q J Nucl Med. 45(1):78-83, 2001
16. Hamdy NA et al: The palliative management of skeletal metastases in prostate cancer: use of bone-seeking radionuclides and bisphosphonates. Semin Nucl Med. 31(1):62-8, 2001
17. Han SH et al: 186Re-etidronate. Efficacy of palliative radionuclide therapy for painful bone metastases. Q J Nucl Med. 45(1):84-90, 2001

PALLIATION OF METASTATIC BONE PAIN

IMAGE GALLERY

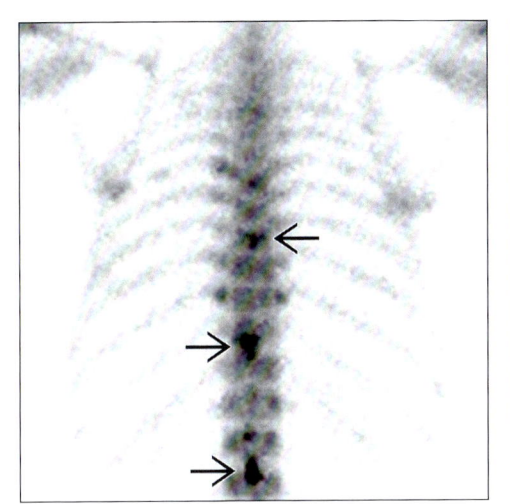

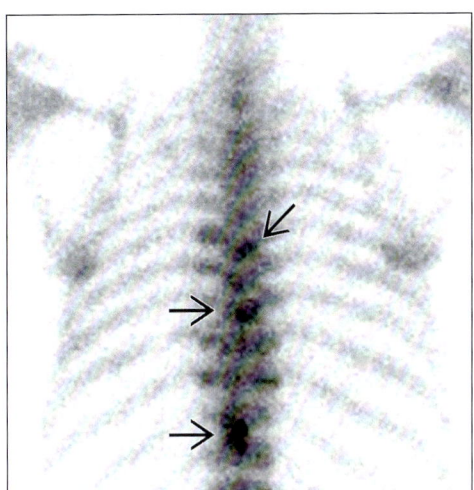

(Left) Posterior Tc-99m MDP bone scan shows multiple bone metastases ➔, corresponding to pain. *(Right)* Posterior Sm-153 image (same patient as previous) following treatment shows uptake in bone lesions ➔. The low-energy gamma emission (103 keV) from Sm-153 allows imaging if desired.

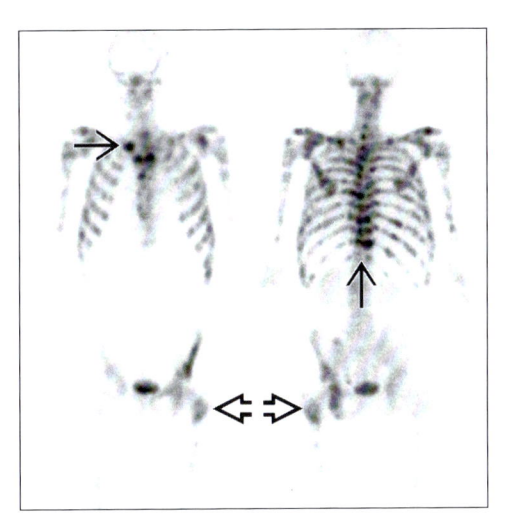

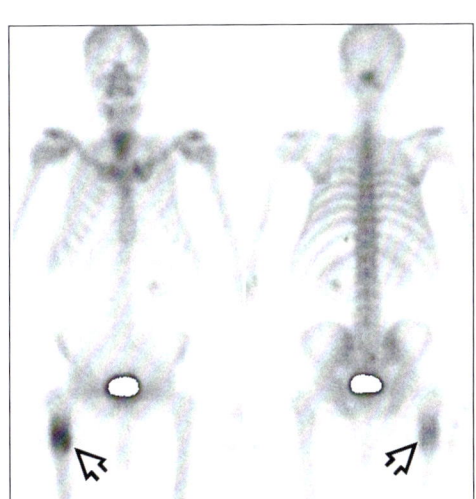

(Left) Tc-99m MDP bone scan in patient with bone pain caused by diffuse metastases ➔. Femoral lesion ⇨ can be simultaneously treated with external beam radiation due to pathologic fracture risk. *(Right)* Tc-99m MDP bone scan shows metastasis in right femur ⇨. Although symptomatic, because it is a solitary lesion, external beam radiation is preferred palliative measure.

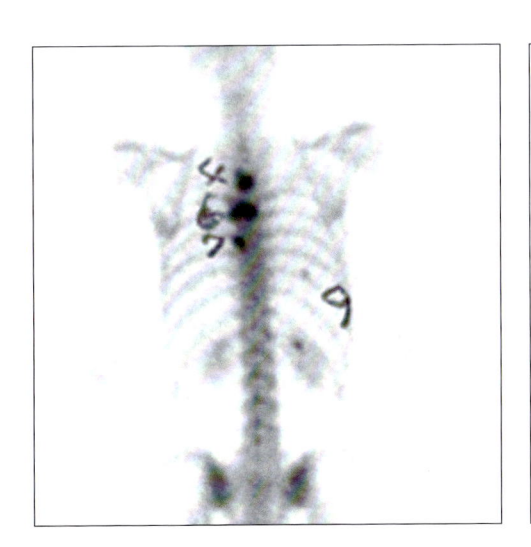

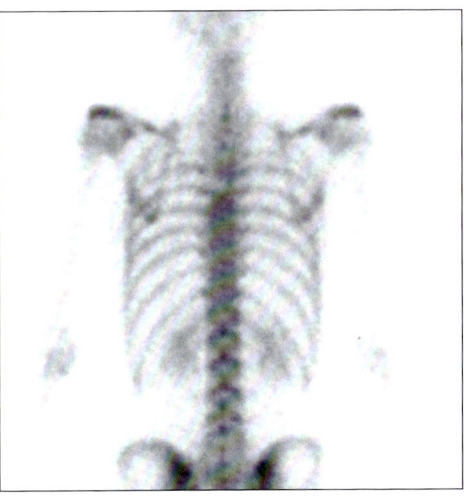

(Left) Posterior Tc-99m MDP bone scan shows multiple metastases (numbers denote vertebral, rib level) in patient with diffuse bone pain treated with Sm-153 (Courtesy Cytogen Corp). *(Right)* Posterior Tc-99m MDP bone scan (same patient as previous) shows no residual uptake in metastases. Treatment is considered palliative, however it may also decrease tumor burden (Courtesy Cytogen Corp).

CELLULITIS

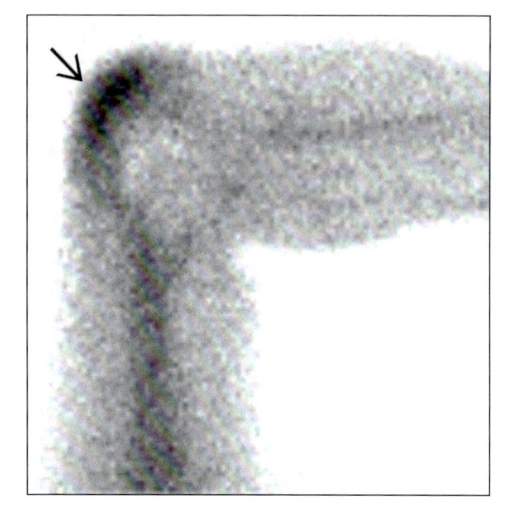

Blood pool phase bone scan shows soft tissue uptake ➔ at olecranon process, compatible with cellulitis. Delayed phase images were also positive, diagnosing osteomyelitis. See next image.

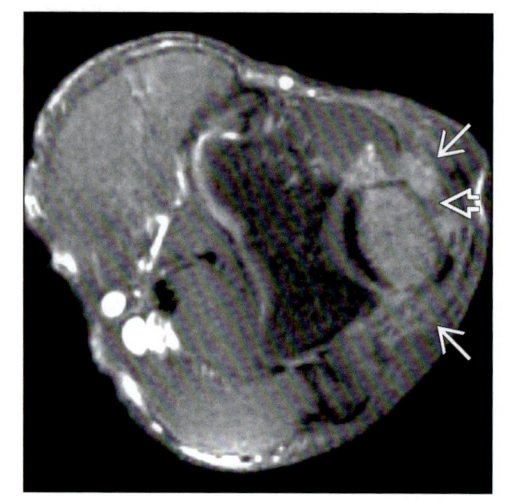

Axial gadolinium T1 C+ MR with fat-suppression in the same patient as previous image, confirms cellulitis ➔ in soft tissues as well as osteomyelitis ➔ of olecranon process.

TERMINOLOGY

Definitions
- Acute infection in connective tissues of deeper layers of dermis; may then extend to soft tissues beneath skin

IMAGING FINDINGS

General Features
- Best diagnostic clue
  - Often clinical diagnosis based on inflammatory response to infection
    - Redness
    - Tenderness
    - Pain
    - Edema
  - Nuclear medicine
    - Increased activity in soft tissue, evident on vascular phases of Tc-99m diphosphonate bone scan, Ga-67 scintigraphy, In-111 white blood cell (WBC) scintigraphy, FDG PET
- Location
  - Can occur anywhere
    - More commonly lower legs and face (erysipelas)
  - Orbital cellulitis
    - Infection of soft tissues posterior to septum
  - Periorbital cellulitis
    - Infection outside of septum
- Size
  - Can be large or small area
    - Size reflects severity
- Morphology
  - Borders not well-demarcated
  - May have lymphangitic streaking

Nuclear Medicine Findings
- Tc-99m diphosphonate three phase bone scan
  - Distinguish cellulitis from osteomyelitis with bone scan
  - Cellulitis
    - Angiographic phase: Diffuse uptake in soft tissue
    - Equilibrium blood pool phase: Diffuse uptake in soft tissue
    - Delayed (mineral) phase: Often mild bone uptake due to hyperemia → fades by 24 h
  - Osteomyelitis

DDx: Other Causes of Uptake on Vascular Phase of Bone Scan

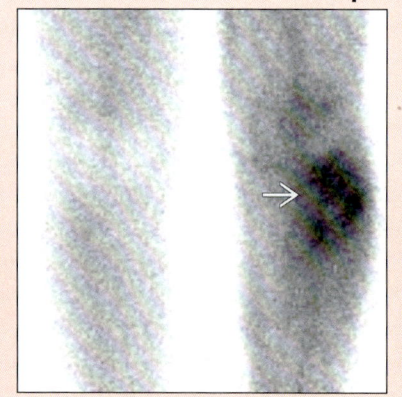

Tumor

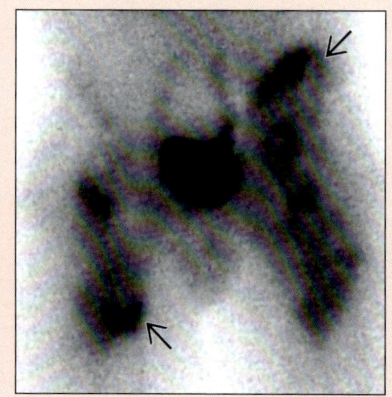

Heterotopic Ossification

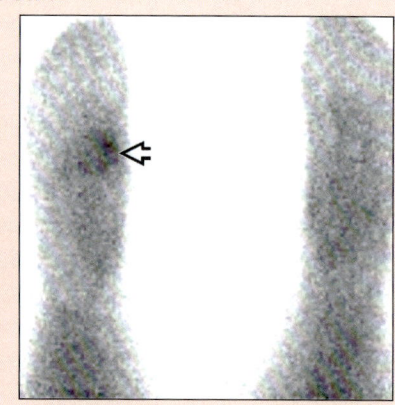

Acute Fracture

CELLULITIS

Key Facts

Terminology
- Acute infection in connective tissues of deeper layers of dermis; may then extend to soft tissues beneath skin

Imaging Findings
- Distinguish cellulitis from osteomyelitis with bone scan
- Delayed image of bone scan (6-24 hours) useful to rule out/diagnose osteomyelitis if large amount of hyperemia on initial phases
- Increased uptake of labeled WBC in soft tissues = cellulitis
- Correlate In-111 WBC scan with Tc-99m MDP bone scan to localize area of infection
- SPECT or SPECT/CT may also help localize cellulitis from osteomyelitis
- Increased uptake on Ga-67 with cellulitis, but not with lymphedema

Top Differential Diagnoses
- Neoplasm
- Fracture
- Necrotizing Fasciitis

Clinical Issues
- Important to distinguish cellulitis from osteomyelitis
- Unless cellulitis severe or complicated, clinical improvement begins within 24 to 48 hours

Diagnostic Checklist
- Delayed bone scan images at 6-24 hours with cellulitis to further evaluate for osteomyelitis
- Additional imaging with CT, MR, ultrasound for complicated cases

---

- ↑ Activity in bone on vascular and delayed (mineral) phases
- Bone uptake does not fade at 24 h
- Delayed image of bone scan (6-24 hours) useful to rule out/diagnose osteomyelitis if large amount of hyperemia on initial phases
- Indium-111 WBC scintigraphy
    - Cellulitis
        - Increased uptake of labeled WBC in soft tissues = cellulitis
    - Osteomyelitis
        - Increased uptake in bone; no corresponding Tc-99m sulfur colloid uptake
        - May have superimposed cellulitis
    - Correlate In-111 WBC scan with Tc-99m MDP bone scan to localize area of infection
        - May be difficult to distinguish soft tissue from bone uptake on WBC scintigraphy
        - Dual acquisition of Tc-99m (140 keV) and In-111 (171, 247 keV) windows differentiates osseous from extraosseous uptake
        - SPECT or SPECT/CT may also help localize cellulitis from osteomyelitis
- Ga-67 scintigraphy
    - Ga-67 may help distinguish chronic lymphedema from cellulitis
        - Increased uptake on Ga-67 with cellulitis, but not with lymphedema
    - SPECT or SPECT/CT may help localize

Imaging Recommendations
- Best imaging tool
    - Imaging typically not needed unless severe or in critical location (e.g., orbit)
    - Radiographs
        - Soft tissue gas, edema or foreign body
    - Ultrasound
        - Helpful in emergent situation
        - Rule out abscess
        - Guides percutaneous drainage or aspiration
    - CT
        - Evaluate for abscess
        - Rule out foreign body
        - Differentiate periorbital cellulitis from orbital cellulitis
        - Help diagnose necrotizing fasciitis
    - MR
        - Help diagnose necrotizing fasciitis (facial enhancement)
        - Best examination to diagnose osteomyelitis
- Protocol advice
    - Tc-99m MDP three phase bone scan
        - Spot views over area of interest for angiographic, blood pool, and delayed phases
        - Delayed images as needed
        - Comparison 100K images at 4, 24 h may allow better assessment of fading/increasing activity
- Additional nuclear medicine imaging options
    - PET/CT
        - May be useful to differentiate soft tissue infection from osteomyelitis
        - Accompanying CECT can provide valuable information
        - Not reimbursable by medicare

DIFFERENTIAL DIAGNOSIS

Neoplasm
- Soft tissue and osseous tumors
- Hyperemia causes increased tracer accumulation

Fracture
- Correlation with clinical history is best differentiating factor
- Small Brodie abscess with adjacent cellulitis can be indistinguishable from a stress fracture on bone scan and radiographs

Necrotizing Fasciitis
- MR will show increased signal in deep tissues
- Definitive diagnosis with surgery
- Much higher morbidity, mortality rate than cellulitis
- Often times need immediate surgical debridement

CELLULITIS

PATHOLOGY

General Features
- Genetics
  - Inherited diseases which increase risk
    - Hyper-immunoglobulin E syndrome
    - Chronic granulomatous disease
- Etiology
  - Associated with breaks in skin
    - Following surgery, lymphadenectomy
    - Post-traumatic
    - Foreign body
    - Peripheral vascular disease, diabetes mellitus
    - Drug users
  - May not always have skin injury
  - Most commonly a bacterial infection
    - Vast majority gram-positive microorganisms: Staphylococcus, streptococcus
    - Infants: Group B streptococcus
    - Remainder mostly gram-negative bacilli, especially in immunocompromised
    - E. coli cellulitis can lead to nephrotic syndrome
  - Rare to be caused by fungus, even if immunocompromised
- Epidemiology: US: 2-3 cases per 100 people each year
- Associated abnormalities
  - Immunocompromised patients at higher risk
    - Diabetes mellitus
    - Chronic steroid therapy
    - Chemotherapy
    - HIV
  - Edema predisposes
    - Lymphedema
    - Chronic venous stasis

Microscopic Features
- Inflammatory WBCs
- Edema
- Bacteria
- Fungus (rare)

CLINICAL ISSUES

Presentation
- Most common signs/symptoms
  - Usually acute
    - Swelling
    - Pain
    - Redness
    - Increased WBC count
- Other signs/symptoms: Possible history of recent skin injury or surgery

Demographics
- Age
  - More common 45-64 years
  - Erysipelas
    - 6 months - 3 years
    - > 50 years
- Gender: M = F

Natural History & Prognosis
- Important to distinguish cellulitis from osteomyelitis
- Unless cellulitis severe or complicated, clinical improvement begins within 24 to 48 hours
- Excellent prognosis for uncomplicated cases
- Complications
  - Gangrene
  - Sepsis
  - Lymphangitis
  - Meningitis

Treatment
- Antibiotics
  - Oral, if mild
  - Intravenous, if severe
  - Choice of antibiotic depends on infection source
  - Routinely given for 7 to 14 days
- Surgery
  - For necrosis, gangrene
- Abscess drainage
  - Percutaneous or incision and drainage

DIAGNOSTIC CHECKLIST

Consider
- Delayed bone scan images at 6-24 hours with cellulitis to further evaluate for osteomyelitis
- Additional imaging with CT, MR, ultrasound for complicated cases
  - Ultrasound useful to rule out abscess (fast, easy, no radiation)
- Not all soft tissue uptake = cellulitis (e.g., sarcoma, septic arthritis)

Image Interpretation Pearls
- Cellulitis typically has soft tissue uptake on angiographic and blood pool images, minimal bone uptake on delayed images

SELECTED REFERENCES

1. Bar-Shalom R et al: SPECT/CT using 67Ga and 111In-labeled leukocyte scintigraphy for diagnosis of infection. J Nucl Med. 47(4):587-94, 2006
2. Palestro CJ et al: Combined labeled leukocyte and technetium 99m sulfur colloid bone marrow imaging for diagnosing musculoskeletal infection. Radiographics. 26(3):859-70, 2006
3. Grimbacher B et al: Hyper-IgE syndromes. Immunol Rev. 203:244-50, 2005
4. Keidar Z et al: The diabetic foot: initial experience with 18F-FDG PET/CT. J Nucl Med. 46(3):444-9, 2005
5. Khanna G et al: Imaging of chronic granulomatous disease in children. Radiographics. 25(5):1183-95, 2005
6. Fugitt JB et al: Necrotizing fasciitis. Radiographics. 24(5):1472-6, 2004
7. Swartz MN: Clinical practice. Cellulitis. N Engl J Med. 350(9):904-12, 2004
8. Suga K et al: Ga-67-avid massive cellulitis within a chronic lymphedematous limb in a survivor of Hodgkin's disease. Clin Nucl Med. 26(9):791-2, 2001
9. Dupuy A et al: Risk factors for erysipelas of the leg (cellulitis): case-control study. BMJ. 318(7198):1591-4, 1999
10. Hopper KD et al: CT and MR imaging of the pediatric orbit. Radiographics. 12(3):485-503, 1992

CELLULITIS

IMAGE GALLERY

Typical

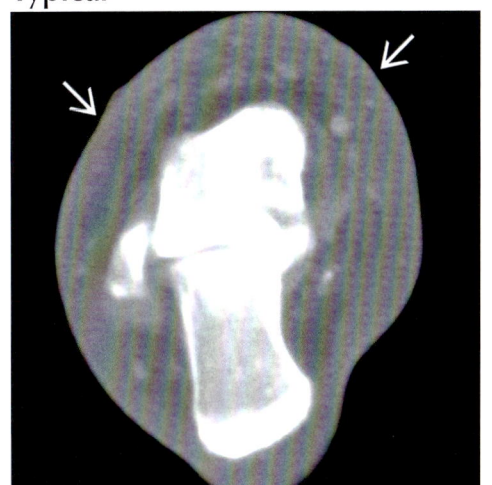

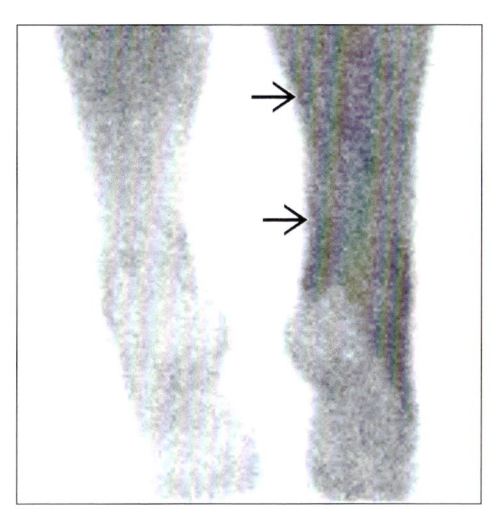

(Left) Axial CECT of right ankle shows edema in subcutaneous tissues ➡, compatible with cellulitis. Bone scan was performed to evaluate for osteomyelitis. See next image. **(Right)** Posterior blood pool phase bone scan in the same patient as previous image, shows increased uptake ➡ in right lower leg and foot. See next image.

Typical

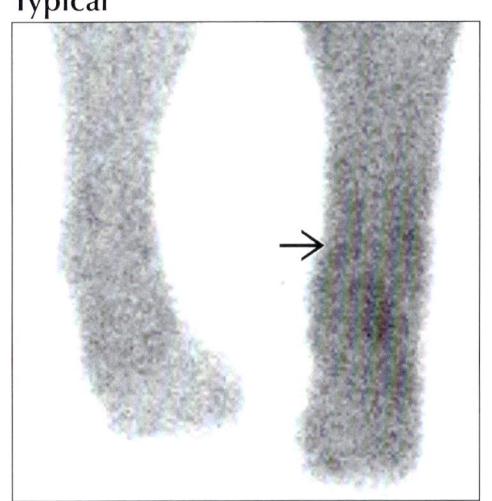

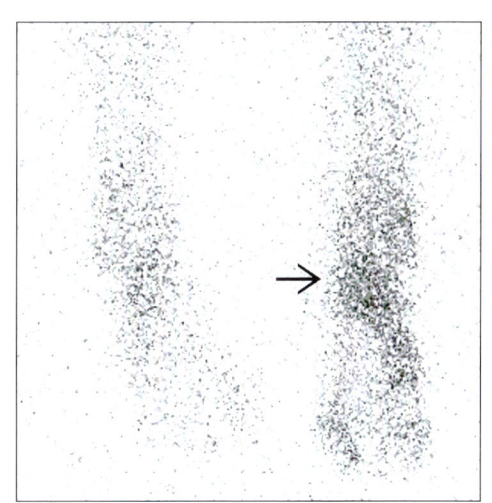

(Left) Posterior delayed phase bone scan in the same patient as previous image, shows uptake in soft tissues ➡, confirming cellulitis. Given generalized poor bone uptake, the patient was re-imaged at 24 hours. See next image. **(Right)** Posterior bone scan at 24 hours in the same patient as previous image, shows mild uptake in the right foot bones ➡, but less than on soft tissue phases, compatible with increased delivery of tracer to bone due to hyperemia. Often fades by 24 h.

Typical

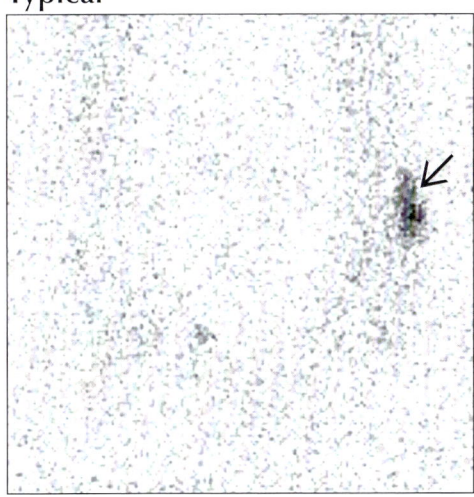

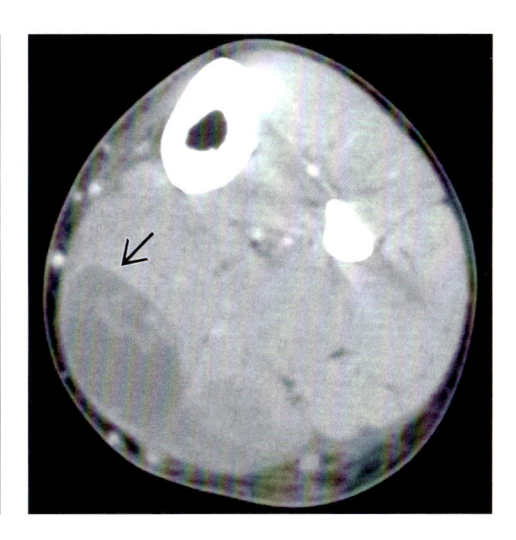

(Left) Anterior labeled leukocyte scintigraphy shows uptake in lateral left ankle ➡ in a patient with erythema and swelling, consistent with cellulitis. For most precise anatomic localization, this study could be compared to bone scan. **(Right)** Axial CECT shows large abscess ➡ in subcutaneous tissues of posteromedial left leg. Cross-sectional imaging is useful to exclude abscess and fasciitis, which is difficult to evaluate on a labeled leukocyte scan.

OSTEOMYELITIS, APPENDICULAR

Plantar angiographic phase bone scan of the feet in a patient with diabetic foot ulcer shows hypervascularity about left great toe ⇒, suspicious for osteomyelitis.

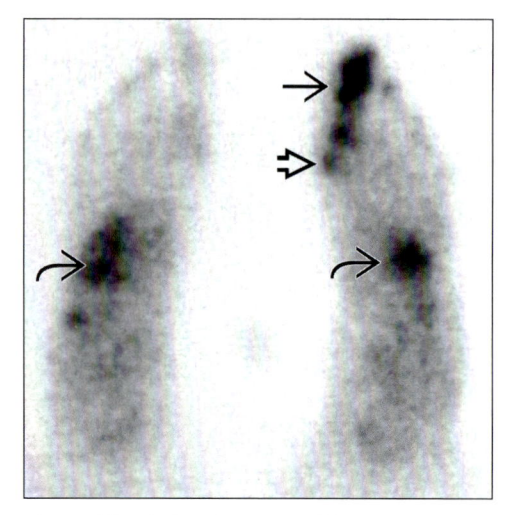

Plantar delayed phase bone scan of feet in same patient at left shows ↑ activity in phalanges ⇒ and medial sesamoid ⇒ of left great toe, indicating osteomyelitis. Note Charcot changes ⇒.

TERMINOLOGY

Definitions
- Osteomyelitis: Local or generalized suppurative process causing progressive destruction of bone
- Aggressive bone lesion with one or more of the following: Periosteal reaction, soft-tissue swelling, subperiosteal abscess, draining sinus

IMAGING FINDINGS

General Features
- Best diagnostic clue
  - Biopsy with cultures and sensitivities = gold standard for diagnosis
  - MR: Marrow edema ↑ T2, loss of fat signal ↓ T1, contrast enhancement ↑T1
  - When MR is contraindicated
    - 3-phase bone scan: Increased activity on angiographic, blood pool, and delayed phases
    - Tagged white blood cell (WBC) and Ga-67 scans: Tracer accumulation corresponding to bone
- Location
  - Adults: Feet (diabetics), arthroplastic components, surgically revised joints
  - Lower extremities > upper extremities, tibia > femur
  - Fracture sites, especially open fractures
  - Brodie abscess (indolent subacute osteomyelitis): Classically metaphyseal although may be epiphyseal or in metaphyseal equivalent

Nuclear Medicine Findings
- Tc-99m methylene diphosphonate 3-phase bone scan
  - Classic appearance on 3-phase bone scan: Increased activity on all 3 phases
  - Occasionally photopenic on bone scan: Marrow thrombosis, ↑ intramedullary pressure (particularly in children)
  - Useful for imaging of larger regions or whole body (angiographic phase must be targeted, however) or for patients with contraindications to MR
  - May be falsely negative in neonates and infants
- Tagged WBC and Ga-67 scans: Tracer accumulation corresponding to bone in region of suspicion

Imaging Recommendations
- Best imaging tool

DDx: Mimics of Osteomyelitis on Bone Scan

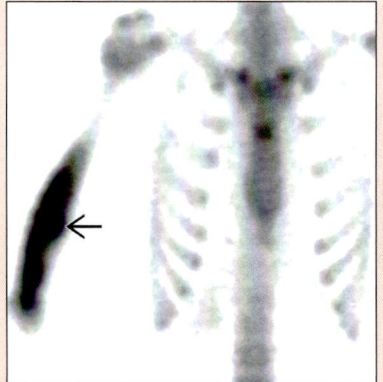

Ewing Sarcoma

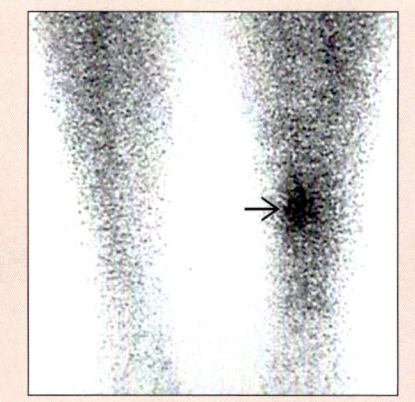

Osteoid Osteoma

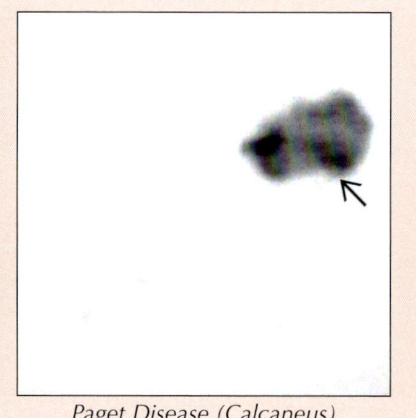

Paget Disease (Calcaneus)

OSTEOMYELITIS, APPENDICULAR

Key Facts

Terminology
- Osteomyelitis: Local or generalized suppurative process causing progressive destruction of bone

Imaging Findings
- Classic appearance on 3-phase bone scan: Increased activity on all 3 phases
- Occasionally photopenic on bone scan: Marrow thrombosis, ↑ intramedullary pressure (particularly in children)
- Tagged WBC and Ga-67 scans: Tracer accumulation corresponding to bone in region of suspicion
- In-111 or Tc-99m HMPAO WBCs localize to areas of infection
- Tc-99m sulfur colloid (SC) marrow mapping has similar uptake to WBC scan in chronic inflammation or red marrow
- Ga-67 scintigraphy: Depicts distribution of infection/inflammation (Fe surrogate), may be helpful in chronic osteomyelitis

Top Differential Diagnoses
- Arthropathy
- Healing Trauma
- Ewing Sarcoma
- Paget Disease: Osteitis Deformans
- Osteoid Osteoma

Clinical Issues
- Clinical and laboratory findings are frequently inaccurate, typical findings may or may not be present, diagnosis can be difficult
- Blood cultures: Positive in ~ 50% of patients with osteomyelitis

---

- CE MR: 90-95% sensitivity/specificity in patients with pristine bone
  - ↑ T2 (marrow edema), ↓ T1 (fat signal), cortical disruptions (↑ T2), contrast enhancement (↑ T1)
  - Local and subperiosteal fluid (abscess), devitalized bone (sequestra), sinus tracts, periosteal reaction
  - Requires targeted imaging of suspicious region
  - Contraindications: Adjacent prosthesis, coexistent degenerative changes, neuropathic joint, standard MR contraindications
- Tc-99m 3-phase bone scan if MR contraindicated: > 95% sensitivity and specificity in patients with pristine bone
  - Widely available, rarely contraindicated
  - If non-pristine bone, may require tagged WBC scan for optimal diagnosis
  - In cases of coexistent bone abnormalities such as arthropathy, trauma, noninfectious process or surgical change, specificity poor (~ 33%)
  - Arthroplasties/prostheses may be 3-phase positive due to normal hyperemic healing, osteoblastic remodeling for ≥ 12 months
- Protocol advice
  - 3-phase bone scan
    - Adult dose: 20-25 mCi (740-925 MBq) Tc-99m MPD IV
    - Angiographic phase: 2-second planar images for 60 seconds in anterior and posterior projections over region of interest
    - Blood pool phase: Static planar image over area of concern, anterior/posterior projections
    - Mineral/delayed phase: Whole body or spot image in anterior/posterior projections, lateral/oblique projections as needed
    - Delayed: 8 h and 24 h images demonstrate progressive uptake; hyperemic delivery of tracer to bone due to cellulitis fades
    - SPECT may be useful in specific applications
    - SPECT improves spatial resolution, distinguishing soft tissue from bone involvement
- Additional nuclear medicine imaging options
  - Tagged WBC scan
    - In-111 or Tc-99m HMPAO WBCs localize to areas of infection
    - Improves differentiation of aseptic inflammation, cellulitis, osteomyelitis: Estimated accuracy 92%
    - When coexistent arthropathy/trauma/structural deformity present, WBC scan necessary
    - If WBC scan positive, perform Tc-99m SC marrow map to exclude WBC accumulation in reticuloendothelial system elements (red marrow, chronic inflammation)
    - Can be performed concurrently if using In-111 labeled WBCs
    - Tc-99m HMPAO WBC scan: Better imaging characteristics, however requires Tc-99m SC marrow map later if (+) (same imaging energy); ↑ blood pool may result in false +
    - Areas of WBC activity which are not concordant on Tc-99m SC are positive for osteomyelitis (discordant pattern)
    - If WBC activity has matching (concordant) Tc-99m SC activity, the study is negative for osteomyelitis
    - Concordant activity associated with infiltration of chronic granulomatous cells (e.g., neuropathic arthropathy, surgical changes)
    - WBC scan also recommended to evaluate treatment response
    - False (+) in recently "violated" bone (e.g., fracture, postsurgical) due to localization in marrow elements
  - Tc-99m sulfur colloid (SC) marrow mapping has similar uptake to WBC scan in chronic inflammation or red marrow
  - Ga-67 scintigraphy: Depicts distribution of infection/inflammation (Fe surrogate), may be helpful in chronic osteomyelitis
    - When compared with bone scan, Ga-67 uptake should greater uptake or = uptake of different size (larger or smaller)
- Correlative imaging features
  - Plain film: Limited sensitivity and specificity
    - Normal initially, recognition may take 2-3 weeks

OSTEOMYELITIS, APPENDICULAR

- Loss of cortical margins, periosteal reaction, erosions, soft tissue swelling, sequestra, involucra, sclerosis (late)
○ Ultrasound has limited role
  - Subperiosteal fluid (pus) is diagnostic
  - Also soft tissue swelling, periosteal thickening, periosteal elevation > 2 mm

DIFFERENTIAL DIAGNOSIS

Arthropathy
- Neuropathic, osteoarthritic, rheumatoid, gout: Concordant WBC and SC marrow map avoid diagnosis of osteomyelitis

Healing Trauma
- Clinical history of fracture, surgery

Ewing Sarcoma
- Invades soft tissues with absent or insignificant inflammatory changes, edema or cellulitis

Paget Disease: Osteitis Deformans
- Trabecular disorganization and thickening, lysis and sclerosis with "blade of grass" boundary at leading edge

Osteoid Osteoma
- Small, focal, with central nidus of osteosclerosis
- Pain at night, relieved by aspirin

PATHOLOGY

General Features
- Etiology
  ○ Usually bacterial, may be polymicrobial
  ○ Most common cause: Extension of cellulitis or traumatic direct inoculation in adolescents/adults
    - Intraosseous extension via Volkmann (transverse) and Haversian (longitudinal) canals
    - Penetrating trauma, decubitus ulcers, wounds
    - Bacteroides fragilosa: Common in diabetics
    - Pseudomonas aeruginosa: IV drug users
  ○ Septic arthritis, prosthesis failure
- Epidemiology
  ○ Diabetes mellitus
    - Up to 1/4 of all diabetics will suffer severe foot morbidity during their lifetimes
    - Especially with ulcerations, wounds and penetrating injuries of feet
  ○ IV drug users
    - Osteomyelitis occurs in unusual locations
  ○ More common in patients with AIDS, immune suppression, sickle cell anemia
  ○ Orthopedic procedures, arthroplasties, open fractures predispose
- Associated abnormalities
  ○ Cellulitis, infected open wound, sinus tract, frank drainage of pus through skin (advanced cases)
  ○ Brodie abscess: Cavitary, usually metaphyseal, collection of necrotic debris, WBCs

Microscopic Features
- Inflammation, edema, suppuration with infiltration of neutrophils, lymphocytes

CLINICAL ISSUES

Presentation
- Most common signs/symptoms
  ○ Bone pain, erythema, swelling, fluctuance, fever, nausea, malaise, sweats, chills
    - Pain may be absent in advanced neuropathy
    - Fever and adenopathy often absent or mild
  ○ ↑ WBC count, erythrocyte sedimentation rate
  ○ Clinical and laboratory findings are frequently inaccurate, typical findings may or may not be present, diagnosis can be difficult
  ○ Blood cultures: Positive in ~ 50% of patients with osteomyelitis
- Other signs/symptoms
  ○ Adjacent abscess, local extension into joint, fistula
  ○ Pathologic fracture

Demographics
- Gender: M:F = 2:1

Natural History & Prognosis
- Good prognosis assuming adequate therapy
  ○ May result in structural deformity or growth disturbance especially with inadequate treatment
- Chronic osteomyelitis more likely recalcitrant, especially in diabetics and in tissue with poor blood supply, peripheral vascular disease

Treatment
- Eradication through IV antibiotic therapy, wound hygiene, surgical debridement, amputation
  ○ Chronic osteomyelitis requires surgical intervention

DIAGNOSTIC CHECKLIST

Consider
- Cellulitis, degenerative arthropathy, traumatic change

Image Interpretation Pearls
- Both bone scan and MR are sensitive but nonspecific if osteomyelitis suspected with coexisting arthropathy/trauma/structural deformity
  ○ WBC scan useful
- WBC scan with Tc-99m SC discordance is > 90% sensitive, specific for osteomyelitis

SELECTED REFERENCES

1. El-Maghraby TA et al: Nuclear medicine methods for evaluation of skeletal infection among other diagnostic modalities. Q J Nucl Med Mol Imaging. 50(3):167-92, 2006
2. Filippi L et al: Usefulness of Hybrid SPECT/CT in 99mTc-HMPAO-Labeled Leukocyte Scintigraphy for Bone and Joint Infections. J Nucl Med. 47(12):1908-13, 2006
3. Segura AB et al: What is the role of bone scintigraphy in the diagnosis of infected joint prostheses? Nucl Med Commun. 25(5):527-32, 2004

OSTEOMYELITIS, APPENDICULAR

IMAGE GALLERY

Typical

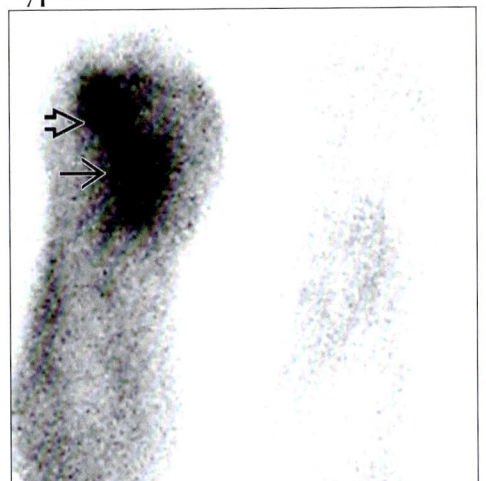

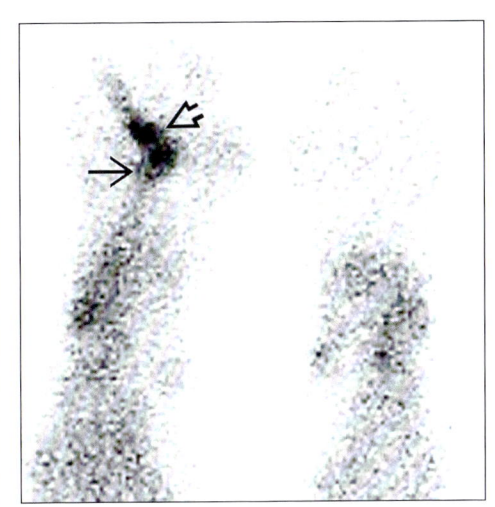

(Left) Plantar blood pool phase bone scan shows ↑ activity about the second and third metatarsals ➔ extending into the third digit ▷, indicating cellulitis, suspicious for osteomyelitis. *(Right)* Plantar delayed phase bone scan in same patient at left shows tracer accumulation in head of right third metatarsal ➔, and proximal phalanx of third digit ▷, indicating osteomyelitis.

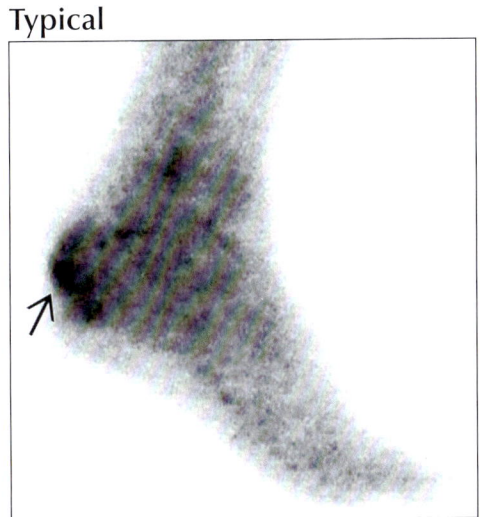

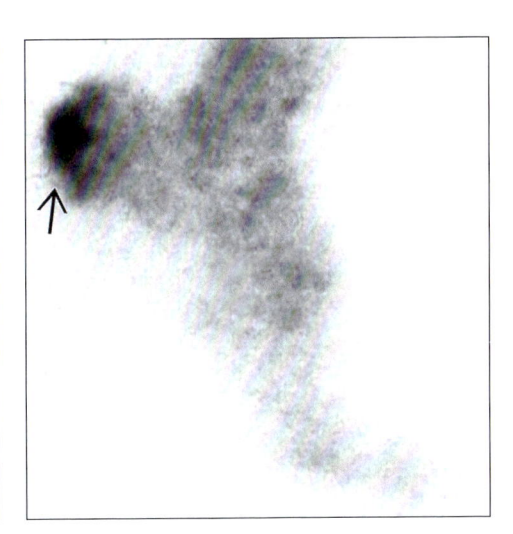

Typical

(Left) Right lateral blood pool phase bone scan shows ↑ activity in posterior right calcaneus ➔ in diabetic patient with heel ulcer. *(Right)* Right lateral delayed phase bone scan in same patient at left shows ↑ activity in posterior calcaneus ➔, indicating osteoblastic activity from osteomyelitis.

Typical

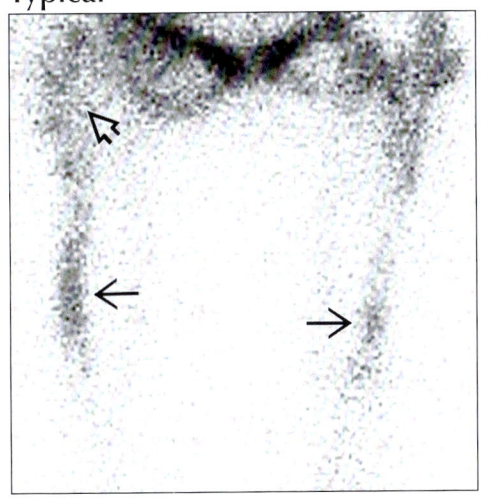

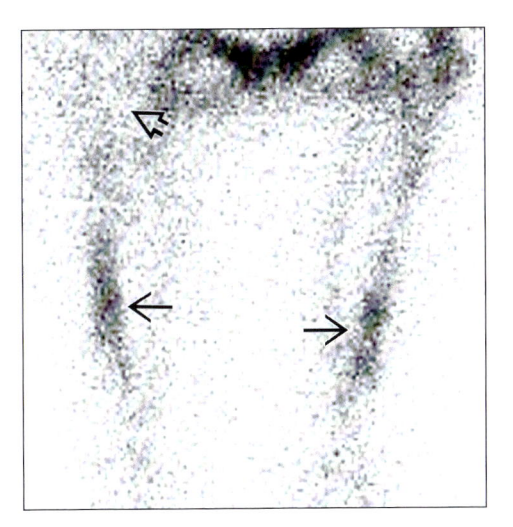

(Left) Anterior In-111 WBC scan shows leukocyte aggregation in proximal right ▷ and bilateral mid femurs ➔, necessitating Tc-99m SC marrow map. *(Right)* Anterior Tc-99m SC marrow map in same patient at left shows presence of reticuloendothelial system cells (red marrow) in mid femurs ➔. Absence of activity in proximal right femur is consistent with osteomyelitis ▷.

OSTEOMYELITIS, APPENDICULAR

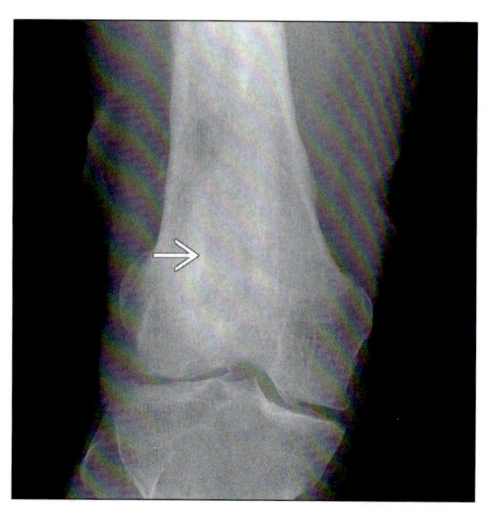

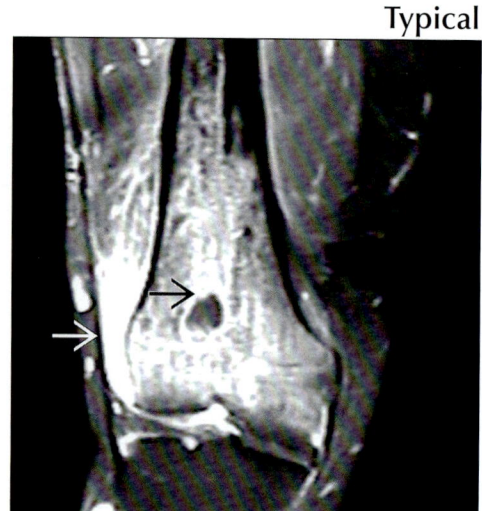

(Left) Anterior radiograph shows lucent medullary lesion ➡ at site of Brodie abscess. See next 3 images. *(Right)* Coronal T2 weighted MR in same patient as previous image shows fluid signal lateral to distal femoral condyle ➡ and at site of Brodie abscess in intramedullary region ➡.

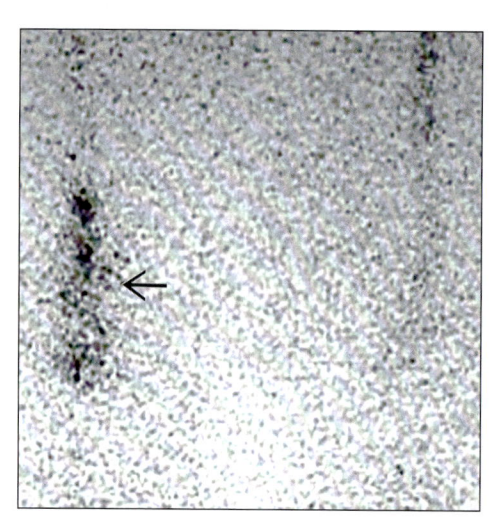

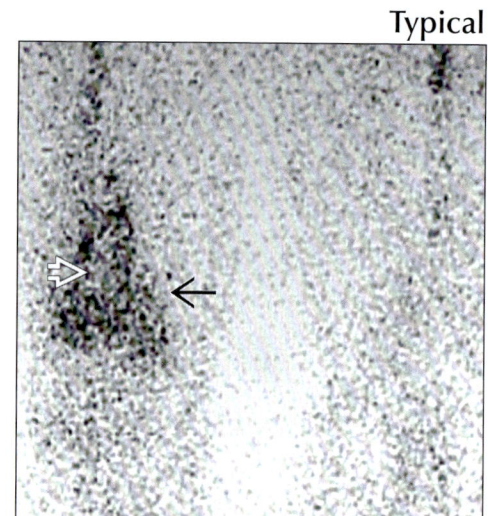

(Left) Anterior In-111 WBC scan in same patient as previous image shows linear accumulation ➡ in distal right femur corresponding to lucent region on plain radiograph. See corresponding marrow map (next image). *(Right)* Anterior Tc-99m SC scan in same patient as previous image shows red marrow distribution ➡. Focal photopenia ➡ corresponds to WBC accumulation in Brodie abscess. This discordance indicates osteomyelitis.

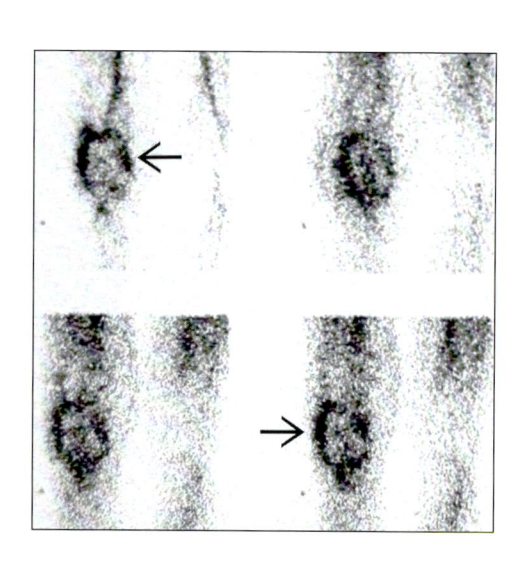

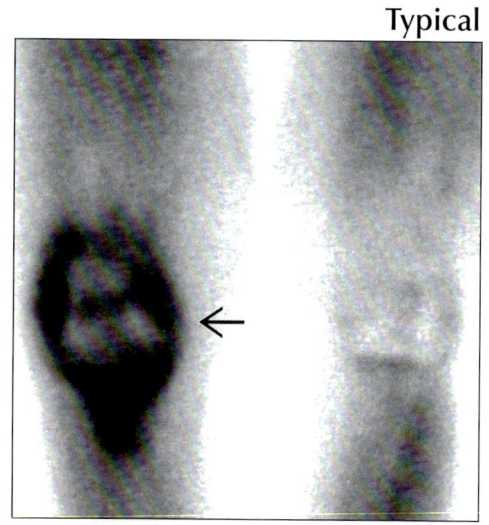

(Left) Anterior angiographic phase bone scan shows ↑ flow about the right knee ➡, concerning for post-operative changes, cellulitis or osteomyelitis. See next image. *(Right)* Anterior blood pool phase bone scan in same patient at left shows hyperemia about the right knee arthroplasty ➡. See next image.

OSTEOMYELITIS, APPENDICULAR

Typical

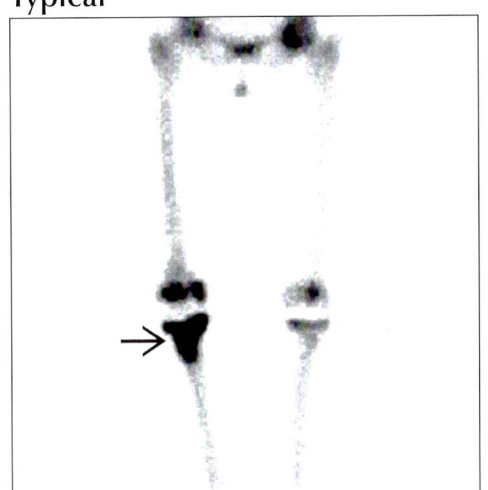

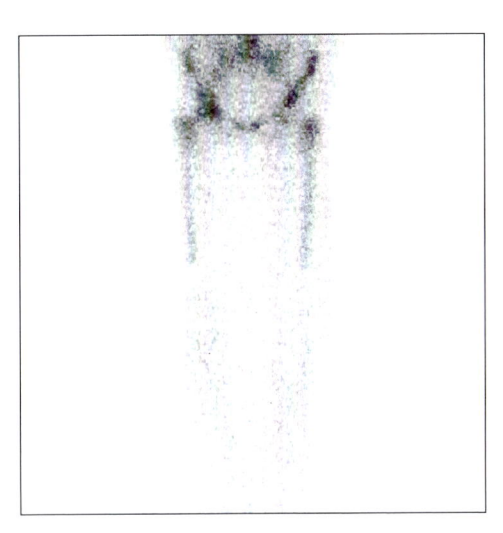

(Left) Anterior delayed phase bone scan in same patient as previous image shows extensive osteoblastic activity about the right knee arthroplasty ➔, particularly adjacent to tibial component, prompting In-111 WBC scan. See next image. (Right) Anterior In-111 WBC scan in same patient as previous image shows no abnormal activity, excluding osteomyelitis and indicating cellulitis/postsurgical changes.

Typical

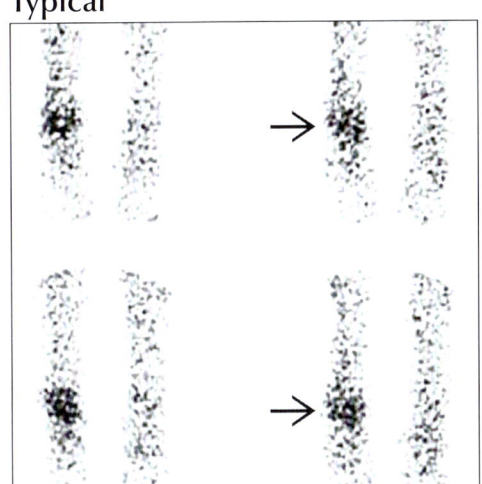

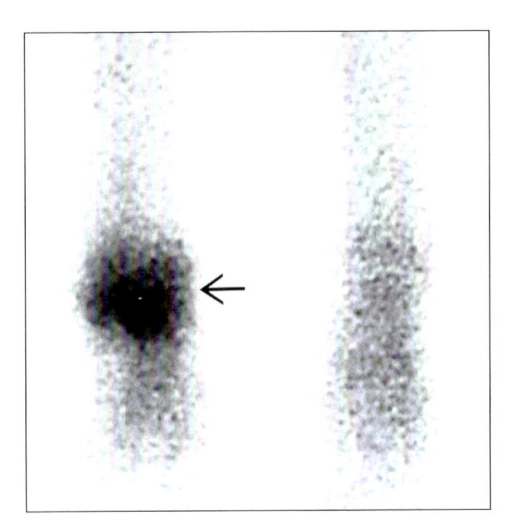

(Left) Anterior angiographic phase bone scan shows increased blood flow to the right ankle region ➔ in patient with pain, fever, ↑ white cell count. See next image. (Right) Anterior blood pool phase bone scan in same patient at left shows ↑ activity about the right ankle ➔ indicating hyperemia in soft tissues.

Typical

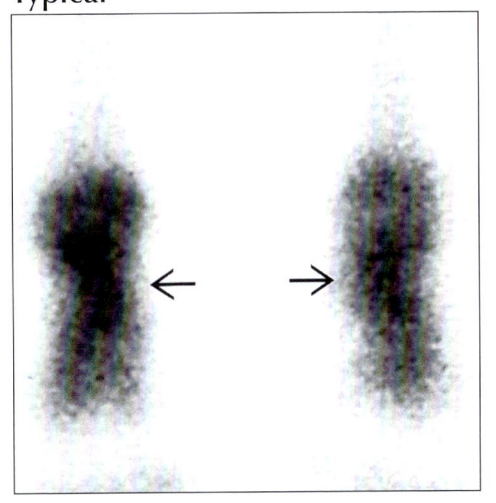

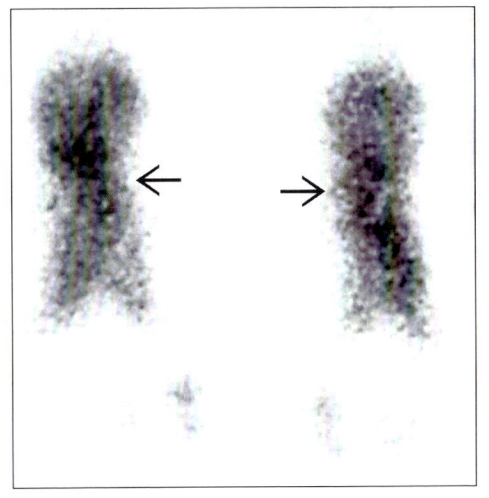

(Left) Anterior delayed phase bone scan at 4 h in same patient at left shows ↑ tracer accumulation about both ankles ➔, indicating symmetric increased osteoblastic activity without osteomyelitis. (Right) Anterior delayed phase bone scan at 24 h ("4th phase") in same patient at left shows improved visualization of bones ➔ with symmetric activity, excluding osteomyelitis.

OSTEOMYELITIS, AXIAL

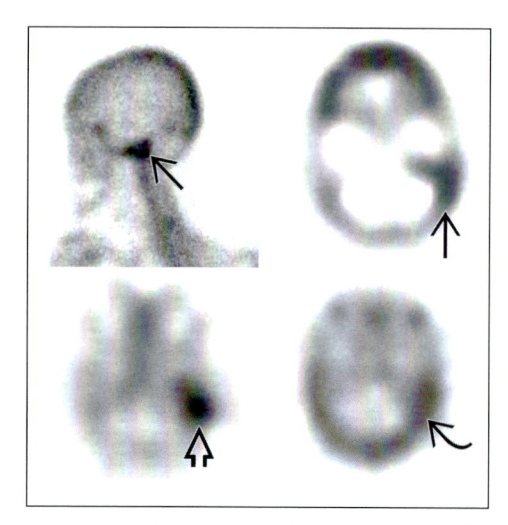

Increased activity in temporal bone on bone scan ➔ and gallium scan ➔ in a patient with malignant otitis externa. Post-therapy gallium scan shows good treatment response ➔.

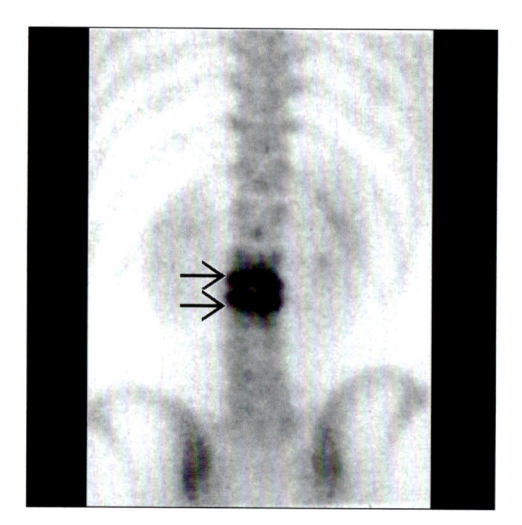

Posterior bone scan shows increased activity in endplates of two adjacent vertebral bodies ➔. This appearance is characteristic of discitis or discogenic sclerosis.

TERMINOLOGY

Definitions
- Acute or chronic bone infection from hematogenous, contiguous, traumatic, iatrogenic sources

IMAGING FINDINGS

General Features
- Best diagnostic clue
  - MR: Edema (↑ T2), enhancement with contrast (↑ T1); loss of fat signal without contrast (↓ T1)
  - Increased activity localizing to bone on three phase bone scan, labeled leukocyte scintigraphy, Ga-67 scintigraphy
    - Bone scan more sensitive than radiography/CT, possibly also MR in early infection (within 48 hours of symptoms); SPECT increases sensitivity

Nuclear Medicine Findings
- PET: Likely ↑ sensitivity; not currently reimbursed for infection imaging
- Bone Scan
  - Three phase bone scan
    - Infection: Positive on all three phases of bone scan (nonspecific)
    - No hyperemia on first phase: High negative predictive value for infection
- Ga-67 Scintigraphy: Positive for infection if higher activity than bone scan or equal uptake but different shape
- Labeled Leukocyte Scintigraphy
  - High positive predictive value
  - Photopenia/false negative in 25% spinal osteomyelitis
  - Localizes to normal marrow elements in absence of infection: Requires Tc-99m sulfur colloid marrow map (shows absent uptake in osteo)

Imaging Recommendations
- Best imaging tool
  - CEMR
  - Nuclear medicine: Three-phase bone scan, Ga-67, labeled leukocyte scintigraphy

DDx: Mimics of Axial Osteomyelitis

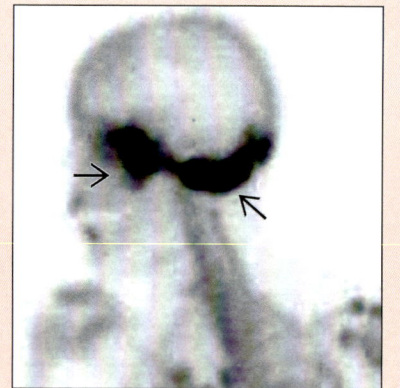

Fibrous Dysplasia 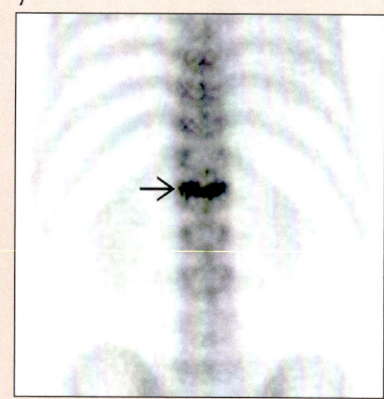 | *Compression Fracture* 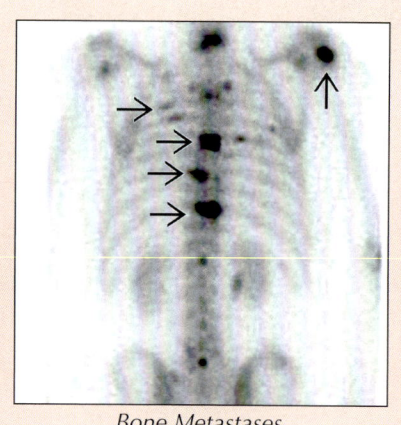 | *Bone Metastases*

OSTEOMYELITIS, AXIAL

Key Facts

Terminology
- Acute or chronic bone infection from hematogenous, contiguous, traumatic, iatrogenic sources

Imaging Findings
- Increased activity localizing to bone on three phase bone scan, labeled leukocyte scintigraphy, Ga-67 scintigraphy

Top Differential Diagnoses
- Neoplasm
- Fracture
- Discitis/Discogenic Sclerosis

Diagnostic Checklist
- Negative first phase of three phase bone scan: High negative predictive value for osteomyelitis

DIFFERENTIAL DIAGNOSIS

Neoplasm
- Primary can show ↑ activity on three phase bone scan, Ga-67
- Metastases: Multiple, scattered bone lesions

Fracture
- Acute: Increased activity on three-phase bone scan
- Chronic: Increased activity on delayed images
- Spinal compression: Increased activity in (usually superior) vertebral endplate

Discitis/Discogenic Sclerosis
- Increased activity in adjacent endplates of two vertebral bodies around disc

PATHOLOGY

General Features
- Etiology
  - Mechanism
    - Head and neck: Osteoradionecrosis, odontogenic, chronic sinusitis, malignant external otitis
    - Spine/pelvis: Hematogenous spread, contiguous extension, trauma, iatrogenic
  - Organisms: S. aureus, epidermis; gram negatives (immunocompromised)
  - Risk factors: Diabetes, end-stage renal disease, immunocompromise, trauma, surgery

CLINICAL ISSUES

Demographics
- Age
  - Peak incidence: 5th decade
  - Second most common age: 2nd decade
- Gender: M > F; 1.5-3:1

Treatment
- IV antibiotics, debridement

DIAGNOSTIC CHECKLIST

Image Interpretation Pearls
- Negative first phase of three phase bone scan: High negative predictive value for osteomyelitis
- Bone scan + Ga-67: Infection if Ga-67 uptake > bone scan, or if similar uptake but different size/shape region (larger or smaller); useful with chronic infection
- Labeled leukocyte scintigraphy
  - Can be false negative/photopenic in spinal osteomyelitis
  - Can be false positive in areas of expanded marrow (compare images to Tc-99m sulfur colloid which localizes in area of noninfected marrow)

SELECTED REFERENCES
1. Palestro CJ et al: Radionuclide imaging in orthopedic infections. Semin Nucl Med. 27(4):334-45, 1997

IMAGE GALLERY

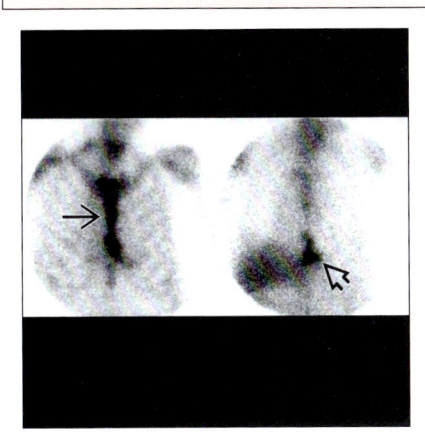

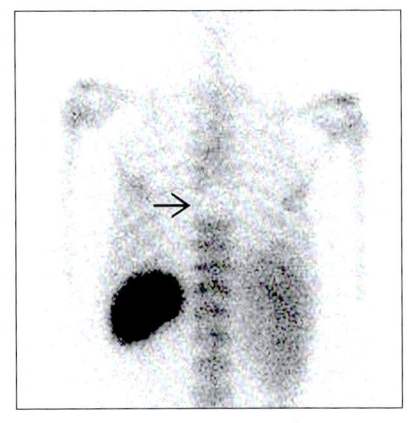

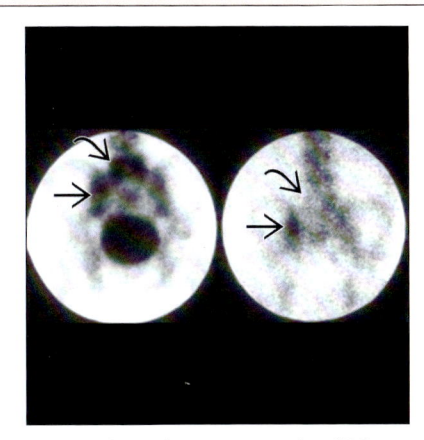

(Left) Anterior bone scan following median sternotomy infection shows expected ↑ activity ➔. Ga-67 scan shows ↑ activity in xiphoid ➔, consistent with osteomyelitis. (Center) Posterior labeled leukocyte scintigraphy shows photopenia ➔ in known spinal osteomyelitis. Labeled leukocyte scan is often falsely negative in spinal osteomyelitis. (Right) Posterior bone scan (Lt. panel) shows ↑ activity in L5 ➔, left SI joint ➔, consistent with infection. Corresponding labeled WBC scan (Rt. panel) shows photopenia in L5 (false negative) and ↑ activity in left SI.

OSTEOMYELITIS, TEMPORAL BONE

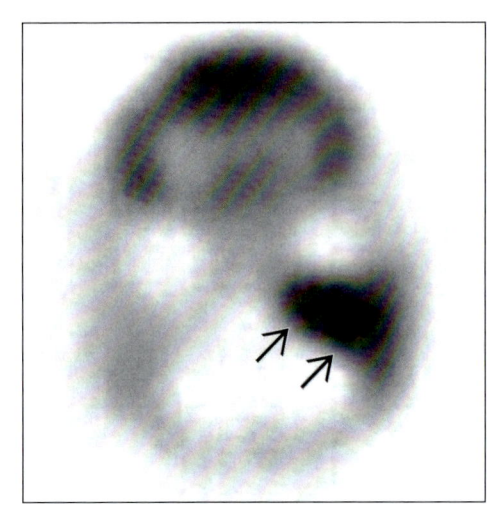

Axial Tc-99m MDP SPECT of the skull shows increased uptake in the left temporal bone ➡, extending to the petrous apex. Patient was recently treated for malignant otitis externa. See next image.

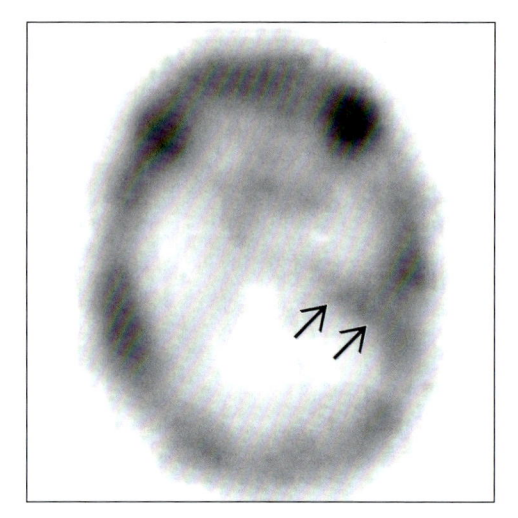

Axial Ga-67 SPECT of the skull performed within a few days of previous bone scan. Temporal bone uptake of Ga-67 ➡ is < < than on corresponding bone scan (no active infection). Mild uptake = bony remodeling.

TERMINOLOGY

Abbreviations and Synonyms
- Malignant otitis externa

Definitions
- Otitis external extending aggressively to adjacent bone, meninges, vessels, cranial nerves

IMAGING FINDINGS

General Features
- Best diagnostic clue: Uptake on Ga-67 SPECT > Tc-99m diphosphonate SPECT = active infection
- Location: External auditory canal, mastoid air cells, petrous apex, temporal mandibular joint
- CT: Preferable > MR for bone erosions, initial dx
- MR: Better definition of soft tissue abnormalities
- Abnormalities on CT/MR may persist despite Rx

Nuclear Medicine Findings
- Active infection: Uptake of Ga-67 > bone scan; or = uptake but different shape
- Ga-67 SPECT at 6-8 weeks: Marked ↓ in Ga-67 uptake = infection resolved
- Mild bone scan, Ga-67 uptake may persist: Bony remodeling, healing

Imaging Recommendations
- Best imaging tool
  - CT, MR: Initial diagnosis (CT preferable)
  - Ga-67/bone scan SPECT combined imaging: Assessment of disease activity
  - Follow-up Ga-67 6-8 weeks following treatment: Confirmation of therapeutic response

DIFFERENTIAL DIAGNOSIS

Fibrous Dysplasia
- Sclerosis on CT, lack of ↑ sed rate

Malignancy
- Ga-67 uptake ↑: Lymphoma, melanoma

Isolated Mastoiditis
- Imaging findings isolated to mastoid sinus

DDx: Mimics of Temporal Bone Osteomyelitis

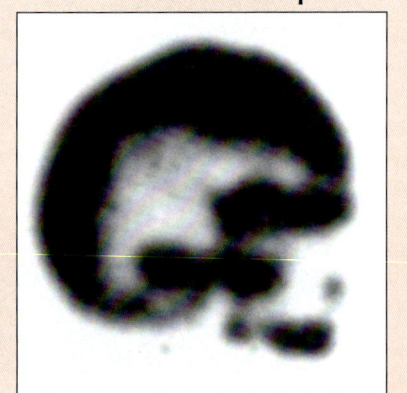

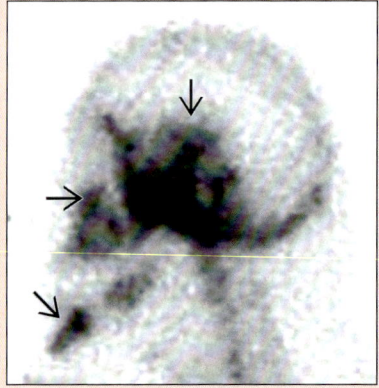

Paget Disease *Fibrous Dysplasia* *TMJ Arthritis*

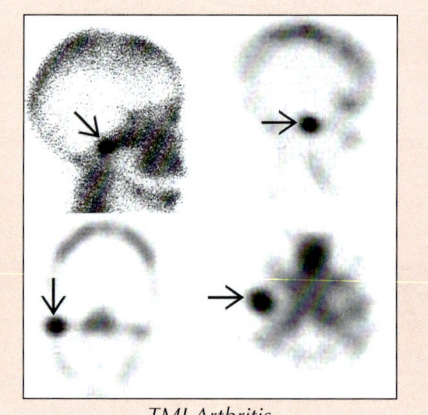

OSTEOMYELITIS, TEMPORAL BONE

Key Facts

Terminology
- Otitis external extending aggressively to adjacent bone, meninges, vessels, cranial nerves

Imaging Findings
- CT, MR: Initial diagnosis (CT preferable)
- Ga-67/bone scan SPECT combined imaging: Assessment of disease activity
- Follow-up Ga-67 6-8 weeks following treatment: Confirmation of therapeutic response

Top Differential Diagnoses
- Fibrous Dysplasia
- Malignancy
- Isolated Mastoiditis
- Temporal Mandibular Joint Degenerative Disease

Pathology
- Etiology: Pseudomonas aeruginosa most common pathogen
- Epidemiology: Most common in elderly diabetics

Temporal Mandibular Joint Degenerative Disease
- Pain, uptake on nuclear scans confined to TMJ

PATHOLOGY

General Features
- Etiology: Pseudomonas aeruginosa most common pathogen
- Epidemiology: Most common in elderly diabetics

CLINICAL ISSUES

Presentation
- Unrelenting otalgia, headache, purulent otorrhea, ↑ sed rate, ↑ WBC count, fever
- Granulation tissue in external auditory canal

Natural History & Prognosis
- Begins as granulation tissue at bone/cartilage interface
- Most commonly: Infection spreads via fissures of Santorini to soft tissues inferior to the temporal bone
- May progress to chondritis, osteomyelitis extending posteriorly into mastoid, anteriorly into temporomandibular joint, medially to petrous apex

Treatment
- Extended IV antibiotics → oral, surgical debridement in complicated cases

DIAGNOSTIC CHECKLIST

Consider
- Ga-67 + bone scan SPECT to assess disease activity
- Follow-up Ga-67 6-8 weeks post therapy

SELECTED REFERENCES

1. Prasad KC et al: Osteomyelitis in the head and neck. Acta Otolaryngol. 127(2):194-205, 2007
2. Djalilian HR et al: Treatment of culture-negative skull base osteomyelitis. Otol Neurotol. 27(2):250-5, 2006
3. Chang PC et al: Central skull base osteomyelitis in patients without otitis externa: imaging findings. AJNR Am J Neuroradiol. 24(7):1310-6, 2003
4. Sreepada GS et al: Skull base osteomyelitis secondary to malignant otitis externa. Curr Opin Otolaryngol Head Neck Surg. 11(5):316-23, 2003
5. Sun SS et al: Simultaneous Tc-99m MDP and Ga-67 citrate uptake of benign lymphoid hyperplasia in the mastoid region. Clin Nucl Med. 26(9):797, 2001
6. Ohashi T et al: Atypical osteomyelitis of the temporal bone. Acta Otolaryngol Suppl. 522:99-103, 1996
7. Chandler JR et al: Osteomyelitis of the base of the skull. Laryngoscope. 96(3):245-51, 1986
8. Noyek AM et al: The clinical significance of radionuclide bone and gallium scanning in osteomyelitis of the head and neck. Laryngoscope. 94(5 Pt 2 Suppl 34):1-21, 1984
9. Strashun AM et al: Malignant external otitis: early scintigraphic detection. Radiology. 150(2):541-5, 1984
10. Parisier SC et al: Nuclear scanning in necrotizing progressive "malignant" external otitis. Laryngoscope. 92(9 Pt 1):1016-9, 1982

IMAGE GALLERY

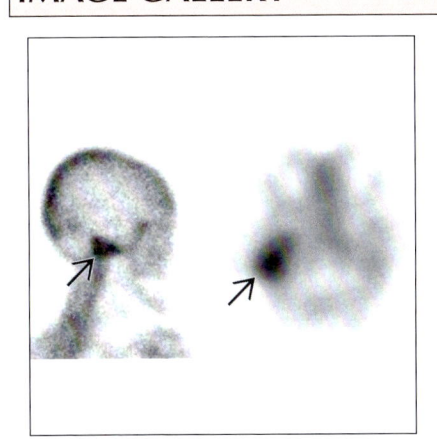

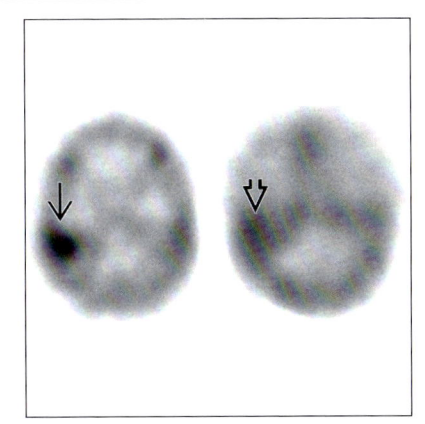

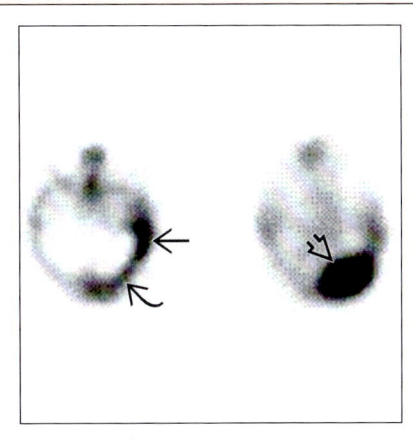

(Left) Lateral planar (lt) and SPECT (rt) Tc-99m MDP shows ↑ uptake in the right mastoid ➔ in patient with malignant otitis externa. See next image. (Center) Corresponding Ga-67 SPECT (lt) shows ↑ uptake in more anterior/apical petrous portion of the temporal bone ➔ (continuing infection). Follow-up Ga-67 SPECT (rt) 8 wks later shows infection resolved ➔. (Right) Axial Tc-99m MDP SPECT (lt) in patient with malignant otitis externa shows spread to left mastoid ➔ and calvarium ➔. Ga-67 SPECT (rt) shows intense uptake in an epidural abscess ➔.

OSTEOMYELITIS, FEET

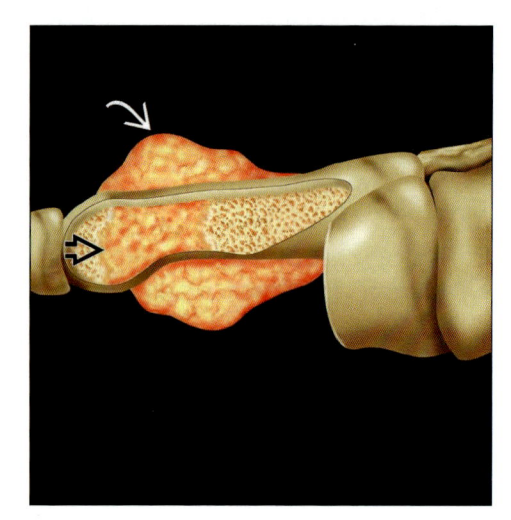

Sagittal graphic shows osteomyelitis of the metatarsal with involvement of bone ⊵ and adjacent soft tissue ⇨.

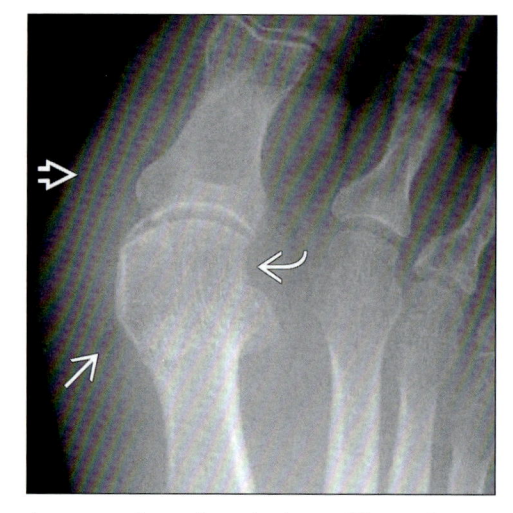

Anteroposterior radiograph shows diffuse soft tissue swelling ⊵, air in soft tissues ➡, and destructive changes in medial metatarsal head ⊵ in a patient with diabetic foot ulcer and osteomyelitis.

TERMINOLOGY

Abbreviations and Synonyms
- Diabetic foot, pedal osteomyelitis

Definitions
- Infection in osseous structures of foot, usually from contiguous spread of adjacent infection

IMAGING FINDINGS

General Features
- Best diagnostic clue: Cortical destruction adjacent to ulceration
- Location
  - Most common in 1st and 5th metatarsals, followed by calcaneus
  - Neuropathic joint involves midfoot

Nuclear Medicine Findings
- PET
  - F-18 FDG uptake at sites of inflammation due to increased glycolysis in inflammatory cells
  - Preliminary results show high sensitivity
- Bone Scan
  - Three phase bone scan
    - Angiographic phase: Regional hyperperfusion
    - Immediate static phase: Focal hyperemia
    - Delayed phase: Focal bony uptake on delayed images
    - 3-phase bone scan for osteomyelitis: Sensitivity 90%, specificity 46%, accuracy 65%
  - Four phase bone scan may increase specificity (accuracy ~ 85%)
    - With osteomyelitis, degree of bone uptake should increase at 24 hours
- Labeled Leukocyte Scintigraphy
  - Adds specificity: Labeled leukocytes usually do not accumulate at areas of new bone formation without infection
    - False positive may occur in neuropathic joint
  - In-111 labeled white blood cell (WBC) scan: Comparable to bone scan for accurate localization
    - Sensitivity 86%, specificity 74%, accuracy 74%
  - Tc-HMPAO WBC scan: Higher anatomic detail than with In-111 WBC
    - Sensitivity 86%, specificity 85%, accuracy 85%

DDx: Mimics of Osteomyelitis of Foot on Bone Scan

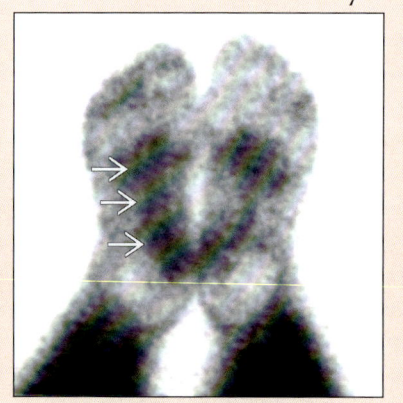

Plantar Fasciitis 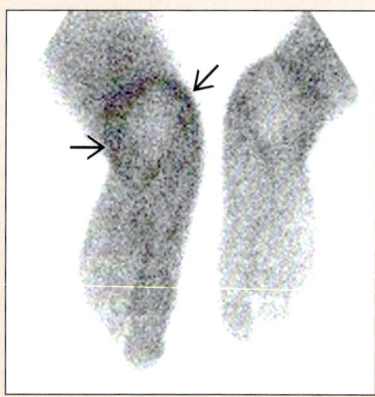 | *Cellulitis* 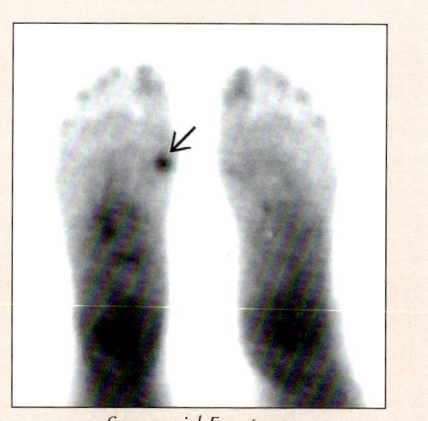 | *Sesamoid Fracture*

OSTEOMYELITIS, FEET

Key Facts

Terminology
- Infection in osseous structures of foot, usually from contiguous spread of adjacent infection

Imaging Findings
- 3-phase bone scan for osteomyelitis: Sensitivity 90%, specificity 46%, accuracy 65%
- Four phase bone scan may increase specificity (accuracy ~ 85%)
- In-111 labeled white blood cell (WBC) scan: Comparable to bone scan for accurate localization
- Tc-HMPAO WBC scan: Higher anatomic detail than with In-111 WBC
- Osteomyelitis in violated bone: Region of interest + on WBC scan and - on Tc-99m sulfur colloid scintigraphy

Top Differential Diagnoses
- Neuropathic Osteoarthropathy (Charcot Joint)
- Fracture
- Cellulitis
- Arthritis
- Osteonecrosis

Diagnostic Checklist
- Prompt diagnosis important
- Classic findings of infection often absent
- Multiple studies often necessary
- Negative bone scan: High negative predictive value for absence of infection
- WBC scintigraphy: ↑ Specificity of bone scan
- Tc-99m sulfur colloid marrow scintigraphy: May be necessary to determine distribution of normal marrow elements in violated bone, Charcot joint

---

- Tc-99m sulfur colloid scintigraphy
  - May be used in conjunction with labeled WBCs to delineate areas of bone marrow distribution, which takes up labeled WBCs
  - Evaluate images for discordant uptake
    - Osteomyelitis in violated bone: Region of interest + on WBC scan and - on Tc-99m sulfur colloid scintigraphy
    - No osteomyelitis: Region of interest + on WBC scan and + on Tc-99m sulfur colloid scintigraphy
  - Adds specificity in areas of altered bone marrow distribution (sensitivity 100%, specificity 94%)

Radiographic Findings
- Classic triad: Bone demineralization, cortical erosion, periosteal reaction
- Requires 30-50% bone loss before radiographically evident
- Plain films may not be + until several weeks after infection onset
- Accuracy for early diagnosis: 30-50%

CT Findings
- May demonstrate cortical destruction, bony sequestrum, periosteal reaction
- Soft tissue evaluation limited

MR Findings
- T1WI: Low marrow signal
- T2WI: High marrow signal
- Abnormal marrow signal, cortical destruction
- Contrast-enhancement to assess soft tissue infection, sinus tracts
- Sensitivity 90%, specificity 74%

Imaging Recommendations
- Best imaging tool
  - Plain film, complemented by radionuclide exams and/or MR
    - Used to identify sites of soft tissue air and bone changes
  - Three-phase bone scan
    - Useful in screening exams in patients with low probability of infection
    - High negative predictive value
    - Used in equivocal cases on plain film, MR
  - Labeled WBC scintigraphy
    - Useful as adjunct to bone scan
  - Tc-99m sulfur colloid scintigraphy
    - Useful in violated bone with altered marrow
- Protocol advice
  - Three or four phase Tc-99m MDP bone scan
    - Clinical history, exam: Physical inspection of foot invaluable for image correlation
    - Dose: 20-30 mCi Tc99-MDP (740 MBq-1.11 GBq)
    - Angiographic phase: Flow images of 30 frames, 1-3 seconds per frame; plantar positioning of feet over camera
    - Blood pool phase: Within 10 minutes of injection, 200-300K counts/image; plantar images, plus lateral (or medial) view
    - Delayed phase: 3-4 hours, 150-250K counts/image; plantar images, plus lateral (or medial) view
    - 4th phase: In patients with severe vascular disease, may need more delayed image (6-24 hours)
  - Labeled WBC scintigraphy
    - Dose: 0.5 mCi (18.5 MBq) In-111 labeled WBC; 10-20 mCi (370-740 MBq) Tc-99m HMPAO
    - Foot positioned similarly to bone scan
    - Injection to image time: 24 hours for In-111; 4-8 hours for Tc-99m HMPAO
    - Counts: 10-20 minutes per image for In-111; 800K or 5-10 minutes for Tc-99m HMPAO
    - Photopeak selection: 173 and 247-keV for In-111; 140 keV for Tc-99m HMPAO
    - Superior imaging quality with Tc-99m HMPAO
    - Bone scan may not be necessary for violated bone (combine with Tc-99m sulfur colloid scintigraphy)
  - Tc-99m sulfur colloid scintigraphy
    - Dose: 8-10 mCi (296-370 MBq) Tc-99m sulfur colloid
    - Imaging time: 20 minutes post injection
    - Position feet similarly to labeled WBC images, bone scan

OSTEOMYELITIS, FEET

- Use in violated bone, neuropathic joint (identifies sites of expanded bone marrow)
- F-18 FDG PET: Role currently evolving

DIFFERENTIAL DIAGNOSIS

Neuropathic Osteoarthropathy (Charcot Joint)
- ↑ Activity on bone scan
- Fractures common, which induces bone marrow expansion ⇒ false + labeled WBC studies
- Add Tc-99m sulfur colloid "marrow map" to delineate marrow distribution

Fracture
- Positive on immediate and delayed imaging
- Should not accumulate labeled white cells

Cellulitis
- Positive on flow and immediate static images
- No focal delayed uptake

Arthritis
- Plain film: Osteophytes, joint space narrowing
- Delayed bone scan images positive
- Inflammatory arthritis: May be positive on flow imaging

Osteonecrosis
- May involve talus or metatarsal head
- Bone scan findings depend on stage of disease: Initially photopenic, followed by increased uptake during reparative phase

PATHOLOGY

General Features
- Etiology
  - Diabetics have multiple risk factors
    - Sensory neuropathy ⇒ ↓ perception of trauma, leading to repetitive injury, ulcers, ligamentous injury, altered weight bearing
    - Autonomic neuropathy ⇒ dry, cracked skin, predisposing to ulceration
    - Peripheral vascular disease associated with infection progression, impaired healing
    - Diabetic immunopathy ⇒ poor healing
    - Motor neuropathy ⇒ muscle atrophy and foot deformity
  - Multiorganism infection common
  - Distal disease associated with adjacent ulcer
  - Proximal and midfoot disease associated with Charcot joint
- Epidemiology
  - Forefoot: 90% from contiguous infection (foot ulcer)
  - Midfoot: Charcot joint ± infection
- Associated abnormalities
  - Septic arthritis in 30%
  - Soft tissue abscess, sinus tract not uncommon

Gross Pathologic & Surgical Features
- Areas of suppuration, necrosis, dead bone (sequestrum)
- Periosteal elevation, abscess
- Pyogenic arthritis
- Adjacent draining soft tissue tracts

Microscopic Features
- Acute inflammatory reaction
- After one week, chronic inflammatory cells predominate

CLINICAL ISSUES

Presentation
- Most common signs/symptoms
  - Often asymptomatic
  - Traditional signs of infection may be absent (erythema, warmth, purulent discharge)
  - WBC count and erythrocyte sedimentation rate (ESR) may be misleading
- Other signs/symptoms: Charcot neuropathic arthropathy: Swollen, unstable foot, effusion

Demographics
- Age: Older population

Natural History & Prognosis
- Early and aggressive treatment of osteomyelitis essential in avoiding amputation
- Diabetes: Leading cause of nontraumatic lower extremity amputation

Treatment
- IV antibiotics
- Wound debridement, revascularization, amputation

DIAGNOSTIC CHECKLIST

Consider
- Prompt diagnosis important
- Classic findings of infection often absent
- Multiple studies often necessary

Image Interpretation Pearls
- Osteomyelitis: ↑ Activity in site of clinical concern on angiographic, immediate static and delayed phase bone scan images (sensitive but nonspecific)
- Negative bone scan: High negative predictive value for absence of infection
- WBC scintigraphy: ↑ Specificity of bone scan
- Tc-99m sulfur colloid marrow scintigraphy: May be necessary to determine distribution of normal marrow elements in violated bone, Charcot joint

SELECTED REFERENCES

1. Morrison WB et al: Work-up of the diabetic foot. Radiol Clin North Am. 40(5):1171-92, 2002
2. Turpin S et al: Role of scintigraphy in musculoskeletal and spinal infections. Radiol Clin North Am. 39(2):169-89, 2001

OSTEOMYELITIS, FEET

IMAGE GALLERY

Typical

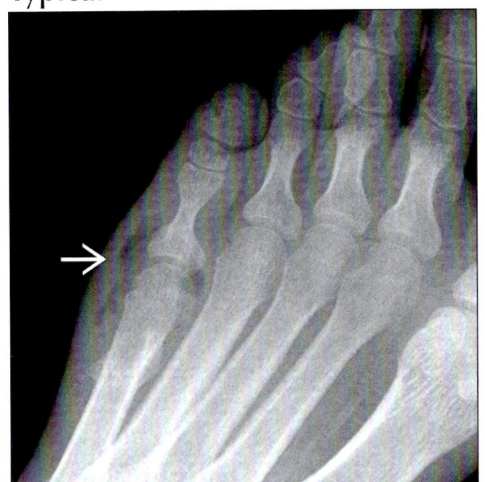

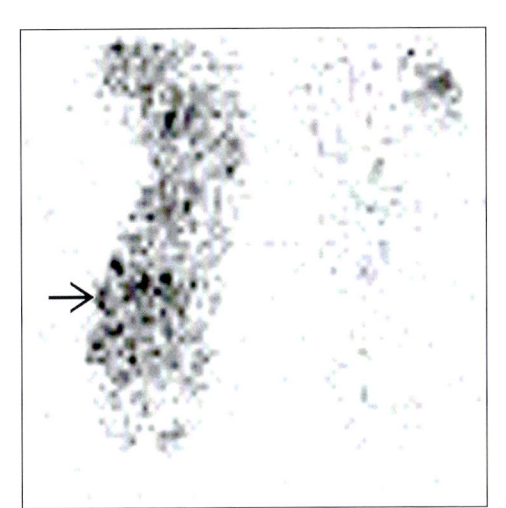

(Left) Radiograph shows subcutaneous gas about the fifth metatarsal ➡ in a diabetic patient with cellulitis. Same as next five images. **(Right)** Plantar angiographic phase bone scan in same patient as previous image, shows diffuse hyperperfusion to right foot ➡. See next image.

Typical

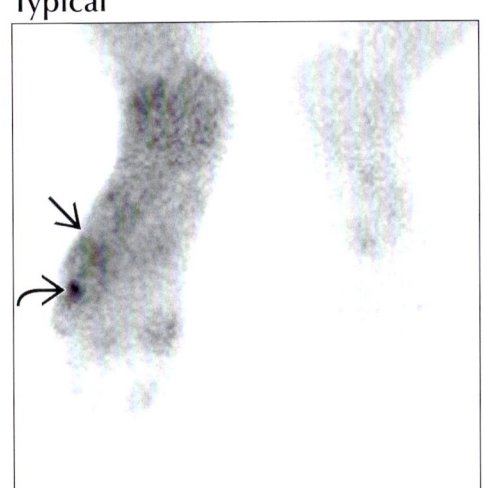

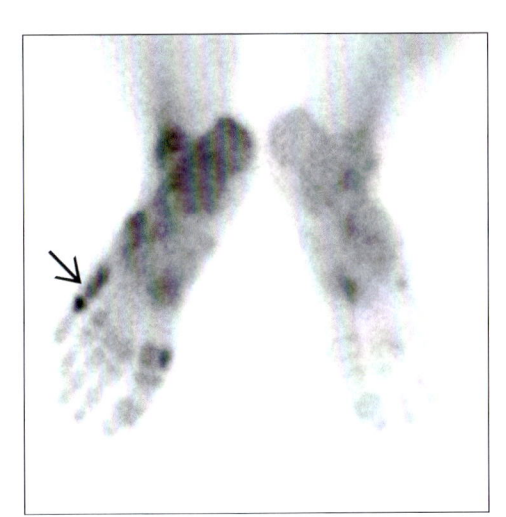

(Left) Plantar equilibrium blood pool image in same patient shows diffuse hyperemia ➡ and focal activity at 5th metatarsal ➡. See next image. **(Right)** Plantar delayed bone scan shows focal uptake along 5th metatarsal head and shaft ➡, consistent with osteomyelitis. See next image.

Typical

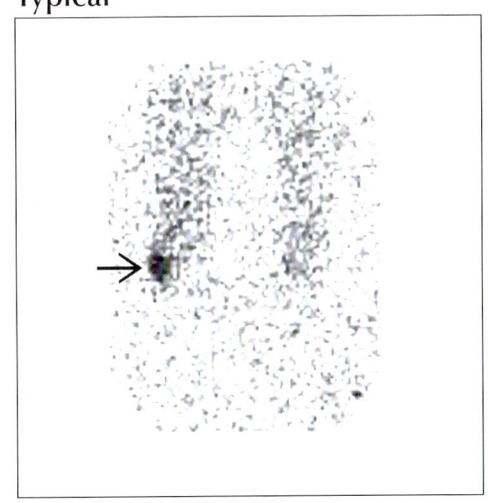

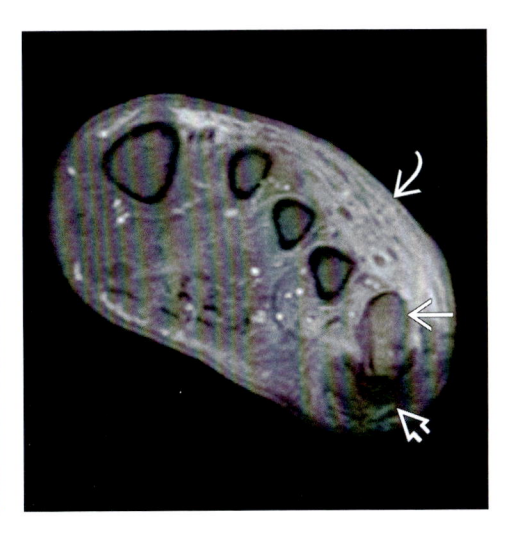

(Left) Labeled leukocyte scintigraphy shows focal WBC localization in region of right 5th metatarsal ➡, confirming diagnosis of osteomyelitis. See next image. **(Right)** T1WI shows 5th metatarsal enhancement ➡ and soft tissue enhancement in adjacent cellulitis ➡, consistent with osteomyelitis. Focal hypointensity represents abscess ➡. (Courtesy P. Wasserman, DO).

OSTEOMYELITIS, PEDIATRIC

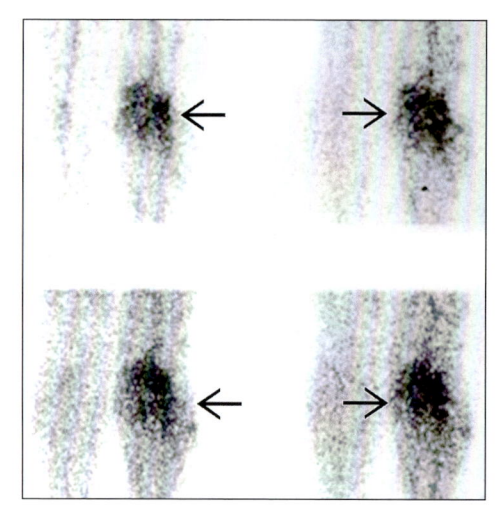

Anterior sequential vascular phase bone scan of a child, shows typical findings of hyperemia surrounding the left knee ➔, secondary to inflammation. See next image.

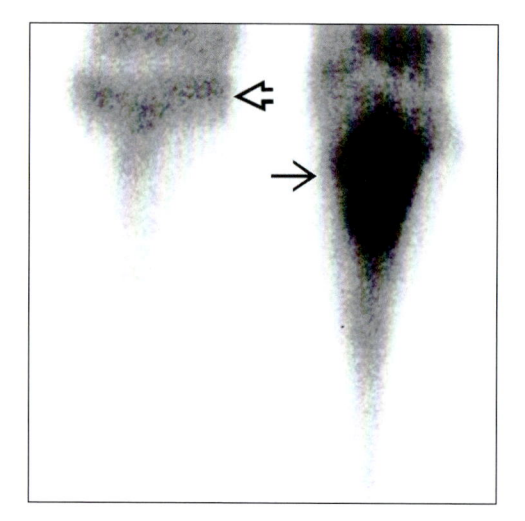

Anterior delayed phase imaging of the same patient as left, shows extensive osteoblastic activity in the proximal left tibia ➔, indicating osteomyelitis. Normal activity in right physis ⇨.

TERMINOLOGY

Abbreviations and Synonyms
- Central osteitis, bacterial osteitis

Definitions
- Infection of bone
- Osteo = bone, myelo = marrow, itis = inflammation

IMAGING FINDINGS

General Features
- Best diagnostic clue
  - MR findings of marrow edema, enhancing/necrotic tissues, subperiosteal abscess
  - Clinical and laboratory findings contributory
    - Needle aspiration allows diagnosis, pathogen identification in < 2/3 of cases
    - Blood cultures allow pathogen identification in 1/3 to 1/2 of cases
  - 3 phase bone scan can have limited sensitivity in pediatric population
    - Should not be relied on to rule out osteomyelitis
  - Lesions can be hyper-, hypo- or isointense to surrounding bone
- Location
  - Usually in long bones: Tibia, femur, humerus
    - < 50% of newborn cases multifocal
  - Foot (especially following puncture injury)
  - Rarely smaller bones, including vertebra (usually older child, mean 7.5 years old), patella, dens, ribs

Nuclear Medicine Findings
- Three-phase Tc-99m MDP bone scan
  - Pediatric osteomyelitis is complex and lesions can show increased, decreased, or similar activity relative to other bony structures
  - Scintigraphy should not play a primary role in acute pediatric musculoskeletal pain cases
  - Widely available, sensitive, but limited specificity
    - Bone scan is true positive in as few as 30% of cases
  - As problem solving tool: Allows whole body evaluation for possible multifocal osteomyelitis

Radiographic Findings
- Conventional X-ray: First study of choice
  - Plain radiographs often initially negative, limited sensitivity early in disease

DDx: Mimics of Pediatric Osteomyelitis on Bone Scan

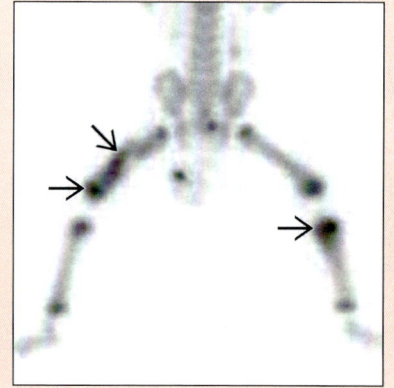

Fractures (NAT) 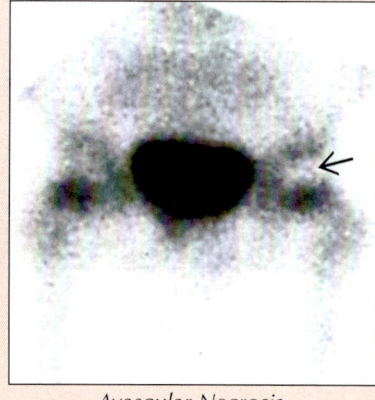 | *Avascular Necrosis* 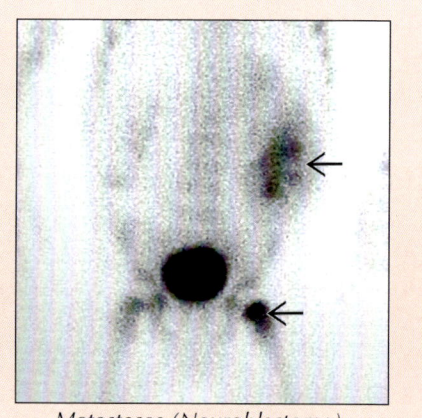 | *Metastases (Neuroblastoma)*

OSTEOMYELITIS, PEDIATRIC

Key Facts

Imaging Findings
- Usually in long bones: Tibia, femur, humerus
- Conventional X-ray: First study of choice
- X-rays useful in excluding other underlying conditions including fracture, dislocation, tumor
- CT more sensitive than X-ray, less sensitive than MR
- MR for targeted scanning, occasionally utilized in whole body evaluation
- MR sensitivity ~ 95%
- Scintigraphy should not play a primary role in acute pediatric musculoskeletal pain cases
- Bone scan is true positive in as few as 30% of cases
- As problem solving tool: Allows whole body evaluation for possible multifocal osteomyelitis

Top Differential Diagnoses
- Trauma, Fracture, Joint Derangement
- Septic Arthritis
- Toxic Synovitis
- Cellulitis
- Neoplasm
- Rheumatologic Disease
- Avascular Necrosis, Metabolic Bone Disease

Clinical Issues
- Localized, constant pain; fever; erythema
- Limp, guarding, refusal to bear weight
- Positive bone or blood cultures
- Age: Most common is < 5 years
- Gender: Male predominant
- Up to 10% recur, may develop chronic osteomyelitis
- Growth plate disturbance, bone growth delay, joint destruction and chronic arthritis more common with delayed diagnosis, inadequate therapy

---

  - Early findings include soft tissue swelling, edema/fluid, obliteration of fat planes
  - Later findings of bone destruction: Erosion, demineralization, periosteal reaction
  - Inexpensive, easily acquired
  - X-rays useful in excluding other underlying conditions including fracture, dislocation, tumor

CT Findings
- Similar constellation of manifestations as plain radiographs: Soft tissue swelling, edema/fluid, bony demineralization, periosteal reaction
- CT more sensitive than X-ray, less sensitive than MR
  - However, easier to acquire, less time consuming than MR

MR Findings
- Marrow edema: T1 hypointense, T2 hyperintense
- Contrast-enhancing tissues represent vascular components of involved parenchyma
  - Nonenhancing tissues indicate devitalized parenchyma and necrotic fluid collections
- Subperiosteal fluid collections/microabscesses
- MR for targeted scanning, occasionally utilized in whole body evaluation
  - MR sensitivity ~ 95%
  - Nonspecific in cases of underlying bony abnormality such as trauma/arthropathy

Ultrasonographic Findings
- Edema, fluid collection, abscess, cortical disruption
- Ultrasound may be useful, particularly in newborns/infants where high frequency transducers have excellent sonic access

Imaging Recommendations
- Protocol advice
  - Whole body 3 phase bone scintigraphy
    - Tc-99m MDP dose: Adjust to as low as 2 mCi, (74 MBq), according to pediatric patients dosing algorithms, i.e., ages < 12 y use Webster's rule: (Age + 1/Age + 7) x Adult dose (~ 30 mCi)
    - Hydrate patient prior to procedure to promote soft tissue washout, improves target to background
    - Inject in extremity away from sites of interest to prevent false positives secondary to endovascular pooling, venous valvular adherence
    - Targeted angiographic and blood pool images
    - Image at 3-4 hrs (up to 24 hrs in difficult cases)
    - Best target to background ratio at 6-12 hours
    - Place detector as close as possible to subject, especially with smaller patients
    - Empty bladder prior to imaging, Foley catheter may be useful, sit on detector views if bladder activity remains an issue
    - Protect camera from urine contamination
    - Spot images: ~ 3 minutes each (5-600 k counts)
    - Whole body scan: Table advance at 10 cm/min
    - Pinhole images critical for joints with companion views of asymptomatic side
    - SPECT adds accuracy, preferably with CT or MR fusion
    - May need sedation for optimal imaging
- Additional nuclear medicine imaging options
  - In 111 white blood cell (WBC) scan has limited utility in pediatric population
    - High splenic dosimetry (can be > 30 rads)
  - Tc 99m HMPAO WBC scan preferred
    - Vascular phase, image at 4 hours and 24 h
    - Especially in vertebral osteomyelitis, WBC scan can show focal photopenia
    - If violated bone, can use Tc-99m sulfur colloid marrow map to exclude normal marrow

DIFFERENTIAL DIAGNOSIS

Trauma, Fracture, Joint Derangement
- Including nonaccidental trauma
- Bone scan may be insensitive in flat bones, metaphyses

Septic Arthritis
- Joint effusion with distension of capsule

OSTEOMYELITIS, PEDIATRIC

- Bright on T2WI MR; fluid density on CT or conventional radiography
- Bone scan: May be cold early, hot later
- May be associated with joint subluxation
- Loss of articular cartilage, subsequent cortical erosions

Toxic Synovitis
- Self-limited synovitis of hip, unilateral
- More common than septic hip, Legg-Calve-Perthes or slipped capital femoral epiphyses
- M > F, low grade temp (< 101° F), otherwise healthy
- Diagnosis of exclusion

Cellulitis
- Positive on vascular phase; negative on delayed phase of three-phase bone scan
- Mimics false negative osteomyelitis on bone scan

Neoplasm
- Neuroblastoma, osteosarcoma, Ewing sarcoma, acute myelocytic/leukocytic leukemia

Rheumatologic Disease
- Joint space narrowing, subchondral cysts (particularly hands, wrists, feet)
- Elevated ESR, HLA-B27, IgA /IgM rheumatoid factor

Thrombophlebitis
- May coexist with osteomyelitis in up to 30% of cases

Avascular Necrosis, Metabolic Bone Disease
- Sickle cell disease, bone infarct, vaso-occlusive crises
  - Diffuse increased osteoblastic remodeling secondary to marrow expansion, especially epiphyseal
  - Infarcts acutely photopenic/normal with increased healing osteoblastic activity 2-10 days later
- Avascular necrosis: Legg-Calve-Perthe, sickle cell disease, renal failure, steroids
  - Cold (early) to hot (late) on bone scan

Chronic Recurrent Multifocal Osteomyelitis
- Scattered lytic/sclerotic long bone, clavicular lesions
- Intermittently recurrent
- Glucocorticoid and anti-inflammatory treatments; antibiotic therapies ineffective

PATHOLOGY

General Features
- Etiology
  - Usually hematogenous spread in children
    - Penetrating trauma, local wound extension
  - Classically Staph A, Strep pneumonia/pyogenes
    - Newborns: Staph A, group B Strep, Gram-enteric bacteria (E. coli, Proteus mirabilis, Enterobacter)
    - Penetrating injury through shoe: Pseudomonas A
    - Fungus, mycobacteria (including TB) also occur
- Associated abnormalities
  - Immunosuppression: Diabetes mellitus, sickle cell
  - Increased risk of DVT, usually local
  - Disseminated infection
  - Increased risk for septic arthritis, especially neonates

Gross Pathologic & Surgical Features
- Intramedullary, cortical, subperiosteal purulence/abscesses: Medullary, superficial, localized or diffuse
- Bone necrosis, demineralization, cortical collapse, formation of sequestra/abscesses

CLINICAL ISSUES

Presentation
- Most common signs/symptoms
  - Localized, constant pain; fever; erythema
  - Limp, guarding, refusal to bear weight
  - Positive bone or blood cultures
- Other signs/symptoms
  - Joint pain, however ↓ ROM may also accompany soft tissue swelling
  - Elevated ESR, procalcitonin, C-reactive protein
    - Leukocytosis present in < 50%, may be normal especially chronic osteomyelitis
  - Draining wound/fistula indicates chronic infection

Demographics
- Age: Most common is < 5 years
- Gender: Male predominant

Natural History & Prognosis
- Up to 10% recur, may develop chronic osteomyelitis
- Growth plate disturbance, bone growth delay, joint destruction and chronic arthritis more common with delayed diagnosis, inadequate therapy

Treatment
- Aspiration prior to antibiotic initiation
- Antibiotic therapy, usually 4-8 weeks, initially IV
- Surgical resection as necessary
  - Poor vascular supplies limit antibiotic delivery
- Adjuvant hyperbaric oxygen therapy
- Imaging useful to evaluate treatment response

DIAGNOSTIC CHECKLIST

Image Interpretation Pearls
- Bone destruction and inflammatory changes are hallmarks of osteomyelitis

SELECTED REFERENCES

1. Crary SE et al: Venous thrombosis and thromboembolism in children with osteomyelitis. J Pediatr. 149(4):537-41, 2006
2. Dimaala J et al: Odontoid osteomyelitis masquerading as a C2 fracture in an 18-month-old male with torticollis: CT and MRI features. Emerg Radiol. 12(5):234-6, 2006
3. Mellado Santos JM: Diagnostic imaging of pediatric hematogenous osteomyelitis: lessons learned from a multi-modality approach. Eur Radiol. 16(9):2109-19, 2006
4. Pineda C et al: Imaging of osteomyelitis: current concepts. Infect Dis Clin North Am. 20(4):789-825, 2006
5. Frank G et al: Musculoskeletal infections in children. Pediatr Clin North Am. 52(4):1083-106, ix, 2005
6. Stott NS: Review article: Paediatric bone and joint infection. J Orthop Surg (Hong Kong). 9(1):83-90, 2001

OSTEOMYELITIS, PEDIATRIC

IMAGE GALLERY

Typical

Typical

Typical

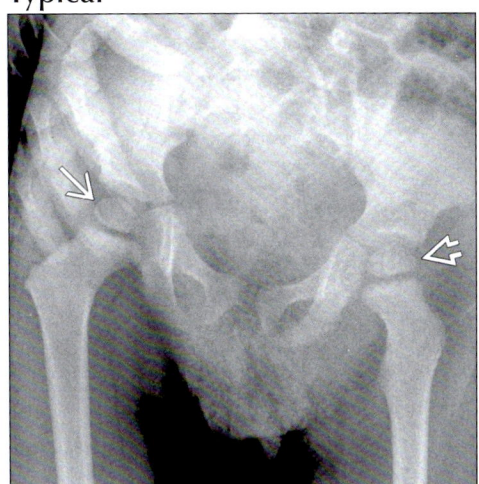

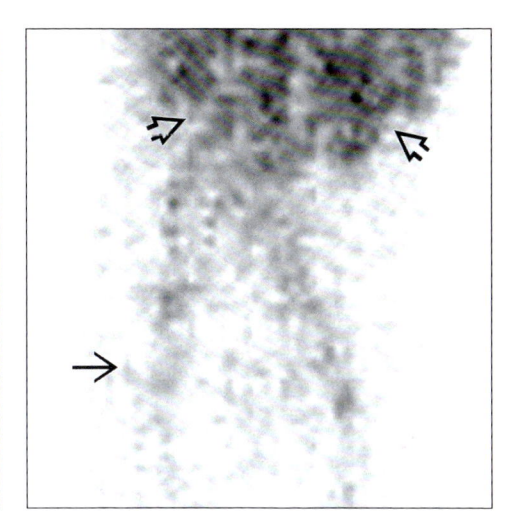

(Left) Anteroposterior radiograph shows demineralization of right femoral epiphyses ➡ in patient with right hip pain, clinical concern for osteomyelitis. Normal left femoral epiphysis ➡. See next 3 images. *(Right)* Anterior Tc-99m MDP angiographic phase image in the same patient as left shows trace hyperemia over the right hip ➡. Normal visceral ➡ activity. See next image.

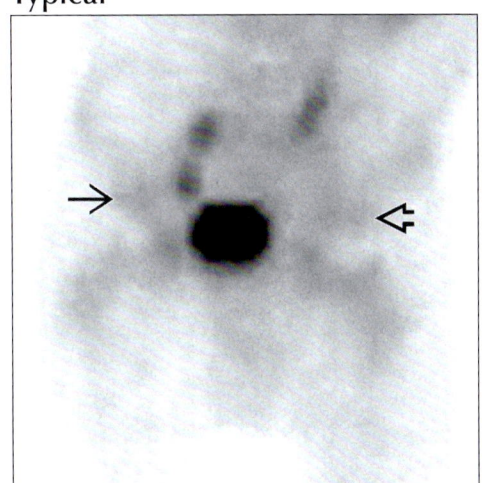

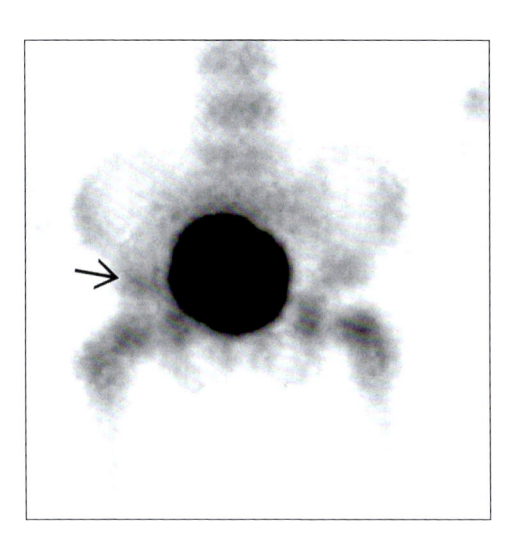

(Left) Anterior blood pool phase bone scan in the same patient as previous shows faintly increased tracer in right acetabulum ➡ when compared to the left ➡, nonspecific. See next image. *(Right)* Anterior delayed phase bone scan in the same patient as left, shows minimal increased tracer in right femoral head ➡. Ultimate diagnosis: Osteomyelitis and septic hip. Illustrates insensitivity of bone scan.

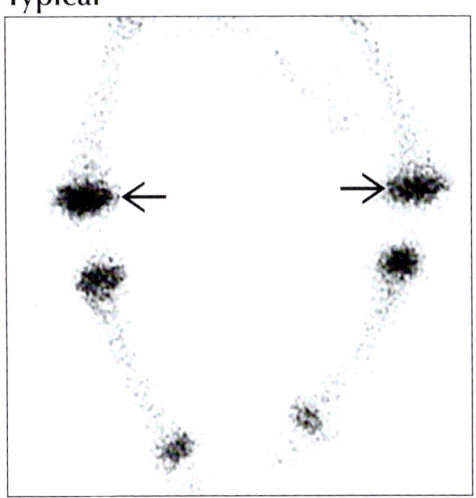

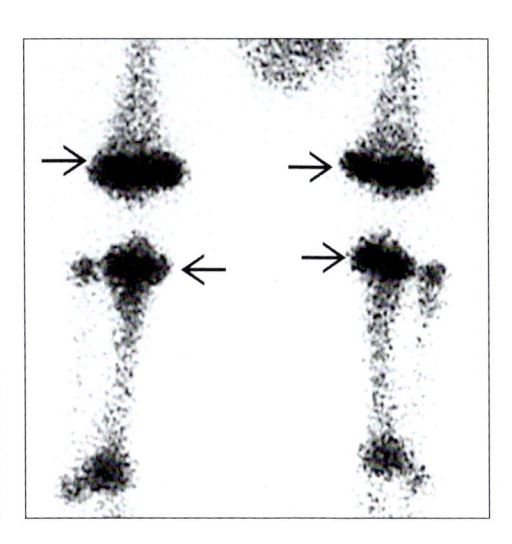

(Left) Anterior delayed phase bone scan shows external rotation of legs ➡, with resulting superimposition of tibias and fibulas, which limits evaluation in a pediatric patient with knee pain. See next image. *(Right)* Anterior bone scan in the same patient as left shows correct positioning, revealing normal symmetric femoral, tibial and fibular growth plate activity ➡.

OSTEOMYELITIS, PEDIATRIC

Typical

(Left) Anterior delayed phase bone scan shows externally rotated knees and lower extremities in a patient with right knee pain. Note decreased right ankle/foot activity ➡ secondary to disuse. See next image. *(Right)* Anterior pinhole views in the same patient as previous shows increased tracer activity at medial right femoral epiphysis ➡, consistent with osteomyelitis. Illustrates importance of bilateral pinhole views.

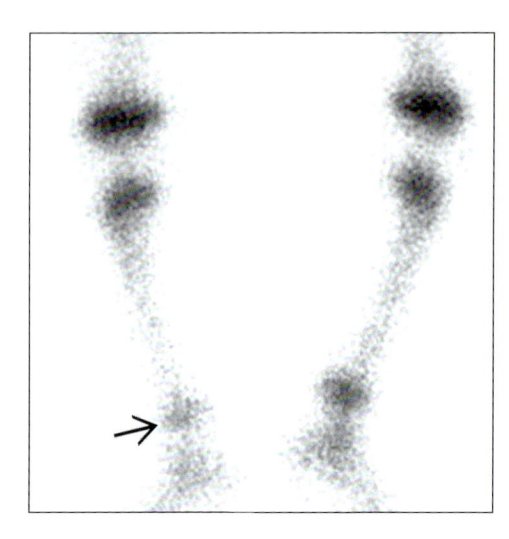

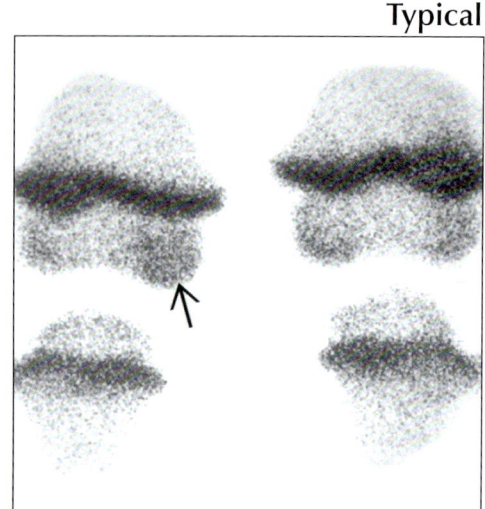

Typical

(Left) Anterior bone scan Tc-99m MDP bone phase imaging shows osteomyelitis with faintly increased tracer accumulation in the right humeral diaphysis ➡. See next image. (Courtesy C. Benton, MD). *(Right)* Anterior T1 contrast-enhanced, fat-suppressed MR of the right humerus in the same patient as left, shows enhancement of the periosteum ➡ and marrow ➡. (Courtesy C. Benton, MD).

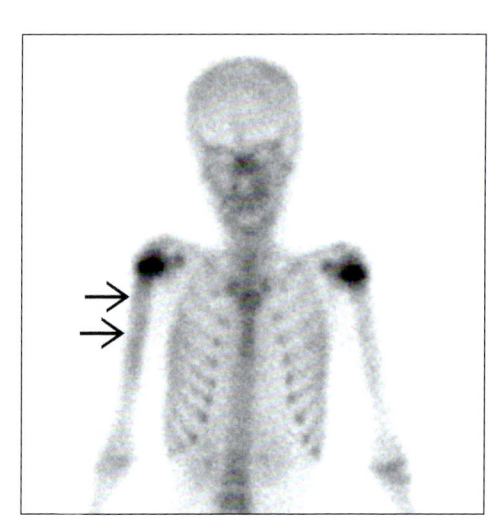

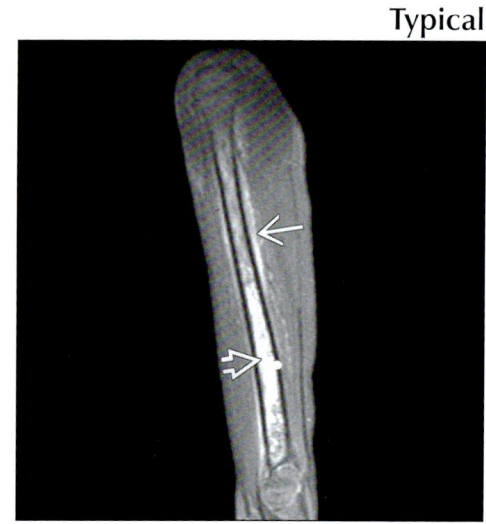

Typical

(Left) Anterior bone scan shows increased tracer in the right femoral head and acetabulum ➡, in a pediatric patient with new onset of limp and right hip pain. Normal left hip ➡. See next image. *(Right)* Axial T2WI MR of the same patient as left, shows increased signal within the right femoral head ➡, adjacent medial acetabulum ➡, and lateral joint space ➡. See next image.

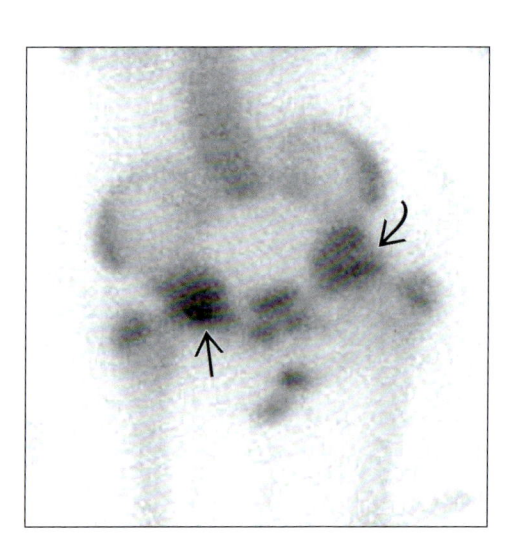

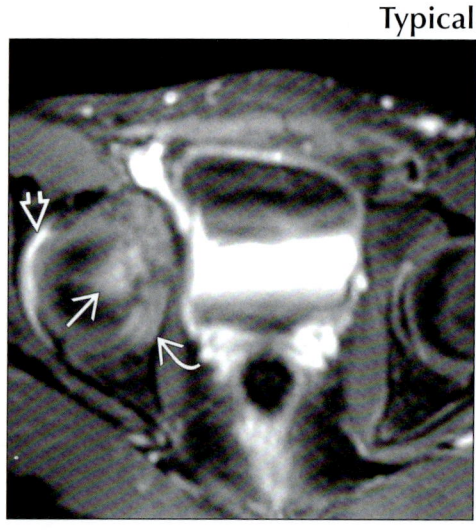

OSTEOMYELITIS, PEDIATRIC

Typical

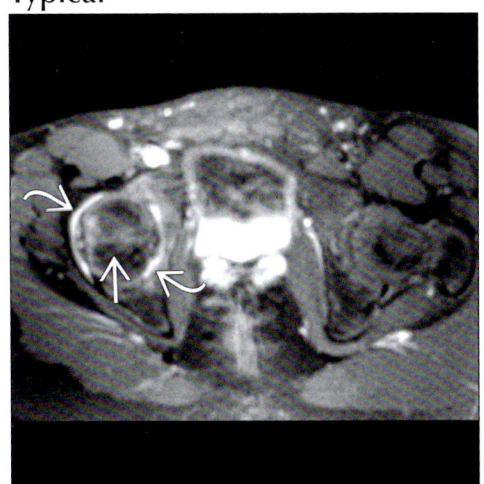

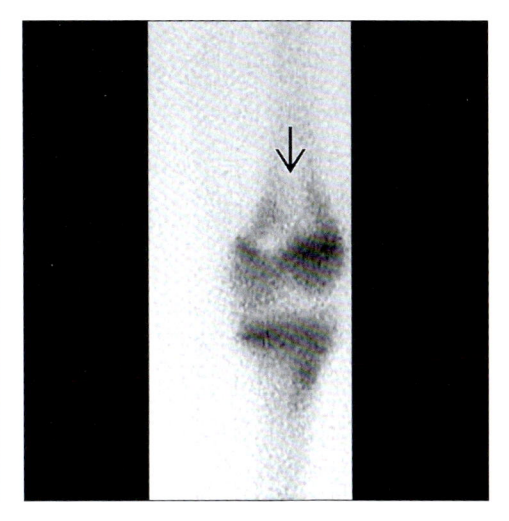

(Left) Axial T2WI MR in the same patient as left, shows further right femoral head marrow edema ➔ and joint fluid ➔, indicating osteomyelitis and septic arthritis of right hip. *(Right)* Anterior bone scan shows photopenic region in distal left femoral diaphysis and diametaphysis ➔, demonstrating osteomyelitis presenting as a "cold" defect.

Typical

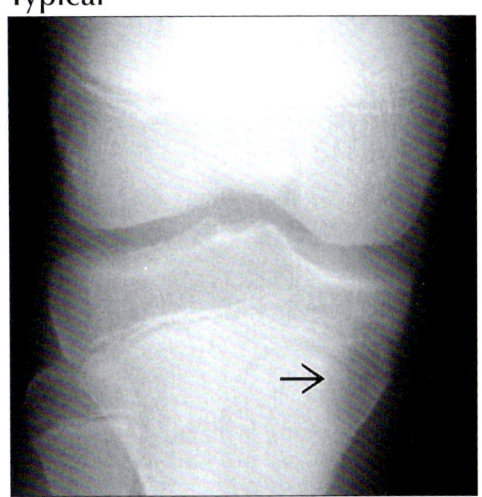

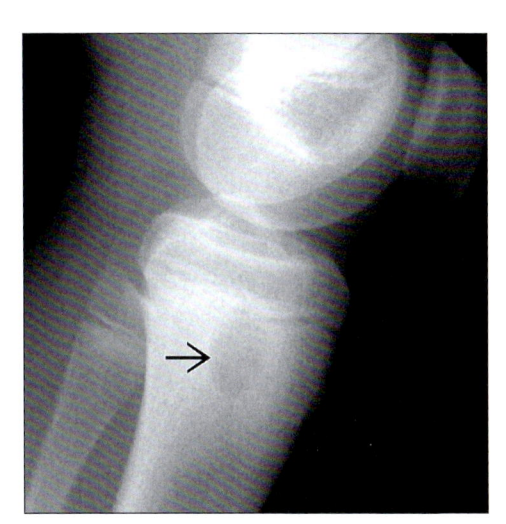

(Left) Anterior posterior radiograph shows lucent demineralization of the proximal medial metaphysis ➔. Same as next 3 images. (Courtesy C. Anton, MD). *(Right)* Lateral radiograph of the same patient as previous, shows lytic lesion ➔. Brodie abscess (subacute osteomyelitis) was found at surgery. (Courtesy C. Anton, MD).

Typical

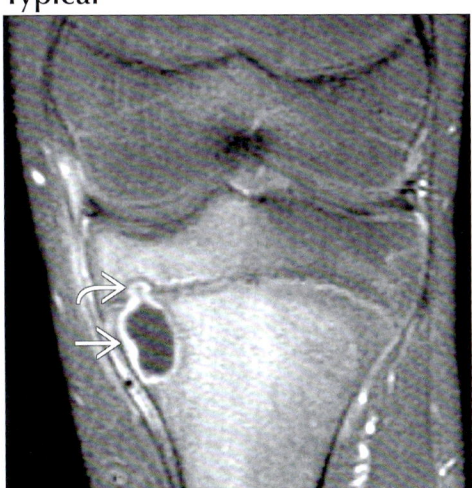

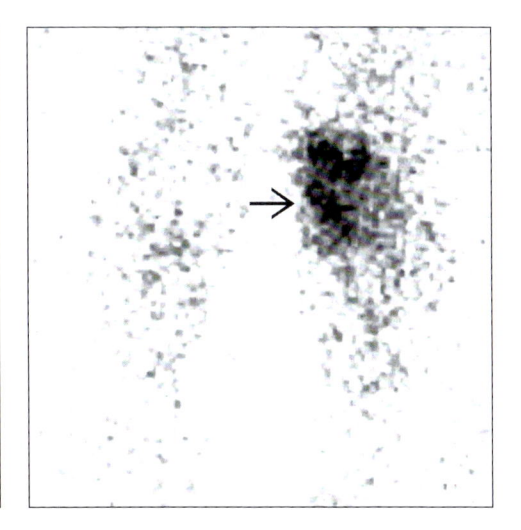

(Left) Coronal T2 C+ MR in the same patient as previous shows proximal tibial metaphyseal lesion showing marginal enhancement ➔ perforating into epiphysis ➔. (Courtesy C. Anton, MD). *(Right)* Anterior In-111 WBC scan in same patient as previous, shows increased tracer accumulation about the proximal tibia and knee ➔ in region of subacute osteomyelitis.

HYPERPARATHYROIDISM

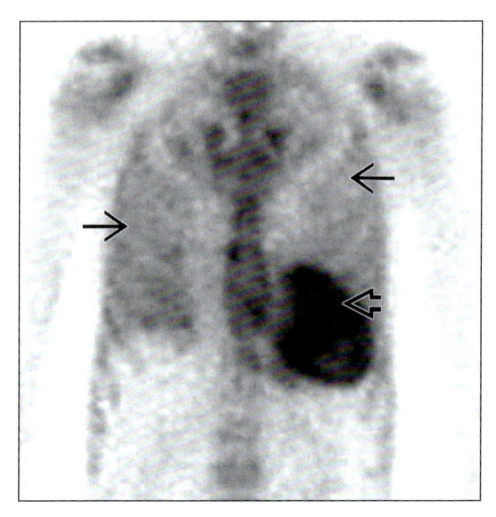

Anterior bone scan shows uptake in lungs ➡ and heart ➡ due to soft tissue calcification in a patient with primary HPT.

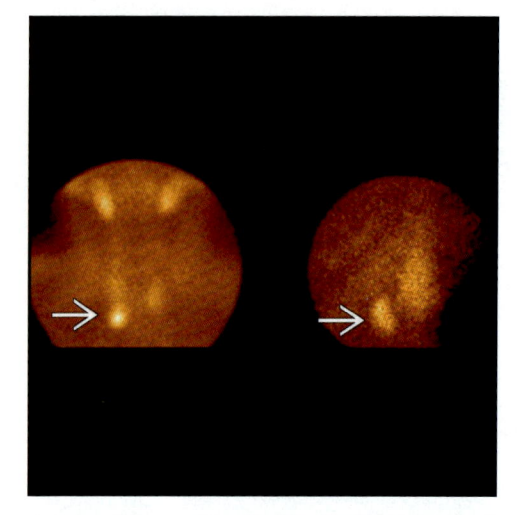

Anterior (left panel) and right lateral (right panel) Tc-99m MIBI scan of the neck at 90 min post injection shows parathyroid adenoma ➡ posterior to the inferior aspect of the right thyroid lobe.

TERMINOLOGY

Abbreviations and Synonyms
- Hyperparathyroidism (HPT)

Definitions
- Primary HPT
  - Over-production of parathyroid hormone (PTH) by parathyroid adenoma (80%), hyperplasia (20%), carcinoma (rare)
    - Hypercalcemia, hypophosphatemia results
- Secondary HPT (renal osteodystrophy)
  - Hypersecretion of PTH by hyperplastic parathyroid glands due to end-organ resistance to the hormone
- Tertiary HPT
  - Long-standing secondary HPT ⇒ autonomous parathyroid function/adenoma

IMAGING FINDINGS

General Features
- Best diagnostic clue
  - Clinical diagnosis
    - History: ± Renal failure
    - Symptoms: Moans, groans, stones, bones
    - Laboratory values: Hypercalcemia, elevated parathyroid hormone
  - Radiography: Effects of osteoclastic resorption of bone
    - Subperiosteal resorption (lacy cortical thinning) classically at radial side of middle phalanges of index, middle fingers
    - Brown tumors: Microfracture ⇒ hemorrhage, macrophages, fibrous replacement of bone
    - Pathologic fractures
  - Bone scan
    - Superscan (axial and appendicular skeleton)
    - Increased activity in brown tumors
    - Organ/soft tissue uptake
  - Tc-99m sestamibi (MIBI) scintigraphy
    - Used to localize parathyroid adenoma in patients with primary HPT
    - Classically, focal increased activity in expected region of parathyroid gland(s) that persists after thyroid washout

DDx: Mimics of HPT on Bone Scan

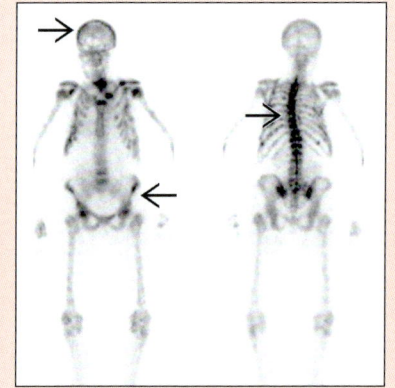

Diffuse Metastatic Disease

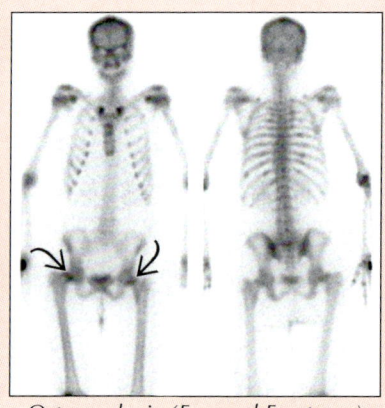

Osteomalacia (Femoral Fractures)

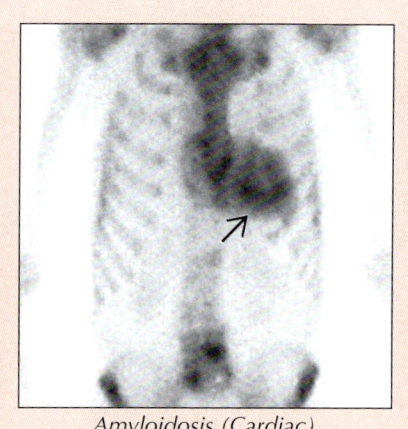

Amyloidosis (Cardiac)

HYPERPARATHYROIDISM

Key Facts

Terminology
- Primary HPT
- Secondary HPT (renal osteodystrophy)
- Tertiary HPT

Imaging Findings
- Superscan: Absent renal, soft tissue activity; diffusely ↑ uptake in axial and appendicular skeleton (vs. axial predominance with metastatic disease)
- Brown tumors: Increased activity in expansile bone lesion in patient with HPT
- Soft tissue uptake on bone scan: Lung, stomach, kidneys, heart, pancreas due to soft tissue calcification

Top Differential Diagnoses
- Malignancy
- Osteomalacia
- Osteoporosis
- Other Nonosseous Uptake on Bone Scan

Clinical Issues
- Usually asymptomatic: Suspect in patients with hypercalcemia on routine blood chemistry analysis
- In outpatients, 1° HPT is most common cause of hypercalcemia
- In inpatients, malignancy is most common cause of hypercalcemia (1° HPT is second)

Diagnostic Checklist
- Differential diagnosis for superscan, soft tissue uptake on bone scan includes HPT
- Consider HPT in patient with sites of focal increased bone activity (brown tumors) and superscan

Nuclear Medicine Findings
- Bone Scan
  - Superscan: Absent renal, soft tissue activity; diffusely ↑ uptake in axial and appendicular skeleton (vs. axial predominance with metastatic disease)
  - Brown tumors: Increased activity in expansile bone lesion in patient with HPT
  - Soft tissue uptake on bone scan: Lung, stomach, kidneys, heart, pancreas due to soft tissue calcification
- Tc-99m MIBI Scintigraphy
  - Primary HPT: Focal increased activity in parathyroid adenoma that persists after thyroid washout
    - Early anterior images: Thyroid and parathyroid adenoma evident
    - Late anterior images: Parathyroid adenoma retains tracer; however, up to 40% of parathyroid adenomas washout concurrently with thyroid
    - Lateral early and late images help localize adenoma in anteroposterior plane, in relation to thyroid gland
    - SPECT: Useful to localize adenoma in three dimensions, localize ectopic parathyroid adenomas

Radiographic Findings
- Subperiosteal resorption (lacy cortical thinning)
  - Classically at radial side of middle phalanges of index, middle fingers
  - High specificity for hyperparathyroidism, practically diagnostic
- Tapering resorption of distal clavicles
- Femoral calcar, medial tibial plateau, rib rarefaction
- Tuft resorption, acro-osteolysis
- Brown tumor (osteitis fibrosa cystica)
  - Facial bones (esp. mandible), long bones, ribs
- Salt and pepper calvarium
- Long bone bowing
- Vertebral insufficiency fractures
- Resorption at SI joints and symphysis pubis
- Reactive osteoblastic sclerosis of vertebral endplates ("rugger jersey")
  - More common in 2° HPT

Imaging Recommendations
- Best imaging tool
  - Radiography: 21-35% sensitive
    - Radiographs of hands most commonly utilized imaging modality for evaluation/surveillance
    - Subperiosteal resorption, (lacy cortical thinning), has high specificity, practically diagnostic
  - Bone scintigraphy: 20-50% sensitive to stigmata of hyperparathyroidism
    - Allows whole body imaging
  - Tc-99m MIBI scintigraphy
    - Pre-operative localization of parathyroid adenoma in patients with primary HPT
    - Allows minimally invasive surgery for resection of parathyroid adenoma

DIFFERENTIAL DIAGNOSIS

Malignancy
- Bone metastases
  - Prostate, breast, lung, bladder cancer; lymphoma, leukemia
  - Superscan: Uptake tends to spare distal extremities, usually not as uniform as HPT
- Hypertrophic pulmonary osteoarthropathy
  - Classically seen in lung cancer; however, possible with many cancers
- Paraneoplastic syndrome, usually producing parathormone related protein (PTHrP)
  - Bronchogenic carcinoma, neuroectodermal tumor, renal cell carcinoma
  - Hypercalcemia in cancer patients usually result of PTHrP, not metastases themselves

Osteomalacia
- Normal collagen matrix with absence of osteoid mineralization
  - Insufficient calcium, phosphorus or both
  - Often hot at rib ends, scattered fractures, generalized increased uptake on bone scan

HYPERPARATHYROIDISM

Osteoporosis
- Deficit of otherwise normal bone secondary to Increased turnover
- No subperiosteal resorption or brown tumors

Other Nonosseous Uptake on Bone Scan
- Tumor, metastases, pleural effusion, autoinfarcted spleen, amyloidosis, calcific pericarditis, myositis ossificans, free pertechnetate (gastric, thyroid), etc.

PATHOLOGY

General Features
- Etiology
  - Primary HPT
    - Parathyroid adenoma(s) in ~ 80%
    - Parathyroid hyperplasia in ~ 20%
    - Parathyroid carcinoma rare
  - Secondary HPT
    - Usually in setting of renal failure, abnormal phosphate metabolism (hyperphosphatemia), ↓ intestinal calcium/vitamin D absorption
    - Ineffective PTH action at end organ ⇒ hyperparathyroidism without hypercalcemia
  - Tertiary HPT
    - Autonomous parathyroid function
    - Usually in setting of renal failure
    - History of chronic hypocalcemia/chronic parathyroid stimulation, usually after suffering from chronic 2° hyperparathyroidism
    - Loss of normal feedback control loop, parathyroid glands become insensitive to blood PTH levels
- Epidemiology
  - Adult population affected
    - ~ 1:500 women/yr
    - ~ 1:2,000 men/yr
- Associated abnormalities
  - Multiple endocrine neoplasia (MEN) syndromes
    - Type I (Wermer syndrome)
    - Type IIA (Sipple disease)

Microscopic Features
- Increased mitochondria in oxyphil cells of adenomatous parathyroid glands

CLINICAL ISSUES

Presentation
- Most common signs/symptoms
  - Usually asymptomatic: Suspect in patients with hypercalcemia on routine blood chemistry analysis
    - In outpatients, 1° HPT is most common cause of hypercalcemia
    - In inpatients, malignancy is most common cause of hypercalcemia (1° HPT is second)
    - 1°, 3° HPT associated with hypercalcemia
    - 2° HPT associated with hypocalcemia
  - Moans, groans, stones and bones
    - Psychic moans: Neuropsychiatric symptoms (e.g., memory loss, depression)
    - Abdominal groans: Nausea, vomiting, dyspepsia, constipation
    - Stones: Nephrolithiasis/renal colic
    - Bones: Bone pain, pathologic fracture
- Other signs/symptoms
  - Gastric ulcers
  - Pancreatitis
  - Muscular weakness/hypotonicity

Demographics
- Age
  - 40-60 yrs, average 55 yrs at diagnosis
    - Consider MEN, esp. in patients < 30 yrs
- Gender: M:F ~ 1:4

Natural History & Prognosis
- Bone scan and radiography after definitive therapy demonstrate restorative mineralization of bone matrix which continues for 6-12 months or longer

Treatment
- Resection of adenomatous gland(s) in 1° HPT and refractory 3° HPT
  - Successful in > 90% when performed by an experienced team
  - Cervical exploration being replaced by microinvasive, focally targeted approaches after localization (e.g., with Tc-99m MIBI scintigraphy)
- Medical therapy: Calcitriol (a metabolite of vitamin D) may blunt PTH release in 2° or 3° HPT associated with chronic renal failure

DIAGNOSTIC CHECKLIST

Consider
- Tc-99m MIBI scintigraphy for optimal pre-operative localization of parathyroid adenoma in patients with primary HPT

Image Interpretation Pearls
- Differential diagnosis for superscan, soft tissue uptake on bone scan includes HPT
- Consider HPT in patient with sites of focal increased bone activity (brown tumors) and superscan

SELECTED REFERENCES

1. Fleischer J et al: Oxyphil parathyroid adenoma: a malignant presentation of a benign disease. J Clin Endocrinol Metab. 89(12):5948-51, 2004
2. Manaster BJ et al: The Requisites, Musculoskeletal Imaging, Second Ed. Mosby, Inc. 401-4, 2002
3. Demirkol MO et al: Intense skeletal lesions in a patient with primary hyperparathyroid disease. Clin Nucl Med. 26(8):727-8, 2001
4. Morrone LF et al: Maxillary brown tumor in secondary hyperparathyroidism requiring urgent parathyroidectomy. J Nephrol. 14(5):415-9, 2001
5. Fouda MA: Primary hyperparathyroidism: King Khalid University Hospital Experience. Ann Saudi Med. 19(2):110-5, 1999
6. Huraib S et al: Long-term effect of intravenous calcitriol on the treatment of severe hyperparathyroidism, parathyroid gland mass and bone mineral density in haemodialysis patients. Am J Nephrol. 17(2):118-23, 1997

HYPERPARATHYROIDISM

IMAGE GALLERY

Typical

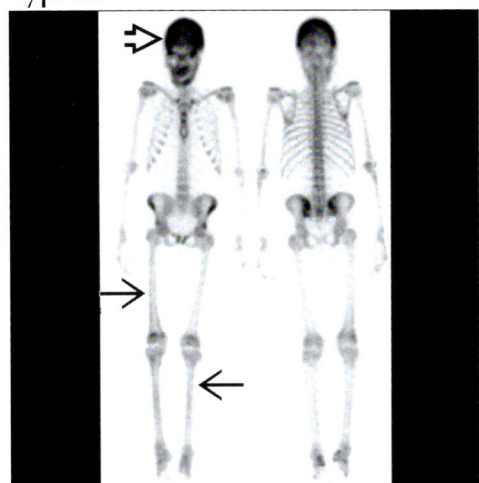

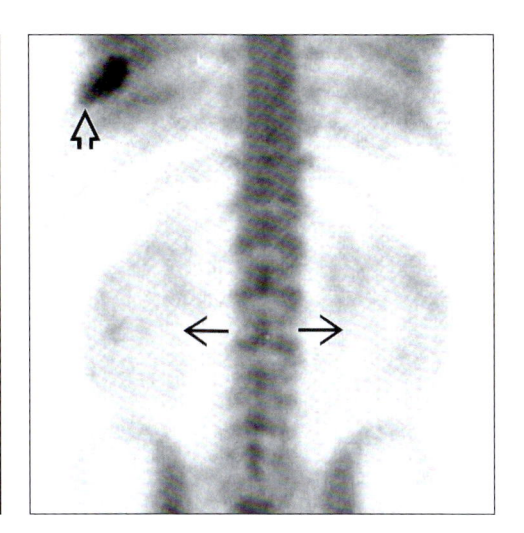

(**Left**) Anterior and posterior bone scan shows superscan, characterized by diffusely increased uptake in calvarium ⊳, axial and appendicular skeleton → with absent soft tissue and renal activity, typical of secondary HPT. (**Right**) Posterior bone scan shows increased uptake in a posterior left rib ⊳ in a patient with HPT. Note polycystic kidneys without normal tracer excretion in collecting systems → due to renal failure. See next image.

Typical

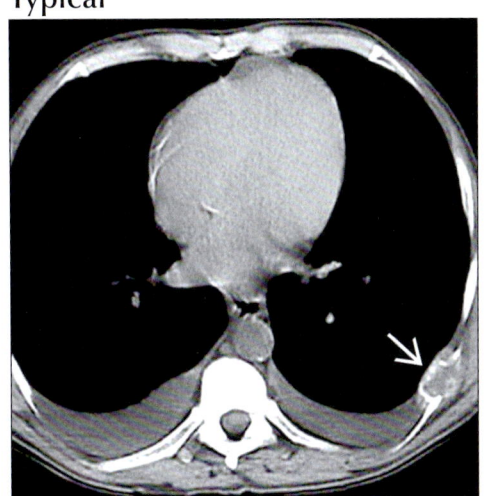

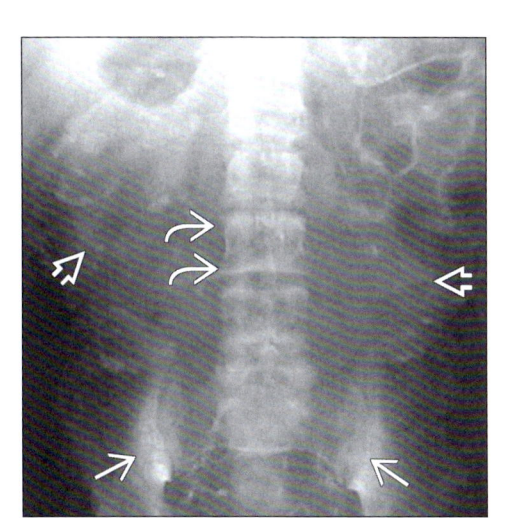

(**Left**) Axial NECT in the same patient as previous image shows expansile, peripherally sclerotic rib lesion →, consistent with ossifying brown tumor of HPT. (**Right**) Anterior posterior radiograph of lumbar spine shows coarse renal calcifications in polycystic kidneys →, rugger jersey spine →, and subchondral iliac sclerosis/resorption → due to secondary HPT.

Typical

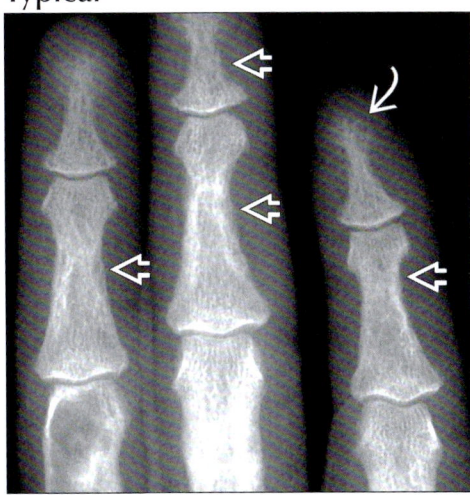

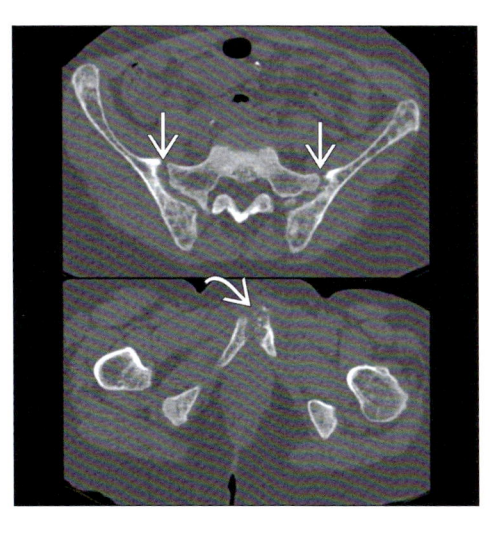

(**Left**) Posteroanterior radiograph shows subperiosteal resorption at the radial aspect of middle and distal phalanges ⊳, prominent tuft resorption →. (Courtesy B. Manaster, MD). (**Right**) Axial CT shows mixed sclerotic/lucent pattern of HPT with subcondral resportion of SIA → and pubic symphysis →.

OSTEOMALACIA

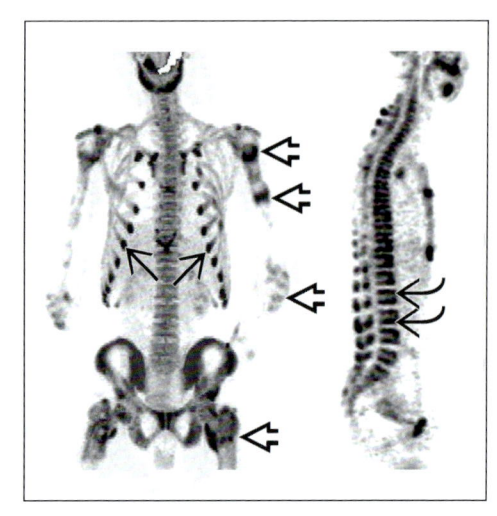

FDG PET shows findings of renal osteodystrophy (osteomalacia & hyperparathyroidism): ↑ FDG uptake at anterior rib ends ➡, vertebral endplates ➡, fractures & Looser zones ➡. (Courtesy J. Hoffman, MD).

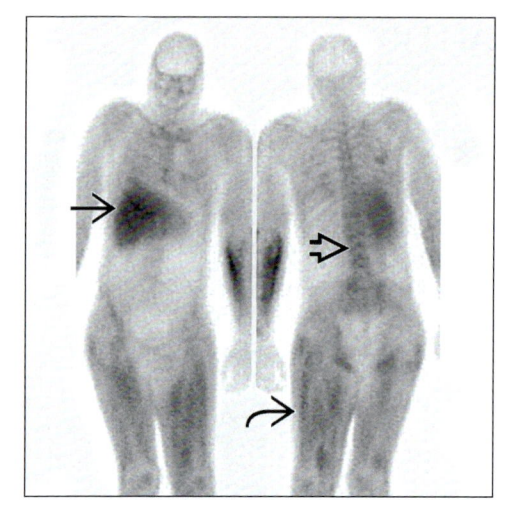

Ant and post Tc-99m MDP bone scan shows findings of osteomalacia from severe aluminum toxicity (2° long term hemodialysis + aluminum antacids): Poor bone uptake ➡, diffuse soft tissue ➡ and liver ➡ uptake.

TERMINOLOGY

Abbreviations and Synonyms
- Osteomalacia: "Soft bones"

Definitions
- Osteomalacia: Incomplete mineralization of normal osteoid following closure of growth plates
  - Osteomalacia: Typically involves trabecular & cortical bone
- Rickets: Incomplete mineralization of normal osteoid in immature skeleton
  - Rickets: Manifestation of osteomalacia in children
  - Rickets: Primarily involves growth plates, metaphyseal zones of provisional calcification
- Renal osteodystrophy: Combined features of osteomalacia, secondary hyperparathyroidism and osteoporosis

IMAGING FINDINGS

General Features
- Best diagnostic clue
  - Plain film, CT: Smudgy, coarsened, demineralized bone; Looser zones, insufficiency fractures
  - Bone scan: Accentuation of anterior ends of all ribs in an adult; uptake in fractures, Looser zones
- Location
  - Most common location for Looser zones
    - Medial aspect of proximal femurs
    - Pubic bones
    - Dorsal aspect of proximal ulnae
    - Distal scapulae & ribs

Nuclear Medicine Findings
- Bone scan (Tc-99m diphosphonate)
  - Increased bone scan uptake at all anterior rib ends in adult: Similar to normal pediatric pattern
  - Focal bone scan uptake: Fractures, Looser zones
  - Bone scan findings of osteomalacia may coexist with bone scan findings of secondary hyperparathyroidism in spectrum of renal osteodystrophy
    - Metastatic calcification: Most typically lungs, stomach, heart (any combination)

DDx: Bone Scan Mimics of Osteomalacia

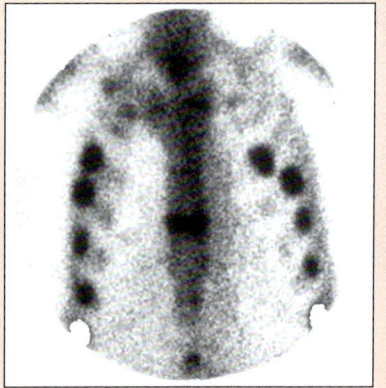

Anterior Rib Fractures (CPR) 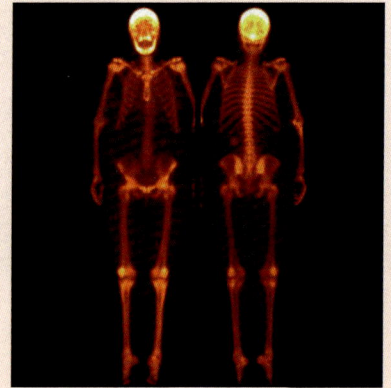   *Hyperparathyroidism* 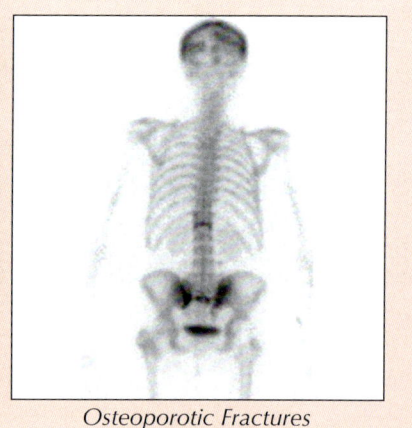   *Osteoporotic Fractures*

OSTEOMALACIA

Key Facts

Terminology
- Osteomalacia: Incomplete mineralization of normal osteoid following closure of growth plates
- Osteomalacia: Typically involves trabecular & cortical bone
- Rickets: Incomplete mineralization of normal osteoid in immature skeleton
- Rickets: Manifestation of osteomalacia in children
- Rickets: Primarily involves growth plates, metaphyseal zones of provisional calcification
- Renal osteodystrophy: Combined features of osteomalacia, secondary hyperparathyroidism and osteoporosis

Imaging Findings
- Plain film, CT: Smudgy, coarsened, demineralized bone; Looser zones, insufficiency fractures
- Bone scan: Accentuation of anterior ends of all ribs in an adult; uptake in fractures, Looser zones
- Bone scan findings of osteomalacia may coexist with bone scan findings of secondary hyperparathyroidism in spectrum of renal osteodystrophy
- Aluminum osteomalacia: ↓ uptake by bones; diffuse ↑ uptake by soft tissues, liver
- FDG PET: May show similar pattern to that on bone scan; may identify tumor in oncogenic osteomalacia

Pathology
- Normal osteoid
- Reduced calcification (especially in new bone)

Diagnostic Checklist
- Osteomalacia may coexist with findings of secondary hyperparathyroidism in renal osteodystrophy

---

  - Superscan pattern of metabolic bone disease: Uniform increased uptake involving all bones, including hands and feet; skull may be particularly "hot"; "striped tie" sternum; absence of renal, bladder, normal soft tissue activity
  - Tumoral calcinosis
 - Rickets: Difficult to diagnose on bone scan due to normal growth plate activity; multiple insufficiency fractures may mimic non-accidental trauma on bone scan
 - Aluminum osteomalacia: ↓ uptake by bones; diffuse ↑ uptake by soft tissues, liver
- FDG PET: May show similar pattern to that on bone scan; may identify tumor in oncogenic osteomalacia

Radiographic Findings
- Most typical radiographic finding: Lucent, smudgy, coarsened trabecula
- Radiographic findings may show nonspecific osteopenia
- Pathologic fractures: Tend to be transverse
- Looser zones
  - Wide linear transverse lucencies (pseudofractures)
    - Perpendicular to cortex of bone
    - Extend incompletely across width of bone
  - Typically along concave aspect of bone
- Rickets
  - Undermineralization of osteoid at growth plates: Frayed metaphyses

MR Findings
- Evaluate soft tissues for ligament rupture
- Non-radiographically apparent fractures

DIFFERENTIAL DIAGNOSIS

Osteoporosis
- Normal mineralization, reduced osteoid
- Radiographically: Lacks coarsened trabecular, smudgy appearance seen with osteomalacia
- Bone scan findings are usually negative until compression fractures occur

Multiple Myeloma
- May mimic osteoporosis
- Multiple "punched out" lytic lesions: May be inapparent or appear as "cold defects" on bone scan
- Often normal bone scan until insufficiency fractures occur

Hyperparathyroidism
- Differs from osteomalacia in that hyperparathyroidism shows proportionate loss of mineral and osteoid matrix

Stress or Fatigue Fractures
- Typical stress fractures are along convex aspect of bone

Mimics of Rickets
- Metaphyseal dysplasia (type Schmid)
  - May mimic rickets radiographically
  - Growth plate widening but mineralization
  - Inborn error of enchondral ossification
  - Laboratory values normal
- Hypophosphatasia
  - May mimic rickets radiographically

Metastatic Disease
- May mimic multiple fractures of osteomalacia

PATHOLOGY

General Features
- Genetics
  - Vitamin D dependent rickets type 1: 1α hydroxylase deficiency
  - X-linked hypophosphatemic rickets (vitamin D resistant rickets): PHEX mutation
  - Autosomal dominant hypophosphatemic rickets: FGF23 mutation
  - Autosomal recessive hypophosphatemic rickets: DMP1 mutation
  - Hereditary hypophosphatemic rickets with hypercalciuria: NaPi2c mutation
- Etiology

OSTEOMALACIA

- Vitamin D abnormalities
  - Dietary vitamin D-deficiency
  - Dietary calcium deficiency (rare in developed countries)
  - Liver disease: Interferes with hydroxylation of prohormone vitamin D
  - Biliary disease: Related to malabsorption of vitamin D
  - Vitamin D dependent rickets type 1 and type 2 (vitamin D resistance)
  - GI malabsorption
  - Premature infants with prolonged parenteral nutrition, low birth weight
  - Copper deficiency in premature infants
- Hypophosphatemia: Includes many renal tubular defects
  - X-linked hypophosphatemic rickets (vitamin D resistant rickets)
  - Autosomal dominant hypophosphatemic rickets
  - Autosomal recessive hypophosphatemic rickets
  - Hereditary hypophosphatemic rickets with hypercalciuria
  - Renal phosphate loss: Fanconi syndrome, Dent disease, cadmium toxicity, heavy metal poisoning
  - Excessive antacid intake
- Oncogenic osteomalacia
  - FG23 secretion
  - Also vitamin D-refractory
  - Often due to small, benign mesenchymal soft tissue or bone tumors: Hemangioma, hemangiopericytoma, nonossifying fibroma, giant cell tumor, etc.
  - Normocalcemic, decreased serum HPO_4^- and alkaline phosphatase
  - Responds to tumor resection
- Toxicities
  - Drugs: Fluoride, diphosphonates (especially etidronate), Imatinab, Dilantin, phenobarbital
  - Other: Parenteral aluminum, aluminum containing antacids
- Other
  - Hypophosphatasia: Alkaline phosphatase deficiency; various forms of severity
  - Chronic acidosis
- May be a component of spectrum of findings in renal osteodystrophy
  - Osteomalacia
  - Secondary hyperparathyroidism
  - Rickets (skeletally immature)
  - Osteoporosis
- Associated abnormalities
  - Typical laboratory values
    - Decreased serum and urine Ca^{++}
    - Decreased serum and urine HPO_4^-
    - Elevated serum alkaline phosphatase
  - Laboratory values may vary with etiology

Microscopic Features
- Normal osteoid
- Reduced calcification (especially in new bone)
- Aluminum staining

CLINICAL ISSUES

Presentation
- Most common signs/symptoms: Non-radiating symmetrical bone pain: First in lower lumbar spine, next to thighs, spreading to arms, ribs

Demographics
- Age
  - Any age
  - Inherited disorders frequently in childhood, infancy

Treatment
- Highly dependent on cause of osteomalacia
  - May include parenteral vitamin D and calcium
  - Parenteral nutrition
  - Calcitriol & phosphate supplements (X-linked hypophosphatemic rickets)
  - Orthopedic surgery for fixation/stabilization
  - Identify and excise tumor in case of oncogenic osteomalacia

DIAGNOSTIC CHECKLIST

Consider
- Osteomalacia may coexist with findings of secondary hyperparathyroidism in renal osteodystrophy

SELECTED REFERENCES

1. Amin H et al: Osteomalacia and secondary hyperparathyroidism after kidney transplantation: Relationship to vitamin D deficiency. Am J Med Sci. 333(1):58-62, 2007
2. Casari S et al: A case of oncogenic osteomalacia detected by 111In-pentetreotide total body scan. Clin Exp Rheumatol. 21(4):493-6, 2003
3. Chun KA et al: Osteoblastoma as a cause of osteomalacia assessed by bone scan. Ann Nucl Med. 17(5):411-4, 2003
4. Akaki S et al: Flare response seen in therapy for osteomalacia. J Nucl Med. 39(12):2095-7, 1998
5. Ryan PJ et al: Bone scintigraphy in metabolic bone disease. Semin Nucl Med. 27(3):291-305, 1997
6. McAfee JG: Radionuclide imaging in metabolic and systemic skeletal diseases. Semin Nucl Med. 17(4):334-49, 1987
7. Karsenty G et al: Value of the 99mTc-methylene diphosphonate bone scan in renal osteodystrophy. Kidney Int. 29(5):1058-65, 1986
8. Botella J et al: The bone scan in patients with aluminium-associated bone disease. Proc Eur Dial Transplant Assoc Eur Ren Assoc. 21:403-9, 1985
9. Drueke T et al: Dialysis osteomalacia: clinical aspects and physiopathological mechanisms. Clin Nephrol. 24 Suppl 1:S26-9, 1985
10. Fogelman I et al: Diphosphonates in the evaluation of metabolic bone disease. Clin Rheumatol. 1(1):41-4, 1982
11. Fogelman I et al: A comparison of bone scanning and radiology in the evaluation of patients with metabolic bone disease. Clin Radiol. 31(3):321-6, 1980
12. Singh BN et al: Unusual bone scan presentation in osteomalacia: symmetrical uptake--a suggestive sign. Clin Nucl Med. 3(7):292-5, 1978
13. Sy WM et al: Bone scan in chronic dialysis patients with evidence of secondary hyperparathyroidism and renal osteodystrophy. Br J Radiol. 48(575):878-84, 1975

OSTEOMALACIA

IMAGE GALLERY

Typical

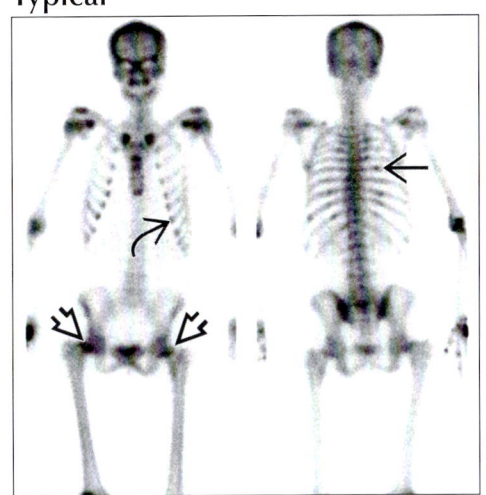

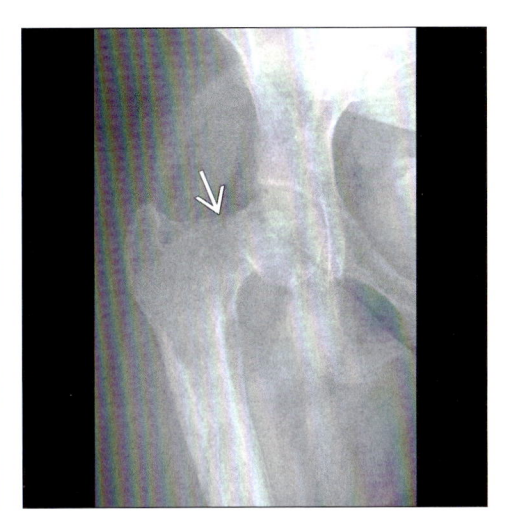

(Left) Typical findings of adult osteomalacia (due to small hemangiopericytoma) on Tc-99m bone scan: Uptake at all anterior rib ends ➔ and numerous rib ➔ and femoral neck ➔ fractures. Same patient as next 3 images. *(Right)* AP radiograph of right hip shows smudgy, coarsened trabecula, poor mineralization, femoral neck fracture ➔ with varus angulation in a patient with oncogenic osteomalacia.

Typical

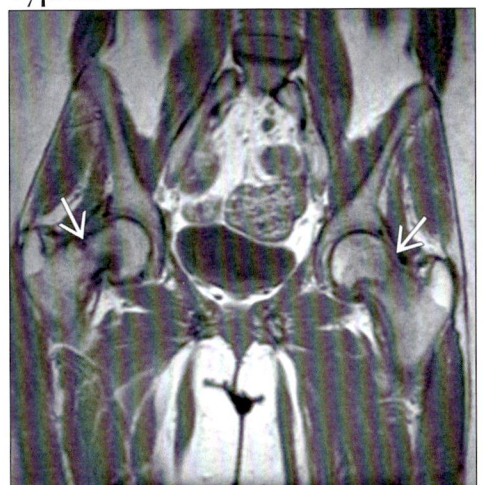

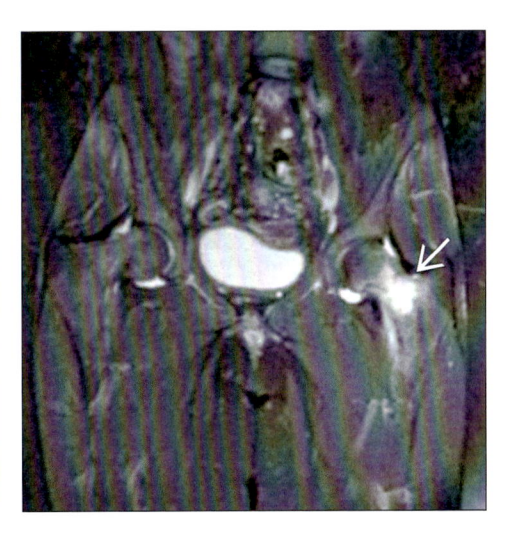

(Left) T1 MR AP pelvis in patient with oncogenic osteomalacia shows linear decreased signal due to bilateral femoral neck fractures ➔. The right femoral neck fracture is associated with varus angulation. *(Right)* T2 MR in same patient with oncogenic osteomalacia as previous 3 images shows increased signal 2° edema associated with left femoral neck fracture ➔, suggesting acuity.

Variant

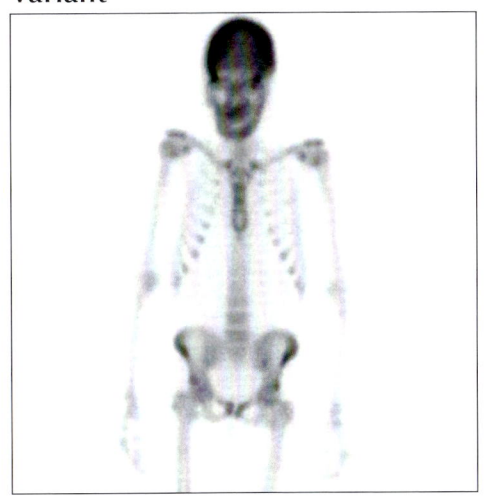

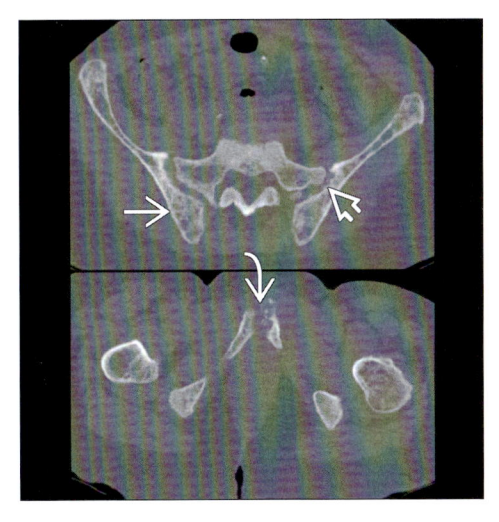

(Left) AP planar Tc-99m bone scan shows findings of renal osteodystrophy: Increased uptake at all rib ends (2° osteomalacia); increased cranial uptake and homogeneous diffuse "superscan" appearance (2° hyperparathyroidism). See next image. *(Right)* Axial CT pelvis shows smudgy coarsened trabecula and poor mineralization ➔ (osteomalacia); subperiosteal bone resorption at pubic symphysis ➔ & SIA joints ➔ (hyperparathyroidism).

HYPERTROPHIC OSTEOARTHROPATHY

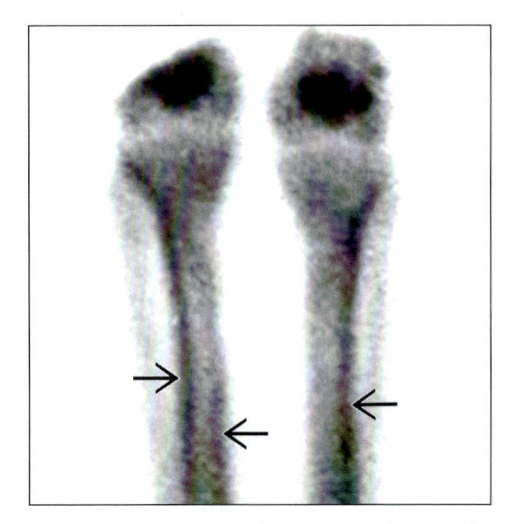

Anterior Tc-99m MDP bone scan shows thin, symmetric, linear increased tracer accumulation along the tibias ⇒, indicating active osteoblastic periosteal reaction due to HOA.

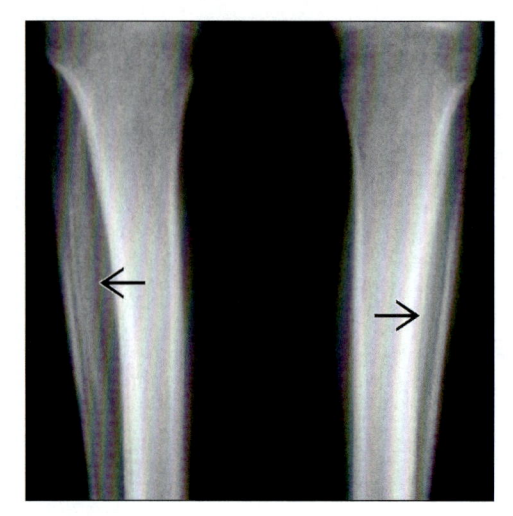

Anterior posterior plain film of proximal tibiae/fibulae shows elevated uniform and symmetric laminated-appearing periosteal reactions ⇒, typical for HOA.

TERMINOLOGY

Abbreviations and Synonyms
- Primary hypertrophic osteoarthropathy (HOA): Rare
  - Pachydermoperiostitis, Touraine-Solente-Gole syndrome
- Secondary HOA: More common
  - Hypertrophic pulmonary osteoarthropathy (HPOA), pulmonary hypertrophic osteoarthropathy (PHOA), secondary HOA, Pierre Marie-Bamberger syndrome, steoarthopathia hypertrophicans

Definitions
- Diffuse periosteal reaction of long bones in response to underlying thoracic, cardiac or abdominal disease, or as an inherited disorder

IMAGING FINDINGS

General Features
- Best diagnostic clue: Tc-99m (diphosphonate) bone scan shows symmetric ↑ activity of diaphyseal, metaphyseal surfaces of long bones
- Location
  - Distal femur, tibia/fibula and radius/ulna most common
  - Usually distal long bone, diffuse, symmetric
  - Localized HOA associated with vascular graft infections, affects corresponding vascular territories
- Morphology
  - Periosteal reactions on conventional imaging
    - May be smooth initially becoming irregular or "onionskin" with time
  - Acro-osteolysis more common in patients with primary HOA and right-to-left shunts

Imaging Recommendations
- Best imaging tool
  - Plain films initially
    - Periosteal reactions of diaphyses, then metaphyses (also epiphyses in primary HOA)
    - Acro-osteolysis occurs in more advanced disease
    - CXR to evaluate potential thoracic pathology
    - CT/MR may be utilized for additional characterization as needed
  - Skeletal scintigraphy for evaluation and surveillance

DDx: Mimics of HOA on Bone Scan: Other Causes of Cortical Uptake

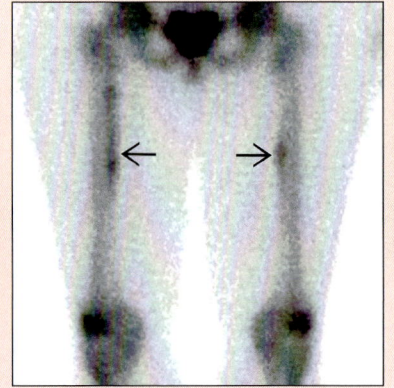

Adductor Strain/Avulsion 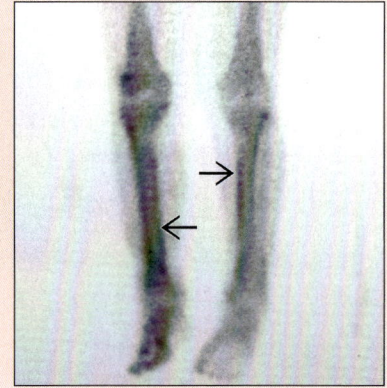   *Venous Stasis* 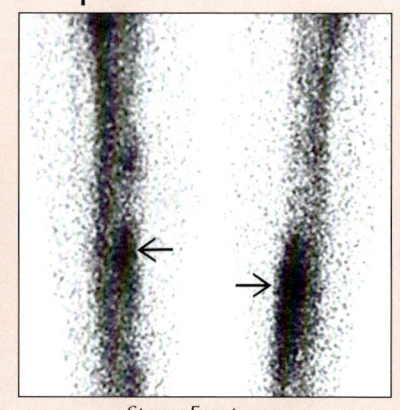   *Stress Fractures*

HYPERTROPHIC OSTEOARTHROPATHY

Key Facts

Imaging Findings
- Best diagnostic clue: Tc-99m (diphosphonate) bone scan shows symmetric ↑ activity of diaphyseal, metaphyseal surfaces of long bones
- Distal femur, tibia/fibula and radius/ulna most common
- Skeletal scintigraphy for evaluation and surveillance
- Linear increased tracer accumulation = periosteal reaction

Top Differential Diagnoses
- Skeletal Metastases
- Thyroid Acropachy
- Paget Disease
- Venous Insufficiency
- Hypervitaminosis A
- Infantile Cortical Hyperostosis
- Camurati-Engelmann Disease
- Stress Fracture

Pathology
- Primary HOA: Autosomal dominant
- Secondary HOA: No significant genetic correlation
- Epidemiology: Secondary HOA accounts for ≥ 95% of HOA
- Pulmonary disease associated with secondary HOA: Classically bronchogenic carcinoma or pulmonary metastases

Diagnostic Checklist
- Tc-99m MDP bone scan to evaluate therapy response
- Consider secondary HOA in patients undergoing bone scintigraphy for malignancy staging workup

---

- Linear increased tracer accumulation = periosteal reaction
- Rapid resolution with response of malignancy to chemotherapy
- Protocol advice
    - Tc-99m MDP whole body bone scintigraphy: 20-25 mCi (740-925 MBq) IV (adults)
    - Pediatric: Adjust dose to as low as 2 mCi (74 MBq) according to pediatric dosing algorithms (e.g., ages < 12 y use Webster rule: (Age+1/age+7) x adult dose)
    - Hydrate patient to promote soft tissue washout, improve target to background
    - Image at 3-4 h (5-7 h in patients with poor cardiac output or renal failure to clear soft tissues); can image up to 24 h if necessary
    - Whole body single pass scan: 1 million count anterior/posterior planar images; static (spot, 500k count) images of areas of interest (arms, legs)

DIFFERENTIAL DIAGNOSIS

Skeletal Metastases
- Seeding of intramedullary spaces by viable, replicating ectopic neoplastic cells
- Predominantly focal lesions located in regions of red marrow
    - Spine, ribs, sternum, pelvis, proximal portions of femora and humeri
- Superscan can show diffuse, homogeneous bone uptake, not the cortical pattern of long bones seen in HOA

Thyroid Acropachy
- History of thyroid ablation or resection for thyrotoxicosis (Graves disease)
- Clubbing with metacarpal/metatarsal and phalangeal fluffy "hair on end" periosteal reaction
- Unlikely to involve tibia/fibula, radius/ulna

Paget Disease
- Coarse trabecular remodeling and bony expansion on correlative plain film or CT examination
- More common in pelvis, spine, skull

Venous Insufficiency
- Usually confined to lower extremities, below knees
- Decreased corresponding soft tissue clearance

Hypervitaminosis A
- Thick, wavy, long bone diaphyseal periostitis
- Infants and preadolescents

Infantile Cortical Hyperostosis
- Proliferative hyperostosis of infancy, Caffey disease
    - Distinguished by mandibular involvement
    - Also involves tibia, ulna, clavicle
    - Age < 6 months
    - Self limiting: Recovery by 2-3 years

Camurati-Engelmann Disease
- Progressive diaphyseal dysplasia
- Increased osteoblastic tracer activity throughout bone rather than cortical distribution as in HOA

Stress Fracture
- Due to overuse, repetitive stress
- Often tibial, metatarsal

PATHOLOGY

General Features
- Genetics
    - Primary HOA: Autosomal dominant
        - However ~ 2/3 of cases appear sporadically, mechanism unclear
    - Secondary HOA: No significant genetic correlation
- Etiology
    - Secondary HOA: Associated with any of a number of chronic conditions, 90% of which are intrathoracic (primary disease process may not be pulmonary)
        - Mechanism unclear: Hypotheses include humoral factors including vascular endothelial growth factor, circulating toxins, irritants, autoimmune

HYPERTROPHIC OSTEOARTHROPATHY

- Alternative considerations include neurogenically mediated alterations and increases in peripheral blood supply
- Epidemiology: Secondary HOA accounts for ≥ 95% of HOA
- Associated abnormalities
  - Classically, neoplastic or infectious thoracic disease associated with secondary HOA (although cardiac, abdominal processes not uncommon)
  - Pulmonary disease associated with secondary HOA: Classically bronchogenic carcinoma or pulmonary metastases
    - ≥ 80% of cases associated with bronchogenic carcinoma
    - Pleural mesothelioma: Secondary HOA in ≤ 50%
    - Other: Chronic obstructive pulmonary disease, pleural fibroma, chronic infection, cystic fibrosis, Hodgkin lymphoma, interstitial fibrosis
  - Cardiac disease, particularly with right-to-left shunt
    - Includes patent ductus arteriosis (PDA) with pulmonary hypertension
  - Less common with chronic extrathoracic diseases
    - Chronic inflammatory processes: Ulcerative colitis, endograft infection, Whipple disease
    - Bowel disease: Crohn disease, lymphoma, bacillary and amebic dysentery
    - Liver disease: Cirrhosis (alcoholic, biliary, other), hepatopulmonary syndrome
    - Neoplasm: Esophageal, pancreatic, gastric, nasopharyngeal cancer

Microscopic Features
- Edema and neoangiogenesis of subperiosteum with elevation
- Osteoblastic activation and subsequent mineralization

CLINICAL ISSUES

Presentation
- Most common signs/symptoms
  - Extremity swelling, skin thickening, digital clubbing, "mushrooming" of tufts, erythema, arthralgias extending from joint into adjacent bone
    - Tibiotalar, knee, radiocarpal joint pain most common
    - Usually symmetric
- Other signs/symptoms
  - Joint effusions and synovitis: Rheumatoid arthritis also in differential
  - Primary HOA
    - Leonine facies: Ptosis and thickening of skin with furrowing resulting in a "lion-like" appearance
    - Cutis vertices gyrata (convolutional cranial skin folds, "bulldog scalp")
    - Hyperhidrosis, seborrhea, acne

Demographics
- Age
  - Primary HOA: Usually presents in childhood or adolescence
  - Secondary HOA: Age distribution coincident with development of underlying disease process
- Gender
  - Primary HOA: M > F, reported 9:1
    - More common in people of African descent
  - Secondary HOA: No gender prevalence beyond that of underlying disease processes

Natural History & Prognosis
- Primary HOA: Generally self-limiting disease with stabilization by 3rd-4th decades, then asymptomatic
- Secondary HOA: Prognosis depends on underlying pathology, not HOA

Treatment
- Treatment of primary HOA: Symptomatic
  - NSAIDs, analgesics for symptomatic relief
  - Pamidronate, bisphosphonates
- Treatment of secondary HOA: Depends on underlying illness/pathology
  - Surgery, radiation therapy, chemotherapy, antibiotics, immune modulators
  - Improvement occurs spontaneously with effective treatment
  - Octreotide has seen reported success, hypothetically secondary to potent vascular endothelial growth factor antagonism
  - Improvement can be seen radiographically within weeks of therapy
    - Resolution of diffuse periosteal reaction within months
    - Arthropathy may improve sooner than periosteum
  - Recurrent disease may result in recurrent clinical and imaging findings

DIAGNOSTIC CHECKLIST

Consider
- Tc-99m MDP bone scan to evaluate therapy response
- Consider secondary HOA in patients undergoing bone scintigraphy for malignancy staging workup

SELECTED REFERENCES

1. Alonso-Bartolome P et al: Hypertrophic osteoarthropathy secondary to vascular prosthesis infection: report of 3 cases and review of the literature. Medicine (Baltimore). 85(3):183-91, 2006
2. Altman RD et al: Hypertrophic osteoarthropathy. In: Harris ED Jr, ed. Kelly's Textbook of Rheumatology. 7th ed. Philadelphia, Elsevier Saunders, 1749-50, 2006
3. Hemady N et al: A patient with dyspnea and swollen, painful wrists. Am Fam Physician. 74(11):1909-11, 2006
4. Strobel K et al: Pulmonary hypertrophic osteoarthropathy in a patient with nonsmall cell lung cancer: Diagnosis with FDG PET/CT. Clin Nucl Med. 31(10):624-6, 2006
5. Angel-Moreno Maroto A et al: Painful hypertrophic osteoarthropathy successfully treated with octreotide. The pathogenetic role of vascular endothelial growth factor (VEGF). Rheumatology (Oxford). 44(10):1326-7, 2005
6. Cannavo SP et al: Pierre Marie-Bamberger syndrome (secondary hypertrophic osteoarthropathy). Int J Dermatol. 44(1):41-2, 2005
7. Suzuma T et al: Pamidronate-induced remission of pain associated with hypertrophic pulmonary osteoarthropathy in chemoendocrine therapy-refractory inoperable metastatic breast carcinoma. Anticancer Drugs. 12(9):731-4, 2001

HYPERTROPHIC OSTEOARTHROPATHY

IMAGE GALLERY

Typical

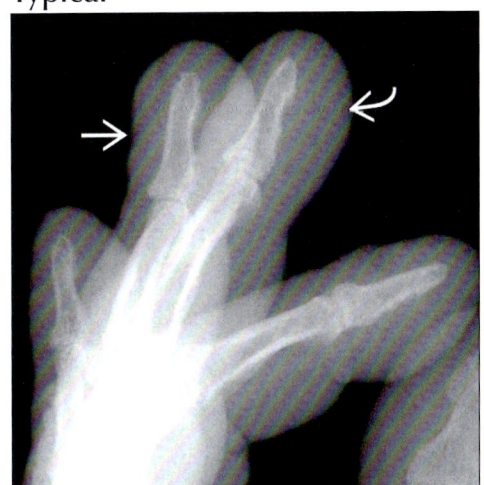

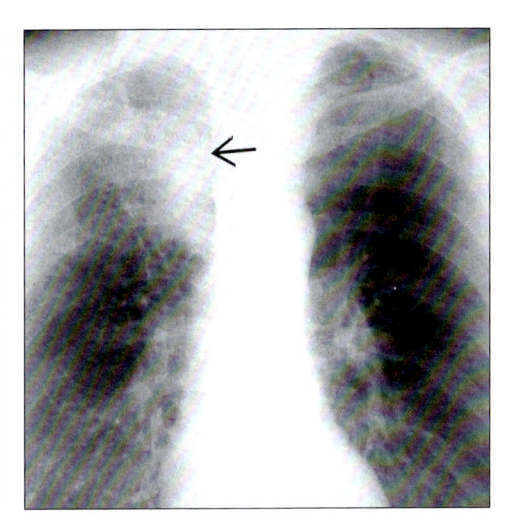

(Left) Lateral radiograph shows marked clubbing of digits with flattening of nail bed angle ➔ and marked soft tissue swelling ➔, prompting chest evaluation. See next image. *(Courtesy B. Manaster, MD).* **(Right)** Posterior anterior chest radiograph in same patient as previous shows right upper lobe lung mass ➔, biopsy-proven bronchogenic carcinoma. *(Courtesy B. Manaster, MD).*

Typical

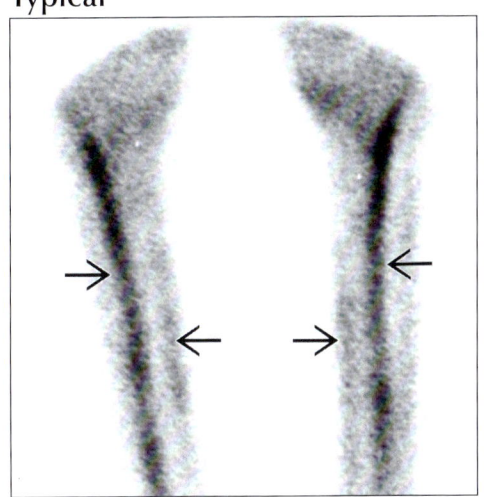

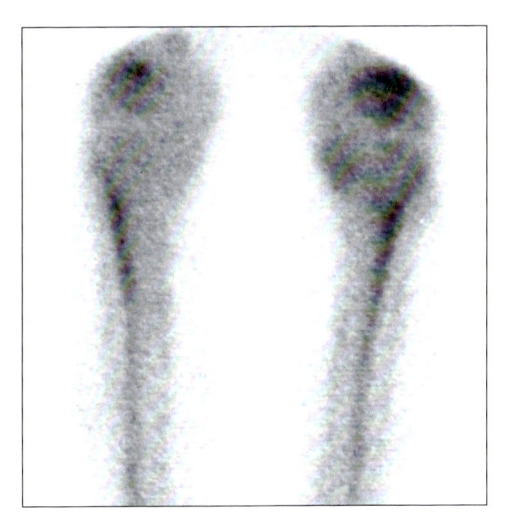

(Left) Anterior Tc-99m MDP bone scan shows symmetric increased tracer uptake corresponding to tibial diaphyseal cortices ➔ in patient with secondary HOA due to bronchogenic cancer. See next image. **(Right)** Anterior Tc-99m MDP bone scan (same patient as previous image) 4 weeks after chemotherapy, shows significant resolution of diaphyseal osteoblastic reaction.

Typical

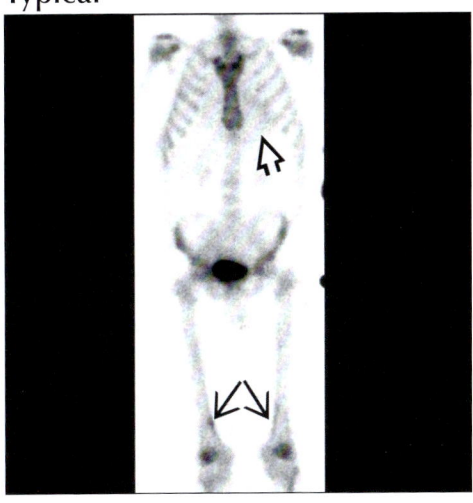

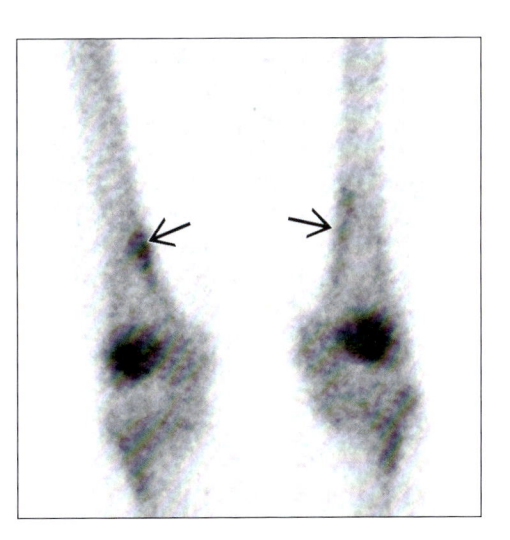

(Left) Anterior and posterior Tc-99m MDP bone scan shows mild focal uptake at medial cortices of the femoral diaphyses ➔. Note incidental malignant pericardial effusion ➔. **(Right)** Anterior Tc-99m MDP bone scan spot image of same patient at left illustrates typical location of earliest scintigraphic changes of HOA: Medial diaphyseal cortices of distal femurs ➔.

HYPERTROPHIC OSTEOARTHROPATHY

Typical

(Left) Anterior radiograph shows typical early periosteal reaction ➔, consistent with HOA. This finding should prompt further evaluation for etiology. See next image. *(Courtesy K. Sanders, MD).*
(Right) Anterior Tc-99m MDP bone scan shows subtle linear increased activity in periosteal reactions in the medial femurs ➔, prompting survey for intrathoracic disease.

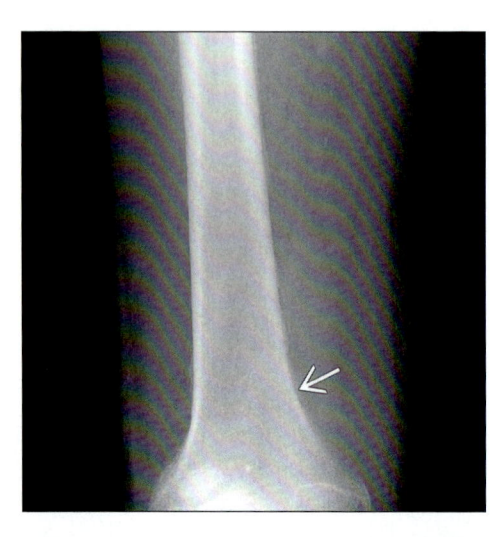

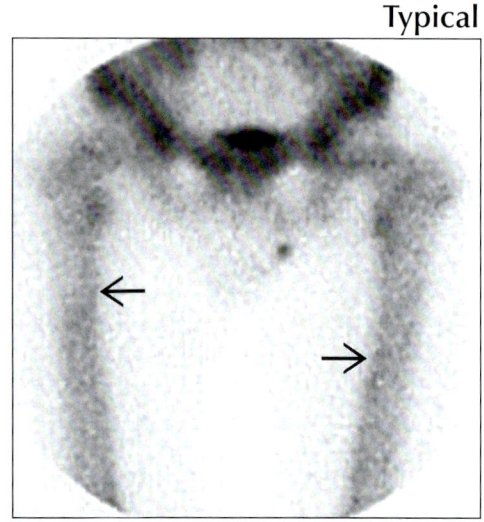

Typical

(Left) Anteroposterior radiograph of hand shows extensive, exuberant periosteal elevation and ossification ➔ in patient with primary HOA. *(Courtesy B. Manaster, MD).*
(Right) Anteroposterior radiograph of distal radius and ulna in a patient with primary HOA shows marked periosteal reactions ➔. *(Courtesy B. Manaster, MD).*

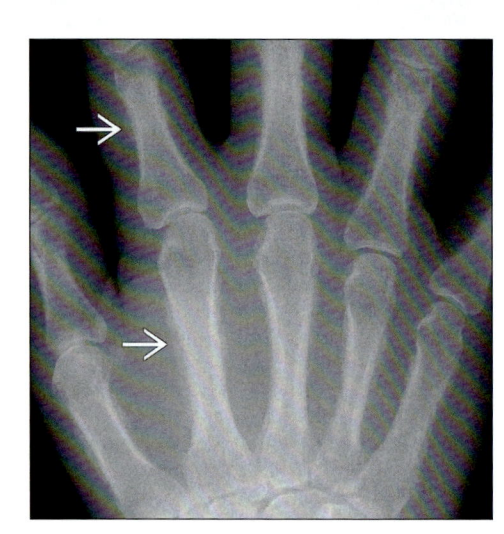

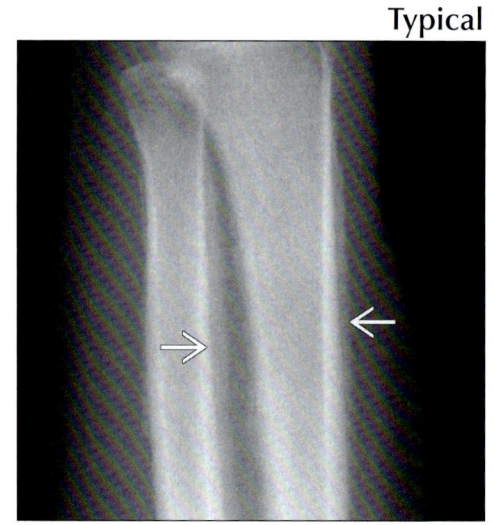

Typical

(Left) Anteroposterior radiograph of same patient at left shows typical periosteal reaction of fibula ➔, while tibial periosteal reaction has become ossified ➔. *(Courtesy B. Manaster, MD).*
(Right) Anterior Tc-99m MDP bone scan in same patient at left shows increased cortical tracer activity ➔ indicating HOA. *(Courtesy B. Manaster, MD).*

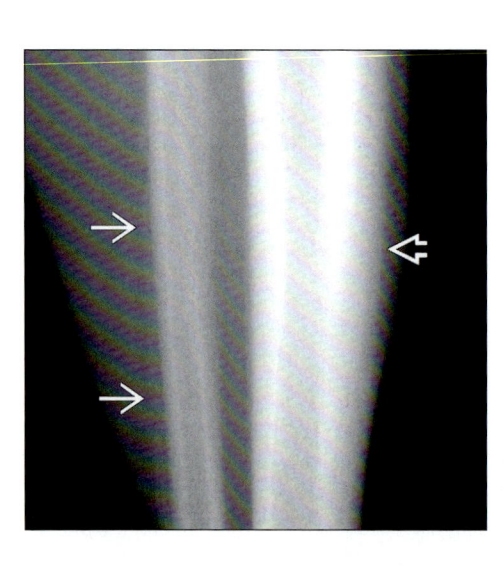

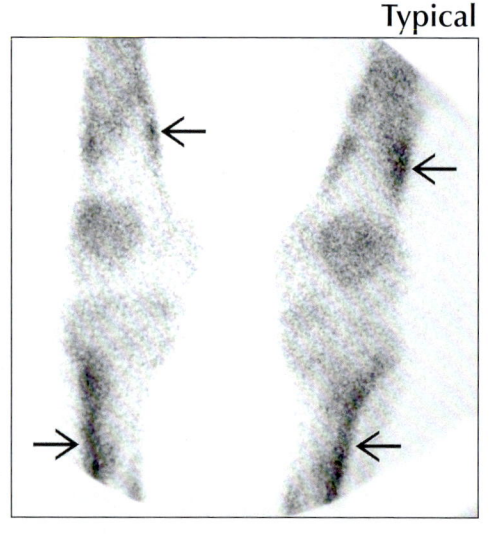

HYPERTROPHIC OSTEOARTHROPATHY

Typical

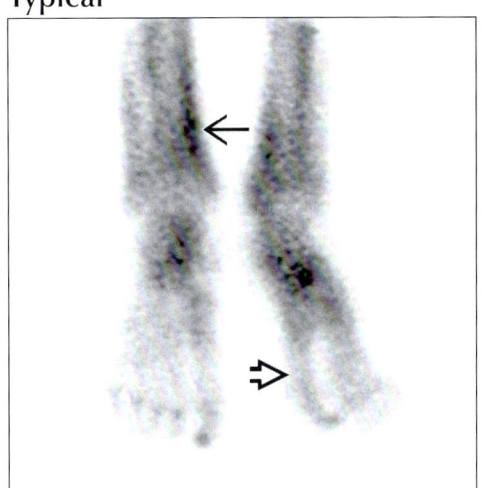

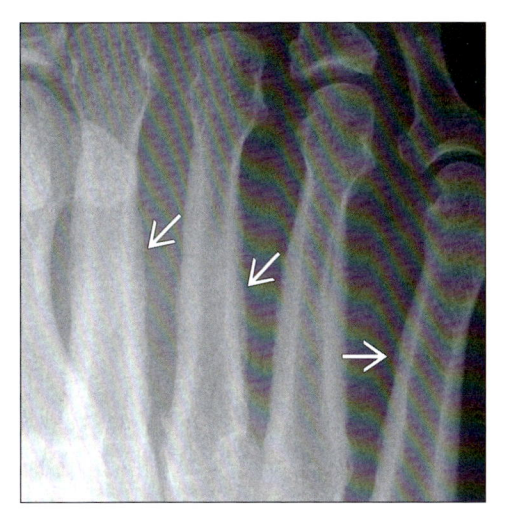

(Left) Anterior Tc-99m MDP mineral phase scintigraphy shows abnormal cortical tracer accumulation of the tibias ➔ extending into the first metatarsals ⇨, consistent with HOA. (Right) Anteroposterior radiograph shows wavy periosteal reaction in metatarsals ➔. The differential diagnosis includes HOA. (Courtesy B. Manaster, MD).

Typical

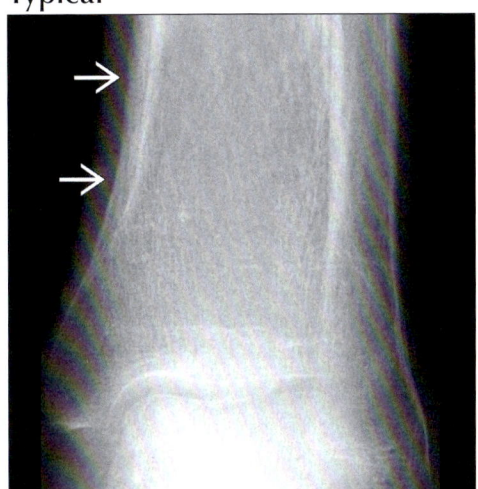

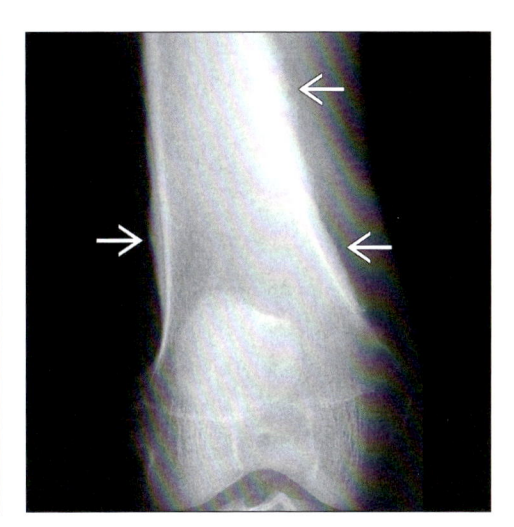

(Left) Anteroposterior radiograph in patient with lung cancer and distal femur pain due to HOA showing periosteal reaction ➔. (Courtesy B. Manaster, MD). (Right) Anteroposterior radiograph shows periosteal reaction about distal femur ➔ in patient with knee pain. Subsequent thoracic evaluation revealed lung cancer. (Courtesy B. Manaster, MD).

Typical

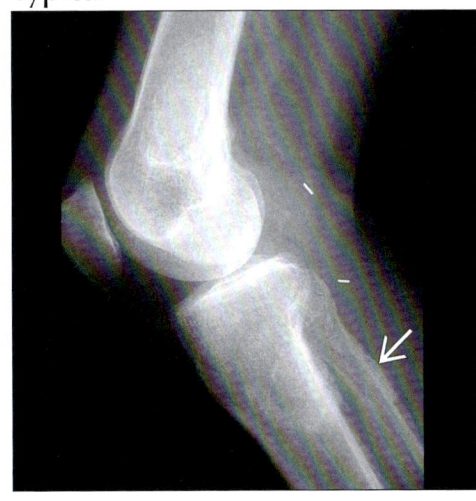

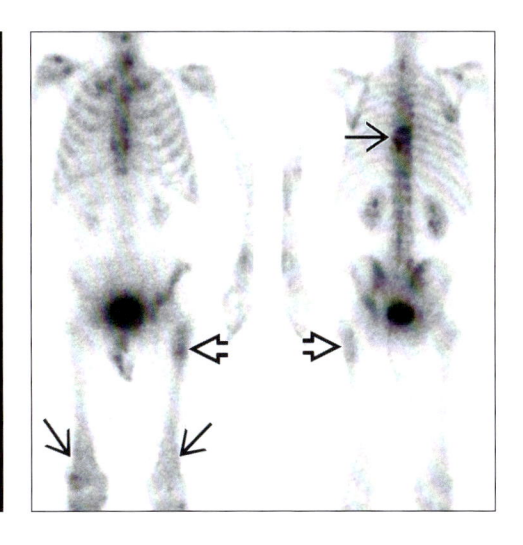

(Left) Lateral radiograph of knee shows periosteal reaction of fibula ➔ prompting thoracic imaging that subsequently led to diagnosis of bronchogenic carcinoma. (Courtesy B. Manaster, MD). (Right) Anterior and posterior Tc-99m MDP bone scan of patient with bronchogenic carcinoma shows metastatic disease of thoracic spine ➔ and left femur ⇨. Very subtle early changes of HOA in distal femurs.

PAGET DISEASE

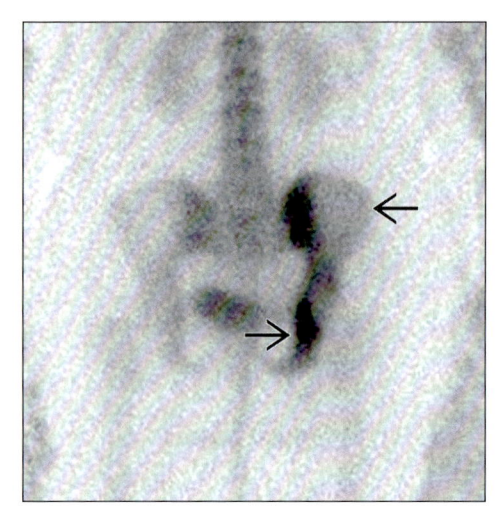

Anterior and posterior bone scan in patient with back pain shows increased activity in majority of right hemipelvis ➡. See next image.

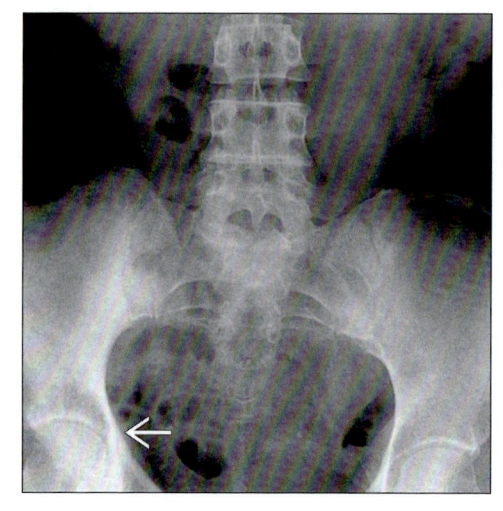

AP radiograph in same patient as previous shows sclerosis in right hemipelvis and iliopectineal line thickening ➡, consistent with PD.

TERMINOLOGY

Abbreviations and Synonyms
- Paget disease (PD) of bone; osteitis deformans; osteoporosis circumscripta (skull)

Definitions
- Disorder of abnormal/excessive bone remodeling characterized by coarse trabeculae, sclerosis, and expansion of one or more bones
- Active disease begins with osteolytic phase followed by sclerotic or mixed active phase; inactive or quiescent phase demonstrates sclerotic lesions
- Although thickened, abnormal bone weaker and bone deformity or fracture common

IMAGING FINDINGS

General Features
- Best diagnostic clue: Intense activity & expansile appearance of entire affected bone on bone scan
- Location
  - Predominantly axial skeleton, proximal femur
    - Pelvis (30-75%) > vertebra (30-75%) > skull (25-65%) > proximal long bones (esp. femur)
    - May affect any bone
    - Ribs, fibula, hands, feet uncommon
  - Polyostotic > monostotic (10-35%)
- Morphology
  - Lytic phase often ⇒ large, geographic lesion
  - Sclerotic or mixed phase: Coarse, thick trabeculae in expanded bone

Nuclear Medicine Findings
- Bone Scan
  - Intensely ↑ bone scan uptake can be seen in all areas of active disease even before radiographic change
    - Uptake may be particularly intense in lytic phase
    - Inactive or quiescent phase should show no increased uptake
  - Angiographic images from three-phase bone scan show increased blood flow with intensity closely correlating with level of disease activity
  - Disease deterioration or recurrence often found on bone scan before lab value changes
  - Worsening lesion on bone scan raises possibility of superimposed primary or metastatic tumor

DDx: Paget Disease of Bone

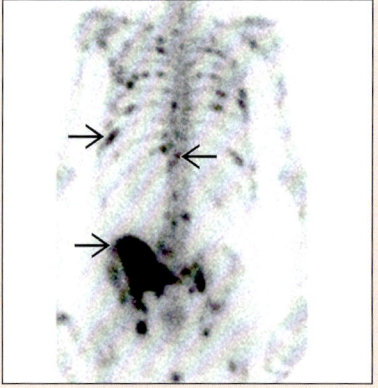

Bone Metastases

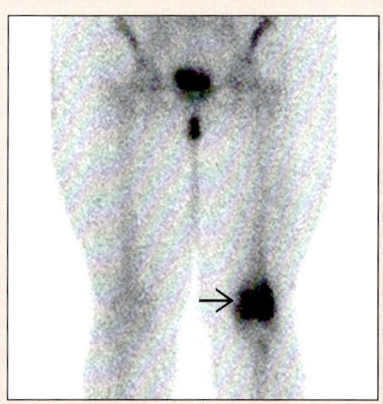

Primary Bone Tumor (Giant Cell)

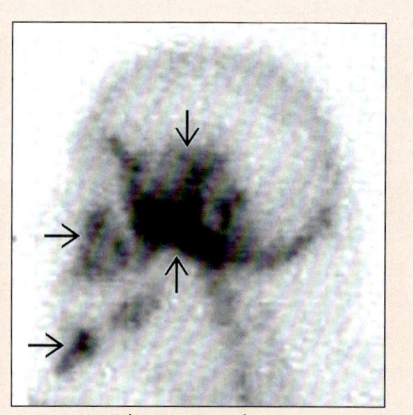

Fibrous Dysplasia

PAGET DISEASE

Key Facts

Terminology
- Paget disease (PD) of bone; osteitis deformans; osteoporosis circumscripta (skull)
- Disorder of abnormal/excessive bone remodeling characterized by coarse trabeculae, sclerosis, and expansion of one or more bones
- Although thickened, abnormal bone weaker and bone deformity or fracture common

Top Differential Diagnoses
- Bone Metastases
- Primary Bone Tumor
- Fibrous Dysplasia (FD)

Clinical Issues
- Asymptomatic ~ 90%
- Painful extremities, bowing long bones, secondary osteoarthritis
- ↑ Serum alkaline phosphatase, ↑ urinary and serum hydroxyproline
- Malignant degeneration rare (generally < 1%)

Diagnostic Checklist
- Bone scan most sensitive test to detect PD
- Whole body bone scan: Diagnose, assess extent of PD
- Focal increased activity over background of affected bone: Consider fracture, malignant degeneration
- Bone metastases vs. PD can be difficult differential diagnosis
- New sites in patient with long-standing PD suggest metastatic disease
- Radiographic, MR, biopsy correlation may be necessary to distinguish PD from metastases

---

- Labeled Leukocyte Scintigraphy
  - PD can cause increased uptake in absence of infection; Tc-99m sulfur colloid marrow map can confirm presence of expanded bone marrow
  - Photopenic defects can also occur with PD (hypocellularity with sclerosis)
- Thallium-201 & Ga-67 Scintigraphy
  - Currently, not typically utilized for PD
  - Uptake usually of similar intensity to bone scan
  - Occasionally more accurate than bone scan alone in monitoring disease
    - Development of malignancy will show ↑ accumulation while successful therapy shows resolution
- FDG PET
  - FDG uptake: Usually absent in benign disease
  - Mild uptake possible but marked uptake unusual
  - Intense uptake requires exclusion of superimposed malignancy, although PD is known cause of false positive on PET

Radiographic Findings
- Skull: Osteoporosis circumscripta, focal cotton wool densities, & cranial thickening, especially in frontal bone, with inner and outer table involvement
  - Cementomas in mandible and maxilla may affect teeth
- Spine: "Picture frame" vertebra or ivory vertebra; compression fracture; PD typically involves both body and posterior elements of same level
- Pelvis: Iliopubic/ilioischial thickening, unilateral extensive lesion common, acetabuli protrusio
- Long bones: Epiphyseal predominance with advancing wedge or flame-shaped osteolysis, deformity common

CT Findings
- Bone CT: Characteristic patterns similar to radiographs: Lysis followed by irregular coarsened trabeculae in expansile lesion

MR Findings
- Useful for evaluating neurological complications of disease or malignant degeneration
- Normal marrow signal until disease very advanced; mildly increased T1 and low T2 signal, unless tumor or fracture present, causing contrast-enhancement or increased signal on T2 WI

Imaging Recommendations
- Best imaging tool
  - Bone scan most sensitive modality for whole body skeletal survey
    - Diagnose PD
    - Identify multiple sites
    - Identify quiescent disease
- Protocol advice
  - Delayed whole body images at 2-3 hours following 20-25 mCi (740-925 MBq) Tc-99m MDP IV
  - SPECT to increase sensitivity (e.g., spine)

DIFFERENTIAL DIAGNOSIS

Bone Metastases
- Most frequently differential concern encountered in work-up of PD
- Can mimic lytic or sclerotic phases of PD as intense uptake on bone scan can create a falsely expanded appearance of bone

Primary Bone Tumor
- Primary bone tumors such as osteosarcoma and chondrosarcoma typically show markedly increased uptake on bone scan
- Benign tumors such as giant cell tumor, aneurysmal bone cyst, and occasionally enchondromas may also have + bone scan, although most benign tumors show background activity
- Radiographic correlation often diagnostic

Fibrous Dysplasia (FD)
- Benign developmental disorder leading to fibro-osseous tissue replacing medullary spaces of one or more bones
- Favored sites of FD: Ribs, skull, femur

PAGET DISEASE

- Rib and distal extremity involvement more common than in PD; spine and pelvic FD less common
- Bone scan: Moderate to intense radiotracer accumulation
- FDG PET: Usually negative or minimal activity
- Presentation usually differs from PD: Young adults/teens, may be associated with cutaneous cafe-au-lait spots and endocrine abnormalities
- FD has widely variable X-ray appearance, bubbly lesions may be differentiated from PD but sclerotic lesions have similar appearance

PATHOLOGY

General Features
- Genetics
  - Up to 40% have positive family history; 15-20% have 1st degree relative affected
  - Certain genetic mutations such as 1/p62 gene found in familial form and some sporadic cases
- Etiology
  - Proposed viral or slow viral etiology (controversial)
  - Some relation to paramyxovirus described, measles-like particles and respiratory syncytial virus antigens both found in some cases
- Epidemiology
  - Incidence varies with geography: Greater in some cold climate countries and populations with ancestors from Great Britain
  - Rare: Asia, India, Scandinavia
- Associated abnormalities
  - Metastases may coexist, possibly increased blood flow causes increased susceptibility
  - Malignant degeneration
  - Giant cell tumors: Lytic lesion usually confined to facial bones
  - Plasma cell myeloma possibly associated

Microscopic Features
- 1: Giant osteoclasts with more numerous nucleoli and intranuclear inclusion bodies ⇒ osteolysis
- 2: Osteoblasts recruited for compensatory bone formation ⇒ deposition of disorganized lamellar bone
- 3: Marrow spaces fill with fibrous connective tissue, blood vessels ⇒ hypervascularity
- 4: Hypocellularity may ensue ⇒ regions of sclerotic bone only

CLINICAL ISSUES

Presentation
- Most common signs/symptoms
  - Asymptomatic ~ 90%
  - Painful extremities, bowing long bones, secondary osteoarthritis
  - Neurological complications: Deafness, spinal cord compression
  - High output CHF: Likely due to hyperemia in affected bones rather than arteriovenous malformations as previously thought
- Laboratory findings
  - ↑ Serum alkaline phosphatase, ↑ urinary and serum hydroxyproline
    - Levels usually reflect disease status
    - Lower levels in patients with monostotic PD
  - Calcium, phosphorus and acid phosphatase usually normal

Demographics
- Age
  - Rare < 40 yrs, incidence increases with age
    - Affects up to 4% of people > 55 yrs and 10% of those > 80 yrs
    - Rare juvenile form may occur
- Gender: M > F (1.8:1)

Natural History & Prognosis
- Many patients asymptomatic, requiring no treatment
- Lasting remission may be achieved
- Malignant degeneration rare (generally < 1%)
  - While risk low, it is ↑ in widespread disease (up to 5-10%)
  - 1° tumors: Osteosarcoma (50-60%) > fibrosarcoma (20-25%) > chondrosarcoma (10%)
  - Investigate worsening pain and soft tissue mass or developing lytic area, especially if previously sclerotic

Treatment
- Bisphosphonates (e.g., alendronate) first-line
  - Binds onto bone matrix and inhibits osteoclast number and demineralization
- Calcitonin may be used briefly to inhibit bone reabsorption; inhibitory effects on osteoclasts often incomplete, relapse common
- Plicamycin (Mithramycin): Inhibits RNA synthesis and osteoclast action; side effects common (renal/liver failure, bone marrow suppression)
- Osteotomy or surgical decompression of vertebral disease may be required for severe cases

DIAGNOSTIC CHECKLIST

Consider
- Bone scan most sensitive test to detect PD
- Whole body bone scan: Diagnose, assess extent of PD
- Focal increased activity over background of affected bone: Consider fracture, malignant degeneration
- Bone metastases vs. PD can be difficult differential diagnosis
  - New sites in patient with long-standing PD suggest metastatic disease
  - Radiographic, MR, biopsy correlation may be necessary to distinguish PD from metastases

SELECTED REFERENCES
1. Cook GJ et al: Fluorine-18-FDG PET in Paget's disease of bone. J Nucl Med. 38(9):1495-7, 1997
2. Bahk YW et al: Bone pathologic correlation of multimodality imaging in Paget's disease. J Nucl Med. 36(8):1421-6, 1995
3. Fogelman I et al: The role of bone scanning in Paget's disease. Metab Bone Dis Relat Res. 3(4-5):243-54, 1981

PAGET DISEASE

IMAGE GALLERY

Typical

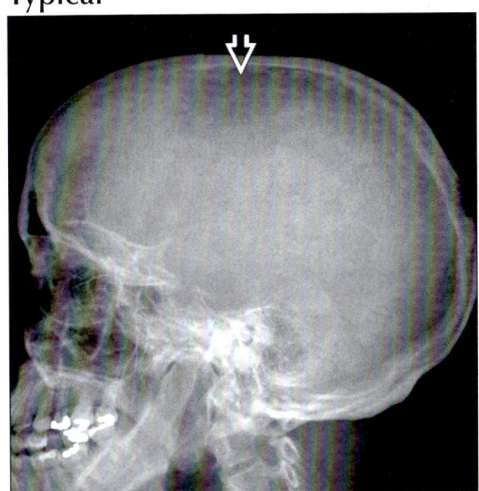

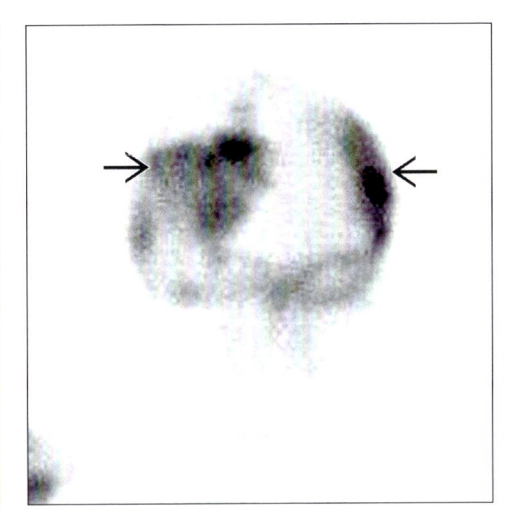

(Left) Lateral skull radiograph shows lytic skull lesion ➔ in patient with osteoporosis circumscripta from PD. (Courtesy R. Lopez, MD). (Right) Anterior bone scan in patient with elevated alkaline phosphatase shows intense geographic activity in skull ➔, at site of PD confirmed by radiography.

Typical

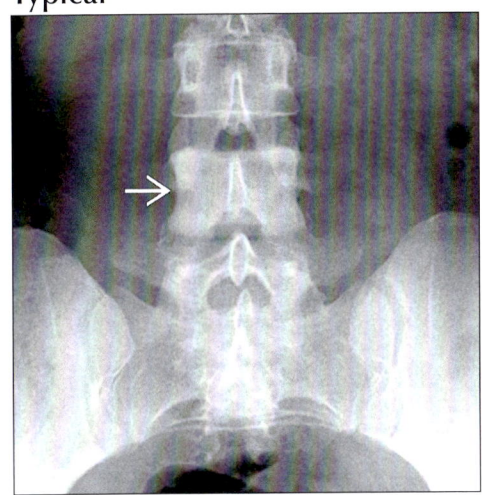

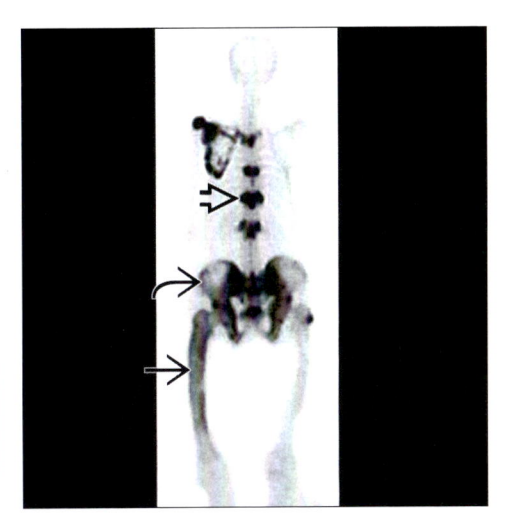

(Left) AP radiograph shows diffuse sclerosis of L4 ➔ causing a mild "ivory vertebra" appearance typical of PD. (Courtesy R. Lopez, MD). (Right) Posterior bone scan shows expansion, bowing and ↑ uptake in femur ➔, ↑ uptake in pelvis ➔, both vertebral body and posterior element of vertebrae ➔, and scapula in patient characteristic of PD.

Typical

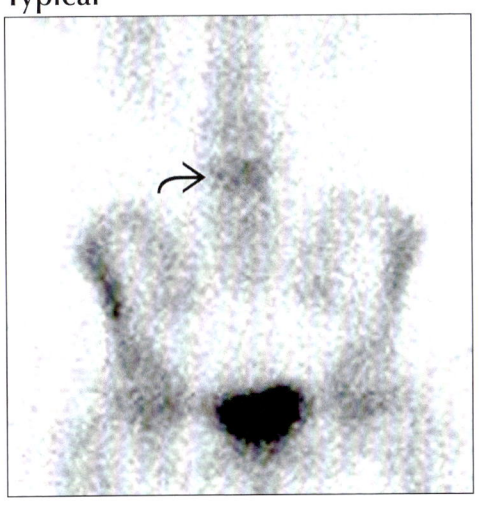

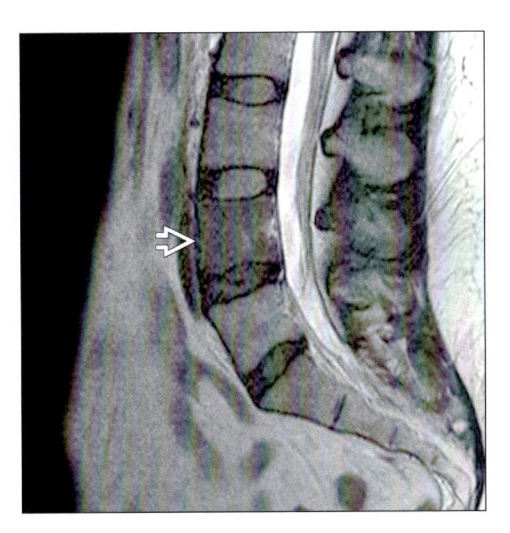

(Left) Anterior and posterior bone scan shows minimal uptake in L4 vertebral body ➔ in patient with stable, treated PD. See next image. (Right) Sagittal T2 MR of same patient as previous image shows low signal in L4 vertebra ➔, typical of advanced or treated PD.

FIBROUS DYSPLASIA

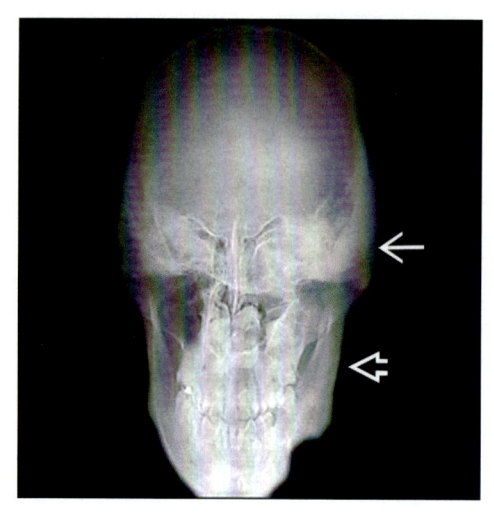

Anterior posterior radiograph shows ground-glass density and expansion of the temporal bone ➡ and mandible ⇨, typical of craniofacial FD. See next image.

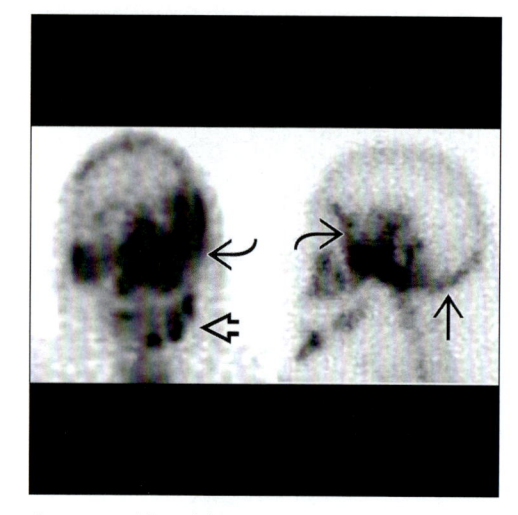

Anterior and lateral bone scan in the same patient as previous image shows increased activity in left skull base ➡, temporal bone ➚ and mandible ⇨.

TERMINOLOGY

Abbreviations and Synonyms
- Fibrous dysplasia (FD), Lichtenstein-Jaffe disease, fibrous osteodystrophy
- McCune Albright syndrome: FD, cafe au lait spots, endocrinopathy

Definitions
- Fibrous tissue occupying normal medullary spaces
  - Weaker than normal bone
  - At risk for pain, pathologic fracture, bone deformity
  - Monostotic, polyostotic, craniofacial, cherubic

IMAGING FINDINGS

General Features
- Best diagnostic clue
  - Radiograph or CT: Lucent tumor-like lesion
    - Homogeneous, ± expansion, endosteal scalloping
    - Dense sclerotic margin = "rind sign"
    - Typically ellipsoid, no periosteal reaction
- Location
  - Monostotic: Ribs > femur > facial bones
  - Polyostotic: Diaphyseal or metaphyseal femur > tibia > pelvis > foot > ribs, skull, facial bones
  - Craniofacial: Bones of sinuses > temporal, occipital
  - Cherubic: Bilateral maxilla and mandible, symmetric

Imaging Recommendations
- Best imaging tool
  - First line: Plain film radiography for diagnosis
    - Expansile, radiolucent, ground-glass appearance
- Imaging findings
  - Bone scan: Uptake is variable
    - Specificity too low to diagnose FD with bone scan
    - Useful to identify monostotic vs. polyostotic FD
    - Increased activity in pathologic fracture
  - Ga-67 scintigraphy: Increased activity in FD lesions
  - FDG PET: Increased uptake in active phase of FD
  - CT: No mineral cortex nor soft tissue mass; active lesions enhance
  - MR: Homogeneous ↓ T1; T2 variable; active lesions enhance

DDx: Mimics of Fibrous Dysplasia

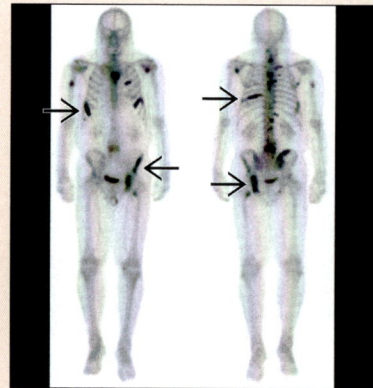

Bone Metastases

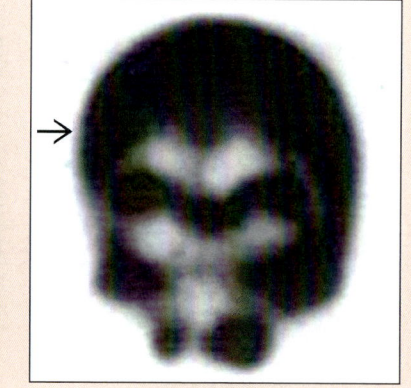

Paget Disease

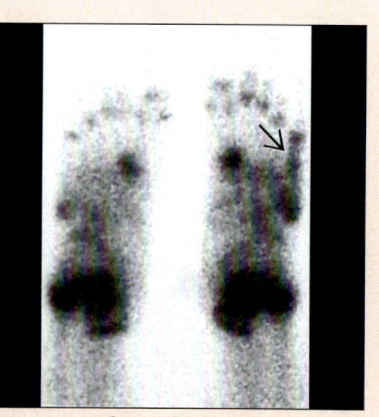

Stress Fracture

FIBROUS DYSPLASIA

Key Facts

Terminology
- Fibrous tissue occupying normal medullary spaces
- At risk for pain, pathologic fracture, bone deformity
- Monostotic, polyostotic, craniofacial, cherubic

Top Differential Diagnoses
- Paget Disease
- Osteogenesis Imperfecta
- Bone Tumors

Clinical Issues
- Pain, pathologic fracture
- Bone enlargement, expansion, deformity
- Cranial nerve impingement

Diagnostic Checklist
- Significantly ↑ activity on bone scan with acute pain: Pathologic fracture, malignant degeneration

DIFFERENTIAL DIAGNOSIS

Paget Disease
- Lytic, osteogenic, then sclerotic, flame-shaped, extending toward diaphysis

Osteogenesis Imperfecta
- Deformed, often curvaceous, long bones with moderate diaphyseal uptake

Bone Tumors
- Primary tumors; metastases (mimic polyostotic FD)

Neurofibromatosis
- Intramedullary lesions rare
- Smooth cafe au lait spots ("coast of California")

PATHOLOGY

General Features
- Genetics
  - Linked to genetic mutation of 20q13.2-13.3
  - Cherubism: Autosomal dominant, variable
- Associated abnormalities
  - Calvarial and facial asymmetry, exophthalmos
  - Craniofacial form: Leontiasis ossea ⇒ leonine facies
  - Femur: Coxa vara, shepherd's crook

Microscopic Features
- Fibrous, immature collagen matrix containing cystic fluid collections punctuating irregular trabeculae
- Defective osteoblastic maturation, poor mineralization

CLINICAL ISSUES

Presentation
- Most common signs/symptoms
  - Pain, pathologic fracture
  - Bone enlargement, expansion, deformity
  - Cranial nerve impingement

Demographics
- Age: Most < 15 yrs.; monostotic often > 30 yrs.

Natural History & Prognosis
- Usually benign/self limiting, occasional malignant degeneration (e.g., osteosarcoma, fibrosarcoma)

DIAGNOSTIC CHECKLIST

Consider
- Significantly ↑ activity on bone scan with acute pain: Pathologic fracture, malignant degeneration

SELECTED REFERENCES
1. Nakahara T et al: Use of SPECT in evaluation of fibrous dysplasia of the skull. Clin Nucl Med. 29(9):554-9, 2004
2. Zhibin Y et al: The role of radionuclide bone scintigraphy in fibrous dysplasia of bone. Clin Nucl Med. 29(3):177-80, 2004

IMAGE GALLERY

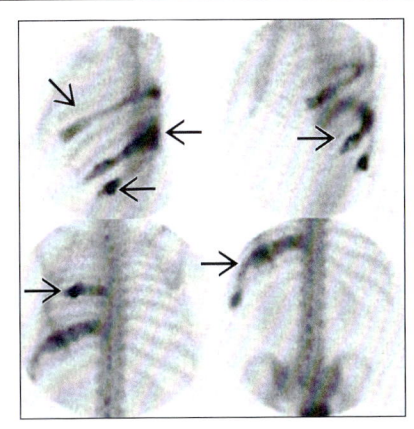

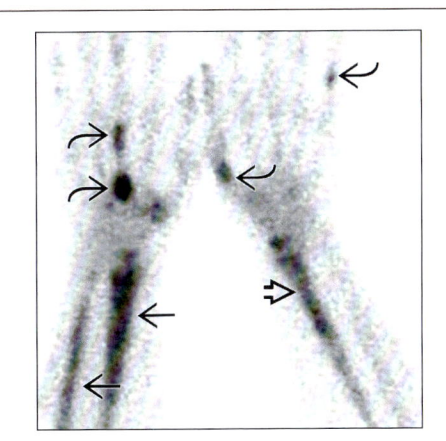

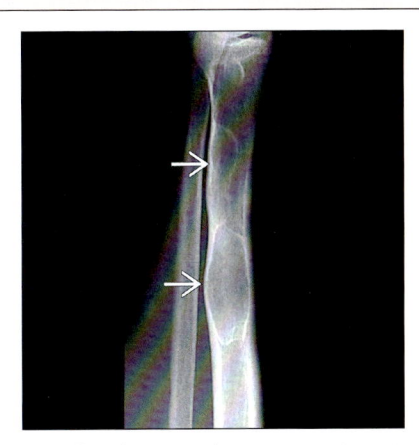

(Left) Posterior and oblique bone scan of ribs shows multiple expansile lesions in ribs of left hemithorax ➡, indicating polyostotic FD. (Center) Palmar bone scan of wrists shows increased activity in right radius and ulna ➡, bilateral hands ➡, and left radius ➡ in a patient with polyostotic FD. See next image. (Right) Forearm radiograph in the same patient as previous shows lytic, expansile, intramedullary lesions of FD ➡. Note characteristic thickened, sclerotic margins ("rind sign").

MELORHEOSTOSIS

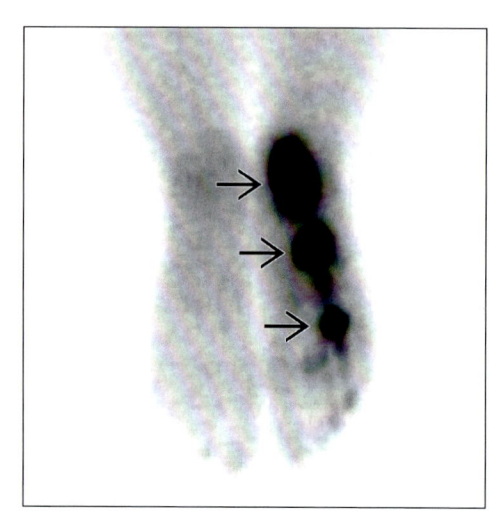

Delayed plantar bone scan shows marked uptake along the fourth ray ➔ of right foot in patient with melorheostosis. See next image.

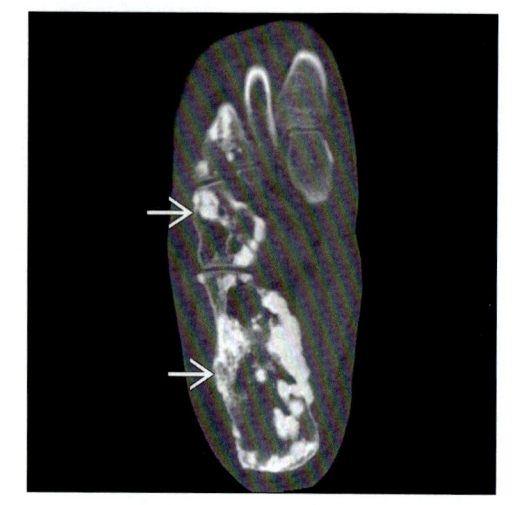

Bone CT of the foot in the same patient as previous image, shows sclerotic densities ➔ corresponding to increased activity on bone scan.

TERMINOLOGY

Abbreviations and Synonyms
- Leri disease

Definitions
- Rare, benign, sclerosing bone dysplasia demonstrating dense bone formation, typically along cortex of tubular bones
  - Frequently associated with scleroderma like skin change, pain, vascular change

IMAGING FINDINGS

General Features
- Best diagnostic clue
  - Well-circumscribed, undulating areas of cortical sclerosis on radiographs
    - Often referred to as "dripping candle wax" pattern on plain film
- Location
  - May involve inner or outer cortical surface
  - Almost always unilateral, often monostotic
  - Affects tubular bones of extremities, most commonly long bones, occasionally hands and feet
    - Axial skeleton involvement rare
  - May be regional, crossing joints in a ray, following a sclerotome
    - When present, this pattern is highly characteristic

Nuclear Medicine Findings
- Bone Scan
  - Bone scan: Increased blood flow on angiographic, blood pool, and delayed images
  - Mild to moderately avid Tc-99m MDP accumulation localizing only to areas of sclerosis
  - Uptake closely corresponds to radiographic abnormality distribution
  - Scintigraphic abnormalities most often nonspecific, should be correlated with radiographs
  - Scintigraphy not necessary for diagnosis, most often found incidentally
- Thallium-201
  - Tl-201 not typically utilized in melorheostosis as radiographs pathognomonic
  - Could be used where concern for malignant degeneration exists

DDx: Mimics of Melorheostosis on Bone Scan

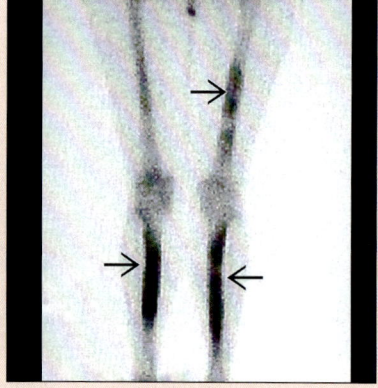

Progressive Diaphyseal Dysplasia

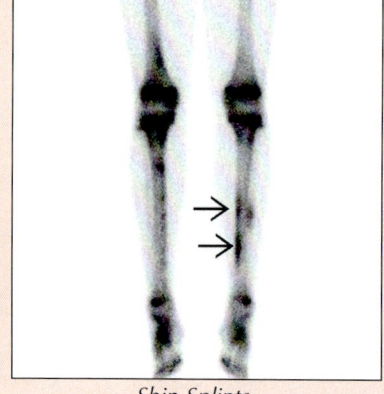

Shin Splints

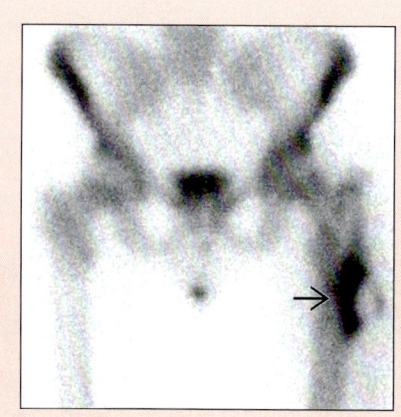

Tumor: Osteosarcoma

MELORHEOSTOSIS

Key Facts

Terminology
- Rare, benign, sclerosing bone dysplasia demonstrating dense bone formation, typically along cortex of tubular bones
- Frequently associated with scleroderma like skin change, pain, vascular change

Imaging Findings
- Well-circumscribed, undulating areas of cortical sclerosis on radiographs
- Often referred to as "dripping candle wax" pattern on plain film
- Affects tubular bones of extremities, most commonly long bones, occasionally hands and feet
- Axial skeleton involvement rare
- May be regional, crossing joints in a ray, following a sclerotome
- Bone scan: Increased blood flow on angiographic, blood pool, and delayed images
- Mild to moderately avid Tc-99m MDP accumulation localizing only to areas of sclerosis
- Uptake closely corresponds to radiographic abnormality distribution
- Best imaging tool: Radiographic appearance usually sufficiently characteristic to make diagnosis

Top Differential Diagnoses
- Tumor
- Stress Fracture
- Paget Disease
- Mixed Sclerosing Osteodystrophy
- Osteopoikilosis
- Osteopathia stria

- Will typically show increased accumulation in areas of malignancy
- Can complement MR, allowing whole body scanning and possibly better tumor margin detection, discriminating signal changes from edema

Radiographic Findings
- Pattern of distribution on radiographs useful for differentiating hyperostoses
- Dense cortical sclerosis without osseous destruction

CT Findings
- Dense cortical sclerosis typical although cancellous involvement may be present
- Soft tissue mass may be associated with abnormal bone
- CT work-up not necessary for areas of hyperostosis

MR Findings
- T1WI: Sclerotic bone shows low signal
- T2WI
  - Sclerotic regions show decreased signal
  - No marked marrow edema or destruction typical of malignancy
  - High-signal, soft-tissue mass may be discovered adjacent to affected bone
- MR useful when clinical change raises possibility of malignant degeneration
- May discover incidental abnormality when MR performed for painful extremity
- MR not required for initial evaluation of lesion discovered on radiograph

Imaging Recommendations
- Best imaging tool: Radiographic appearance usually sufficiently characteristic to make diagnosis
- Protocol advice
  - Clinical history of painful extremities warrants performance of three-phase bone scan
    - 20 mCi (740 MBq) Tc-99m MDP intravenously
    - Perform dynamic angiographic images 2 sec/frame for 1 minute of affected extremity
    - Blood pool/soft-tissue phase images of all affected immediately follow
    - Delayed osseous phase images 2-3 hours after injection of whole body with spot views of affected region
  - Perform correlation with radiographs to confirm diagnosis

DIFFERENTIAL DIAGNOSIS

Tumor
- Bone scan: Sclerotic metastasis may show increased accumulation, distribution is usually scattered
- Primary bone tumors such as osteosarcoma can be difficult to discriminate from benign melorheostosis scintigraphically

Stress Fracture
- May involve bones in a "ray" (e.g., in the foot), but radiographs will not show dense sclerosis

Paget Disease
- Scintigraphic uptake often more intense and more commonly in axial skeleton
- Usually affects an entire bone

Mixed Sclerosing Osteodystrophy
- Must identify more than one pattern of hyperostosis, which may rarely coexist, in same patient
- Other hyperostotic disorders found superimposed include osteopoikilosis, osteopathia stria
- Unlike melorheostosis, these other bone disorders do not generally show increased activity on bone scan
- Osteopoikilosis
  - Rare, frequently familial sclerosing bone dysplasia
  - Characterized by numerous rounded sclerotic densities or numerous bone islands
  - Often spares axial locations most commonly involved in metastatic disease (e.g., spine)
  - Typical locations involve shoulders and hips but can arise anywhere

MELORHEOSTOSIS

- Usually normal radiotracer uptake on bone scan and PET
- Osteopathia stria
  - Autosomal dominant or sporadic disorder causing dense linear striations of endochondral bone
  - Most often occurs in metaphysis
- These other sclerosing bone disorders do not generally show increased activity on bone scan, unlike melorheostosis
- Mixed sclerosing dysplasias may involve intramembranous and endochondral ossification sites

PATHOLOGY

General Features
- Etiology
  - Unknown etiology generally without hereditary features
    - In cases where melorheostosis overlaps with other inherited sclerosing dysplasias, a genetic component is possible, but not well-established
  - Sclerotome distribution raises possibility of etiologies such as damage of a single nerve root
- Associated abnormalities
  - Linear scleroderma
  - Mesenchymal tumors: Arteriovenous malformation, hemangioma, glomus tumor
  - Mixed sclerosing bone dystrophy: Rare coexistence of more than one pattern of hyperostosis in same patient
    - These coexisting processes may include osteopathia stria & osteopoikilosis
  - Neurofibromatosis, tuberous sclerosis
  - Other bone tumors such as osteosarcoma or metastases may rarely develop in an affected bone

Microscopic Features
- Increased angiogenesis and abundant osteoid
- Numerous osteoclasts

CLINICAL ISSUES

Presentation
- Most common signs/symptoms
  - May be asymptomatic
  - Often presents with pain and swelling of affected joints
  - Skin changes: Subcutaneous edema, erythema, abnormal pigmentation
- Other signs/symptoms
  - Deformity from muscle contractures and atrophy
  - Growth disturbances from abnormal growth plate fusion or contractures

Demographics
- Age
  - Frequently diagnosed in childhood or young adulthood but may manifest at anytime
  - Onset usually insidious, frequently diagnosed in young adulthood but may manifest any time
- Gender: M = F

Natural History & Prognosis
- Chronic, sometimes debilitating disease
- Symptoms typically progress over time with episodes of exacerbation and remission
- Rarely associated with other bone malignancy such as giant cell tumor or osteosarcoma

Treatment
- Medical therapy for symptom control
- Surgical treatment of soft tissue complications
- Infrequently, advanced cases require joint replacement or amputation

DIAGNOSTIC CHECKLIST

Consider
- Diagnosis of melorheostosis before unnecessary biopsy of associated soft tissue mass frequently seen
- Perform radiographs when bone scan shows abnormal uptake in a linear pattern in long bones or a sclerotome distribution

Image Interpretation Pearls
- Melorheostosis causes a positive bone scan unlike other benign sclerosing etiologies

SELECTED REFERENCES

1. McCay T et al: Multifocal melorheostosis. Clin Nucl Med. 31(8):504-5, 2006
2. Shivanand G et al: Melorheostosis with scleroderma. Clin Imaging. 28(3):214-5, 2004
3. Freyschmidt J: Melorheostosis: a review of 23 cases. Eur Radiol. 11(3):474-9, 2001
4. Judkiewicz AM et al: Advanced imaging of melorheostosis with emphasis on MRI. Skeletal Radiol. 30(8):447-53, 2001
5. Kalbermatten NT et al: Progressive melorheostosis in the peripheral and axial skeleton with associated vascular malformations: imaging findings over three decades. Skeletal Radiol. 30(1):48-52, 2001
6. Nishiyama Y et al: Diagnostic value of TI-201 and three-phase bone scintigraphy for bone and soft-tissue tumors. Clin Nucl Med. 25(3):200-5, 2000
7. Greenspan A et al: Bone dysplasia series. Melorheostosis: review and update. Can Assoc Radiol J. 50(5):324-30, 1999
8. Spieth ME et al: Radionuclide imaging in forme fruste of melorheostosis. Clin Nucl Med. 19(6):512-5, 1994
9. Mahoney J et al: Demonstration of increased bone metabolism in melorheostosis by multiphase bone scanning. Clin Nucl Med. 16(11):847-8, 1991
10. Drane WE: Detection of melorheostosis on bone scan. Clin Nucl Med. 12(7):548-51, 1987
11. Eugenidis N et al: Demonstration of melorheostosis by bone scan. Eur J Nucl Med. 4(1):75-6, 1979
12. Murray RO et al: Melorheostosis and the sclerotomes: a radiological correlation. Skeletal Radiol. 4(2):57-71, 1979
13. Younge D et al: Melorheostosis in children. Clinical features and natural history. J Bone Joint Surg Br. 61-B(4):415-8, 1979
14. Whyte MP et al: 99mTc-pyrophosphate bone imaging in osteopoikilosis, osteopathia striata, and melorheostosis. Radiology. 127(2):439-43, 1978

MELORHEOSTOSIS

IMAGE GALLERY

Typical

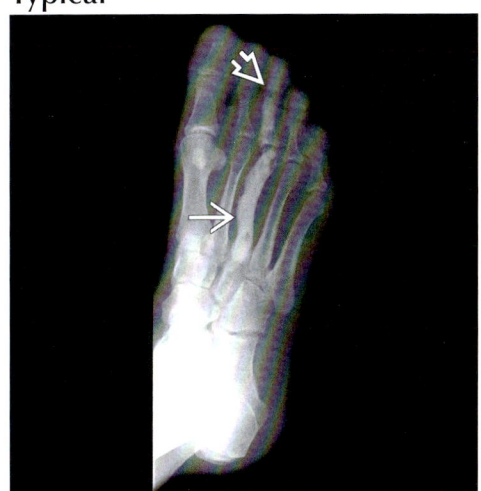

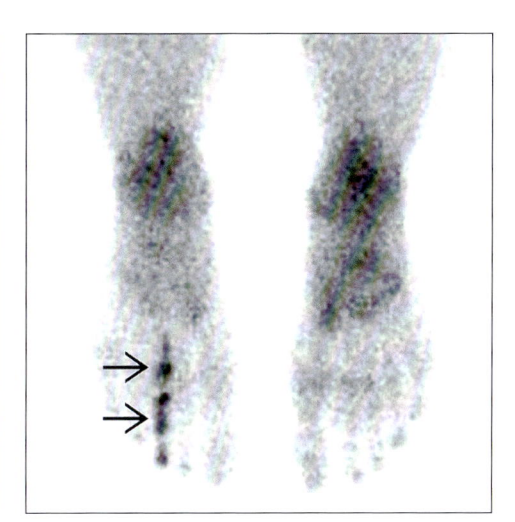

(Left) Radiograph of the foot shows dense sclerosis in the third metatarsal ➡ and phalanges ➡, typical of melorheostosis. See next image. *(Right)* Plantar bone scan in the same patient as previous image, shows moderate uptake in the third ray ➡. This appearance could be confused with stress fractures.

Typical

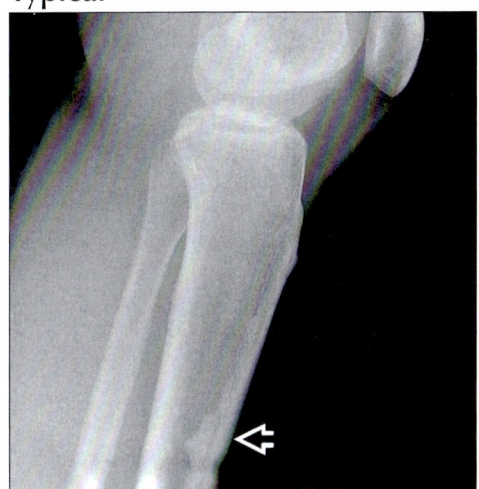

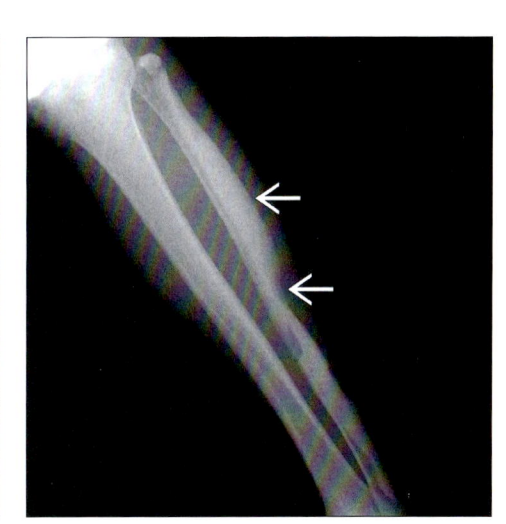

(Left) Right lateral radiograph of the knee in a patient with leg pain shows well-marginated, undulating area of cortical sclerosis ➡ from melorheostosis. *(Right)* Anterior radiograph shows diffuse sclerosis of the fibula ➡ causing bone deformity in a patient with melorheostosis. (Courtesy M. Pitt, MD).

Typical

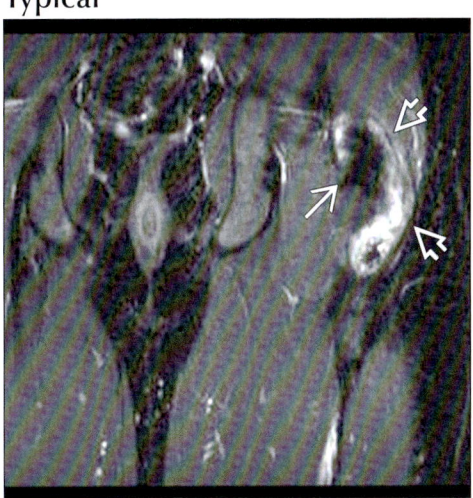

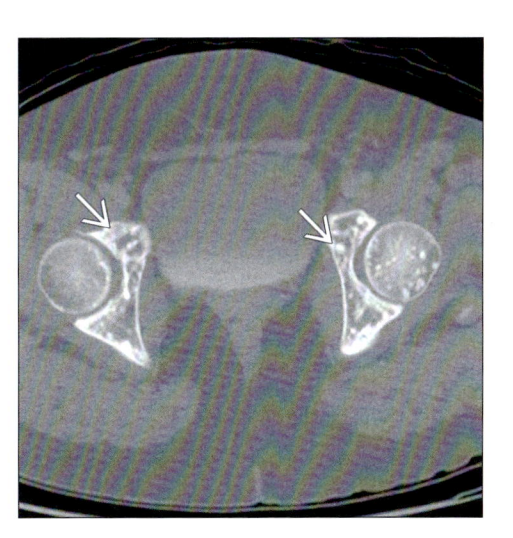

(Left) Coronal STIR MR with soft tissue high-signal ➡ around low-signal melorheostosis ➡ in the left greater trochanter, which might be confused with sarcoma or infection. (Courtesy M. Pitt, MD). See next image. *(Right)* Axial hip CT reveals multiple sclerotic "bone island" densities ➡ from osteopoikilosis, another benign sclerotic bone dysplasia which can simultaneously occur with melorheostosis.

MULTIPLE ENCHONDROMATOSES

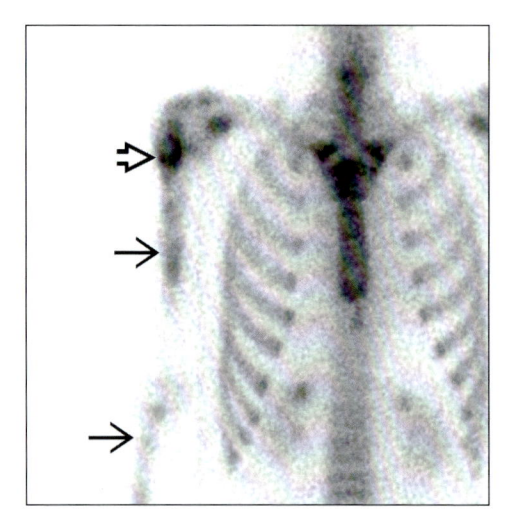

Anterior bone scan in a patient with Ollier disease shows increased activity in right upper extremity. Note intense focus of activity in proximally, due to fracture. See next image.

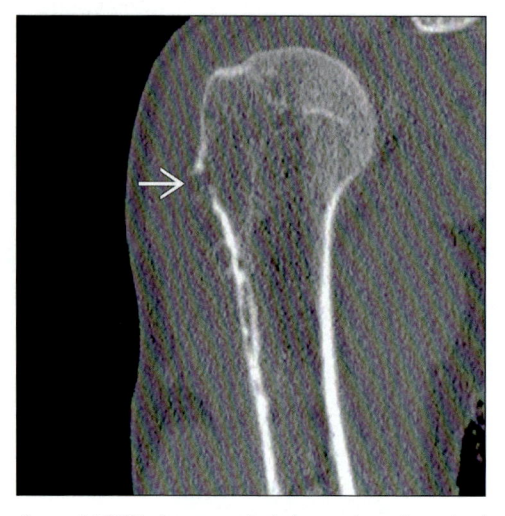

Coronal NECT shows cortical destruction of proximal humerus, corresponding to intense uptake on bone scan. This proved to be sarcomatous transformation of enchondroma in Ollier disease.

TERMINOLOGY

Definitions
- Multiple enchondromatoses: Syndromes with multiple benign intraosseous cartilaginous tumors
- Ollier disease
  - Multiple enchondromas
    - Typically asymmetric involvement of half of body
    - Bilateral involvement may occur
- Maffucci syndrome
  - Multiple enchondromas
  - Soft tissue hemangiomas, less commonly lymphangiomas
  - Unilateral involvement of hands and feet
- Metachondromatosis
  - Multiple enchondromas and osteochondromas

IMAGING FINDINGS

General Features
- Best diagnostic clue
  - Bone scan
    - Ollier disease: Increased activity in multiple bone lesions, misshapen bone, limb length discrepancy
    - Maffucci syndrome: Increased activity in multiple bone and soft tissue lesions, misshapen bone and soft tissue, limb length discrepancy
    - Metachondromatosis: Increased uptake in multiple bone lesions
- Location
  - Near growth plate in metaphysis, but may extend into diaphysis
  - Asymmetric distribution
  - Predilection for long and short tubular bones
    - May form in any bone formed by endochondral ossification
  - Common sites
    - Phalanges
    - Femur
    - Tibia
- Size
  - Variable
    - Usually < 3 cm
- Morphology
  - Depends on stage of evolution
  - Benign lesions well-defined

DDx: Mimics of Multiple Enchondromatoses

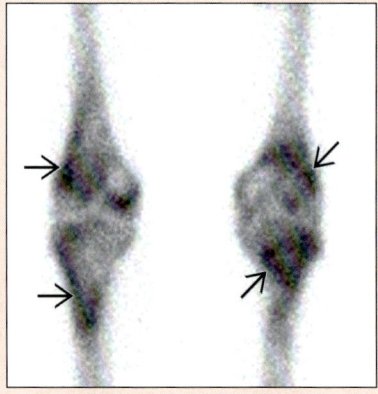

Multiple Bone Infarcts 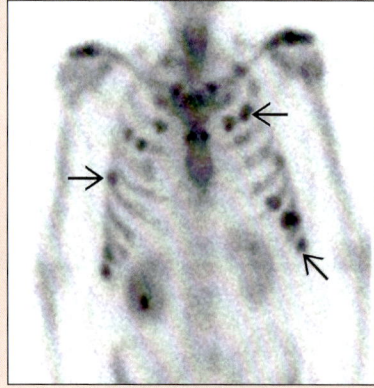 | Bone Metastases 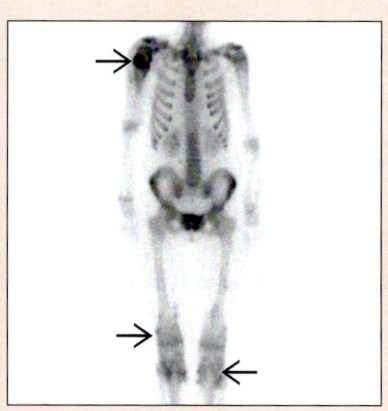 | Osteochondromatosis (MHE)

MULTIPLE ENCHONDROMATOSES

Key Facts

Terminology
- Multiple enchondromatoses: Syndromes with multiple benign intraosseous cartilaginous tumors

Imaging Findings
- Ollier disease: Increased activity in multiple bone lesions, misshapen bone, limb length discrepancy
- Maffucci syndrome: Increased activity in multiple bone and soft tissue lesions, misshapen bone and soft tissue, limb length discrepancy
- Metachondromatosis: Increased uptake in multiple bone lesions

Top Differential Diagnoses
- Bone Infarcts
- Trauma
- Multiple Hereditary Osteochondromatosis (Multiple Hereditary Exostoses, MHE)
- Bone Metastases

Clinical Issues
- Usually painless
- Multiple palpable bony masses on fingers or toes
- Unilateral or asymmetric shortening of extremities

Diagnostic Checklist
- Bone scan to identify all sites of multiple enchondromas
- Serial bone scans to identify increasing activity: Suspicious for malignant degeneration
- Bone scan to evaluate bony etiology of acute pain: Increased activity may represent pathologic fracture or malignant degeneration

---

  - Radiolucent lesion with punctate calcification
- **Imaging Recommendations**
- Best imaging tool
  - Plain films: First line study for diagnosis
    - Well-demarcated lesions with expansile remodeling
    - Cortex often thinned
    - Endosteal scalloping common
    - Internal matrix: Arc and ring configuration of cartilage
    - Soft tissue hemangiomas associated with subcutaneous calcified phleboliths in Mafucci syndrome
    - Cortical break, soft tissue mass, or rapid growth suggests malignant transformation
  - MR
    - T1WI: Low to intermediate signal
    - T2WI: Low to intermediate signal
    - Calcification results in signal void on both sequences
    - Enhancement, edema, soft tissue mass in malignant degeneration
- Protocol advice
  - Bone scan
    - Whole body planar imaging: Anterior and posterior
    - Palmar views of hands, plantar views of feet
    - Spot views of areas of interest, individual enchondromas (e.g., painful sites)
    - Three phase bone scan of acutely painful lesions: Chondrosarcoma may be hypervascular on first phase
- Imaging findings
  - CT
    - Cortex may be thinned but intact
    - Identify chondroid matrix
  - Bone scan
    - Primary diagnosis
    - Evaluate polyostotic sites
    - Evaluate for increased activity on serial bone scans (suggest malignant degeneration, pathologic fracture)
    - Visualization on bone scan depends on status of ossification
    - Chondrosarcoma has increased uptake in comparison with benign lesions

DIFFERENTIAL DIAGNOSIS

Bone Infarcts
- Well-defined sclerotic lesions
- Serpiginous borders
- Bone scan findings variable
  - Acute: Photopenic
  - Healing: Increased uptake
  - Often several lesions of variable activity, denoting various phases of healing

Trauma
- Accidental, nonaccidental
- Plain films: Multiple fractures
- Bone scan shows multiple areas increased uptake
  - Multiple sites of variable increased uptake suggest nonaccidental trauma (signifies various stages of bone healing)

Multiple Hereditary Osteochondromatosis (Multiple Hereditary Exostoses, MHE)
- Similar bone scan findings to multiple enchondromatoses
  - Variable uptake in benign lesions
  - Increased uptake in sarcomatous transformation
- Radiography used to differentiate osteochondromas from enchondromas
  - Osteochondromas have bony protuberance pointing away from joint, covered by cartilaginous cap

Bone Metastases
- Multiple sites of increased activity in patient with primary neoplasm
- Axial > appendicular skeleton

MULTIPLE ENCHONDROMATOSES

PATHOLOGY

General Features
- Genetics
  - Both Ollier disease and Maffucci syndrome nonfamilial
  - Metachondromatosis is autosomal dominant
- Epidemiology
  - Ollier syndrome: 1/100,000
  - Mafucci syndrome: Rare
- Associated abnormalities
  - Growth deformities
  - Leg length discrepancy

Gross Pathologic & Surgical Features
- Multiple oval-shaped cartilaginous nodules in osseous portions of bone
  - Blue-white hyaline cartilage mixed with yellow calcific foci
- Enchondromas may undergo gradual calcification or ossification
- Differentiation between osteochondroma and low-grade chondrosarcoma difficult
  - May require biopsy
- Hemangiomas in Mafucci syndrome appear as blue subcutaneous nodules

Microscopic Features
- Derangement of cartilaginous growth
- Migration of cartilaginous rests from epiphysis into metaphysis
- Cartilaginous rests develop into intraosseous chondromas
- Variable degree of cellularity and chondrocyte phenotype
- Calcification common

CLINICAL ISSUES

Presentation
- Most common signs/symptoms
  - Usually painless
  - Multiple palpable bony masses on fingers or toes
  - Unilateral or asymmetric shortening of extremities
- Other signs/symptoms
  - Limp secondary to leg length discrepancy
  - May become apparent at onset of walking
  - Mildly delayed bone age
  - Acute pain: Malignant transformation, pathologic fracture
  - Enlarging lesion after puberty: Malignant transformation

Demographics
- Age
  - Presents early, first decade of life
    - Rarely observed at birth
- Gender: M:F = 1:1

Natural History & Prognosis
- Ollier disease
  - Sarcomatous transformation in 25-30%
- Mafucci syndrome
  - Higher incidence of soft tissue tumors
    - CNS
    - Ovarian
    - Pancreatic
  - Varying reports of sarcomatous transformation (15-56%)
  - Soft tissue hemangioma may transform into vascular sarcoma (3-5%)
- Extent of disease variable
  - Slight involvement to severe, generalized disease
- Tendency towards spontaneous arrest at maturity

Treatment
- Asymptomatic
  - No treatment required
- Surgery may be necessary for complications
  - Pathologic fractures
  - Correction of angular deformities
    - Osteotomy
    - Limb-lengthening procedures
  - Malignant transformation
- Vascular lesions of Mafucci syndrome
  - Sclerotherapy
  - Irradiation
  - Surgical resection

DIAGNOSTIC CHECKLIST

Consider
- Bone scan to identify all sites of multiple enchondromas
- Serial bone scans to identify increasing activity: Suspicious for malignant degeneration
- Bone scan to evaluate bony etiology of acute pain: Increased activity may represent pathologic fracture or malignant degeneration

SELECTED REFERENCES

1. Martson A et al: Extensive limb lengthening in Ollier's disease: 25-year follow-up. Medicina (Kaunas). 41(10):861-6, 2005
2. Kaya H et al: Bilateral symmetrical Ollier disease and Tc-99m MDP bone scintigraphy. Clin Nucl Med. 29(7):456, 2004
3. Loder RT et al: Determination of bone age in children with cartilaginous dysplasia (multiple hereditary osteochondromatosis and Ollier's enchondromatosis). J Pediatr Orthop. 24(1):102-8, 2004
4. Nguyen BD: Ollier disease with synchronous multicentric chondrosarcomas: scintigraphic and radiologic demonstration. Clin Nucl Med. 29(1):45-7, 2004
5. Trikha V et al: Ollier's disease: characteristic Tc-99m MDP scan features. Clin Nucl Med. 28(1):56-7, 2003
6. Zwenneke Flach H et al: Best cases from the AFIP. Maffucci syndrome: radiologic and pathologic findings. Armed Forces Institutes of Pathology. Radiographics. 21(5):1311-6, 2001
7. Gruning T et al: Bone scan appearances in a case of Ollier's disease. Clin Nucl Med. 24(11):886-7, 1999
8. Chew DK et al: Ollier's disease: varus angulation at the lower femur and its management. J Pediatr Orthop. 18(2):202-8, 1998
9. Minami M et al: Bone scintigraphy in Maffucci syndrome. Radiat Med. 2(1):49-55, 1984

MULTIPLE ENCHONDROMATOSES

IMAGE GALLERY

Typical

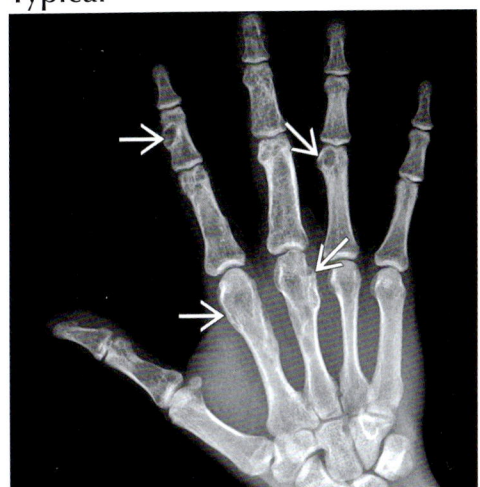

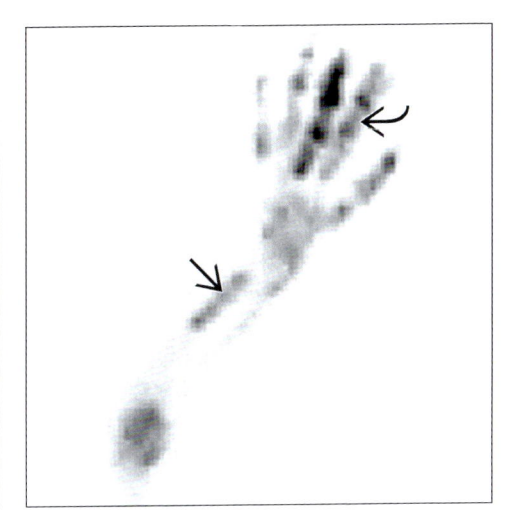

(Left) Radiograph shows multiple, well-circumscribed enchondromas ➡ involving phalanges and metacarpals of the right hand in a patient with Ollier disease. (Right) Bone scan of upper extremities shows multiple sites of involvement of the right ulna ➡ and phalanges ➡ in a patient with Ollier disease. The multiple enchondromas resulted in shortening deformity of the forearm.

Typical

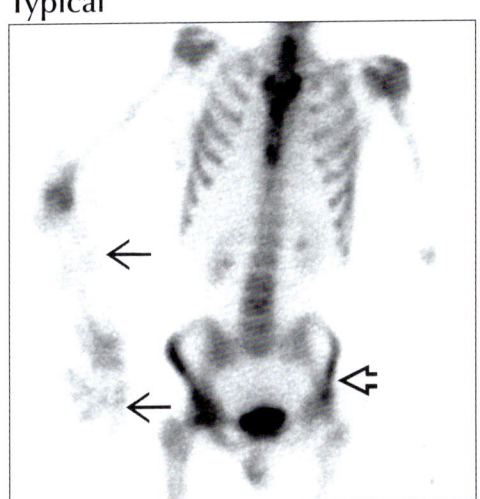

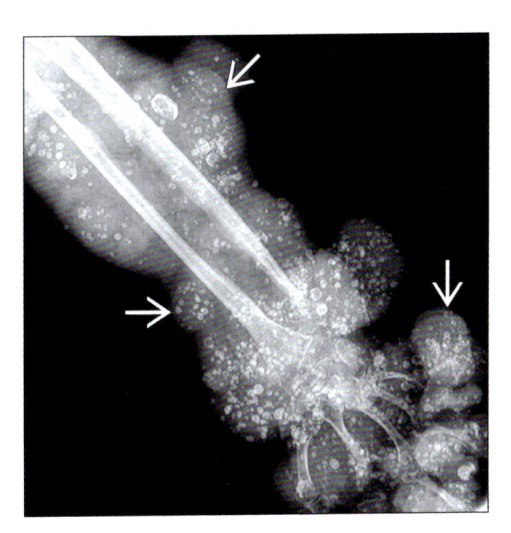

(Left) Bone scan shows mildly increased activity in soft tissues of the right upper extremity ➡ corresponding to large, deforming hemangiomas in Mafucci syndrome. Hypoplasia of left iliac bone is due to growth disturbance due to enchondromas ➡. See next. (Right) Anteroposterior radiograph multiple phleboliths ➡ in deforming hemangiomas of Mafucci syndrome.

Typical

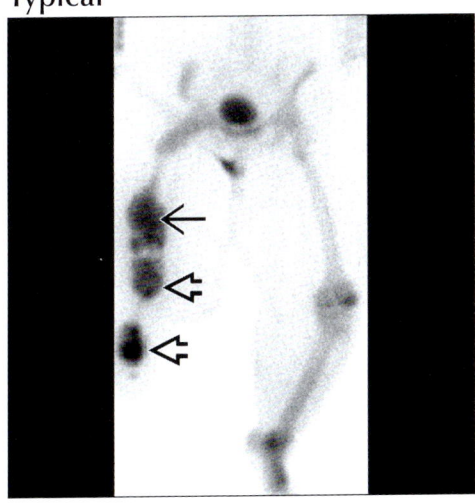

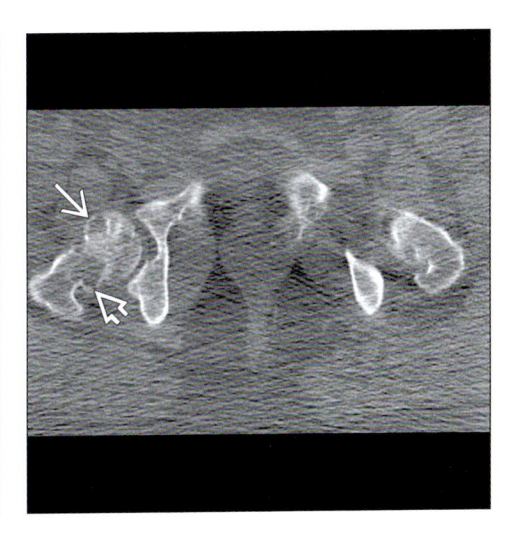

(Left) Bone scan shows severe involvement in a patient with Ollier disease. Multiple enchondromas in distal femur ➡ and proximal tibia ➡ resulted in severe growth disturbance. (Right) NECT shows well-circumscribed enchondroma of the right femoral head ➡ and neck ➡ in a patient with Ollier disease.

MULTIPLE HEREDITARY EXOSTOSES

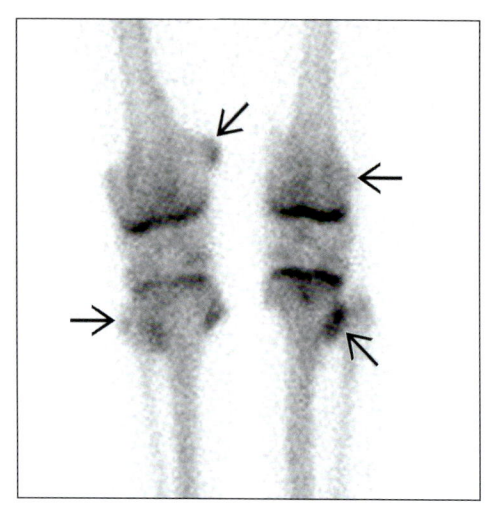

Anterior bone scan shows multiple bony excrescences ➔, extending from lower extremities in a patient with multiple hereditary exostosis. See next image.

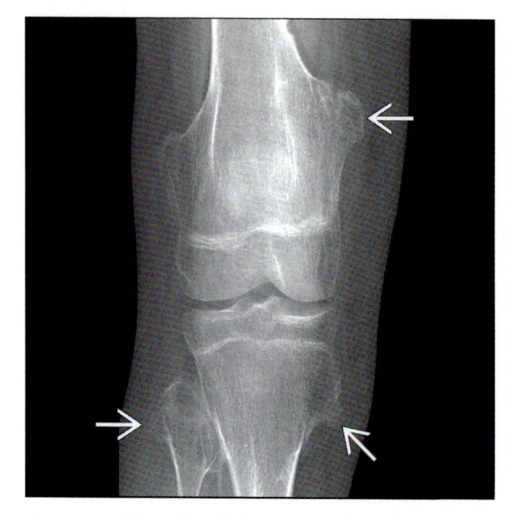

Anterior radiograph of the same patient as previous image, shows sites of sessile exostoses ➔ about the right knee.

TERMINOLOGY

Abbreviations and Synonyms
- Multiple hereditary exostoses (MHE), hereditary multiple exostosis (HME), familial osteochondromatosis, diaphyseal aclasis, multiple osteomatosis

Definitions
- Developmental disease characterized by multiple osteochondromas throughout skeleton
- Genetic basis
  - 2/3 of patients with MHE have family history

IMAGING FINDINGS

General Features
- Best diagnostic clue
  - Tc-99m MDP bone scan: Variable uptake in multiple bony excrescences
  - Radiography: Continuity of exostosis with underlying bone cortex and medullary canal = osteochondroma
  - Associated cartilaginous cap best seen on MR or CT
- Location
  - Involvement of all bones except calvarium above skull base reported
  - Incidence of bone involvement in patients with MHE
    - Scapula and rib: 40%
    - Humerus: 50-98%
    - Elbow: 35-40%
    - Wrist: 30-60%
    - Hands: 20-30%
    - Pelvis: 5-15%
    - Hips: 30-50%
    - Knees: 70-98%
    - Ankles: 25-54%
    - Feet: 10-25%
- Size: Variable, but usually between 1 and 10 cm
- Morphology
  - Sessile
    - Broad based
    - Diameter greatest at base, contiguous with cortex
  - Pedunculated
    - Diameter increases following a tapered stalk
    - Usually points away from joint

DDx: Mimics of Exostoses

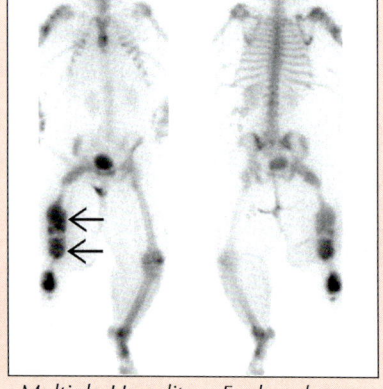

Multiple Hereditary Enchondromas

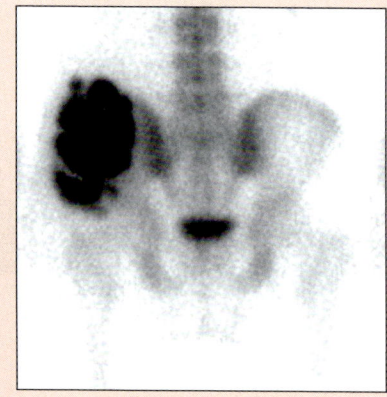

Chondrosarcoma

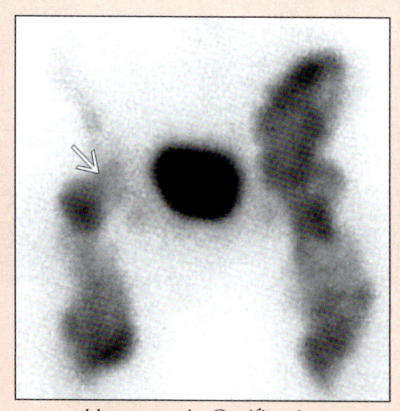

Heterotopic Ossification

MULTIPLE HEREDITARY EXOSTOSES

Key Facts

Terminology
- Developmental disease characterized by multiple osteochondromas throughout skeleton
- 2/3 of patients with MHE have family history

Imaging Findings
- Involvement of all bones except calvarium above skull base reported
- Variable activity in multiple bony excrescences on bone scan
- Degree of radiotracer uptake on bone scan directly correlates with degree of endochondral bone formation
- More uptake in younger patients, but uptake may persist beyond skeletal maturity
- Quiescent lesions (no uptake) more common in older patients
- Increased activity with malignant degeneration, fracture, post-surgical
- Bone scan: Cannot reliably differentiate between osteochondroma and chondrosarcoma
- Bone scan: High negative predictive value for absence of malignant degeneration

Clinical Issues
- Pain
- Bone deformity
- Fracture: Usually at base
- Vascular compromise
- Neurologic symptoms
- Bursae formation
- Osteochondroma may undergo malignant transformation

Nuclear Medicine Findings
- Tc-99m MDP bone scan
  - Variable activity in multiple bony excrescences on bone scan
  - Degree of radiotracer uptake on bone scan directly correlates with degree of endochondral bone formation
  - More uptake in younger patients, but uptake may persist beyond skeletal maturity
  - Quiescent lesions (no uptake) more common in older patients
  - Increased activity with malignant degeneration, fracture, post-surgical
    - Bone scan: Cannot reliably differentiate between osteochondroma and chondrosarcoma
    - Bone scan: High negative predictive value for absence of malignant degeneration

Imaging Recommendations
- Best imaging tool
  - Plain films diagnostic
    - Skeletal survey to include extremities, chest, pelvis
- Protocol advice
  - Dose: 20-30 mCi (740 MBq-1.11 GBq) Tc-99m MDP IV in adults; 250-300 µCi/kg (9-11 MBq/kg) IV in children
  - Whole body anterior/posterior scan for skeletal survey
  - High resolution spot views over areas of concern
- Correlative imaging features
  - Radiography
    - Cartilage covered exostosis on external surface of bone
    - Varying calcification of cartilage cap
    - Undertubulation of long bones (Erlenmeyer flask deformity)
    - Malignant degeneration: Development of soft tissue mass or thick, bulky cartilaginous cap
  - CT
    - NECT: Demonstrate continuity of cortical and medullary bone with exostosis
    - May show thickness of cartilaginous cap
    - Valuable with complex anatomy (e.g., pelvis, spine)
  - MR
    - T1WI: Intermediate signal
    - T2 WI: Cartilaginous cap displays high signal intensity, band of low signal (perichondrium) surrounds cap
    - Evaluate bursae

DIFFERENTIAL DIAGNOSIS

Solitary Osteochondroma
- Monostotic lesion
- Older population in contrast to MHE

Multiple Enchondromatosis
- Multiple areas of varying uptake on scintigraphy
- Often have bone deformities and limb-length discrepancy

Chondrosarcoma
- More intense uptake on scintigraphy
- Radiography: Bone destruction, growth in size after skeletal maturity
- Often associated with pain

PATHOLOGY

General Features
- Genetics
  - Autosomal dominant
    - In females may have incomplete penetrance
  - Three distinct loci: Chromosome 8, 11, 19
    - Mutations in ETX1 (8q24.1) and EXT2 (11p13): Regulate chondrocyte maturation, differentiation
- Etiology
  - Fragment of epiphyseal growth plate cartilage herniates through periosteal bone surrounding growth plate
    - Continues to grow and undergoes endochondral ossification

MULTIPLE HEREDITARY EXOSTOSES

- Results in subperiosteal excrescence with overlying cartilaginous cap
- Epidemiology
  - 1:50,000 to 1:100,000 in Western population
  - Higher incidence (100-1,310 per 100,000) in isolated populations
    - Chamorros (Guam)
    - Ojibway Indian community of Pauingassi (Manitoba, Canada)

Gross Pathologic & Surgical Features

- Cartilage cap
  - Shiny bluish gray surface
  - Thickness
    - Young patients: 1 to 3 cm
    - Adults: Absent to a few mm
  - Lobulated surface, cauliflower-like, ± calcifications

Microscopic Features

- Cartilage cap merges with underlying bone
- Covered with thin layer of fibrous tissue that functions as perichondrium
- Cap resembles growth plate (columns of chondrocytes that mature)
- Endochondral ossification leads to medullary bone, typically with yellow marrow

CLINICAL ISSUES

Presentation

- Most common signs/symptoms
  - Pain
  - Bone deformity
    - Most commonly first noticed on conspicuous sites such as tibia or scapula
    - Osseous bowing and malalignment
    - Limb-length discrepancy
    - Valgus deformities of knees, ankles
    - Asymmetry of pectoral, pelvic girdles
    - Bowing of radius with radial deviation of wrist
    - Subluxation of radiocapitellar joint
    - Extrinsic pressure on adjacent bone
    - Short stature
    - Amount of involvement and deformity of forearm and distal leg measures overall disease extent
- Other signs/symptoms
  - Fracture: Usually at base
  - Vascular compromise
    - From vessel displacement, stenosis, or occlusion from adjacent osteochondroma
    - Pseudoaneurysms reported due to pressure effects
  - Neurologic symptoms
    - Peripheral: Compression, entrapment neuropathy
    - Central (skull, spine): Cranial nerve deficits, radiculopathy, spinal stenosis, cauda equina syndrome, myelomalacia
  - Bursae formation
    - Between osteochondroma and surrounding soft tissue (exostosis bursata), especially at sites of friction (scapula, hip, shoulder)
    - Bursae may exhibit inflammatory or infectious change

Demographics

- Age
  - Exostoses diagnosed in first decade in > 80% of patients with MHE
  - Almost all patients diagnosed by 12 years
- Gender: M:F = 1.5:1

Natural History & Prognosis

- Patients with limited, small lesions may remain asymptomatic
- Lesions enlarge while physes open, tend to stop growing with skeletal maturity
- Spontaneous regression occasionally
- Short stature common (most heights 0.5-1.0 standard deviations below mean)
- Osteochondroma may undergo malignant transformation
  - Most are low-grade chondrosarcomas
    - Long-term survival good (70-90%)
    - Worse prognosis with dedifferentiated lesions
  - Prevalence in MHE 3-5% (vs. 1% in solitary osteochondromas)
  - Continued lesion growth and hyaline cartilage cap > 1.5 cm suggests malignant transformation
  - Occurs at earlier age in MHE patients (average age 25-30 years) than in patients with isolated osteochondromas (average age 50-55 years)
  - Metastases unusual (3-7%)
    - Most often to lungs

Treatment

- Treatment based on severity, complications
- Small lesions followed, supportive care
- Surgery
  - Osteochondroma resection
    - Resected at base, including overlying perichondrium to reduce recurrence
    - Overall recurrence rate 2%
  - Correction of associated deformities
- Multiple surgeries common (average 2.7 per patient)
- Continued clinical and radiographic surveillance necessary throughout life
- In case of malignant transformation
  - Wide surgical resection and limb salvage
  - Local recurrence depends on margin adequacy

DIAGNOSTIC CHECKLIST

Consider

- Skeletal survey in suspected cases
- Continued growth or onset of pain in adults: Suspect malignancy

SELECTED REFERENCES

1. Epstein DA et al: Bone scintigraphy in hereditary multiple exostoses. AJR Am J Roentgenol. 130(2):331-3, 1978

MULTIPLE HEREDITARY EXOSTOSES

IMAGE GALLERY

Typical

Typical

Typical

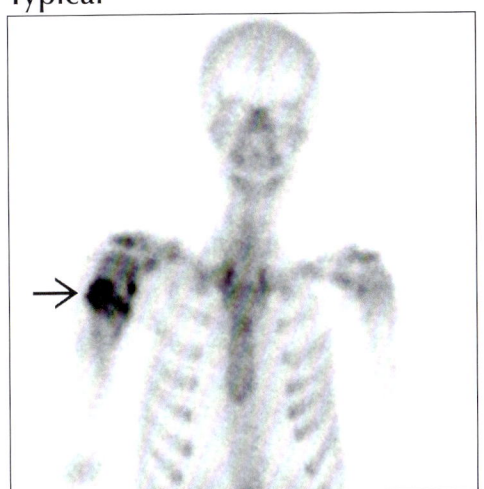

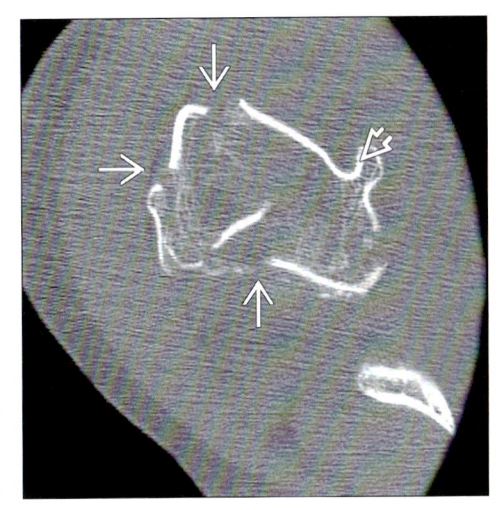

(Left) Anterior bone scan shows intense uptake in humeral fracture ➡ through the base of the osteochondroma in a patient with MHE. See next image. (Right) NECT in the same patient as previous image, shows a fracture of the proximal humerus ➡ corresponding to intense uptake on the bone scan. Note adjacent small osteochondroma ➡.

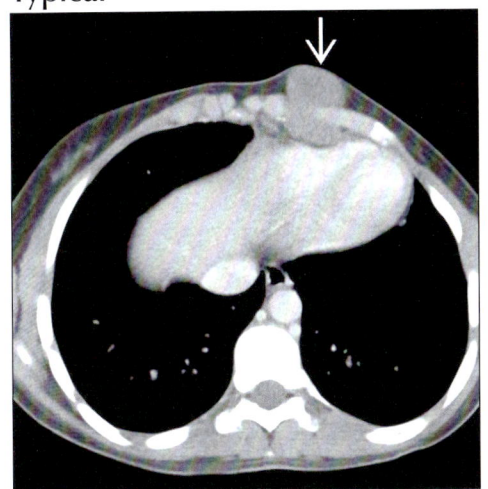

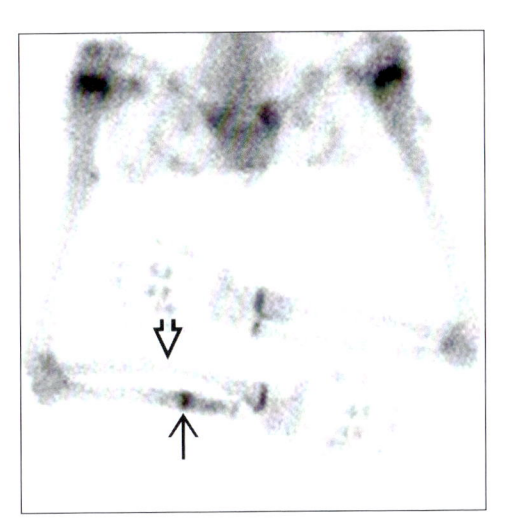

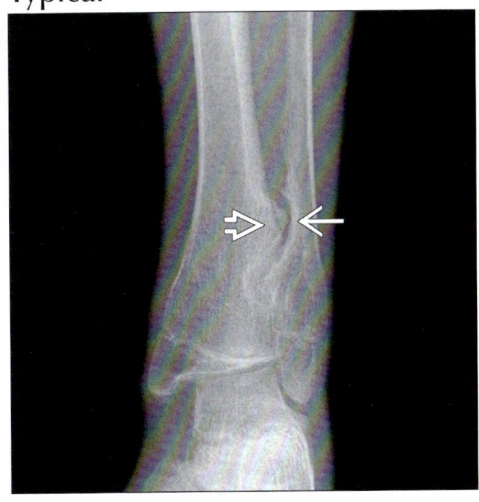

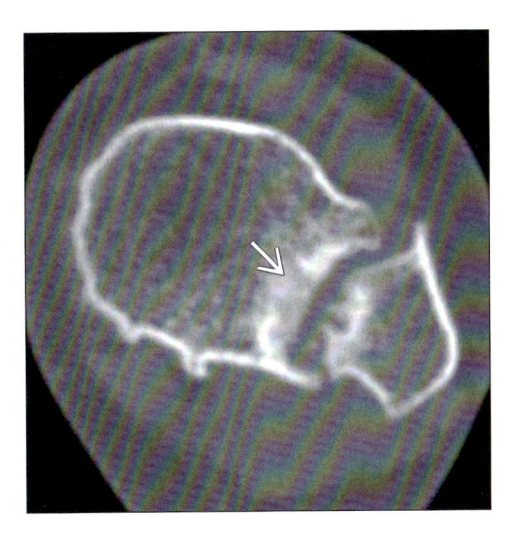

(Left) Axial CECT shows a soft tissue, chest wall mass ➡ in a 14 year old girl with MHE. Pathology revealed low grade chondrosarcoma. (Right) Spot views of forearms on bone scan shows bowing of radius ➡ and post-surgical change in ulna ➡, performed to lengthen ulna and relieve radial deformity.

(Left) Posterior radiographs of the right ankle show osteochondroma of the distal tibia ➡ with scalloping of the fibula ➡. Pressure effects can involve bones, nerves or vascular structures. See next image. (Right) NECT in the same patient as previous image, shows interdigitation of the lesion ➡ along the syndesmotic ligament.

OSSEOUS NECROSIS

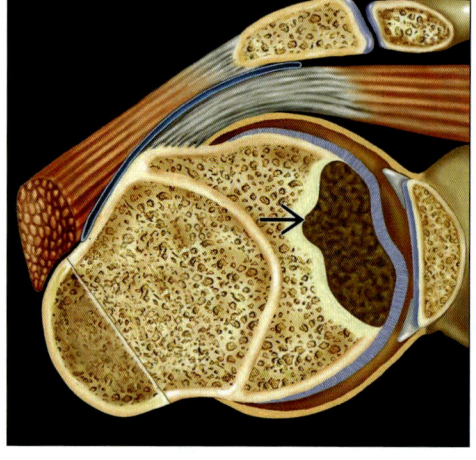

Graphic of shoulder shows avascular necrosis of humeral head ➔. The humeral and femoral heads are most common sites of AVN.

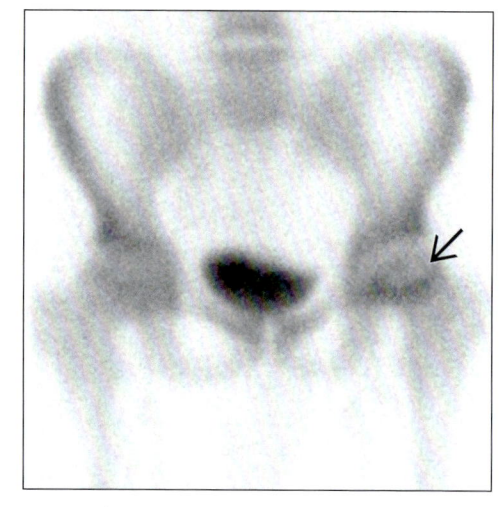

Anterior bone scan shows central photopenic defect with reactive rim of left femoral head ➔ in 15 year old boy with history of steroid use and acute hip pain. This is an early bone scan finding of AVN.

TERMINOLOGY

Abbreviations and Synonyms
- Avascular necrosis (AVN), aseptic necrosis, bone infarct, osteonecrosis, osseous necrosis, ischemic necrosis

Definitions
- Ischemic death of trabecular bone and marrow

IMAGING FINDINGS

General Features
- Best diagnostic clue: MR: T1 peripheral, geographic ↓ signal; T2 ↓ signal peripheral border, ↑ signal inner border
- Location
  - Femoral head, humeral head most common
  - Scaphoid
  - Knee: Medial femoral condyle (Blount disease) in pediatrics; idiopathic osteonecrosis (elderly females)
  - Lunate (Kienbock disease)
  - Tarsal navicular (Köhler disease)
  - Talus
  - Proximal tibia
  - Vertebrae
  - Small bones hands and feet
  - Pelvis
  - Metatarsal head (Freiberg disease)
- Morphology: Humeral/femoral head: Linear/wedge-shaped photopenia

Nuclear Medicine Findings
- Bone Scan
  - Bone scan 80-85% sensitive with use of SPECT
  - Vascular phase
    - Photopenic defect
    - May have donut sign due to surrounding hyperemia, adjacent synovitis
    - SPECT imaging helpful in unmasking hyperemia from avascular area
  - Reparative phase
    - Photopenia diminishes
    - Increased activity due to osteoblastic response
  - May see involvement of multiple joints in patients with underlying disease (e.g., sickle cell disease)
- Tc-99m Sulfur Colloid

DDx: Clinical Mimics of AVN

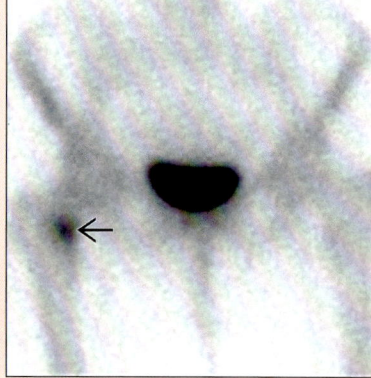

Stress Fracture

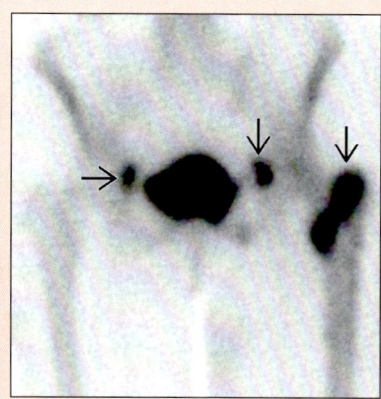

Insufficiency Fractures

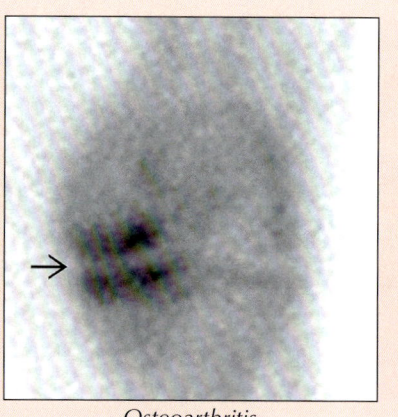

Osteoarthritis

OSSEOUS NECROSIS

Key Facts

Terminology
- Ischemic death of trabecular bone and marrow

Imaging Findings
- Best diagnostic clue: MR: T1 peripheral, geographic ↓ signal; T2 ↓ signal peripheral border, ↑ signal inner border
- Morphology: Humeral/femoral head: Linear/wedge-shaped photopenia
- Bone scan 80-85% sensitive with use of SPECT
- May see involvement of multiple joints in patients with underlying disease (e.g., sickle cell disease)

Top Differential Diagnoses
- Fracture
- Transient Osteoporosis
- Infection
- Bone Tumor
- Bursitis
- Osteoarthritis

Clinical Issues
- Pain, initially with sudden onset
- Warmth, tenderness, erythema sometimes seen with acute infarct
- Male > female (up to 8x in most locations)
- Spontaneous osteonecrosis knee: Elderly females
- Symptomatic disease may lead to structural failure and severe secondary arthritis
- Asymptomatic disease may resolve
- AVN of hip: Increased risk of involvement of opposite hip

- Defines distribution of viable red bone marrow ("marrow map"), reticuloendothelial system
- Symptomatic sites of AVN: Decreased activity immediately after vaso-occlusive event
- Asymptomatic sites of AVN: Decreased activity in area of old bone infarct
- Useful in identifying patients with expanded marrow, such as sickle cell patients
- Limitations of use of Tc-99m sulfur colloid in AVN
  - Developmental regression of red marrow in extremeties (distal to proximal): Adult pattern is axial and proximal appendicular
  - Elderly: May lose red marrow signal in proximal femurs, humeri; may be asymmetrical
  - Loss of red marrow signal with infection, trauma
- Dose: 8-10 mCi (296-370 MBq), image 20-30 min post injection

Radiographic Findings
- Early subchondral lucency → sclerosis → collapse → secondary degenerative change

CT Findings
- Osteopenia → subchondral lucency → sclerosis
- Less sensitive than MR

MR Findings
- T1WI: Hypointense peripheral band outlining central region
- T2WI: Hyperintense inner border (granulation tissue) parallel to hypointense periphery (sclerosis, fibrosis)

Imaging Recommendations
- Best imaging tool
  - MR usually most sensitive
    - First line evaluation
  - Bone scan more sensitive than plain film
    - Useful in identifying multiple sites of involvement
    - If MR indeterminate
- Protocol advice
  - Dose: Tc-99m MDP bone scan
    - Pediatrics: (Age + 1/Age + 7) x adult dose
    - Adult: 20-30 mCi (740 MBq-1.11 GBq)
    - Inject away from site of interest
  - Angiographic, static and delayed planar images
    - Anterior and posterior images
    - High resolution or pinhole collimator
    - Symmetric positioning of both affected and unaffected opposite region
    - Beware bladder artifact; due to high counts in bladder, backprojection reconstruction artifact can ⇒ loss of counts in adjacent bones, may simulate AVN of hip
  - SPECT
    - Increases sensitivity through improved spatial resolution and enhanced tissue contrast
    - If imaging hip, empty bladder first

DIFFERENTIAL DIAGNOSIS

Fracture
- History of trauma, weakened bone
- Hyperemia and delayed increased uptake

Transient Osteoporosis
- Bone marrow edema syndrome: Femoral head and neck
- Most common in third and fourth decades, may be seen in 3rd trimester of pregnancy
- Hyperemia and diffuse increased uptake of radiotracer
  - Involves femoral head, neck, intertrochanteric region
  - Acetabulum spared
- Resolves over 10-12 month period

Infection
- Acute hematogenous osteomyelitis (pediatric) and chronic post-traumatic osteomyelitis (adult)
- Pain and fever
- Positive uptake of radiotracer on three phase bone scan
- Often involves both sides of joint

Bone Tumor
- Metastasis

OSSEOUS NECROSIS

- ○ Medullary marrow replaced
- ○ Most often from lung, breast, prostate, renal and thyroid malignancies
- ○ Typically increased uptake; extensively lytic or anaplastic lesions may have decreased uptake
- Primary bone tumor: Chondrosarcoma, osteosarcoma
  - ○ Intense increased uptake

Bursitis
- Inflammation of bursa
- Associated with overuse
- Diffuse hyperemia and increased uptake in area of bursa

Osteoarthritis
- Increased uptake in weight bearing location
- Older population
- Increased uptake in periarticular distribution

PATHOLOGY

General Features
- Etiology
  - ○ Traumatic
    - Disrupted blood supply at time of injury
    - Follows subcapital femoral neck fracture (60-75%), dislocation of hip joint (25%), scaphoid fracture (30-40% in cases with nonunion)
    - Slipped capital femoral epiphysis (15-40%)
    - Anatomic factors may predispose
    - Kienbock disease more common with ulna minus variant wrist
  - ○ Non-traumatic
    - Corticosteroids (endogenous or exogenous use)
    - Alcohol abuse
    - Idiopathic (spontaneous osteonecrosis knees, Legg-Calve-Perthes, Freiberg disease)
    - Pancreatitis: Fat emboli
    - Organ transplant
    - Sickle cell anemia
    - Anti phospholipid antibodies
    - Vasculitis: SLE, collagen-vascular disease, prior radiation
    - HIV infection
    - Caisson disease: Nitrogen bubbles occlude arterioles
    - Gaucher disease
    - Coagulopathy

Gross Pathologic & Surgical Features
- Depends on stage of infarct
- Pale bone marrow with varying degrees of necrosis
- Cystic degeneration in area of infarct
- Secondary osteoarthritis after structural failure and collapse of articular surface

Microscopic Features
- Early
  - ○ Cellular ischemia with death of hematopoietic cells, osteocytes and lipocytes
- Repair
  - ○ Necrotic debris in intertrabecular spaces
  - ○ Ingrowth of mesenchymal cells and capillaries
  - ○ Vascular granulation tissue separates dead bone from adjacent live bone
  - ○ Mesenchymal cells differentiate into osteoblasts
  - ○ Eventual new layers of bone formation

CLINICAL ISSUES

Presentation
- Most common signs/symptoms
  - ○ Clinical features depend on age of disease
    - Pain, initially with sudden onset
    - Warmth, tenderness, erythema sometimes seen with acute infarct
- Other signs/symptoms: May be asymptomatic

Demographics
- Age
  - ○ Depends on underlying disease
    - Sickle cell disease: Presents in first decades of life
    - Legg-Calve-Perthes: Young boys
    - AVN of hip: 20-50 years
- Gender
  - ○ Male > female (up to 8x in most locations)
  - ○ Spontaneous osteonecrosis knee: Elderly females

Natural History & Prognosis
- Symptomatic disease may lead to structural failure and severe secondary arthritis
- Asymptomatic disease may resolve
- AVN of hip: Increased risk of involvement of opposite hip

Treatment
- Treat underlying disease
- Idiopathic: Treat conservatively and symptomatically
  - ○ Hydration, analgesics
- Conservative
  - ○ Lower extremities: No weight-bearing
  - ○ Analgesics
- Decompression: With or without bone-grafting
- Osteotomy: Moves area of necrosis away from site of maximum weight bearing
- Joint replacement: For advanced disease
- Diphosphonate therapy

DIAGNOSTIC CHECKLIST

Consider
- Bone scan more sensitive than plain films
  - ○ Use high resolution/pinhole collimators or SPECT for most sensitive bone scan
  - ○ Bone scan less sensitive than MR in most cases
- Bone scan used to identify multiple sites of involvement in patients with risk factors

SELECTED REFERENCES
1. Kim KY et al: The diagnostic value of triple head single photon emission computed tomography (3H-SPECT) in avascular necrosis of the femoral head. Int Orthop. 17(3):132-8, 1993

OSSEOUS NECROSIS

IMAGE GALLERY

Typical

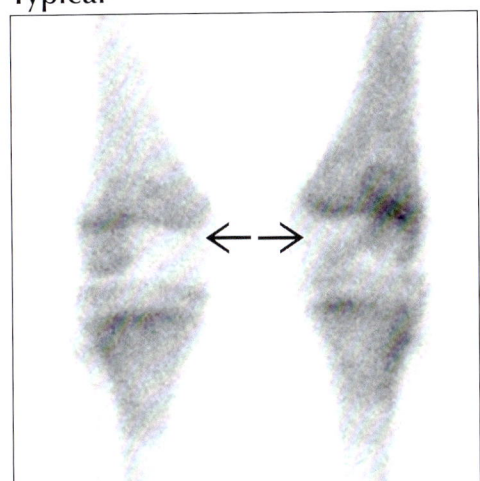

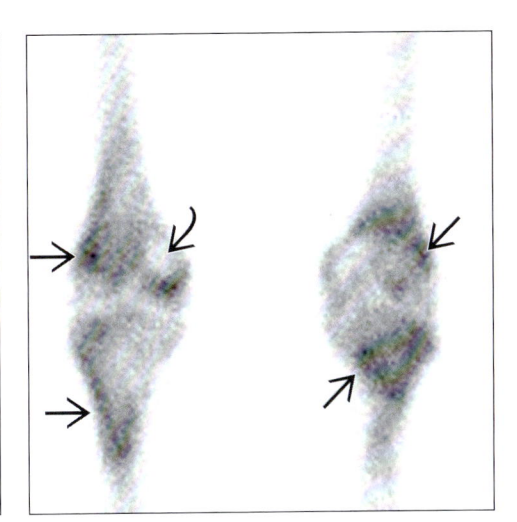

(Left) Anterior bone scan of the knees in a patient with a history of steroid use and acute knee pain shows photopenic defects in the medial femoral condyles ⇨, consistent with early phase AVN. *(Right)* Anterior bone scan of the knees in a patient with sickle cell disease shows multiple bone infarcts in various phases. Note early phase photopenia ⇨ as well as foci of increased activity ⇨ indicative of reparative phase.

Typical

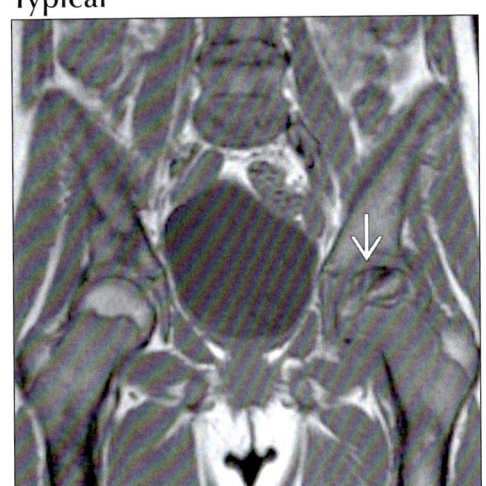

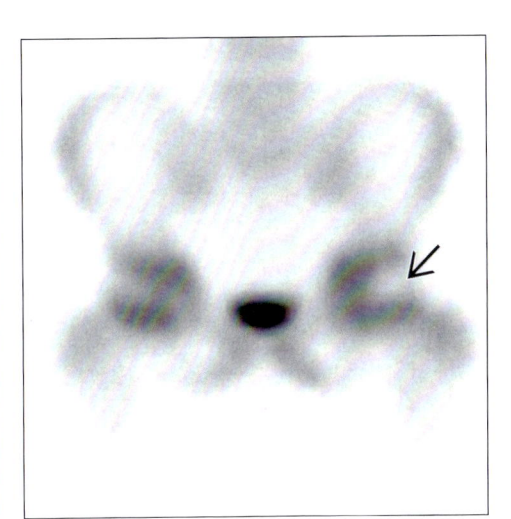

(Left) Coronal MR shows altered marrow signal in the left femoral epiphysis ⇨, typical appearance of AVN. *(Right)* Anterior bone scan shows photopenic AVN in the left femoral epiphysis ⇨ in a young boy with early Legg-Calve-Perthes disease.

Typical

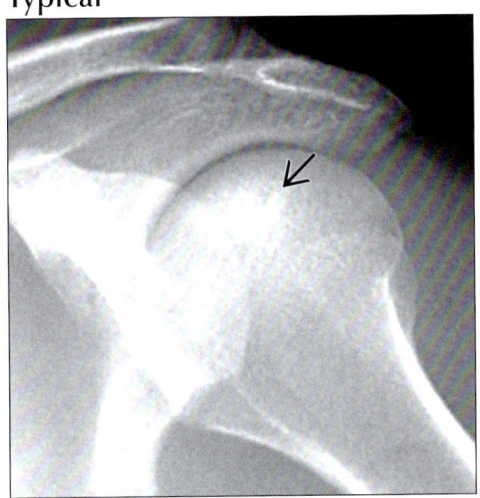

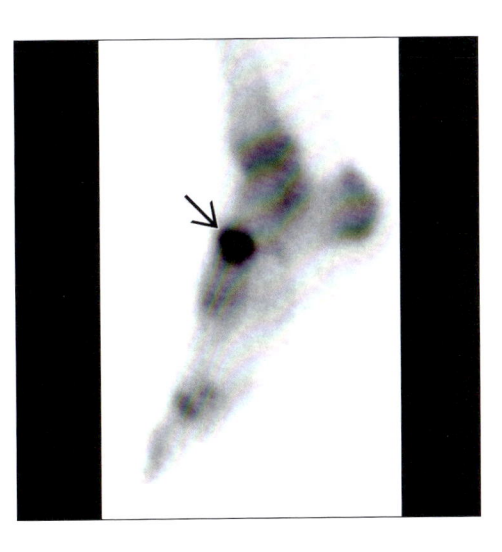

(Left) Radiograph shows area of sclerosis ⇨ in a sickle cell patient with prior humeral head infarction. *(Right)* Bone scan of the feet shows increased activity in the left navicular ⇨ in a patient with advanced Köhler disease (AVN of tarsal navicular).

LEGG-CALVE PERTHES DISEASE

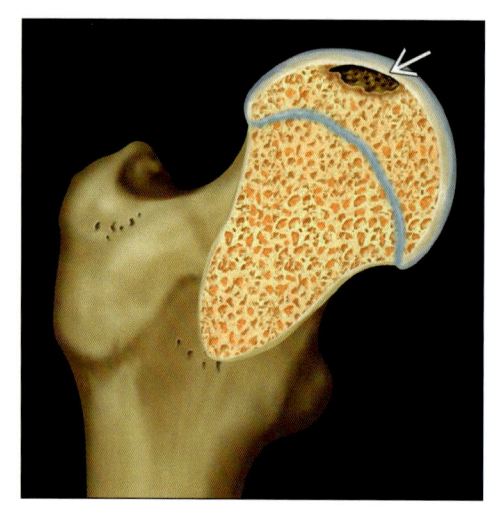

Coronal graphic shows subchondral necrosis ➔ in proximal superior lateral aspect of the epiphysis in early Legg-Calve Perthes disease.

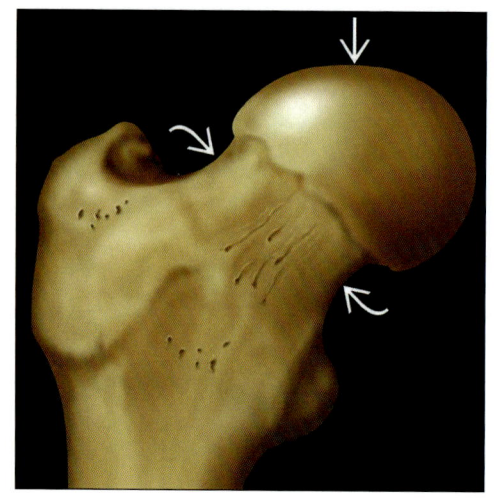

Coronal graphic shows late changes of Legg-Calve Perthes disease, with flattening of the femoral head (coxa plana) ➔ and shortening/thickening of the femoral neck (coxa magna) ➔.

TERMINOLOGY

Definitions
- Legg-Calve Perthe (LCP) disease: Avascular or ischemic necrosis of proximal femoral epiphysis

IMAGING FINDINGS

General Features
- Best diagnostic clue: Photopenic defect in lateral aspect of proximal femoral epiphysis on bone scan

Nuclear Medicine Findings
- Bone Scan
  - Early phase: Photopenic defect in proximal femoral epiphysis, especially laterally
  - Healing phase: Revascularization
    - Lateral stripe sign: Increased activity along lateral aspect of epiphysis; better prognosis
  - Healing phase: Neovascularization
    - Base filling or mushroom pattern (extension of activity through growth plate into base of epiphysis); worse prognosis
  - After healing: Joint space may be widened due to small epiphysis or cartilage hypertrophy

Radiographic Findings
- Radiography
  - Effusion; flat, sclerotic capital epiphysis; metaphyseal irregularity; joint space widening
  - Relatively insensitive: Radiographic changes can be delayed up to 5 months after ischemia onset

MR Findings
- T1WI: Hypointense intraarticular effusion, irregularity along periphery of ossific nucleus, linear hypointensity traversing femoral ossification center
- T2WI: Physeal cartilage ± hyperintense in early stage, hyperintense joint effusion

Imaging Recommendations
- Best imaging tool: Bone scan is highly sensitive (98%) and specific (95%) for LCP
- Protocol advice
  - Position patient symmetrically
  - Magnified, pinhole, SPECT images useful
  - Static anterior and posterior images

DDx: Other Causes of Hip Pain in Children

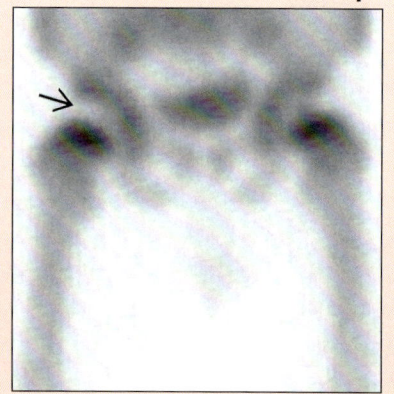

Early Septic Joint (Cold)

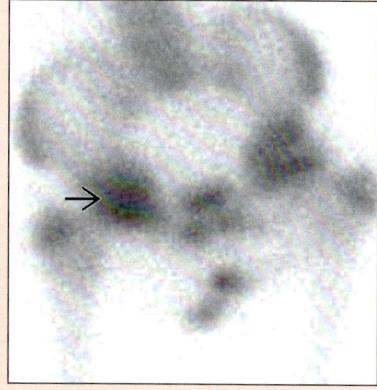

Late Septic Joint/Osteomyelitis (Hot)

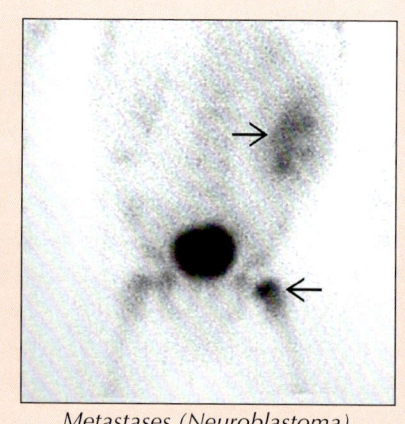

Metastases (Neuroblastoma)

LEGG-CALVE PERTHES DISEASE

Key Facts

Imaging Findings
- Best diagnostic clue: Photopenic defect in lateral aspect of proximal femoral epiphysis on bone scan
- Best imaging tool: Bone scan is highly sensitive (98%) and specific (95%) for LCP

Top Differential Diagnoses
- Toxic Synovitis
- Septic Hip
- Juvenile Chronic Arthritis (JCA)
- Juvenile Osteonecrosis
- Slipped Capital Femoral Epiphysis
- Osteoid Osteoma

Clinical Issues
- Most common signs/symptoms: Limp; groin pain, referred thigh or knee pain
- Age: 3-12 years; median 7 years
- Gender: M:F = 4-5:1

DIFFERENTIAL DIAGNOSIS

Toxic Synovitis
- Bone scan: Mild diffuse ↑ uptake throughout hip joint

Septic Hip
- Bone scan: Early may be cold (↑ pressure); later diffusely ↑ uptake through out hip joint on all phases

Juvenile Chronic Arthritis (JCA)
- Bone scan: ↑ Flow and accumulation in around joint

Juvenile Osteonecrosis
- Similar bone scan findings to LCP

Slipped Capital Femoral Epiphysis
- Bone scan: ↑ Uptake in hip joint due to synovitis; decreased uptake in epiphysis due to avascular necrosis

Osteoid Osteoma
- Positive three phase bone scan in focal bone lesion

PATHOLOGY

General Features
- Etiology: Insufficiency of capital epiphyseal blood supply with physis acting as a barrier
- Epidemiology
  - 1:1,200 children < 15 years
  - 15 to 20% bilateral

CLINICAL ISSUES

Presentation
- Most common signs/symptoms: Limp; groin pain, referred thigh or knee pain

Demographics
- Age: 3-12 years; median 7 years
- Gender: M:F = 4-5:1

DIAGNOSTIC CHECKLIST

Image Interpretation Pearls
- Bone scan: Confirm high-quality, magnified, pinhole or SPECT images of hips
- Early phase on bone scan: Photopenia in lateral femoral capital epiphysis
- Healing phase on bone scan: Increased uptake laterally or through epiphyseal plate

SELECTED REFERENCES

1. Comte F et al: Confirmation of the early prognostic value of bone scanning and pinhole imaging of the hip in Legg-Calve-Perthes disease. J Nucl Med. 44(11):1761-6, 2003
2. Connolly LP et al: Assessing the limping child with skeletal scintigraphy. J Nucl Med. 39(6):1056-61, 1998

IMAGE GALLERY

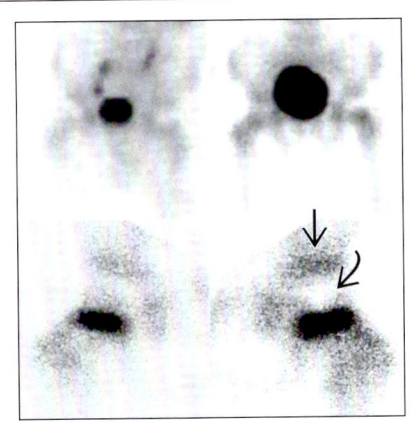

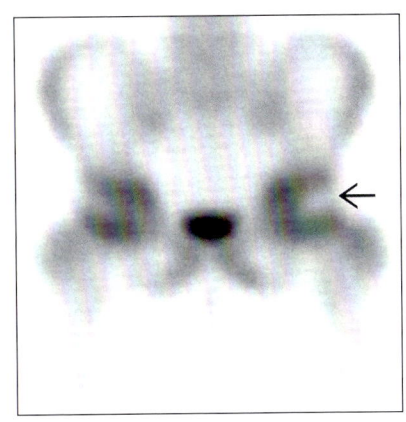

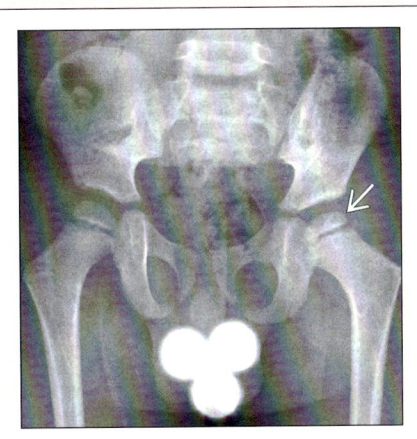

(Left) Three phase bone scan shows improved sensitivity for detection of LCP on pinhole (lower) vs. standard (upper) views. Note photopenia of lateral femoral epiphysis ➔, uptake in acetabulum (associated synovitis) ➔. *(Center)* Bone scan shows photopenia ➔ of the lateral aspect of the left femoral epiphysis in early LCP. See next image. *(Right)* Early LCP may show slight sclerosis of femoral head ➔. Later findings: Fragmentation and collapse → reconstitution with coxa plana/magna deformity → late degenerative change.

JOINT PROSTHESES, PAINFUL

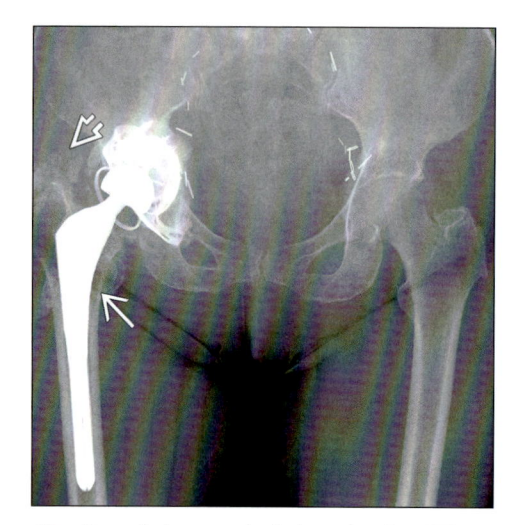

AP radiograph shows total right hip arthroplasty ➡ with no loosening or displacement in patient with acute right hip pain. Note heterotopic bone ➡. See next image.

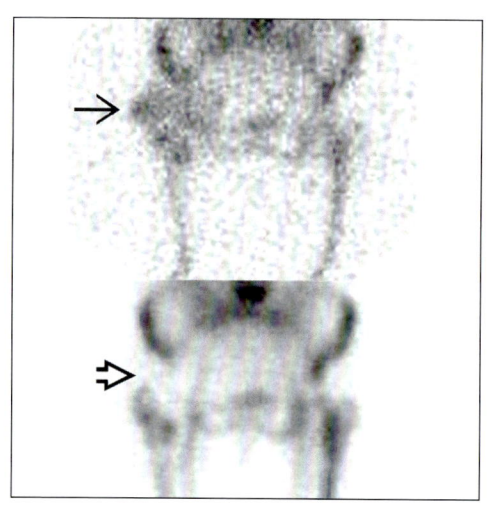

Labeled leukocyte scan shows ↑ activity ➡ around right hip prothesis. Tc-99m sulfur colloid marrow map shows no correlative marrow uptake ➡. Discordant findings support diagnosis of infection.

TERMINOLOGY

Definitions
- Acute, subacute, chronic pain after arthroplasty due to several etiologies (e.g., infection, loosening, fracture)

IMAGING FINDINGS

General Features
- Location
  - Hip, knee most common
  - Shoulder, elbow, wrist, metacarpophalangeal, ankle

Nuclear Medicine Findings
- Bone scan: All joint prostheses show ↑ activity initially
  - Up to 20% continue to have ↑ activity at 1 year
  - Hip prostheses: Mildly ↑ activity in marrow space distally common due to normal marrow elements
  - Knee prostheses commonly show persistently ↑ activity (esp. medial tibial component)

Imaging Recommendations
- Best imaging tool
  - Three phase bone scan: Evaluate hyperemia, blood pool, delayed uptake in painful joint
    - Prosthetic joint infection: + On all phases of three phase bone scan, diffusely increased uptake about prosthesis
    - Loosening: ± On first two phases, focal increased activity at prosthesis/joint interface on delayed image
    - Fracture: ± On first two phases, depending on chronicity; focal periprosthetic ↑ uptake on delayed image
  - Labeled leukocyte scintigraphy: + In infection; however, in violated bone, labeled leukocytes may localize in normal marrow elements
    - Tc-99m sulfur colloid scintigraphy: Marrow in unusual locations post-surgery; + uptake in normal, uninfected marrow elements

DIFFERENTIAL DIAGNOSIS

Prosthetic Joint Infection
- Infection rate, by prosthesis: Shoulder < 2%, hip < 1%, knee < 1%

DDx: Other Causes of Painful Joints

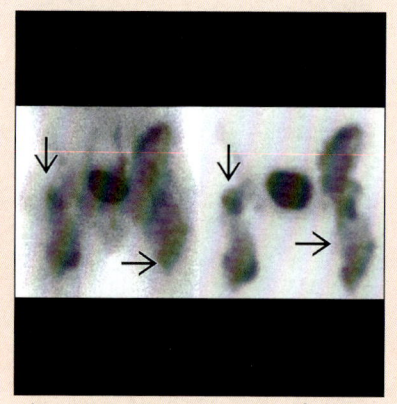

Immature Heterotopic Ossification

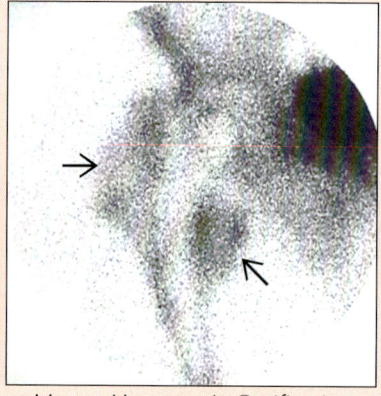

Mature Heterotopic Ossification

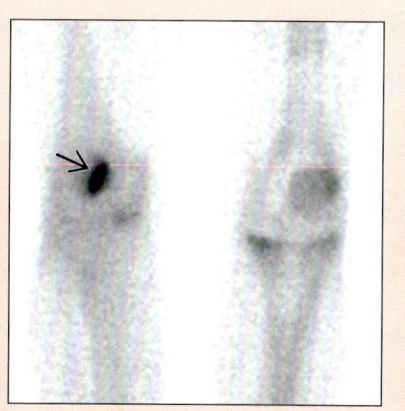

Patellar Fracture

JOINT PROSTHESES, PAINFUL

Key Facts

Imaging Findings
- Prosthetic joint infection: + On all phases of three phase bone scan, diffusely increased uptake about prosthesis
- Loosening: ± On first two phases, focal increased activity at prosthesis/joint interface on delayed image
- Fracture: ± On first two phases, depending on chronicity; focal periprosthetic ↑ uptake on delayed image
- Labeled leukocyte scintigraphy: + In infection; however, in violated bone, labeled leukocytes may localize in normal marrow elements

Top Differential Diagnoses
- Prosthetic Joint Infection
- Prosthetic Joint Loosening
- Heterotopic Ossification
- Periprosthetic Fracture, Stress Fracture

- Rx with IV antibiotics, prosthesis removal, arthrodesis; or prosthesis removal, IV antibiotics, revision arthroplasty
- Early: < 3 months after prosthesis placement; delayed: 3-24 months (difficult to distinguish from loosening); late: > 24 months
- Bone scan: Diffuse amount of uptake along all/most of bone-prosthesis interface

Prosthetic Joint Loosening
- Loss of prosthetic fixation; due to wear, osteolysis
- Differentiating joint loosening from infection often requires aspiration and culture
- Bone scan: Compared to infection, more focal regions of uptake along bone-prosthesis interface

Heterotopic Ossification
- Primitive cells in periprosthetic soft tissue ⇒ osteoblasts ⇒ lamellar bone
- Bone scan: Increased activity in soft tissues surrounding prosthesis

Periprosthetic Fracture, Stress Fracture
- More common with associated osteoporosis, rheumatoid arthritis, prior revision
- Hip: Fracture common distal to femoral stem of prosthesis tip along lateral cortex
- Bone scan: Focal increased activity

Synovitis, Bursitis
- Inflammation of synovial structures, soft tissue, bursae
- Bone scan: Positive on first 2 phases of bone scan; both may show superficial, mild uptake on 3rd phase

Dislocation/Abnormal Prosthetic Alignment
- Dislocation in < 2% of hip arthroplasties
- Radiograph diagnosis

Arthrofibrosis
- Excessive scar tissue ⇒ decreased range of motion

CLINICAL ISSUES

Presentation
- Most common signs/symptoms
  - Infection: Acute, chronic pain; ± intermittent fever, erythema, leukocytosis
  - Loosening: Chronic pain, more with weight-bearing
  - Fracture: Acute onset pain, may become chronic

DIAGNOSTIC CHECKLIST

Consider
- Normal angiographic (first) phase on bone scan: High negative predictive value for excluding infection

SELECTED REFERENCES
1. Love C et al: Role of nuclear medicine in diagnosis of the infected joint replacement. Radiographics. 21(5):1229-38, 2001

IMAGE GALLERY

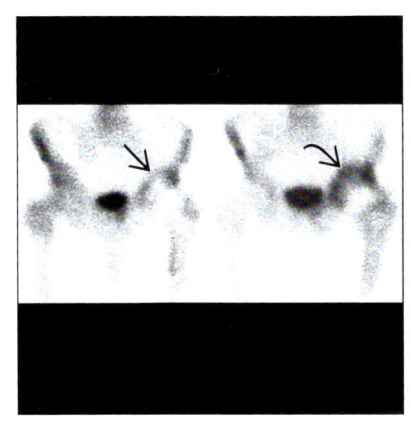

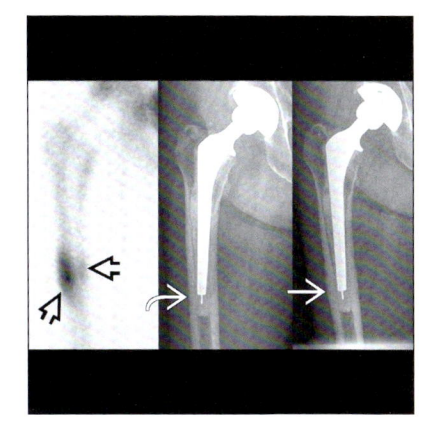

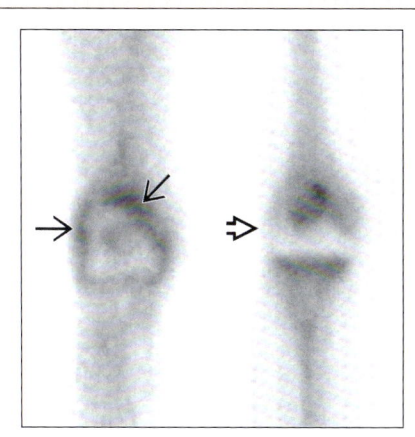

(Left) Baseline ➔ and 2 yr ➔ bone scans show interval development of uptake around acetabular component, consistent with loosening. Infection typically involves both components. (Center) Anterior bone scan shows ↑ uptake at tip of femoral prosthesis ➔. Radiographs at baseline ➔ and at time of bone scan shows progressive cortical thickening ➔ 2° to stress fx. (Right) Anterior bone scan shows hyperemia around joint capsule on blood pool image ➔ but no abnormal bone uptake on delayed image ➔. Findings support synovitis/bursitis.

FAILED BACK SURGERY SYNDROME

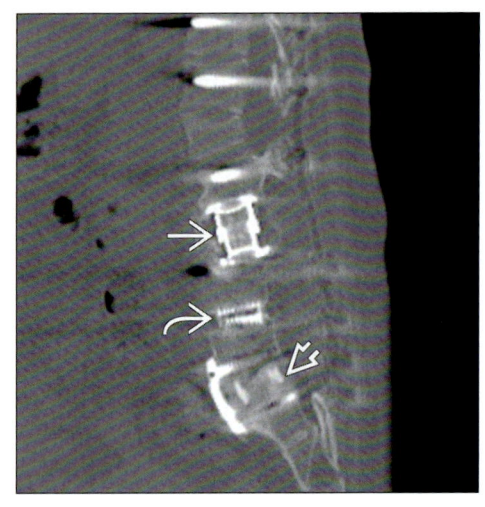

Sagittal CT of the LS spine shows stress cage ➡, intervertebral fusion cage ➡, and bone strut graft ➡. See next image.

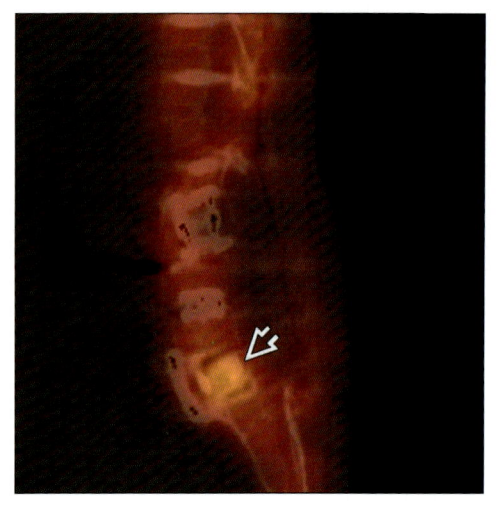

Sagittal fused Tc-99m MDP SPECT/CT shows ↑ uptake within bone block spacer ➡, consistent with ongoing incorporation of the graft. This is not an abnormal finding.

TERMINOLOGY

Abbreviations and Synonyms
- Failed back surgery syndrome (FBSS)

Definitions
- Persistent or recurrent pain despite back surgery to relieve pain or neurological compromise

IMAGING FINDINGS

General Features
- Best diagnostic clue
  - Focal ↑ uptake on SPECT corresponding to bony abnormality on CT or MR
    - Accurate localization: Optimized by fusion of SPECT to CT or MR (dedicated camera or off-line fusion of separate study)
- Location
  - Levels above and below fusion: ↑ Biomechanical forces at facets, unfused disc spaces
  - Within fusion: Pseudarthrosis, fracture, hardware failure, infection, foreign body reaction
  - Long spinal rods: Toggling at attachment sites of hooks, screws

Nuclear Medicine Findings
- Conventional 3 phase bone scan + SPECT (best if fused to CT, MR)
  - Marked hyperemia on vascular phase images should raise concern for infection
  - Following spinal fusion
    - Pseudoarthroses of bony fusion: Band of uptake through fusion mass; bony defect may be "cold" with uptake along adjacent margins
    - Disc fusion material may undergo foreign body reaction, fusion failure: ↑ Uptake at bone/fusion interface; uptake within graft may be indistinguishable from active graft incorporation
    - Facets/discs above or below level of fusion: ↑ Biomechanical forces; focal ↑ uptake on bone scan
    - Pedicle screws may transgress or erode into facet joints: Creates severe inflammation, mechanical instability, widening and subluxation, intense uptake on bone scan
    - Pedicle screws may become loose: Focal uptake around screw due to toggling effect

DDx: Mimics of Failed Back Surgery Syndrome

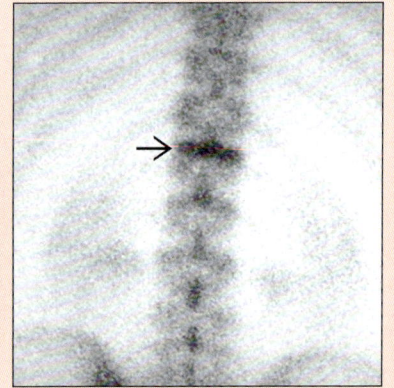

Benign Compression

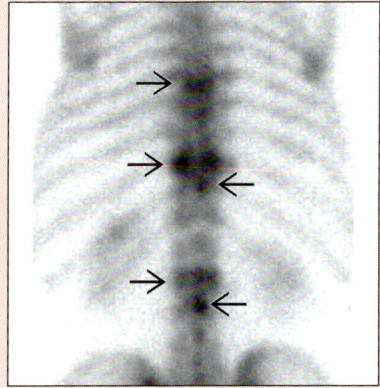

Paget Disease

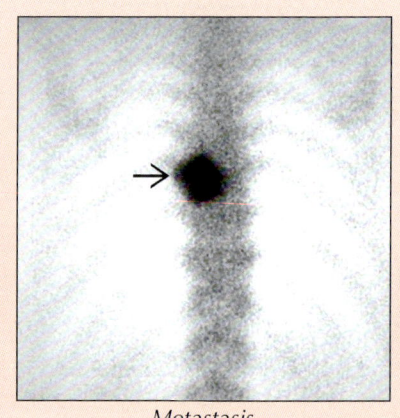

Metastasis

FAILED BACK SURGERY SYNDROME

Key Facts

Terminology
- Persistent or recurrent pain despite back surgery to relieve pain or neurological compromise

Imaging Findings
- Levels above and below fusion: ↑ Biomechanical forces at facets, unfused disc spaces
- Within fusion: Pseudarthrosis, fracture, hardware failure, infection, foreign body reaction
- Long spinal rods: Toggling at attachment sites of hooks, screws
- Conventional 3 phase bone scan + SPECT (best if fused to CT, MR)
- Large number of non-diagnostic In-111 WBC scans for post-operative spinal infection
- Ga-67: Perform in conjunction with conventional bone scan (BS)
- MR: Exclude neurogenic cause; synovial facet abnormalities often predict SPECT positivity
- SPECT fused to CT or MR fusion: Identify sites of abnormal bony remodeling
- High correlation with improvement following targeted therapy based on SPECT bone scan
- NECT: Best bony definition for SPECT coregistration; identify fracture, pseudoarthrosis, prosthetic complications
- Precise "line-up" of SPECT to CT or MR
- Attenuation correction of SPECT with SPECT/CT not advisable

Pathology
- Epidemiology: FBSS occurs in 10-40% of patients following back surgery

---

- Following rodding or scoliosis or fixation for stabilization
  - Hooks may "cut out" or create stress remodeling at sites of attachment; may impinge on adjacent bone
  - Loose screws: Exert toggle effect, ↑ uptake in surrounding bone
  - Mild-moderate multilevel uptake at sites of laminar hooks, pedicle screw: Common during 1st post-operative year, thereafter decreases
- Impending pedicle or pars fracture: Focal ↑ uptake on bone scan; often becomes "cold" after fracture with stress-remodeling/uptake at other site in vertebral ring
- In-111 leukocyte (WBC) scan
  - Must be performed in conjunction with Tc-99m sulfur colloid "marrow map"
  - Large number of non-diagnostic In-111 WBC scans for post-operative spinal infection
  - Critical issues limiting use of In-111 WBC scan to dx post-surgical spinal infection
    - Labeled WBCs normally localize to red marrow of vertebrae: Reticuloendothelial cells remove damaged labeled WBCs; labeled monocytes in equilibrium between between blood & marrow
    - Tc-99m sulfur colloid also normally localizes to red marrow of vertebrae: Define distribution of normal reticuloendothelial cells
    - Infection ≥ 48 h: Normal red marrow is replaced by granulocytes, inflammatory cell & debris; "cold" on Tc-99m sulfur colloid marrow scan
    - Surgery (even discectomy) often devascularizes red marrow: "Cold" vertebrae on In-111 WBC
    - Spinal infection: 25% of documented cases are "cold" on WBC scan; devascularization of vertebrae → ↓ vascular entry of WBCs into site of infection
  - Positive for infection: In-111 WBC scan hot or warm, Tc-99m sulfur colloid scan cold; sensitivity 60%
  - Indeterminate for infection: In-111 WBC scan cold, Tc-99m sulfur colloid scan cold (can be seen with normal post-operative spine or infection)
- Ga-67 scintigraphy
  - Ga-67: Perform in conjunction with conventional bone scan (BS)
  - Compare magnitude of Ga-67 uptake to that on BS: Compare each to surrounding normal region of bone
    - Ga-67 uptake > BS uptake: Positive for spinal osteo
    - Ga-67 uptake = BS uptake, but different sized region (larger or smaller): Positive for spinal osteo
    - Ga-67 uptake < BS uptake: Negative for spinal osteo
    - Ga-67 uptake = BS uptake (same sized region): Indeterminate for spinal osteo
  - With documented osteomyelitis: Ga-67 scan indeterminate > 50% of cases; few false- and false+

Imaging Recommendations
- Best imaging tool
  - MR: Exclude neurogenic cause; synovial facet abnormalities often predict SPECT positivity
  - SPECT fused to CT or MR fusion: Identify sites of abnormal bony remodeling
    - High correlation with improvement following targeted therapy based on SPECT bone scan
  - NECT: Best bony definition for SPECT coregistration; identify fracture, pseudoarthrosis, prosthetic complications
  - Suspected infection (hardware precluding MR)
    - In-111 WBC/Tc-99m marrow map: If negative, proceed to Ga-67/Tc-99m bone scan
- Protocol advice
  - Tc-99m bone scan (BS)
    - Best approach: Conventional three phase bone scan plus directed SPECT, fusion of SPECT to CT or MR
    - Angiographic phase over site of pain, blood pool images of entire spine: ↑ Hyperemia may signify infection, ↑ inflammatory process
    - Planar images of entire spine: Identify "worst" sites for SPECT

FAILED BACK SURGERY SYNDROME

- SPECT imaging of region of pain: Improved contrast; shows abnormalities not on planar images
- SPECT fusion to CT or MR is critical: Dedicated SPECT/CT camera; "off-line" fusion of SPECT to separate CT or MR
- Optimized image quality of SPECT/CT or MR fusion: Reconstruct SPECT over same region as CT, MR
- Precise "line-up" of SPECT to CT or MR
- Attenuation correction of SPECT with SPECT/CT not advisable
- Additional nuclear medicine imaging options
  - FDG PET: Increased uptake in areas of inflammation, active bony remodeling
  - NaF PET: May replace conventional BS in future; improved image quality over conventional BS; not currently FDA approved or reimbursed

DIFFERENTIAL DIAGNOSIS

Metastatic Disease
- Cancer history, correlate with CT/MR findings

Paget Disease
- Expanded bone, coarsened trabecula, ↑↑ elevated alkaline phosphatase, involvement of both vertebral body and posterior element

Occult Fracture
- Linear uptake across superior endplate, loss of vertebral height, underlying osteoporosis, sacral insufficiency fracture

PATHOLOGY

General Features
- Etiology
  - Instability
  - Stenosis: Central, lateral
  - Recurrent disc herniation, disruption
  - Missed lesions, wrong level
  - Intraneural fibrosis/epidural scar
  - Arachnoiditis
  - Reflux sympathetic dystrophy
  - Muscle spasm/soft tissue disfunction
  - Facet syndrome
  - Pseudarthrosis
  - Metallic implant reaction
  - Occult fracture
- Epidemiology: FBSS occurs in 10-40% of patients following back surgery
- Associated abnormalities: Often psychologically debilitating

CLINICAL ISSUES

Presentation
- Most common signs/symptoms: Recurrent back pain, radicular pain, numbness, weakness
- Other signs/symptoms: Depression, anxiety

Treatment
- Physical therapy
- Targeted facet injection: Anesthetics, steroids
- Neuromodulation: Spinal cord stimulation
- Medications
  - Anti-inflammatories
  - Analgesics
    - Potential for substance abuse, narcotic dependency
  - Neuropathic pain may respond to antidepressants (e.g., tricyclics), anti-epileptics
  - Treatment of accompanying depression, anxiety
- Epidural anesthetics, steroids
- Repeat surgery

DIAGNOSTIC CHECKLIST

Consider
- MR or CT myelogram: Identify neural, soft tissue etiology of FBSS
- BS SPECT/CT or SPECT/MR fusion: Identify osseous etiology of FBSS

Image Interpretation Pearls
- Targeting facet injections to "hot spots" on BS: Improvement in pain score, cost-savings > clinically-driven targeted therapy

SELECTED REFERENCES

1. Guyer RD et al: Failed back surgery syndrome: diagnostic evaluation. J Am Acad Orthop Surg. 14(9):534-43, 2006
2. Hazard RG: Failed back surgery syndrome: surgical and nonsurgical approaches. Clin Orthop Relat Res. 443:228-32, 2006
3. Kim KY et al: Magnetic resonance image-based morphological predictors of single photon emission computed tomography-positive facet arthropathy in patients with axial back pain. Neurosurgery. 59(1):147-56; discussion 147-56, 2006
4. Pneumaticos SG et al: Low back pain: prediction of short-term outcome of facet joint injection with bone scintigraphy. Radiology. 238(2):693-8, 2006
5. Salgado R et al: Imaging of the postoperative spine. Semin Roentgenol. 41(4):312-26, 2006
6. Skaf G et al: Clinical outcome of surgical treatment of failed back surgery syndrome. Surg Neurol. 64(6):483-8, discussion 488-9, 2005
7. Onesti ST: Failed back syndrome. Neurologist. 10(5):259-64, 2004
8. Sanders WP et al: Imaging of the postoperative spine. Semin Ultrasound CT MR. 25(6):523-35, 2004
9. Schofferman J et al: Failed back surgery: etiology and diagnostic evaluation. Spine J. 3(5):400-3, 2003
10. Talbot L: "Failed back surgery syndrome". BMJ. 327(7421):985-6, 2003
11. Slipman CW et al: Etiologies of failed back surgery syndrome. Pain Med. 3(3):200-14; discussion 214-7, 2002
12. Van Goethem JW et al: Review article: MRI of the postoperative lumbar spine. Neuroradiology. 44(9):723-39, 2002
13. Waguespack A et al: Etiology of long-term failures of lumbar spine surgery. Pain Med. 3(1):18-22, 2002
14. Anderson VC et al: Failed back surgery syndrome. Curr Rev Pain. 4(2):105-11, 2000

FAILED BACK SURGERY SYNDROME

IMAGE GALLERY

Typical

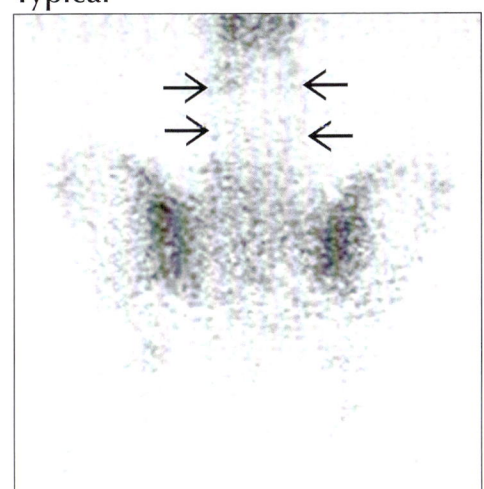

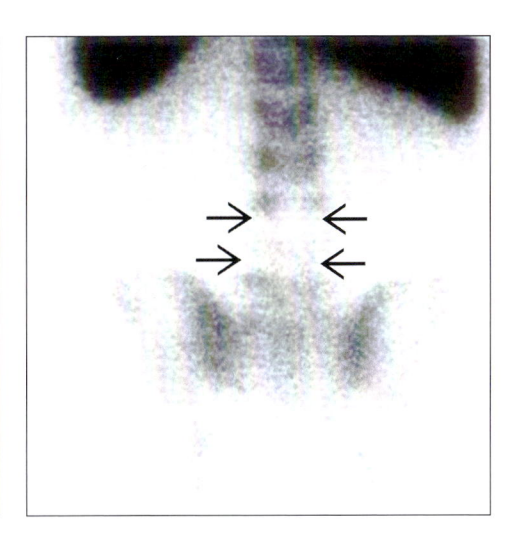

(Left) Posterior planar In-111 WBC scan of the lower lumbar spine and pelvis shows photopenic defect at L3-L4 ➡, consistent with normal post-surgical loss of normal red marrow. However, osteomyelitis is not excluded. See next image. *(Right)* Posterior planar Tc-99m sulfur colloid scan of the LS spine and pelvis shows cold defects ➡ concordant with In-111 WBC scan, typical with post-surgical change. Osteomyelitis is not ruled out.

Typical

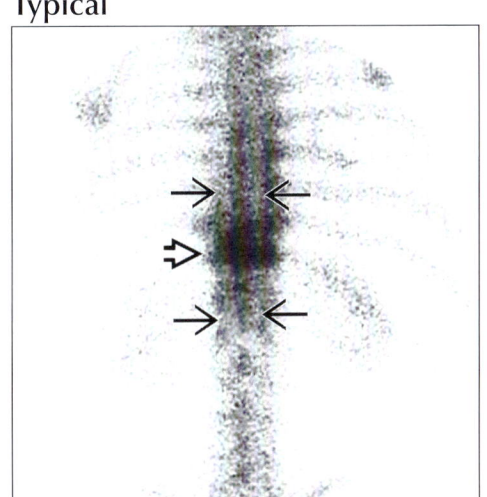

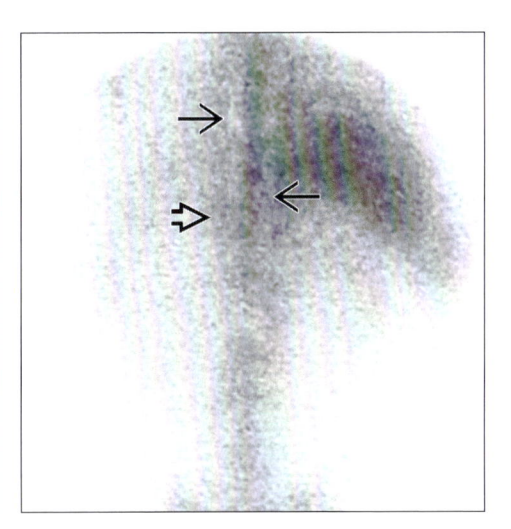

(Left) Posterior planar Tc-99m MDP scan of the TL spine shows photopenic defects corresponding to rods ➡. There is ↑ tracer uptake at the thoracolumbar junction ➡. See next image. *(Right)* Posterior planar Ga-67 scan of the TL spine shows photopenic defects corresponding to rods ➡. Uptake of Ga-67 < Tc-99m at the thoracolumbar junction ➡. Therefore, osteomyelitis is unlikely.

Typical

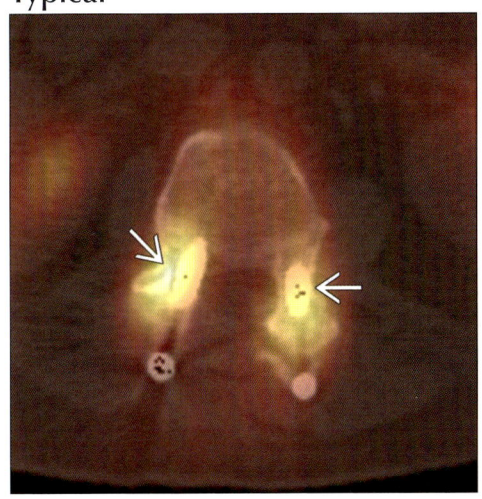

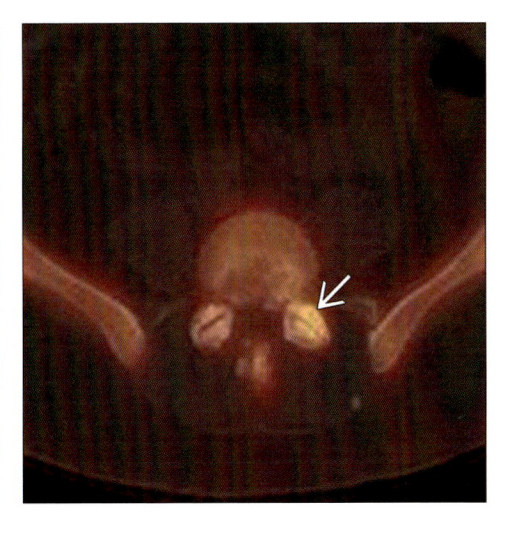

(Left) Axial fused Tc-99m MDP SPECT/CT shows intense uptake around pedicle screws ➡, which is consistent with abnormal remodeling due to loosening (fracture or infection also considered). *(Right)* Axial fused Tc-99m MDP SPECT/CT shows mild increased uptake in left L5/S1 facet joint ➡, consistent with degenerative change.

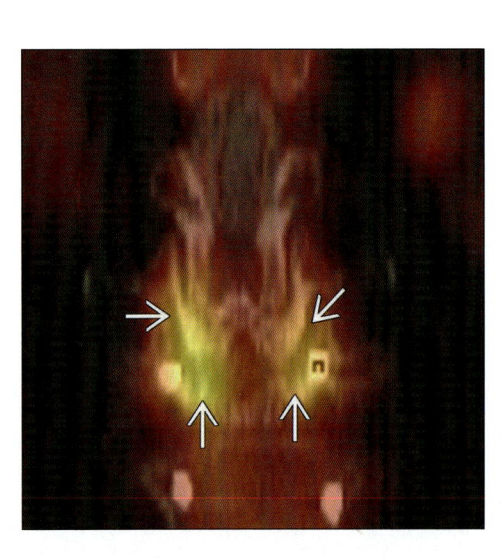

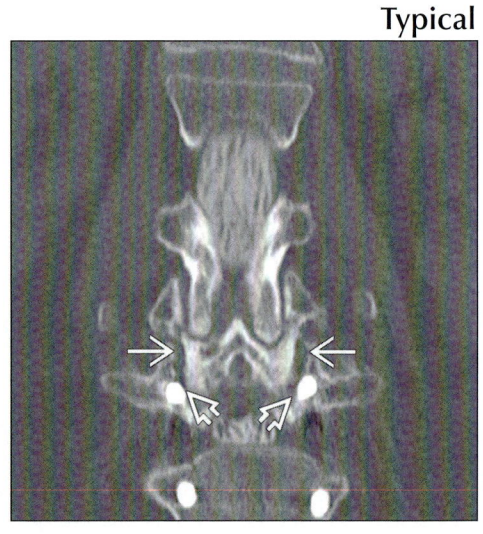

FAILED BACK SURGERY SYNDROME

(Left) Posterior planar Tc-99m MDP scan shows intense uptake at endplates of L1/2 disc space ⇨, above level of long fusion ➡. Worsened discogenic sclerosis above or below fusion mass is a common outcome of fusion. *(Right)* Posterior planar Tc-99m MDP scan shows well-healed fusion mass at L4/5 ➡, with bilateral increased uptake at level above ➡, hard to localize on planar views. See next 4 images.

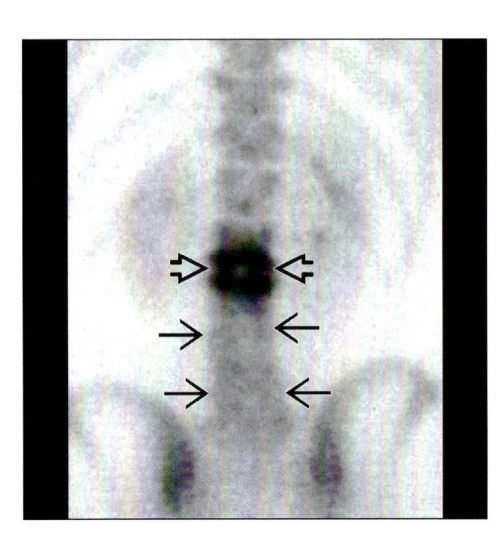

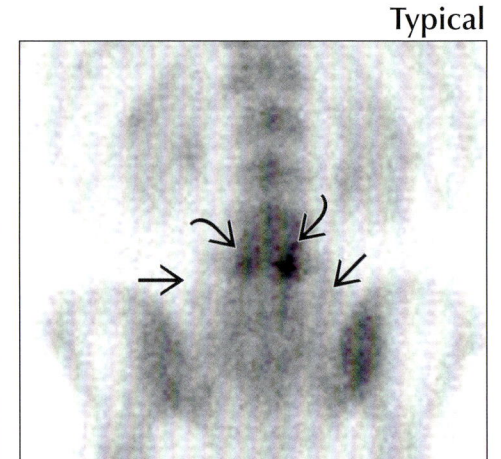

(Left) Axial fused Tc-99m MDP SPECT/CT shows intense increased uptake in facet joints (rt > lt) ➡, consistent with abnormal bony remodeling. *(Right)* Axial CT myelogram of the LS spine shows widening and erosion of facet joints ➡, transgressed by pedicle screws ➡, which causes intense inflammatory reaction, pain, weakening of facets and build up of inflammatory/scar tissue ➡. See next 2 coronal images.

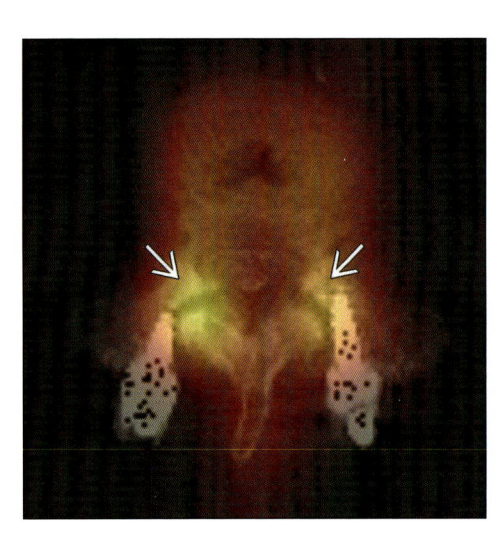

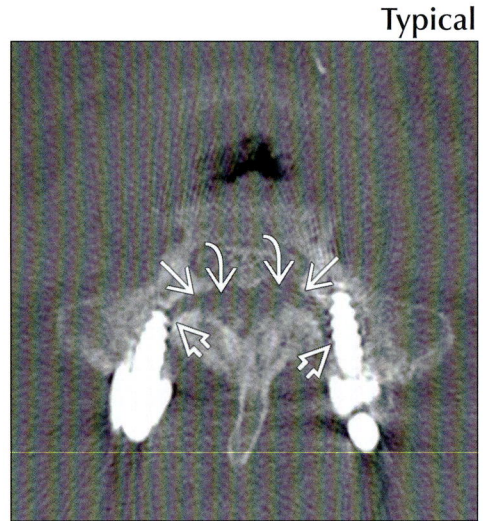

(Left) Coronal fused Tc-99m MDP SPECT/CT shows intense increased uptake in facet joints (rt > lt) ➡, consistent with abnormal bony remodeling. *(Right)* Coronal CT myelogram of the LS spine shows widening and erosion of facet joints ➡, and confirms entry of pedicle screws into the facet joints ➡, creating severe inflammation, joint laxity.

FAILED BACK SURGERY SYNDROME

Typical

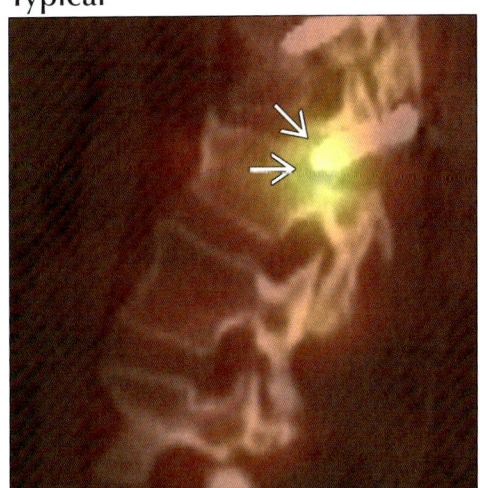

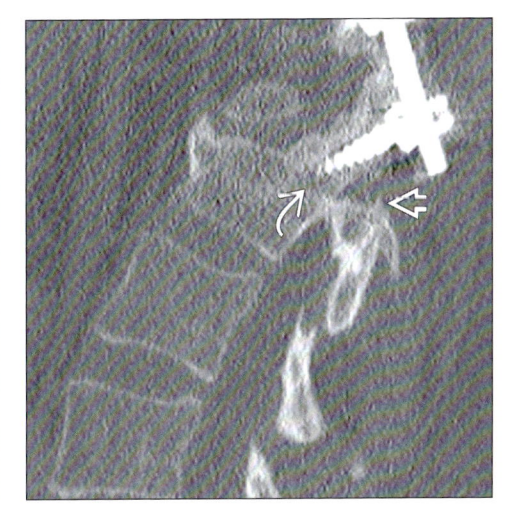

(Left) Sagittal fused Tc-99m MDP SPECT/CT shows intense uptake around the tip of the pedicle screw ➡, consistent with fracture or loosening. See next image. (Right) Sagittal CT of the LS spine shows fracture of the posterior element ➡, with suggestion of extension to the tip of the pedicle screw ➡ at the site of increased uptake on SPECT.

Typical

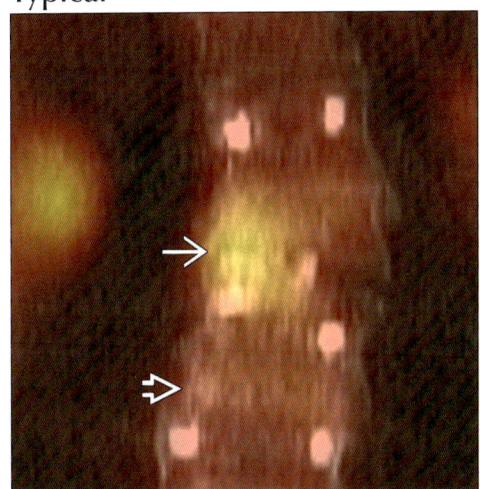

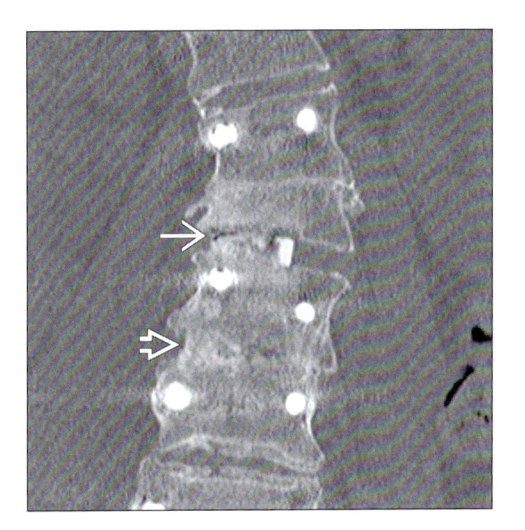

(Left) Coronal fused Tc-99m MDP SPECT/CT shows increased uptake at the level of the fused disc space ➡, due to failed fusion/pseudarthrosis. There is no abnormal uptake at the fused level below ➡. See next image. (Right) Coronal CT of the LS spine shows lucency along the superior aspect of the disc fusion at the site of SPECT uptake ➡, consistent with failed fusion/pseudoarthrosis. Note solid fusion at the level below ➡. See next 2 images.

Typical

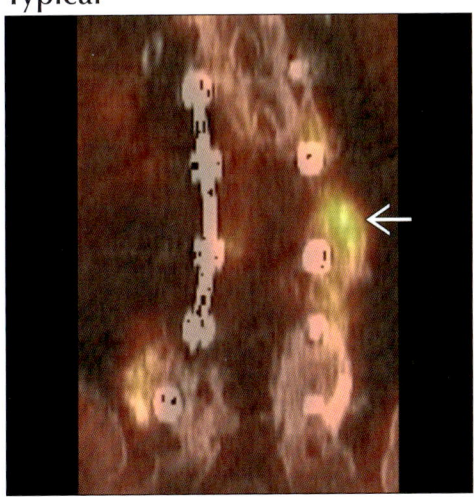

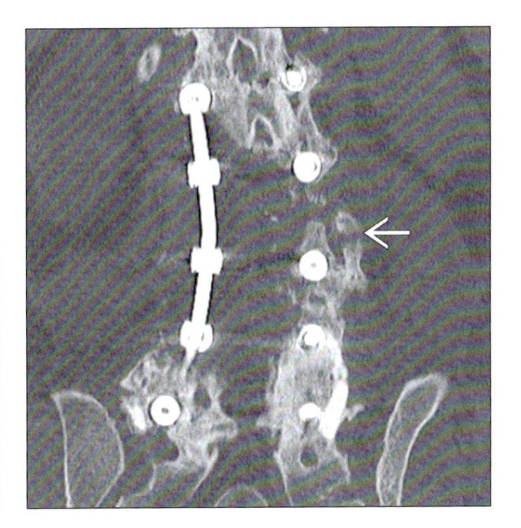

(Left) More posterior coronal fused Tc-99m MDP SPECT/CT shows increased uptake through the posterior fusion mass at the site of pseudoarthrosis ➡. See next image. (Right) Coronal CT of the LS spine shows defect in the posterior fusion mass at the site of SPECT uptake ➡, consistent with failed fusion/pseudarthrosis.

INSUFFICIENCY FRACTURE

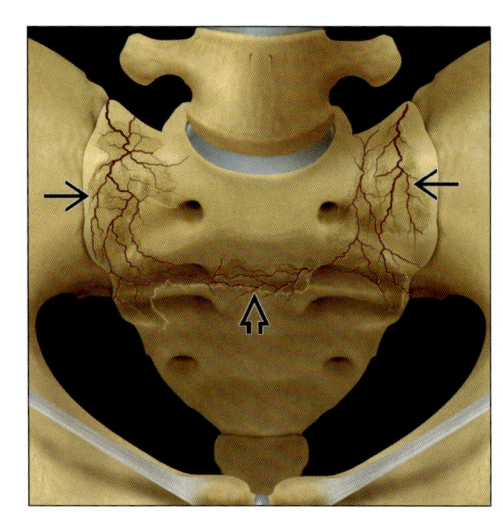

Coronal graphic shows typical sacral insufficiency fracture, which includes bilateral vertical sacral ala fractures ➔ and horizontal connecting sacral body fracture ⇨.

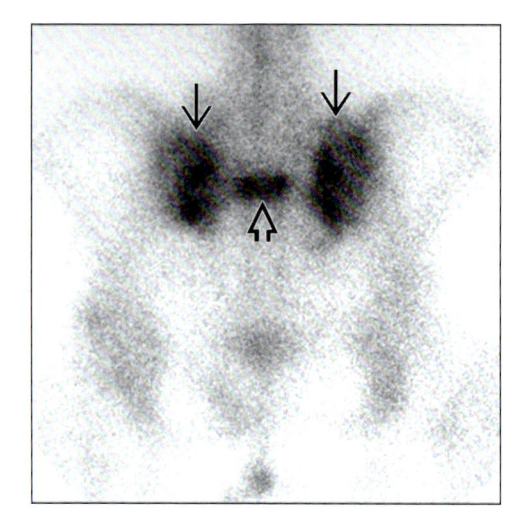

Bone scan of posterior pelvis shows typical "H" ("Honda", "butterfly") pattern of sacral insufficiency fracture, with both vertical ➔ and horizontal ⇨ components.

TERMINOLOGY

Definitions
- Stress fracture (fx)
  - Insufficiency fracture
    - Normal stress on bone demineralized due to osteoporosis or metabolic bone disease
  - Fatigue fracture
    - Repetitive stress on normal bone
  - Note: "Pathologic fracture" is a term usually reserved for fx through bone focally weakened by tumor or infection

IMAGING FINDINGS

General Features
- Best diagnostic clue
  - Linear increased uptake on delayed (mineral phase) of bone scan
    - Highly sensitive; specific if typical in pattern and distribution
- Location
  - Sacrum: Unilateral or bilateral
  - Other pelvic girdle (pubic ring, ilium)
  - Vertebral bodies: Thoracolumbar junction (lower thoracic to upper lumbar) most common
  - Proximal femur: Femoral neck most common
  - Calcaneus
- Size
  - Initially small, well-defined, linear, often incomplete
  - Progresses to linear area of uptake extending through entire width of bone
  - Advanced cases are wider, may progress to complete or displaced fracture
- Morphology
  - Sacrum
    - Unilateral (vertical through ala)
    - Bilateral (vertical through both ala +/- horizontal component through sacrum) - called "H", "butterfly", or "Honda" sign
    - May be associated with pubic ring fractures due to altered biomechanics
  - Vertebral body
    - Superior endplate only, progressing in severity to involve entire vertebral body
  - Proximal femur
    - Linear transverse uptake, neck most common

DDx: Vertebral Insufficiency Fracture

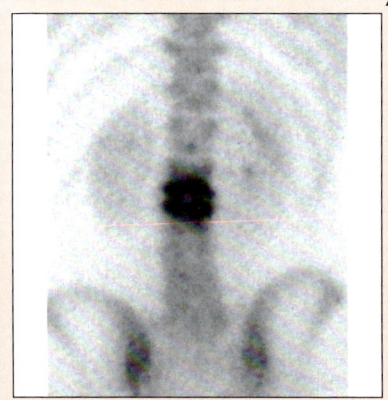

Discitis

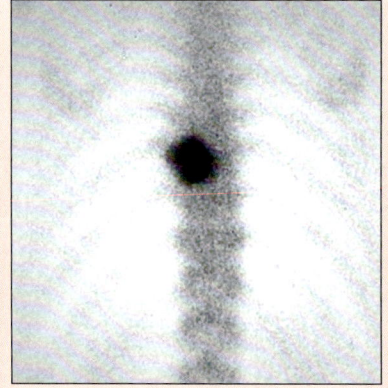

Metastasis

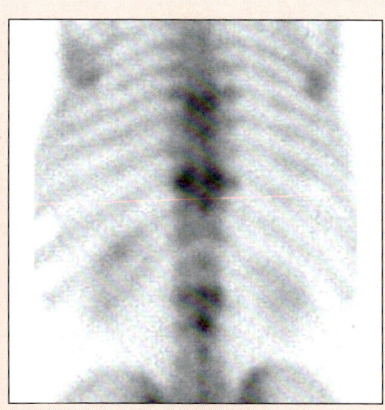

Paget Disease

INSUFFICIENCY FRACTURE

Key Facts

Terminology
- Insufficiency fracture
- Normal stress on bone demineralized due to osteoporosis or metabolic bone disease

Imaging Findings
- Bone scan: Increased uptake in linear pattern on delayed images; positive blood pool in acute cases
- Bone scan positive by 72 h, but geriatric patients may require > 1 week for precise localization
- Sacral: Unilateral (vertical through ala); bilateral "H" sign (vertical through both ala +/- horizontal component through sacrum)
- Vertebral body: Linear uptake of superior endplate progressing to complete vertebral body involvement
- Proximal femur: Linear transverse uptake; neck most common site

- Bone scan: Highly sensitive; specific if typical pattern
- Consider MR as first choice if event < 72 hours old, or < 1week in very elderly patient
- Consider CT to define trabecular destruction

Clinical Issues
- Absent to minimal velocity trauma
- Symptoms > physical signs
- Age: Average age 72 years (females), 59 years (males)
- Gender: 92% female

Diagnostic Checklist
- Hyperemia on vascular phase images in more acute cases
- Linear increased uptake on bone scan corresponding to sclerotic line or band on plain radiograph
- CT or MR in non-typical cases

- Calcaneus
  - Fracture usually along weight bearing portion of posterior calcaneus (tuberosity)

Nuclear Medicine Findings
- Bone Scan
  - Bone scan: Increased uptake in linear pattern on delayed images; positive blood pool in acute cases
  - Bone scan positive by 72 h, but geriatric patients may require > 1 week for precise localization
  - Sacral: Unilateral (vertical through ala); bilateral "H" sign (vertical through both ala +/- horizontal component through sacrum)
  - Vertebral body: Linear uptake of superior endplate progressing to complete vertebral body involvement
  - Proximal femur: Linear transverse uptake; neck most common site

Radiographic Findings
- Radiography
  - Insensitive; ± osteopenia
  - Vertebral body: Loss of vertebral body height, superior endplate density, preservation of disc space
  - Proximal femur: Sclerotic or lucent transverse band, +/- angular deformity of femoral neck
  - Sacrum: Sclerotic linear bands
  - Calcaneus: Sclerotic band along tuberosity

CT Findings
- NECT
  - Indicated when MR not available and bone scan inconclusive
  - Linear sclerosis
  - Fx difficult to identify if in plane of scan

MR Findings
- T1WI
  - Hypointense linear band
  - ± Visualized hypointense fx line
- T2WI
  - Hyperintense marrow edema
  - Hypointense fx line; high-resolution images may be required to identify fx

- No trabecular destruction
- ± Adjacent soft tissue edema (no mass)

Imaging Recommendations
- Best imaging tool
  - Bone scan: Highly sensitive; specific if typical pattern
  - Bone scan also identifies associated fractures in other regions due to altered biomechanics
  - Consider MR as first choice if event < 72 hours old, or < 1week in very elderly patient
  - Consider CT to define trabecular destruction
- Protocol advice
  - Bone scan
    - 3 phase: Recommended, positive vascular phase helpful in identifying more acute fx
    - Delayed (mineral phase): Use high-resolution collimator, obtain high count images, place camera close to patient, empty urinary bladder
    - SPECT: Helpful in complex spinal cases
  - MR: Include PD FSE coronal
  - CT: 2-4 mm slices, bone algorithm, sagittal and coronal reformatting

DIFFERENTIAL DIAGNOSIS

Sacral Insufficiency Fracture
- Overuse vs. indirect trauma
- Muscle +/- myotendinous tears or strains
- Degenerative sacroiliac (SIA) joint disease
- L5/S1 disc disease
- Osteitis condensans ilii (mechanical stress induced osteosclerosis in the ilium involving inferior 1/3 of the SIA joint)

Vertebral Body Insufficiency Fracture
- Degenerative or traumatic disc disease
- Discitis
- Spondylolisthesis, spondylolysis
- Muscle strain

INSUFFICIENCY FRACTURE

Proximal Femoral Fracture
- Trochanteric bursitis
  - Hyperintensity parallel to greater trochanter on FS PD FSE or STIR
- Iliopsoas bursal inflammation = groin pain + findings anterior to hip + lateral to neurovascular structures
- Septic joint

All Sites
- Metastatic disease
  - Bone scan or PET can assess other sites of disease
  - May require CT documentation of loss of normal trabecular morphology
- Arthritis
  - Arthritis and insufficiency fracture may coexist in older patients

PATHOLOGY

General Features
- Etiology
  - Normal force applied to demineralized bone
  - Postmenopausal osteoporosis
  - Disuse osteopenia
  - Steroid, drug-induced osteopenia
  - Metabolic bone disease
  - Testicular atrophy/testosterone deficiency (males)
  - Prior radiation to region

Microscopic Features
- Osteoclastic resorption > osteoblastic activity
- Microfractures
- Reduced bone mineral density

CLINICAL ISSUES

Presentation
- Most common signs/symptoms: Pain with weight-bearing or ambulation
- Other signs/symptoms: Pain with pelvic or hip fractures may be difficult to localize
- Clinical Profile
  - Absent to minimal velocity trauma
  - Back, hip, gluteal, groin pain
  - May be non-ambulatory
  - Point tenderness over fracture site
  - Gait abnormality
  - Limited range of motion
  - Symptoms > physical signs

Demographics
- Age: Average age 72 years (females), 59 years (males)
- Gender: 92% female

Natural History & Prognosis
- Majority heal with conservative treatment
- May progress to complete fx without treatment
- Healing: Slow process (2-5 months)
- Complications: Related to prolonged immobilization
- Additional insufficiency fractures due to altered biomechanics

Treatment
- Conservative
  - Analgesics
  - Bed rest
  - Reduced weight-bearing
  - Physical therapy (range-of-motion, gait training, muscle strengthening/stretching)
- Plasty
  - Interventional radiologic technique
  - For vertebral and sacral fractures
  - Percutaneous injection polymethylmethacrylate
  - Nearly instantaneous relief of pain
- Hardware
  - Displaced, complete femoral neck fractures

DIAGNOSTIC CHECKLIST

Consider
- Hyperemia on vascular phase images in more acute cases
- Linear increased uptake on bone scan corresponding to sclerotic line or band on plain radiograph
- CT or MR in non-typical cases

SELECTED REFERENCES

1. Blake SP et al: Sacral insufficiency fracture. Br J Radiol. Review, 77(922):891-6, 2004
2. Soubrier M et al: Insufficiency fracture. A survey of 60 cases and review of the literature. Joint Bone Spine. Jun;70(3):209-18, 2003
3. Boissonnault WG et al: Differential diagnosis of a sacral stress fracture. J Orthop Sports Phys Ther. 32(12):613-21, 2002
4. Garant M: Sacroplasty: A new treatment for sacral insufficiency fracture. J of Vasc Interventional Radiol. 12(12):1265-7, 2002
5. Kawaguchi S et al; Insufficiency fracture of the spine: a prospective analysis based on radiographic and scintigraphic diagnosis. : J Bone Miner Metab. 19(5):312-6, 2001
6. Connolly JF: Fractures and dislocations: Closed management. 1st ed. Philadelphia PA, WB Saunders, 471-2, 1995
7. Blomlie V et al: Radiation induced insufficiency fractures of the sacrum: Evaluation with MR imaging. Radiology. 188:241-44, 1993
8. Abe H et al: Radiation-induced insufficiency fractures of the pelvis: Evaluation with 99mTc-methylene diphosphonate scintigraphy. AJR. 158:599-602, 1992
9. Daffner RH et al: Stress fractures: Current concepts. AJR. 159:245-52, 1992
10. Peh WC et al: Tarlov Cysts; Another cause of sacral insufficiency fractures? Clin Radiol. 46:329-30, 1992
11. Brahme SK et al: Magnetic resonance appearance of sacral insufficiency fractures. Skeletal Radiol. 19:489-493, 1990
12. Cooper KL et al: Insufficiency fractures of the sacrum. Radiology. 156:15-20, 1985
13. Schneider R et al: Unsuspected sacral fractures: Detection by radionuclide bone scanning. AJR. 144:337-41, 1985

INSUFFICIENCY FRACTURE

IMAGE GALLERY

Variant

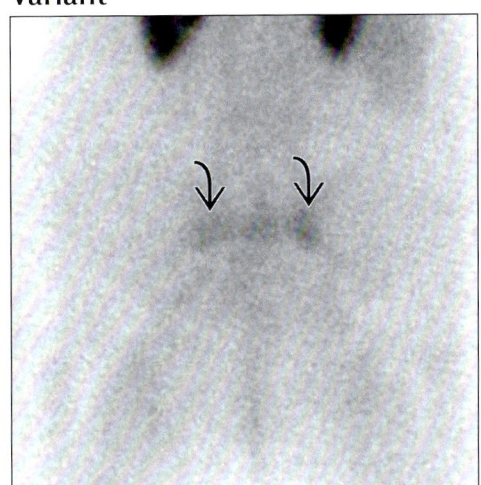

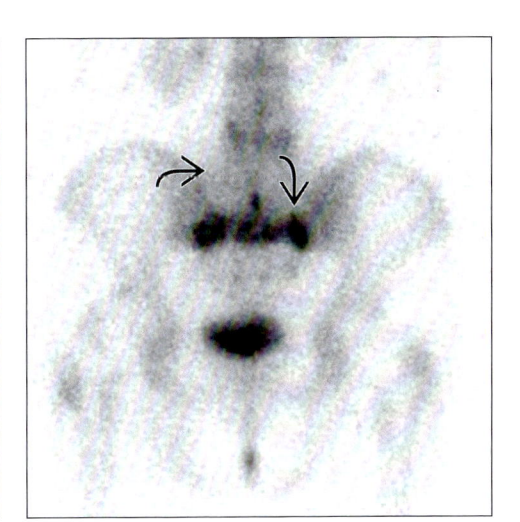

(Left) Early blood pool image of bone scan of the posterior pelvis with hyperemia of transverse sacral insufficiency fracture ➔, indicating an acute fracture. See delayed image (right). (Right) Delayed planar bone scan of the pelvis demonstrates transverse sacral insufficiency fracture ➔ with incomplete vertical components at outer margins of the horizontal fracture.

Typical

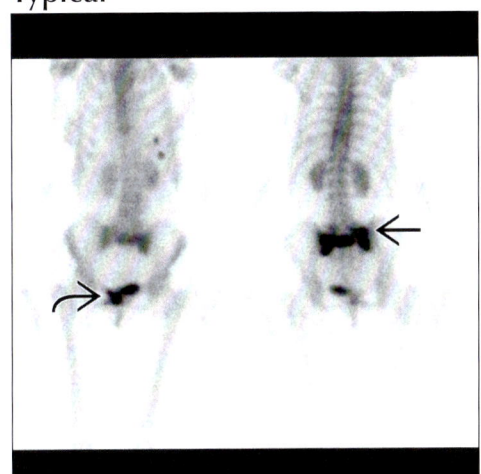

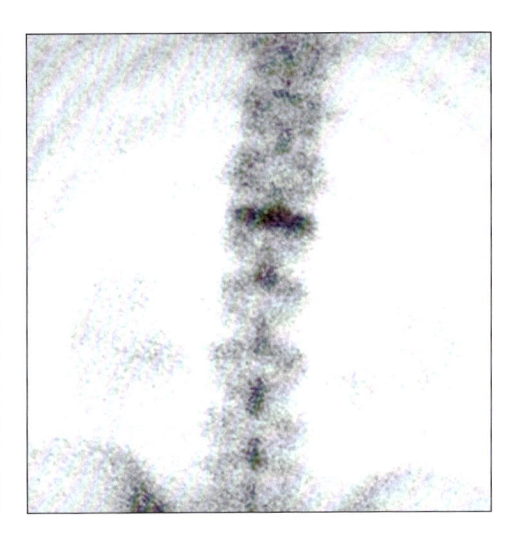

(Left) Bone scan anterior and posterior bone scan in an elderly, osteoporotic woman shows insufficiency fractures of the pubis ➔ and sacrum ➔. (Right) Bone scan of thoracolumbar spine with activity confined to superior endplate, with preservation of disc space, typical of insufficiency compression fracture of vertebra.

Typical

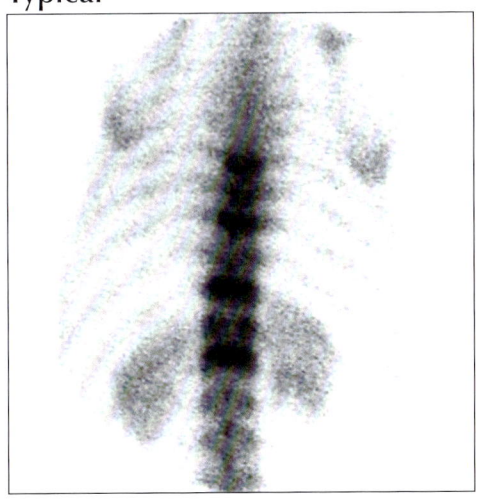

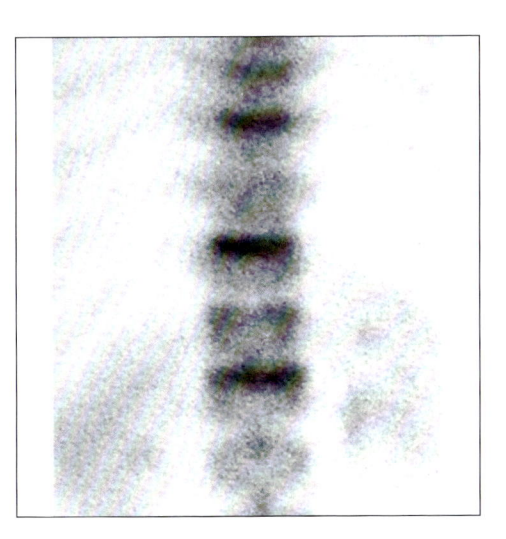

(Left) Posterior bone scan of the thoracolumbar spine with multilevel uptake. Images were obtained with general purpose collimator. See mag acquisition with high-resolution collimator at right. (Right) Bone scan in same patient as left acquired with magnification using high resolution collimator. Multi-level uptake is confined to superior endplates, confirming insufficiency fractures.

INSUFFICIENCY FRACTURE

(Left) Bone scan of the foot with uptake along the posterior calcaneal tuberosity ➡, the typical pattern seen in insufficiency fractures of the calcaneus. See plain radiograph at right. *(Right)* Plain radiograph companion to the bone scan at right. There is sclerosis parallel to the plane of the calcaneal tuberosity ➡. This pattern is typical of a calcaneal stress fracture.

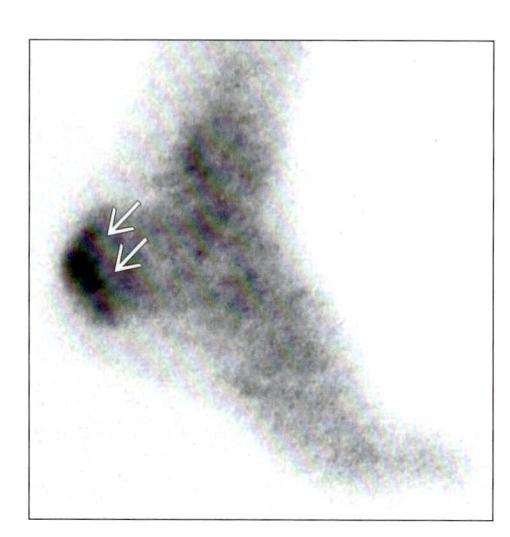

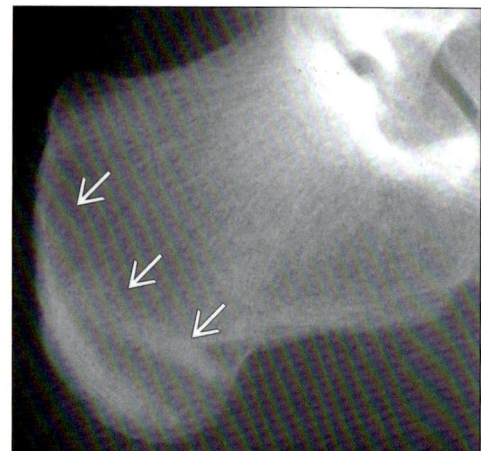

(Left) Bone scan of 24 year old female with osteomalacia (note hot anterior rib ends). Bilateral proximal femur and posterior rib uptake suggesting insufficiency fractures. See detail pelvis (right), and radiograph and MR (below). *(Right)* Bone scan of anterior pelvis (whole body scan previous image) confirming transverse uptake of both femoral necks, typical for insufficiency fractures. See radiograph and MR (next).

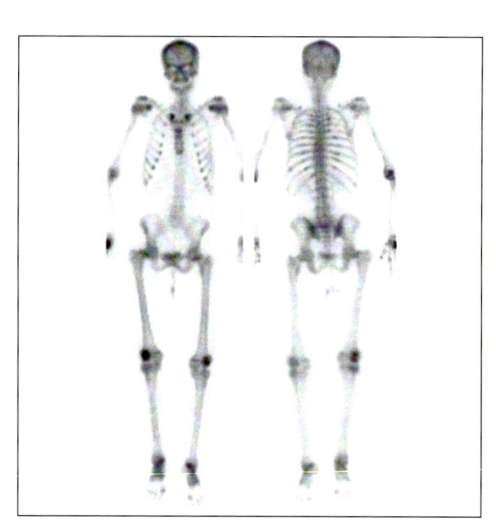

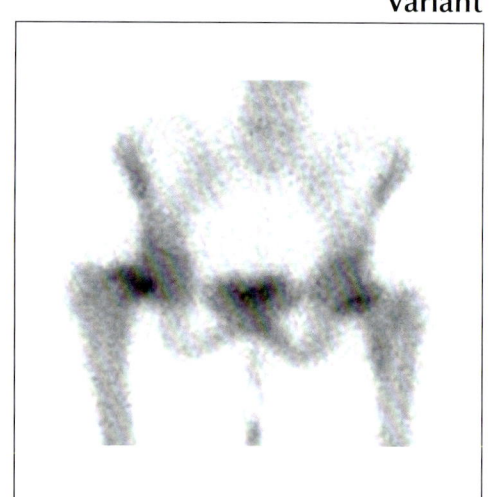

(Left) Radiograph of the pelvis from above patient with smudgy trabecular density of osteomalacia, angled right femoral neck fracture, and no obvious fracture of left femoral neck. See MR (next image). *(Right)* T2 MR from patient on left and above, with fracture line and edema of left femoral neck confirming acute insufficiency fracture. Angled right femoral neck fracture is subacute.

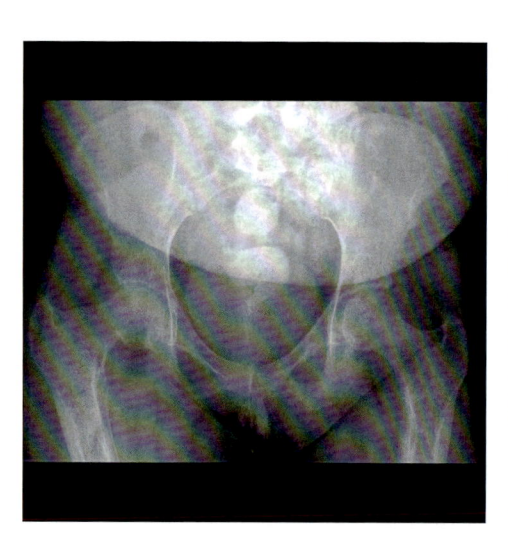

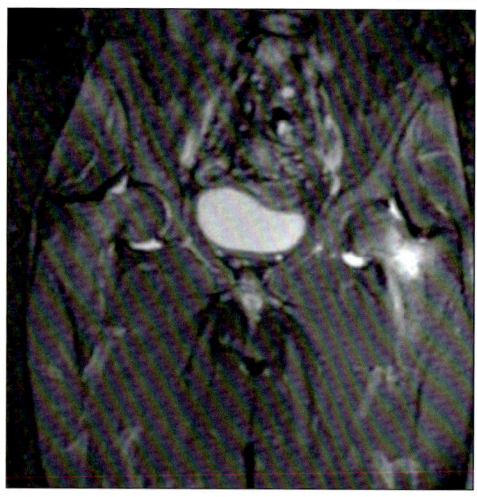

INSUFFICIENCY FRACTURE

Variant

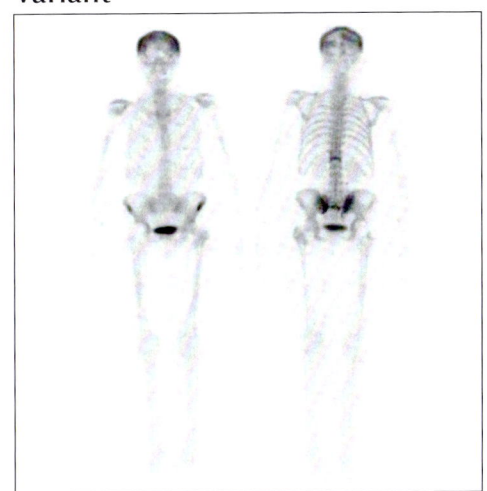

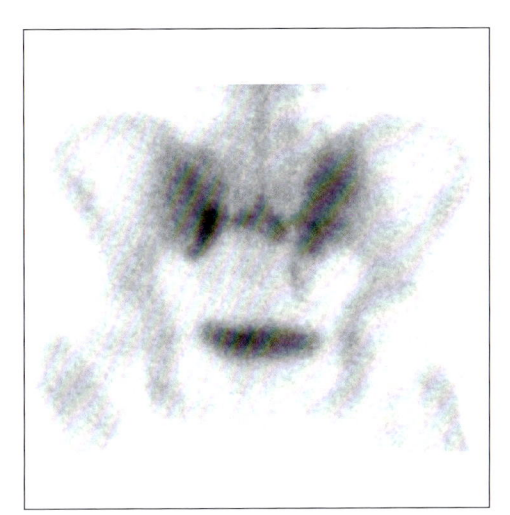

(Left) Whole body bone scan with insufficiency fractures of the sacrum and upper lumbar spine. Osteopenia and hot calvarium is suggestive of multiple myeloma. See next five images. *(Right)* Bone scan of the posterior pelvis confirms sacral insufficiency fracture.

Variant

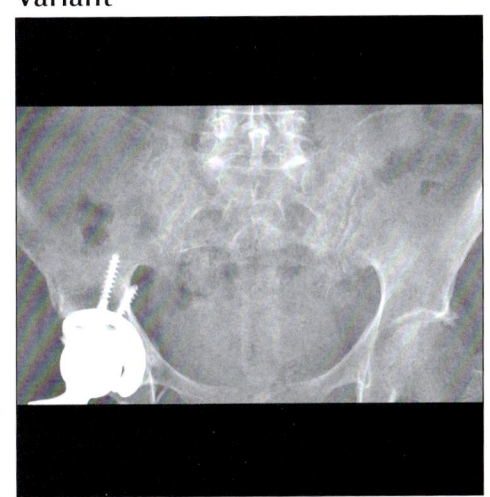

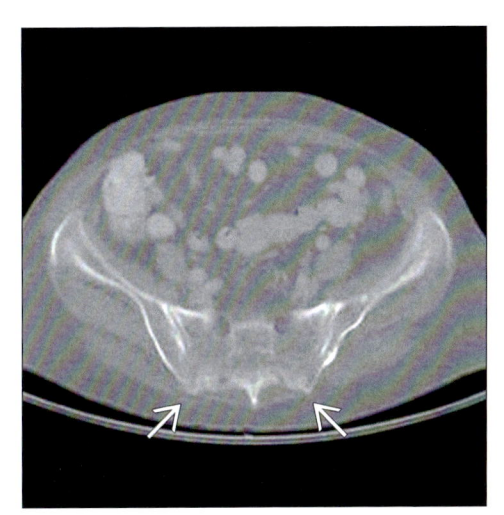

(Left) Radiograph of the pelvis demonstrates osteopenia. The sacrum is difficult to evaluate but suggests sclerosis. See CT (right). *(Right)* CT of the pelvis shows subtle sclerosis of the mid sacrum is consistent with sacral insufficiency fracture ➡. See next image for calvarium.

Variant

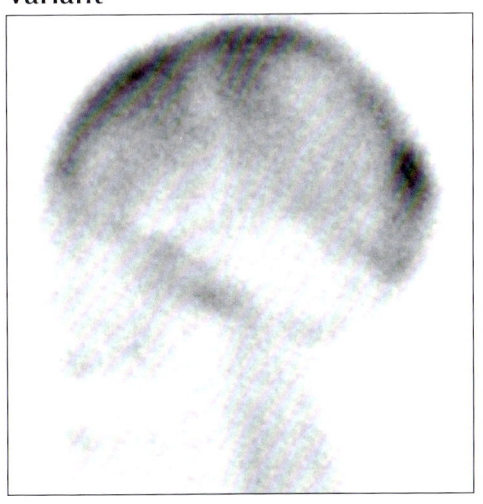

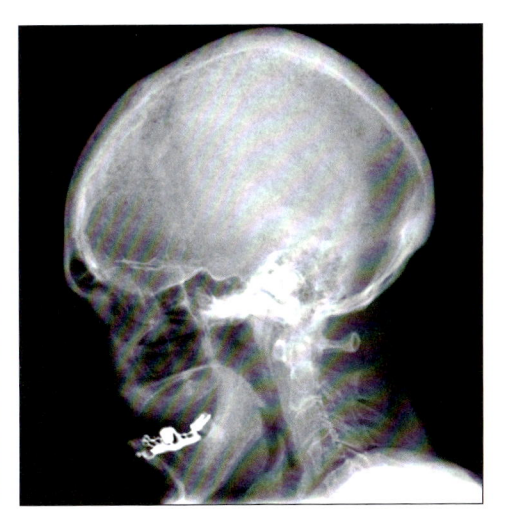

(Left) Bone scan of lateral skull with "hot" cranium, consistent with multiple myeloma (differential: Hyperostosis, myelodysplasia, hyperparathyroidism, Paget's and hemoglobinopathy). See right. *(Right)* Lateral radiograph of the skull with subtle salt-and-pepper pattern of small punched out lesions, consistent with multiple myeloma.

FRACTURE

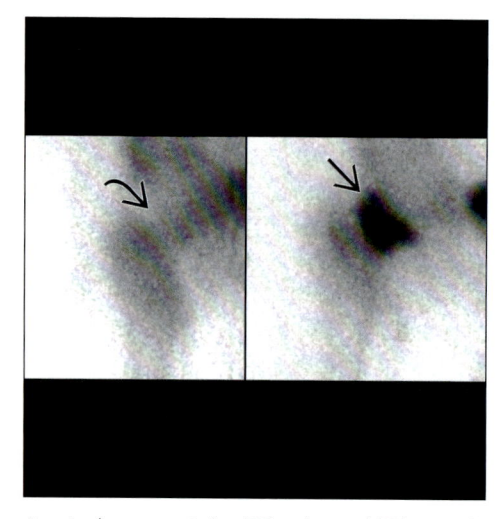

Anterior bone scan 3 days ➡ and 1 week ➡ post right femoral neck fracture in an elderly patient. Scan at 3 days shows vague uptake around photopenic ➡ fracture, which becomes (+) at 1 week ➡.

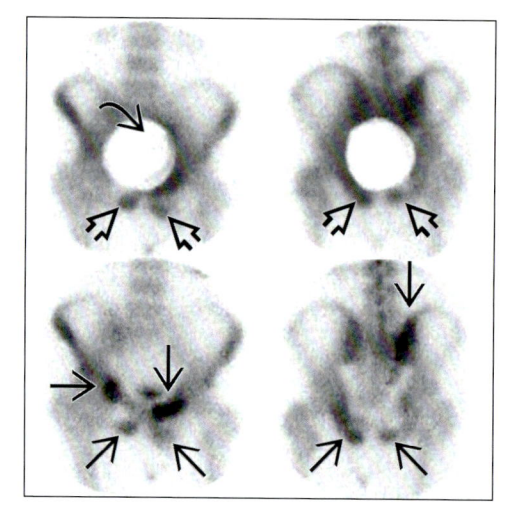

Bone scan of anterior and posterior pelvis suggests bilateral ischial fractures ➡. Bladder catheterization and removal of lead shield ➡ reveals many more fractures ➡.

TERMINOLOGY

Definitions
- Cortical disruption of bone due to abnormal stress to normal bone or normal stress to abnormal bone

IMAGING FINDINGS

Nuclear Medicine Findings
- Tc-99m MDP bone scan
  o Acute fractures: 80% abnormal at 24 h, 95% at 72 h, 98% at 1 week (longer in elderly)
    - Usually positive on three phase bone scan
    - In elderly: Uptake poorly localized until ≥ 1 week
    - In pediatrics: Skull, metaphyseal/epiphyseal, skull & acute long bone fractures may be poorly seen
    - Toddler, trampoline fractures in children: ↑ Uptake usually bilateral, although asymmetric
    - Return to normal: 2/3 x 1 yr, 90% x 2 yrs
  o Non/delayed union: Intense uptake at fracture site > 1 yr may indicate delayed union; photopenic defect at fracture site portends nonunion
  o Acute pathologic fractures: Larger region of uptake due to tumor, extension of uptake along periosteum
  o Transverse fractures of large long bones: May signify weak bone
- FDG PET: Increased uptake in acute, subacute fractures

Imaging Recommendations
- Best imaging tool
  o Plain radiography: First line imaging modality
  o NECT
    - Characterize complex, subtle or nondisplaced fractures
    - Evaluate articular integrity, hematomas
  o MR
    - Identify fractures not evident by plain radiography or CT
    - Characterize soft tissue and cartilage injury
    - Define underlying pathology (e.g., tumor)
  o Bone scan
    - Identify additional or remote fractures, occult fractures with bone scan when other modalities fail
    - Identify polyostotic/metastatic process with bone scan when underlying tumor suspected

DDx: Mimics of Spinal Fractures

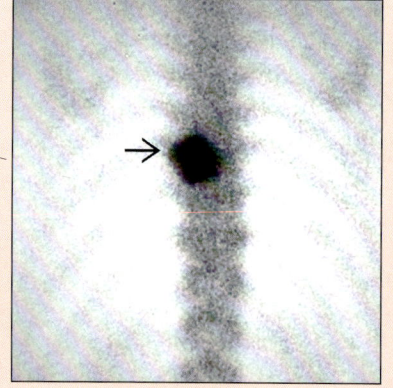

Metastasis

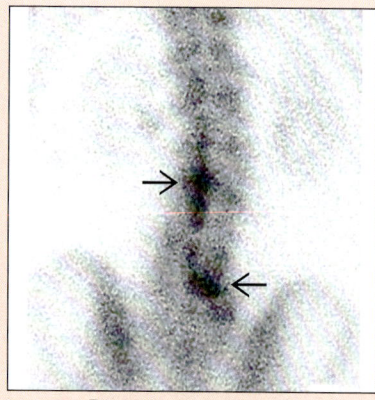

Degenerative Disease

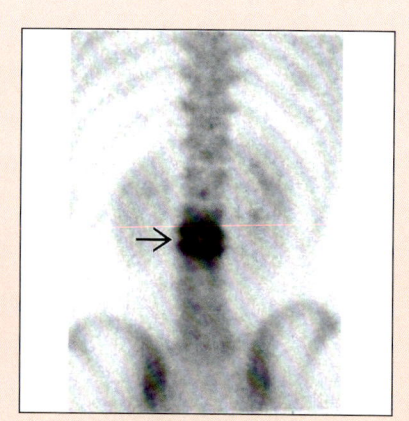

Discitis or Discogenic Sclerosis

FRACTURE

Key Facts

Imaging Findings
- Identify additional or remote fractures, occult fractures with bone scan when other modalities fail
- Identify polyostotic/metastatic process with bone scan when underlying tumor suspected
- Bone scan can be first line imaging for sports-related stress fractures
- Planar images of region of interest, whole body scan
- SPECT to increase sensitivity in spine

Top Differential Diagnoses
- Bone Tumor
- Osteomyelitis

Diagnostic Checklist
- Bone scan relatively insensitive with acute fractures in elderly, pediatric patients
- Increased activity in fracture: 2/3 return to normal on bone scan by 1 yr, 90% by 2 yrs

---

- Bone scan can be first line imaging for sports-related stress fractures
- Protocol advice
  - Hydrate patient prior to procedure; inject in extremity away from sites of interest; empty bladder, catheterize if needed
  - Three phase bone scan preferred; delayed image at 3-4 hours, longer if necessary to clear background
  - Planar images of region of interest, whole body scan
  - SPECT to increase sensitivity in spine

DIFFERENTIAL DIAGNOSIS

Bone Tumor
- Correlative imaging to exclude underlying process (MR, CT)
- Bone scan to evaluate for polyostotic process

Osteomyelitis
- Bone scan first (vascular) phase "hotter" with infection than for fracture

PATHOLOGY

General Features
- Etiology
  - Trauma, overuse, nonaccidental trauma
  - Pathologic: Osteoporosis, primary or metastatic malignancy, cyst, infection, inherited bone disorders

CLINICAL ISSUES

Treatment
- Anatomic reduction: Traction, surgical, manual
- Immobilization: Casting, hardware, external fixation

DIAGNOSTIC CHECKLIST

Image Interpretation Pearls
- Bone scan relatively insensitive with acute fractures in elderly, pediatric patients
- Increased activity in fracture: 2/3 return to normal on bone scan by 1 yr, 90% by 2 yrs

SELECTED REFERENCES

1. Lee E et al: Role of radionuclide imaging in the orthopedic patient. Orthop Clin North Am. 37(3):485-501, viii, 2006
2. Connolly LP et al: Skeletal scintigraphy in the multimodality assessment of young children with acute skeletal symptoms. Clin Nucl Med. 28(9):746-54, 2003
3. Shon IH et al: F-18 FDG positron emission tomography and benign fractures. Clin Nucl Med. 28(3):171-5, 2003
4. Greenspan A et al: A musculoskeletal radiologist's view of nuclear medicine. Semin Nucl Med. 27(4):372-85, 1997
5. Holder LE: Bone scintigraphy in skeletal trauma. Radiol Clin North Am. 31(4):739-81, 1993
6. Murray IP: The role of SPECT in the evaluation of skeletal trauma. Ann Nucl Med. 7(1):1-9, 1993
7. McDougall IR et al: Complications of fractures and their healing. Semin Nucl Med. 18(2):113-25, 1988

IMAGE GALLERY

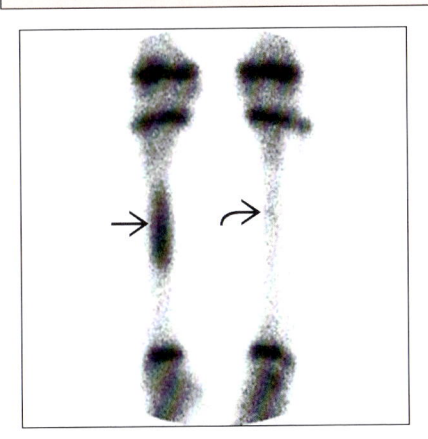

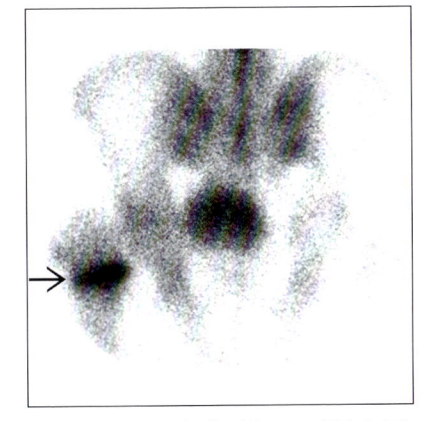

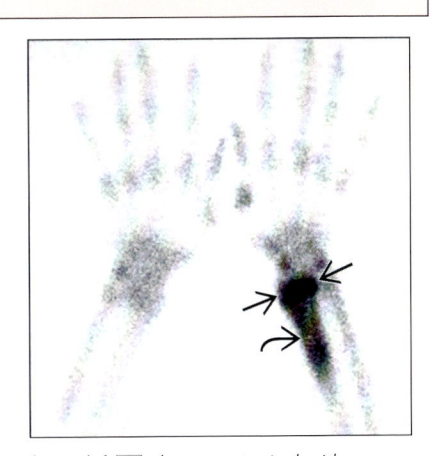

(Left) Anterior bone scan of lower legs in a 5 year old with right, mid, tibial fracture ➔. Subtle uptake on left ➔ also seen, typical with trampoline and toddler type fractures. (Center) Posterior bone scan of pelvis shows left transverse subtrochanteric fracture ➔. Subtrochanteric location and transverse orientation suggest underlying weak bone, severe osteoporosis in this case. (Right) Bone scan of hands and distal forearms shows transverse fracture of distal radius ➔. Extension of uptake more proximally ➔ suggests underlying tumor.

TRAUMA, NON-ACCIDENTAL

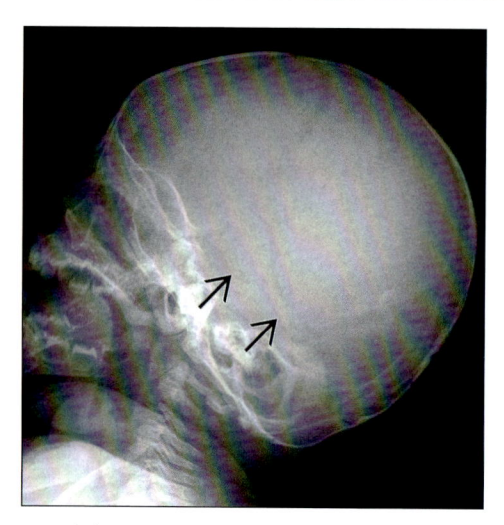

Lateral plain radiograph of skull shows linear fracture of temporal bone ➡ in a child with suspected NAT. See next image.

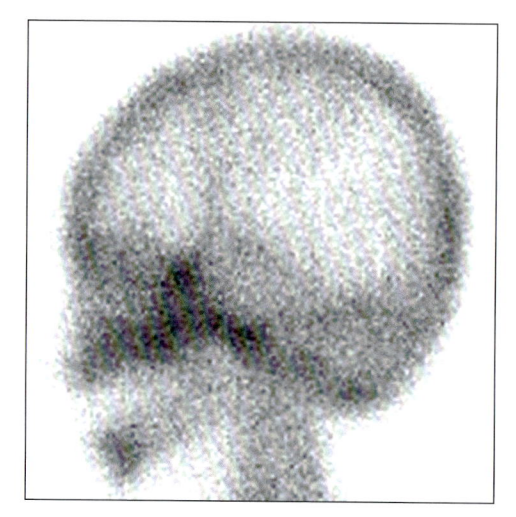

Lateral bone scan of skull in same patient as previous shows normal activity in temporal bone. Bone scan is often insensitive for skull fractures in children.

TERMINOLOGY

Abbreviations and Synonyms
- Nonaccidental trauma (NAT), nonaccidental injury, child/intimate partner/elder abuse

Definitions
- Willful and deliberate act resulting in physical injury

IMAGING FINDINGS

General Features
- Best diagnostic clue
  - Bone injury on bone scan: Variably increased activity in multiple fractures of varying ages
    - Rib: Most frequent site overall
    - Metaphyseal, juxtametaphyseal (bucket-handle)
    - Spiral or oblique long-bone fracture suspicious for NAT in young person
    - Skull: Low sensitivity, specificity of bone scan in children due to immature sutures
  - Soft tissue/visceral injury on bone scan: Local hyperemia or soft tissue uptake

Nuclear Medicine Findings
- Whole body bone scan
  - Multiple fractures of varying ages
    - Children: Potentially can be positive 24 hr after acute injury, return to normal by ~ 4 mos
  - Elderly: In older (60+) individuals fracture may not be positive until ≥ 1 wk after event
  - Fractures of long bones (humerus or femur)
  - Long diaphyseal areas of uptake: Subtle early sign can precede periosteal elevation
  - Metaphyseal corner or "beaking" sign: Proper windowing, pinhole views of both extremities to ↑ sensitivity

Imaging Recommendations
- Best imaging tool
  - Radiography: Skeletal survey first-line
    - May be negative in early injury
    - More sensitive than bone scan for pediatric skull fractures
  - Whole body bone scan: Evaluate for radiographically occult lesions if NAT suspected
  - CT: Head/soft tissue/visceral injury

DDx: Mimics of Non-Accidental Trauma

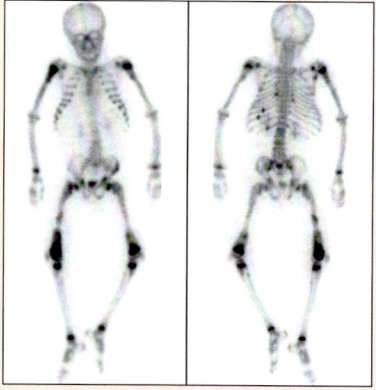

Osteogenesis Imperfecta

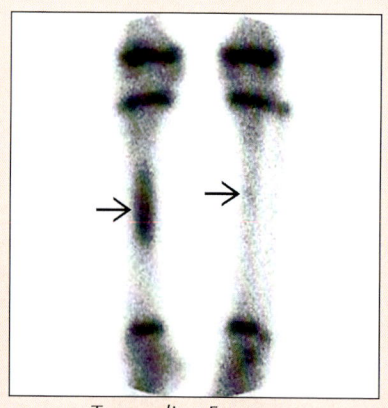

Trampoline Fractures

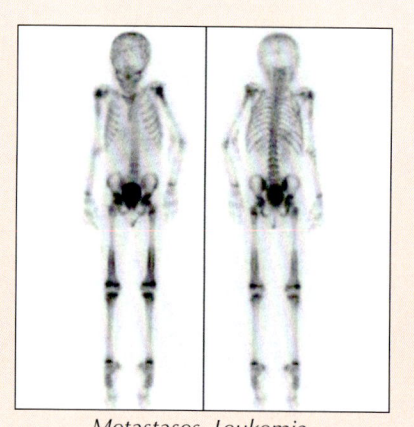

Metastases, Leukemia

TRAUMA, NON-ACCIDENTAL

Key Facts

Terminology
- Willful and deliberate act resulting in physical injury

Imaging Findings
- Bone injury on bone scan: Variably increased activity in multiple fractures of varying ages
- Soft tissue/visceral injury on bone scan: Local hyperemia or soft tissue uptake

Clinical Issues
- History inconsistent with findings
- Suspicion of NAT by primary healthcare provider

Diagnostic Checklist
- Especially in pediatrics, right-to-left asymmetry on bone scan suggests pathology (nonspecific)
- High index of suspicion for NAT: Multiple fractures of varying age on bone scan in any age group

DIFFERENTIAL DIAGNOSIS

Osteogenesis Imperfecta
- Genetic disorder; Incidence of 1 in ~ 15,000; weak, fragile bones ⇒ fracture

Osteoporosis
- Nutritional, age-related, metabolic bone disease
- Fracture, insufficiency fracture; can be of varying ages

Syndrome of Congenital Insensitivity to Pain
- Extremely rare; recurrent fracture, neuropathic joints, osteomyelitis

Caffey Disease
- Rare; presents in infants, children
- Periosteal new bone formation, cortical thickening; multifocal, commonly diaphyseal long bone

Neoplasm
- Metastatic disease may mimic multifocal trauma

PATHOLOGY

General Features
- Associated abnormalities: Developmental, growth delays

CLINICAL ISSUES

Presentation
- Most common signs/symptoms
  - Multiple healing fractures of various ages
  - History inconsistent with findings
  - Suspicion of NAT by primary healthcare provider

Demographics
- Gender
  - Pediatrics: In general, no sex predilection
  - Intimate partner: More likely women

DIAGNOSTIC CHECKLIST

Image Interpretation Pearls
- Especially in pediatrics, right-to-left asymmetry on bone scan suggests pathology (nonspecific)
- High index of suspicion for NAT: Multiple fractures of varying age on bone scan in any age group

SELECTED REFERENCES

1. Kemp AM et al: Which radiological investigations should be performed to identify fractures in suspected child abuse? Clin Radiol. 61(9):723-36, 2006
2. Hobbs CJ: ABC of child abuse. Fractures. BMJ. 298(6679):1015-8, 1989
3. Worlock P et al: Patterns of fractures in accidental and non-accidental injury in children: a comparative study. Br Med J (Clin Res Ed). 293(6539):100-2, 1986

IMAGE GALLERY

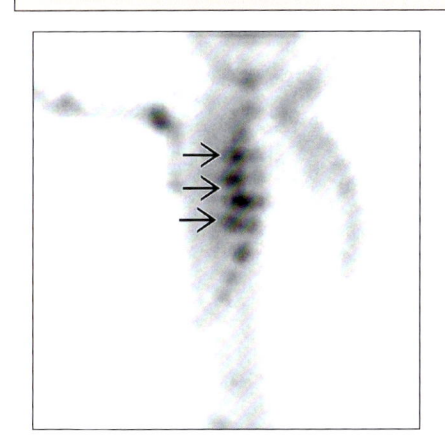

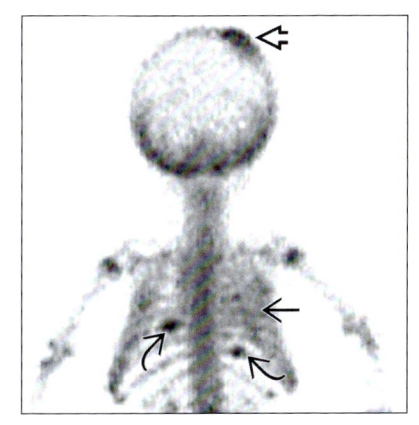

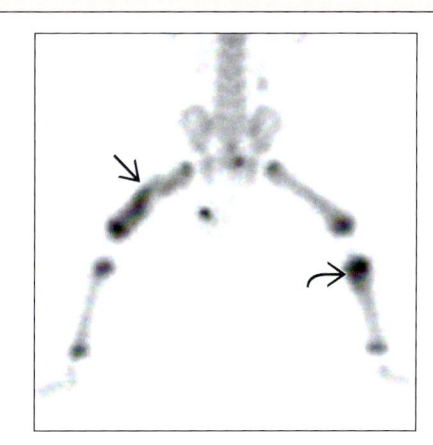

(Left) RAO bone scan shows increased uptake in five adjacent anterior right ribs ➡, consistent with acute rib fractures. Bone scan is insensitive for subacute/old rib fractures in children. *(Center)* Posterior bone scan in NAT shows old ➡ and new ➡ rib fractures, as well as skull fracture ➡. *(Right)* Anterior bone scan in a child shows ↑ activity in mid to distal right femur ➡, left proximal tibia ➡ due to fractures from NAT.

STRESS FRACTURE

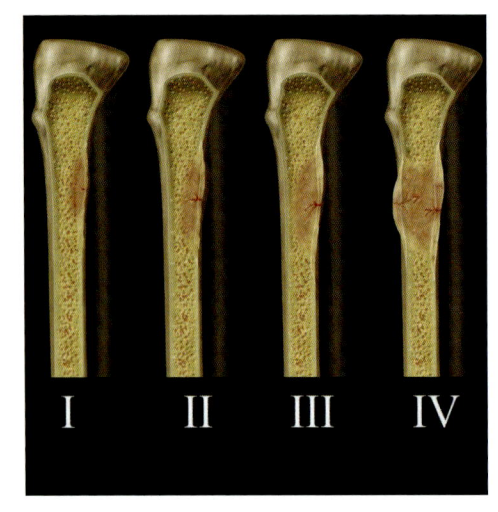

Graphic of the proximal tibia shows spectrum of stress fractures, depicting grades I-IV. Progressive involvement can be seen in advanced or inadequately treated stress fractures.

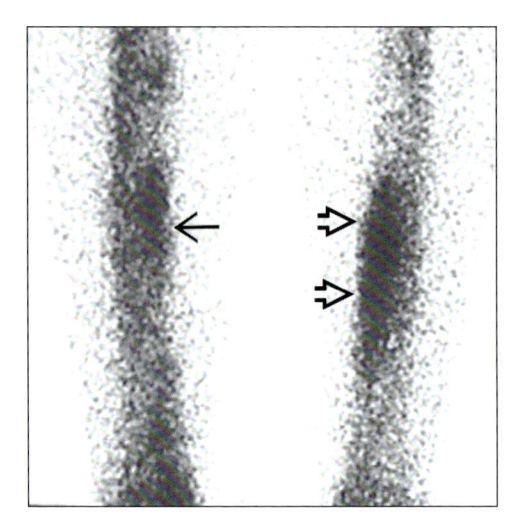

Anterior mineral phase Tc-99m bone scan shows typical right mid tibial stress fracture ➡. Activity spanning mid and distal left tibia indicates more advanced contralateral stress fracture ⇨.

TERMINOLOGY

Abbreviations and Synonyms
- Fatigue fracture

Definitions
- Stress reaction in bone leading to fracture
- Skeletal trauma secondary to repetitive loading overcoming intrinsic repair rates, resulting in a spectrum of progressive bone disruption ranging from micro damage stress reaction to complete fracture
- Stress fracture: Abnormal stress or overuse imposed on otherwise normal bone
- Stress fracture differs from insufficiency fracture: Physiologic stress overwhelming abnormal (insufficient) bone
  - Underlying metabolic or other bony deficiency
- Partial or complete fracture
  - Grade I: Less than 25% of cortex
  - Grade II: 25-50% cortical involvement
  - Grade III: 50-75% cortical involvement
  - Grade IV: > 75% cortical involvement

IMAGING FINDINGS

General Features
- Best diagnostic clue
  - MR: T1WI hypointensity
  - Tc-99m MDP three-phase bone scan: Focal uptake on vascular and delayed phases
- Location
  - Most often lower extremity secondary to stress of weight-bearing, especially in fatigue fractures
    - Most common: Tibial shaft (posteromedial cortex of distal third); running, activity requiring rapid decelerations/stops
    - Anterior tibial stress fractures uncommon: African-American athletes, marching in sand, telemark skiers; mimics direct contusion
    - Tarsal bones: Calcaneus (vertically oriented, parallel to physeal scar), talus, navicular
    - Metatarsals, particularly 2nd and 3rd: Walking, marching, endurance sports, ballet
    - Fibula: Marathon running, jumping, ballet

DDx: Mimics of Stress Fracture on Bone Scan

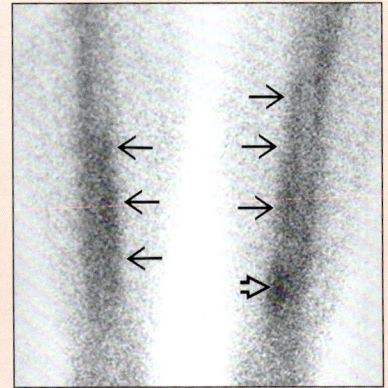

Shin Splints (with Small Stress Fx) 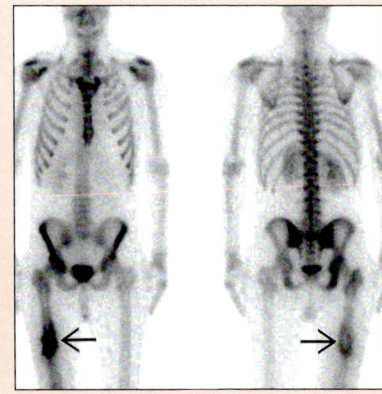 *Pathologic Fracture* 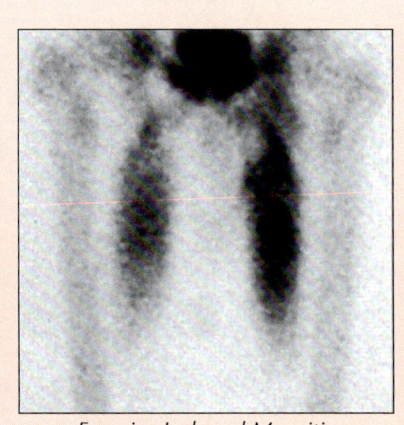 *Exercise-Induced Myositis*

STRESS FRACTURE

Key Facts

Terminology
- Stress fracture: Abnormal stress or overuse imposed on otherwise normal bone

Imaging Findings
- Typically positive on all 3 phases
- Angiographic and blood pool phase positivity may become less conspicuous after 2-4 weeks
- Delayed phase abnormality can persist for ≥ 6-12 months
- Usually focal, fusiform or oval configuration of increased activity
- Focal activity (e.g., < 1/5th length of tibia)
- Whole body scan: Evaluate for other abnormalities, no additional radiation
- SPECT recommended to increase sensitivity, especially when evaluating spine

Top Differential Diagnoses
- Shin Splints/Tibial Periostitis
- Joint Derangement, Trauma, Avulsion
- Neoplasm: Benign or Malignant
- Pathologic fracture

Clinical Issues
- Chronic skeletal pain with weight-bearing or repetitive use in absence of trauma
- Symptoms may be vague and mimic other etiologies
- Age: ↑ With age (↓ bone density)
- Gender: M:F = 1:2
- Prognosis generally very good providing early recognition, appropriate therapy, compliance
- Resolution may take 1-18 months or more

- Spine: Pars, pedicles; spondylolysis may occur in young athletes (L5 > L4 > L3); may be incomplete or unilateral; younger patients more likely asymptomatic
- Sacrum: More common than other pelvic sites; "H" configuration due to vertical and horizontal fractures implies insufficiency fracture
- Pelvis: Pubic rami/symphysis pubis, also iliac or supra-acetabular
- Femur: Most common in medial femoral neck/intertrochanteric region; distal femur most common posteriorly (lateral images helpful)
- Sesamoids: Running, jumping; ddx sesamoiditis
- Occasionally humerus, radius, ulna, scapula, rib

Nuclear Medicine Findings
- Tc-99m MDP three-phase bone scan: Sensitivity 75-95%, limited specificity
  - Clinical history important for interpretation
  - Allows whole body imaging
  - Typically positive on all 3 phases
  - Angiographic and blood pool phase positivity may become less conspicuous after 2-4 weeks
  - Delayed phase abnormality can persist for ≥ 6-12 months
  - Early bone scan limited in patients with osteoporosis (may require 48-72 hours to mount osteoblastic response)
  - Usually focal, fusiform or oval configuration of increased activity
  - Focal activity (e.g., < 1/5th length of tibia)
  - Areas of asymptomatic uptake in athletes: Stress-induced remodeling; may or may not progress to stress fractures

Radiographic Findings
- First-line imaging
- Low sensitivity (10-15%) initially, useful to exclude other pathologies
- Delayed imaging improves accuracy
- Sclerosis, periosteal thickening, callous formation after 2 weeks or more
- Occasionally reveals discrete, visible fracture

CT Findings
- CT: Findings similar to those on radiography, best sensitivity to osteopenia

MR Findings
- High sensitivity 85-95%, high specificity
- Increased fat-suppressed T2, PD or STIR signal on MR: Bone edema suggestive but nonspecific
- Focal, linear low-density fracture delineation may be revealed on T1WI, corresponding to T2 abnormalities
- Stress fracture may be obscured by coexistent marrow changes in anorexia nervosa

Imaging Recommendations
- Best imaging tool: MR: High sensitivity, specificity; advantages include evaluation of adjacent soft tissues, tendons, ligaments; no ionizing radiation
- Protocol advice
  - Tc-99m MDP three-phase bone scan
    - Hydrate patient prior to procedure to promote soft tissue washout, improves target to background
    - 20-25 mCi (740-925 MBq) Tc-99m diphosphonate IV, inject away from area of interest
    - Angiographic and blood pool phases over area of interest
    - Delayed image at 3-4 hours, 2-3 hours longer in patients with poor cardiac output or renal failure
    - Best target-to-background ratio at 6-12 hours, can image up to 24 hours in difficult cases
    - Whole body scan: Evaluate for other abnormalities, no additional radiation
    - SPECT recommended to increase sensitivity, especially when evaluating spine

DIFFERENTIAL DIAGNOSIS

Shin Splints/Tibial Periostitis
- Microavulsion of Sharpey fiber attachments
- Linear, superficial posterior medial tibial cortex, ≥ 1/3 of tibial length
- Angiographic phase hyperemia absent/minimal

STRESS FRACTURE

Soft Tissue Pathology
- Strains, sprains, contusions, myositis, tendinopathies, neuropathies, compartment syndromes
- Bone may be positive on angiographic and blood pool phases, then negative on mineral phase

Joint Derangement, Trauma, Avulsion
- Suspected on radiography; MR characterizes

Neoplasm: Benign or Malignant
- Radiography often suspicious for diagnosis
- Pathologic fracture
  - Local loss of skeletal integrity secondary to underlying bone lesion
  - More commonly metaphyseal
  - Sclerotic, lytic, or permeative, associated mass, endosteal scalloping by CT
  - Well-defined T1 signal changes in pathologic bone, associated mass, endosteal scalloping, T2 changes nonspecific

PATHOLOGY

General Features
- Etiology
  - Wolff law: Bone remodels in response to stress
  - Overuse overwhelms accommodative remodeling
    - Osteoclastic activity may precede adequate osteoblastic reparatory remodeling by weeks
- Epidemiology
  - Up to 10% of sports medicine cases, frequently overlooked
  - More common in females and non-athletes who undertake new or increased activities
    - In females, high-impact activities (running, cheerleading, gymnastics) have higher correlation with stress fractures
  - Typically occur in situations of normal, healthy patients with overuse activity patterns
  - Insufficiency fractures may occur secondary to metabolic bone disorders
    - Senile osteopenia
    - Postmenopausal osteopenia, osteoporosis
    - Previously irradiated bone
    - Vitamin D, phosphate disorders
    - Hyperparathyroidism
    - Chronic renal disease
    - Aluminum, fluoride, heavy metal toxicity
- Associated abnormalities
  - Osteoporosis, eating disorders, amenorrhea may be present in women
  - Spondylolysis, spondylolisthesis

Microscopic Features
- Microdamage with reactive osteoclastic/osteoblastic remodeling

CLINICAL ISSUES

Presentation
- Most common signs/symptoms
  - Chronic skeletal pain with weight-bearing or repetitive use in absence of trauma
  - Symptoms may be vague and mimic other etiologies
  - Stress fracture may be initial presentation in anorexia nervosa

Demographics
- Age: ↑ With age (↓ bone density)
- Gender: M:F = 1:2

Natural History & Prognosis
- Prognosis generally very good providing early recognition, appropriate therapy, compliance
  - Resolution may take 1-18 months or more
- Insufficiency fractures have compromised bone initially, less inclined to heal
- Complications: Delayed union/nonunion (not uncommon), avascular necrosis, pseudoarthrosis

Treatment
- Rest, rehabilitation, bracing, surgery in advanced/complicated cases

DIAGNOSTIC CHECKLIST

Consider
- DDx: Strains, sprains, contusions, derangements, periostitis

Image Interpretation Pearls
- Stress fracture: Positive three-phase imaging with appropriate history
- Areas of asymptomatic uptake in athletes: Stress-induced remodeling; may or may not progress to stress fractures

SELECTED REFERENCES

1. Berger FH et al: Stress fractures in the lower extremity The importance of increasing awareness amongst radiologists. Eur J Radiol. 62(1):16-26, 2007
2. Lee E et al: Role of radionuclide imaging in the orthopedic patient. Orthop Clin North Am. 37(3):485-501, viii, 2006
3. Sofka CM: Imaging of stress fractures. Clin Sports Med. 25(1):53-62, viii, 2006
4. Tins B et al: Marrow changes in anorexia nervosa masking the presence of stress fractures on MR imaging. Skeletal Radiol. 35(11):857-60, 2006
5. Fayad LM et al: Distinction of long bone stress fractures from pathologic fractures on cross-sectional imaging: how successful are we? AJR Am J Roentgenol. 185(4):915-24, 2005
6. Gaeta M et al: CT and MR imaging findings in athletes with early tibial stress injuries: comparison with bone scintigraphy findings and emphasis on cortical abnormalities. Radiology. 235(2):553-61, 2005
7. Lee SW et al: Fatigue stress fractures of the pubic ramus in the army: imaging features with radiographic, scintigraphic and MR imaging findings. Korean J Radiol. 6(1):47-51, 2005
8. Connolly LP et al: Young athletes with low back pain: skeletal scintigraphy of conditions other than pars interarticularis stress. Clin Nucl Med. 29(11):689-93, 2004

STRESS FRACTURE

IMAGE GALLERY

Typical

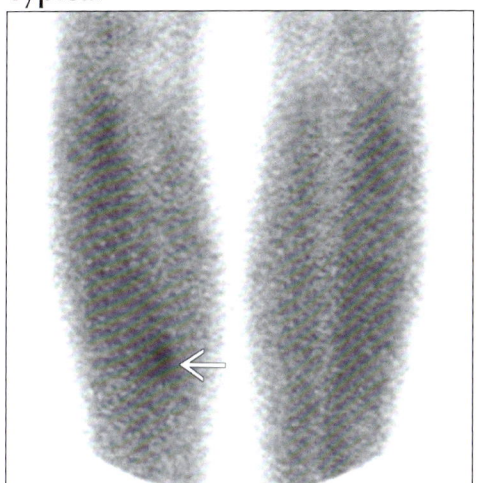

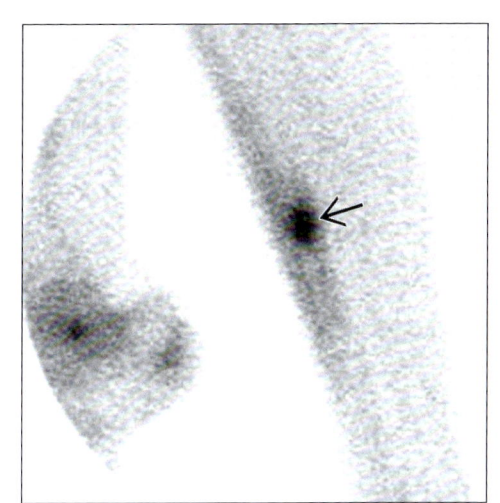

(Left) Anterior blood pool phase bone scan shows hyperemia at junction of mid and distal thirds of right tibia ➡. Patient was a runner with leg pain. See next image. *(Right)* Right medial delayed phase bone scan in same patient shows typical posteromedial cortical tracer accumulation in right tibia ➡, confirming a grade II/III stress fracture.

Typical

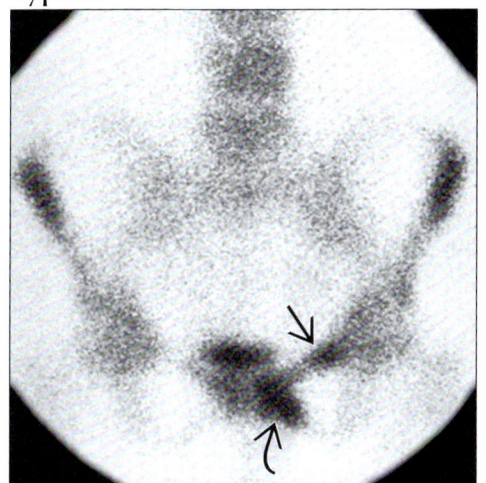

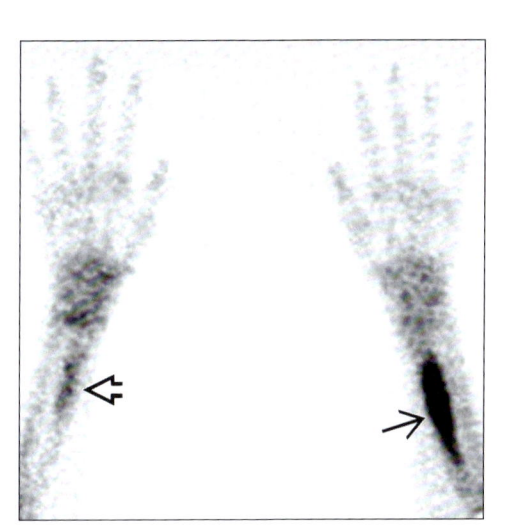

(Left) Anterior mineral phase Tc-99m bone scan shows increased activity at the left superior ➡ and inferior ➡ pubic rami in a patient with pubic stress fracture. *(Right)* Bilateral palmar delayed phase bone scan shows increased activity in distal radial diaphyses, left ➡ greater than right ➡, indicating stress fractures in a gymnast.

Typical

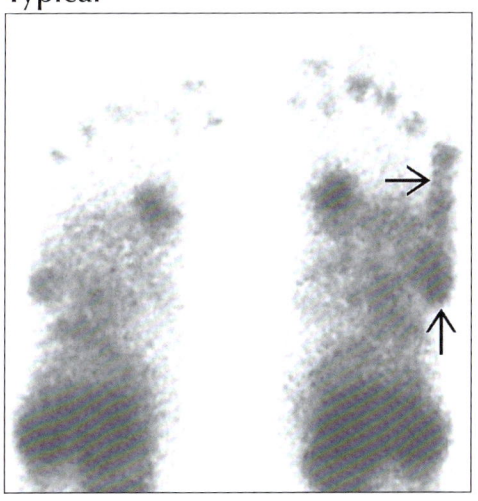

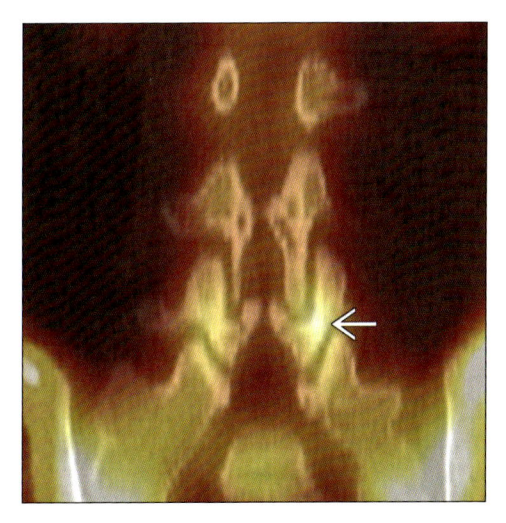

(Left) Plantar delayed phase bone scan shows increased activity along left 5th metatarsal ➡ indicating stress fracture in skeletally immature patient with open growth plates. See next image. *(Right)* Coronal post acquisition fusion of CT and SPECT studies shows uptake at left L5 pars interarticularis stress fracture ➡, demonstrating value of SPECT-CT fusion.

ARTHRITIS, NON-INFECTIOUS

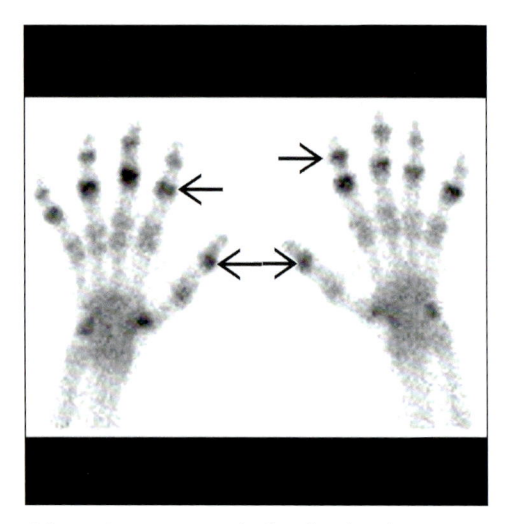

Palmar bone scan of the hands demonstrates distribution of uptake typical of osteoarthritis: DIP and PIP joints ➔ and base of thumbs, with relative sparing of wrists and MCP joints.

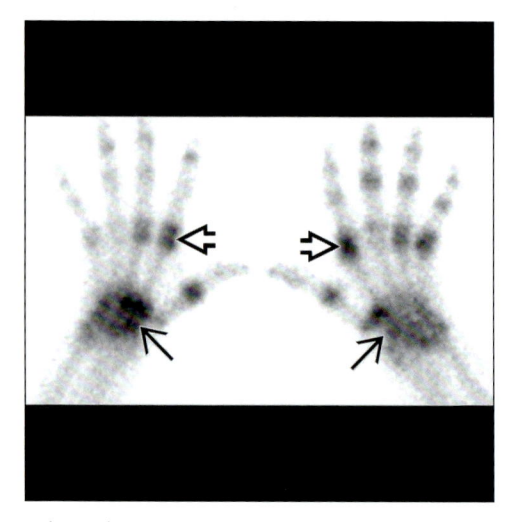

Palmar bone scan of the hands demonstrates distribution of uptake typical of rheumatoid arthritis: Wrists ➔ and MCP ⇨ joints.

TERMINOLOGY

Abbreviations and Synonyms
- Osteoarthritis (OA), degenerative joint disease (DJD), degenerative arthritis, hypertrophic arthritis, osteoarthropathy
- Inflammatory arthropathy
  - Rheumatoid
    - Rheumatoid arthritis
    - Systemic lupus erythematosus
    - Scleroderma
    - Juvenile rheumatoid arthritis
  - Seronegative spondyloarthropathies
    - Ankylosing spondylitis
    - Psoriatic arthritis
    - Reactive arthritis (Reiter syndrome)
  - Metabolic-induced arthritides
    - Gout
    - Calcium pyrophosphate crystal deposition (CPPD) disease/pseudogout
    - Hemochromatosis

Definitions
- Deterioration of joints leading to compromise of function with eventual loss of integrity

IMAGING FINDINGS

General Features
- Best diagnostic clue: Increased activity in joint articulations on bone scan
- Location
  - OA
    - Distal interphalangeal (DIP) joints
    - Proximal interphalangeal (PIP) joints
    - Carpal metacarpal (CMC) joints
    - Metatarsal phalangeal (MTP) joints
    - Hips
    - Knees
    - Spinal facets
  - Inflammatory: Variable, etiology dependent
    - Rheumatoid (e.g., bilateral wrists, feet)
    - Seronegative (e.g., spine, SI joints)
    - Metabolic (e.g., great toe)

DDx: Mimics of Non-Infectious Arthritis on Bone Scan

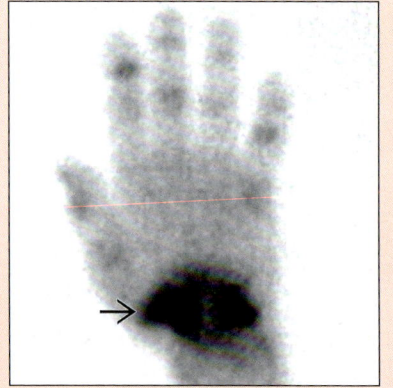

Septic Arthritis

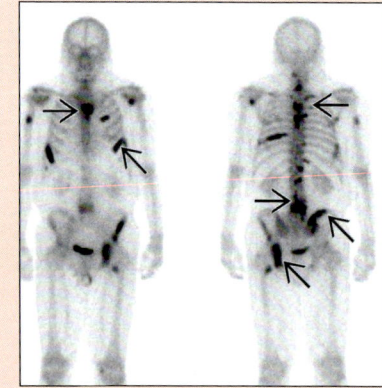

Bone Metastases

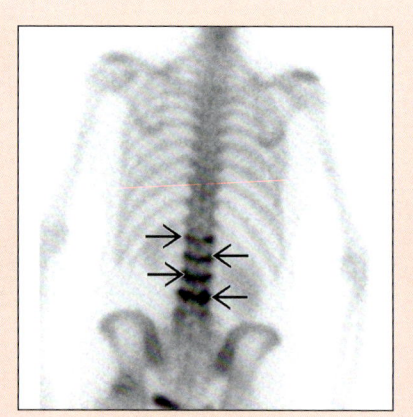

Insufficiency Fractures

ARTHRITIS, NON-INFECTIOUS

Key Facts

Terminology
- Osteoarthritis (OA), degenerative joint disease (DJD), degenerative arthritis, hypertrophic arthritis, osteoarthropathy
- Inflammatory arthropathy
- Seronegative spondyloarthropathies
- Metabolic-induced arthritides

Imaging Findings
- Best diagnostic clue: Increased activity in joint articulations on bone scan
- Increased activity on PET about affected joints due to inflammatory response

Top Differential Diagnoses
- Trauma
- Neoplasm
- Osteomyelitis, Septic Arthritis
- Bone Infarction, Avascular Necrosis

Diagnostic Checklist
- Bone scan for whole-body evaluation of arthritides, confirmation of diagnosis
- Bone scan to confirm presence of radiographically occult joint disease
- Bone SPECT and SPECT/CT useful for localizing radiographically occult lesions in spine, postsurgical spine evaluation
- Bone scan spot views of palmar hands, plantar feet for best evaluation
- Bone metastases and arthritides can be confused: Plain film/CT/MR correlation valuable
- Arthritis can be positive on bone scan and FDG PET

Nuclear Medicine Findings
- Bone Scan: Increased activity about affected joints due to osteoblastic response
- PET
  - Increased activity on PET about affected joints due to inflammatory response

Imaging Recommendations
- Best imaging tool
  - Plain radiography: First-line study in workup of arthritides
    - Less sensitive than bone scan or MR
  - Bone scan
    - Useful for whole-body evaluation of arthritides, confirmation of diagnosis
    - Useful to confirm presence of radiographically occult joint disease
    - Non-infectious arthritis often incidental finding on whole body imaging for bone metastases, can be difficult to distinguish from metastases
    - SPECT and SPECT/CT useful for localizing radiographically occult lesions in spine, postsurgical spine evaluation
    - Active osteoblastic activity of arthritides can be three phase bone scan positive
  - MR: Modality of choice for evaluation of localized inflammatory arthritides
- Protocol advice
  - Bone scan
    - Whole body bone scan for skeletal survey
    - Spot views: Palmar hands, plantar feet; others as needed
    - SPECT: Preferred for characterizing vertebral lesions

DIFFERENTIAL DIAGNOSIS

Trauma
- Fracture, subluxation, avulsion
- Plain films often indicated for clarification after lesions identified on bone scan
- CT may be necessary particularly in spine, pelvis, ribs, sternum

Neoplasm
- Primary vs. metastatic
- Can be difficult to distinguish multifocal metastatic disease from degenerative change
  - Joints commonly affected by degenerative change
  - Spine metastases can mimic spine OA
    - Metastases more common in vertebral body; OA involves endplates and facets

Osteomyelitis, Septic Arthritis
- Periarticular increased activity on all phases of three phase bone scan
- Clinically suggestive picture with symptoms including fever, elevated WBC, constant pain, erythema

Bone Infarction, Avascular Necrosis
- Vascular compromise preceding collapse and subsequent degenerative arthritis
- MR useful in equivocal cases

PATHOLOGY

General Features
- Genetics
  - OA: Hereditary component
  - Rheumatoid: Associated with HLA-DRB1, 18q21 region of RNFRSR11A gene
  - Seronegative spondyloarthropathies: HLA-B27
- Etiology
  - Forces exceeding normal stresses on an otherwise healthy joint
  - Cartilaginous decline with subsequent underlying bony compromise
    - Initiated by chondral insult secondary to loose bodies, osteochondral defects, synovial and synovial fluid pathology
  - Underlying bony failure because of inherent compromise, vascular disruption, metabolic derangement, inflammation

ARTHRITIS, NON-INFECTIOUS

- Autoimmune disease
- Systemic metabolic disease (e.g., gout)
- Epidemiology
  - OA
    - Most common joint disorder
    - 1/3 people > 65 yrs have radiographically positive knee OA
  - Rheumatoid arthritis
    - Prevalence up to 1.5% of people in North America
  - Seronegative spondyloarthropathies
    - Prevalence < 1%
- Associated abnormalities
  - OA
    - Overweight
    - Prior injury
    - Sports
    - Developmental anomalies
  - Rheumatoid arthritis
    - Anemia
    - Pulmonary nodules
    - Amyloidosis
    - Inflammatory heart conditions
    - Ocular
    - Neurological
  - Seronegative spondyloarthropathies
    - Ulcerative colitis
    - Crohn disease

Gross Pathologic & Surgical Features

- Articular cartilaginous degeneration
- Osteophytosis (marginal bone hypertrophy)
- Synovial hypertrophy and inflammation

CLINICAL ISSUES

Presentation

- Most common signs/symptoms
  - OA
    - Joint pain, swelling, tenderness, stiffness, decreased range of motion, joint effusion
    - Hands, knees common
    - Long term: Joint deformity
    - Laboratory: Positive C reactive protein
  - Rheumatoid arthritis
    - Morning stiffness, soft-tissue swelling, symmetric arthritis, hands affected
    - Long term: Swan neck deformity
    - Laboratory: Positive rheumatoid factor
  - Seronegative spondyloarthropathies
    - Chronic pain, stiffness
    - Laboratory: Negative rheumatoid factor
    - Reactive: Associated with preceding infection (usually genital, gastrointestinal), uveitis, urethritis

Demographics

- Age
  - OA
    - Incidence increases with age
  - Rheumatoid arthritis
    - Peak 4th to 6th decades
  - Seronegative spondyloarthropathies
    - Younger population (~ 20-40 yrs)
- Gender
  - OA
    - Male = female
  - Rheumatoid arthritis
    - M:F = 1:2.5
  - Seronegative spondyloarthropathies
    - M > F

Treatment

- Medical therapy
  - Anti-inflammatory drugs
  - Anti-rheumatoid agents (e.g., methotrexate)
  - Antibiotics
- Physical therapy
  - Non-weight bearing exercise: Swimming, bicycling
  - Weight training
  - Flexibility, stretching exercises
- Surgery
  - Arthroplasty
  - Osteotomy
  - Arthrodesis

DIAGNOSTIC CHECKLIST

Consider

- Bone scan for whole-body evaluation of arthritides, confirmation of diagnosis
- Bone scan to confirm presence of radiographically occult joint disease
- Bone SPECT and SPECT/CT useful for localizing radiographically occult lesions in spine, postsurgical spine evaluation
- Bone scan spot views of palmar hands, plantar feet for best evaluation

Image Interpretation Pearls

- Bone metastases and arthritides can be confused: Plain film/CT/MR correlation valuable
- Arthritis can be positive on bone scan and FDG PET

SELECTED REFERENCES

1. O'Shea F et al: The challenge of early diagnosis in ankylosing spondylitis. J Rheumatol. 34(1):5-7, 2007
2. Goerres GW et al: F-18 FDG whole-body PET for the assessment of disease activity in patients with rheumatoid arthritis. Clin Nucl Med. 31(7):386-90, 2006
3. Houseni M et al: Facet joint arthropathy demonstrated on FDG-PET. Clin Nucl Med. 31(7):418-9, 2006
4. Palosaari K et al: Bone oedema predicts erosive progression on wrist MRI in early RA--a 2-yr observational MRI and NC scintigraphy study. Rheumatology (Oxford). 45(12):1542-8, 2006
5. Punzi L et al: Value of C reactive protein in the assessment of erosive osteoarthritis of the hand. Ann Rheum Dis. 64(6):955-7, 2005
6. Wunder A et al: Molecular imaging: novel tools in visualizing rheumatoid arthritis. Rheumatology (Oxford). 44(11):1341-9, 2005
7. Guermazi A et al: Imaging of bone erosion in rheumatoid arthritis. Semin Musculoskelet Radiol. 8(4):269-85, 2004
8. Mohana-Borges AV et al: Monoarticular arthritis. Radiol Clin North Am. 42(1):135-49, 2004
9. Manaster BJ et al: The Requisites, Musculoskeletal Imaging, Second Ed., Mosby. 105-187, 2002

ARTHRITIS, NON-INFECTIOUS

IMAGE GALLERY

Typical

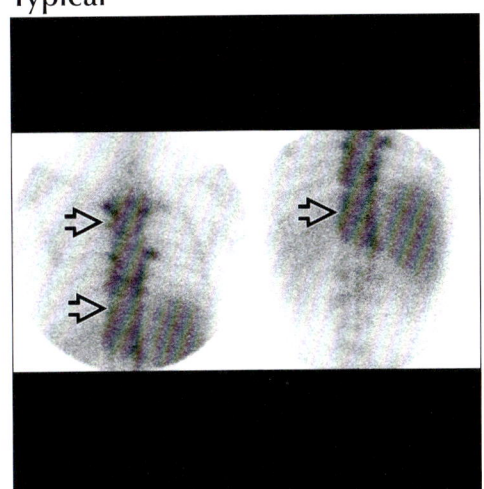

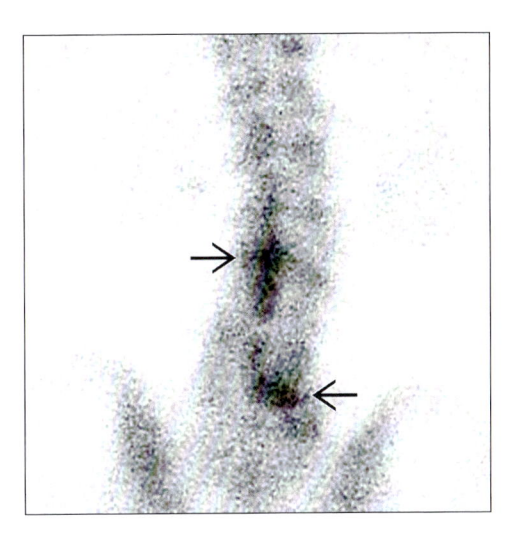

(Left) Posterior bone scan of the thoracic and upper lumbar spine demonstrates multilevel confluent uptake ⇒ typical of active bone bridging due to ankylosing spondylitis. *(Courtesy J. Hoffman, MD).* *(Right)* Posterior bone scan of the lumbar spine demonstrates increased uptake at disc spaces of the concave aspects of alternating lateral curvatures ⇒, typical of degenerative scoliosis.

Typical

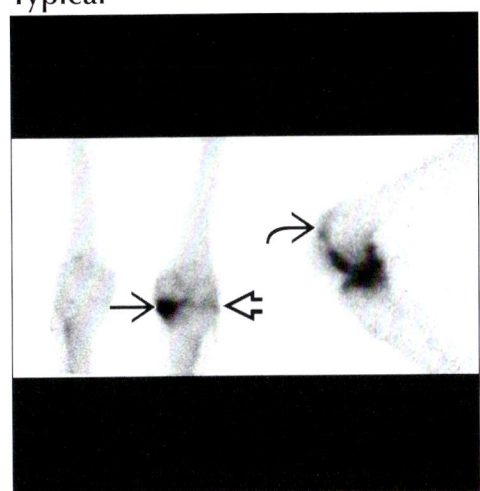

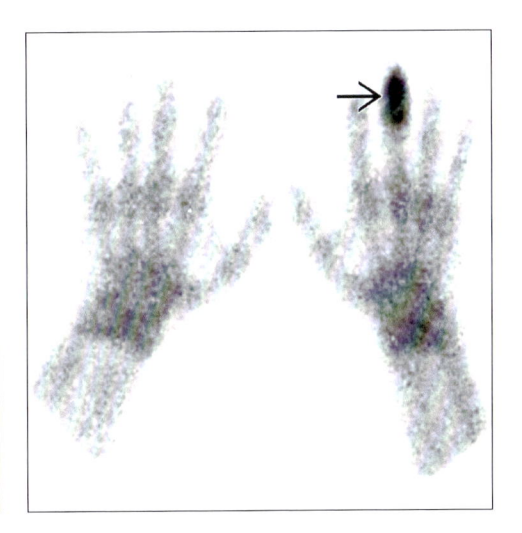

(Left) Anterior and left lateral bone scan of the knees shows marked uptake of the medial compartment ⇒, and mild uptake of the lateral ⇒ and patellofemoral ⇒ compartments, typical of degenerative joint disease. *(Right)* Palmar bone scan of the hands shows intense uptake in the third DIP joint and adjacent bones ⇒ due to acute gouty arthropathy. On bone scan, this is indistinguishable from septic joint with osteomyelitis.

Typical

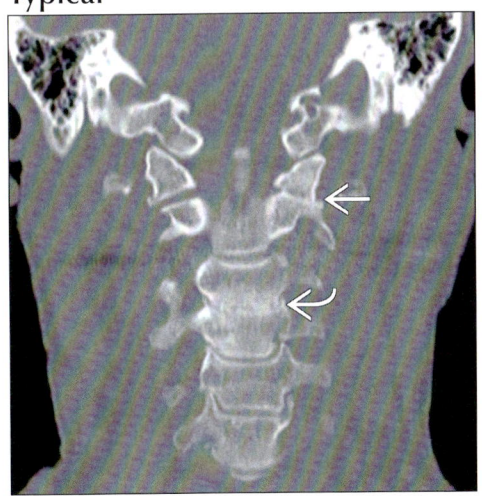

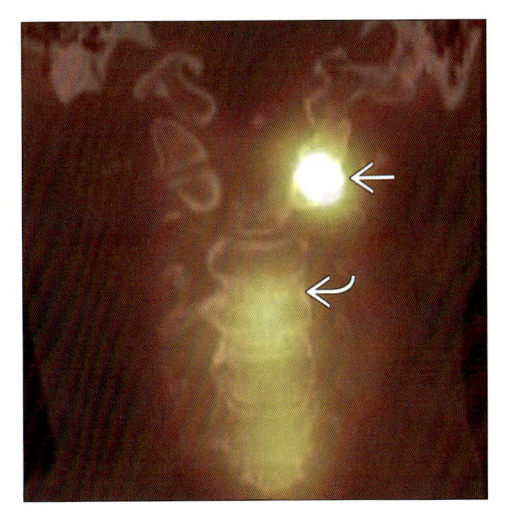

(Left) Coronal NECT shows degenerative changes, most severe in left C1/C2 ⇒ and C3/C4 endplates ⇒ in patient with chronic neck pain. See next image. *(Right)* Coronal bone scan SPECT/CT shows increased activity at left C1/C2 ⇒ indicating the site of bone remodeling. Mildly increased activity in mid cervical endplates ⇒ is comparatively quiescent.

COMPLEX REGIONAL PAIN SYNDROME

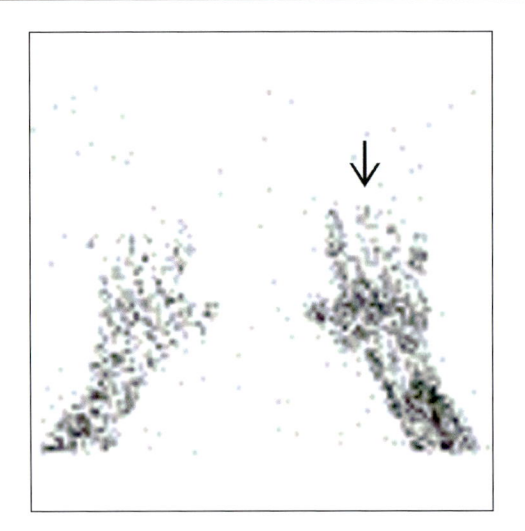

Palmar angiographic phase of bone scan in a patient with CRPS shows classical finding of increased blood flow to involved hand ➔. See next image.

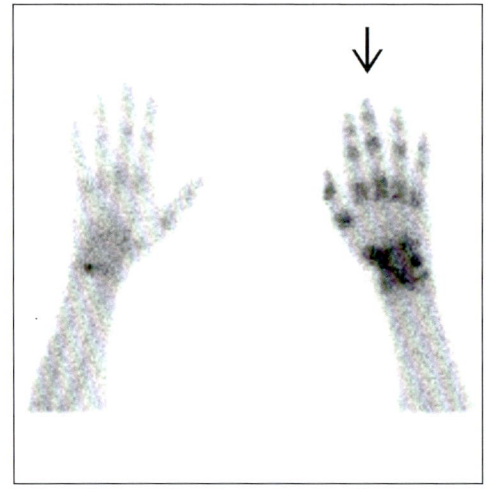

Palmar delayed images of bone scan in a patient with CRPS show classical periarticular activity in hand of the involved extremity ➔.

TERMINOLOGY

Abbreviations and Synonyms
- Complex regional pain syndrome (CRPS)
- Reflex sympathetic dystrophy (RSD)
- Sudeck atrophy (SA)
- Causalgia

Definitions
- Painful disorder of extremities
  - Usually due to injury, surgery, vascular event
  - Usually unilateral; bilateral in ~ 25%
- Once thought to be mediated by sympathetic nervous system (not proven)
- Current thought: Likely neurological disorder affecting vascular system, pain receptors
  - CRPS type 1
    - No detectable nerve lesion
    - "Reflex sympathetic dystrophy"
  - CRPS type 2
    - Detectable nerve lesion
    - "Causalgia"
- Staging
  - Stage 1: Extremity pain characterized by aching, throbbing, burning, cold/touch intolerance, swelling
    - Early, hyperemic stage
    - Pain, sensory abnormalities predominate
  - Stage 2: Muscle wasting, ↑ soft tissue edema, brawny skin, ↑ pain, vasomotor abnormalities
    - Dystrophic stage
    - 3-6 months after onset of stage 1
    - May last weeks, months
  - Stage 3: ↓ Range of motion, digit/joint contracture, waxy skin, brittle, ridged nails, vasomotor abnormalities, ↓ pain
    - Atrophic stage
    - Permanent

IMAGING FINDINGS

General Features
- Best diagnostic clue
  - Tc-99m MDP bone scan: Classically, increased periarticular activity in affected limb on delayed images
    - Periarticular activity increases distally

DDx: Mimics of CRPS

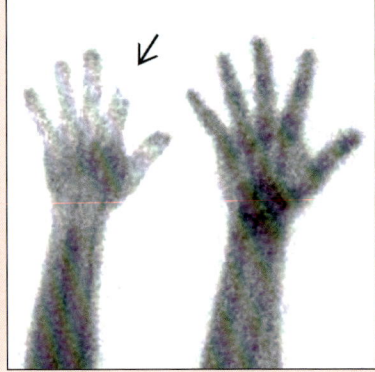

Vasospasm (Raynaud)

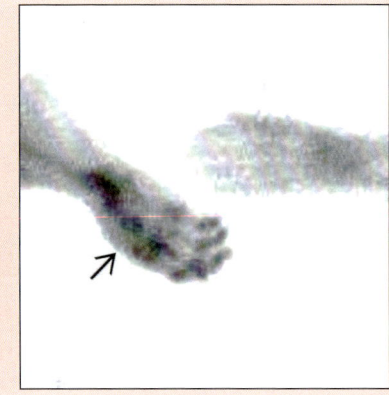

Contracture

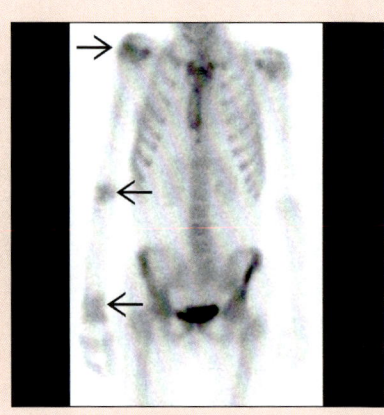

Disuse

COMPLEX REGIONAL PAIN SYNDROME

Key Facts

Terminology
- Complex regional pain syndrome (CRPS)
- Painful disorder of extremities
- Usually due to injury, surgery, vascular event
- Usually unilateral; bilateral in ~ 25%
- Stage 1: Extremity pain characterized by aching, throbbing, burning, cold/touch intolerance, swelling
- Stage 2: Muscle wasting, ↑ soft tissue edema, brawny skin, ↑ pain, vasomotor abnormalities
- Stage 3: ↓ Range of motion, digit/joint contracture, waxy skin, brittle, ridged nails, vasomotor abnormalities, ↓ pain

Imaging Findings
- Tc-99m MDP bone scan: Classically, increased periarticular activity in affected limb on delayed images
- Periarticular activity increases distally

Clinical Issues
- Burning, stinging pain
- Vasomotor instability
- Hyperesthesia
- Skin changes (thickened, waxy), hair loss

Diagnostic Checklist
- Bone scan to look for signs of "classic" CRPS findings
- High intensity uptake on bone scan suggests better prognosis, positive response to therapy
- Early bone scan in patient with suspected CRPS to effect early therapy if positive
- Palmar and plantar delayed planar images to best display periarticular activity

---

- Location
  - Upper, lower extremities most common
  - Face reported
  - Usually unilateral; bilateral in ~ 25%

Nuclear Medicine Findings
- Three-phase bone scan: "Classic" findings
  - Angiographic phase: Hyperemia in affected limb
  - Blood pool phase: Increased periarticular activity when compared with unaffected limb
  - Delayed phase: Increased periarticular activity in affected limb; abnormal activity increases distally
- Stage 1: Usually normal bone scan
- Stage 2: Hyperemia on angiographic phase, increased periarticular activity on blood pool and delayed phase
  - Decreased blood flow can be seen, suggests vasospasm, more common in children
- Stage 3: Hyperemia on angiographic phase, increased periarticular activity on blood pool and delayed phase

Radiographic Findings
- Osteopenia most common, especially subchondral
- Less common: Joint destruction, sclerosis, osteophytosis
- Radiography helpful in stage 2, 3

CT Findings
- Stage 3: Focal areas of osteoporosis

MR Findings
- Stage 2: Soft tissue edema, tissue contrast-enhancement, thickened skin, muscle atrophy
- Stage 3: Muscle atrophy, thickened skin

Imaging Recommendations
- Best imaging tool
  - Three-phase bone scan
    - Stage 1: 25% sensitivity
    - Stage 2: 85% sensitivity
    - Stage 3: > 95% sensitivity
- Protocol advice
  - 20-30 mCi (740-1110 MBq) Tc-99m MDP IV
  - Mechanical issues associated with radiotracer injection (e.g., hyperemia can be caused by tourniquet release) can compromise study
    - If evaluating upper extremity, attempt injection in lower extremity
    - If evaluating lower extremity, inject radiotracer in upper extremity
  - Three phase bone scan: Always include opposite side for same time (not counts)
    - Excellent planar images of hands (palmar) and feet (plantar) required for optimal periarticular evaluation
    - Angiographic phase: Include distal aspect of affected and unaffected extremity
    - Immediate static (blood pool) phase: Include entire extremity (e.g., shoulders to tips of fingers), affected and unaffected extremity
    - Delayed: Include entire extremity (e.g., shoulders to tips of fingers), affected and unaffected extremity
  - Whole body scan
    - May be useful for imaging both extremities at once
    - Likely need spot views of most distal extremity nevertheless

DIFFERENTIAL DIAGNOSIS

Disuse
- Post-traumatic, stroke
- Bone scan: Increased periarticular uptake early in disuse is more pronounced proximally, rather than distally (in CRPS); uptake decreased in chronic disuse

Neuropathy
- Nerve impingement, Pancoast syndrome
- Bone scan: Typically normal

Vascular
- Vasculitis, Raynaud syndrome, venous thrombosis, arteriovenous fistula, frostbite

COMPLEX REGIONAL PAIN SYNDROME

- RSD: Can mimic CRPS with patchy uptake on blood pool; asymmetrical uptake on delayed images

Bone Disorder
- Migratory osteolysis
- Bone scan: Increased uptake in early stages

PATHOLOGY

General Features
- Genetics
  o HLA-A3, HLA-B7, HLA-DR2(15) implicated
  o HLA-DR2(15) associated with poor treatment response
- Etiology
  o Peripheral nerve-mediated inflammation and pain
  o Central nervous system likely has role as well
- Epidemiology
  o Usually precipitating event
    - Soft tissue injury: Cause of 40% of CRPS cases in one study
    - Fracture: Cause of 25% of CRPS cases in one study
    - Myocardial ischemia: 5-20% of these patients have CRPS
    - Stroke: 10-20% of patients with hemiplegia
    - Knee: Arthroscopic surgery most common predisposition
    - Vascular intervention: Reports after arteriovenous graft, hemodialysis
  o In ~ 35% of patients with CRPS, no precipitating event apparent
- Associated abnormalities
  o Emotional disturbances
  o Fibromyalgia
  o Sleep disorders

Gross Pathologic & Surgical Features
- Edema
- Muscle atrophy
- Thickened, waxy skin
- Hair loss

Microscopic Features
- Mast cells, neutrophils, macrophages in affected limb
- Inflammatory cytokines in affected limb
- Fibroblasts, macrophages, Schwann cells in affected nerves

CLINICAL ISSUES

Presentation
- Most common signs/symptoms
  o Burning, stinging pain
  o Vasomotor instability
    - Color, temperature, sweating asymmetry
  o Hyperesthesia
- Other signs/symptoms
  o Swelling
  o ↓ Range of motion
  o Skin changes (thickened, waxy), hair loss
  o Osteopenia

Demographics
- Age
  o Adults
    - Usually 30-60 years
    - Mean age 49 years
  o Children < 18 yrs
    - Lower extremity predominance (5:1 vs. adults)
    - CRPS 1: Girls > boys
    - CRPS 2: Girls = boys
    - Incidence highest ~ puberty
- Gender: Females > males
- Ethnicity: CRPS I may be more common in Caucasians

Natural History & Prognosis
- Children
  o Respond well to intensive physical therapy (cure rate of 90% without medications)
  o Recurrence rate: 30-50%
- Adults
  o Recurrence rate: 2% per patient-year
- High intensity uptake on bone scan suggests better prognosis, positive response to therapy
- Early diagnosis and treatment important to prevent permanent sequelae

Treatment
- Physical therapy (particularly with children)
- Medication
  o Tricyclic antidepressants
  o NSAIDs
  o Steroids
  o Anticonvulsants
  o Bisphosphonates
  o Opioids
- Nerve manipulation
  o Sympathetic blocks
  o Transcutaneous electrical nerve stimulation (TENS)
  o Spinal cord stimulation
  o Sympathectomy (not common)

DIAGNOSTIC CHECKLIST

Consider
- Bone scan to look for signs of "classic" CRPS findings
  o Patient may respond well to course of steroids
- High intensity uptake on bone scan suggests better prognosis, positive response to therapy
- Early bone scan in patient with suspected CRPS to effect early therapy if positive
- Palmar and plantar delayed planar images to best display periarticular activity

SELECTED REFERENCES

1. Harden RN et al: Diagnosis of complex regional pain syndrome: signs, symptoms, and new empirically derived diagnostic criteria. Clin J Pain. 22(5):415-9, 2006
2. Wilder RT: Management of pediatric patients with complex regional pain syndrome. Clin J Pain. 22(5):443-8, 2006
3. Intenzo CM et al: The role of nuclear medicine in the evaluation of complex regional pain syndrome type I. Clin Nucl Med. 30(6):400-7, 2005

COMPLEX REGIONAL PAIN SYNDROME

IMAGE GALLERY

Typical

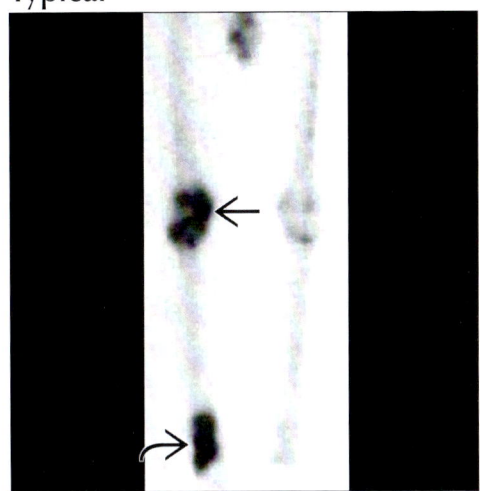

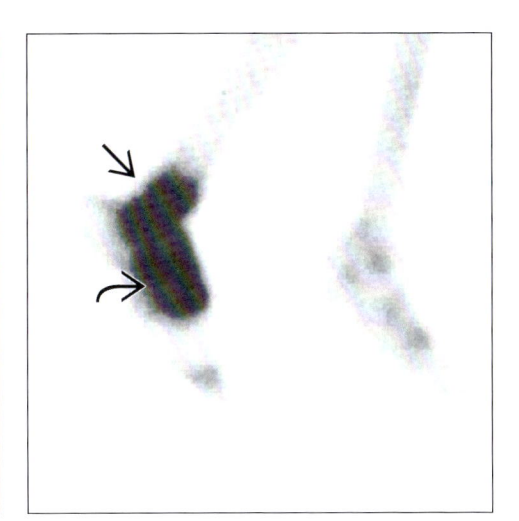

(Left) Anterior delayed phase bone scan in a patient with right lower extremity pain and no history of injury, shows increased periarticular activity about the right knee ➔ and ankle/foot ➔. See next image. (Right) Spot view bone scan of feet in the same patient as previous image shows markedly increased periarticular activity in right ankle ➔ and midfoot ➔. Markedly positive bone scan suggests this patient would have good response to therapy.

Typical

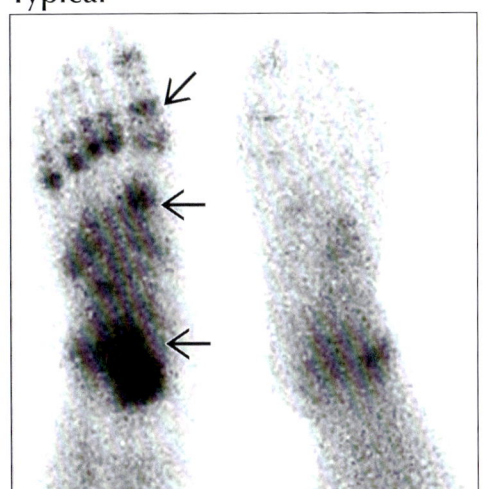

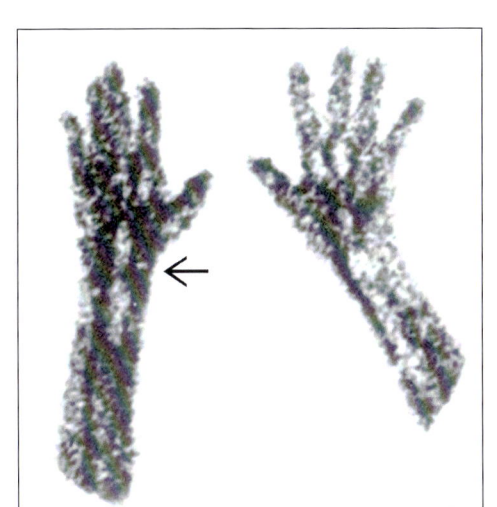

(Left) Plantar bone scan of feet in patient with burning lower extremity pain after minor injury shows increased activity ➔ in a periarticular distribution in right foot, classic findings of CRPS. Note how plantar image show distal joints exceptionally well. (Right) Palmar angiographic phase bone scan shows increased blood flow ➔ in painful right upper extremity. See next image.

Typical

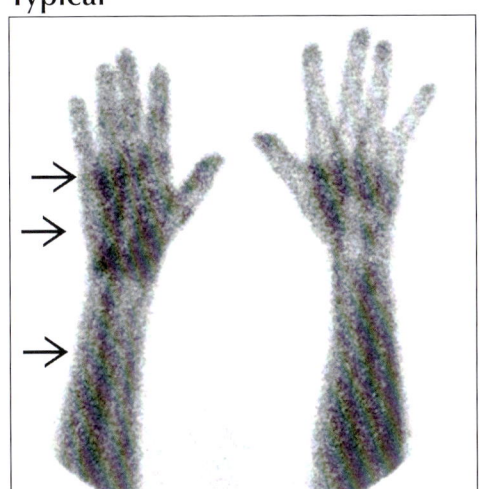

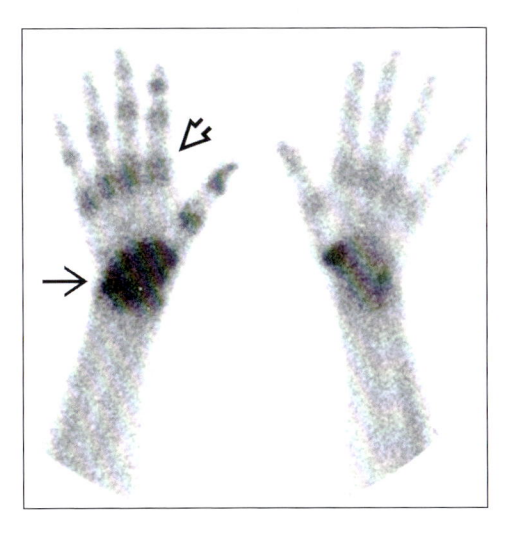

(Left) Palmar blood pool phase bone scan in the same patient as previous image, shows increased activity throughout right upper extremity ➔ when compared to left. See next image. (Right) Palmar delayed phase bone scan in the same patient as previous image, shows increased activity about joints of right wrist ➔ and hand ➔, classic findings of CRPS.

HIP PAIN

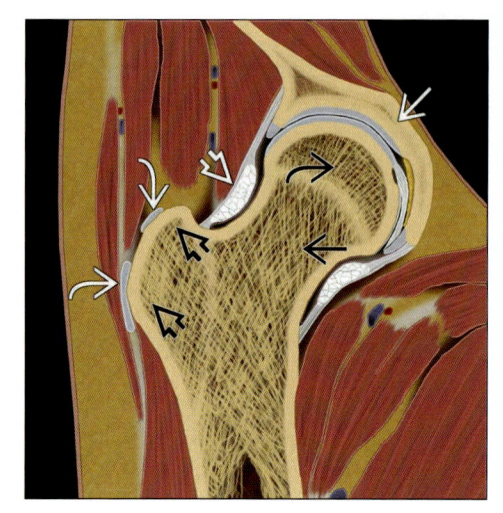

Coronal graphic shows hip anatomy: Femoral head, and neck, greater and lesser trochanters, acetabulum, bursae, and capsule.

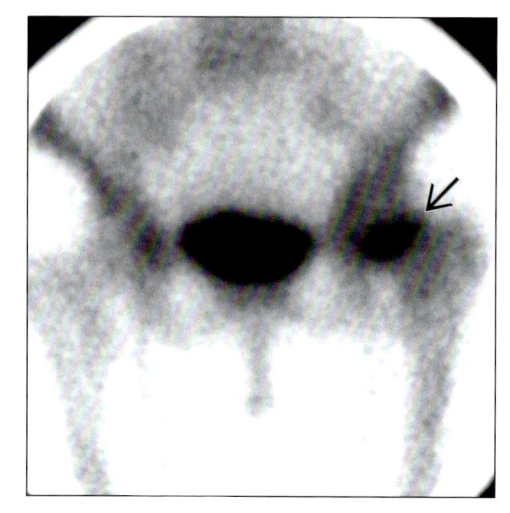

Anterior bone scan shows radiographically occult fracture of left femoral neck in a patient with hip pain. (Courtesy J. Ball, MD).

TERMINOLOGY

Definitions
- Pain in hip caused by variety of traumatic, nontraumatic etiologies
- May originate from vicinity of hip (osseous structures, surrounding bursa or tendinous attachments) or be referred from lower spine or knee

IMAGING FINDINGS

Nuclear Medicine Findings
- Bone Scan: Focal or diffusely increased activity on bone scan in osseous structures of hip, surrounding bursa, muscles, tendons, or soft tissues

Imaging Recommendations
- Best imaging tool
  - Plain films: First-line study
  - Nuclear medicine: Three phase bone scan to localize radiographically occult lesions
- Protocol advice
  - Adult: 20-30 mCi (740-1110 MBq) Tc-99m MDP IV
  - Pediatric: (Age + 1/age + 7) x adult dose
  - Angiographic phase: Anterior and posterior dynamic image over hips
  - Blood pool phase: Static anterior, posterior images
  - Delayed phase: Anterior and posterior planar images from lumbar spine to knees
  - Converging, pinhole, SPECT images as needed
- Additional nuclear medicine imaging options
  - Labeled leukocyte scintigraphy or Ga-67 scintigraphy if suspected infection
  - Tc-99m sulfur colloid marrow map may be needed as adjunct if violated bone (e.g., hip prosthesis)

DIFFERENTIAL DIAGNOSIS

Fracture
- Stress
  - ↑ Uptake on flow, blood pool, delayed images
  - Stress fracture of femoral neck
    - Compressive: Inferior margin of femoral neck
    - Tensile stress: Superior border of femoral neck
- Insufficiency

DDx: Other Conditions Associated with Hip Pain

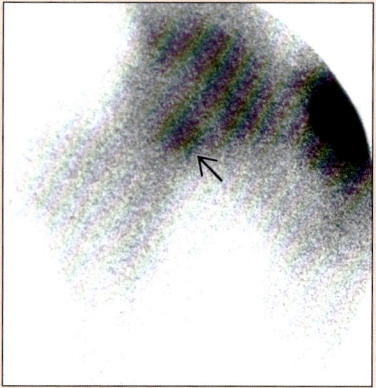

Osteoid Osteoma

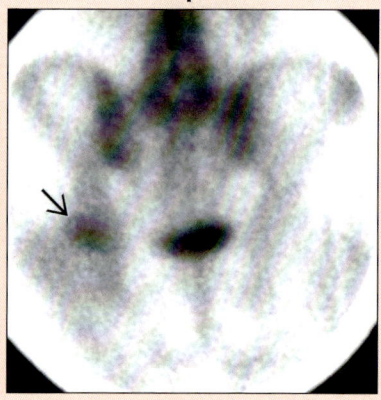

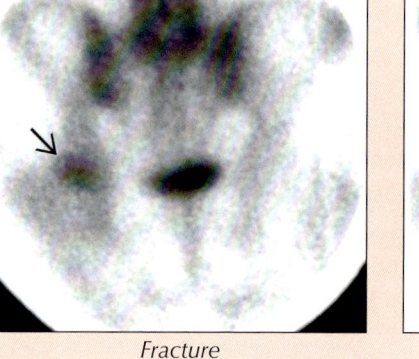

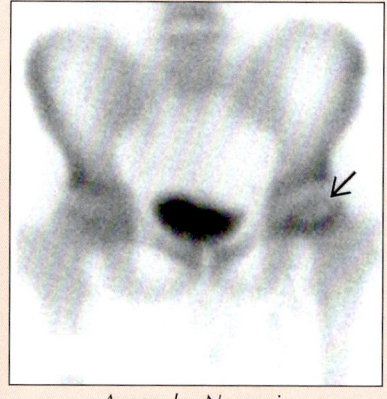

Fracture

Avascular Necrosis

HIP PAIN

Key Facts

Terminology
- Pain in hip caused by variety of traumatic, nontraumatic etiologies
- May originate from vicinity of hip (osseous structures, surrounding bursa or tendinous attachments) or be referred from lower spine or knee

Imaging Findings
- Plain films: First-line study
- Nuclear medicine: Three phase bone scan to localize radiographically occult lesions
- Labeled leukocyte scintigraphy or Ga-67 scintigraphy if suspected infection
- Tc-99m sulfur colloid marrow map may be needed as adjunct if violated bone (e.g., hip prosthesis)

Clinical Issues
- Young: Avulsion injury and stress fractures in athletes
- Older: Osteoarthritis, metastasis, insufficiency fractures
- In one study, 14% of > 6,000 respondents over age 60 reported hip pain in previous 6 week period

Diagnostic Checklist
- Bone scan for investigation of radiographically occult hip pain
- Include lumbar spine and knees in images, as pain from these sites can be referred to hip
- Correlate bone scan with radiographs, MR to add specificity
- Labeled leukocyte scintigraphy if infection suspected

  - May involve femoral neck, acetabulum, sacrum, ilium, pubic bones
  - Positive 2-3 weeks before radiographic changes evident
  - Occurs in osteoporotic patients and patients with predisposing metabolic or endocrine factors (steroids, rheumatoid arthritis, radiation therapy)
- Post-traumatic, occult fracture
  - Bone scan sensitivity high, increases after 48 hours (sensitivity 93%, specificity 95%)
  - Approximately 50% of patients with clinical suspicion of fracture and negative plain films will have occult fracture on radionuclide exam or MR
  - False negative: Study performed too early; fracture through avascular bone
  - False positive: Acetabular curtain osteophytes

Bursitis
- Trochanteric bursitis most common
  - Focal increased uptake on superior and lateral side of greater trochanter
- Associated with overuse

Arthritis/Synovitis
- Degenerative osteoarthritis
  - Insidious onset groin and thigh pain, worse in mornings and exacerbated by axial loading; stiffness
  - Increased uptake on delayed images in areas of active subchondral bone and active osteophytes
- Rheumatoid arthritis
  - Hip pain and morning stiffness
  - Bone scan sensitive, but not specific
    - Hyperemia and diffuse increased uptake
    - Joints with increased activity likely to develop erosions
- Synovitis
  - May be inflammatory or infectious
  - Periarticular hyperemia; ± effusion

Avulsion Injury
- Common in young athletes

- Ischium, greater and lesser trochanter, anterior-superior iliac spine, anterior-inferior iliac spine, iliac crest
  - Bony or cartilaginous failure secondary to force applied by musculoskeletal unit
- Early findings: Focal hyperemia, intense uptake on three-phase bone scan
- Later: Less intense uptake

Avascular Necrosis (AVN)
- Early findings: Photopenia (day 7 to 10)
- Reparative phase: Increased uptake (1 to 3 weeks)
- Sensitivity 78-91% (85-95% with SPECT)

Primary Bone Tumor
- Benign
  - Osteoid osteoma: Vascular nidus surrounded by focal sclerosis displaying increased uptake
  - Giant cell tumor: May display uniformly increased uptake or rim of increased uptake with photopenic center
  - Unicameral bone cyst: Normal uptake or photopenia unless complicated by fracture
  - Aneurysmal bone cyst: Hyperemia, doughnut pattern of uptake
- Malignant
  - Plasmacytoma, chondrosarcoma, Ewing sarcoma, osteosarcoma, fibrosarcoma, malignant fibrous histiocytoma
  - Increased uptake in area of tumor, metastases

Metastatic Disease
- Lung, prostate, breast, renal cell, thyroid most common primaries for osseous metastases
- Typically multiple sites of increased uptake in axial skeleton distribution
  - May have solitary site of involvement
- Aggressive lytic lesions may appear cold

Paget Disease
- Involvement of pelvis common, often unilateral
- Typically painless

HIP PAIN

- Bone scan: Most sensitive test to demonstrate Paget disease (usually increased uptake, misshapen bone)

Transient Osteoporosis
- Self-limited diffuse bone marrow edema of femoral head and neck
- Bone scan: Hyperemia and diffusely increased uptake
  - Involves femoral head, neck, intertrochanteric region
  - Acetabulum spared

Acetabular Labral Tear
- Hyperemia, increased uptake in superior/superomedial acetabulum ("eyebrow pattern")

Enthesopathy
- Reactive periostitis at site of muscle attachment
- Increased uptake on bone scan

Rhabdomyolysis
- Soft tissue uptake after extensive exercise (e.g., long distance runners)

Osteomyelitis
- Increased uptake on all phases of three phase bone scan
- Labeled leukocyte scintigraphy adds specificity

Fibrous Dysplasia
- Intense hyperemia and intense uptake with well-delineated margins
- Bone scan determines activity and extent of involvement

Pediatric Population Variants
- Legg-Calve-Perthes disease
  - Disrupted blood supply to capital femoral epiphysis
  - Limp; groin, thigh, knee pain; boys 3-12 yrs
  - Initial photopenia, then ↑ uptake with healing
- Juvenile osteonecrosis
  - AVN with identifiable etiology (e.g., sickle cell disease, thalassemia)
- Slipped capital femoral epiphysis
  - Affects boys in early adolescence
  - Early: Widening or ovaling of affected physis with increased uptake on bone scan
  - Mid: Loss of activity in physis secondary to growth plate disruption
  - Late: May progress to chondrolysis with increased uptake in acetabular roof

Painful Hip Prosthesis
- In first year after surgery the pattern of periprosthetic uptake is variable; sequential scans may be necessary
- Aseptic loosening: Increased uptake at acetabular component or tip of femoral component on bone scan
- Dislocation: Radiographic diagnosis
- Infection: Diffuse periprosthetic activity on three phase bone scan (nonspecific)
  - Lack of hyperemia on first phase of three-phase bone scan = high negative predictive value

PATHOLOGY

General Features
- Epidemiology: High incidence of hip pain in population > 60 yrs

CLINICAL ISSUES

Presentation
- Most common signs/symptoms
  - Lateral hip pain increased by pressure: Bursitis
  - Increasing pain after weight bearing, improves with rest: Osteoarthritis
  - Constant pain: Inflammation, infection, neoplastic
  - Pain worse at night, relieved by aspirin: Osteoid osteoma
  - Lateral hip pain, extending down leg and over a wide area: L4/5 nerve entrapment

Demographics
- Age
  - Young: Avulsion injury and stress fractures in athletes
  - Older: Osteoarthritis, metastasis, insufficiency fractures
    - In one study, 14% of > 6,000 respondents over age 60 reported hip pain in previous 6 week period

Treatment
- Conservative: Rest, non-weight bearing activity, physical therapy
- Medical: NSAIDs, steroids, IV antibiotics
- Surgical
  - Core decompression: Transient osteoporosis, AVN
  - Fixation: Hip fracture
  - Hip prosthesis: End stage degenerative disease
  - Wide surgical excision: Tumor
  - Debridement: Infection
- Radiation
  - Metastatic disease: External beam radiation, beta-emitting agents (e.g., samarium, strontium)

DIAGNOSTIC CHECKLIST

Consider
- Bone scan for investigation of radiographically occult hip pain
  - Include lumbar spine and knees in images, as pain from these sites can be referred to hip
- Correlate bone scan with radiographs, MR to add specificity
- Labeled leukocyte scintigraphy if infection suspected

SELECTED REFERENCES

1. Williams TR et al: Acetabular stress fractures in military endurance athletes and recruits: incidence and MRI and scintigraphic findings. Skeletal Radiol. 31(5):277-81, 2002
2. Moreno AJ et al: Bone scan manifestation of transient osteoporosis of the hip. Clin Nucl Med. 26(10):872-3, 2001
3. Fernandez-Ulloa M et al: Orthopaedic nuclear medicine: the pelvis and hip. Semin Nucl Med. 28(1):25-40, 1998

HIP PAIN

IMAGE GALLERY

Typical

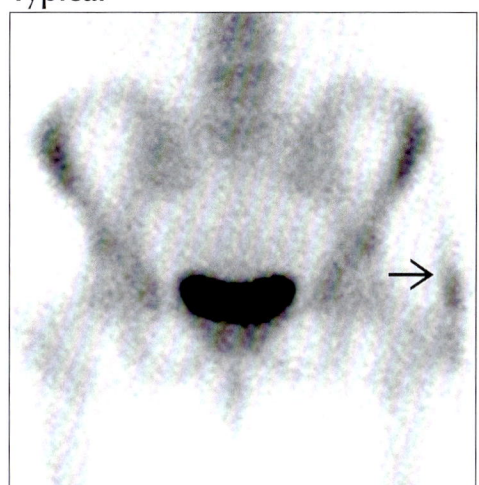

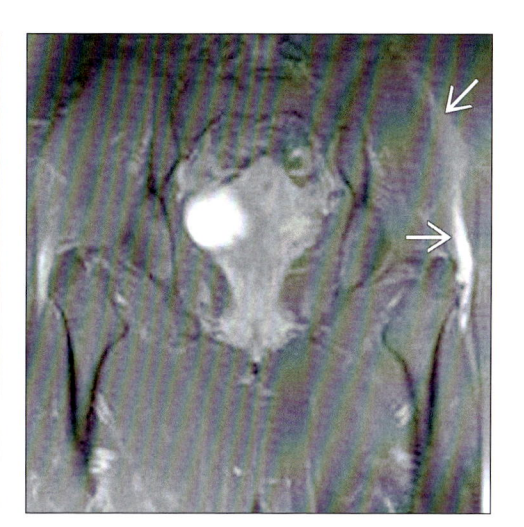

(Left) Bone scan shows focal accumulation at greater trochanter ➡ with soft tissue activity extending superiorly in a patient with gluteus medius avulsion. See next image. *(Right)* T2WI MR in the same patient as previous image, shows increased signal ➡ corresponding to abnormal soft tissue activity on bone scan.

Typical

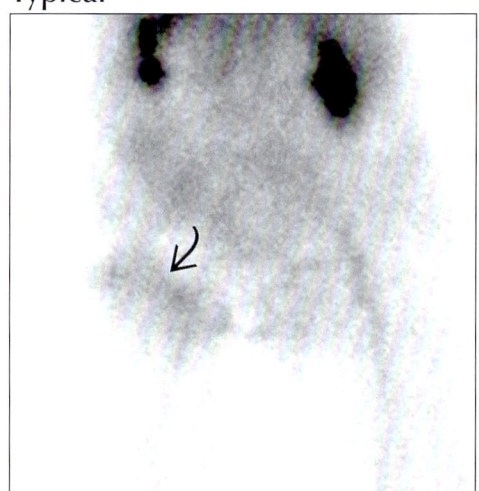

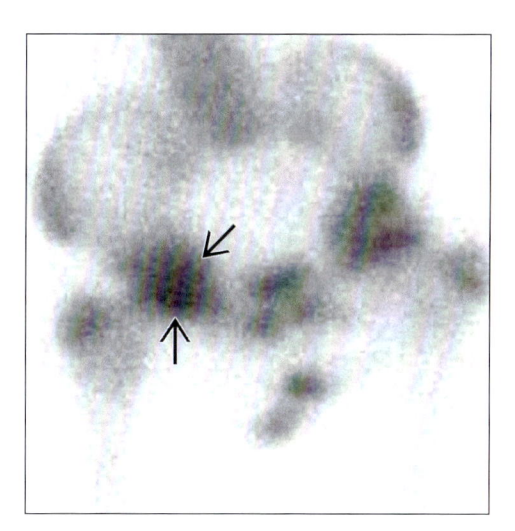

(Left) Anterior blood pool phase bone scan shows hyperemia of right hip ➡ in a young patient with hip pain, intermittent fever, and increased white blood cell count. See next image. *(Right)* Anterior delayed bone scan in the same patient as previous image, shows diffuse increased activity in right hip ➡. Biopsy confirmed osteomyelitis.

Typical

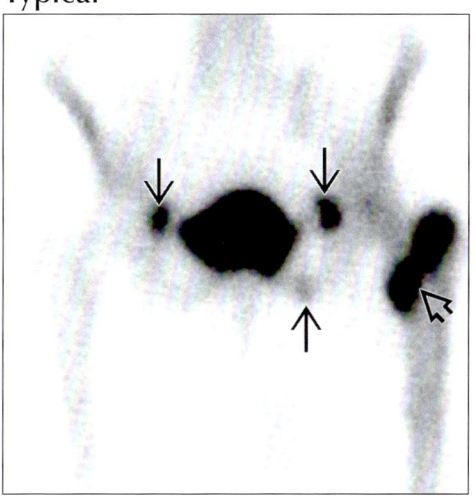

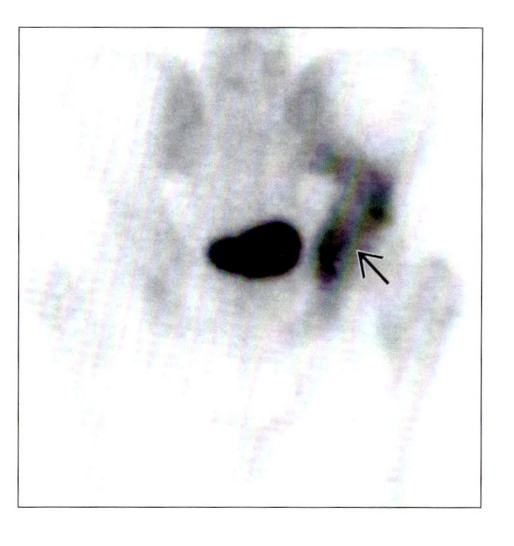

(Left) Anterior bone scan shows postsurgical left intertrochanteric fracture ➢. Additional pelvic insufficiency fractures were radiographically occult ➡. *(Right)* Posterior bone scan in a patient with lung cancer and right hip pain shows diffuse increased activity in right acetabulum ➡, site of solitary bone metastasis.

WRIST PAIN

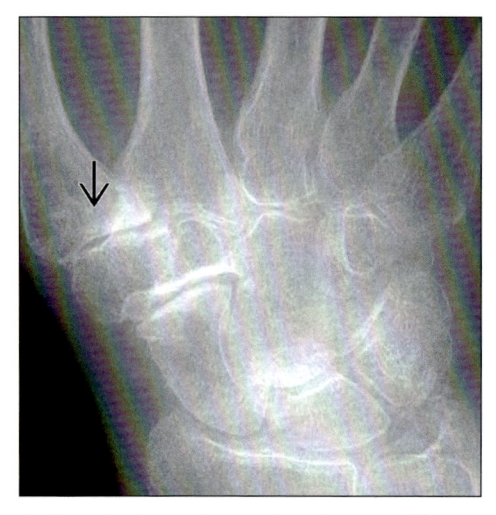

Radiograph shows degenerative changes, with joint space narrowing and adjacent sclerosis ➡, involving base of first metacarpal in a patient with osteoarthritis. (Courtesy B. Manaster, MD, PhD).

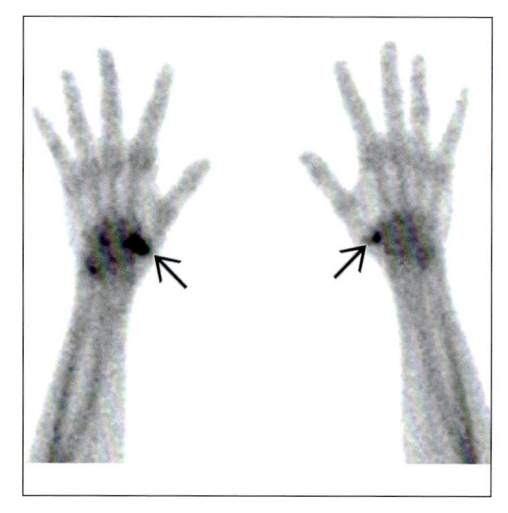

AP bone scan of the hands (same patient as previous image) shows bilateral degenerative osteoarthritis at the first metacarpal-carpal articulation ➡.

TERMINOLOGY

Definitions
- Acute or chronic pain in region of carpals

IMAGING FINDINGS

General Features
- Best diagnostic clue
  - Bone scan: Increased activity in site of trauma, osteoarthritis, tumor, etc., nonspecific
    - Bone scan: Focuses site of further workup (radiography, CT, MR) to determine etiology

Imaging Recommendations
- Best imaging tool
  - Radiography: First-line study for wrist pain
  - Three phase bone scan: Localizes source of pain, focuses further work-up and differential diagnosis in radiographically occult lesions
- Protocol advice
  - Three phase, whole body, spot view delayed bone scans useful, depending on clinical scenario
  - Adult dose: 20-30 mCi (740 MBq-1.11 GBq) Tc-99m MDP IV
  - Pediatric dose: (Age+1/age+7) x adult dose (as low as 2 mCi) Tc-99m MDP IV
  - Inject in arm opposite from site of interest; if complex regional pain syndrome suspected, inject in foot vein
    - Do not apply tourniquet: Results in reactive hyperemia upon release/injection
  - Image in neutral palmar position; add ulnar/radial deviation or lateral view as necessary
  - Tape hands to camera prevent movement
  - Place gauze between fingers to separate
  - High resolution collimator
  - Symmetric positioning important, especially in children when comparing epiphyseal activity
  - Flow images: Palmar position, dynamic, 3 sec/frame x 40
  - Blood pool images: Palmar position, static image
  - Delayed image: 500K counts, label right vs. left, obtain ~ 3 hours post injection
    - May need delayed imaging in diabetic or vasculopathic patients

DDx: Mimics of Hand/Wrist Pathology on Bone Scan

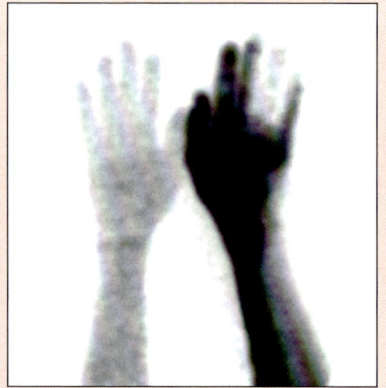

Intra-Arterial Injection

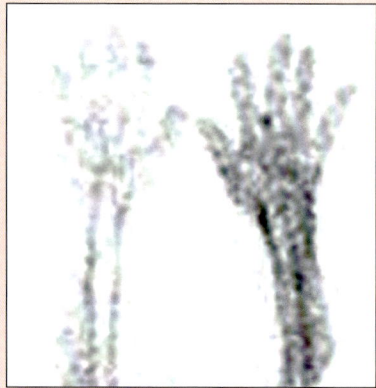

Reactive Hyperemia (Tourniquet)

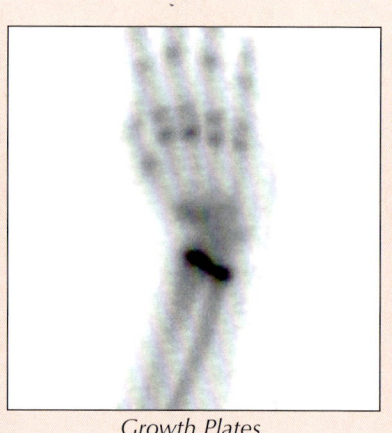

Growth Plates

WRIST PAIN

Key Facts

Imaging Findings
- Radiography: First-line study for wrist pain
- Three phase bone scan: Localizes source of pain, focuses further work-up and differential diagnosis in radiographically occult lesions

Top Differential Diagnoses
- Occult Fracture
- Osteomyelitis
- Arthritis/Synovitis
- Bone Infarction
- Osteoarthritis
- Reflex Sympathetic Dystrophy (RSD), Regional Pain Syndrome
- Myositis/Tendinitis
- Ganglion Cyst
- Radial/Ulnar Artery Thrombosis
- Soft Tissue Vascular Mass
- Tumor
- Fibrous Dysplasia

Clinical Issues
- Young: Overuse in sports (gymnastics, softball, weight lifting, football, rugby, golf, tennis)
- Adults: Repetitive use injury, often occupational (typist, cashier, painting, use of vibratory tools, sewing, meat processor, computer operator)
- Seniors: Degenerative changes

Diagnostic Checklist
- Correlate bone scan with history, physical examination, and prior studies
- High resolution, palmar images for optimal bone scan

DIFFERENTIAL DIAGNOSIS

Occult Fracture
- Most common: Scaphoid (85%)
  - Pain with palpation anatomic snuff box
  - Often from forward fall
  - Most common in scaphoid waist
  - Waist and proximal pole fractures most at risk for avascular necrosis (AVN) and nonunion
- Second most common: Distal radius
  - From forward fall on outstretched hand
  - Dorsiflexion, hyperextension
- Less common: Hook of hamate fracture (1.5%)
  - Soreness in palm
  - Direct blow or fall on outstretched wrist
- Bone scan: Acute fracture shows ↑ activity on all phases of three phase bone scan

Osteomyelitis
- Bone scan: ↑ Activity on all phases of three phase bone scan
  - May add 24 hr image (4th phase) to increase specificity for osteomyelitis if positive
- Add labeled leukocyte scintigraphy in violated (trauma, surgery) bone
  - Tc-99m HMPAO labeled leukocyte scintigraphy preferred for extremities, in children
- Often from trauma, laceration, bite, penetrating injury; hematogenous or contiguous spread

Arthritis/Synovitis
- Diffuse ↑ activity on all phases of three phase bone scan periarticular distribution
- May be secondary to infection, rheumatoid arthritis, ankylosing spondylitis, reactive arthritis (Reiter syndrome), systemic lupus erythematosus
- Whole body bone scan may reveal extent of disease

Bone Infarction
- Kienbock disease: AVN of lunate
  - From interruption of blood supply to anatomically susceptible lunate
  - Related to trauma and negative ulnar variance
  - Dorsal tenderness about lunate
- Scaphoid AVN
  - Follows fracture with disruption of blood supply to proximal pole
- ↓ Uptake on flow, blood pool, delayed images with early AVN
- ↑ Activity on delayed bone scan in healing phase

Osteoarthritis
- Degenerative osteoarthritis: Most intense uptake at base of thumb, often involves DIP
- Normal flow and blood pool images, ↑ uptake on delayed imaging of three phase bone scan
- Plain film: Joint space narrowing, sclerosis
- Wrist pain with activity

Reflex Sympathetic Dystrophy (RSD), Regional Pain Syndrome
- Either ↑ or ↓ uptake on flow and blood pool images in extremity
- ↑ Uptake in periarticular distribution on delayed images, increases distally
- Present with pain, swelling, vasomotor instability

Myositis/Tendinitis
- De Quervain tenosynovitis: First extensor compartment
  - ↑ Uptake on all phases of three phase bone scan along distal radius, abductor pollicis longus, extensor pollicis brevis
  - Wrist pain, radial side
  - Racquet sports, golf, occupational overuse; repetitive activities lead to increased friction and inflammation
  - Most common stenosing tenosynovitis in athletes
- Extensor carpi ulnaris tendinitis
  - Repetitive activities using ulnar deviation
  - Second most frequent site of stenosing tenosynovitis in upper extremity
  - Pain dorsally at distal ulna

WRIST PAIN

Ganglion Cyst
- Homogeneous fluid-filled cyst in communication with scapholunate interval
- Common cause of wrist pain with soft tissue mass
- Usually normal bone scan

Radial/Ulnar Artery Thrombosis
- Decreased flow to affected distribution on angiographic phase images

Soft Tissue Vascular Mass
- Transient ↑ activity on flow, blood pool images of three phase bone scan
- No abnormal bone uptake on delayed image

Tumor
- Chondroid tumors
  - Osteochondroma, enchondroma, chondroblastoma, chondromyxoid fibroma: Rare
  - Varying degrees of uptake on bone scan
- Bone island
  - Failure of mature trabeculae to resorb and remodel
  - Normal to mildly ↑ uptake on bone scan
- Osteoid osteoma
  - Pain, worse at night, relieved by anti-inflammatory drugs
  - Marked ↑ uptake on bone scan, double density sign
- Osteoblastoma
  - Larger lesion (> 2 cm)
  - ↑ Uptake of radiotracer
- Giant cell
  - Expansile lytic lesion in metaphysis, extends to articular surface
  - ↑ Flow, hyperemia, may see doughnut sign on delayed image with peripherally ↑ activity
- Unicameral/aneurysmal bone cyst
  - Unicameral
    - Often asymptomatic, may present with pathologic fracture
    - Bone scan may be normal or display ↑ peripheral uptake and ↓ central radiotracer uptake
  - Aneurysmal bone cyst
    - Present with progressive pain and swelling
    - Bone scan: Doughnut sign, with ↑ peripheral uptake and photopenic center
- Sarcoma
  - Rhabdomyosarcoma: Most common soft tissue tumor in children
    - ↑ Uptake on flow, blood pool images
  - Osseous sarcomas
    - ↑ Uptake all 3 phases
    - Whole body bone scan for metastasis

Fibrous Dysplasia
- May present in wrist or hand (rare)
- ↑ Uptake on all phases of three phase bone scan
- Monostotic and polyostotic forms: Whole body bone scan to determine activity and extent of involvement

CLINICAL ISSUES

Presentation
- Most common signs/symptoms
  - Challenging clinical differential diagnosis due to complexity of carpus
  - May present with pain on movement (sprain, radiocarpal arthritis, fracture)
  - Swelling
    - Localized: Ganglion cyst
    - Diffuse: Complex regional pain syndrome
  - Morning stiffness: Rheumatoid arthritis
  - Focal pain
    - Base of thumb: Osteoarthritis
    - Dorsolateral pain: De Quervain tenosynovitis
- Other signs/symptoms: Wrist pain: 14% of ER visits

Demographics
- Age
  - Young: Overuse in sports (gymnastics, softball, weight lifting, football, rugby, golf, tennis)
  - Adults: Repetitive use injury, often occupational (typist, cashier, painting, use of vibratory tools, sewing, meat processor, computer operator)
  - Seniors: Degenerative changes
- Gender: Women: More prone to osteoarthritis and rheumatoid arthritis

Natural History & Prognosis
- Early diagnosis helpful in preventing complications
- If traumatic injury, understand mechanism of injury

Treatment
- Overuse: Correct workplace ergonomics
- Fracture: Immobilization to prevent complications
- Surgery: Tumors, some fractures may require fixation, ganglion cyst
- Osteoarthritis: Anti-inflammatories, physical therapy
- Infection: Antibiotics, debridement

DIAGNOSTIC CHECKLIST

Consider
- Bone scan to evaluate radiographically occult disease, focus differential diagnosis, direct further workup
- Correlate bone scan with history, physical examination, and prior studies
- High resolution, palmar images for optimal bone scan

SELECTED REFERENCES
1. Nagle DJ: Evaluation of chronic wrist pain. J Am Acad Orthop Surg. 8(1):45-55, 2000
2. Vande Streek P et al: Upper extremity radionuclide bone imaging: the wrist and hand. Semin Nucl Med. 28(1):14-24, 1998
3. Patel N et al: High-resolution bone scintigraphy of the adult wrist. Clin Nucl Med. 17(6):449-53, 1992
4. Maurer AH: Nuclear medicine in evaluation of the hand and wrist. Hand Clin. 7(1):183-200, 1991
5. Linn MR et al: Imaging the symptomatic wrist. Orthop Clin North Am. 21(3):515-43, 1990

WRIST PAIN

IMAGE GALLERY

Typical

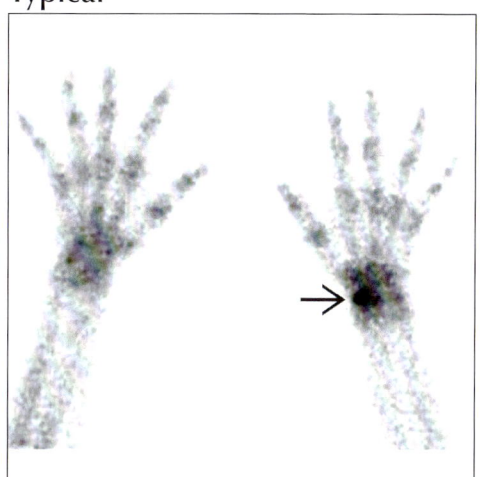

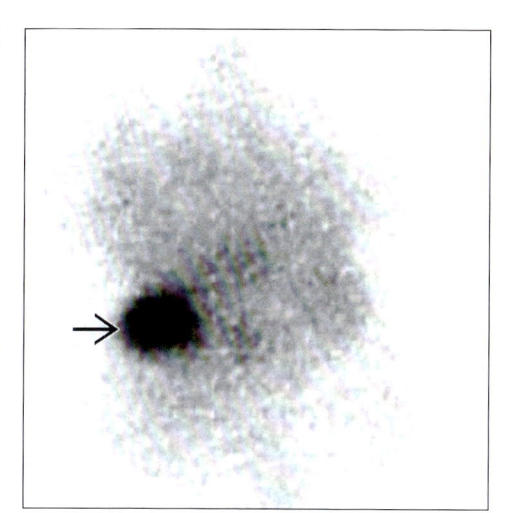

(Left) AP bone scan of the hands in a patient who fell on outstretched hand. Intense uptake in the mid radial aspect of the wrist ➡ is due to a fracture of the scaphoid. See next 2 images. *(Right)* Pinhole bone scan of the wrist better delineates focal intense uptake due to a fracture of the scaphoid ➡.

Typical

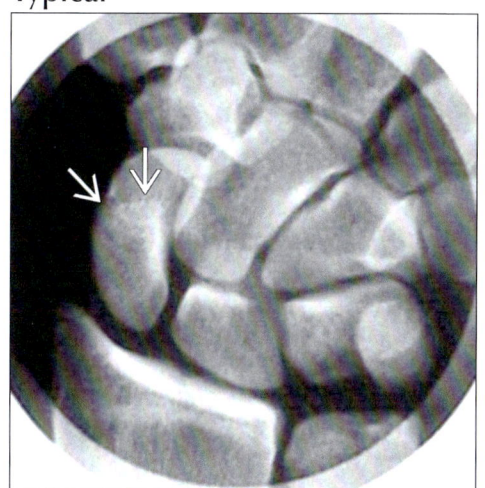

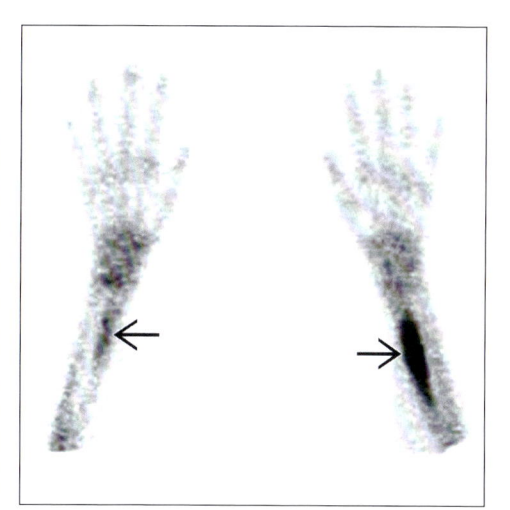

(Left) Scaphoid views of the wrist confirm a transverse fracture of the scaphoid ➡. Initial radiographs 7 days previous were negative. *(Right)* AP bone scan of the hands and forearms in a gymnast with bilateral forearm/wrist pain shows bilateral radial uptake ➡ due to stress fractures, which were radiographically inapparent.

Typical

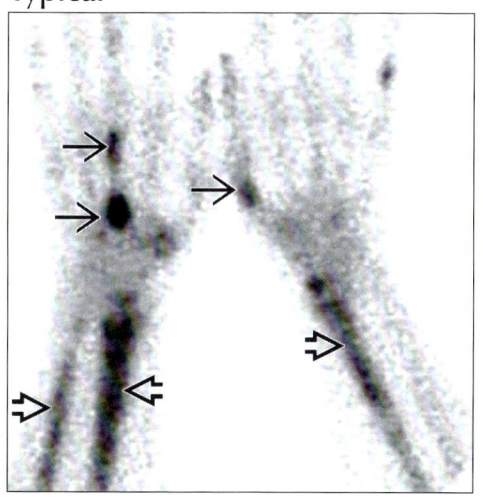

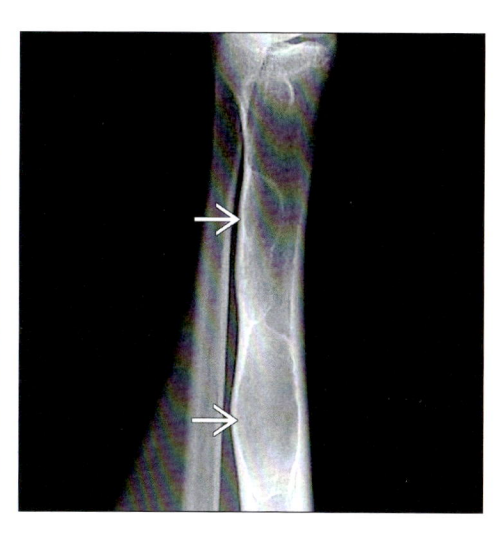

(Left) AP bone scan of both hands and forearms demonstrates multiple sites of uptake in the hands ➡ and forearms ➡ in a patient with fibrous dysplasia. See next image. *(Right)* Plain radiograph of the distal forearm shows well-circumscribed, non-aggressive appearing bone lesions ➡ with a ground-glass matrix typical of fibrous dysplasia.

WRIST PAIN

(Left) AP bone scan of the hands, wrists shows linear uptake ⮕ across distal radius due to fracture. Extension of activity ⮕ more proximally is due to underlying bone tumor (was not radiographically apparent). *(Right)* Oblique bone scan of hands, wrists shows increased uptake in distal radius, with central photopenia (doughnut sign) ⮕. The patient is an 11 year old with aneurysmal bone cyst. See next image.

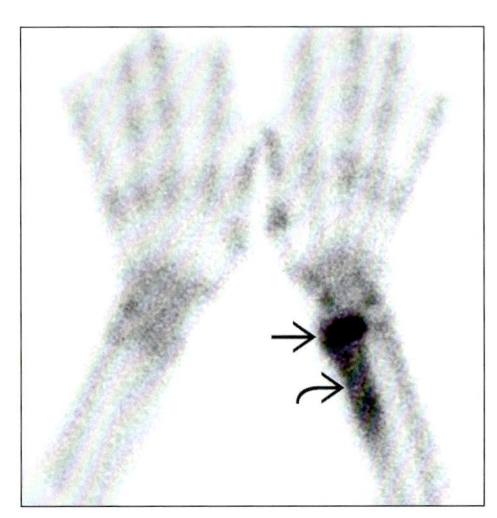

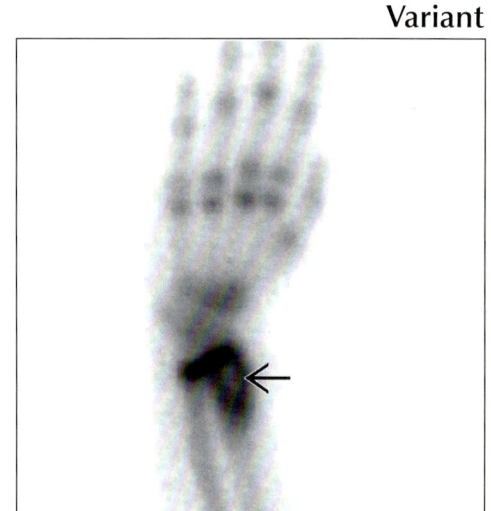

(Left) Axial MR of the wrist in the same patient as previous image, shows a fluid-fluid level ⮕ centrally, corresponding to photopenic area of bone scan. *(Right)* Increased uptake in DIP ⮕ and PIP ⮕ joints, with sparing of CMP joints and carpus. This is a typical pattern seen with erosive osteoarthritis.

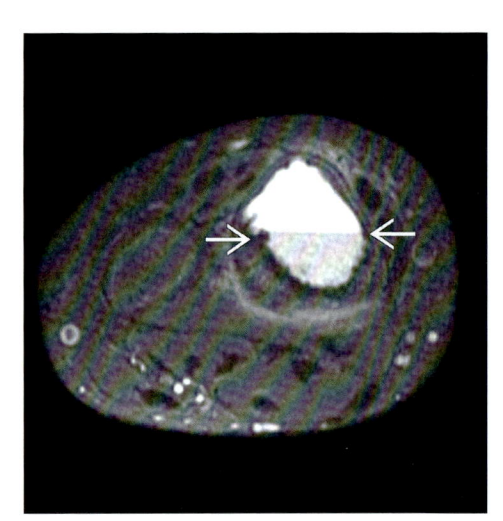

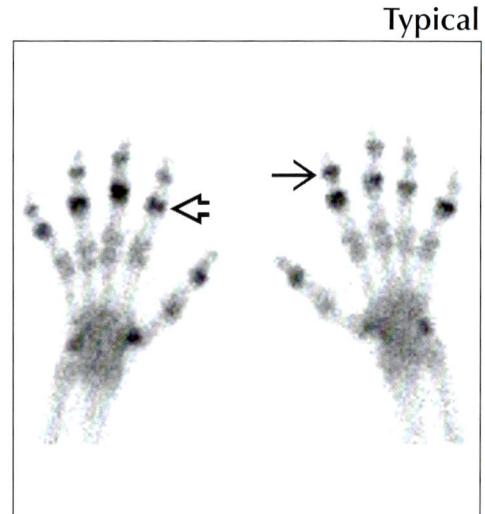

(Left) AP bone scan of the hands and wrists shows bilateral uptake in CMP joints ⮕ and wrist ⮕ in a patient with very early rheumatoid arthritis (RA). Although bilateral, RA is often not symmetrical on bone scan. *(Right)* AP bone scan of the hands and wrists in a patient with advanced RA showing typical distribution in wrists ⮕ and CMP joints ⮕. Note ↓ uptake in fused CMC joints ⮕. Disease activity often better reflected by bone scan than plain film.

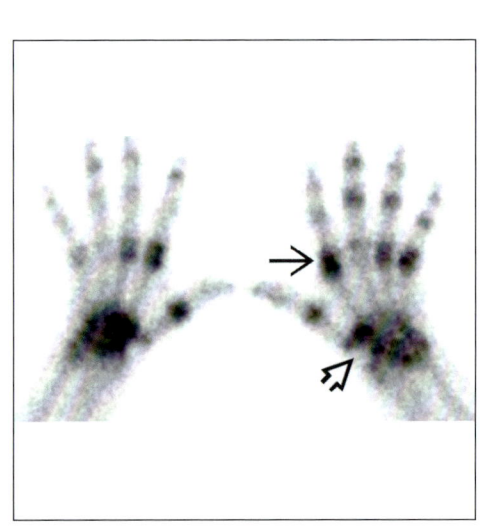

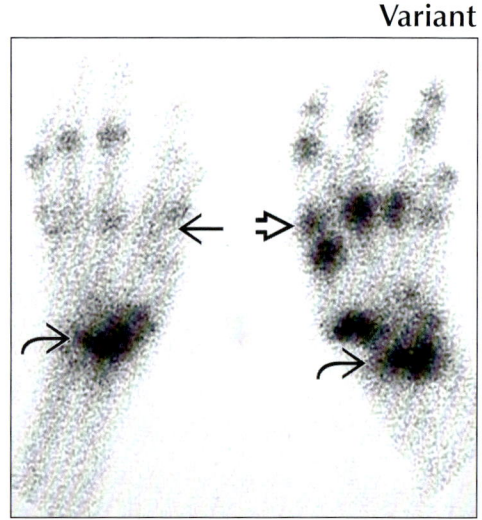

WRIST PAIN

Variant

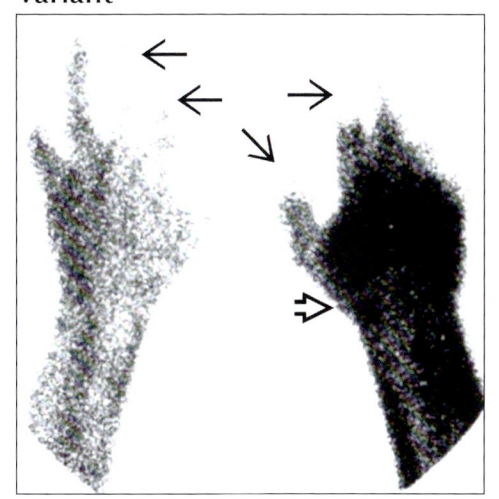

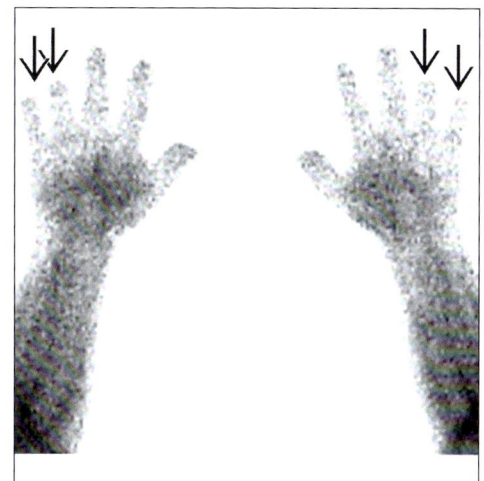

(Left) AP blood pool image from a bone scan in a patient with frostbite injury showing absent perfusion to several digits ➡ and reactive hyperemia ⮕ to more proximal tissues. *(Right)* Bone scan AP blood pool images of the hands in patient with carpal tunnel syndrome (CTS) 2° growth hormone Rx for Turner syndrome (note short 4th an 5th digits ➡). Bone scan is typically normal in CTS.

Variant

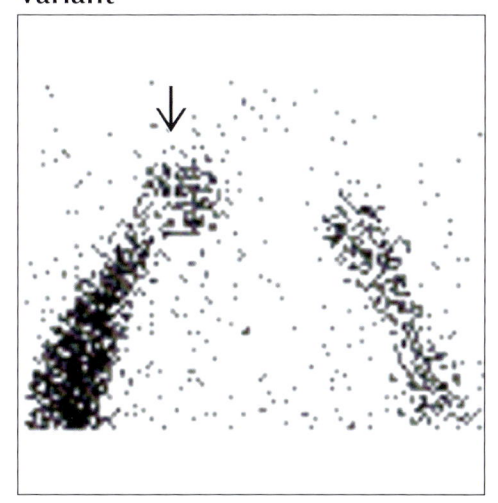

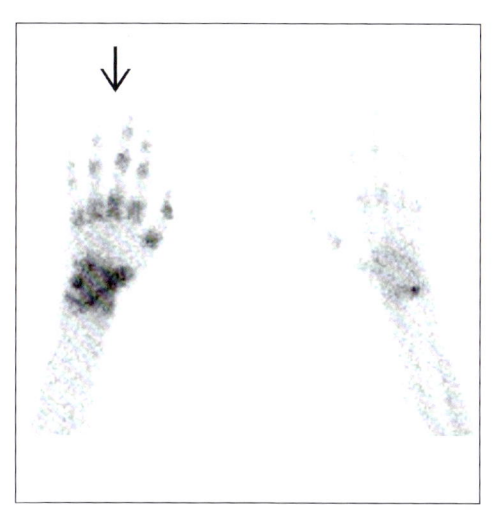

(Left) Angiographic phase of bone scan in RSD shows increased uptake in affected arm/hand ➡. Blood flow may either be ↑ or ↓ in regional pain syndrome (RSD). See next image. *(Right)* AP bone scan of hands wrists shows periarticular uptake in involved extremity ➡, typical of regional pain syndrome (RSD). Discrepancy between abnormal/normal side typically increases distally.

Typical

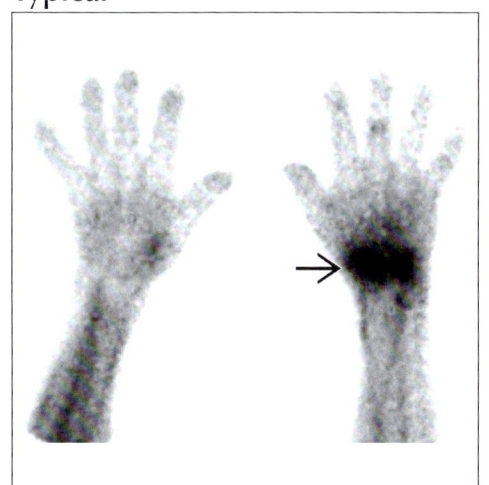

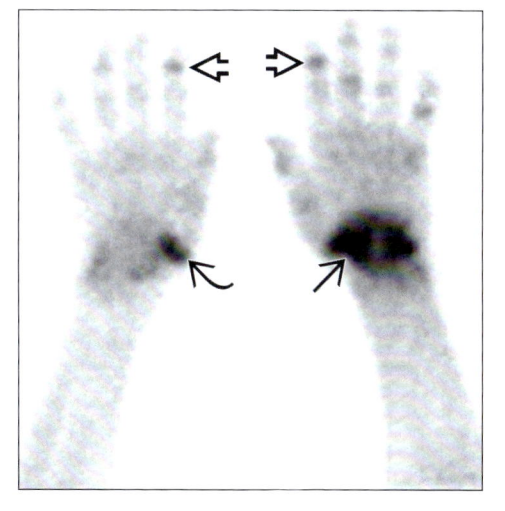

(Left) AP blood pool images of bone scan shows intense hyperemia ➡ due to sporotrichosis of the wrist from rose thorn puncture 6 weeks previous. See next image. *(Right)* AP bone scan shows intense uptake throughout carpus due to sporotrichosis ➡. Note also osteoarthritis of the 1st carpometacarpal joint ➡ and several distal interphalangeal joints ⮕.

CALCANEAL PAIN

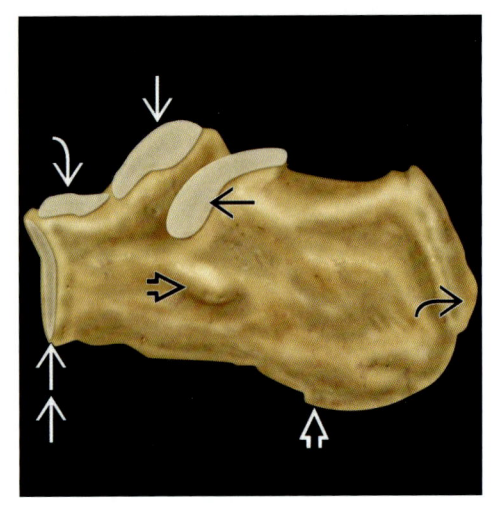

Graphic of lateral calcaneus. Superior anterior, middle, posterior facets (articulate with talus). Cuboid articular surface, peroneal tubercle, lateral process, tuberosity.

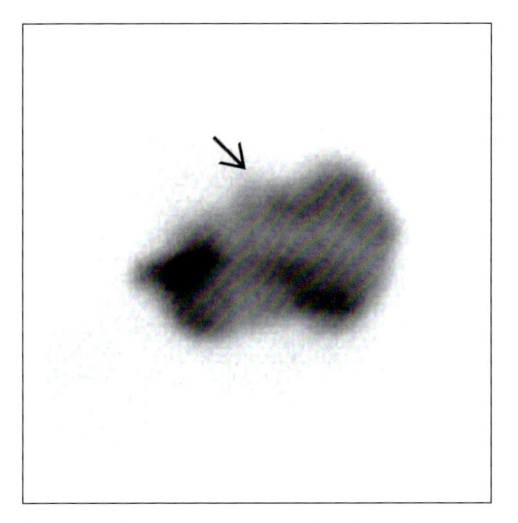

Right medial bone scan of the foot shows increased activity in entire calcaneus in a patient with Paget disease of the calcaneus.

TERMINOLOGY

Definitions
- Calcaneus: Largest tarsal bone
  - Superior
    - Anterior, middle, posterior facets articulate with talus
  - Anterior
    - Cuboid articular surface
  - Lateral
    - Peroneal tubercle
  - Medial
    - Sustentaculum tali
  - Posterior
    - Lateral process
    - Calcaneal tuberosity

IMAGING FINDINGS

General Features
- Best diagnostic clue
  - Focal increased activity on bone scan
- Clinical history, location of abnormality, correlative imaging increase specificity of findings

Imaging Recommendations
- Best imaging tool
  - First line: Radiograph
    - If positive, quick, widely available, inexpensive diagnosis
  - Radiographically occult pain: Tc-99m MDP three-phase bone scan
    - Bone scan more sensitive than radiographs/CT, particularly early in process
    - Focuses search for abnormality in specific area
    - Specificity of bone scan ↑ with radiographic/CT correlation
- Protocol advice
  - Tc-99m MDP three-phase bone scan
    - Pediatric dose: (Age + 1/age + 7) x adult dose, as low as 2 mCi
    - Adult dose: 20-20 mCi (740 MBq - 1.11 GBq) Tc-99m MDP IV
  - Angiographic phase: Dynamic plantar images
  - Blood pool phase: Plantar and lateral or medial static images

DDx: Tendonitis Producing Calcaneal Pain

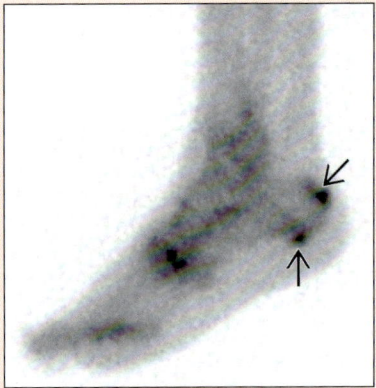

Achilles Tendonitis 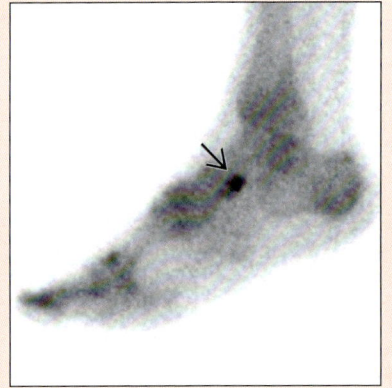 | *Tibialis Posterior Tendonitis* 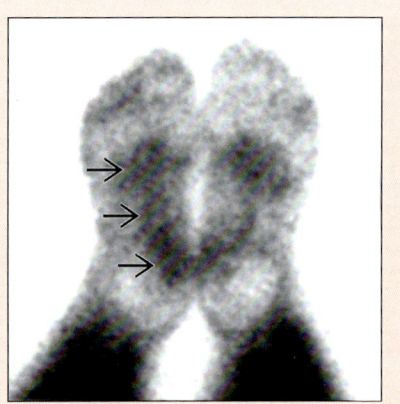 | *Plantar Fasciitis*

CALCANEAL PAIN

Key Facts

Terminology
- Calcaneus: Largest tarsal bone

Imaging Findings
- Radiographically occult pain: Tc-99m MDP three-phase bone scan
- Bone scan more sensitive than radiographs/CT, particularly early in process
- Specificity of bone scan ↑ with radiographic/CT correlation
- Plantar view preferred over anterior views of feet
- Medial or lateral view allows comparison/correlation with plantar view
- In diabetic, vascular disease patients, static images may need to be longer (~ 15 min) and later (4-24 hrs) for adequate bone visualization

Top Differential Diagnoses
- Fracture, Stress Fracture
- Tendonitis
- Diabetic Neuropathic Arthropathy
- Osteomyelitis
- Tarsal Coalition
- Subtalar Synovitis
- Periosteal Contusion
- Neoplasm
- Metabolic Bone Disease

Clinical Issues
- Localized pain
- Inability to bear weight
- Acute trauma
- Repetitive use
- Diabetes mellitus

- Delayed phase (~ 3 hrs): Plantar and lateral or medial static images
- Fourth phase: 24 hr image if poor bone uptake on delayed phase (e.g., vascular disease, diabetes mellitus)
- Plantar view preferred over anterior views of feet
  - Feet closer to collimator than with anterior images ⇒ improved resolution
  - Feet can be secured to collimator with tape, reducing motion artifact
- Medial or lateral view allows comparison/correlation with plantar view
- In diabetic, vascular disease patients, static images may need to be longer (~ 15 min) and later (4-24 hrs) for adequate bone visualization

DIFFERENTIAL DIAGNOSIS

Fracture, Stress Fracture
- Calcaneal fracture
  - ~ 2% of all fractures
  - Most common in men 30-60 years
  - Commonly caused by axial loading
    - Fall from height > 14 feet (rock climbers, roofers)
    - Automobile accidents
  - Intra-articular
    - ~ 75% of calcaneal fractures
    - Involve posterior facet
    - Shear, compression
  - Extra-articular
    - ~ 25% of calcaneal fractures
    - Fractures that do not involve posterior facet
- Stress fractures often bilateral (athletes)
- Sever disease: Overuse injury in children; growth plate may be displaced
- Bone scan
  - Intense focal uptake in acute fracture, decreases with healing
  - Often used to identify stress fracture
- CT
  - Excellent for displaced calcaneal fractures
  - Insensitive for stress fractures

Tendonitis
- Achilles tendonitis
  - Plantar flexor muscle weakness
  - ↑ Dorsiflexion
  - Bone scan: ↑ Activity at calcaneal tuberosity, along tendon
  - Calcaneal spur often accompanies
- Plantar fasciitis
  - Strain of plantar fascia
  - Prolonged pronation, jumping, obesity
  - Bone scan: ↑ Activity along plantar fascia, at lateral process
  - Calcaneal spur often accompanies
- Tibialis posterior tendonitis
  - Pronated flatfoot
  - Bone scan: ↑ Uptake
    - Medial aspect of navicular bone
    - Near tibialis posterior tendon insertion
    - Often bilateral

Diabetic Neuropathic Arthropathy
- Small muscle wasting
- Decreased sensation
- Weight maldistribution
- Bone scan: ↑ Activity on delayed imaging in midfoot, variable activity on 1st, 2nd phases
- MR: Collapse of midfoot arch
  - Bony prominence replacement
- Radiography
  - Early changes nonspecific
    - Soft tissue swelling
    - Loss of joint space
  - Forefoot: Bone resorption
    - Metatarsal head disappearance
  - Hindfoot: Osseous fragmentation
    - New bone formation

Osteomyelitis
- Hematogenous spread of bacteria
- Soft tissue infection spread
- Local inoculation following surgery or trauma

CALCANEAL PAIN

- Most common in posterior or inferior surface
- Bone scan: Best early diagnosis
  - ↑ Activity on all three phases with appropriate history
- Radiography: Periosteal reaction, osteolysis, sequestra

Tarsal Coalition
- Ossification present at birth
- Tarsal joint motion limited
- Bone scan: ↑ Uptake at coalition, often bilateral
- Radiography: Asymmetry of subtalar joint, tarsal beaking, "C" sign
- CT: Joint space narrowing, osseous bridging, sclerosis

Subtalar Synovitis
- Hypertrophic synovium, articular destruction
- Localized nodular synovitis, benign synovioma, posttraumatic synovitis
- Localized pain, erythema, swelling, palpable mass
- Bone scan: ↑ uptake in bone or joint
  - Often ↑ uptake in talus
- CT: Define bone response, soft-tissue nature of lesion
  - Soft-tissue invasion with destruction of subtalar joint

Periosteal Contusion
- High-energy trauma vs. repeated subthreshold loading
- Bone scan: Markedly ↑ tracer uptake in all three phases
- MR: ↓ Signal on T1WI, ↑ signal on T2WI

Neoplasm
- Benign, malignant
- Bone scan
  - Usually increased activity
  - Decreased activity with aggressively lytic bone metastases
  - Double density sign: Osteoid osteoma
- Radiographs, CT, MR: Adds to specificity of bone scan findings, narrowing differential diagnosis

Metabolic Bone Disease
- Paget disease of bone
  - Usually involves entire bone
  - Bone scan: ↑ Uptake
    - Uptake may decrease with treatment, duration of disease
- Osteoporosis ⇒ insufficiency fracture

CLINICAL ISSUES

Presentation
- Most common signs/symptoms
  - Localized pain
  - Inability to bear weight
  - History
    - Acute trauma
    - Repetitive use
    - Athletics
    - Open wound
    - Diabetes mellitus
    - Obesity
    - Osteoporosis

Demographics
- Age
  - Children: Sever disease most frequent cause of heel pain (8-13 years)
  - Adults: Chronic ailments, fractures

Natural History & Prognosis
- Fracture: Intra-articular fracture morbidity higher than extra-articular
- Tendinitis: Generally favorable prognosis
- Diabetic neuropathic arthropathy: Chronic pain, loss of range of motion
- Osteomyelitis: Good, unless complication (e.g., vascular disease, diabetes mellitus)
- Tarsal coalition: May resolve spontaneously; can lead to chronic pain
- Subtalar synovitis: Early diagnosis, surgery important for resolution; may recur
- Periosteal contusion: Self-limiting
- Paget disease of bone: Can lead to pain, bone deformity, neurological deficits, fractures
  - May be asymptomatic

Treatment
- Fracture
  - Usually nonsurgical (extra-articular) such as casting, no weight-bearing, physical therapy
  - If intra-articular, greater likelihood of open reduction and internal fixation
- Stress fracture: Limit weight-bearing activities
  - Usually self-limiting if compliance with conservative therapy
- Tendonitis: Generally conservative
  - Immobilization
  - Anti-inflammatory medications
  - Shoe inserts
  - Physical therapy
  - Local anesthetic injections
  - Surgery rare except in cases of completely ruptured tendon (e.g., Achilles)
- Diabetic neuropathic arthropathy
  - Prevention with tight blood sugar control
  - Symptomatic management
- Osteomyelitis: Long term IV antibiotics
- Tarsal coalition: Severe disease can require surgery
- Periosteal contusion: Self-limiting
- Subtalar synovitis: Arthroscopic synovectomy
- Paget disease of bone: Bisphosphonates

DIAGNOSTIC CHECKLIST

Consider
- Bone scan to determine etiology of radiographically occult calcaneal pain

SELECTED REFERENCES

1. Loutfi I et al: Cases of abnormal triple-phase bone scan in the foot. Semin Nucl Med. 24(3):251-3, 1994
2. Prather JL et al: Scintigraphic findings in stress fractures. J Bone Joint Surg Am. 59(7):869-74, 1977

CALCANEAL PAIN

IMAGE GALLERY

Typical

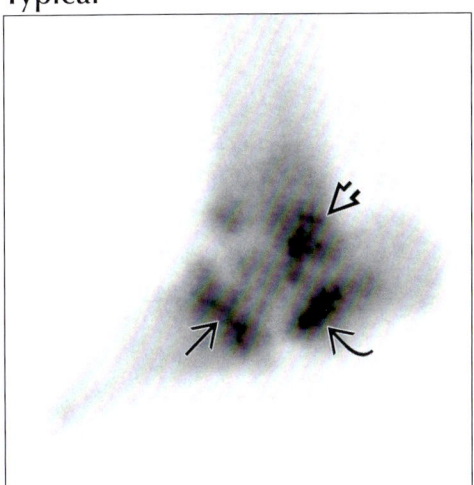

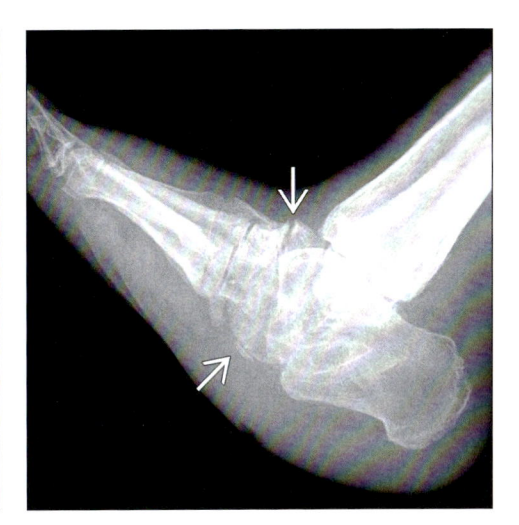

(Left) Bone scan shows increased uptake in the calcaneocuboid ⮕, tibiotalar ⮕, and talonavicular ⮕ joints in a patient with diabetic neuropathic arthropathy (Charcot joint). See next image. *(Right)* Right foot radiograph shows collapse of bones in mid foot ⮕, consistent with Charcot joint. Compare to bone scan in previous image.

Typical

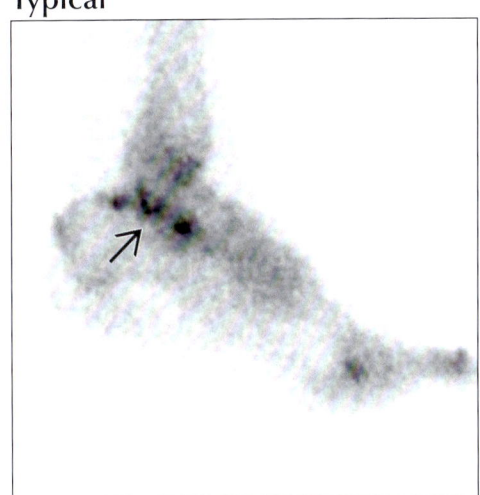

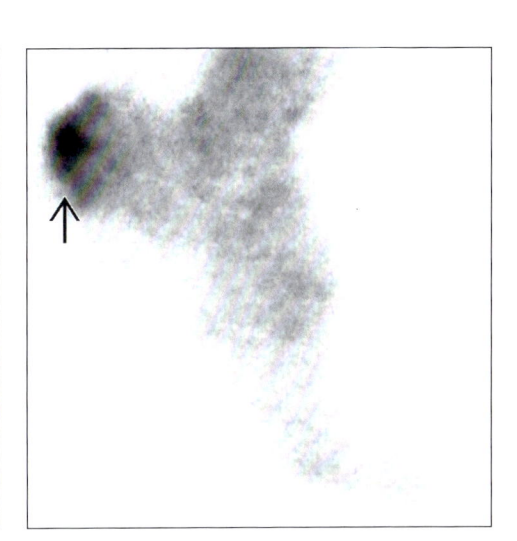

(Left) Medial bone scan of the left foot performed for foot pain shows increased activity at subtalar joint ⮕, consistent with tarsal coalition or subtalar degenerative change. *(Right)* Medial bone scan of the left foot shows increased activity in posterior calcaneus ⮕, in a patient with pressure ulcer on heel and negative radiographs, consistent with osteomyelitis.

Typical

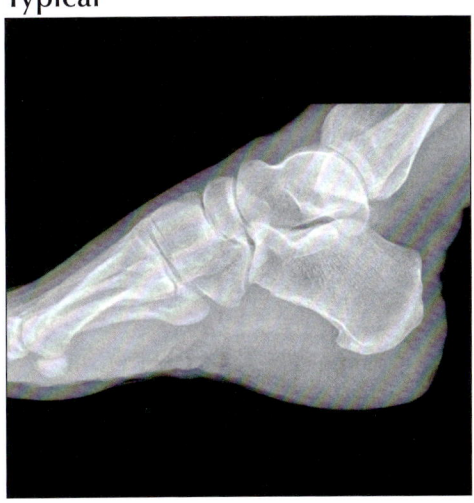

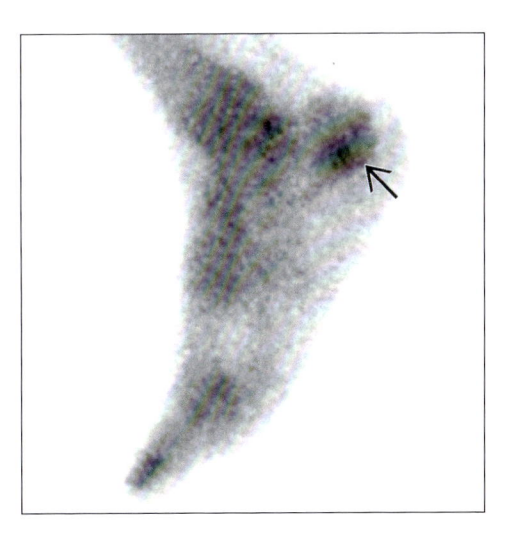

(Left) Radiograph of the right foot in a patient with heel pain after mis-step on stairs shows no calcaneal abnormality. See next image. *(Right)* Medial bone scan of the right foot in the same patient as previous image, shows increased activity in calcaneus ⮕, consistent with acute fracture.

KNEE PAIN

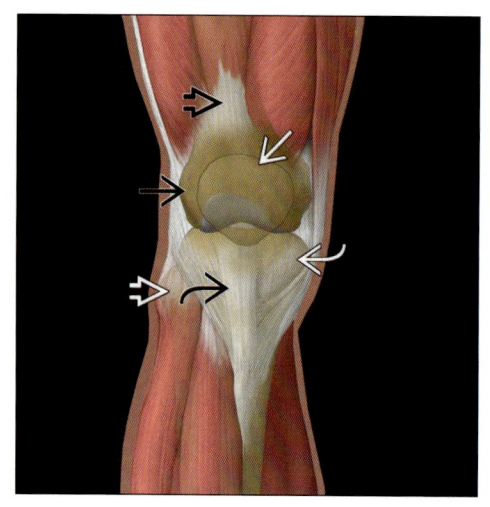

Anterior graphic shows bones of the right knee: Femoral condyle ⇨, patella ➡, tibial plateau ➡, fibular head ➡. Note the quadriceps ➡ and patellar ➡ tendons.

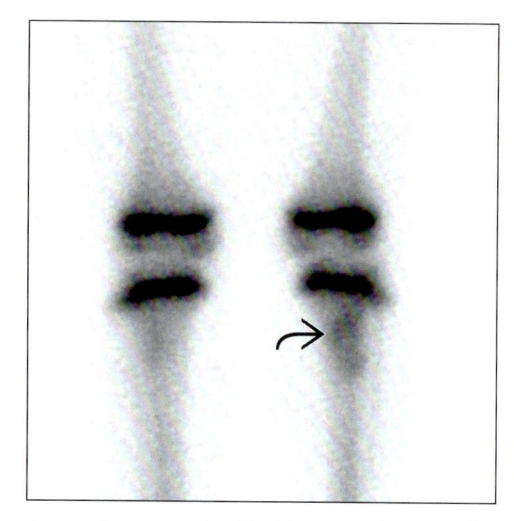

Anterior bone scan of child with suspected osteomyelitis shows increased activity at left tibial neck ⤳, consistent with infection.

TERMINOLOGY

Definitions
- Bones
  - Provide structure
  - Lateral, medial femoral condyle
  - Lateral, medial tibial condyle
  - Fibular head
  - Patella
- Ligaments
  - Attach bone to bone
  - Anterior, posterior cruciate ligament
  - Medial, lateral collateral ligament
  - Iliotibial band
- Tendons
  - Attach muscle to bone
  - Quadriceps, patellar
- Menisci
  - Cartilaginous pads between femur, tibia
  - Lateral, medial
- Bursae
  - Provide gliding surface between muscles, tendons, ligaments
  - Fluid-filled sacs (several)
- Muscles
  - Flex, extend, slightly rotate knee joint
  - Quadriceps, hamstrings

IMAGING FINDINGS

General Features
- Best diagnostic clue
  - Tc-99m MDP three-phase bone scan
    - Increased activity in many etiologies
    - High sensitivity
    - Variable specificity, depending on etiology
    - Correlative imaging increases specificity of findings
  - First-line: Radiography
  - MR: For highest specificity of etiology of knee pain

Nuclear Medicine Findings
- Bone Scan
  - Osteoarthritis: Increased activity in active osteophyte formation, degenerative change
  - Fracture, stress fracture: Increased activity
  - Patellofemoral pain syndrome: Uptake in proximal tibia and patella

DDx: Common Causes of Knee Pain: Other Imaging Modalities

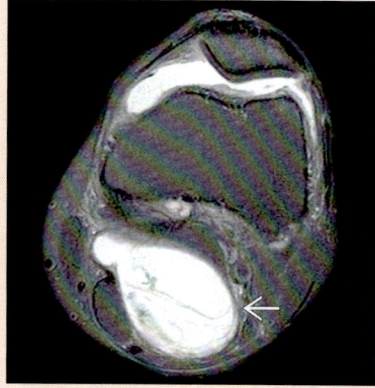

Popliteal Cyst

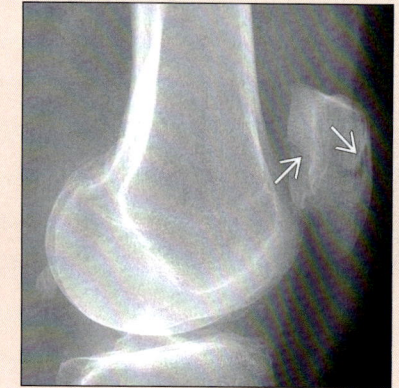

Patella Fracture

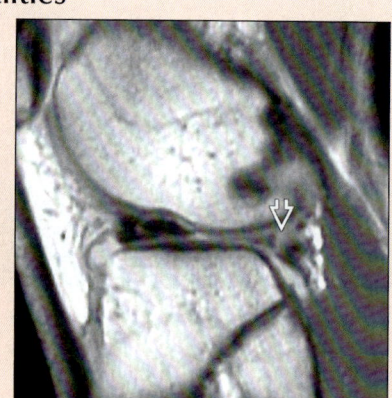

Meniscus Tear

KNEE PAIN

Key Facts

Imaging Findings
- Tc-99m MDP three-phase bone scan
- Increased activity in many etiologies
- High sensitivity
- Correlative imaging increases specificity of findings
- Angiographic and blood pool phases: Anterior images over knees
- Delayed phase: Hips to feet plus spot images over knees (anterior extended; lateral flexed)
- SPECT imaging can ↑ sensitivity, localization
- If poor uptake of tracer (e.g., diabetic patients), 24 hr images can ↑ sensitivity

Clinical Issues
- Children: Patellar malalignment, tendon injury (sports), meniscal tear, tibial apophysitis, referred pain, osteochondritis dessicans
- Young adults (18-30 yrs): Meniscal tear, tendon injury (sports), bursitis, overuse injury, septic arthritis
- Adults (30-50 yrs): Meniscal tear, tendon injury (sports), bursitis, tendinitis, autoimmune, patellofemoral pain syndrome
- Older adults: Osteoarthritis, sports-related tendon injury, tendinitis, bursitis, popliteal cyst, crystal-induced inflammatory arthropathy

Diagnostic Checklist
- Bone scan for nontraumatic knee pain, radiographically occult knee pain
- Imaging hips to feet (especially in children) to identify non-knee etiology of pain
- Anterior extended and lateral flexed images of knees useful on bone scan

---

  - Ligamentous injury: May be positive at ligament insertion site
  - Popliteal cyst: May be normal, mildly increased
  - Meniscal tear: Increased activity in tibial plateau
  - Iliotibial band syndrome: Increased activity in lateral tibial condyle
  - Infection: Three-phase positive
  - Bursitis: Increased activity in adjacent bone

Radiographic Findings
- Radiography
  - Osteoarthritis: Joint space narrowing, sclerosis, osteophytes
  - Fracture, stress fracture: Acute, subacute, remote; stress fracture often negative
  - Patellofemoral pain syndrome: Patellar tilt, patella alta, patella baja
  - Ligamentous injury: Widening of joint space, fracture of proximal bones
  - Popliteal cyst: Soft tissue mass, calcification
  - Meniscal tear: Usually normal
  - Iliotibial band syndrome: Rule out fractures, otherwise negative
  - Infection: Osteolysis, prosthetic migration
  - Bursitis: Likely normal

CT Findings
- Bone CT
  - Osteoarthritis: Joint space narrowing, sclerosis, osteophytes
  - Fracture, stress fracture: Cortical disruption
  - Patellofemoral pain syndrome: Patellar subluxation, tilt
  - Ligamentous injury: MCL, LCL tears visible
  - Popliteal cyst: Fluid-filled mass
  - Meniscal tear: Low resolution, poor specificity
  - Iliotibial band syndrome: Bony fragments 2° to avulsion
  - Infection: Cortical destruction, osteolysis
  - Bursitis: Fluid-filled mass

MR Findings
- Osteoarthritis: Joint effusion, osteophytes in patellofemoral compartment
- Fracture, stress fracture: Hypointense fracture, edema
- Patellofemoral pain syndrome: Patellar tilt, lateralization of tibial tubercle
- Ligamentous injury: Edema, hyperintense signal, torn ligament
- Popliteal cyst: Hyperintense mass behind medial femoral condyle
- Meniscal tear: Signal intensity, articular findings increase with severity
- Iliotibial band syndrome: Fluid collection, thickened band
- Infection: Edema, enhancement, abscess
- Bursitis: Fluid collection, hypointense signal

Imaging Recommendations
- Best imaging tool
  - Radiography, MR for acute knee pain
  - Bone scan for nontraumatic knee pain, radiographically occult knee pain
- Protocol advice
  - 25-30 mCi (925 MBq - 1.11 GBq) Tc-99m MDP IV
  - Three-phase bone scan
    - Angiographic and blood pool phases: Anterior images over knees
    - Delayed phase: Hips to feet plus spot images over knees (anterior extended; lateral flexed)
    - SPECT imaging can ↑ sensitivity, localization
    - If poor uptake of tracer (e.g., diabetic patients), 24 hr images can ↑ sensitivity
  - In adults, knee pain likely traumatic, osteoarthritis, use injuries to knee
  - In children, knee pain often due to knee pathology; however, image hips to feet in case of referred, poorly localized pain

KNEE PAIN

DIFFERENTIAL DIAGNOSIS

Osteoarthritis
- Caused by cartilage breakdown
- Frequency increases with age

Patellofemoral Pain Syndrome
- Also called chondromalacia patella
- Due to subluxation of patella
- Anterior knee pain
- Treatment: Strengthen quadriceps

Ligamentous Injury
- Medial collateral ligament
  - Often associated with ACL injury
  - Valgus stress mechanism
  - Swelling, medial knee pain
- Lateral collateral ligament
  - Varus stress mechanism
  - Rarely fully severed
  - Swelling, lateral knee pain
- Anterior cruciate ligament
  - Mechanism: Medial twisting of weight-bearing leg
  - Most common ligamentous injury
  - 70% have associated meniscal injuries
- Posterior cruciate ligament
  - Mechanism: Lateral twisting of weight-bearing leg, direct contact to anterior knee, hyperextension

Fracture, Stress Fracture
- Fractures often associated with soft tissue injury
- Stress fracture due to repeated high impact activity

Knee Effusion
- Normally diagnosed by palpitation
- Causes include overuse, systemic disease, trauma
- Usually drained before further imaging

Bursitis
- Mechanism: Repetitive, extended kneeling or squatting
- Obvious deep, painful swelling, decreased range

Popliteal Cyst
- Also called Baker cyst
- Painful, fluid-filled mass on posterior aspect of knee joint
- Most common in adults 55-70 years and children 4-7 years

Meniscal Tear
- Most common cause of knee pain
- Commonly medial meniscus

Iliotibial Band Syndrome
- Common in cyclists, long distance runners
- Usually diagnosed with physical examination

Infection
- Puncture wounds, surgery, prostheses

Neoplasm
- Benign, malignant
- Usually increased activity on bone scan, nonspecific

- Correlative radiography, CT, MR for specificity, diagnosis

PATHOLOGY

General Features
- Epidemiology
  - Most common musculoskeletal complaint
  - 30% of adults experience knee pain

CLINICAL ISSUES

Presentation
- Most common signs/symptoms
  - Pain
  - Swelling
  - Crepitus
  - ↓ Mobility

Demographics
- Age
  - Children: Patellar malalignment, tendon injury (sports), meniscal tear, tibial apophysitis, referred pain, osteochondritis dessicans
  - Young adults (18-30 yrs): Meniscal tear, tendon injury (sports), bursitis, overuse injury, septic arthritis
  - Adults (30-50 yrs): Meniscal tear, tendon injury (sports), bursitis, tendinitis, autoimmune, patellofemoral pain syndrome
  - Older adults: Osteoarthritis, sports-related tendon injury, tendinitis, bursitis, popliteal cyst, crystal-induced inflammatory arthropathy
- Gender: Knee pain more common in women

Treatment
- Treatment depends on etiology

DIAGNOSTIC CHECKLIST

Consider
- Bone scan for nontraumatic knee pain, radiographically occult knee pain
- Imaging hips to feet (especially in children) to identify non-knee etiology of pain
- Anterior extended and lateral flexed images of knees useful on bone scan

SELECTED REFERENCES

1. Christian SR et al: Imaging of anterior knee pain. Clin Sports Med. 25(4):681-702, 2006
2. Etchebehere EC et al: Orthopedic pathology of the lower extremities: scintigraphic evaluation in the thigh, knee, and leg. Semin Nucl Med. 28(1):41-61, 1998
3. Ryan PJ et al: A prospective comparison of clinical examination, MRI, bone SPECT, and arthroscopy to detect meniscal tears. Clin Nucl Med. 23(12):803-6, 1998
4. Murray IP et al: SPECT for acute knee pain. Clin Nucl Med. 15(11):828-40, 1990
5. Hejgaard N et al: Bone scan in the patellofemoral pain syndrome. Int Orthop. 11(1):29-33, 1987

KNEE PAIN

IMAGE GALLERY

Typical

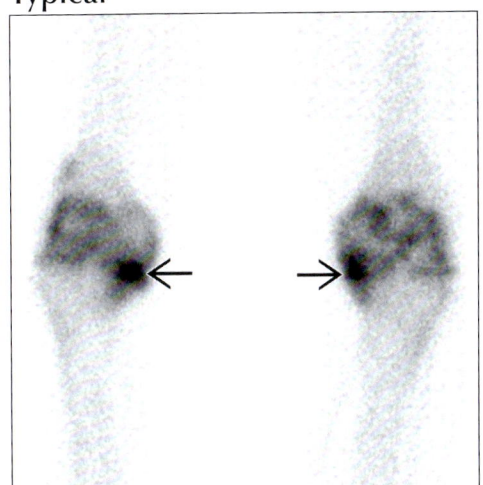

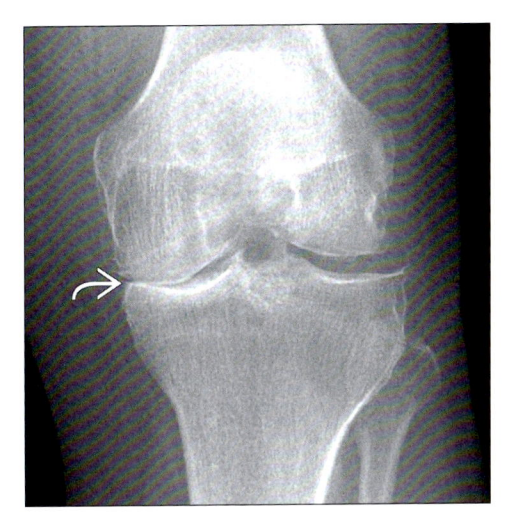

(Left) Anterior bone scan of 64 year old patient with bilateral knee pain shows increased uptake, most severe in the medial compartments ⇒, signifying active bony remodeling of osteoarthritis. See next image. (Right) Anterior radiograph in the same patient as previous image, shows bone-on-bone contact in the medial compartment of the left knee ⇒, signifying severe degenerative osteoarthritis.

Typical

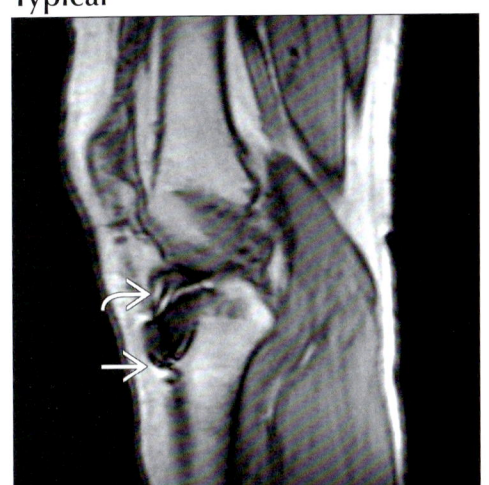

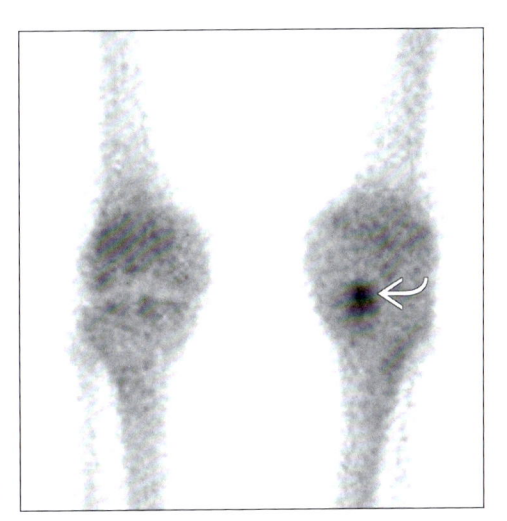

(Left) Left lateral MR of 59 year old patient with knee and hip pain shows wavy contour of the ACL ⇒, signifying ACL injury. Metallic artifact ⇒ is due to ACL repair. (Right) Anterior bone scan in the same patient as previous image, shows increased uptake in the medial left tibial plateau ⇒, signifying ACL injury post repair.

Typical

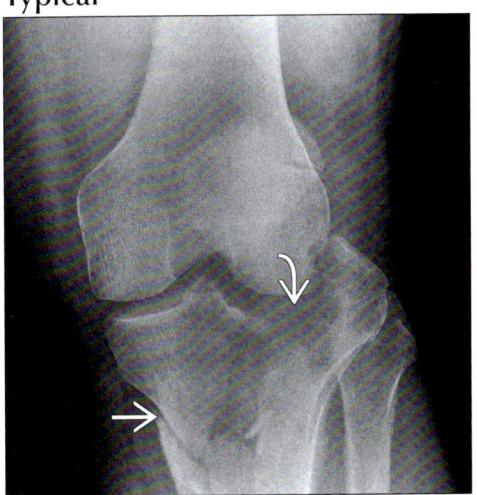

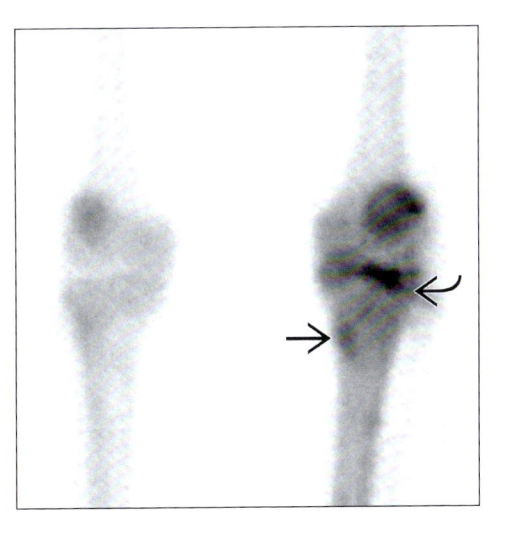

(Left) Anterior radiograph of 33 year old patient who fell from a height of four feet onto the left heel, shows comminuted fracture of the left tibial metaphysis ⇒ and lateral plateau ⇒. (Right) Anterior bone scan in the same patient as previous image, with pain at 1 year shows ↑ activity in the left proximal tibia ⇒, signifying ongoing remodeling. Note patellar uptake ⇒, consistent with chondromalacia.

HETEROTOPIC OSSIFICATION

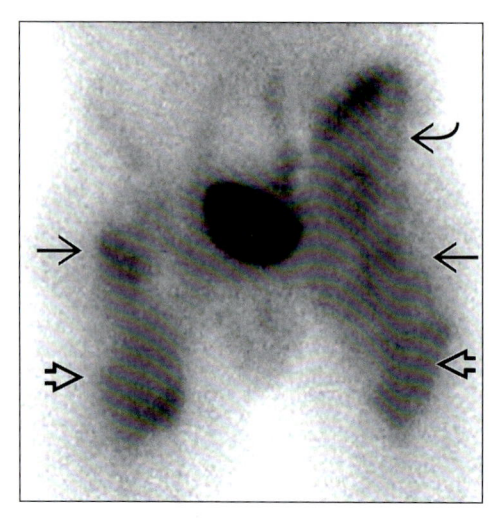

Anterior Tc-99m MDP blood pool phase bone scan shows extensive increased activity about bilateral hips ➡, proximal femurs ➡, and left hemipelvis ➡ in paraplegic patient. See next image.

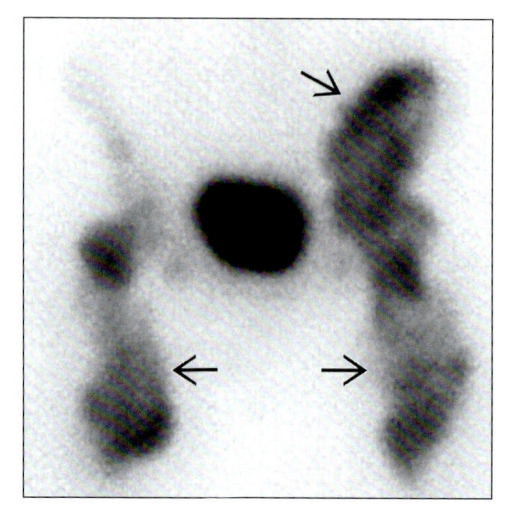

Anterior Tc-99m MDP delayed phase bone scan in same patient as left, shows similar distribution of tracer ➡ indicating heterotopic ossification that is not yet mature.

TERMINOLOGY

Abbreviations and Synonyms
- Preferred terminology: Heterotopic ossification (HO)
  - Ectopic ossification, myositis ossificans circumscripta/traumatica
  - Atraumatic HO, fibrodysplasia ossificans progressiva, Munchmeyer disease, myositis ossificans atraumatica

Definitions
- Extraskeletal osteogenesis
  - Typically (though not necessarily) in muscle
    - Also tendons, fascia (fasciitis ossificans), subcutaneous fat

IMAGING FINDINGS

General Features
- Best diagnostic clue: Amorphous, ill-defined, immature, soft-tissue bone formation, subsequent ossific maturation
- Location
  - Heterotopic ossification
    - Thighs: Contusion, crush injury
    - Tends to be diaphyseal in thigh (differential dx: Osteosarcoma, frequently metadiaphyseal)
    - Hips: Arthroplasty, neurologic impairment
    - Most common postsurgically about hip flexors
    - Upper extremities: Elbows, shoulders, brain injury
    - Knees: Spinal cord injury
  - Fibrodysplasia ossificans progressiva
    - Spreads from axial to appendicular, proximal to distal, cranial to caudal: Sternocleidomastoid, paraspinous, masticators, shoulder, pelvic muscles
    - Causes progressive limitation
- Morphology: Thickened muscle/fascia with edema (CT/MR), amorphous calcification, ossific maturation

Nuclear Medicine Findings
- Tc-99m MDP three-phase and whole body bone scan
  - Positive on angiographic, blood pool, delayed bone scan phases during formation, maturation
  - Moderately positive on delayed phase only when lesion becomes stable: Useful to monitor maturation
  - At maturation (6 months to 2 years), lesion matches or is similar to normal bone on bone scan

DDx: Other Causes of Soft Tissue Uptake on Bone Scan

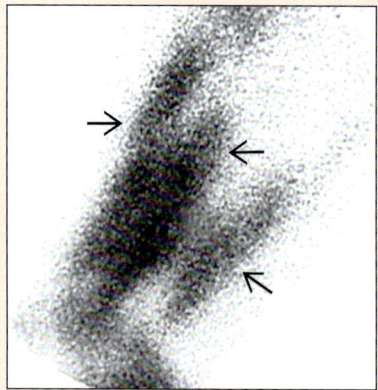

Myositis

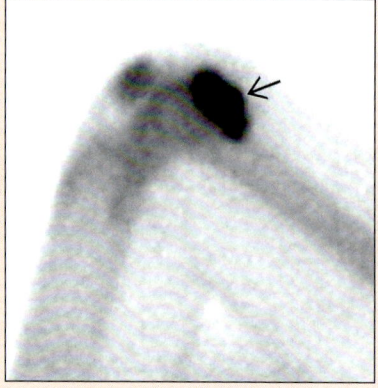

Parosteal Osteosarcoma

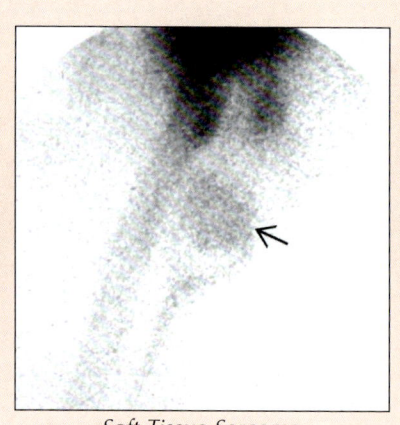

Soft Tissue Sarcoma

HETEROTOPIC OSSIFICATION

Key Facts

Terminology
- Extraskeletal osteogenesis

Imaging Findings
- Best diagnostic clue: Amorphous, ill-defined, immature, soft-tissue bone formation, subsequent ossific maturation
- Thighs: Contusion, crush injury
- Hips: Arthroplasty, neurologic impairment
- Upper extremities: Elbows, shoulders, brain injury
- Knees: Spinal cord injury
- Plain radiography: May show immature amorphous ill-defined bone by 2-6 weeks
- CT/MR: Soft tissue mass with peripheral calcification/bone formation
- Positive on angiographic, blood pool, delayed bone scan phases during formation, maturation
- At maturation (6 months to 2 years), lesion matches or is similar to normal bone on bone scan
- Ga-67 scintigraphy: May be incidentally + on imaging performed for infectious processes

Top Differential Diagnoses
- Deep Venous Thrombosis
- Extraskeletal (Parosteal) Osteosarcoma, Synovial Sarcoma, Chondrosarcoma
- Tumoral Calcinosis
- Hematoma

Diagnostic Checklist
- Use 3-phase bone scan to follow maturation course
- Plain film correlation for bone scan findings if HO diagnosis not established

---

- Ga-67 scintigraphy: May be incidentally + on imaging performed for infectious processes
- WBC, Tc-99m sulfur colloid scans: May be positive in mature HO due to red marrow/reticuloendothelial

Radiographic Findings
- Plain radiography: May show immature amorphous ill-defined bone by 2-6 weeks
  - If typical recommend 30 day repeat radiography
  - Subsequent imaging shows progressive ossific maturation/demarcation at ~ 6 weeks
  - 6-12 weeks: Lamellar bone develops at the boundaries of the involved tissue
- Brooker classification for hip HO
  - I: Islands of bone in soft tissue
  - II: Bone spurs with ≥ 1 cm between opposing surfaces
  - III: Spurs with ≤ 1 cm space
  - IV: Ankylosis

CT Findings
- CT/MR: Soft tissue mass with peripheral calcification/bone formation
  - Organization occurs with maturation as above
  - Central fat may be present in mature HO

Ultrasonographic Findings
- Ultrasound: Usually incidental finding of vascular US for DVT
  - Look for HO concurrently with venous survey
  - Increasingly organized, echogenic margins, central hypoechogenicity: Maturing bone
  - Sheetlike calcification is considered specific
  - Very operator dependent

Imaging Recommendations
- Best imaging tool
  - Plain radiographs: First-line imaging modality
    - Inexpensive, widely available, well-tolerated
    - Evaluates underlying bony conditions, excludes many other causes
  - Tc-99m MDP three-phase and whole body bone scan
    - More sensitive than other imaging modalities, particularly early in disease
    - Used to follow HO maturation
- Protocol advice
  - Tc-99m MDP bone scan
    - Adult dose: 20-25 mCi (740-925 MBq) IV adults
    - Pediatric dose: As low as 2 mCi (74 MBq) Tc-99m MDP; Webster's rule for patients < 12 yrs: (Age + 1/age + 7) x adult dose
    - Hydrate patient prior to procedure to improve soft tissue washout, ↑ target to background
    - Inject in extremity away from site of interest to prevent pooling, venous valvular adherence, subsequent false positives
    - Angiographic phase: Dynamic images over area of interest during radiotracer injection
    - Blood pool phase: Static image over area of interest
    - Delayed phase: Image at 3-4 hours postinjection, 2-3 hours longer in patients with poor cardiac output or renal failure, 24 hours in difficult cases
    - Whole body scan: 1 million count anterior/posterior planar images; then static (spot, 500k count) images of areas of interest
    - SPECT may be used in regions of suspicion, fusion to CT/MR useful for specific localization

DIFFERENTIAL DIAGNOSIS

Deep Venous Thrombosis
- May coexist secondary to local compression
- Pain, erythema, swelling, similar patient population

Extraskeletal (Parosteal) Osteosarcoma, Synovial Sarcoma, Chondrosarcoma
- Histology of HO easily mistaken for (osteo)sarcoma; ideally diagnosis established without biopsy
- HO should have soft tissue plane separating lesion from adjacent bone
- Osteosarcoma ossifies from center, opposite of HO

HETEROTOPIC OSSIFICATION

Tumoral Calcinosis
- Globular juxta-articular soft tissue calcifications, encapsulated granulomatous hydroxyapatite

Hematoma
- May be present prior to heterotopic ossification
- Nonenhancing centrally (in contrast to HO)
- Progressive evolution of blood products on MR, dystrophic calcification may occur
- Spontaneous resorption, persistence/enlargement requiring drainage, or abscess formation may occur

PATHOLOGY

General Features
- Genetics
  - Fibrodysplasia ossificans progressiva (FOP), Munchmeyer disease
    - Autosomal dominant, rare, childhood onset
    - May be linked to a bone morphogenic protein receptor gene defect
- Etiology
  - Myositis ossificans traumatica, no significant genetic linkage, most often secondary to trauma
    - Blunt trauma, crush injuries, infection, burns, surgery, immobilization
    - Often hip arthroplasty, ORIF of femur/elbow fractures
    - CNS injury, compromise, (25% or more), including: Poliomyelitis, Guillain-Barré
    - Electrical rhabdomyolysis
    - Common in patients with previous HO
  - FOP, Munchmeyer disease
    - Atraumatic, idiopathic
- Associated abnormalities
  - Post-traumatic form
    - "DISH, ankylosing spondylitis, Paget disease"
  - Hereditary form, FOP
    - Shortening/segmentation abnormalities of digits (great-toe), metatarsals, metacarpals, spine

Gross Pathologic & Surgical Features
- Undifferentiated centrally, mature peripheral bone
  - Progressive from center to periphery
  - Central tissues sufficiently undifferentiated to complicate histologic distinction vs. osteosarcoma
  - Marginal tissues show mature osteoid matrix
  - If biopsy performed, sample peripheral, central and intermediate regions of lesion to help establish characteristic zonal maturation

Microscopic Features
- Mesenchymal stem cells develop into spindle cells then osteoblasts
- Osteoblasts produce woven bone with progressive organization ultimately forming lamellated bone surrounding trabecular bone
- Microscopic bone formation starts around 1 week, lamellated bone ~ 6 weeks, mature ~ 6-24 months

CLINICAL ISSUES

Presentation
- Most common signs/symptoms
  - Post-traumatic/non-hereditary: Pain, swelling, hard palpable mass, edema, contractures
  - Progressive limitation/restriction of motion

Demographics
- Gender: M:F is 2:1 in patients with central cord insult

Natural History & Prognosis
- Lesions may persist permanently, resolution may occur, particularly lesions induced by local damage
  - Neurologically induced lesions unlikely to resolve
- Malignant degeneration to osteosarcoma mentioned in the literature but incidence may be skewed by formidable histologic interpretations

Treatment
- Pharmaceutical prevention: NSAIDs, (indomethacin prophylaxis), diphosphonate therapy (etidronate)
  - Variable success, indomethacin most common
    - Ectopic bone formation decreased, function and pain not significantly different, ↑ complications
- Physical rehabilitation, range of motion therapy
- External beam radiation
- Surgical intervention
  - After maturation has been established to minimize recurrence
  - 3-phase bone scans allow maturation surveillance

DIAGNOSTIC CHECKLIST

Consider
- Use 3-phase bone scan to follow maturation course
- Plain film correlation for bone scan findings if HO diagnosis not established

Image Interpretation Pearls
- Vascular (angiographic) and blood pool phases may be more intense than delayed phase images in early HO
- Conventional modalities should demonstrate peripheral to central ossification, central fat in mature lesions

SELECTED REFERENCES
1. Crundwell N et al: Non-neoplastic conditions presenting as soft-tissue tumours. Clin Radiol. 62(1):18-27, 2007
2. Fransen M et al: Safety and efficacy of routine postoperative ibuprofen for pain and disability related to ectopic bone formation after hip replacement surgery (HIPAID): randomised controlled trial. BMJ. 333(7567):519, 2006
3. Karunakar MA et al: Indometacin as prophylaxis for heterotopic ossification after the operative treatment of fractures of the acetabulum. J Bone Joint Surg Br. 88(12):1613-7, 2006
4. Banovac K et al: Prevention and treatment of heterotopic ossification after spinal cord injury. J Spinal Cord Med. 27(4):376-82, 2004
5. Yin KS et al: Refractory heterotopic ossification with complications. J Spinal Cord Med. 24(2):119-22, 2001

HETEROTOPIC OSSIFICATION

IMAGE GALLERY

Typical

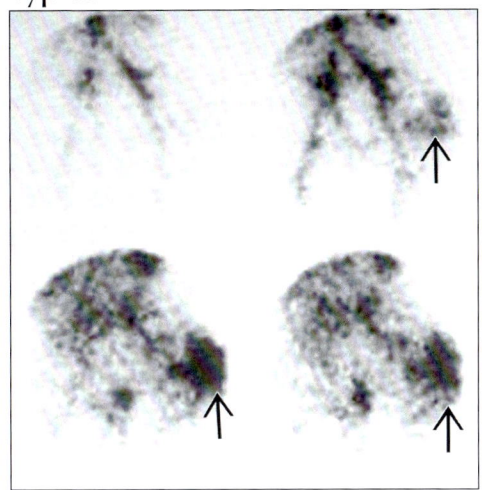

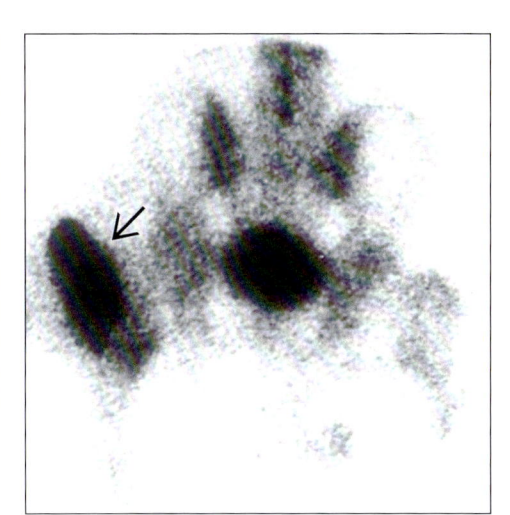

(Left) Anterior Tc-99m MDP angiographic phase bone scan shows vascular blush and washout ➡ adjacent to left hip, typical of early heterotopic ossification. Same as next image. *(Right)* Posterior Tc-99m MDP delayed phase bone scan in same patient as previous image, shows increased activity adjacent to left greater trochanter ➡ indicating actively forming heterotopic ossification.

Typical

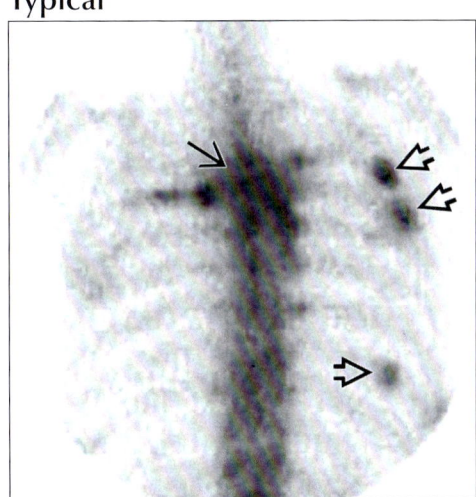

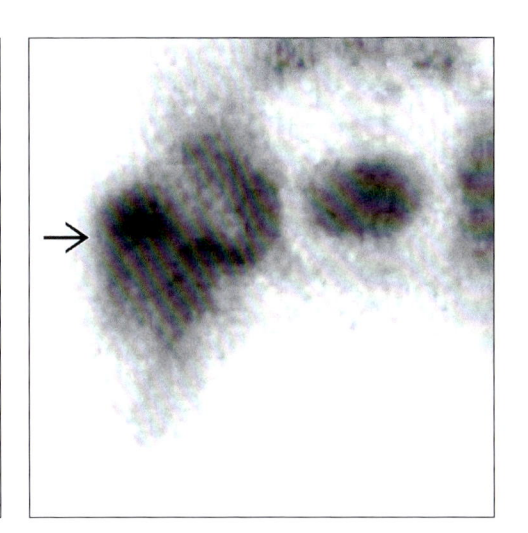

(Left) Posterior Tc-99m MDP bone scan shows post-traumatic changes of T4 ➡ and rib fractures ⇨ in patient with spinal cord injury due to motor vehicle accident. See next image. *(Right)* Anterior Tc-99m MDP bone scan in same patient at left shows tracer accumulation about right hip ➡, indicating heterotopic ossification. See next image.

Typical

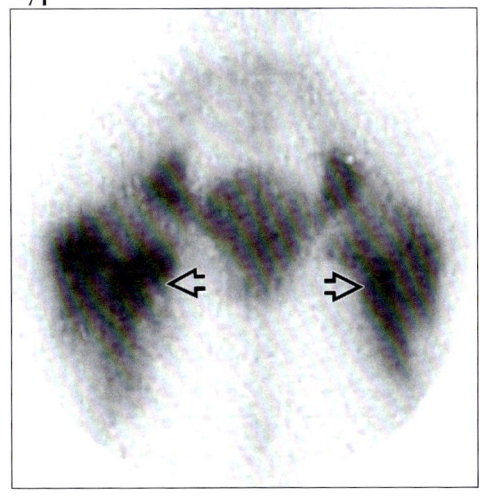

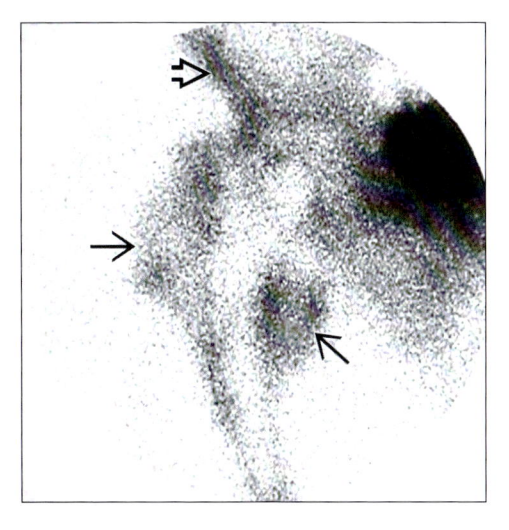

(Left) Tc-99m MDP bone scan of previous patient in "tail-on-detector" view shows bilateral hip heterotopic ossification ⇨. *(Right)* Anterior Tc-99m MDP bone scan of the right hip in a patient with a right total hip arthroplasty shows mature heterotopic ossification ➡, similar in uptake to adjacent normal regions of bone ⇨.

HETEROTOPIC OSSIFICATION

(Left) Anterior and posterior Tc-99m MDP bone scan shows abnormal tracer in soft tissues of left hip ⇒ indicating moderate, immature heterotopic ossification. (Right) Tc-99m MDP angiographic phase bone scan in head injury patient with right elbow pain shows increased activity over right elbow ⇒. See next 6 images.

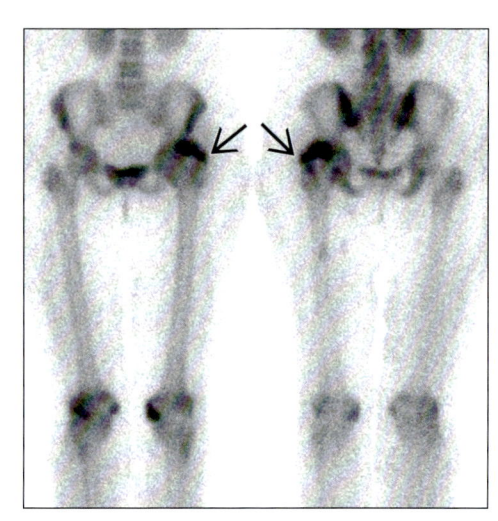

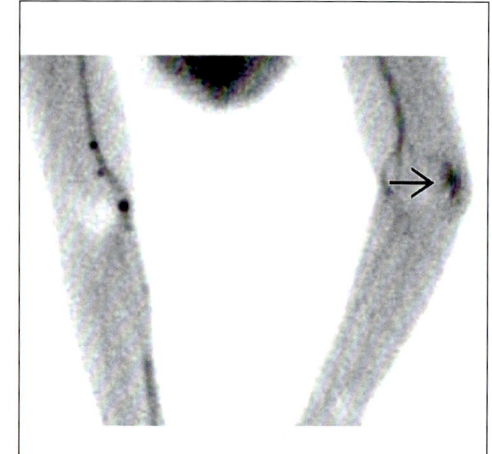

(Left) Anterior Tc-99m MDP blood pool phase bone scan in same patient as previous image, shows intense increased activity over right elbow ⇒ indicating actively forming heterotopic ossification. (Right) Tc-99m MDP bone scan shows tracer about right elbow ⇒, increased in relation to normal bone. This is consistent with actively forming HO. Note uptake in calvarium ⇒ (trauma).

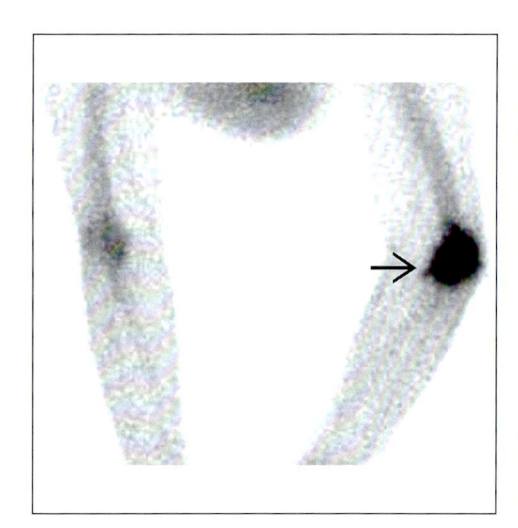

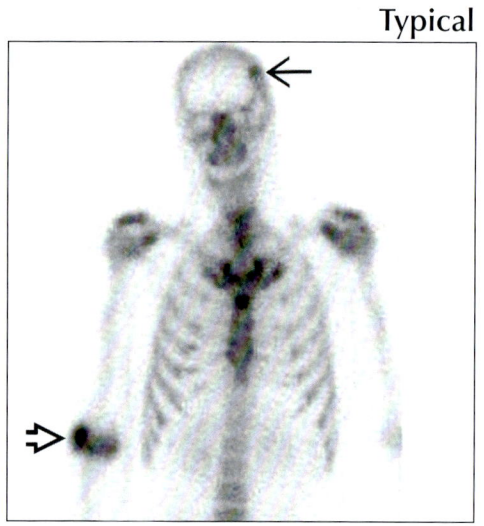

(Left) Lateral radiograph of right elbow taken at same time as previous bone scan in patient with pain and swelling shows no definite ossification. (Right) Radiograph of right elbow shows small areas of vague soft tissue ossification ⇒ signifying early heterotopic ossification.

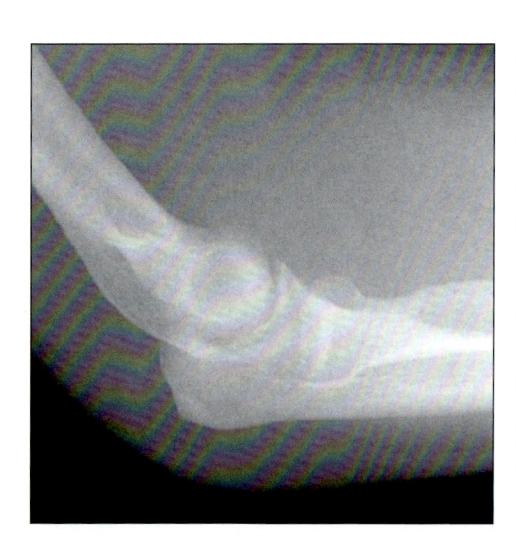

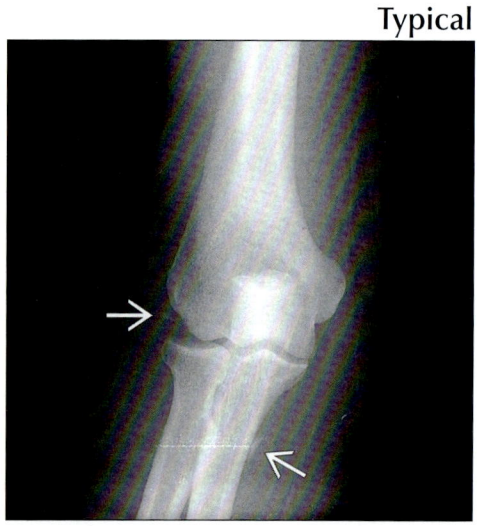

HETEROTOPIC OSSIFICATION

Typical

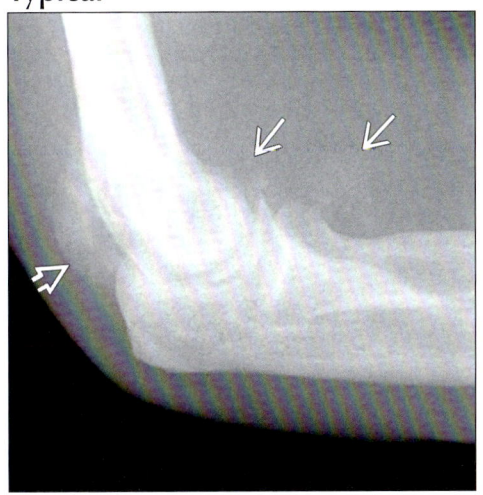

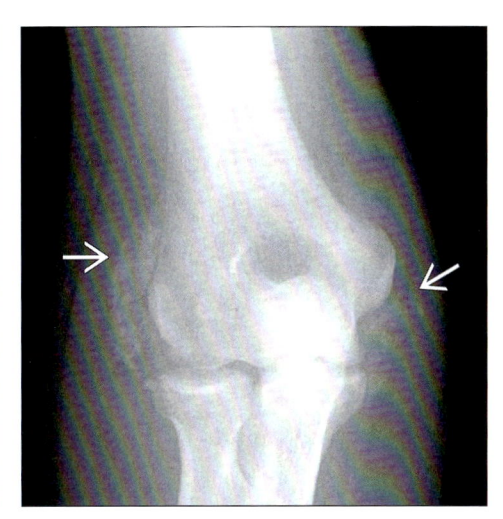

(Left) Right lateral radiograph 6 weeks later in same patient as previous images shows ongoing maturation of heterotopic ossification anterior ➡ and posterior ➡ to right elbow. *(Right)* Anterior posterior radiograph of right elbow in same patient as previous images, shows extent of maturing heterotopic ossification about the joint ➡ in a distribution corresponding to previous bone scan.

Typical

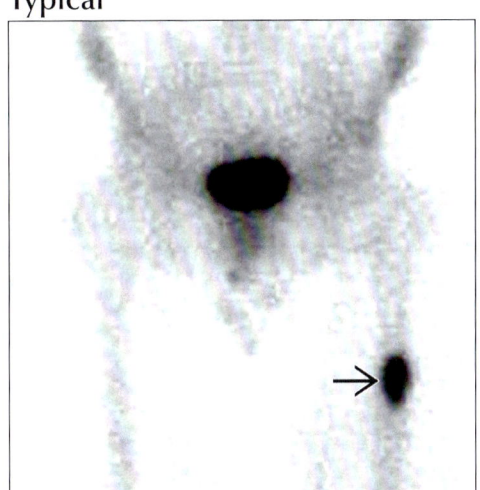

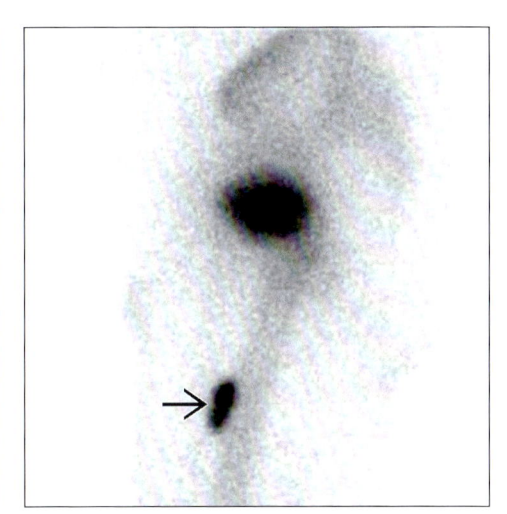

(Left) Tc-99m MDP bone scan in patient with lung cancer shows an incidental, elongated left mid-femoral diaphyseal lesion ➡, suspicious for metastatic lesion. Same as next 3 images. *(Right)* Left lateral Tc-99m MDP bone scan of same patient as previous image, shows tracer accumulation anterior and adjacent to femoral cortex ➡, likely heterotopic ossification. See next.

Typical

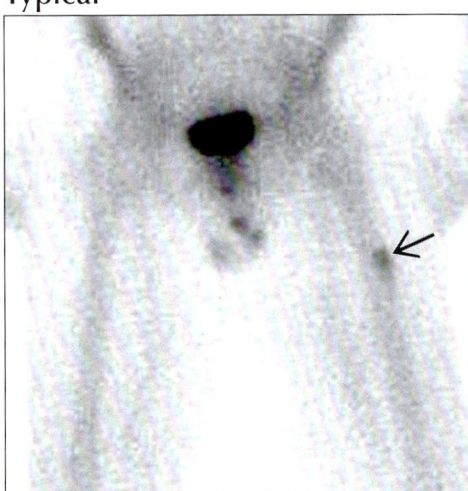

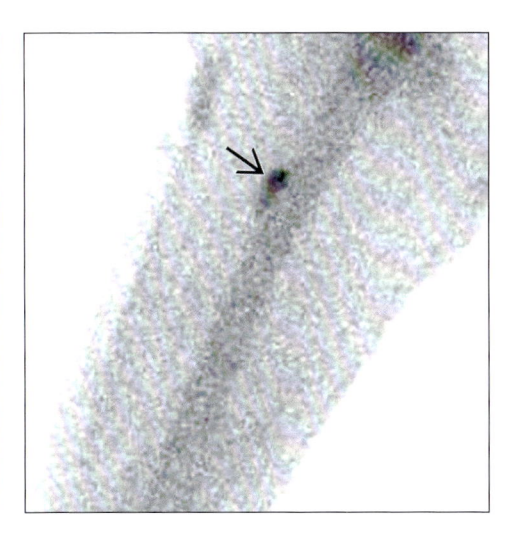

(Left) Anterior Tc-99m MDP bone scan 8 weeks later in same patient as previous image, shows marked interval decrease in activity ➡ relative to prior bone scan. *(Right)* Left lateral Tc-99m MDP bone scan shows similar decrease indicating resolving heterotopic ossification ➡ likely the result of occult trauma.

SKELETAL MUSCLE DISORDERS

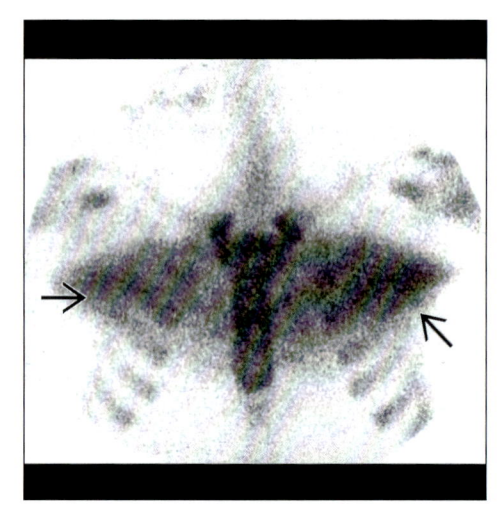

Anterior bone scan of chest shows increased uptake in pectoralis muscles ➔ in a patient who performed recent strenuous exercise (weight-lifting).

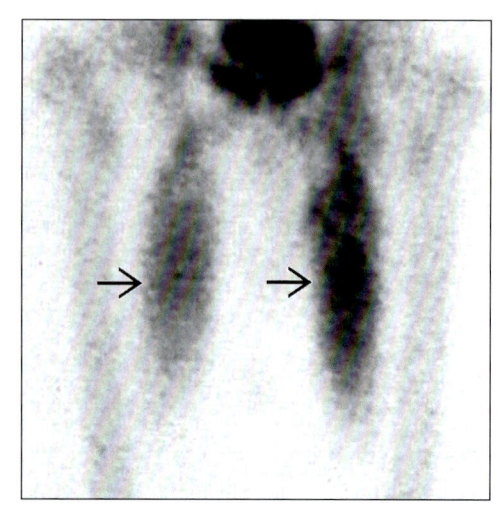

Anterior bone scan of thighs shows intense uptake in adductor muscles ➔ in patient following long horseback ride (English saddle, repetitive posting).

TERMINOLOGY

Abbreviations and Synonyms
- Myositis: Polymyositis, dermatomyositis, inclusion body myositis
- Rhabdomyolysis

Definitions
- Inflammatory, ischemic, metabolic or traumatic disorders of skeletal muscle
- Myositis: Inflammatory disease of skeletal muscle
- Rhabdomyolysis: Breakdown of muscle fibers releasing muscle fiber contents into circulation

IMAGING FINDINGS

General Features
- Best diagnostic clue: Focal ↑ muscle uptake on bone scan indicates muscle injury

Nuclear Medicine Findings
- Tc-99m bone scan (diphosphonate or pyrophosphate)
  - ↑ Uptake indicates muscle injury: Many causes
  - Symmetrically "hot" renal cortex on bone scan often associated with muscle injury (renal myoglobin deposition)
    - "Hot kidneys" on bone scan: Not predictive of rhabdomyolysis-induced renal insufficiency
  - Exercise-induced rhabdomyolysis
    - Bone scan uptake in specific muscles may occur within a week of strenuous exercise
  - Electrical current injury to muscle
    - Uptake in muscle groups indicates passage of electrical current through muscle
    - Uptake in muscles: High risk factor for compartment syndrome
  - Viable vs. necrotic muscle
    - Both show increased uptake on bone scan
    - Absence of perfusion ("cold" defect on early bone scan vascular phase imaging): High likelihood of muscle necrosis, infarction
  - Compartment syndrome: Higher risk if ↑ muscle uptake on bone scan following trauma or infection
  - Myositis ossificans: Heterotopic ossification of muscles

DDx: Mimics of Muscle Uptake of Radionuclides

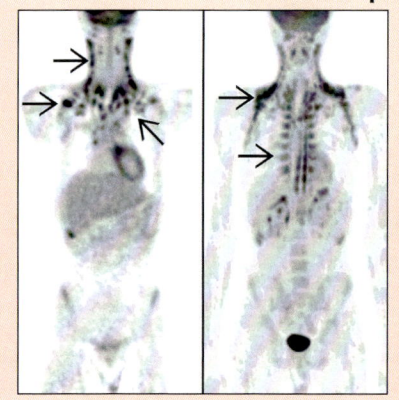

Hypermetabolic Brown Fat

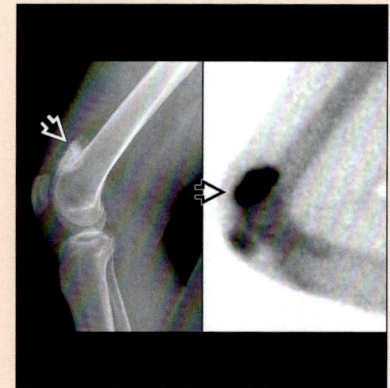

Parosteal Osteosarcoma

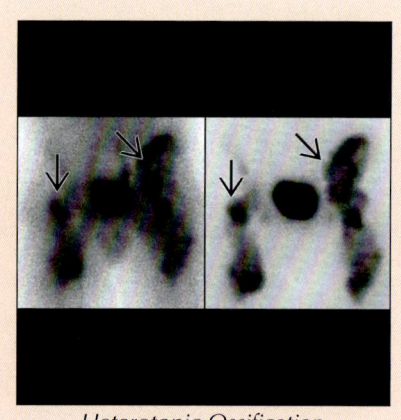

Heterotopic Ossification

SKELETAL MUSCLE DISORDERS

Key Facts

Imaging Findings
- Best diagnostic clue: Focal ↑ muscle uptake on bone scan indicates muscle injury
- Symmetrically "hot" renal cortex on bone scan often associated with muscle injury (renal myoglobin deposition)
- Bone scan uptake in specific muscles may occur within a week of strenuous exercise
- Compartment syndrome: Higher risk if ↑ muscle uptake on bone scan following trauma or infection
- Increased uptake on bone scan in involved muscle groups: Correlates with muscle weakness
- Focal uptake of FDG in muscle groups: Exercise, inflammation, metastases
- Diffuse FDG uptake in all skeletal muscle: Metabolic causes
- Bone scan: Very sensitive for muscle injury, actively forming myositis ossificans
- C+ MR: Best modality for necrotizing fasciitis
- To assess muscle injury: Tc-99m pyrophosphate bone scan preferred over diphosphonate

Top Differential Diagnoses
- Hypermetabolic Brown Adipose Tissue (HBAT)
- Musculoskeletal Tumors
- Tumoral Calcinosis

Diagnostic Checklist
- Bone scan: Increased uptake in skeletal muscle = muscle injury
- FDG PET: Patterns of both generalized and focal muscle uptake less specific for muscle injury

---

- Post-traumatic, burns, neurologic disorders (spinal cord injury, head injury), autosomal dominant disorder (myositis ossificans progressiva)
  - Immature myositis ossificans: Intensely hot on early vascular phase images; uptake on delayed phase greater than normal bone
  - Mature myositis ossificans: No longer hot on vascular phase images; uptake on delayed phase similar to normal bone
- Polymyositis, dermatomyositis: Occurs as primary autoimmune or paraneoplastic disorder
  - Increased uptake on bone scan in involved muscle groups: Correlates with muscle weakness
- Infectious myositis: Group A streptococcal (flesh eating disease), toxic shock, viral, pyomyositis
  - Muscle uptake in group A streptococcal, toxic shock: High likelihood of muscle necrosis, compartment syndrome
- FDG PET
  - Focal uptake of FDG in muscle groups: Exercise, inflammation, metastases
    - Can be indicative of vigorous exercise during preceding 1-2 days prior to FDG injection
    - Can occur with relatively minor muscle activity between FDG injection and scanning (e.g., writing ⇒ forearm muscle uptake)
    - Myositis and metastatic disease to muscle
    - Accessory muscles of respiration: Crying (pediatrics) following FDG injection, ↑ respiratory effort (COPD), hiccups
  - Diffuse FDG uptake in all skeletal muscle: Metabolic causes
    - Elevated insulin: Recent carbohydrate ingestion or insulin administration
    - Hyperthyroidism
    - Other proposed etiologies: Severe cachexia, cachexia plus chronic hypoxia, systemic inflammatory states (especially in elderly)
    - Drugs that may be related: High dose statin therapy, concomitant chemotherapy + protease inhibitor therapy (HIV patients)

Imaging Recommendations
- Best imaging tool
  - Bone scan: Very sensitive for muscle injury, actively forming myositis ossificans
  - C+ MR: Best modality for necrotizing fasciitis
- Protocol advice
  - To assess muscle injury: Tc-99m pyrophosphate bone scan preferred over diphosphonate
    - Slower renal clearance: Remains in blood stream longer to allow longer opportunity for uptake in muscles
  - Early vascular phase imaging advisable to assess muscle viability
- Other imaging options
  - C+ US and C+ MR: Increased perfusion, enhancement in muscle inflammation

DIFFERENTIAL DIAGNOSIS

Hypermetabolic Brown Adipose Tissue (HBAT)
- FDG uptake common due to nonshivering thermogenesis: May maintain core temperature of great vessels, adrenal glands
- Age: Typically < 35 years
- Typical regions of increased FDG uptake in HBAT: Usually bilateral, may be asymmetrical
  - Deep cervical (anterior, posterior cervical, posterior occipital)
  - Supraclavicular, extending into deep, superficial axillae
  - Superior mediastinum around great vessels
  - Intercostal paraspinous
  - Periadrenal, perirenal
- Improved by maintaining patient warmth before and after FDG injection
- Possible improvement by administration of beta blockers, benzodiazepines

Chemotherapy-Induced Adipose Uptake
- FDG uptake in all adipose tissue ("chemo-fat" pattern)

SKELETAL MUSCLE DISORDERS

- Seen while on ↑ dose chemotherapy (e.g., methotrexate, cisplatin), high dose steroids
- Can be associated with bilateral adrenal FDG uptake: Stress response

Musculoskeletal Tumors
- Uptake on bone scan by bone tumors extending into soft tissues may mimic myositis ossificans
  - Osteosarcoma, parosteal osteosarcoma, periosteal osteosarcoma, osteochondroma
- Uptake of bone scan agent in soft tissue sarcomas: Commonly seen on early vascular phase & delayed images

Tumoral Calcinosis
- Periarticular calcification/uptake on bone scan: Most commonly seen with chronic renal tubular disease

PATHOLOGY

General Features
- Etiology
  - Myositis: Polymyositis, dermatomyositis, inclusion body myositis
  - Rhabdomyolysis
    - Severe exertion (e.g., marathon runners)
    - Ischemia (vascular occlusion)
    - Trauma, crush injuries
    - High fever with shaking chills
    - Heat intolerance, heat stroke, malignant hyperthermia
    - Alcoholism with tremors
    - Low phosphate levels
    - Animal toxins (e.g., scorpion bite)
    - Electrical current
    - Infections: Viral, bacterial (e.g., group A streptococcal infection/"flesh eating disease", necrotizing fasciitis)
    - Burn injuries

CLINICAL ISSUES

Presentation
- Most common signs/symptoms
  - Focal or diffuse muscle pain
  - Myositis
    - Trouble rising from a chair
    - Difficulty climbing stairs or lifting arms
    - Fatigue with minor exercise
    - Persistent muscle soreness that does not resolve after a few weeks
    - Trouble swallowing or breathing
  - Rhabdomyolysis
    - Dark urine (myoglobin)
    - Muscle tenderness, stiffness, aching, generalized or focal weakness
- Other signs/symptoms
  - Elevated creatine phosphokinase (CPK)-III: May occur with strenuous exercise of healthy muscle, muscle trauma, muscle disease
  - Other serum elevations: Aldolase, LDH, SGOT, phosphate, myoglobin, potassium
  - Elevated C reactive protein, sedimentation rate: Indicative of underlying inflammatory process
  - Renal insufficiency (rhabdomyolysis)

Natural History & Prognosis
- Rhabdomyolysis can lead to compartment syndrome, muscle necrosis

DIAGNOSTIC CHECKLIST

Image Interpretation Pearls
- Bone scan: Increased uptake in skeletal muscle = muscle injury
- FDG PET: Patterns of both generalized and focal muscle uptake less specific for muscle injury

SELECTED REFERENCES

1. Heffernan E et al: Multiple metastases to skeletal muscle from carcinoma of the esophagus detected by FDG PET-CT imaging. Clin Nucl Med. 31(12):810-1, 2006
2. Jackson RS et al: Prevalence and patterns of physiologic muscle uptake detected with whole-body 18F-FDG PET. J Nucl Med Technol. 34(1):29-33, 2006
3. Chen YK et al: Elevated 18F-FDG uptake in skeletal muscles and thymus: a clue for the diagnosis of Graves' disease. Nucl Med Commun. 25(2):115-21, 2004
4. Chilab S et al: A patient with back pain and unusual appearances on bone scintigraphy. Br J Radiol. 77(921):801-2, 2004
5. Groves AM et al: Extensive skeletal muscle uptake of 18F-FDG: relation to immunosuppressants? J Nucl Med Technol. 32(4):206-8, 2004
6. M Herder GJ et al: Accessory findings on F-18 FDG positron emission tomography in bronchogenic carcinoma. Clin Nucl Med. 28(1):58-9, 2003
7. Kemppainen J et al: Myocardial and skeletal muscle glucose uptake during exercise in humans. J Physiol. 542(Pt 2):403-12, 2002
8. Lim ST et al: Tc-99m MDP three-phase bone scintigraphy in disciplinary exercise-induced rhabdomyolysis. Clin Nucl Med. 25(7):558-9, 2000
9. Buchpiguel CA et al: Cardiac and skeletal muscle scintigraphy in dermato- and polymyositis: clinical implications. Eur J Nucl Med. 23(2):199-203, 1996
10. Elgazzar AH et al: Advanced fibrodysplasia ossificans progressiva. Clin Nucl Med. 20(6):519-21, 1995
11. Delpassand ES et al: Evaluation of soft tissue injury by Tc-99m bone agent scintigraphy. Clin Nucl Med. 16(5):309-14, 1991
12. Maurer AH et al: Diagnosis of traumatic myositis of the intrinsic muscles of the hand by the use of three-phase skeletal scintigraphy. Clin Nucl Med. 15(8):535-8, 1990
13. Guze BH et al: The nuclear medicine bone image and myositis ossificans progressiva. Clin Nucl Med. 14(3):161-2, 1989
14. Sheth KJ et al: Myoglobinuria with acute renal failure and hot kidneys seen on bone imaging. Clin Nucl Med. 9(9):498-501, 1984
15. Matin P et al: Scintigraphic evaluation of muscle damage following extreme exercise: concise communication. J Nucl Med. 24(4):308-11, 1983
16. Steinfeld JR et al: Positive 99mTc-pyrophosphate bone scan in polymyositis. Radiology. 122(1):168, 1977
17. Brown M et al: Radioisotope scanning in inflammatory muscle disease. Neurology. 26(6 PT 1):517-20, 1976
18. Handmaker H et al: The bone scan in inflammatory osseous disease. Semin Nucl Med. 6(1):95-105, 1976

SKELETAL MUSCLE DISORDERS

IMAGE GALLERY

Typical

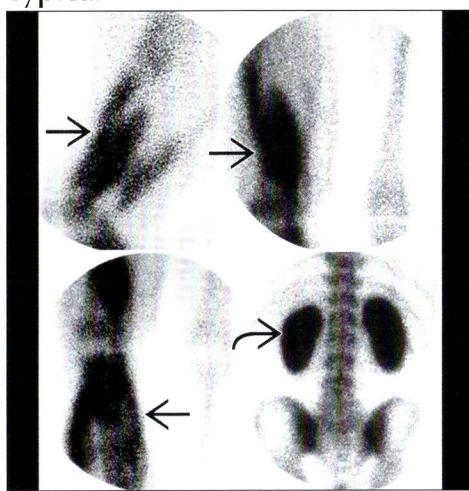

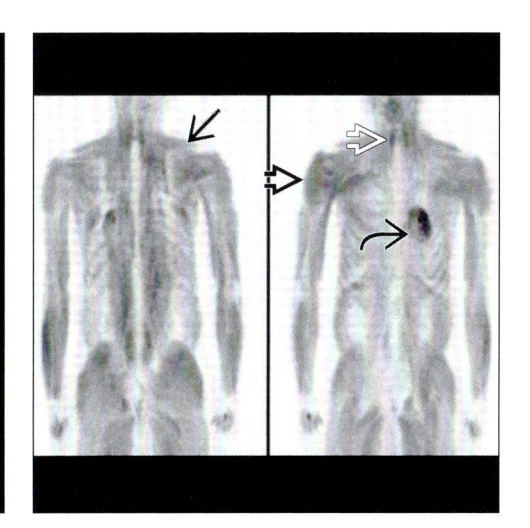

(Left) Bone scan shows increased uptake in multiple muscle groups of the right lower extremity ➡, consistent with muscle injury. Uptake in kidneys ➡ is due to myoglobin deposition. *(Right)* Posterior ➡ and anterior ➡ MIP PET shows diffuse skeletal & myocardial ➡ muscle uptake consistent with insulin response or hyperthyroidism. Note diffusely increased activity in the thyroid ➡.

Typical

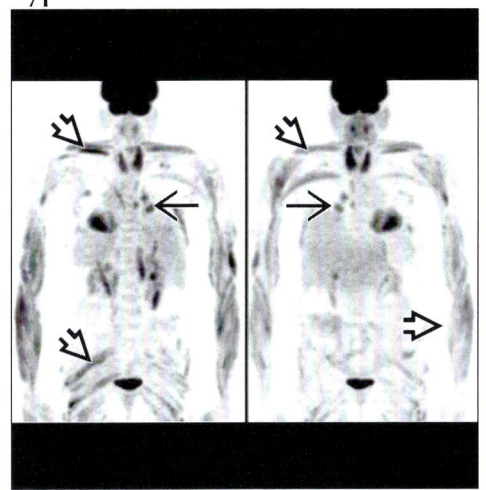

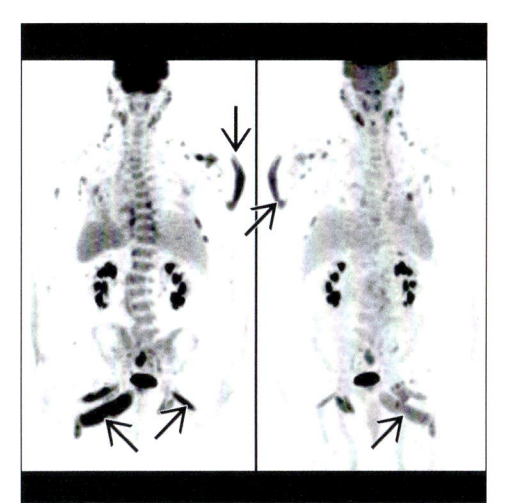

(Left) MIP PET shows ↑ uptake in multiple muscle groups ➡ in a patient with paraneoplastic polymyositis due to small cell lung cancer ➡. *(Right)* MIP PET shows focal increased uptake in several muscle groups ➡ due to biopsy-proven involvement of non-Hodgkin lymphoma (stage four).

Typical

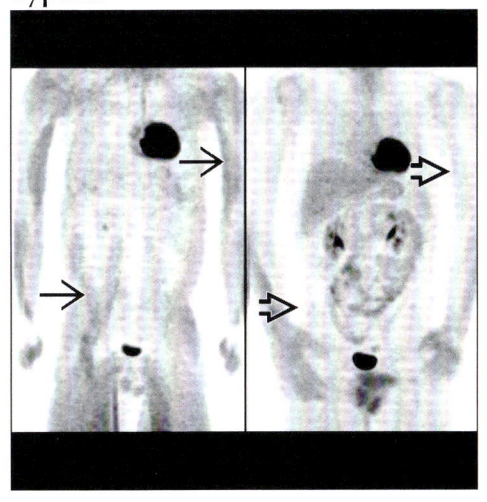

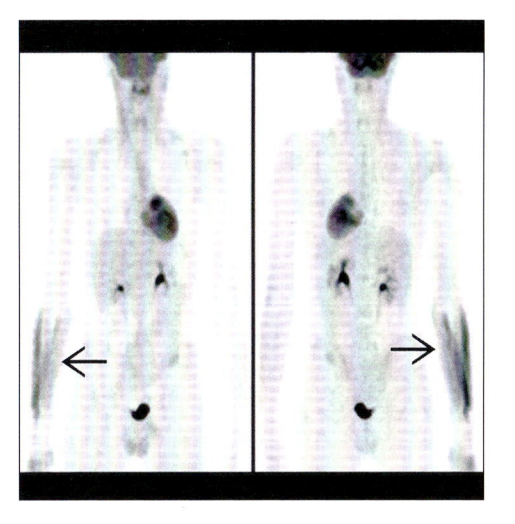

(Left) Anterior MIP PET following carbohydrate ingestion shows increased skeletal muscle uptake ➡, largely resolved in scan following 4 hours of fasting ➡. Insulin drives glucose into skeletal and myocardial muscle. *(Right)* Anterior and posterior MIP PET in a patient who was writing in his journal during interval from FDG injection to imaging shows resultant uptake in muscles of forearm ➡.

AMYLOIDOSIS

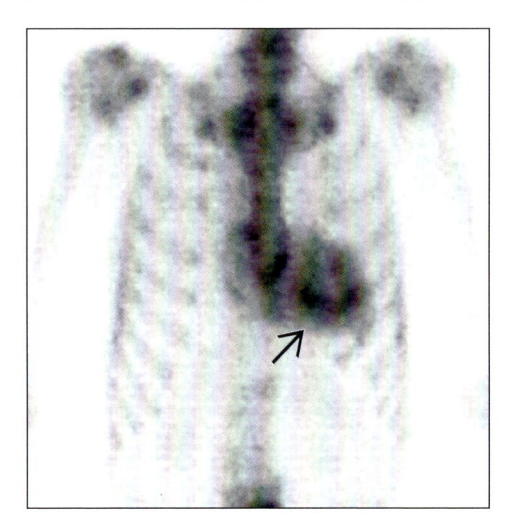

Anterior bone scan shows diffuse myocardial activity in patient with amyloidosis. Myocarditis and other infiltrative cardiac diseases are also differential considerations.

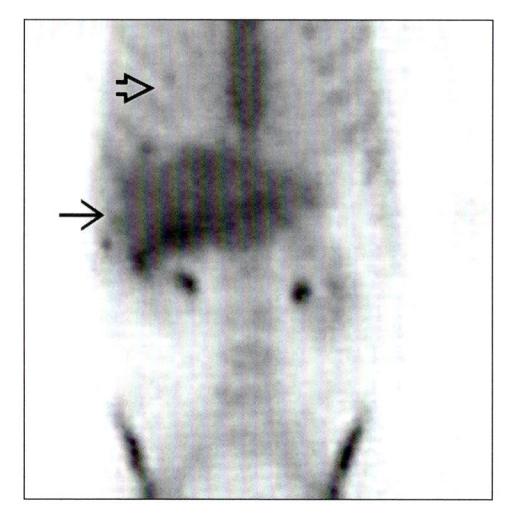

Anterior bone scan shows hepatic faint diffuse lung activity in patient with systemic amyloidosis due to underlying monoclonal gammopathy.

TERMINOLOGY

Definitions
- Based on etiology
  - Amyloidosis (AL) of monoclonal light chain IgG
  - Serum amyloid A (SAA); 2° to inflammation, infection; uncommon in developed countries
  - Amyloid familial transthyretin (AF/ATTR)
  - Amyloid endocrine (AE); medullary thyroid carcinoma-produced calcitonin = precursor
  - Amyloid hemodialysis (AH); β2 microglobulin = precursor
  - Amyloid senile (AS), otherwise idiopathic

IMAGING FINDINGS

General Features
- Best diagnostic clue
  - Incidental visceral activity on Tc-99m MDP bone scan
  - Amyloid-specific tracers investigational
- Location
  - Systemic or localized, diffuse or focal
  - Kidneys, myocardium, lungs, liver, spleen, GI tract, bone, cerebrum, skin, eyes, adrenals, nervous system, vasculature, connective tissue

Imaging Recommendations
- Nuclear medicine imaging options
  - All amyloid-specific radiotracers investigational
  - I-123 serum amyloid P (SAP) scintigraphy
    - Planar and SPECT imaging
    - Sensitivity AL: 90%
    - Sensitivity SAA: 90%
    - Sensitivity ATTR: 48%
  - Tc-99m aprotinin scintigraphy
    - 90 minute planar and SPECT images
    - Kidneys and liver may be false positive, therefore not well evaluated; spleen also variable
  - C-11 Pittsburgh compound B (PIB) PET
    - Binds cerebral amyloid plaques in patients with Alzheimer disease (AD)
    - Amyloid deposition may be result (not cause) of AD; perhaps not best early indicator of AD

DDx: Other Causes of Visceral Uptake on Bone Scan

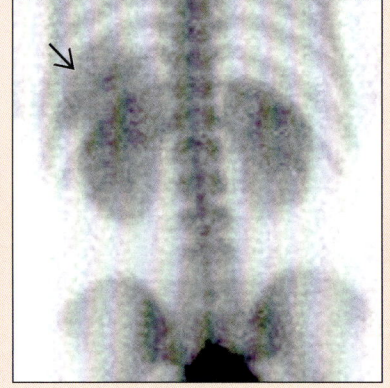

Spleen, Sickle Cell Crisis

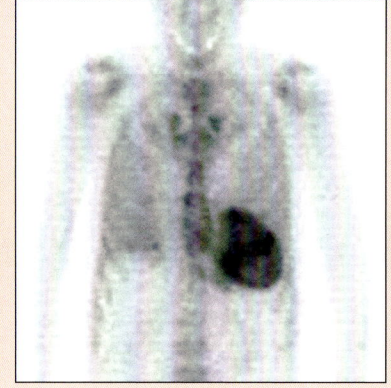

Hyperparathyroidism

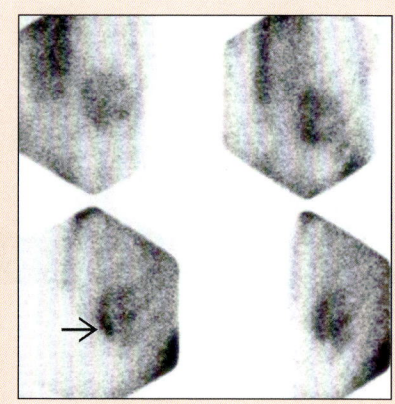

Acute Myocardial Infarction

AMYLOIDOSIS

Key Facts

Imaging Findings
- Incidental visceral activity on Tc-99m MDP bone scan
- Systemic or localized, diffuse or focal

Pathology
- Extracellular fibrillar homologous insoluble proteinaceous sheets of polysaccharide complexes
- Green birefringence/polarized Congo red staining

Clinical Issues
- Most common signs/symptoms: Asymptomatic initially, eventual visceral compromise ⇒ organ failure
- Long-term remissions possible with treatment

Diagnostic Checklist
- Visceral uptake on bone scan: Consider amyloidosis, neoplastic disease, metabolic derangement, infarct, injury or inflammation

DIFFERENTIAL DIAGNOSIS

Primary or Metastatic Neoplastic Disease
- Associated with visceral tumor infiltration secondary to primary malignancy

Metabolic Derangement
- Calcification 2° to hyperparathyroidism or dystrophic calcification (e.g., sickle cell disease)

Infarct, Injury, Inflammation
- Evaluate clinical setting (e.g., myocardial infarction, crush injury, electrocution, strain/overuse)

PATHOLOGY

General Features
- Etiology
  - Plasma cell disorders frequently present
    - Solitary plasmacytoma, multiple myeloma, lymphoma, Waldenstrom macroglobulinemia
  - Underlying inflammatory/infectious disease

Gross Pathologic & Surgical Features
- Infiltration and thickening of tissues by amyloid

Microscopic Features
- Extracellular fibrillar homologous insoluble proteinaceous sheets of polysaccharide complexes
- Green birefringence/polarized Congo red staining

CLINICAL ISSUES

Presentation
- Most common signs/symptoms: Asymptomatic initially, eventual visceral compromise ⇒ organ failure
- Other signs/symptoms: Polyneuropathy, organomegaly, endocrinopathy, monoclonal gammopathy, skin changes (POEMS)

Natural History & Prognosis
- Progressive morbidity, mortality
  - Long-term remissions possible with treatment

Treatment
- Goal: Alleviate proteinaceous precursor production
- Support organ failure

DIAGNOSTIC CHECKLIST

Consider
- Visceral uptake on bone scan: Consider amyloidosis, neoplastic disease, metabolic derangement, infarct, injury or inflammation

SELECTED REFERENCES
1. Hazenberg BP et al: Diagnostic performance of 123I-labeled serum amyloid P component scintigraphy in patients with amyloidosis. Am J Med. 119(4):355, 2006
2. Schaadt BK et al: 99mTc-aprotinin scintigraphy in amyloidosis. J Nucl Med. 44(2):177-83, 2003

IMAGE GALLERY

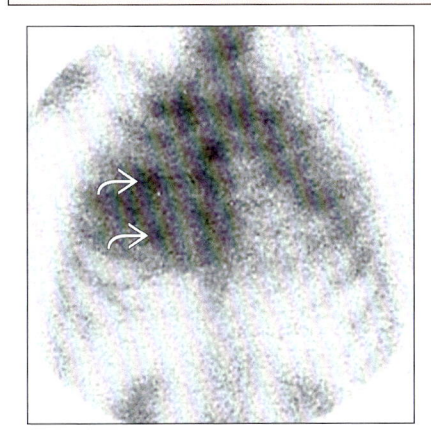

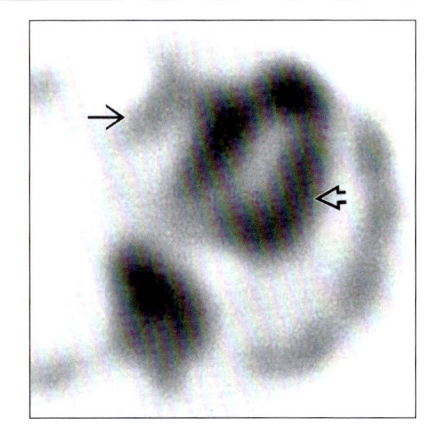

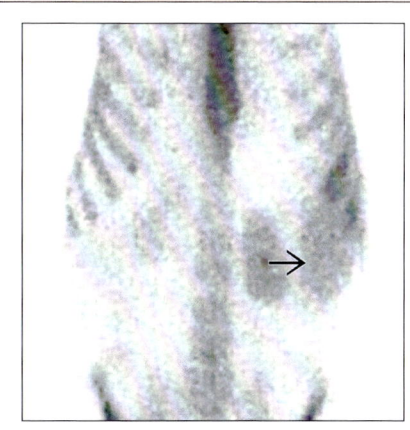

(Left) Anterior bone scan shows diffusely increased activity in lungs with focal parenchymal nodules ➔ in patient with pulmonary amyloidosis. *(Center)* transaxial SPECT bone scan shows tracer accumulation in right ➔ and left ➔ ventricles, consistent with myocardial amyloid deposition. *(Right)* Anterior bone scan shows diffuse activity in spleen ➔ in patient with splenic amyloid.

HEMATOPROLIFERATIVE DISORDERS

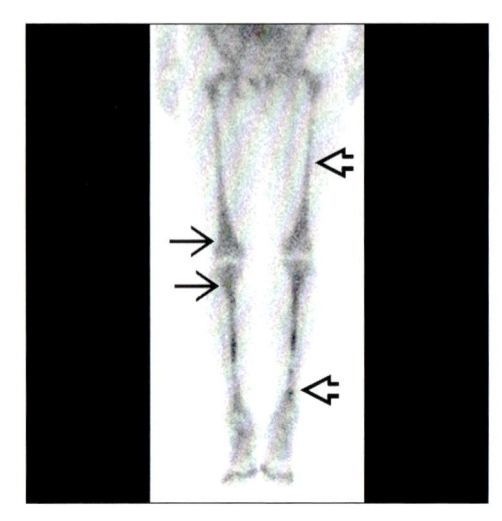

Anterior planar Tc-99m sulfur colloid marrow scan of a patient with myelofibrosis, demonstrates expansion of red marrow into distal long bones, particularly metaphyses. Similar findings seen on WBC scans.

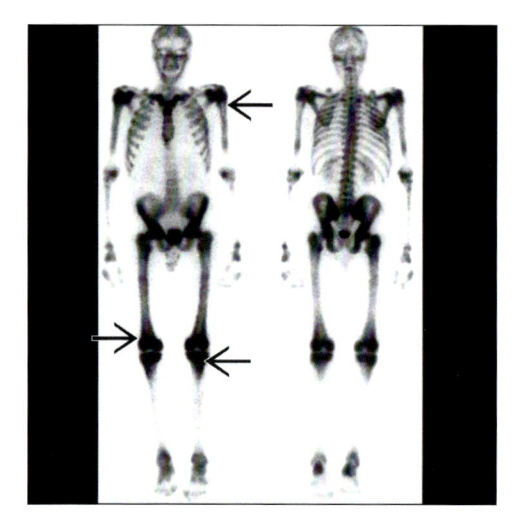

Ant. and post. Tc-99m bone scan of a patient with CML shows marked increased uptake in long bones, particularly metaphyseal regions, 2° to expansion of volume of distribution of red bone marrow.

TERMINOLOGY

Abbreviations and Synonyms
- Myelodysplastic disease
- Myeloproliferative, hematoproliferative disease
- Marrow infiltrative disease
- Marrow hyperplasia

Definitions
- Disorders characterized by expansion of volume of distribution, cellularity, or infiltration of red bone marrow

IMAGING FINDINGS

General Features
- Best diagnostic clue
  - Bone scan or sulfur colloid scan: Increased uptake in metaphyseal regions of distal long bones
  - MR: Increased T1WI signal (< skeletal muscle, intervertebral disc) in metaphyseal regions of distal femurs, proximal tibiae & humeri
- Location
  - Normal red marrow distribution in infant: Involves calvarium and all long bones, including phalanges
  - During maturation: Conversion of red to fatty yellow marrow; typically complete by age 25
  - Normal pattern of conversion: Apophyses, growth plates → long bones (distal → proximal)
  - Normal adult pattern: Red marrow confined to axial skeleton, proximal femurs & humeri
  - Normal adult female variant: Retention of patchy red marrow in femurs, pelvis, humeri (likely due to iron deficiency, menstrual blood loss)
  - Elderly: Further loss of red marrow from proximal long bones, pedicles & posterior elements
  - Basis for pathologic distribution of red marrow
    - Yellow marrow is labile: Reconverts to red marrow with hematoproliferative or infiltrative disease
    - Marrow reconversion (yellow → red): Occurs in reverse order as for conversion (proximal → distal long bones)

Nuclear Medicine Findings
- Tc-99m sulfur colloid marrow scan
  - Normal adult pattern: Uptake in liver, spleen, axial and proximal appendicular bone marrow

DDx: Mimics of Hematoproliferative Disease

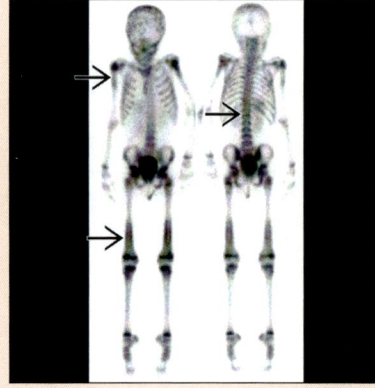

Marrow Metastases (Neuroblastoma) 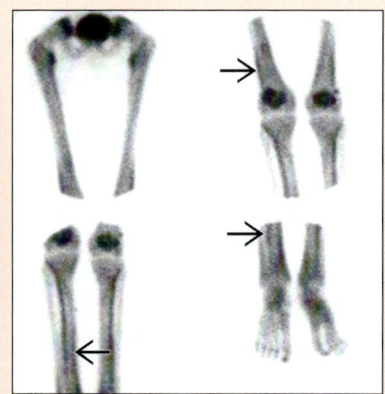 | *Hypertrophic Osteoarthropathy* 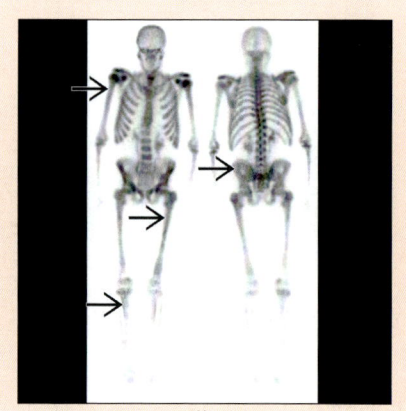 | *Superscan (Diffuse Metastases)*

HEMATOPROLIFERATIVE DISORDERS

Key Facts

Terminology
- Disorders characterized by expansion of volume of distribution, cellularity, or infiltration of red bone marrow

Imaging Findings
- Bone scan or sulfur colloid scan: Increased uptake in metaphyseal regions of distal long bones
- MR: Increased T1WI signal (< skeletal muscle, intervertebral disc) in metaphyseal regions of distal femurs, proximal tibiae & humeri
- Normal red marrow distribution in infant: Involves calvarium and all long bones, including phalanges
- During maturation: Conversion of red to fatty yellow marrow; typically complete by age 25
- Normal adult pattern: Red marrow confined to axial skeleton, proximal femurs & humeri
- Yellow marrow is labile: Reconverts to red marrow with hematoproliferative or infiltrative disease
- Extramedullary hematopoiesis: Sites show uptake on Tc-99m sulfur colloid, In-111 WBC, FDG PET

Top Differential Diagnoses
- Hyperparathyroidism
- Hypertrophic Osteoarthropathy

Pathology
- Stress hematoproliferative disorders
- Myelodysplastic disorders: Myelofibrosis, myeloid metaplasia, mastocytosis, polycythemia vera, essential thrombocytosis, etc.
- Other infiltrative marrow disease: Leukemia, lymphoma, extensive marrow metastases, Gaucher disease, amyloidosis

---

- Marrow reconversion pattern (red to yellow): Uptake extends to distal long bones, especially metaphyses of distal femurs and proximal tibiae & humeri
- Gaucher disease: Uptake in spine and pelvis can be lower (or absent) compared to long bones; marrow reconversion pattern, hepatosplenomegaly
- Sickle cell disease: Marrow reconversion pattern, spleen typically smaller than normal, patchy marrow due to previous infarcts
- Many hematoproliferative or infiltrative marrow diseases also associated with increased hepatosplenomegaly
- Early myelofibrosis: Marrow reconversion pattern
- Late myelofibrosis: Patchy decreased marrow uptake; splenomegaly, focal uptake at sites of extramedullary hematopoiesis
- Labeled WBC scan: Marrow patterns similar to Tc-99m sulfur colloid marrow scan
- Tc-99m diphosphonate bone scan: Marrow expansion pattern shows increased uptake in metaphyseal portions of long bones, especially distal femurs, proximal tibiae and humeri
  - Bone scan in myelofibrosis: Early pattern typical for marrow expansion; late in disease may see patchy decreased uptake in long bones
  - Metastatic disease to marrow: May mimic hematoproliferative marrow expansion pattern on bone scan; even without focal cortical "hot spots"
  - Multiple myeloma: Lesions often cold on bone scan; uptake due to osteopenic compression fractures may mimic osteoporosis, osteomalacia
- FDG PET: Diffuse increased uptake in red marrow, spleen most commonly suggests GCSF, erythropoietin simulation (effect lasts ~ 1 month)
  - FDG PET: Marrow uptake in myeloproliferative, neoplastic, infiltrative marrow disease
  - FDG PET: May show additional sites in suspected solitary plasmacytoma (preferred over Tc-99m sestamibi scan for this purpose)
- Ga-67: Marrow patterns similar to those seen on FDG PET; GCSF, erythropoietin stimulation pattern persists longer than FDG PET (up to 1 yr)
- Extramedullary hematopoiesis: Sites show uptake on Tc-99m sulfur colloid, In-111 WBC, FDG PET

MR Findings
- MR: Signal indicates presence of red (hematopoietic), infiltrative, or yellow (fatty) marrow
  - Normal red (hematopoietic) marrow
    - Normal MR signal on T1WI ≥ intervertebral disc or adjacent skeletal muscle
    - Minimal enhancement with gadolinium contrast
  - Myelodysplastic or infiltrative marrow
    - T1WI MR signal lower than intervertebral disc or skeletal muscle
    - Increased enhancement with gadolinium
  - Exception to the rule: TR weighting > 700 ms (not true T1) seen in several non-pathological conditions
    - Spine of infants
    - Patients with profound chronic anemia (e.g., sickle cell)
    - Transplanted bone marrow
    - Transfused AIDS patients
  - Yellow (fatty) marrow: Fatty signal on all sequences
  - Abnormal conversion of red marrow → yellow marrow
    - Aplastic anemia, post radiation change, some chemotherapies
    - Avascular necrosis: Although tend to occur more commonly in yellow marrow containing bone

Other Modality Findings
- CT, plain radiography
  - Leukemia, marrow metastases (e.g., neuroblastoma): Symmetrical lucent rarefaction of metaphyses
  - Myelofibrosis: Focal or diffuse sclerotic lesions (late manifestation)
  - Mastocytosis: May show focal or diffuse sclerotic lesions, ivory vertebrae
  - Gaucher disease: Erlenmeyer flask deformity of metaphyses, generalized osteopenia

Imaging Recommendations
- Best imaging tool
  - MR

HEMATOPROLIFERATIVE DISORDERS

- Normal red marrow: T1 signal ≥ intervertebral disc, skeletal muscle; minimal enhancement
- Hematoproliferative and infiltrative marrow disease: Marrow reconversion pattern; extension into distal long bones (particularly metaphyses of distal femur, proximal tibiae and humeri)
- Hematoproliferative and infiltrative marrow diseases: Low T1 signal compared to normal intervertebral disc, enhances with gadolinium
- Myelofibrosis: Early stage hypercellular marrow reconversion pattern; late stage low T1, T2 signal from fibrosis
  - Tc-99m sulfur colloid marrow scan: Marrow reconversion pattern, splenomegaly, hepatomegaly
  - Bone scan: Marrow reconversion pattern
- Protocol advice: Tc-99m sulfur colloid marrow scan: SPECT if suspect extramedullary hematopoiesis

DIFFERENTIAL DIAGNOSIS

Hyperparathyroidism
- Diffuse increased uptake on bone scan tends to be diffuse (all bones), primarily cortically based

Hypertrophic Osteoarthropathy
- Increased uptake on bone scan can be more pronounced in metaphyseal region of distal femur, proximal tibia: Tends to be cortically based, not transmedullary
- Periosteal new bone formation on plain film, CT

Paget Disease
- Increased uptake in ends of long bones on bone scan may mimic marrow expansion disease
  - Differs from marrow expansion pattern in that Paget disease is more asymmetrical
  - Associated involvement of hemipelvis or isolated vertebral segments may be characteristic
- Normal fatty marrow signal on MR, although marrow space may be smaller due to cortical thickening
  - Marrow edema usually indicates complication: Fracture, malignant degeneration

Normal Skeletally Immature Patient
- Increased uptake on bone scan in metaphyseal regions is confined to growth plates, should not extend into metaphyses, epiphyses
- Increased uptake on labeled WBC, Tc-99m sulfur colloid in distal long bones (< age 13 yrs)

Arthritis
- Uptake on bone scan centered on articular, not metaphyseal portion of distal long bones

PATHOLOGY

General Features
- Hematoproliferative and infiltrative marrow diseases
  - Stress hematoproliferative disorders
    - Severe reticuloendothelial stimulation (severe sustained infection)
    - Severe or chronic anemia: Thalassemia, sickle cell disease, autoimmune red cell destruction, hereditary spherocytosis
    - Treatment with hemato-/myeloproliferative cytokines (GCSF, erythropoietin): Increased cellularity but not usually reconversion (yellow → red marrow)
  - Myelodysplastic disorders: Myelofibrosis, myeloid metaplasia, mastocytosis, polycythemia vera, essential thrombocytosis, etc.
  - Other infiltrative marrow disease: Leukemia, lymphoma, extensive marrow metastases, Gaucher disease, amyloidosis

CLINICAL ISSUES

Presentation
- Most common signs/symptoms: Vague periarticular pain, spinal pain
- Other signs/symptoms: Variable, depending on cause of underlying disorder: Anemia, bleeding, infections

DIAGNOSTIC CHECKLIST

Image Interpretation Pearls
- Bone scan: Symmetrical metaphyseal uptake in distal long bones suggests hematoproliferative or infiltrative marrow disease

SELECTED REFERENCES

1. Blebea JS et al: Structural and functional imaging of normal bone marrow and evaluation of its age-related changes. Semin Nucl Med. 37(3):185-94, 2007
2. Chhabra A et al: Obscured bone metastases after administration of hematopoietic factor on FDG-PET. Clin Nucl Med. 31(6):328-30, 2006
3. Inoue K et al: Diffuse bone marrow uptake on F-18 FDG PET in patients with myelodysplastic syndromes. Clin Nucl Med. 31(11):721-3, 2006
4. Bredella MA et al: Value of FDG PET in the assessment of patients with multiple myeloma. AJR Am J Roentgenol. 184(4):1199-204, 2005
5. Hung GU et al: Comparison of Tc-99m sestamibi and F-18 FDG-PET in the assessment of multiple myeloma. Anticancer Res. 25(6C):4737-41, 2005
6. Kazama T et al: Effect of colony-stimulating factor and conventional- or high-dose chemotherapy on FDG uptake in bone marrow. Eur J Nucl Med Mol Imaging. 32(12):1406-11, 2005
7. Blodgett TM et al: Diffuse bone marrow uptake on whole-body F-18 fluorodeoxyglucose positron emission tomography in a patient taking recombinant erythropoietin. Clin Nucl Med. 29(3):161-3, 2004
8. Elstrom RL et al: Enhanced marrow [18F]fluorodeoxyglucose uptake related to myeloid hyperplasia in Hodgkin's lymphoma can simulate lymphoma involvement in marrow. Clin Lymphoma. 5(1):62-4, 2004
9. Yao WJ et al: Quantitative PET imaging of bone marrow glucose metabolic response to hematopoietic cytokines. J Nucl Med. 36(5):794-9, 1995
10. Palestro CJ et al: Indium-111-leukocyte imaging in Gaucher's disease. J Nucl Med. 34(5):818-20, 1993

HEMATOPROLIFERATIVE DISORDERS

IMAGE GALLERY

Typical

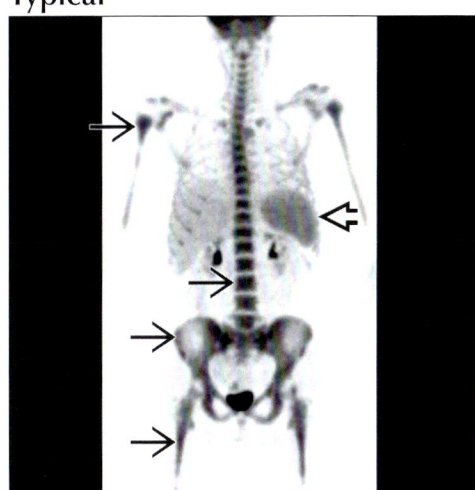

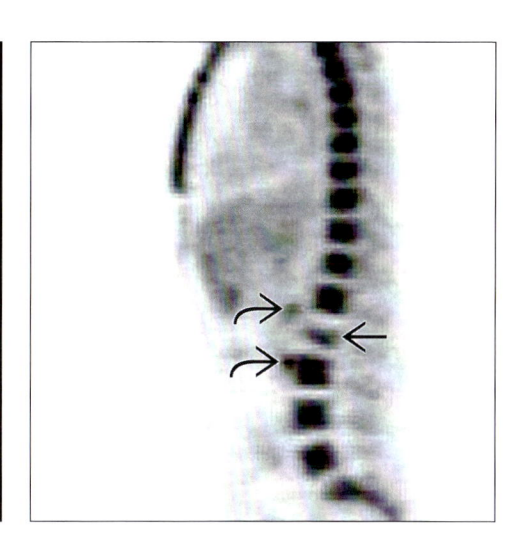

(Left) FDG PET shows typical pattern 2° to treatment with myelo- or hematoproliferative cytokines (GCSF, erythropoietin): Increased uptake in red marrow volume ➔ as well as spleen ➔. (Right) Sagittal FDG PET in a patient on GCSF therapy shows foci of extramedullary hematopoiesis ➔ due to extruded marrow 2° to old L2 compression fracture ➔.

Typical

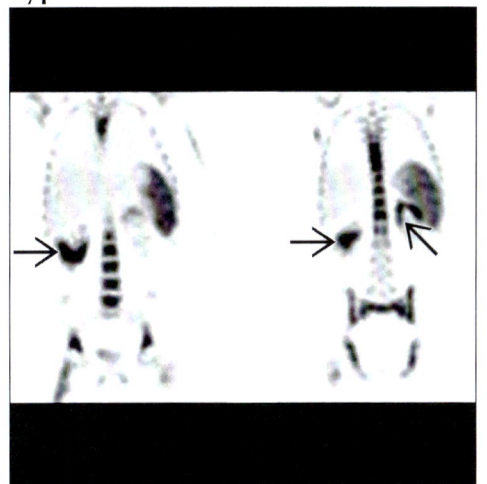

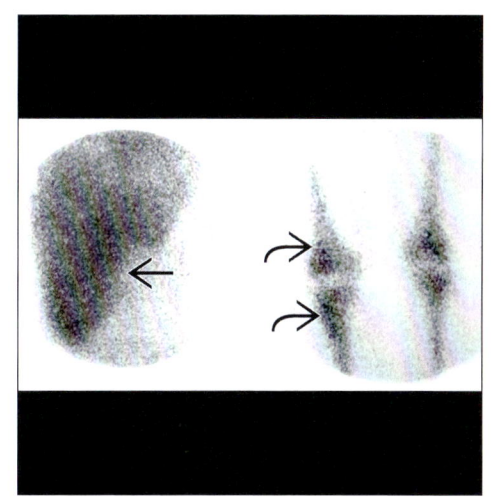

(Left) Coronal FDG PET shows perirenal sites of uptake due to extramedullary hematopoiesis ➔, as well as increased uptake in spleen and bone marrow, in patient undergoing treatment with GCSF. (Right) Anterior In-111 WBC scan shows hepatomegaly ➔ and peripheral marrow expansion ➔, typical of Gaucher disease. Not shown: Reduced uptake in spine & pelvis, also frequently seen in Gaucher disease.

Typical

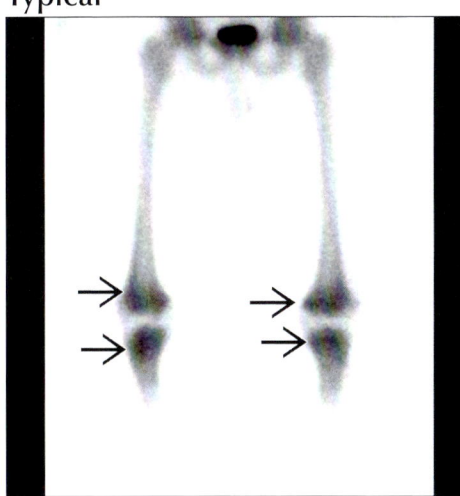

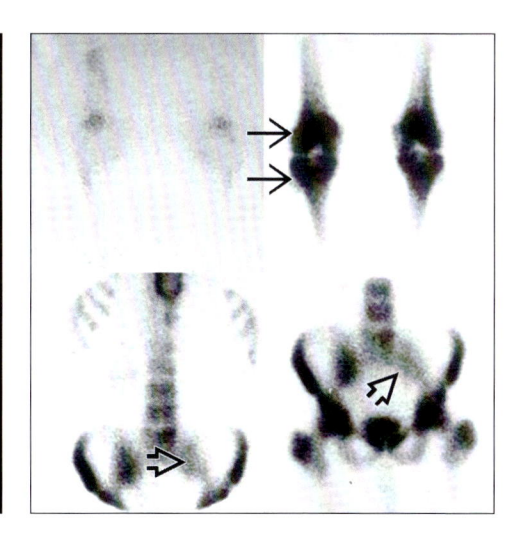

(Left) Anterior bone scan in patient with systemic mastocytosis shows increased uptake in metaphyses ➔ of distal femurs, proximal tibiae, typical of marrow reconversion. (Right) Bone scan of knees at baseline (1), and after development of CML (2), showing progression metaphyseal uptake ➔. Note photopenic attenuation of left SI joint due to splenomegaly ➔.

HEMATOPROLIFERATIVE DISORDERS

(Left) Bone scan shows subtle lytic lesions of sternum ➡, T-11 ➡, and right iliac bone ➡ due to multiple myeloma. See next image. *(Right)* Same patient as previous bone scan. CT shows much more extensive lytic disease (punched out lesions) ➡ than are evident on Tc-99m bone scan, typical of multiple myeloma.

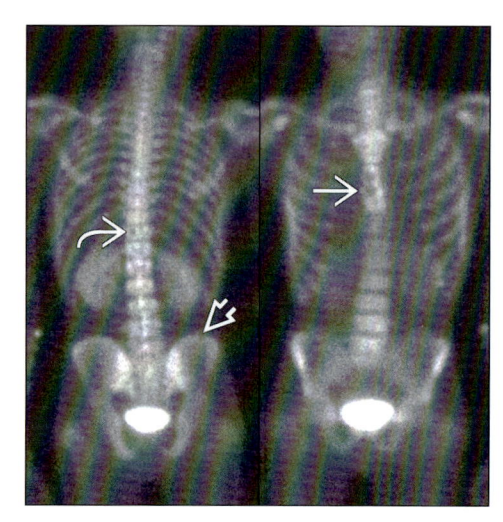

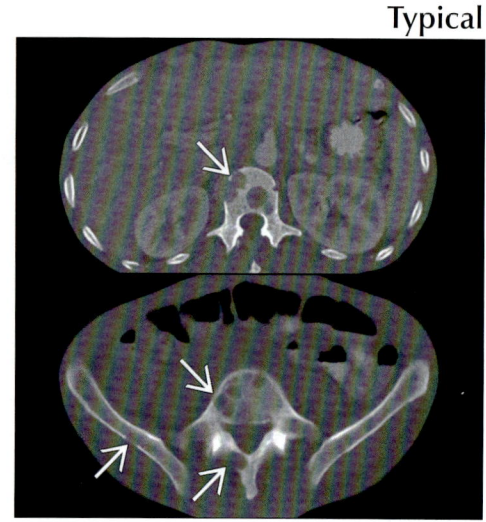

(Left) Anterior bone scan shows nonspecific findings typical of late-stage myelofibrosis: Low level heterogeneous uptake in spine ➡ and long bones ➡ (trauma to right ribs and left patella was incidental). See next image. *(Right)* NECT (coronal reconstructions) show patchy sclerosis of marrow space ➡, ➡ typical of late-stage myelofibrosis.

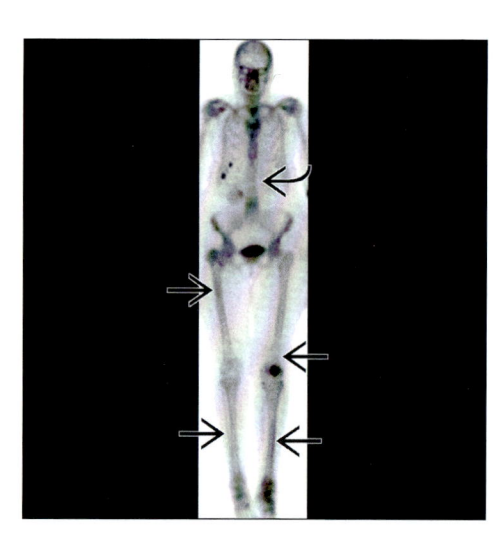

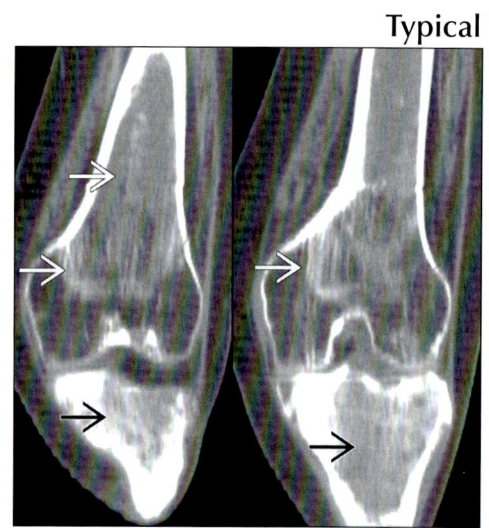

(Left) Anterior Ga-67 scan of chest, post treatment for lymphoma, shows diffuse uptake in bone marrow ➡ typical of GCSF stimulation. See next image. *(Right)* Anterior Ga-67 scan of pelvis, post treatment for lymphoma, shows uptake in bone marrow ➡ typical of GCSF effect. Photopenic regions in pelvis, left proximal femur represent sites of marrow loss ➡ due to treated tumor or radiation.

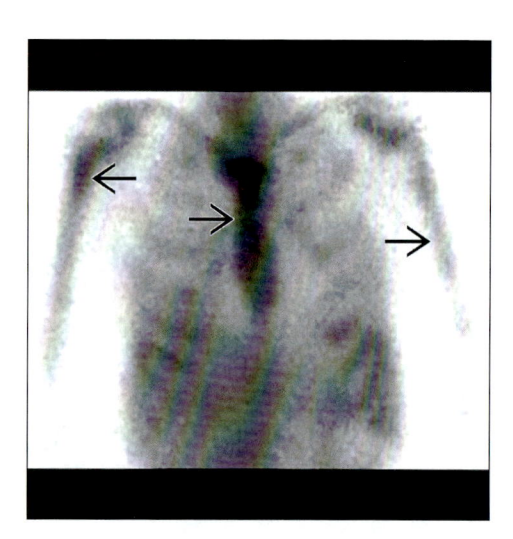

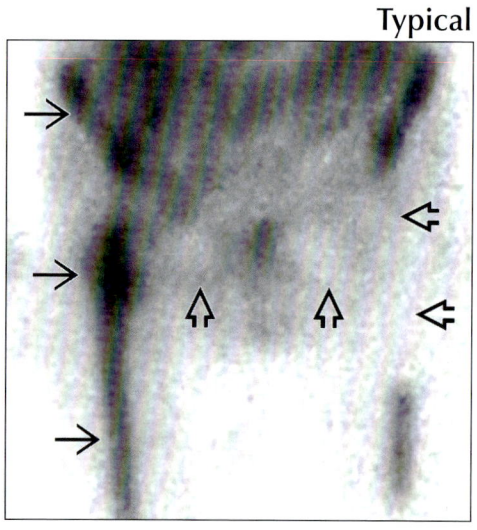

HEMATOPROLIFERATIVE DISORDERS

Typical

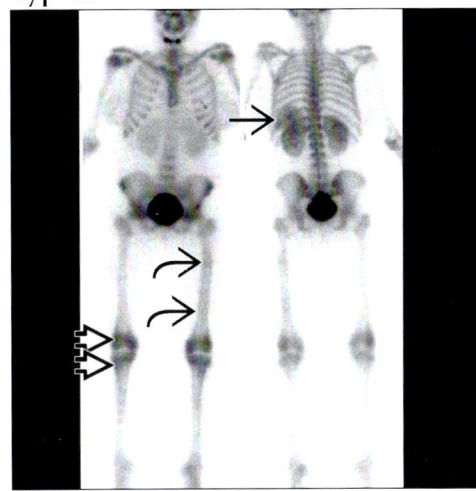

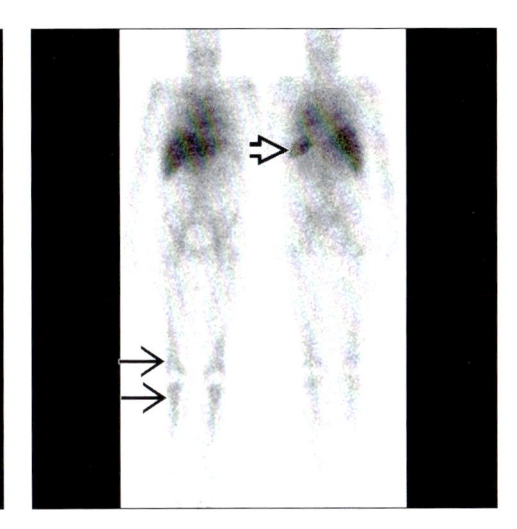

(Left) Bone scan in patient with sickle cell disease shows ↑ uptake in kidneys and spleen ➔ (acute crisis), metaphyseal uptake ➔ (marrow reconversion) and patchy femoral shaft uptake ➔ (acute bone infarct). **(Right)** In-111 WBC scan in patient with sickle cell disease shows small poorly functioning spleen ➔ (normally "hotter" than liver on WBC scan) and ↑ uptake in metaphyses ➔ (distal femurs, proximal tibiae).

Typical

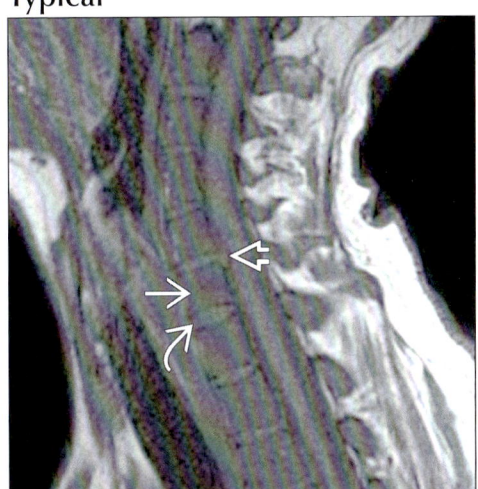

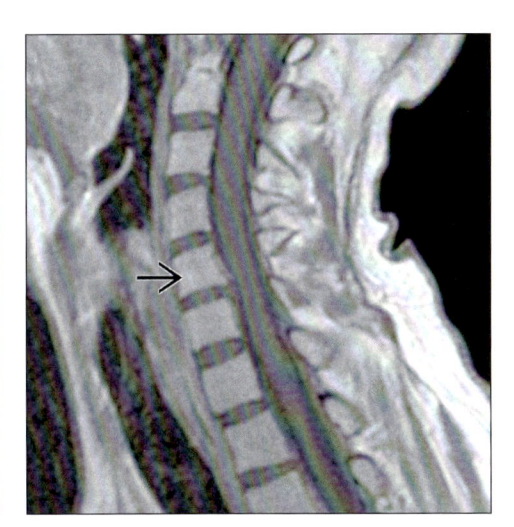

(Left) T1 MR shows diffusely ↓ signal in spine ➔ compared to intervertebral discs ➔. Note incidental disc herniation ➔. Red marrow signal is normally lower than intervertebral disc. See next image. **(Right)** T1 C+ MR in same patient at left shows marked diffuse marrow enhancement ➔. Normal red marrow shows minimal enhancement. Findings suggest hematoproliferative or other infiltrative marrow disease. (Courtesy K. Moore, MD).

Typical

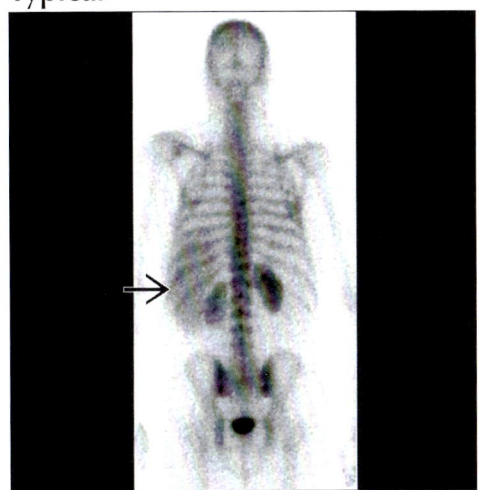

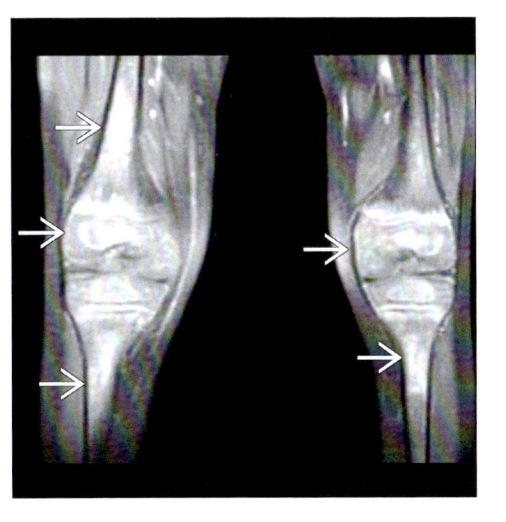

(Left) Posterior bone scan shows ↑ uptake in enlarged spleen ➔, suggesting microinfarction or diffuse siderosis. Patient had late stage myelofibrosis. Note lack of metaphyseal uptake typically seen in early myelofibrosis. **(Right)** Coronal MR shows diffuse marrow infiltrative process ➔ in child with acute lymphoblastic leukemia. Findings also consistent with bilateral symmetrical metastatic marrow disease, such as neuroblastoma.

SICKLE CELL DISEASE, BONE PAIN

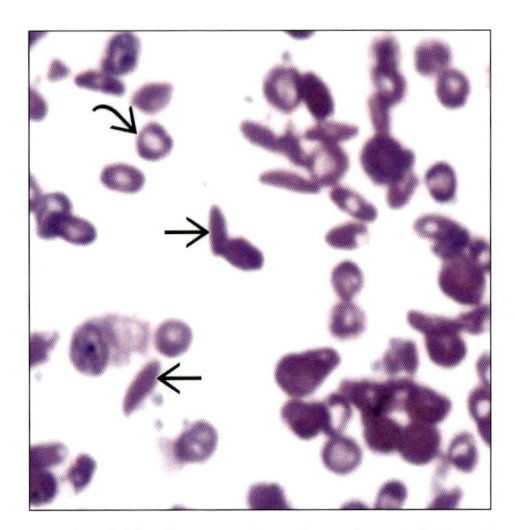

Peripheral blood smear shows hypochromic and sickled red blood cells, hallmark findings of sickle cell disease (SCD).

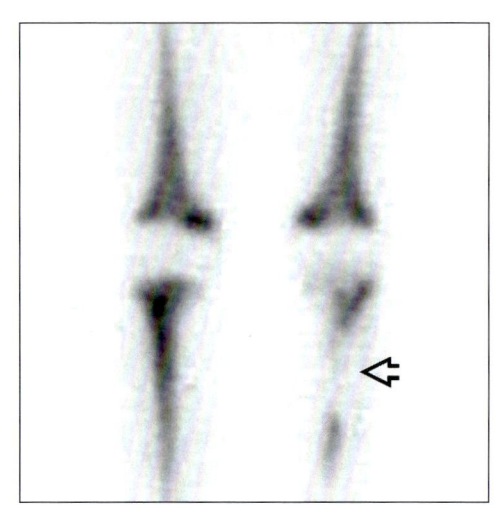

Tc-99m sulfur colloid bone marrow scintigraphy shows photopenic defect in proximal left tibia in patient with SCD and acute leg pain, denoting bone infarction.

TERMINOLOGY

Abbreviations and Synonyms
- Sickle cell disease (SCD), hemoglobinopathy

Definitions
- Genetic disorder of hemoglobin
  - Single base substitution in gene encoding beta-globin subunit
  - Deformed ("sickled") red blood cells
  - Causes wide range of clinical manifestations (e.g., vaso-occlusive crisis ⇒ bone infarction, autosplenectomy ⇒ increased risk of infection)
- Acute musculoskeletal pain in SCD: Bone infarction vs. osteomyelitis
  - Both present with pain, swelling, fever
  - Blood cultures can be negative in up to 50% of cases of acute osteomyelitis
  - Treatments vastly different
    - Bone infarction: Analgesics, hydration
    - Osteomyelitis: Long term antibiotics
  - Early diagnosis important
  - Bone infarction more common than osteomyelitis

IMAGING FINDINGS

General Features
- Best diagnostic clue
  - First line modality: MR
    - T1WI C+: Hypointense in acute bone infarction, may have enhancing rim with healing
    - T1WI C+: Osteomyelitis enhances
  - Nuclear Medicine: Findings on most modalities nonspecific, reserved for problem-solving
    - Bone infarction: ↓ Activity on bone scan; may have no or mild uptake on leukocyte scan
    - Osteomyelitis: ↑ Activity on 3-phase bone scan and leukocyte scan
- Location
  - Bone infarction
    - Axial skeleton and long bones most frequently involved (hematopoietic bone marrow)
    - Most common long bone site: Proximal femur/humerus/tibia, distal femur
  - Osteomyelitis
    - SCD: Hematogenous spread to vascular bone
    - Usually in long bones: Tibia, femur, humerus
- Morphology

DDx: Mimics of Sickle Cell Osteopathy

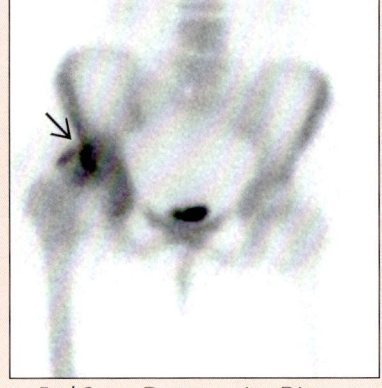

End Stage Degenerative Disease

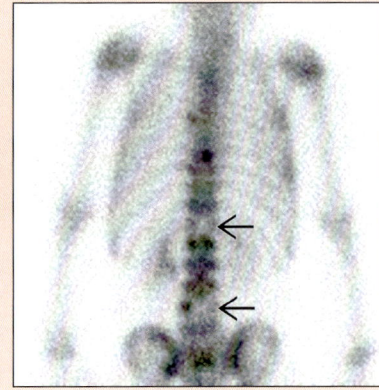

Lytic Bone Metastases

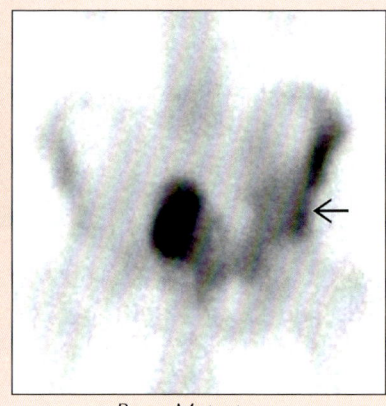

Bone Metastases

SICKLE CELL DISEASE, BONE PAIN

Key Facts

Terminology
- Genetic disorder of hemoglobin
- Causes wide range of clinical manifestations (e.g., vaso-occlusive crisis ⇒ bone infarction, autosplenectomy ⇒ increased risk of infection)
- Acute musculoskeletal pain in SCD: Bone infarction vs. osteomyelitis

Imaging Findings
- First line modality: MR
- Nuclear Medicine: Findings on most modalities nonspecific, reserved for problem-solving

Top Differential Diagnoses
- Sclerotic Bone Tumor
- Lytic Bone Tumor
- Septic Arthritis
- Gout

Clinical Issues
- Bone infarction: Hydration, pain control
- Osteomyelitis: Long term IV antibiotics

Diagnostic Checklist
- For problem-solving, use both bone scan and marrow map to differentiate osteomyelitis and infarction (increased specificity)
- Osteomyelitis: Usually + on bone scan, can be negative; normal or increased uptake on marrow map; usually increased on In-111 WBC, Ga-67
- Bone infarction: Variable activity on bone scan; decreased activity on marrow map; variable activity on Ga-67, In-111 WBC

- Bone infarction: Highly variable; does not extend beyond bone or involve soft tissues
- Osteomyelitis: Can extend beyond bone into soft tissues (cellulitis, edema)

Nuclear Medicine Findings
- Tc-99m MDP bone scan
  - Tracer localizes to regions of osteoblastic activity, hyperemia
  - Bone infarction
    - Acute (days): ↓ Uptake
    - Subacute (1 week): ↑ Uptake
    - Remote (years): Old infarcts can show ↑ activity due to continuing bone remodeling
  - Osteomyelitis
    - ↑ Activity on all phases of three-phase bone scan
    - Occasionally "cold" on third phase of bone scan (especially vertebral osteomyelitis)
  - Whole body scan allows comprehensive skeletal survey for other sites of involvement
    - Generalized ↑ uptake in skeleton often seen 2° to chronic anemia ⇒ marrow expansion
    - Spleen may show uptake 2° to infarction, calcification and fibrosis
    - Asymptomatic increased activity: Old infarction, chronic osteomyelitis, bone remodeling/repair (e.g., treated osteomyelitis, trauma)
- Tc-99m sulfur colloid bone marrow scan ("marrow map")
  - Decreased uptake in either bone infarct or infection: Not specific
  - Tracer localizes in bone marrow reticuloendothelial system
  - Symptomatic sites: ↓ Activity in marrow space immediately following a vaso-occlusive event due to bone marrow edema
  - Asymptomatic regions of ↓ activity = old bone infarction (more commonly seen in older children, adults)
  - Whole body scan allows comprehensive skeletal survey for other sites of involvement
  - Absence of splenic activity often due to autoinfarction, functional asplenia
- Image interpretation: Nuclear medicine findings frequently not specific
  - Osteomyelitis: ↑ Activity on bone scan and WBC scan, ↓ on bone marrow scan
  - Bone Infarction: Variable activity on bone scan, ↓ on bone marrow scan, ↓ or mild ↑ on WBC scan
- WBC scan: Absence of activity suggests infarction; increased uptake may signify either infection or infarction with secondary inflammation

Radiographic Findings
- Plain film: Normal in early bone infarction and osteomyelitis
  - May show periosteal changes (can be seen with bone infarction and osteomyelitis)

MR Findings
- Bone infarction: Marrow edema ± thin rim of enhancement around nonenhancing marrow
- Osteomyelitis: Geographic, irregular marrow enhancement with contrast
- High signal intensity of hematopoietic bone in children can ⇒ false positives
- Diagnosis of acute osteomyelitis: 92% sens, 96% spec
- Can be difficult to distinguish osteomyelitis from bone infarction in some cases

Ultrasonographic Findings
- Osteomyelitis: Subperiosteal fluid collection
- Allows for concurrent aspiration, cultures

Imaging Recommendations
- Best imaging tool: MR: Focal examination of symptomatic site(s)
- Protocol advice
  - Tc-99m MDP bone scan: 30 mCi (1110 MBq) adult dose; pediatric dose: (age +1/age +7) x adult dose
    - Anterior and posterior planar three-phase imaging of focal region
    - Whole body + spot images or spot images only (focused exam)

SICKLE CELL DISEASE, BONE PAIN

- Tc-99m sulfur colloid (filtered) bone marrow map: 10 mCi (370 MBq) adult dose; pediatric dose: (age +1/age +7) x adult dose
  - Ant. and post. planar image at 20-30 min
  - Spot images +/- whole body
- Additional nuclear medicine imaging options
  - In-111 WBC scintigraphy
    - Helpful to differentiate acute osteomyelitis and infarction in equivocal cases
    - Look for areas of ↑ activity discordant to bone or bone marrow scan findings
    - If negative, can exclude infection
  - Ga-67 scintigraphy
    - May show ↓ activity in acute bone infarction
    - Normal activity in healing infarcts
    - If negative, can exclude osteomyelitis
  - PET/CT
    - Case report of role in distinguishing infection vs. infarction, not yet validated

DIFFERENTIAL DIAGNOSIS

Sclerotic Bone Tumor
- Increased uptake on bone scan
- Decreased uptake on bone marrow and WBC scan

Lytic Bone Tumor
- Bone scan can be cold, hot, or cold with warm rim
- Photopenic on bone marrow scan (marrow replacement)

Septic Arthritis
- Positive three phase bone scan with intense periarticular uptake
- Positive In-111 WBC scan

Gout
- Positive periarticular activity on bone scan
- May have positive WBC scan: Intense inflammation

Chronic Inflammation (not infected)
- Increased uptake on bone scan
- Increased uptake on WBC and bone marrow scan (mononuclear cell infiltration)

PATHOLOGY

General Features
- Genetics
  - Autosomal recessive disorder ⇒ instability in RBC morphology in deoxygenated state
  - Amino acid substitution (valine ⇔ glutamate), at sixth position of β-chain in hemoglobin molecule
- Epidemiology
  - Most common: Sub-Saharan Africa, descendants from that region
  - 1 in 12 African-Americans have SC trait (Hb AS)
  - Also found in people of Mediterranean, Indian, Middle Eastern heritage
- Associated abnormalities: Coexisting thalassemia: Includes disorders affecting α hemoglobin as well as β hemoglobin genes

Gross Pathologic & Surgical Features
- Bone infarction: Elongated pale region of bone marrow with hyperemic border sharply demarcated from adjacent bone
- Osteomyelitis: Inflammatory changes, edema, necrosis

Microscopic Features
- Infarction: Cystic spaces due to fat necrosis, focal calcifications, dead trabeculae
  - Late stages: Ingrowth of granulation tissue
- Osteomyelitis: In SCD, usually hematogenous spread of infection, infiltration of white blood cells into bone elements, thrombosis, necrosis

CLINICAL ISSUES

Presentation
- Most common signs/symptoms: Acute pain, fever
- Other signs/symptoms: Acute chest syndrome, jaundice, anemia, infection, stroke, pulmonary hypertension, stunted growth, priapism

Natural History & Prognosis
- Life expectancy for homozygotes ~ 45 years
- Multi-organ damage from chronic vaso-occlusions and hemolysis
- Heterozygotes have more indolent course and near normal life expectancy

Treatment
- Bone infarction: Hydration, pain control
  - Symptoms usually improve < 1 week
- Osteomyelitis: Long term IV antibiotics

DIAGNOSTIC CHECKLIST

Consider
- For problem-solving, use both bone scan and marrow map to differentiate osteomyelitis and infarction (increased specificity)
- Osteomyelitis: Usually + on bone scan, can be negative; normal or increased uptake on marrow map; usually increased on In-111 WBC, Ga-67
- Bone infarction: Variable activity on bone scan; decreased activity on marrow map; variable activity on Ga-67, In-111 WBC

Image Interpretation Pearls
- History, clinical presentation, time course of symptoms important for diagnosis
- Dynamic changes in bone scan appear over time

SELECTED REFERENCES

1. Skaggs DL et al: Differentiation between bone infarction and acute osteomyelitis in children with sickle-cell disease with use of sequential radionuclide bone-marrow and bone scans. J Bone Joint Surg Am. 83-A(12):1810-3, 2001
2. Kim HC et al: Differentiation of bone and bone marrow infarcts from osteomyelitis in sickle cell disorders. Clin Nucl Med. 14(4):249-54, 1989

SICKLE CELL DISEASE, BONE PAIN

IMAGE GALLERY

Typical

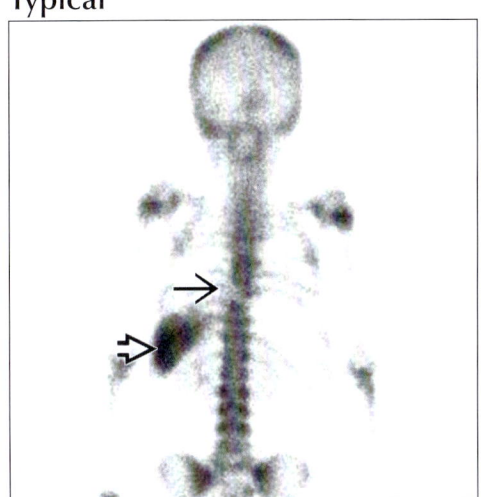

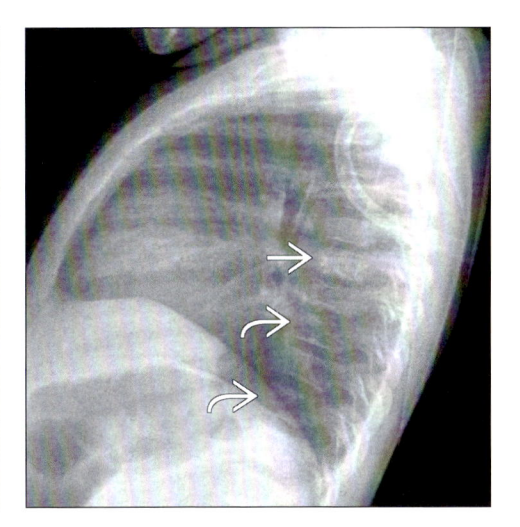

(Left) Posterior bone scan in patient with SCD, shows photopenic defect in thoracic vertebra ➡ denoting bone infarction. Uptake in spleen ⮞ can be due to acute sickle crisis or autoinfarction with calcification. See next image. (Right) Left lateral radiograph in same patient as left, shows corresponding sclerotic vertebral body ➡ with irregular end-plates, indicating remote bone infarction. Note also multilevel biconcave ("fish") vertebrae ➡, typical of SCD.

Typical

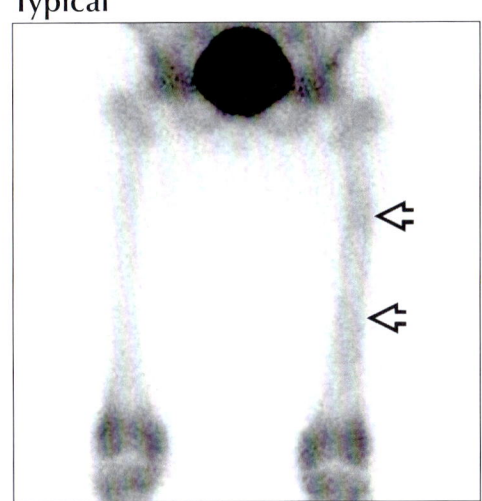

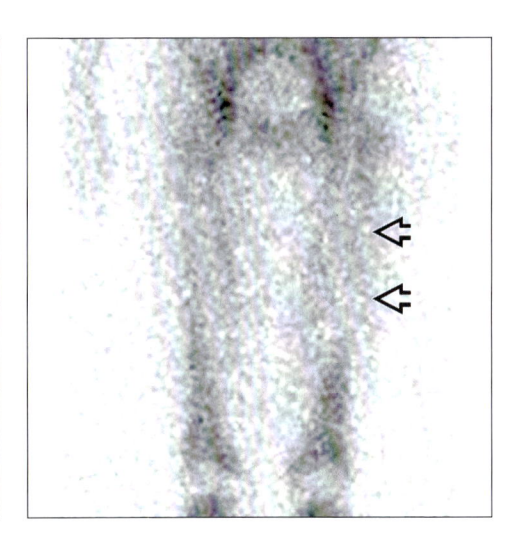

(Left) Anterior bone scan shows heterogeneous uptake in left femur ⮞ in patient with SCD and severe acute femoral pain due to acute bone infarct. See next image. (Right) Anterior labeled leukocyte scintigraphy in same patient as left, shows normal activity in left femur ⮞, supporting the diagnosis of bone infarction rather than osteomyelitis.

Typical

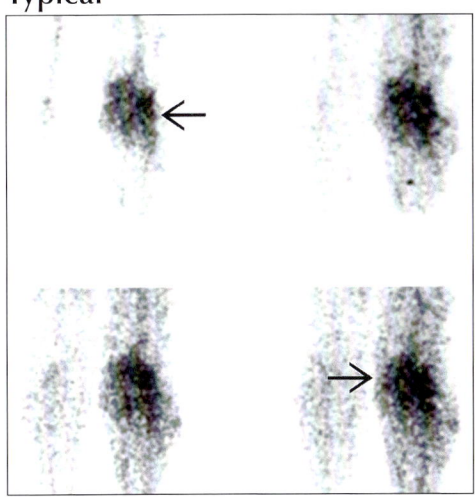

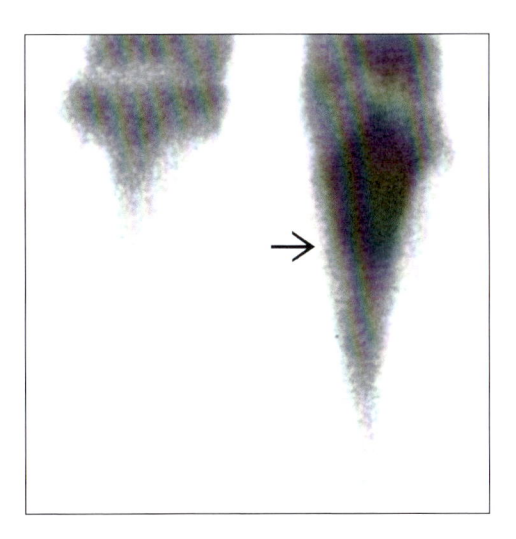

(Left) Anterior angiographic phase bone scan in SCD patient with left shin pain shows increased activity ➡. See next image. (Right) Anterior delayed phase bone scan in same patient as left, shows increased activity in proximal left tibia ➡.

MULTIPLE MYELOMA

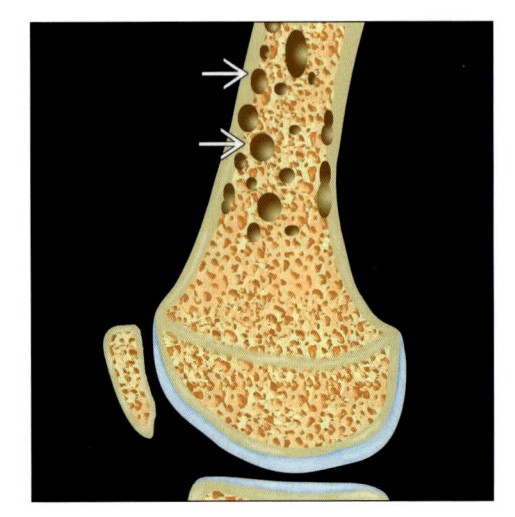

Graphic shows lytic lesions in the distal femur. Multiple myeloma may involve critical weight-bearing bones and result in pathologic fractures.

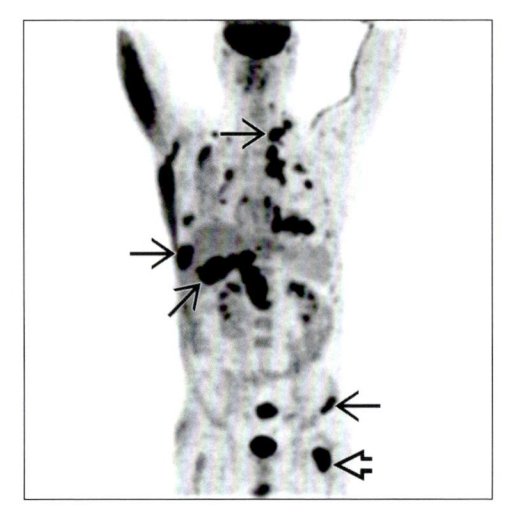

Anterior MIP PET in a patient with multiple myeloma shows numerous hypermetabolic sites. Note focus in left proximal femur, at risk for pathologic fracture.

TERMINOLOGY

Abbreviations and Synonyms
- Multiple myeloma (MM)
- Monoclonal gammopathy of undetermined significance (MGUS)

Definitions
- Cancer of plasma cells in bone marrow
  - Smoldering = inactive
    - Stable protein levels, no end-organ damage
  - Active
    - Elevated protein levels, organ damage

IMAGING FINDINGS

General Features
- Best diagnostic clue: Increased activity in lytic lesion or extramedullary site on PET/CT
- Location
  - Bone marrow and bone (97%)
  - Extramedullary sites
    - Nasopharynx
    - Tonsils
    - Paranasal sinuses
  - Less common: Lung, spleen, liver
- Morphology
  - Usually high levels of bone marrow plasma cells (> 10-15%) and lytic bone lesions
  - Occasionally presents as solid mass in bone or soft tissue (plasmacytoma)

Nuclear Medicine Findings
- Gallium-67 scintigraphy
  - Focal activity in lytic lesions and plasmacytomas
  - Level of Ga-67 correlates with disease activity
  - Markedly ↑ activity in osseous sites where bone scan minimally abnormal/normal indicate fulminant disease with rapid progression, poor prognosis
- Tc-99m MDP bone scan
  - Sensitivity for lesion detection: 75-85%
  - Sensitivity best for cortical lesions with reactive bone formation
  - Poor sensitivity for lytic or trabecular lesions
  - False positives in trauma, infection, degenerative disease
  - Poor test to evaluate status of disease activity

DDx: Common Osseous Lesions Simulating MM

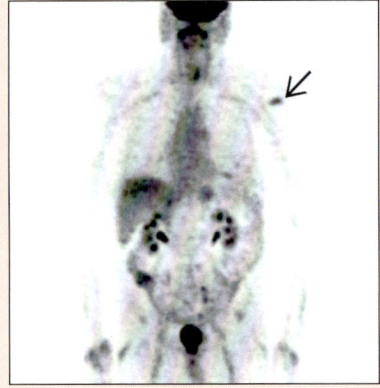

Trauma

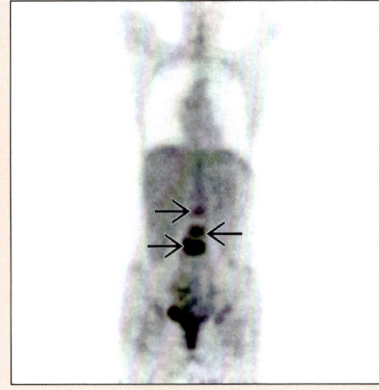

Osteomyelitis

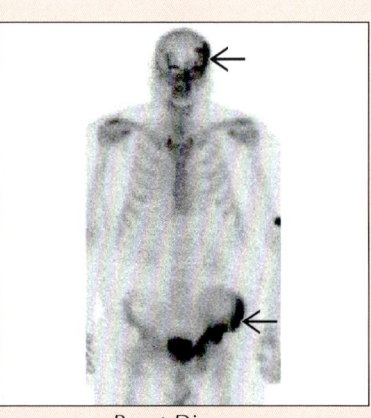

Paget Disease

MULTIPLE MYELOMA

Key Facts

Terminology
- Cancer of plasma cells in bone marrow

Imaging Findings
- Best diagnostic clue: Increased activity in lytic lesion or extramedullary site on PET/CT
- Negative whole body PET in patients with monoclonal gammopathy reliably identifies stable MGUS
- PET provides accurate staging of untreated MM (solitary, multifocal)
- Diffuse marrow uptake on PET usually indicates elevated plasma cell population
- PET useful in radiation therapy planning
- Negative PET 60 days following stem cell transplant = excellent prognosis

Top Differential Diagnoses
- Lytic Skeletal Metastases
- Osteopenia, Osteoporosis
- Other Bone + Soft Tissue Malignancy
- Other Plasma Cell Neoplasms

Clinical Issues
- Osteopenia, back pain, pathologic fracture in 30%
- Pain usually worse supine, at night, not relieved by rest or NSAIDs
- May have fever, weight loss, renal failure
- Clinical findings of > 10% plasma cells in marrow with lytic lesions on X-ray and monoclonal immunoglobulins in blood/urine diagnostic of MM
- Age: Median age at diagnosis: 62 yrs

- Tc-99m sestamibi (MIBI) scintigraphy
  - Activity in tumor correlates with disease activity unless multi-drug resistant tumor
  - Diffuse marrow uptake correlates with diffuse plasma cell increase in marrow (nonspecific, however)
  - Normal uptake in liver, GI tract, kidneys may cause interpretation errors
  - Positive lesion on FDG PET with corresponding negative MIBI suggests multidrug resistance, poor response to chemotherapy
- FDG PET/CT
  - Negative whole body PET in patients with monoclonal gammopathy reliably identifies stable MGUS
  - PET provides accurate staging of untreated MM (solitary, multifocal)
  - Diffuse marrow uptake on PET usually indicates elevated plasma cell population
  - PET exceptionally useful in monitoring disease activity in patients with nonsecretory myeloma
  - Extramedullary FDG activity extremely poor prognostic factor
  - Persistent FDG activity following induction therapy predicts early relapse
  - Patients with relapse often found to have new sites of disease
  - PET useful in radiation therapy planning
  - Negative PET 60 days following stem cell transplant = excellent prognosis

Imaging Recommendations
- Best imaging tool: FDG PET/CT with oral and IV CT contrast
- Protocol advice
  - Whole body scan: Obtain PET/CT from top of head to toes
  - Use oral and IV contrast if renal function is good (creatinine < 1.5)
    - Renal dysfunction common due to high levels of proteins produced by malignant plasma cells which affect renal tubules
  - Marrow stimulant drugs may mask underlying MM lesions
- Correlative imaging features
  - Skeletal survey with radiography
    - Multiple lytic rounded lesions
    - May only demonstrate diffuse osteopenia
    - Subtle X-ray finding: Endosteal scalloping
    - Usually little periosteal reaction
    - Usual sites: Skull, spine, pelvis
    - Preferred initial imaging study
    - Sensitivity limited: 30% demineralization required before lytic lesion detected
  - MR
    - Rounded low signal on T1WI, high signal on T2WI which enhances moderately with gadolinium
    - Diffuse replacement of marrow fat may also be seen on MR
    - MR pattern not specific for MM, can be seen with other malignant and some nonmalignant diseases
    - More sensitive than X-ray or bone scan, equivalent to FDG PET/CT in sensitivity
    - Cannot reliably assess disease activity
    - Provides excellent soft tissue resolution
  - CT
    - Findings similar to X-ray; slightly more sensitive
    - CT useful to guide percutaneous biopsies

DIFFERENTIAL DIAGNOSIS

Lytic Skeletal Metastases
- Breast, prostate, thyroid cancer, renal cell carcinoma

Osteopenia, Osteoporosis
- Increased radiolucency of bone, decreased bone mineral density due to number of causes

Other Bone + Soft Tissue Malignancy
- Lymphoma
- Metastases
- Chondrosarcoma
- Osteosarcoma

MULTIPLE MYELOMA

Other Plasma Cell Neoplasms
- Monoclonal gammopathy of undetermined significance (MGUS)
- Plasma cell leukemia
- Solitary plasmacytoma

PATHOLOGY

General Features
- Genetics: No hereditary basis for MM established
- Etiology
  - Weak radiation exposure link
    - However, higher incidence reported in nuclear industry workers
  - DDT exposure, wood dust exposure, other toxins, herpes virus type 8 weakly linked to MM
- Epidemiology
  - Most common primary bone cancer (3-4 cases/100,000)
  - 1% of all cancers in US
  - 10% of all hematologic malignancies

Microscopic Features
- Histologic variables of plasma cells play a key role in prognosis
  - Six cell types described: Marschalko, small cell, cleaved, polymorphous, asynchronous and blastic
- Proliferation activity prognostic
  - High levels of s-phase plasma cells associated with anemia, hypercalcemia, higher serum beta-2 microglobulins, poor prognosis

Staging, Grading or Classification Criteria
- Durie-Salmon staging system
  - Stage I
    - Small number of myeloma cells
    - Slightly ↓ hemoglobin
    - Plain films with ≤ 1 area of bone involvement
    - Normal calcium
    - Small amount of monoclonal immunoglobulin in blood/urine
  - Stage II
    - Moderate number of myeloma cells
    - Labs and plain films intermediate between stage I and III
  - Stage III
    - Large number of myeloma cells
    - Severely ↓ hemoglobin
    - Hypercalcemia
    - ≥ 3 sites of bone involvement on plain films
    - Large amount of monoclonal immunoglobulin in blood/urine
- International staging system
  - Based on serum beta-2 microglobulin and albumin levels

CLINICAL ISSUES

Presentation
- Most common signs/symptoms
  - Osteopenia, back pain, pathologic fracture in 30%
  - Pain usually worse supine, at night, not relieved by rest or NSAIDs
  - May have fever, weight loss, renal failure
  - Clinical findings of > 10% plasma cells in marrow with lytic lesions on X-ray and monoclonal immunoglobulins in blood/urine diagnostic of MM

Demographics
- Age: Median age at diagnosis: 62 yrs

Natural History & Prognosis
- Five year survival
  - Stage I = 62 months
  - Stage II = 44 months
  - Stage III = 29 months
- Overall median survival: 3 yrs
- Patients with extraosseous disease have poor prognosis (median survival 7 months)

Treatment
- Usually therapy includes alkylating agents and steroids
- Thalidomide often added to regimen to suppress tumor vascularity
- Stem cell transplantation an option

DIAGNOSTIC CHECKLIST

Consider
- FDG PET/CT to stage and establish baseline for monitoring therapy (especially in nonsecretory myeloma)

Image Interpretation Pearls
- Negative FDG PET/CT in patient with monoclonal gammopathy = excellent prognosis
- PET/CT important to localize plasmacytoma, differentiate tumor from normal structures
- FDG PET most accurate test in establishing disease activity

SELECTED REFERENCES

1. Bredella MA et al: Value of FDG PET in the assessment of patients with multiple myeloma. AJR Am J Roentgenol. 184(4):1199-204, 2005
2. Alexandrakis MG et al: Correlation between the uptake of Tc-99m-sestaMIBI and prognostic factors in patients with multiple myeloma. Clin Lab Haematol. 24(3):155-9, 2002
3. Durie BG et al: Whole-body (18)F-FDG PET identifies high-risk myeloma. J Nucl Med. 43(11):1457-63, 2002
4. Van de Berg BC et al: Stage I multiple myeloma: value of MR imaging of the bone marrow in the determination of prognosis. Radiology. 201(1):243-6, 1996
5. Bergsagel D: The incidence and epidemiology of plasma cell neoplasms. Stem Cells. 13 Suppl 2:1-9, 1995
6. Moulopoulos LA et al: Extraosseous multiple myeloma: imaging features. AJR Am J Roentgenol. 161(5):1083-7, 1993
7. Waxman AD et al: Radiographic and radionuclide imaging in multiple myeloma: the role of gallium scintigraphy: concise communication. J Nucl Med. 22(3):232-6, 1981
8. Durie BG et al: A clinical staging system for multiple myeloma. Correlation of measured myeloma cell mass with presenting clinical features, response to treatment, and survival. Cancer. 36(3):842-54, 1975

MULTIPLE MYELOMA

IMAGE GALLERY

Typical

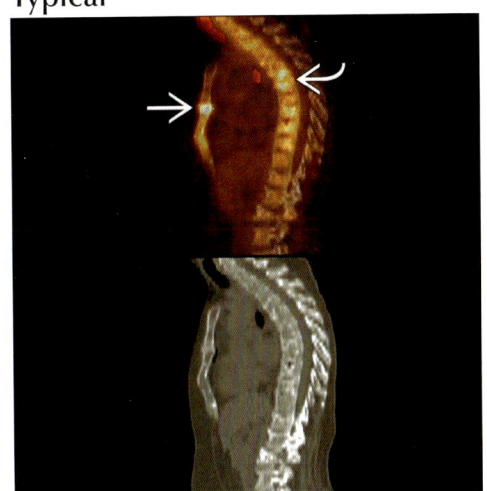

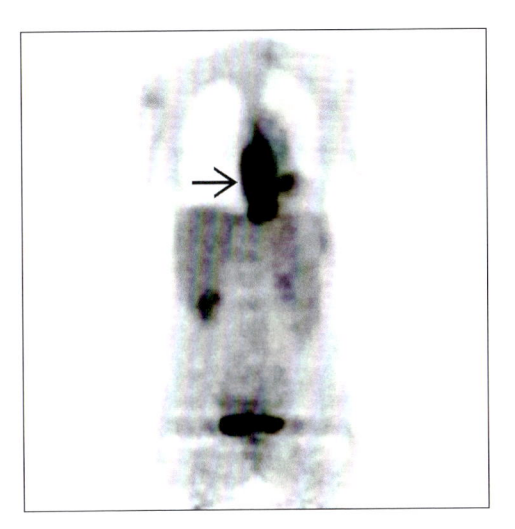

(Left) Fused sagittal PET/CT shows increased activity in sternum ➡ and thoracic spine ➡, lytic lesions in a patient with MM. These lesions are more apparent on PET/CT than on CT alone. *(Right)* Coronal FDG PET shows hypermetabolic esophageal activity ➡ in a patient with dysphagia and monoclonal spike on plasma electrophoresis. Biopsy showed plasma cell infiltrate, consistent with extraosseous plasmacytoma.

Typical

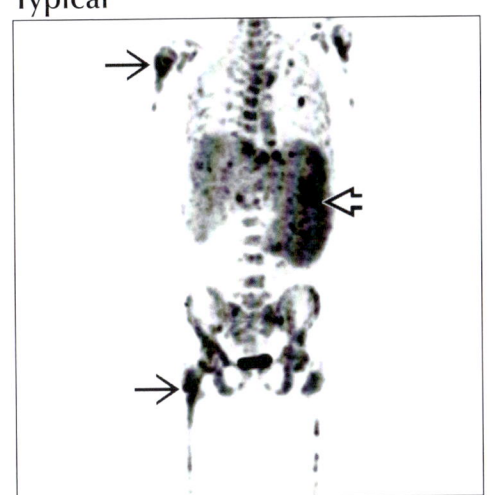

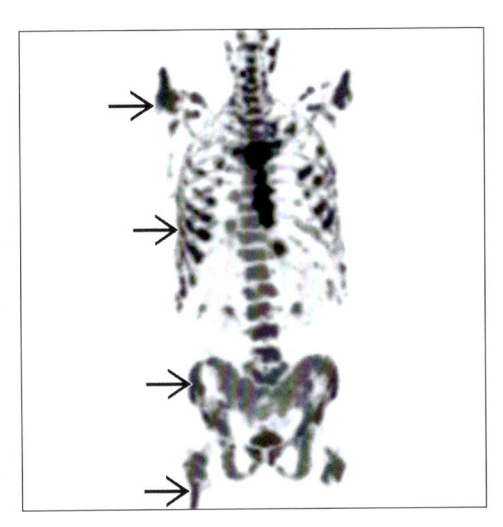

(Left) Baseline MIP PET in a patient with multifocal osseous ➡ and extraosseous MM with extensive splenic involvement ➡. See next image. *(Right)* MIP PET in the same patient as previous image, 8 months later, shows progressive osseous MM ➡. Note little activity in the liver and spleen due to high relative osseous activity.

Typical

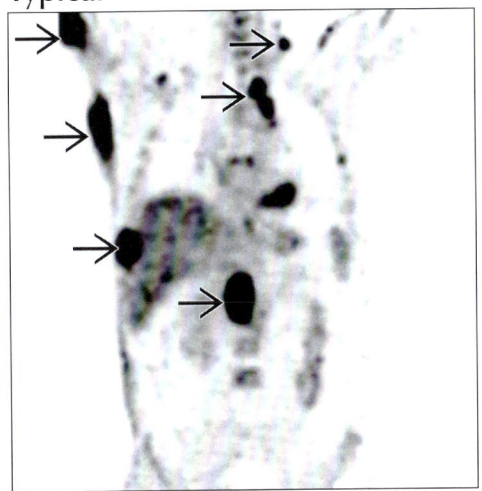

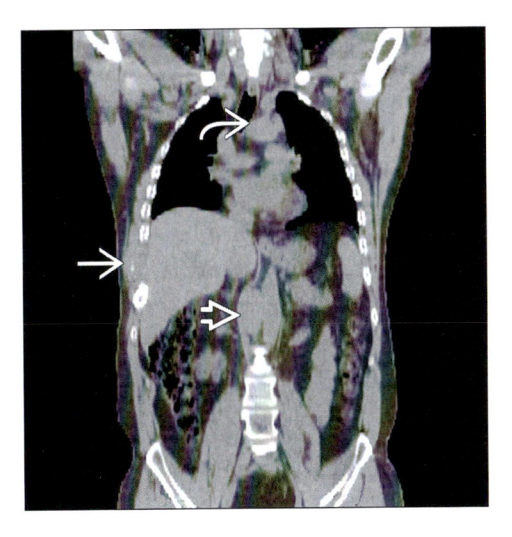

(Left) Coronal PET in a patient with MM shows hypermetabolic activity in multiple soft tissue plasmacytomas ➡ in supraclavicular, muscular, mediastinal, right thorax, and abdominal regions. See next image. *(Right)* Coronal CT in the same patient as previous image shows soft tissue masses in the right lower rib cage ➡, mediastinum ➡, and abdomen ➡. Note difficulty in detecting supraclavicular lesions on CT.

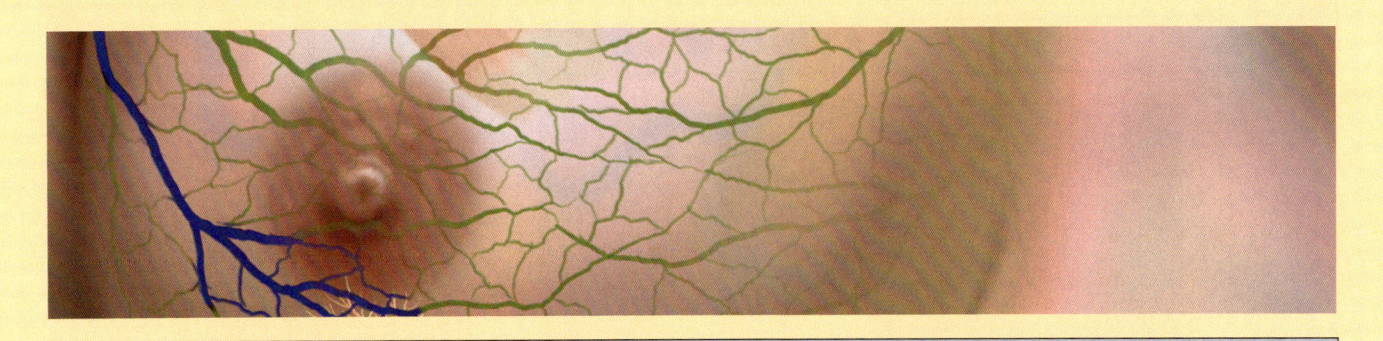

SECTION 2: Vascular and Lymphatics

Lymphatic

Lymphedema	2-2
Sentinel Lymph Node Mapping	2-4

Vascular

Large Vessel Vasculitis	2-8
Atherosclerosis	2-10
Vascular Thrombosis	2-14
Vascular Graft Infection	2-16

LYMPHEDEMA

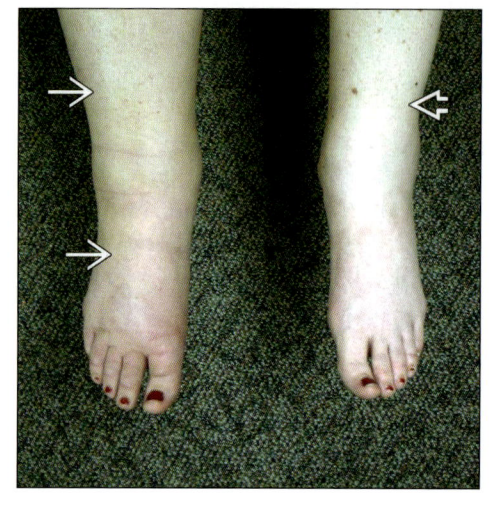

Photograph shows right lower extremity edema ➡ in 38 year old patient with primary lymphedema tarda. Note normal left lower extremity ➡.

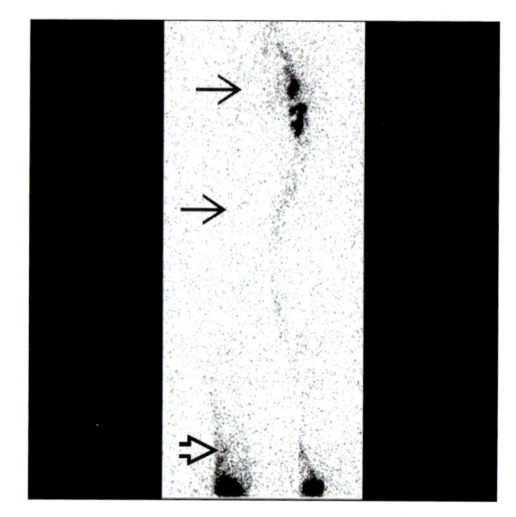

Anterior Tc-99m sulfur colloid LAS shows dermal backflow in right ankle ➡ and nonvisualization of lymphatic channels/regional lymph nodes ➡, consistent with lymphatic dysfunction.

TERMINOLOGY

Abbreviations and Synonyms
- Lymphedema (LE), lymphangioscintigraphy (LAS)

Definitions
- Accumulation of lymphatic fluid causing edema

IMAGING FINDINGS

General Features
- Best diagnostic clue: Tc-99m sulfur colloid LAS shows dermal backflow in extremity

Nuclear Medicine Findings
- Tc-99m Sulfur Colloid
  - Dermal backflow on LAS diagnostic
  - Delayed tracer uptake following injection
  - Asymmetric/absent visualization of lymph nodes, lymphatic trunks
  - Collateral +/- dilated lymphatic channels
  - Interrupted lymphatic channels
  - Lymph nodes of deep lymphatic system visualized

Imaging Recommendations
- Best imaging tool: LAS = standard diagnostic study (vs. contrast lymphangiography)
- Protocol advice
  - 1 mCi (37 MBq) Tc-99m sulfur colloid (SC) in 1 cc normal saline per extremity
  - Ideal particle size: 50-70 nm (filtered)
  - Intradermal injection of dorsum of hands/feet
  - Injection site massage, extremity exercise promotes tracer uptake, improves lymphatic return
  - Tc-99m Sb-SC, Tc-99m albumin colloid, Tc-99m human serum albumin also used

DIFFERENTIAL DIAGNOSIS

Nonlymphatic Causes of Extremity Edema
- Chronic venous insufficiency
- Deep venous thrombosis (DVT)

Primary vs. Secondary LE
- Similar imaging findings
- Clinical history critical for diagnosis

DDx: Extremity Edema

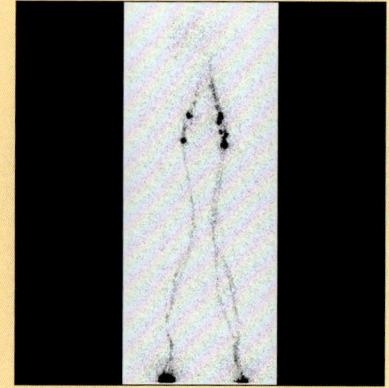

Nonlymphatic Edema: Normal

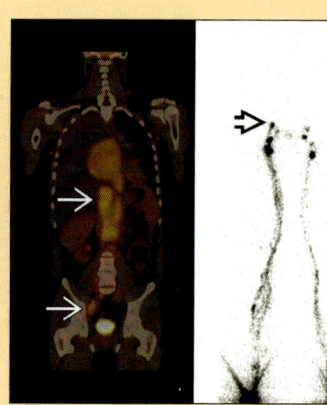

Tumor ⇒ Lymph Obstruction

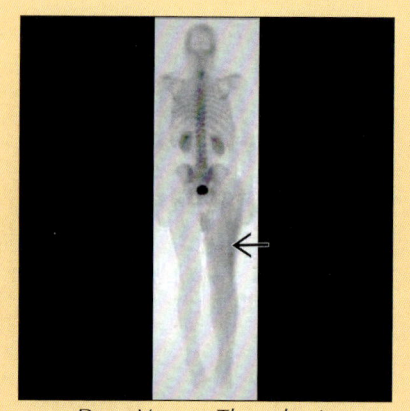

Deep Venous Thrombosis

LYMPHEDEMA

Key Facts

Terminology
- Lymphedema (LE), lymphangioscintigraphy (LAS)
- Accumulation of lymphatic fluid causing edema

Imaging Findings
- Dermal backflow on LAS diagnostic
- Delayed tracer uptake following injection
- Asymmetric/absent visualization of lymph nodes, lymphatic trunks
- Collateral +/- dilated lymphatic channels
- Interrupted lymphatic channels
- Lymph nodes of deep lymphatic system visualized

Pathology
- Primary: Absent or decreased lymphatic channels
- Secondary: Acquired; due to lymphatic obstruction
- Developed countries: Cancer Rx sequelae 1° cause
- Worldwide: Parasitic infection 1° cause
- Fibrosis and lipid deposition in affected lymphatics

PATHOLOGY

General Features
- Etiology
  - Primary: Absent or decreased lymphatic channels
    - Congenital
    - Milroy disease: Autosomal dominant with high penetrance; LE can be present at birth
    - Syndrome-associated: Turner, Klippel-Trenaunay, Noonan, etc.
    - LE precox: Onset of peripheral LE at puberty to 25 years; familial (Meige disease) or sporadic
    - LE tarda: Onset of LE > 30 years
  - Secondary: Acquired; due to lymphatic obstruction
    - Iatrogenic: Lymph node dissection, vascular surgery, radiation therapy
    - Post-infectious (e.g., filariasis)
    - Malignant: Tumor/lymphadenopathy ⇒ obstruction
    - Chronic venous insufficiency
- Epidemiology
  - Developed countries: Cancer Rx sequelae 1° cause
  - Worldwide: Parasitic infection 1° cause
- Associated abnormalities
  - Recurrent soft tissue infection, DVT
  - Chronic LE increases risk of lymphangiosarcoma
    - e.g., Stewart-Treves syndrome (post-mastectomy)

Gross Pathologic & Surgical Features
- Superficial & deep lymphatics throughout body
- Superficial system drains most lymph

Microscopic Features
- Fibrosis and lipid deposition in affected lymphatics

CLINICAL ISSUES

Presentation
- Most common signs/symptoms: Slow onset swelling of affected limb

Treatment
- Microsurgery, liposuction, massage, compression, extremity elevation, hyperthermia, medication
- Late treatment less successful

DIAGNOSTIC CHECKLIST

Consider
- Injection of tracer in dorsum of hands/feet sufficient
- Web-space tracer injection in hands/feet (as with lymphangiography) not necessary

SELECTED REFERENCES

1. Szuba A et al: The third circulation: radionuclide lymphoscintigraphy in the evaluation of lymphedema. J Nucl Med. 44(1):43-57, 2003
2. Williams WH et al: Radionuclide lymphangioscintigraphy in the evaluation of peripheral lymphedema. Clin Nucl Med. 25(6):451-64, 2000

IMAGE GALLERY

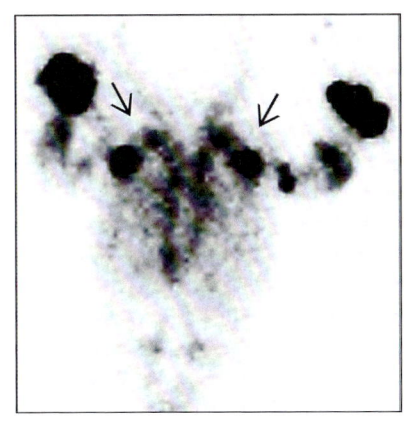

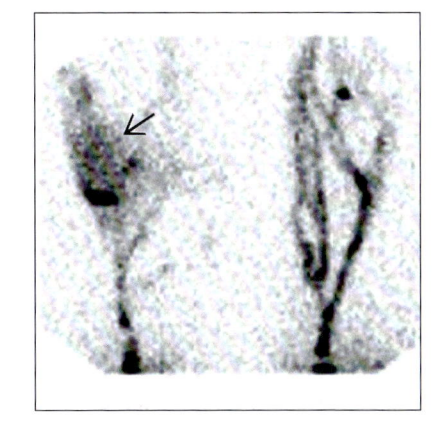

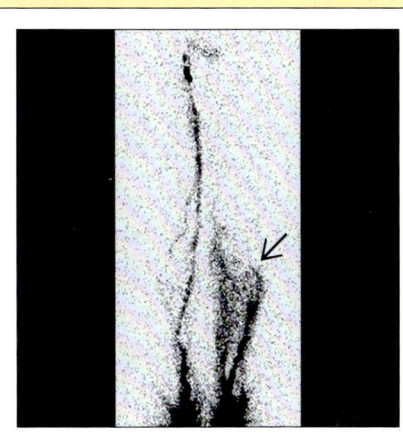

(Left) Anterior Tc-99m sulfur colloid LAS shows tracer pooling in dilated, distorted lymphatic channels ➔ in both upper extremities in 4 month old infant with congenital lymphedema. (Center) Anterior Tc-99m sulfur colloid LAS shows dermal backflow in right calf ➔ in patient with lower extremity edema, consistent with lymphatic obstruction. (Right) Anterior Tc-99m sulfur colloid LAS shows left lower extremity dermal backflow ➔ in 14 year old with primary lymphedema precox.

SENTINEL LYMPH NODE MAPPING

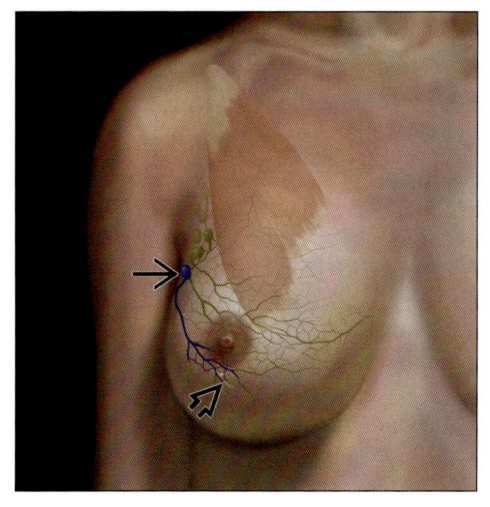

Sketch shows likely lymphatic drainage path and SLN ➔ from subareolar injection site ➔. This injection site is about 90% effective in localizing SLN regardless of site of tumor.

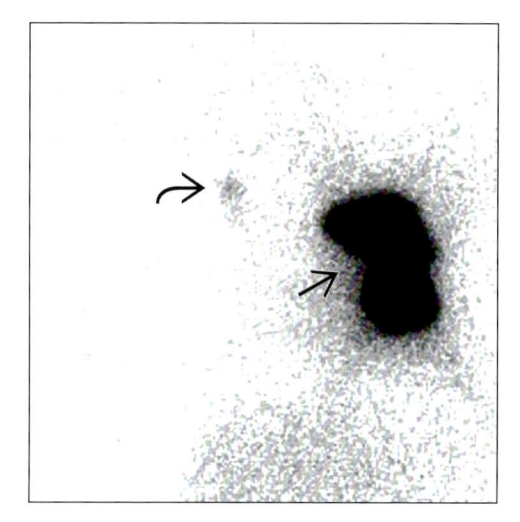

Anterior planar view of combined areolar, intradermal, and peritumoral injection ➔ shows axillary sentinel node ➔.

TERMINOLOGY

Abbreviations and Synonyms
- Sentinel lymph node mapping (SLNM)
- Sentinel lymph node biopsy (SLNB)
- Intraoperative lymphatic mapping (ILM)

Definitions
- Sentinel lymph node (SLN)
  - First lymph node(s) visualized in unique lymphatic drainage basin
  - Usually has metastatic tumor cells prior to other regional lymph nodes
- Sentinel lymph node mapping (SLNM)
  - Radiotracer injected at primary tumor site
  - Pre-operative imaging to define drainage basin(s)
- SLN localization
  - Reduces morbidity of locoregional radical lymphadenectomy (lymphedema, pain)
  - Intra-operative gamma probe detects gamma rays from SLN at surgery: 1-3 nodes "hot" nodes removed at surgery
  - Blue dye injected at surgery; stains SLN blue for visual co-localization with radioactive SLN at surgery

IMAGING FINDINGS

General Features
- Best diagnostic clue
  - SLN mapping > 92% effective in locating SLN
  - Focus of increased activity in regional lymphatic bed
    - First focus with activity that ↑ over time, stays at high level
    - One lymphatic bed can have multiple SLNs (appearing simultaneously)
    - Multiple lymphatic beds can drain single tumor site (each with sentinel node)
- Location
  - Sappey lines: Anatomist from 1800s theorized lymphatic drainage patterns of entire body
  - Head and neck cancer
    - Lymph drainage pattern highly variable, multiple basins
    - Pre-auricular, anterior/posterior cervical, submandibular, supraclavicular, axillary
  - Breast cancer
    - Ipsilateral axilla
    - Clinical significance of internal mammary SLN unclear

DDx: Diagnostic Challenges: SLN Localization

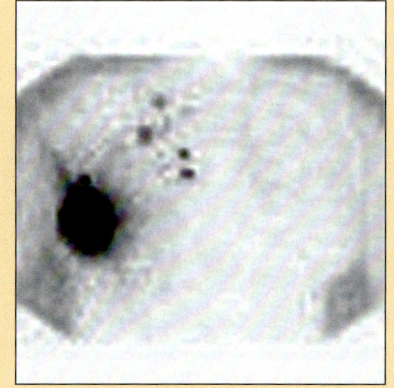

Internal Mammary Nodes

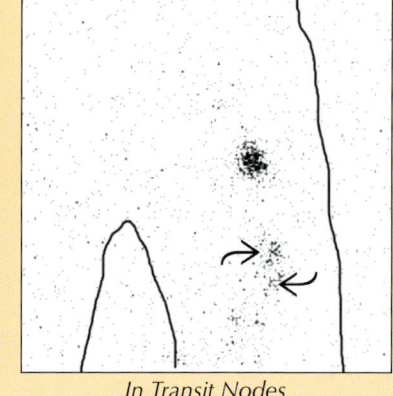

In Transit Nodes

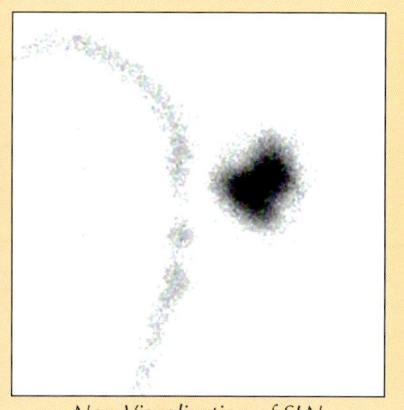

Non Visualization of SLN

SENTINEL LYMPH NODE MAPPING

Key Facts

Terminology
- Sentinel lymph node (SLN)
- First lymph node(s) visualized in unique lymphatic drainage basin
- Usually has metastatic tumor cells prior to other regional lymph nodes
- Sentinel lymph node mapping (SLNM)
- Reduces morbidity of locoregional radical lymphadenectomy (lymphedema, pain)

Imaging Findings
- SLN mapping > 92% effective in locating SLN
- Focus of increased activity in regional lymphatic bed
- First focus with activity that ↑ over time, stays at high level
- One lymphatic bed can have multiple SLNs (appearing simultaneously)
- Multiple lymphatic beds can drain single tumor site (each with sentinel node)
- View dynamically on p-scope: Set at 100% persistence, frequent manual reset
- Truncal and head and neck tumors: Delayed imaging (90 min) to evaluation for additional drainage basins
- Improve orientation: Place sheet source behind patient or "draw" body contour with point source
- Melanoma: Perilesional intradermal injection: 4 quadrant vs. multiple perimeter injections both acceptable

Top Differential Diagnoses
- ~ 20% of sentinel nodes with gross tumor may not visualize on SLN mapping (usually visually abnormal at surgery)

- Torso
  - Lymph drainage pattern highly variable
  - Above L2-umbilical line, axillary drainage more common
  - Below L2-umbilical line, drainage to groin more common
- Pelvic cancer
  - Iliac chain, femoral nodes
- Extremities
  - Arms: Epitrochlear and axillary nodes
  - Legs: Popliteal and groin nodes
- Occasionally drainage used several days in advance to define extent of operative sites
  - Sentinel lymph node localization on day-of or day-before surgery
  - Truncal, head and neck tumors often require surgery at multiple lymphatic drainage basins
- Lymphatic mapping for other indications
  - Lymphoscintigraphy: Generally replaced radiographic lymphangiogram
  - Extremity swelling: To define level of obstruction
  - Chylous ascites or chylous pleural effusion: Define level of interruption of lymph drainage
- Radiation, surgery, bulky nodes: Can also disrupt expected drainage pattern
- Subcutaneous in-transit nodes: Must be marked, may be clinically significant

Nuclear Medicine Findings
- Small, focal site(s) of ↑ activity in regional lymph node bed

Imaging Recommendations
- Best imaging tool
  - Tc-99m sulfur colloid SLN localization/mapping
  - Other tracers (rarely used) include MAA, antimony sulfur colloid
- Protocol advice
  - Can be performed day of, or day before, surgery
  - Tc-99m sulfur colloid
    - 0.4-1 mCi (19-37 MBq) injected at site of primary tumor
    - Filtered or unfiltered sulfur colloid acceptable (proponents for each, no consensus)
    - Injection often painful: Skin nerve endings abundant, quickly subsides
  - SLN marking for surgery
    - Patient in position similar to surgery
    - Patient position during SLN marking must be clearly communicated pre-operatively
    - View dynamically on p-scope: Set at 100% persistence, frequent manual reset
    - Localize SLN with radioactive marker: Capillary tube or cotton swab with Tc-99m pertechnetate (enclosed in barrier to avoid site contamination)
    - Image SLN at two angles, separated by 45° or 90°, mark over anticipated surgical approach
    - Once SLN localized with radioactive marker, mark with indelible marker
    - Cover with transparent dressing (such as Tegaderm™)
  - Images taken: For documentation
    - Lead shield over injection site may facilitate imaging of adjacent LN
    - Truncal and head and neck tumors: Delayed imaging (90 min) to evaluation for additional drainage basins
    - Improve orientation: Place sheet source behind patient or "draw" body contour with point source
  - Intra-operative gamma probe for ILM
    - Ink mark orients surgeon to general SLN site
    - Gamma probe (highly collimated) to detect radioactivity from SLN
    - Highest counts correlate with blue-dyed SLN
    - After successful excision of SLN, counts should drop to 10% above background
  - Melanoma
    - Melanoma: Perilesional intradermal injection: 4 quadrant vs. multiple perimeter injections both acceptable
    - Number of injection sites important: Three minimum based on meta-analysis of pooled data
    - Avoid injecting into inflamed tissue as lymphatics in edematous tissue are altered

SENTINEL LYMPH NODE MAPPING

- Breast cancer
  - Subareolar: 1 injection; 85-100% effective
  - Periareolar (intradermal): 4 injections; 92-100% effective
  - Peritumoral (deep): 4 injections adjacent to solid tumor/biopsy site; ranges from 50-95% effective; sometimes (1-5%) adds additional drainage route such as internal mammary chain or supraclavicular
  - If peritumoral injection follows recent open excision biopsy: Ultrasound guidance to avoid seroma/hematoma
  - Direct tumoral injection has become less common
  - If nonpalpable primary tumor and peritumoral injection desired: Ultrasound or mammographic guidance
  - 1 intradermal injection in skin overlying tumor: Adjunct to second injection technique

DIFFERENTIAL DIAGNOSIS

Skin, Clothing, Bedding Contamination
- May mimic sentinel lymph node

Lymphatic Valves, Channels Seen "End On"
- Clear with time, while nodes increase with time

False Negative Sentinel Lymph Nodes
- Non-functional lymph node "packed" with tumor
- ~ 20% of sentinel nodes with gross tumor may not visualize on SLN mapping (usually visually abnormal at surgery)

PATHOLOGY

Gross Pathologic & Surgical Features
- Tumor involvement may or may not grossly enlarge lymph node

Microscopic Features
- Microscopic detection of tumor may be facilitated by polymerase chain reaction (PCR) for specific tumor genes

CLINICAL ISSUES

Presentation
- Most common signs/symptoms: Palpable enlarged lymph node may or may not be present
- Other signs/symptoms: Advanced nodal spread: Lymphatic obstruction (dermal thickening, lymphedema)

Natural History & Prognosis
- Involvement of regional lymph nodes: Prognostic and treatment implications
  - Breast cancer
  - Skin cancer (melanoma, Merkel cell)
  - Gynecological (ovarian, vulvar), head and neck, colorectal
  - Head and neck cancer
  - Colorectal cancer

DIAGNOSTIC CHECKLIST

Image Interpretation Pearls
- For SLN localization, view on p-scope set at 100% persistence, manual reset frequently
- Focal activity that fades over time: In transit nodes, lymphatic channels "end on", valves
- Head and neck and truncal tumors: Delayed imaging at ≥ 90 minutes identifies additional basins

SELECTED REFERENCES

1. Rossi CR et al: The Impact of Lymphoscintigraphy Technique on the Outcome of Sentinel Node Biopsy in 1,313 Patients with Cutaneous Melanoma: An Italian Multicentric Study (SOLISM-IMI). J Nucl Med. 47(2):234-241, 2006
2. Kaleya RN et al: Lymphatic mapping and sentinel node biopsy: a surgical perspective. Semin Nucl Med. 35(2):129-34, 2005
3. Morton DL et al: Sentinel node biopsy for early-stage melanoma: accuracy and morbidity in MSLT-I, an international multicenter trial. Ann Surg. 242(3):302-11; discussion 311-3, 2005
4. Vijayakumar V et al: A critical review of variables affecting the accuracy and false-negative rate of sentinel node biopsy procedures in early breast cancer. Nucl Med Commun. 26(5):395-405, 2005
5. Alex JC: The application of sentinel node radiolocalization to solid tumors of the head and neck: a 10-year experience. Laryngoscope. 114(1):2-19, 2004
6. Bombardieri E et al: The choice of the correct imaging modality in breast cancer management. Eur J Nucl Med Mol Imaging. 31 Suppl 1:S179-86, 2004
7. Kelley MC et al: Lymphatic mapping and sentinel lymphadenectomy for breast cancer. Am J Surg. 188(1):49-61, 2004
8. Mariani G et al: Radioguided sentinel lymph node biopsy in patients with malignant cutaneous melanoma: the nuclear medicine contribution. J Surg Oncol. 85(3):141-51, 2004
9. Trifiro G et al: Sentinel node detection in pre-operative axillary staging. Eur J Nucl Med Mol Imaging. 31 Suppl 1:S46-55, 2004
10. Celliers L et al: Alternative sites of injection for sentinel lymph node biopsy in breast cancer. ANZ J Surg. 73(8):600-4, 2003
11. Jakub JW et al: Current status of sentinel lymph node mapping and biopsy: facts and controversies. Oncologist. 8(1):59-68, 2003
12. Alazraki NP et al: Sentinel node staging of early breast cancer using lymphoscintigraphy and the intraoperative gamma detecting probe. Radiol Clin North Am. 39(5):947-56, viii, 2001
13. Chung MH et al: Role for sentinel lymph node dissection in the management of large (> or = 5 cm) invasive breast cancer. Ann Surg Oncol. 8(9):688-92, 2001
14. Medina-Franco H et al: Sentinel node biopsy for cutaneous melanoma in the head and neck. Ann Surg Oncol. 8(9):716-9, 2001
15. Reintgen D: Expanding indications for lymphatic mapping and sentinel lymph node biopsy in the breast cancer population. Ann Surg Oncol. 8(9):687, 2001
16. Thelmo MC et al: Micrometastasis to in-transit lymph nodes from extremity and truncal malignant melanoma. Ann Surg Oncol. 8(5):444-8, 2001

SENTINEL LYMPH NODE MAPPING

IMAGE GALLERY

Typical

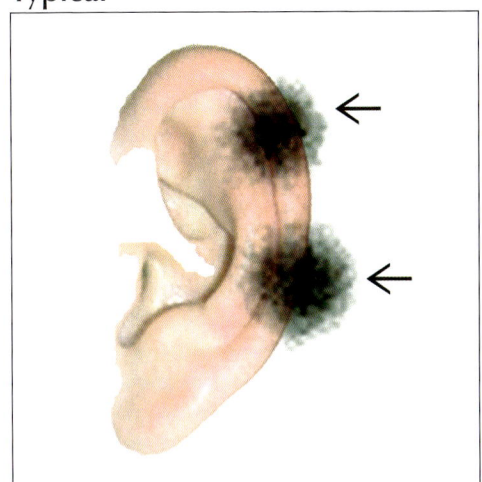

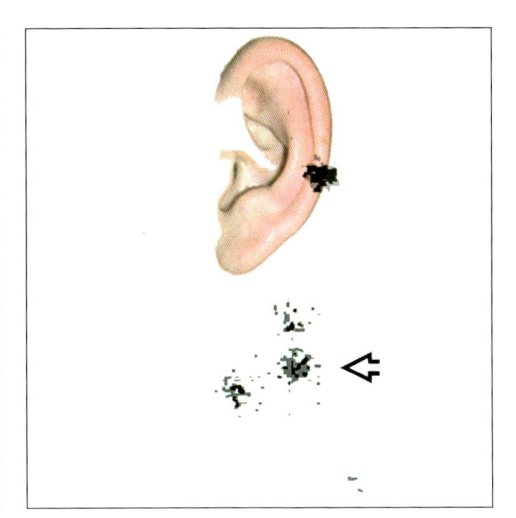

(Left) Melanoma sentinel node image of ear (with superimposed ear) shows only ➡ intradermal injection sites. Same patient as next image. *(Right)* With lead shield over injection site, shows rapid appearance of several nodes, better seen with shield in place. Note the initial sentinel node ⇨. Same patient as previous image.

Typical

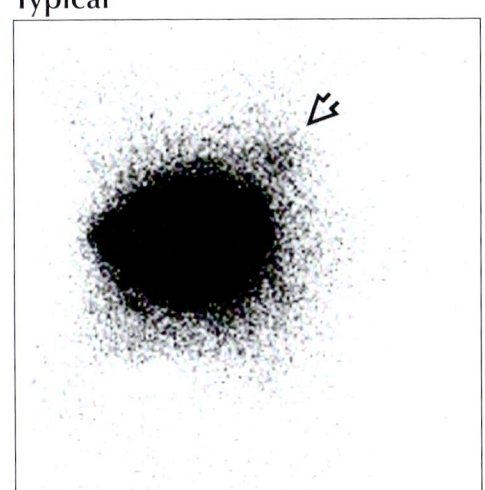

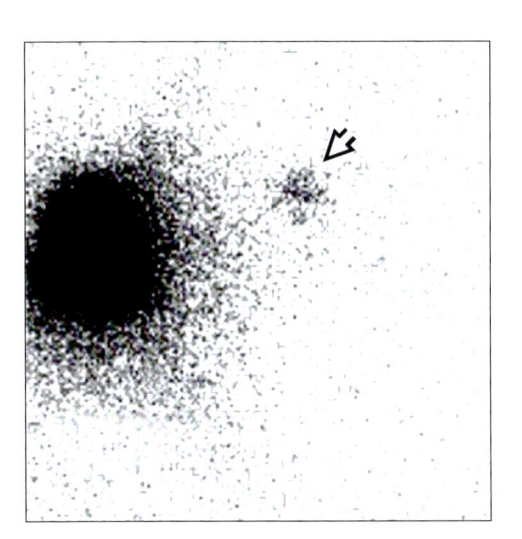

(Left) LAO planar view of breast sentinel node injection suggests sentinel node ⇨ in left axilla. It was totally obscured on AP view. Same patient as next image. *(Right)* Repeat LAO projection with breast held medially shows better localization of sentinel node ⇨ in left axilla.

Variant

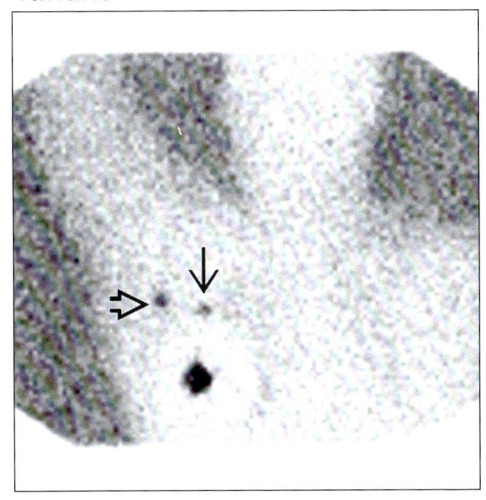

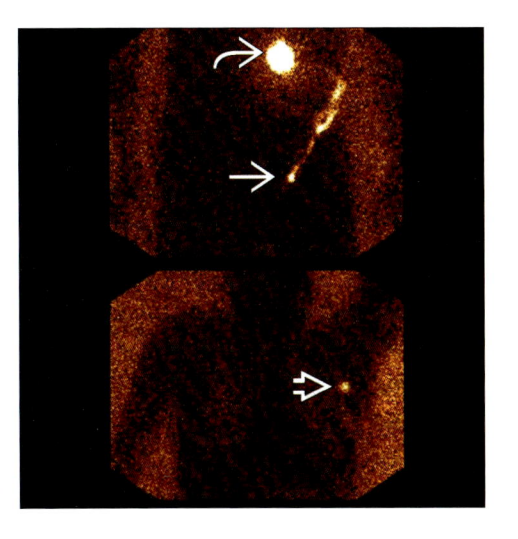

(Left) Anterior planar view shows both axillary node ⇨ and intramammary node ➡. Low level flood source placed behind patient effectively gives body outline. *(Right)* Anterior images of lower and upper trunk following peritumoral injection of waistline melanoma ➡ demonstrates sentinel lymph nodes both in left inguinal ➡ and axillary ⇨ drainage basins.

LARGE VESSEL VASCULITIS

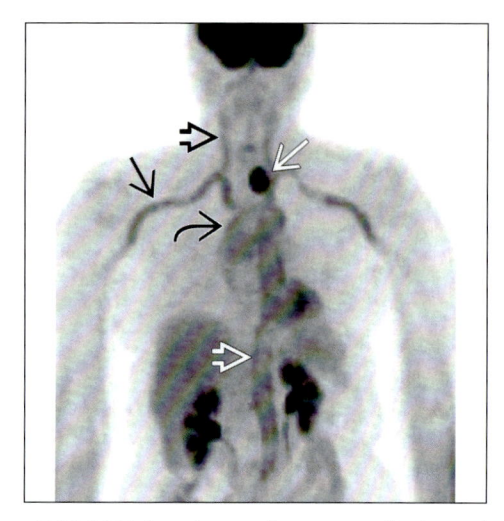

3D FDG PET shows increased activity in walls of carotid ⇨, subclavian → arteries and in dilated ascending aorta ➚, abdominal aorta ⇒ in patient with medullary thyroid cancer ➡.

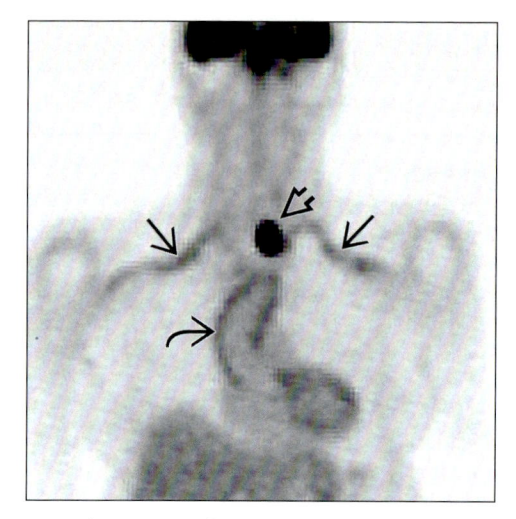

Coronal FDG PET of patient with thyroid cancer ⇨ shows homogeneously increased activity in subclavian arteries → and aorta ➚, signifying large vessel vasculitis.

TERMINOLOGY

Abbreviations and Synonyms
- Giant cell arteritis
- Takayasu arteritis
- Temporal arteritis

Definitions
- Autoimmune-mediated inflammation of aorta, major branch vessels

IMAGING FINDINGS

General Features
- Best diagnostic clue: FDG PET: Homogeneously increased activity in walls of large arteries (aorta, iliac, femoral, subclavian, carotid)
- Location: FDG PET resolution limits detection to larger arteries

Nuclear Medicine Findings
- FDG PET
  - Homogeneous F-18 FDG uptake in arterial walls
  - Activity decreases with effective treatment

Imaging Recommendations
- Best imaging tool: FDG PET/CT
- Protocol advice
  - Image 3 hour post injection (blood pool activity cleared)
  - Low serum glucose (< 150 ng/dl) critical to minimize blood pool activity
- Correlative imaging (CT, MR): Arterial wall thickening, rupture, aneurysm, vascular occlusion sequelae

DIFFERENTIAL DIAGNOSIS

Atherosclerosis
- Mild, heterogeneous activity, skipped regions
- Intense activity: Ulcerated plaques

Vascular Thrombosis
- Increased activity in lumen, not vascular wall

Vascular Grafts
- Mild, diffuse activity; intense, focal if infected

DDx: Mimics of Large Vessel Vasculitis

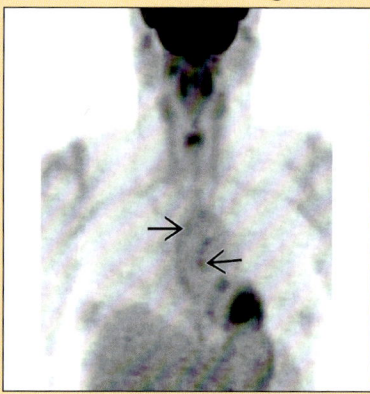

Atherosclerosis

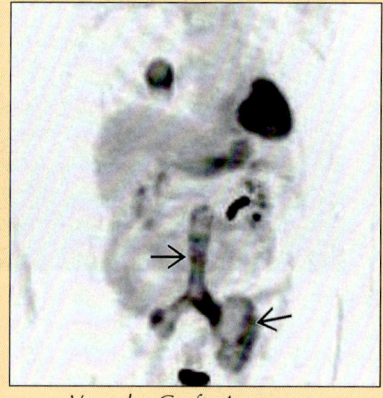

Vascular Graft, Aneurysm

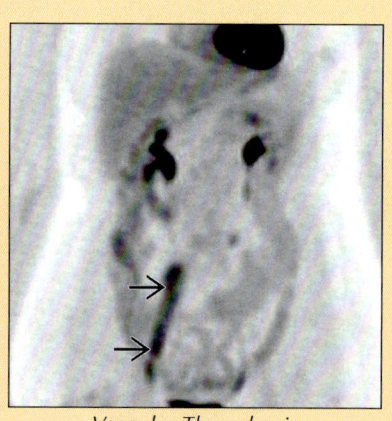

Vascular Thrombosis

LARGE VESSEL VASCULITIS

Key Facts

Imaging Findings
- Best diagnostic clue: FDG PET: Homogeneously increased activity in walls of large arteries (aorta, iliac, femoral, subclavian, carotid)
- Activity decreases with effective treatment
- Image 3 hour post injection (blood pool activity cleared)
- Low serum glucose (< 150 ng/dl) critical to minimize blood pool activity

- Correlative imaging (CT, MR): Arterial wall thickening, rupture, aneurysm, vascular occlusion sequelae

Top Differential Diagnoses
- Atherosclerosis
- Vascular Thrombosis
- Vascular Grafts
- Aneurysm

Aneurysm
- Homogeneous activity; intense, focal if infected

PATHOLOGY

General Features
- Etiology: T-cell response to unidentified antigen
- Epidemiology
  - Giant cell arteritis: Northern European
  - Takayasu: Asian, SE Asian, Mexican, S. American
- Associated abnormalities
  - Polymyalgia rheumatica: 30-40% of patients with giant cell arteritis
  - Associated diseases: Behçet syndrome, rheumatoid arthritis, syphilis, tuberculosis, malignancy

CLINICAL ISSUES

Presentation
- Most common signs/symptoms
  - Systemic: Fever, malaise, weight loss, night sweats, anorexia, depression
  - ↑ Erythrocyte sedimentation rate, C-reactive protein
  - Temporal arteritis: Temporal tenderness, blindness, headache, scalp tenderness, jaw claudication
- Other signs/symptoms
  - Vascular occlusion symptoms (nonpalpable/asymmetric pulses, claudication), rupture, hemorrhage
  - Severe myalgias; neck, shoulder, pelvic muscle stiffness

Demographics
- Age
  - Giant cell arteritis: > 50 years (highest among 75-85 years)
  - Takayasu arteritis: 10-30 years
- Gender: 65% female

Natural History & Prognosis
- Untreated disease ⇒ severe vascular consequences due to occlusion, rupture, hemorrhage

Treatment
- Corticosteroids suppress immune system
- Low-dose aspirin prevents platelet aggregation, luminal occlusion

SELECTED REFERENCES

1. Walter MA et al: The value of [18F]FDG-PET in the diagnosis of large-vessel vasculitis and the assessment of activity and extent of disease. Eur J Nucl Med Mol Imaging. 32(6):674-81, 2005
2. Andrews J et al: Non-invasive imaging in the diagnosis and management of Takayasu's arteritis. Ann Rheum Dis. 63(8):995-1000, 2004
3. Weyand CM et al: Medium- and large-vessel vasculitis. N Engl J Med. 349(2):160-9, 2003
4. Hutson TE et al: Temporal concurrence of vasculitis and cancer: a report of 12 cases. Arthritis Care Res. 13(6):417-23, 2000

IMAGE GALLERY

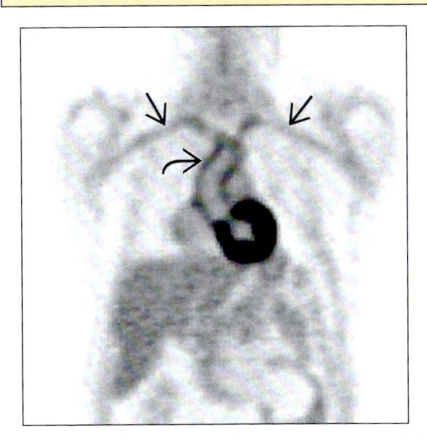

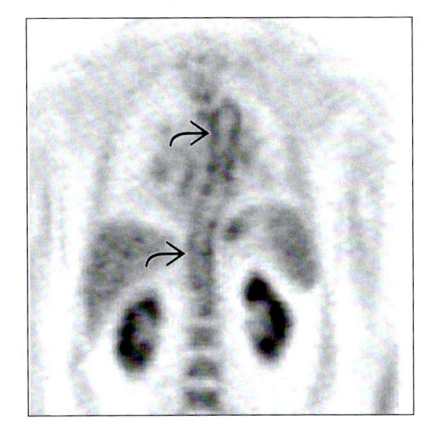

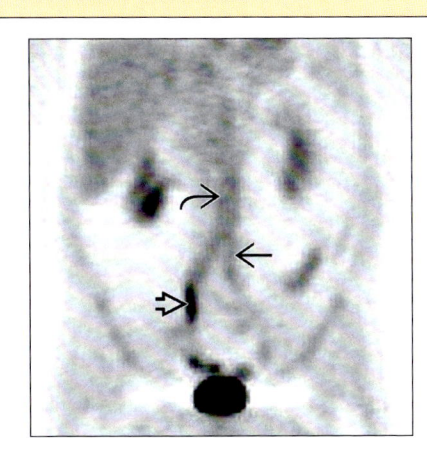

(Left) Coronal FDG PET shows increased activity in subclavian arteries ➔ and ascending aorta ➔ in patient with giant cell arteritis. Same patient as next two images. (Center) Coronal FDG PET shows increased activity in descending thoracic aorta ➔ in patient with giant cell arteritis. (Right) Coronal FDG PET shows increased activity in aorta ➔ and iliac arteries ➔ in patient with giant cell arteritis. Focal activity in right iliac signifies thrombosis ➔.

ATHEROSCLEROSIS

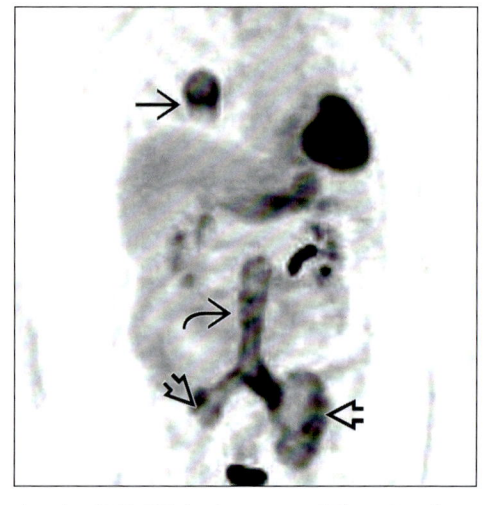

Anterior FDG PET for lung cancer staging shows intense uptake in wall of aorta extending to bilateral iliac artery aneurysms. Same as next patient.

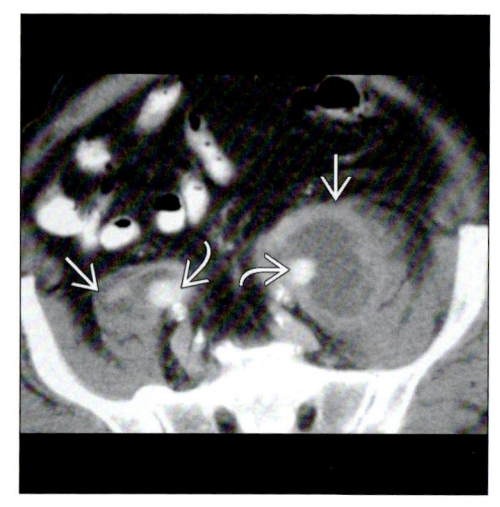

Axial CECT of patient at left shows large aneurysms of iliac arteries and bilateral vascular grafts.

TERMINOLOGY

Abbreviations and Synonyms
- Arteriosclerosis
- Cerebral vascular accident (CVA), stroke
- Coronary artery disease (CAD)

Definitions
- Chronic inflammatory disease of large and medium-sized arteries

IMAGING FINDINGS

General Features
- Best diagnostic clue
  - Advanced disease
    - CT: Arterial wall calcification
    - Contrast angiography: Stenosis
  - Active imaging research to identify
    - Preclinical disease
    - "Vulnerable" or unstable plaque
- Location: Aorta and branch arteries
- Size: Large and medium-sized arteries
- Morphology
  - Stenosis ≥ 50% generally required for clinical significance
  - Focal or diffuse vessel wall calcification
  - Advanced disease: Ectasia, aneurysmal dilatation, rupture, dissection
  - Dissection and rupture: Can occur in heavily calcified vessels without aneurysm

Nuclear Medicine Findings
- FDG PET or PET/CT
  - Youth: No significant FDG uptake in arterial walls
  - Beginning 30s and 40s: Mild diffuse or patchy FDG uptake in vascular walls 2° inflammation
  - Segmental FDG uptake in vascular wall: Usually correspond to areas of greatest calcification
  - Small foci of intense FDG uptake in vascular walls: Suggest ulcerated plaques, thrombogenic foci
- Myocardial perfusion scintigraphy (MPS)
  - Shows perfusion at rest and stress
  - Decreased activity in vascular territory = stenosis

CT Findings
- NECT

DDx: Mimics of Atherosclerosis on FDG PET

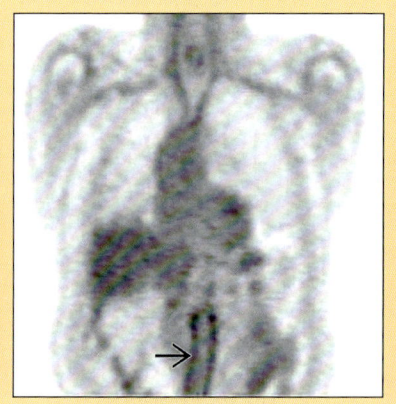

Normal Vascular Graft

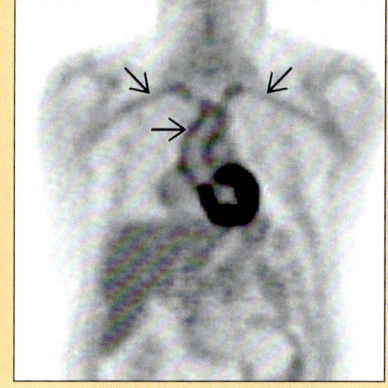

Large Vessel Vasculitis

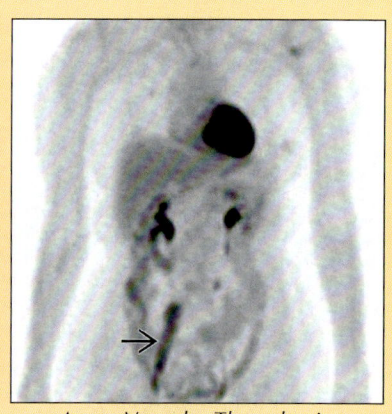

Acute Vascular Thrombosis

ATHEROSCLEROSIS

Key Facts

Terminology
- Chronic inflammatory disease of large and medium-sized arteries

Imaging Findings
- Focal or diffuse vessel wall calcification
- Advanced disease: Ectasia, aneurysmal dilatation, rupture, dissection
- Dissection and rupture: Can occur in heavily calcified vessels without aneurysm
- Youth: No significant FDG uptake in arterial walls
- Beginning 30s and 40s: Mild diffuse or patchy FDG uptake in vascular walls 2° inflammation
- Segmental FDG uptake in vascular wall: Usually correspond to areas of greatest calcification
- Small foci of intense FDG uptake in vascular walls: Suggest ulcerated plaques, thrombogenic foci
- FDG PET: Potential to identify early atherosclerosis, denuded plaque, thrombogenic site (investigational)
- Clinically significant disease: Contrast angiography, MPS, CTA, MRA
- Advanced atherosclerosis/risk stratification: CT, US
- PET: Image 3 hrs after injection to allow clearing of all blood pool activity for optimal vascular evaluation
- PET/CT: Improved ability to localize site of uptake to anatomic structure, calcification

Top Differential Diagnoses
- Large Vessel Vasculitis
- Vascular Thrombosis
- Normal Vascular Graft
- Infected Vascular Graft
- Mycotic Aneurysm

- ○ Electron beam CT (EBCT), multidetector CT (MDCT): Calcium deposition in vascular wall
- ○ Coronary artery calcium score: Risk stratification for CVA, CAD, mortality
- CECT, CTA
  - ○ Method of choice to evaluate peripheral aneurysms (size, location, rupture, dissection)
  - ○ MDCT technique: Alternative to contrast angiography (including chest pain evaluation)
  - ○ Requires IV contrast
  - ○ Limitations: Contrast contraindications (allergy, renal insufficiency), stents, extensive calcifications
  - ○ Direct visualization of atherosclerotic plaques

Angiographic Findings
- Angiography
  - ○ Identifies hemodynamically significant lesions (≥ 50% stenosis), thrombosis, occlusion, ulcerated plaques, collateral vessels
  - ○ Often fails to identify preclinical disease
  - ○ May miss aneurysms due to luminal clot

MR Findings
- Evolving area of investigation atherosclerosis investigation
  - ○ Potential for evaluation of wall, lumen, volume, cap thickness, neovascularity, plaque rupture, plaque composition
  - ○ Protocols: Time of flight and black blood images, gadolinium contrast
  - ○ Iron oxide particles: May identify activated macrophages in actively forming atheroma
  - ○ MR angiography (MRA): Direct visualization of atherosclerotic plaques

Ultrasonographic Findings
- B-mode evaluates vessel walls and lumen
  - ○ Vascular intima media thickness (IMT): Common and internal carotid arteries
    - Normative data well-established: ↑ IMT, IMT progression = risk factors for CVA, CAD
  - ○ Also defines arterial lumen and inter-adventitial diameter
- Brachial artery reactivity: Stiff, atherosclerotic vessels do not react
- Doppler techniques measuring flow ~ percent stenosis (≥ 50% stenosis)
- Intravascular ultrasound (IVUS): Transducer on intravascular catheter tip
  - ○ Advantages: Quantify lumen, wall, plaque characteristics
  - ○ Disadvantages: Minimally invasive, inability to image tight stenosis

Imaging Recommendations
- Best imaging tool
  - ○ FDG PET: Potential to identify early atherosclerosis, denuded plaque, thrombogenic site (investigational)
  - ○ Clinically significant disease: Contrast angiography, MPS, CTA, MRA
  - ○ Advanced atherosclerosis/risk stratification: CT, US
- Protocol advice
  - ○ FDG PET: 10-20 mCi IV
  - ○ PET: Image 3 hrs after injection to allow clearing of all blood pool activity for optimal vascular evaluation
  - ○ PET/CT: Improved ability to localize site of uptake to anatomic structure, calcification

DIFFERENTIAL DIAGNOSIS

Large Vessel Vasculitis
- Diffuse FDG uptake in walls of aorta, iliac, subclavian, femoral, carotid arteries
- ↑ C-reactive protein (CRP) and sedimentation rate indicative of systemic inflammatory condition
- Association with deep temporal scalp tenderness, shoulder and hip girdle myalgias

Vascular Thrombosis
- FDG uptake in lumen, not vascular wall
- FDG uptake likely indicates acute clot (not chronic)

ATHEROSCLEROSIS

Normal Vascular Graft
- Mild, diffuse uptake by graft, minimally accentuated at anastomotic sites

Infected Vascular Graft
- Focal, intense, asymmetric on FDG PET and labeled WBC scintigraphy

Mycotic Aneurysm
- FDG uptake in periphery
- Clinical scenario may indicate infection

PATHOLOGY

General Features
- Genetics
  - Hyperlipidemia
  - Homozygosity for homocystinemia
  - Diseases with possible genetic components: Diabetes, hypertension, obesity
- Etiology
  - Sequence of events
    - Deposition of low density lipids in vascular wall; "fatty streak" begins in childhood
    - Inflammatory mononuclear cells respond, phagocytize lipids (foam cells)
    - Influx of vascular endothelial cells: Deposit extracellular connective tissue (fibrous cap) over lipids, inflammatory cells
    - Growth of fibrous cap ⇒ vascular remodeling ⇒ luminal narrowing, end-organ ischemia
    - Plaque rupture, denudation of endothelium overlying fibrous plaque: Thrombogenic subendothelium and lipid core exposed ⇒ thrombus ⇒ complete occlusion, embolic phenomena
  - Primary risk factors: Diabetes, cigarette smoking, male, hypertension, hyperlipidemia, obesity
  - "Novel" risk factors: Chronic inflammatory conditions, infection, homocysteine, ↑ fibrinogen, ↑ lipoprotein (a), ↑ CRP
- Epidemiology
  - Highest incidence: Developed/developing countries (high fat, refined-carbohydrate diet; cigarettes)
  - Causes > 50% of annual US mortality
  - In US 500,000 per year die from myocardial infarction

Gross Pathologic & Surgical Features
- Intravascular plaque formation, stenosis, obstruction, rupture, aneurysmal dilatation

Microscopic Features
- Deposition of lipids, calcium, cellular debris in arterial intima

CLINICAL ISSUES

Presentation
- Most common signs/symptoms
  - Physical signs depend upon site of involvement
    - Heart: Chest pain
    - Legs: Peripheral vascular disease
    - Brain: Hemiparalysis, dysarthria
  - Often silent until advanced disease

Demographics
- Age: Clinically apparent at 40-70 years
- Gender
  - Premenopausal: M > F
  - Postmenopausal: M = F

Natural History & Prognosis
- Often progresses to fatal event or end-organ failure 2° to ischemia/infarction
- Aggressive treatment improves prognosis

Treatment
- Control of hypertension
- Lower total, low density serum cholesterol
- Control of diabetes
- Dietary: Caloric, saturated fat, cholesterol reduction
- Moderate alcohol intake may be protective
- Exercise, weight reduction: Modifiable risk factors

DIAGNOSTIC CHECKLIST

Image Interpretation Pearls
- Focal intense FDG uptake in vascular wall suggests ulcerated plaque

SELECTED REFERENCES

1. Cordeiro MA et al: Atherosclerotic plaque characterization by multidetector row computed tomography angiography. J Am Coll Cardiol. 47(8 Suppl):C40-7, 2006
2. Davies JR et al: Radionuclide imaging for the detection of inflammation in vulnerable plaques. J Am Coll Cardiol. 47(8 Suppl):C57-68, 2006
3. Desai MY et al: Imaging of atherosclerosis using magnetic resonance: state of the art and future directions. Curr Atheroscler Rep. 8(2):131-9, 2006
4. Fenchel M et al: Atherosclerotic disease: whole-body cardiovascular imaging with MR system with 32 receiver channels and total-body surface coil technology--initial clinical results. Radiology. 238(1):280-91, 2006
5. Jalilian AR et al: Application of radioisotopes in inflammation. Curr Med Chem. 13(8):959-65, 2006
6. Jedryka-Goral A et al: Risk factors for atherosclerosis in healthy employees-a multidisciplinary approach. Eur J Intern Med. 17(4):247-53, 2006
7. Wilensky RL et al: Role of magnetic resonance and intravascular magnetic resonance in the detection of vulnerable plaques. J Am Coll Cardiol. 47(8 Suppl):C48-56, 2006
8. Fuster V et al: Atherothrombosis and high-risk plaque: Part II: approaches by noninvasive computed tomographic/magnetic resonance imaging. J Am Coll Cardiol. 46(7):1209-18, 2005
9. Morasch MD: New diagnostic imaging techniques. Perspect Vasc Surg Endovasc Ther. 17(4):341-50, 2005
10. Nighoghossian N et al: The vulnerable carotid artery plaque: current imaging methods and new perspectives. Stroke. 36(12):2764-72, 2005
11. El-Haddad G et al: Evolving role of positron emission tomography in the management of patients with inflammatory and other benign disorders. Semin Nucl Med. 34(4):313-29, 2004

ATHEROSCLEROSIS

IMAGE GALLERY

Typical

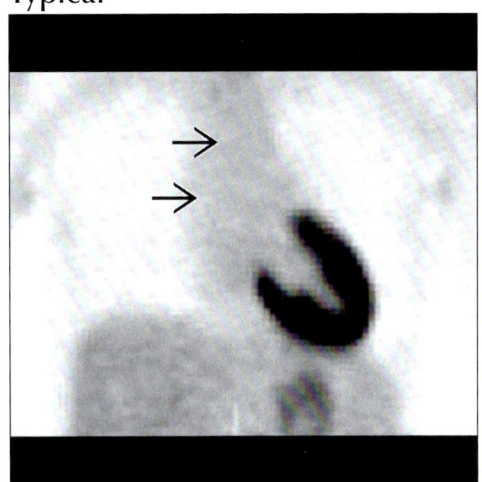

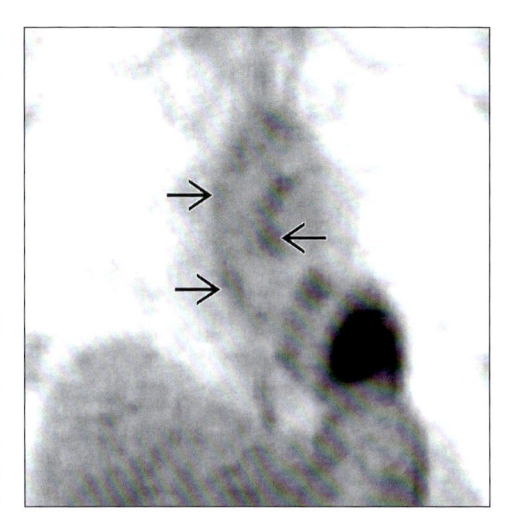

(Left) Coronal FDG PET of chest in young patient shows no increased uptake in aortic wall ➡. By 30-40 years of age, uptake in arterial walls suggests preclinical atherosclerosis. *(Right)* Coronal FDG PET shows patchy uptake in aortic wall ➡, a pattern typical for large-vessel atherosclerosis.

Typical

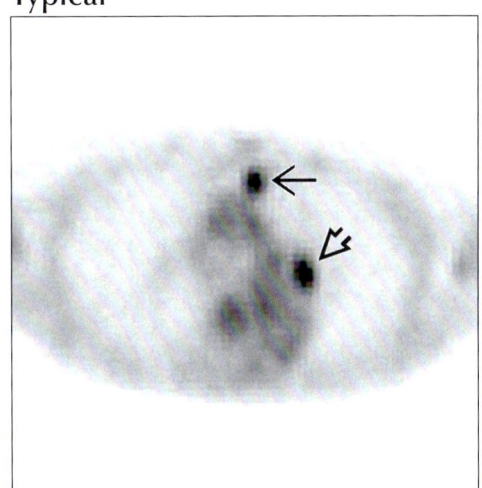

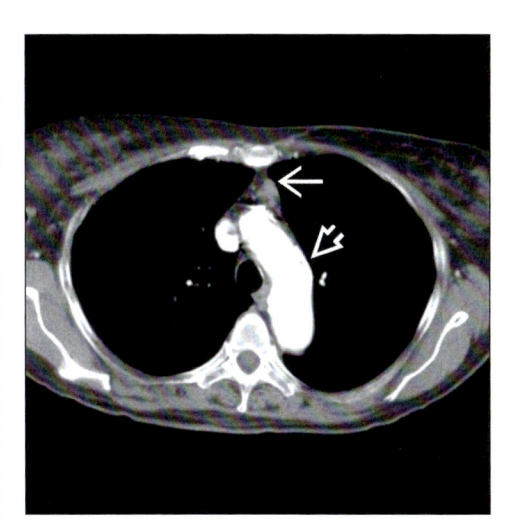

(Left) Axial FDG PET in patient evaluated for thymoma ➡. Intense focal uptake present in aorta ➡. Same as next image. *(Right)* Axial CECT in same patient as previous image shows thymoma ➡. Lateral aortic wall shows focal calcification ➡, likely an ulcerated atherosclerotic plaque.

Other

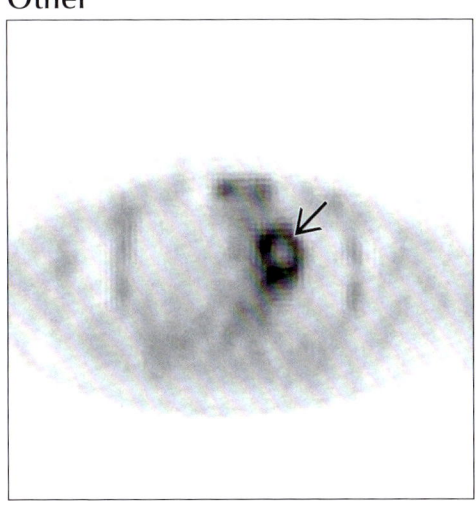

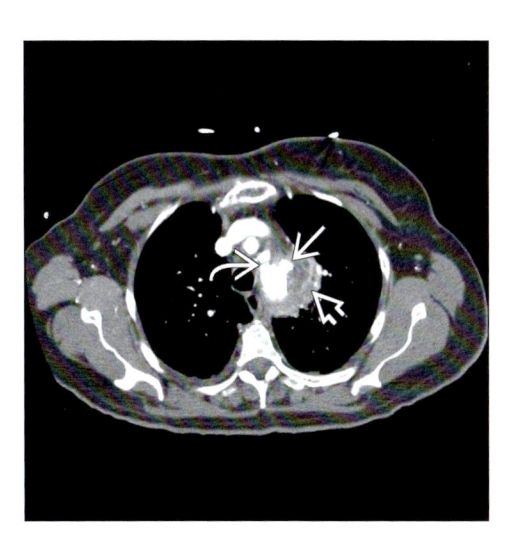

(Left) Axial PET/CT of upper chest shows increased uptake in mass surrounding aortic knob ➡. Same patient as next image. *(Right)* Axial CECT of same patient as previous image shows irregular contour to lumen of aortic knob ➡, peripheral mass ➡, and narrow mouth excrescence of contrast ➡. At surgery, this proved to be mycotic aneurysm.

VASCULAR THROMBOSIS

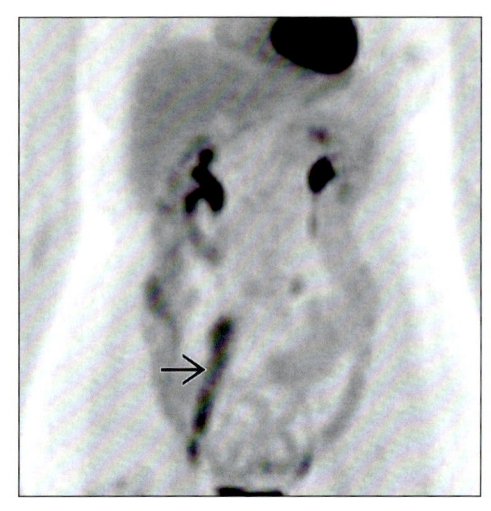

Coronal FDG PET shows intense uptake in right iliac vein ➔ in patient with acute deep venous thrombosis (DVT).

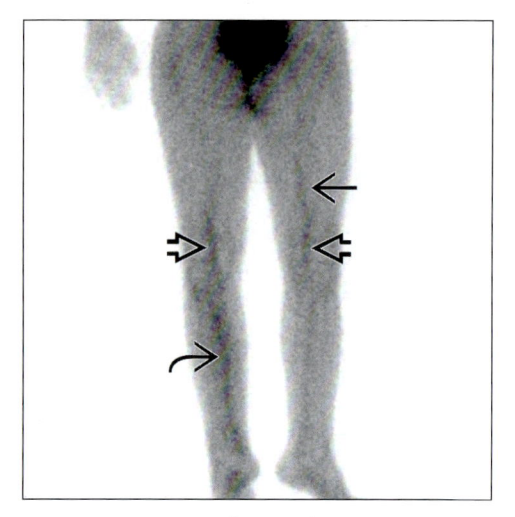

Posterior Tc-99m apcitide scan shows uptake in right femoral ➔, bilateral popliteal ➔ and left calf ➔ veins. Doppler ultrasound confirmed acute DVT.

TERMINOLOGY

Abbreviations and Synonyms
- Deep venous thrombosis (DVT), venothromboembolism (VTE), pulmonary embolism (PE)

Definitions
- Pathologic blood clot formation in blood vessels

IMAGING FINDINGS

General Features
- Best diagnostic clue: Intraluminal filling defect, vascular "cut-off", extensive filling of collateral vessels

Nuclear Medicine Findings
- Tc-99m apcitide (GP IIb/IIIa receptor antagonist, AcuTect): Positive in acute clot (not chronic)
  - 20 mCi Tc-99m apcitide IV, image 30 and 90 minutes post injection
  - Reported sens 73%, spec 67%: Progressive uptake in clot
- FDG PET: Intraluminal hypermetabolic focus
  - Likely positive only in acute clot
- Labeled leukocyte scan: Uptake in acute septic, aseptic clot
- Tc-99m MAA venography: See collaterals, sticks to acute clot
  - Reported sens 88%, spec 96%
  - Tourniquets at ankles, knees; inject 1-2 mCi Tc-99m MAA in dorsal vein of each foot (usually with VQ scan)
  - Early injection phase: Failure to fill deep veins; collaterals seen
  - Delayed Tc-99m MAA images: MAA adheres to acute clot
- Ventilation perfusion scan (VQ scan): Probability of acute PE given pattern

Imaging Recommendations
- Best imaging tool
  - Gold standard: Contrast venography, arteriography, Doppler ultrasound, CTA and MRA (increasingly for central clot)
  - Nuclear medicine: In complicated cases

DDx: Mimics of Acute Deep Venous Thrombosis

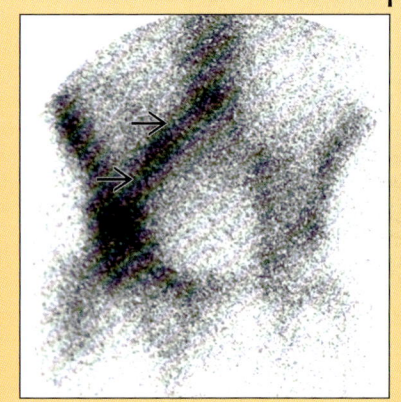

Infected Vascular Graft

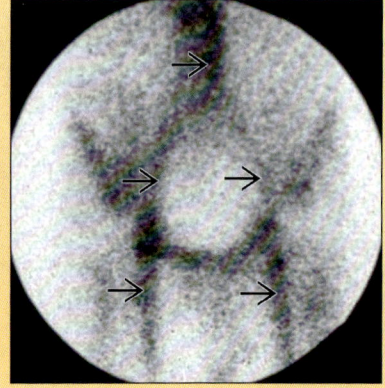

Blood Pool Activity

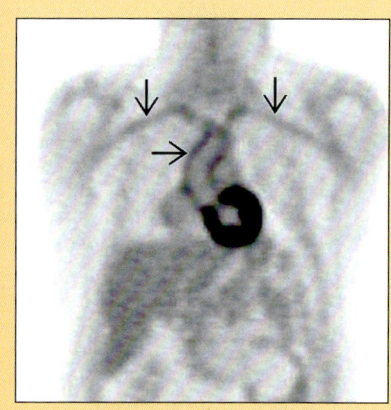

Large Vessel Vasculitis

VASCULAR THROMBOSIS

Key Facts

Imaging Findings
- Tc-99m apcitide (GP IIb/IIIa receptor antagonist, AcuTect): Positive in acute clot (not chronic)
- FDG PET: Intraluminal hypermetabolic focus
- Labeled leukocyte scan: Uptake in acute septic, aseptic clot
- Tc-99m MAA venography: See collaterals, sticks to acute clot

- Gold standard: Contrast venography, arteriography, Doppler ultrasound, CTA and MRA (increasingly for central clot)
- Nuclear medicine: In complicated cases

Top Differential Diagnoses
- Vascular Graft Infection
- Large Vessel Vasculitis
- Blood Pool Activity
- Atherosclerosis

DIFFERENTIAL DIAGNOSIS

Vascular Graft Infection
- WBC scan, FDG PET: Focal or asymmetrical ↑↑ activity

Large Vessel Vasculitis
- FDG PET: Diffusely increased uptake in arterial wall

Blood Pool Activity
- Most problematic with labeled WBC scan, FDG PET

Atherosclerosis
- FDG PET: Focal or patchy uptake in arterial wall

PATHOLOGY

General Features
- Etiology
  - Genetic hypercoagulable conditions
  - Arterial thrombosis: 2° to wall injury/defect (e.g., unstable plaque)
  - Venous thrombosis: Cancer, inflammation, compression, venous stasis
- Epidemiology
  - DVT
    - General population: 1.5:1,000 per year; > 65 years old: 1:100 per year
    - 1/3 will develop PE

CLINICAL ISSUES

Presentation
- Most common signs/symptoms: Extremity swelling, redness, pain
- Other signs/symptoms: Shortness of breath, hemoptysis, pleuritic chest pain, tachycardia (PE)

DIAGNOSTIC CHECKLIST

Image Interpretation Pearls
- Acute thrombosis is an inflammatory lesion: Hot on FDG PET and labeled WBC scans

SELECTED REFERENCES

1. Do B et al: Diagnosis of aseptic deep venous thrombosis of the upper extremity in a cancer patient using fluorine-18 fluorodeoxyglucose positron emission tomography/computerized tomography (FDG PET/CT). Ann Nucl Med. 20(2):151-5, 2006
2. Taillefer R: Radiolabeled peptides in the detection of deep venous thrombosis. Semin Nucl Med. 31(2):102-23, 2001
3. Stevan M et al: Diagnosis of thrombosis of the deep veins of the lower extremities and pelvis and pulmonary thromboembolism using 99Tcm human serum albumin macroaggregates. Nucl Med Commun. 10(3):141-7, 1989
4. D'Alonzo WA Jr et al: Detection of deep venous thrombosis by indium-111 leukocyte scintigraphy. J Nucl Med. 27(5):631-3, 1986

IMAGE GALLERY

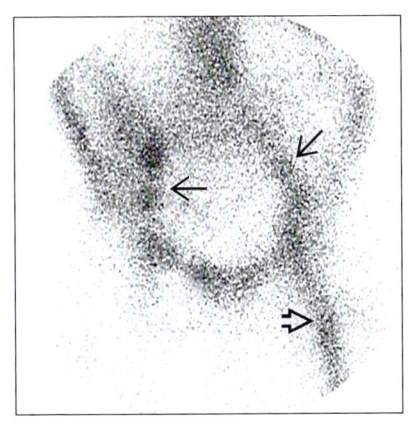

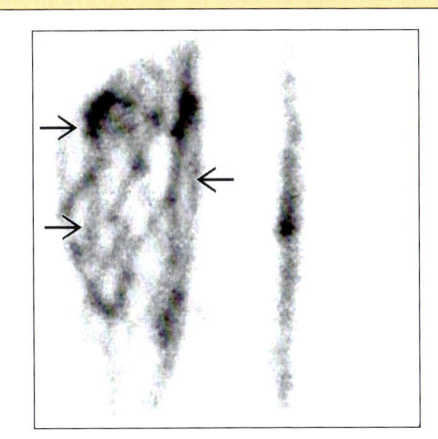

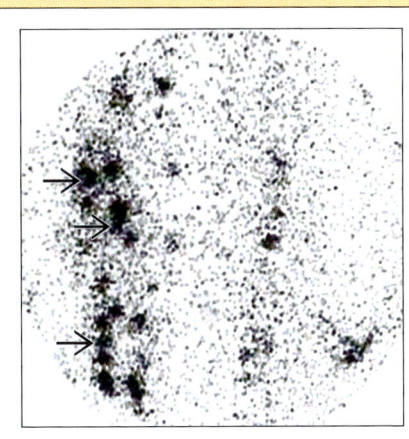

(Left) Anterior planar In-111 WBC scan of the pelvis shows uptake in bilateral iliac ➔ and left femoral ➔ veins. Contrast venography confirmed acute DVT. *(Center)* Anterior lower legs of Tc-99m MAA injection phase images of bilateral foot injection shows collateral filling of right calf veins ➔ in patient with DVT. Same patient as next image. *(Right)* Anterior delayed Tc-99m MAA image of calves with tourniquets applied shows Tc-99m MAA adherent to acute DVT ➔.

VASCULAR GRAFT INFECTION

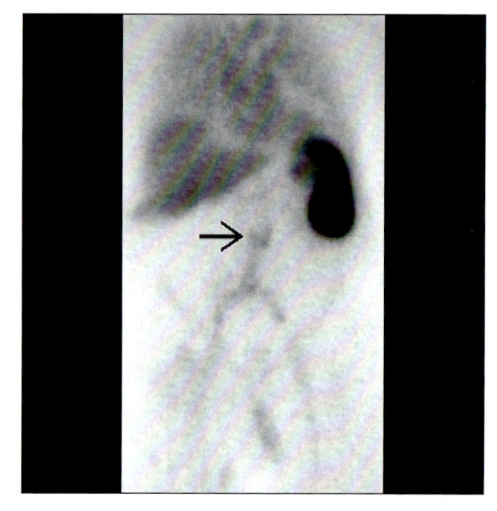

Anterior Tc-99m HMPAO labeled leukocyte scan, 4 hours post injection shows uptake in an infected aorto bi-iliac graft, more prominent at the proximal anastomosis ➡. Same patient as next image.

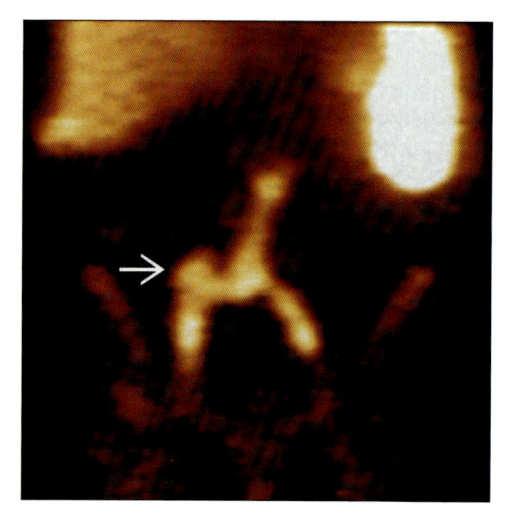

Coronal SPECT of the scan at left confirms marked and asymmetrical uptake in an infected aorto bi-iliac graft. An abscess was also present in the proximal right iliac region ➡.

TERMINOLOGY

Abbreviations and Synonyms
- Aorto bifemoral vascular graft (A-Y graft)

Definitions
- Infected graft: Inflammatory change, phlegmon or abscess associated with bacterial ingrowth into or around vascular graft
- Colonized graft: Bacteria living on/in graft without frank inflammation or pus
- Graft incorporation: Ingrowth of normal host tissues into vascular graft, creating a "pseudoendothelium"
- Graft disincorporation: Loss of pseudoendothelium of host tissues, resulting in "bare graft"

IMAGING FINDINGS

General Features
- Best diagnostic clue: Focal, asymmetric, markedly increased uptake on labeled autologous leukocyte scan
- Location
  - Distribution of vascular graft
  - Proximal and distal anastomoses are most common site of involvement

Nuclear Medicine Findings
- Labeled Leukocyte Scintigraphy
  - Normal
    - Mild homogeneous uptake along distribution of vascular graft is normal
    - Mild diffuse uptake in graft is normal up to one year post-op
    - In some normal patients, mild diffuse uptake in graft can persist indefinitely
  - Colonization
    - Moderate increased uptake along vascular graft inner surface in colonization
    - Colonization often somewhat patchy in nature
  - Abscess or phlegmon
    - Focal, asymmetrical uptake along or near the graft in abscess or phlegmon
    - May extend into adjacent soft tissues
    - Proximal and distal anastomoses are most vulnerable to infection
  - Vascular enteric fistulas

DDx: Labeled Leukocyte Scans: Mimics of Vascular Graft Infections

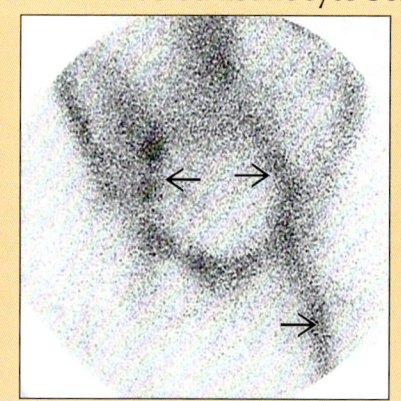

Bilateral DVT

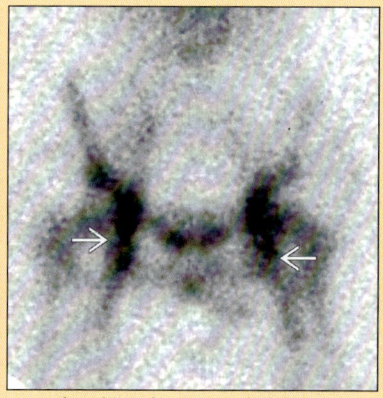

Blood Pool (Large Abdomen)

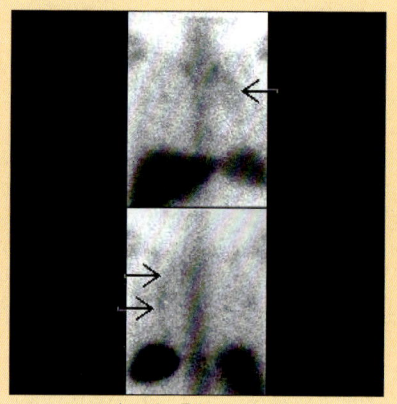

Aortic Dissection

VASCULAR GRAFT INFECTION

Key Facts

Imaging Findings
- Mild homogeneous uptake along distribution of vascular graft is normal
- Mild diffuse uptake in graft is normal up to one year post-op
- Moderate increased uptake along vascular graft inner surface in colonization
- Colonization often somewhat patchy in nature
- Focal, asymmetrical uptake along or near the graft in abscess or phlegmon
- Proximal and distal anastomoses are most vulnerable to infection
- Focal increased uptake at site of fistula (infected, by definition)
- Most common site of vascular enteric fistula is where duodenum crossed aorta
- Best imaging tool: Labeled autologous leukocyte scan

Top Differential Diagnoses
- Normal Blood Pool Activity
- Normal Vascular Graft Activity
- Intravascular Clot
- Normal Bone Marrow Activity in Close Proximity to Vascular Graft

Clinical Issues
- Low grade fever
- Leukocytosis
- Painful swelling around sites of distal anastomoses
- GI bleeding in face of vascular enteric fistulas
- Septic emboli to lower extremities
- Pseudoaneurysms, particularly at sites of distal anastomoses

---

- Focal increased uptake at site of fistula (infected, by definition)
- Most common site of vascular enteric fistula is where duodenum crossed aorta
- Additional sites are between aorta and transverse colon, and between descending colon and iliac graft
- Uptake in bowel due to low grade, intermittent bleeding

Imaging Recommendations
- Best imaging tool: Labeled autologous leukocyte scan
- Protocol advice
  - In-111 generally preferable to Tc-99m exametazime (HMPAO) leukocytes
    - Oblique views are helpful to separate vascular structures from adjacent bone marrow activity, often a problem in the mid-lower lumbar spine and where external iliac vessels crossover pubic bones
  - Tc-99m HMPAO
    - Tc-99m HMPAO leukocytes can be compromised by significant blood pool activity, which can obscure underlying lower grade infection
    - Imaging out to 24 h is desirable
    - Improved SPECT imaging characteristics over In-111 leukocyte
- Additional nuclear medicine imaging options
  - Tc-99m sulfur colloid marrow scan
    - May be necessary to determine if groin activity is bone marrow or vascular graft
    - Dual isotope imaging possible when use with In-111 labeled leukocytes, but not with Tc-99m labeled HMPAO leukocytes
  - F-18 FDG PET
    - Several studies show promising results in identifying graft infections
    - Head-to-head comparison with labeled leukocytes has not been done
    - Normal vascular grafts are often markedly hypermetabolic, which may limit utility of FDG PET for this purpose
    - Many causes of FDG uptake in vessels, including normal blood pool, normal uptake in vascular grafts, aneurysms, pseudoaneurysms, atherosclerosis, vasculitis
- Correlative imaging features
  - CT may show fluid collection around infected graft
    - Nonspecific and can be normal, even long after graft placement (lymphocele)
  - CT may show air around infected graft
    - Highly specific for infected graft, but rarely seen
  - MR may show fluid collection and associated enhancement around graft
    - Fluid collection nonspecific; enhancement more specific
  - Vascular graft: Enteric fistulas
    - Difficult to demonstrate by angiography
    - Often subtle inflammatory change around fistula on CT
    - Direct endoscopic imaging contraindication because can worsen bleeding

DIFFERENTIAL DIAGNOSIS

Normal Blood Pool Activity
- More common with Tc-99m HMPAO, than In-111 labeled leukocytes

Normal Vascular Graft Activity
- Commonly seen in most patients up to one year after graft placement
- In approximately 20% of patients, mild diffuse uptake may persist indefinitely
- Infected graft differs in that it is intense, patchy or asymmetric in uptake

Intravascular Clot
- Labeled leukocytes localize in acute arterial or deep venous thrombosis (DVT)

Normal Bone Marrow Activity in Close Proximity to Vascular Graft
- Oblique images, SPECT may temporally resolve

VASCULAR GRAFT INFECTION

PATHOLOGY

Gross Pathologic & Surgical Features
- Normal graft
  - Inner surface of graft initially consists of bare, or exposed, vascular graft material (e.g. polyester, Gortex)
  - During the first post-operative year, the host tissues grow into the graft material, creating a "pseudoendothelium"
- Colonized graft
  - The pseudoendothelium sloughs off, creating bare areas along graft
- Abscess or phlegmon
  - Tissue inflammation and collections of pus extend around graft material
  - Septic thrombus can form along infected graft surface

Microscopic Features
- Labeled leukocyte preparations
  - Labeled cells include a mixture (1/3 each) white cells, red cells, and platelets
  - Because leukocytes are larger, the bulk of labeled cellular material is leukocyte
- In normal grafts, initial bare graft surface serves as a nidus for platelet and mononuclear cell adhesion
  - This platelet and mononuclear cell adhesion facilitates normal incorporation with host tissues
  - This results in homogeneous uptake of labeled cells along the vascular graft
  - With incorporation, cellular adhesion and uptake on leukocyte scan decrease
- Colonization
  - Disincorporation results in exposed graft material, a nidus for adhesion of labeled cells
- Abscess or phlegmon
  - Focal areas of increased uptake of labeled leukocytes

CLINICAL ISSUES

Presentation
- Most common signs/symptoms
  - Low grade fever
  - Leukocytosis
  - Painful swelling around sites of distal anastomoses
- Other signs/symptoms
  - GI bleeding in face of vascular enteric fistulas
  - Septic emboli to lower extremities
  - Pseudoaneurysms, particularly at sites of distal anastomoses
  - Unusual signs/symptoms
    - Hypertrophic osteoarthropathy (may be unilateral)
    - Pre-tibial swelling

Natural History & Prognosis
- Morbidity and mortality from graft infections is very high
  - Sepsis and septic emboli
  - Amputation due to vascular insufficiency
- Infection less common with endovascular stent grafts

Treatment
- Complete surgical excision of infected and colonized graft with remote reconstruction of distal circulation
  - Preferred treatment in patients who can tolerate the procedure
- Limited local excision with long term antibiotic therapy
  - In patients who are not candidates for more aggressive surgery or distal reconstruction
- Long term antibiotics only
  - Often requires a month or more of broad spectrum, IV antibiotics
  - Difficult to sterilize infected graft because bacteria are living in foreign material
- Arterial allografts
  - Long term durability may be limited
  - Should be considered a short term "bridge transplant"

DIAGNOSTIC CHECKLIST

Consider
- Age of graft (diffuse uptake is normal, especially < 1 year post-op)
- Possibility of vascular thrombotic disease, the most important cause of false positives

Image Interpretation Pearls
- Focal or asymmetrical uptake on labeled leukocyte scan is positive
- Diffuse symmetrical uptake is usually normal
- Other imaging studies are often negative
- Colonization can also cause uptake on leukocyte scan, due to adhesion to disincorporated graft

SELECTED REFERENCES

1. Hart JP et al: Operative strategies in aortic graft infections: is complete graft excision always necessary? Ann Vasc Surg. 19(2):154-60, 2005
2. Turgut H et al: Systemic and local antibiotic prophylaxis in the prevention of Staphylococcus epidermidis graft infection. BMC Infect Dis. 21:5:91, 2005
3. Ducasse E et al: Aortoiliac stent graft infection: current problems and management. Ann Vasc Surg. 18(5):521-6, 2004
4. Soetevent C et al: Vascular graft infection in aortoiliac and aortofemoral bypass surgery: clinical presentation, diagnostic strategies and results of surgical treatment. Neth J Med. 62(11):446-52, 2004
5. Chacko TK et al: Applications of fluorodeoxyglucose positron emission tomography in the diagnosis of infection. Nucl Med Commun. 24(6):615-24, 2003
6. Keidar Z et al: PET/CT using 2-deoxy-2-[18F]fluoro-D-glucose for the evaluation of suspected infected vascular graft. Mol Imaging Biol. 5(1):23-5, 2003
7. Liberatore M et al: Clinical usefulness of technetium-99m-HMPAO-labeled leukocyte scan in prosthetic vascular graft infection. J Nucl Med. 39(5):875-9, 1998
8. Lawrence PF et al: Indium 111-labeled leukocyte scanning for detection of prosthetic vascular graft infection. J Vasc Surg. 2(1):165-73, 1985

VASCULAR GRAFT INFECTION

IMAGE GALLERY

Variant

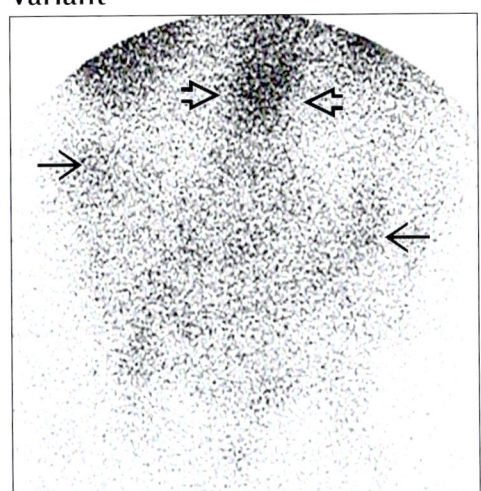

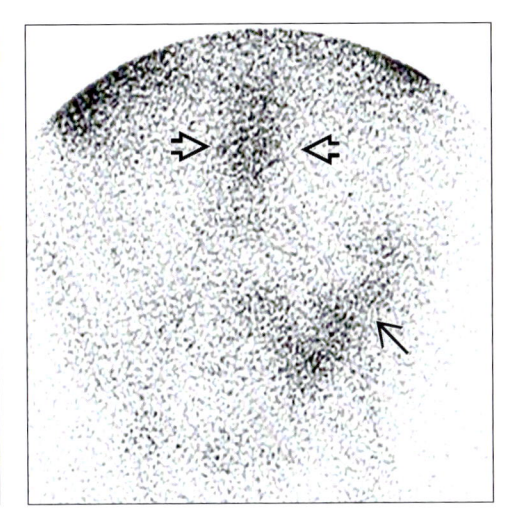

(Left) Anterior abdomen of In-111 labeled leukocyte scan at 24 h in patient with aortic graft, intermittent GI bleed and fever shows diffuse bowel activity ➔ and focus in the mid epigastrium ⇨. See next image. *(Right)* Anterior abdomen at 48 hours shows bowel activity moved through (labeled blood in lumen) ➔. Persistent uptake at infected fistula between aortic graft and transverse duodenum ⇨.

Typical

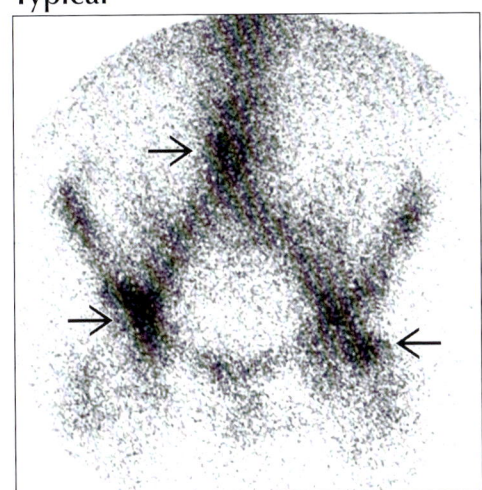

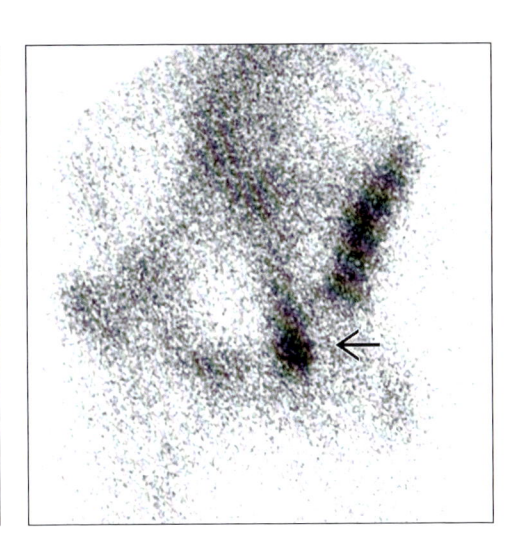

(Left) Anterior abdomen, 24 h In-111 leukocyte scan, shows marked uptake at proximal and distal anastomoses ➔ of an infected A-Y graft. See next image (oblique). *(Right)* Left anterior oblique of scan at left confirms the left inguinal focus is associated with a vascular graft ➔, and not due to bone marrow activity in underlying pubic bone.

Typical

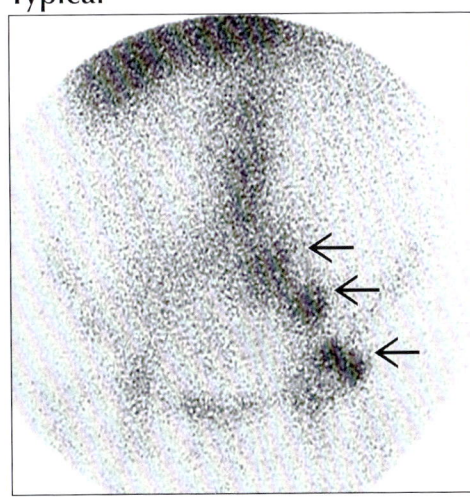

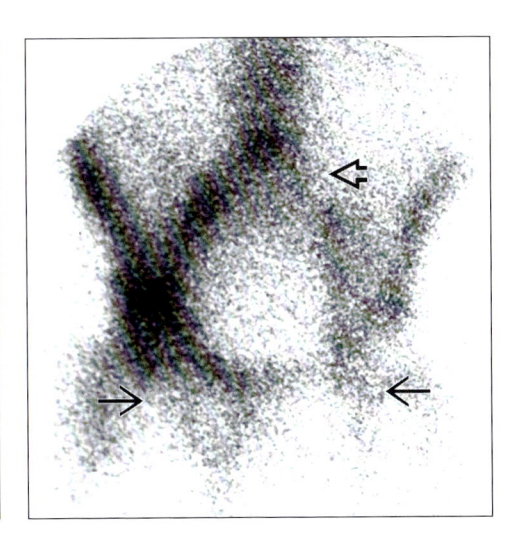

(Left) Anterior labeled leukocyte scintigraphy shows three large foci of intense uptake along the left limb of an A-Y graft ➔, proved at surgery to be abscesses around the infected graft. *(Right)* Anterior labeled leukocyte scintigraphy shows uptake at proximal ⇨ and distal ➔ infected anastamoses of an aorto-bifemoral vascular graft.

VASCULAR GRAFT INFECTION

Variant

(Left) Anterior labeled leukocyte scintigraphy shows intense focal uptake in an infected right limb of an A-Y graft ⇨, mild uptake on left also infected ➔. See next image (post-operative). (Right) Anterior labeled leukocyte scintigraphy post-operatively (same patient as previous) showing no residual infection following removal of infected aorto-bifemoral graft material.

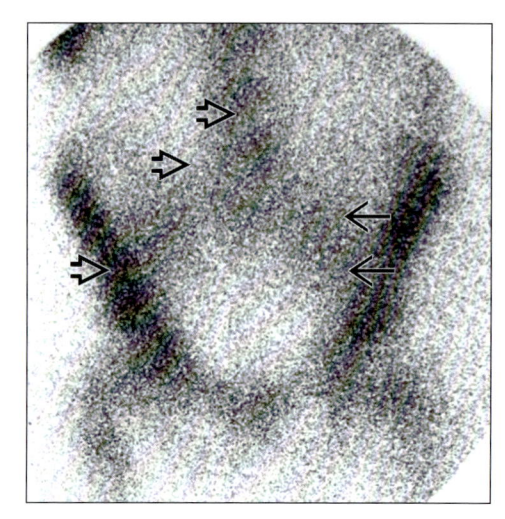

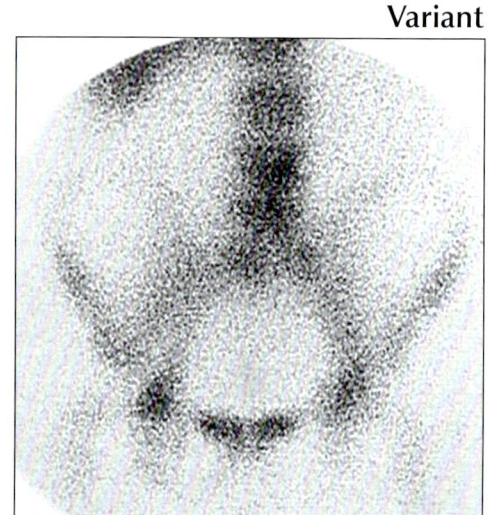

Other

(Left) Anterior MIP image of an FDG PET scan shows uptake in acute deep venous thrombosis involving the right femoral iliac vein ➔. (Right) Anterior MIP of an FDG PET scan demonstrating normal uptake in a non-infected A-Y graft, ➔ and a hypermetabolic periaortic nodal mass due to lymphoma ⇨.

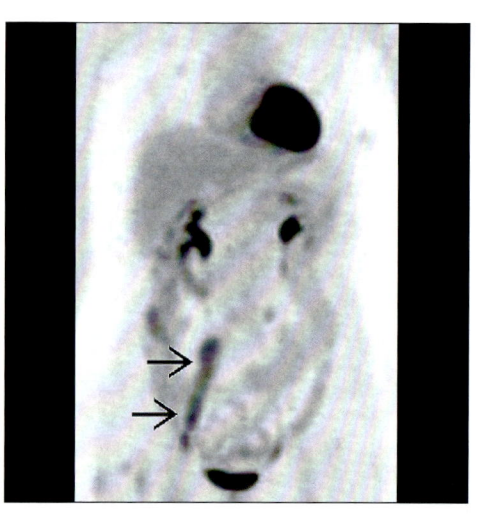

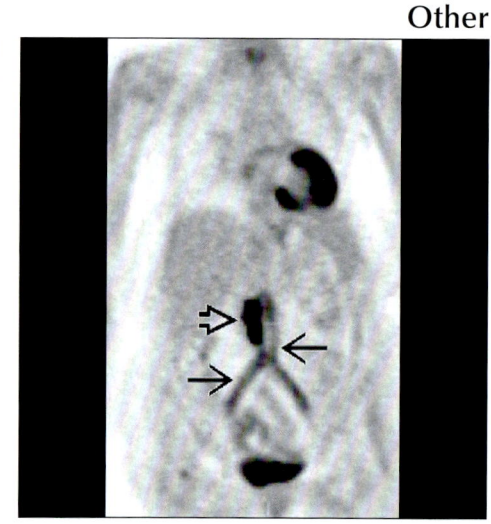

Other

(Left) Anterior MIP of an FDG PET scan showing uptake in a normal, non-infected A-Y graft. Note relatively greater uptake at the proximal anastamosis ➔. This is often normal. (Right) Anterior MIP of an FDG PET scan demonstrates increased blood pool activity ➔ due to elevated glucose or early imaging. Focal uptake in the right groin is a pseudoaneurysm ⇨.

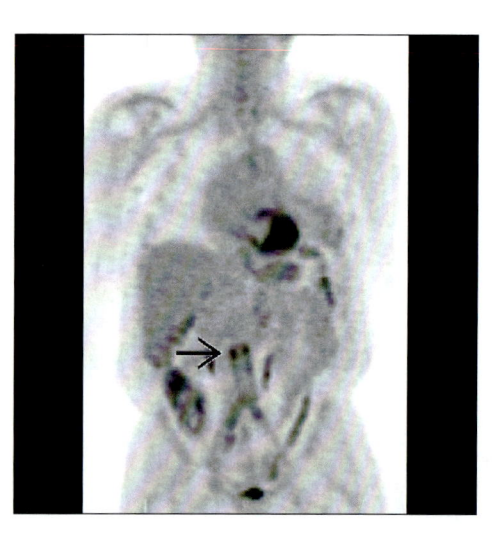

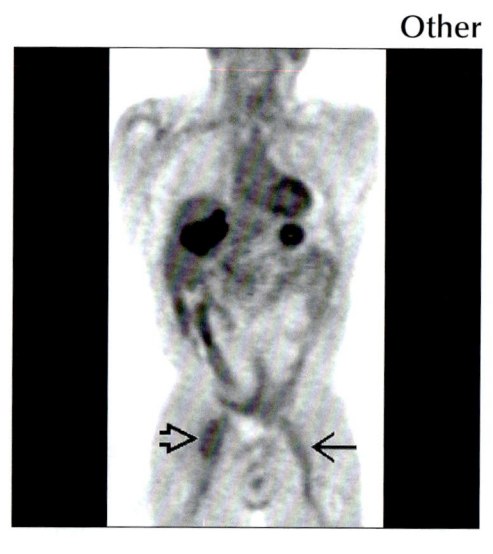

VASCULAR GRAFT INFECTION

Other

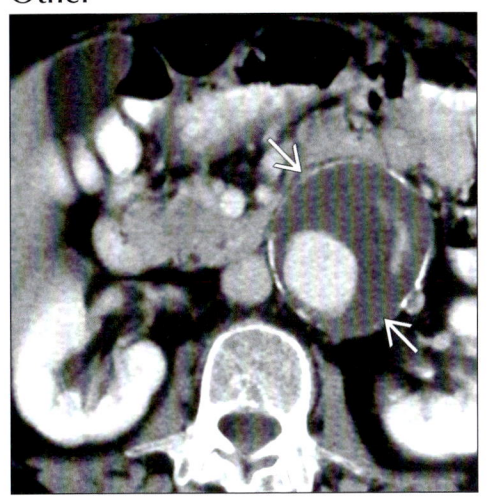

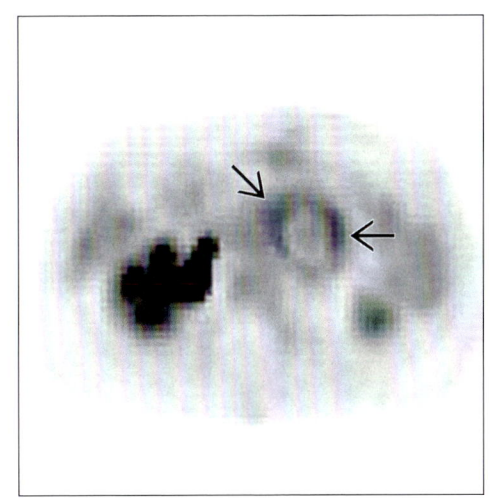

(Left) Axial CECT of the abdomen shows a large abdominal aortic aneurysm ➡. See next image (PET). (Right) Axial FDG PET scan of the abdomen in a patient at left shows uptake in the peripheral portion of the abdominal aortic aneurysm ➡. This is a typical finding in aneurysms, independent of infection.

Other

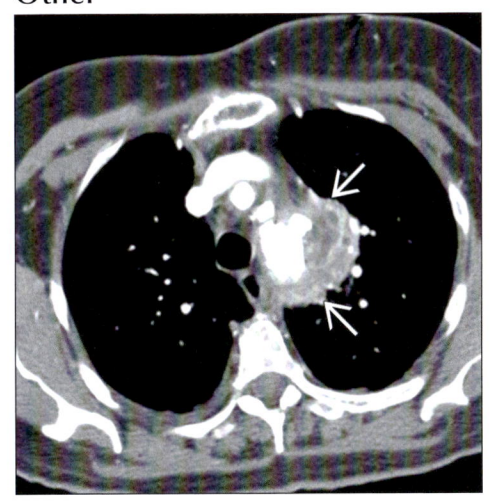

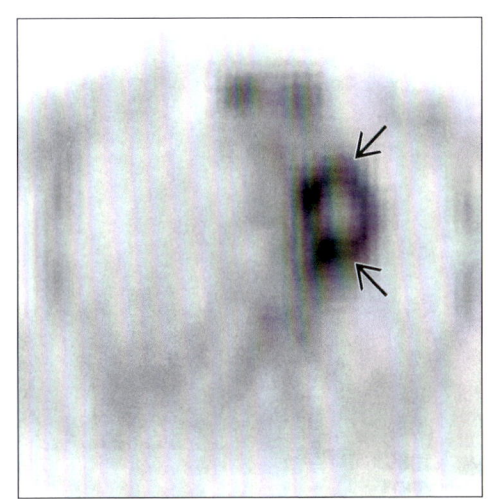

(Left) Axial CECT of the chest shows a mycotic aneurysm of the thoracic aorta ➡. See next image (PET). (Right) Axial FDG PET scan of the chest (same patient as previous image) showing uptake of FDG in a mycotic aneurysm of the aortic arch ➡.

Other

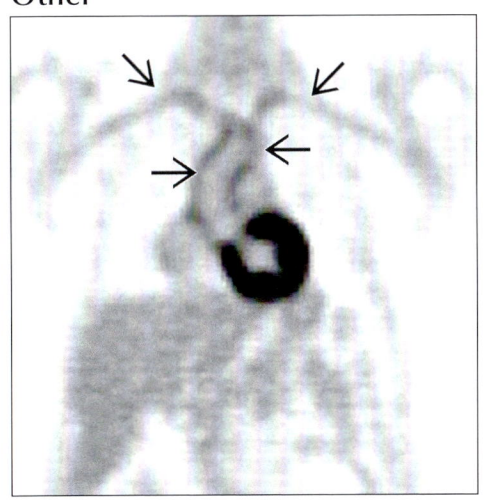

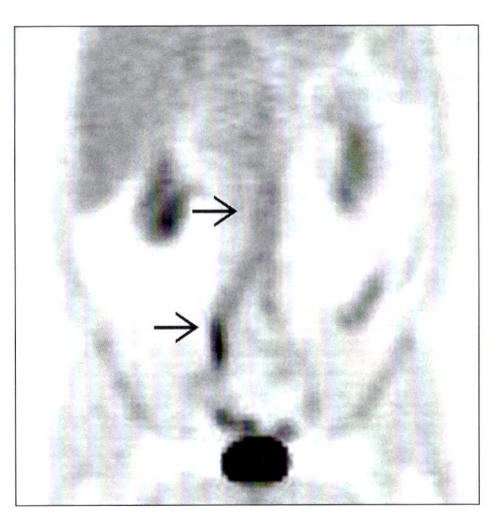

(Left) Coronal FDG PET scan of the chest demonstrates uptake in the walls of vessels due to a large vessel vasculitis ➡. See next image. (Right) Coronal FDG PET scan of the abdomen shows increased uptake in the aorta and iliac arteries ➡ due to a large vessel vasculitis. Same patient as previous image.

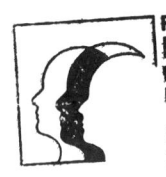

Praxis
Dr. Med. Boris Kirschsieper
Facharzt für Nuklearmedizin
Facharzt für Diagnostische Radiologie

Balger Strasse 50   Tel: (07221) 91 27 94
79532 Baden-Baden   Fax: (07221) 91 27 98

Web: www.Praxis-Kirschsieper.de
E-Mail: info@Praxis-Kirschsieper.de

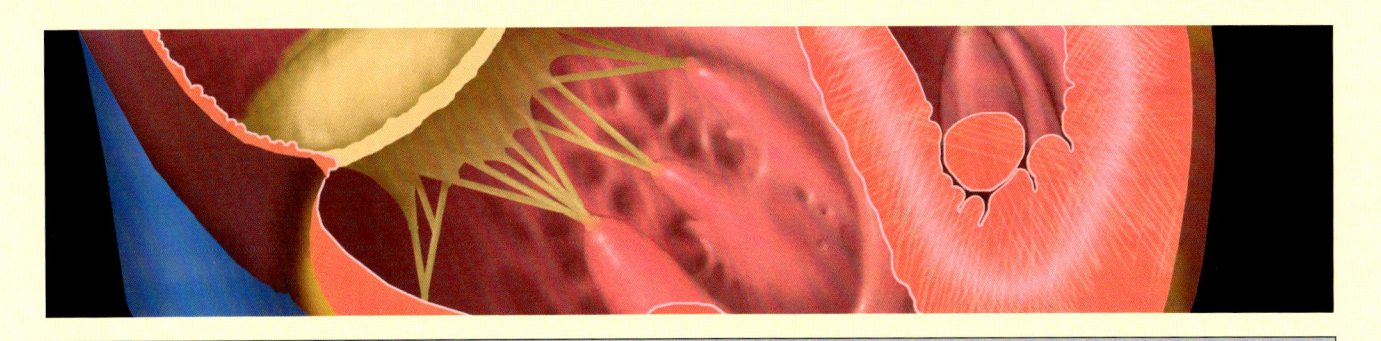

SECTION 3: Cardiovascular

Introduction and Overview
Cardiovascular Overview   3-2

Cardiac
Cardiomyopathy   3-6
Valvular Heart Disease   3-12
Myocardial Ischemia   3-16
Myocardial Viability   3-22
Myocardial Infarction   3-26
Cardiac Transplant   3-32
Left-to-Right Intracardiac Shunts   3-36
Right-to-Left Intracardiac Shunts   3-38

CARDIOVASCULAR OVERVIEW

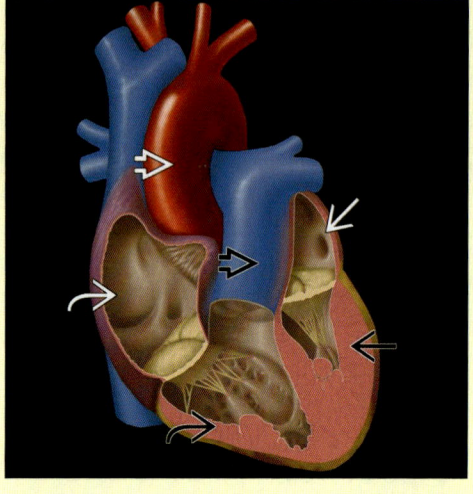

Graphic shows anatomy of heart and great vessels: Left atrium ➡, left ventricle ➡, right atrium ➡, right ventricle ➡, pulmonary artery ➡, aorta ➡.

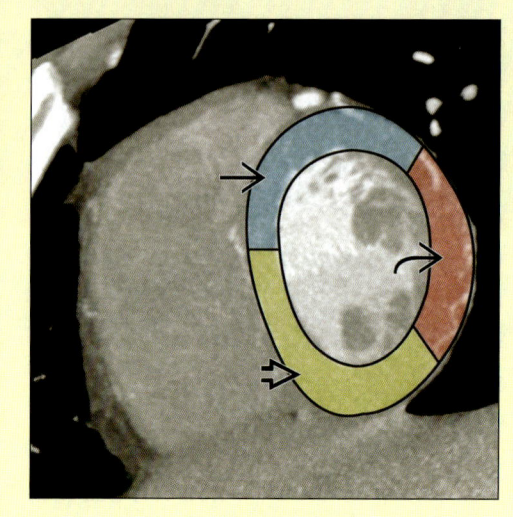

Graphic vascular distribution of left ventricle is shown in short axis: Left anterior descending ➡, circumflex ➡, posterior descending ➡ coronary arteries.

TERMINOLOGY

Abbreviations
- Myocardial perfusion scintigraphy (MPS)
- Radionuclide ventriculography (RNV) = multigated acquisition (MUGA)

IMAGING ANATOMY

General Anatomic Considerations
- Chambers
  - Left ventricle (LV), right ventricle (RV)
  - Left atrium (LA), right atrium (RA)
- Valves
  - Mitral: Bicuspid valve between LA and LV
  - Tricuspid: Between RA and RV
  - Aortic: Three semilunar cusps between LV and aorta
  - Pulmonary: Between RV and PA
- Great vessels
  - Vena cavae: Superior, inferior vena cavae ⇒ RA
  - Pulmonary artery: RV ⇒ lungs
  - Pulmonary veins: Lungs ⇒ LA
  - Aorta: LV ⇒ systemic circulation
- Coronary arteries
  - Left main (LM) ⇒ left anterior descending (LAD), left circumflex (CX)
  - LAD ⇒ septal perforators, diagonal branches
  - CX ⇒ obtuse marginal branches
  - Posterior descending artery (PDA); from right coronary artery (RCA) 85%, CX continuation 15%

Anatomic Relationships
- LAD supplies septum, anterior walls, apex
- CX supplies lateral wall
- PD supplies inferior, inferoseptal walls, apex

CLINICAL PROBLEMS

Coronary Artery Disease: Stress/Rest MPS
- Detection
  - Acute coronary syndrome; acute, chronic angina; atypical chest pain
- Prognosis: Predict probability of cardiac events
- Monitor medical therapy
- Pre-operative evaluation
- Post-coronary artery bypass grafting (CABG)
- Post-myocardial infarction (MI) risk stratification
- Types of stress tests
  - Exercise
    - Preferred in patients without exercise limitations
    - ~ 60% of patients undergoing MPS
    - Contraindicated: Severe aortic stenosis
  - Pharmacologic: Vasodilators
    - Adenosine: Activates adenylate cyclase ⇒ ↓ cAMP, ↓ Ca2+ uptake ⇒ smooth muscle (vascular wall) relaxation; T½ 2 sec; ~ 4 min infusion total
    - Persantine: ↑ Endogenous adenosine; T½ 30-45 min; ~ 7 min infusion total
    - Commonly used with MPS in hospitalized patients (~ 50%)
    - Contraindications: Active asthma, > 1st degree heart block
    - Recommended for patients with pacemakers, left bundle branch block to avoid false (+) on MPS
  - Pharmacologic: Inotrope/chronotropes
    - Dobutamine: β-1 adrenergic agonist; T½ ~ 2 min; infused at increasing doses until target heart rate reached
    - Atropine (anti-muscarinic) commonly used to reach target heart rate
    - Alternative when vasodilator stress contraindicated
    - Contraindications: Arrhythmia, severe aortic stenosis, glaucoma (atropine)

LV Function: RNV (MUGA)
- Cardiotoxic chemotherapy
  - Doxorubicin (Adriamycin) ⇒ oxidative stress, free radical damage to myocytes; fibrosis
  - Dose-dependent (~ 450 mg/m²), yet variable, myotoxicity
  - 2% incidence of heart failure at cumulative doses of ~ 300 mg/m²

CARDIOVASCULAR OVERVIEW

Key Facts

Types of Scans
- Radionuclide ventriculography (RNV)
  - Tc-99m labeled red blood cells
  - Ventricular function
  - Valvular disease
- Myocardial perfusion scintigraphy (MPS)
  - Tl-201, Tc-99m perfusion agents (e.g., tetrofosmin, sestamibi), Rb-82, [N-13]NH4
  - Stress test to diagnose/evaluate coronary artery disease
- Myocardial viability: Tl-201, F-18 FDG
  - Hypoxic yet viable myocardium that would benefit from revascularization
- Research
  - Investigational: Fatty acid, neurotransmitter, receptor imaging

Clinical Scenarios and MPS
- Diabetes mellitus: Diagnose "silent ischemia"; microvascular disease can ⇒ + MPS
- Women: Higher sens/spec than exercise stress
- Morbid obesity
  - MPS often used due to limitations of other modalities
  - Planar imaging if SPECT unachievable
- Pre-operative evaluation
  - Recommended in those with risk factors/signs/symptoms of coronary artery disease
- Acute chest pain
  - Used with clinical history, ECG, laboratory markers to triage patients with chest pain

---

  - Acute (transient) or chronic (progressive LV dysfunction)
  - RNV used due to high accuracy, reproducibility
  - Baseline study, serial studies after/prior to chemo; if clinical change
- Valvular disease
  - First-pass: Stenosis, regurgitation
  - Secondary signs of valvular disease (atrial, ventricular enlargement)
- Cardiomyopathy
  - Ischemic
    - Regional wall motion abnormalities (scar)
  - Nonischemic
    - Diffuse cardiomyopathy (dilated, hypertrophic, restrictive)
- Mental stress ischemia
  - "Broken heart" syndrome; anger/hostility-induced
  - Vascular tone ↑ by sympathetic nervous system, abnormal vasoconstrictor response
  - Can ⇒ reversible perfusion defects, LV dysfunction on MPS

Cardiac Viability: Thallium MPS, FDG PET
- Ischemic vs. nonischemic cardiomyopathy
  - Triage patients appropriately
    - CABG: ~ 15-25% viable (yet underperfused) myocardium
    - CABG: Not useful for patients with > 40% nonviable myocardium
    - Cardiac transplant: Little/no viable myocardium

Valvular Heart Disease: RNV
- Tc-99m labeled red blood cells
- First-pass: Stenosis, regurgitation
- Secondary signs of valvular heart disease (atrial, ventricular enlargement)

CLINICAL SCENARIOS AND MPS

Diabetes Mellitus
- Major risk factor for CAD
- ≤ 20% of diabetic patients with CAD asymptomatic (silent ischemia)
- MPS for diagnosis, prognosis
- Often requires pharmacologic stress 2° comorbidities
- Even with normal coronary arteries, diabetic microvascular endothelial dysfunction can ⇒ + MPS

Women
- CAD leading cause of death in US women
- Exercise ECG stress test in women: 61% sens, 69% spec
- MPS in women: Likely > 83% sens, > 88% spec
- Small heart size may ⇒ false (-) MPS

Morbid Obesity
- Often, other noninvasive tests (echocardiography, MR) unable to be performed due to body habitus
- High rate of false (+) due to soft tissue attenuation
- Many patients also diabetic; microvascular disease can ⇒ perfusion defects in patients with normal coronaries
- Planar MPS if patient too large for SPECT table

Acute Chest Pain
- Emergency department (ED) chest pain evaluation
  - 1/3 presenting with chest pain have cardiac etiology
  - 4-7% with ischemia not admitted to hospital from ED
  - 2-4% with MI missed in ED
- MPS used with clinical history, ECG, laboratory markers to triage patients with chest pain

Operative Risk Assessment
- Evaluate for ischemia, LV function
- Noninvasive stress test recommended in patients with
  - Angina, prior MI, CHF, diabetes
  - Poor functional capacity
  - High-risk surgery: Emergency, prolonged, vascular
- MPS results
  - Very low risk: Normal
  - Low risk: Small fixed or reversible perfusion defects
  - Intermediate risk: Moderate fixed or reversible perfusion defects; small reversible defects with ejection fraction (EF) < 35%

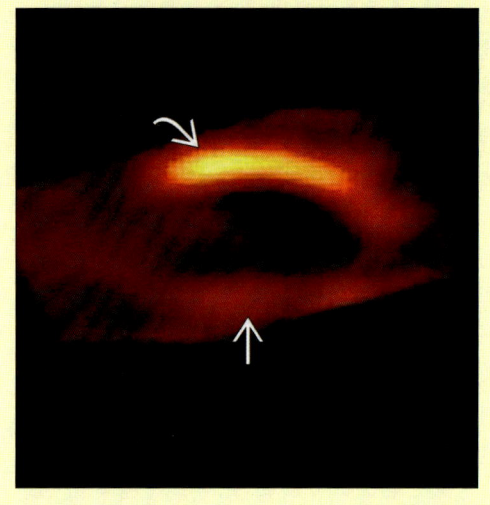

CARDIOVASCULAR OVERVIEW

Vertical long axis MPS shows nearly absent perfusion in inferior wall ➡. Compare this with normal perfusion in anterior wall ➡ (next image).

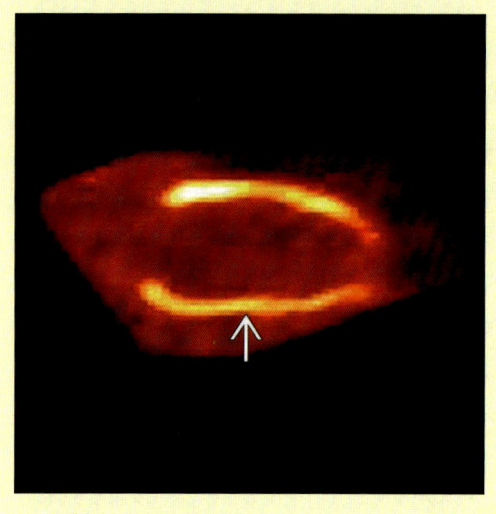

Vertical long axis FDG PET in same patient as previous image shows significant glucose metabolism in inferior wall ➡, signifying underperfused, yet viable myocardium.

- High risk: Moderate fixed or reversible perfusion defects with EF < 35% or diabetes; large reversible perfusion defects

TYPES OF SCANS

Ventricular Function
- RNV, MUGA
  - Tc-99m labeled red blood cells
  - EF, regional wall motion, valvular disease
- Myocardial perfusion scintigraphy SPECT
  - EF, regional wall motion
  - Ventricular volume
  - Tc-99m, Tl-201, Rb-82, [N-13]NH4

Myocardial Perfusion
- Rest and stress studies
- EF, regional wall motion
- Ventricular volume
- Tc-99m, Tl-201, Rb-82, [N-13]NH4

Myocardial Viability
- Tl-201 MPS, FDG PET

Research Imaging Targets
- Angiogenesis, atheromatous plaques, cell death, gene products, hypoxia, inflammation

RADIOPHARMACEUTICALS

Tl-201 Stress Perfusion and Viability
- MPS: Stress and rest (redistribution) SPECT images
  - One dose administered IV at stress: 3 mCi (111 MBq), image at 10 minutes postinjection
  - Rest images: 4 hours postinjection
- Viability: 24 hour image
  - Uptake in myocardium = viability
- Comparison to Tc-99m agents
  - Poorer imaging characteristics (Tl-201 has 69-80 keV = low energy)
  - Tc-99m agents give no viability information

Tc-99m Stress Perfusion Agents
- MPS: Stress and rest SPECT images
  - One dose administered IV at stress: 15-20 mCi (555-740 MBq), image ~ 30 minutes postinjection
  - Second dose administered IV at rest: 30-40 mCi (1.11-1.48 GBq), image ~ 30 minutes postinjection
- Comparison to Tl-201
  - Better imaging characteristics (140 keV)
  - No redistribution of tracer in myocardium (requires 2nd dose of Tc-99m agent)

Tc-99m Labeled Red Blood Cells
- RNV: Gated planar images over heart

PET Perfusion
- PET myocardial perfusion agent
- Improved resolution and attenuation correction vs. SPECT MPS
- Rb-82: On-site generator required
- [N-13]NH4: On-site cyclotron required

F-18 FDG Viability
- Compare to resting perfusion study (SPECT, PET)

Fatty Acid Imaging
- C11-palmitate, I-123-IPPA
- Free fatty acids = primary energy substrate for myocardium in fasting state
- ↓ Myocardial fatty acid uptake ≈ ischemia/hypoxia

Neurotransmission & Receptor
- I-123 MIBG (sympathetic nervous system) SPECT
- Sympathetic/parasympathetic PET tracers

RELATED REFERENCES

1. Klocke FJ et al: ACC/AHA/ASNC guidelines for the clinical use of cardiac radionuclide imaging--executive summary: a report of the American College of Cardiology/American Heart Association Task Force on Practice Guidelines (ACC/AHA/ASNC Committee to Revise the 1995 Guidelines for the Clinical Use of Cardiac Radionuclide Imaging). Circulation. 108(11):1404-18, 2003

CARDIOVASCULAR OVERVIEW

IMAGE GALLERY

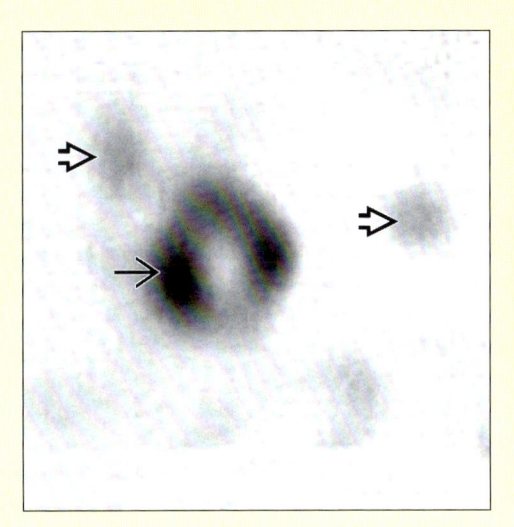

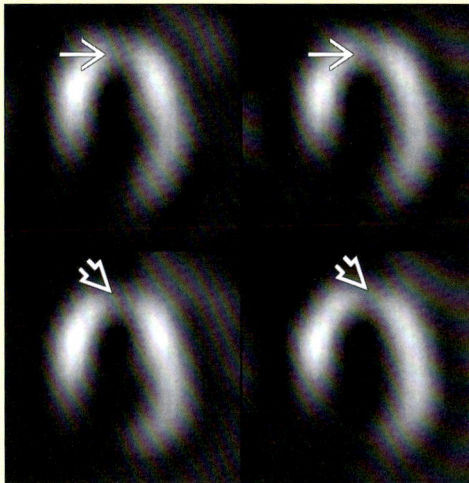

(Left) Short axis MPS shows activity in left ventricle ➡ and in pulmonary renal cell carcinoma metastases ➧. Note: Cardiovascular radiotracers also localize in other benign and malignant entities besides the heart.
(Right) Horizontal long axis MPS shows focally decreased activity in the apex on stress ➡ and rest ➧ images with corresponding normal wall motion, compatible with normal apical thinning (wall motion should be normal).

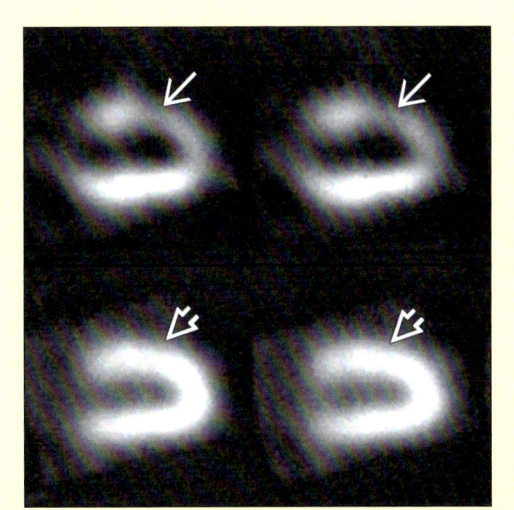

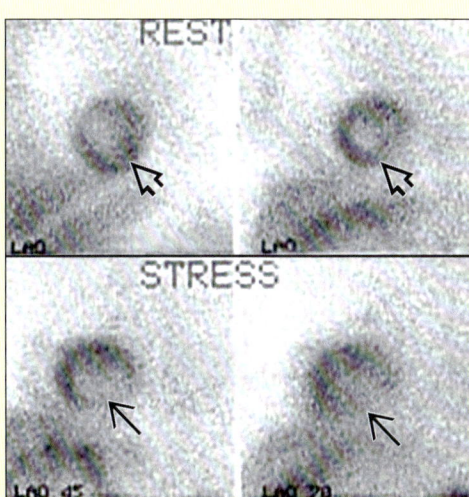

(Left) Vertical long axis MPS shows decreased activity in the anterior wall ➡ on stress that is not evident on rest ➧. This corresponded to an 80% LAD occlusion on cardiac catheterization.
(Right) Planar MPS in morbidly obese patient shows decreased perfusion in the inferior wall on stress ➡ that is not evident on rest ➧, consistent with inducible ischemia.

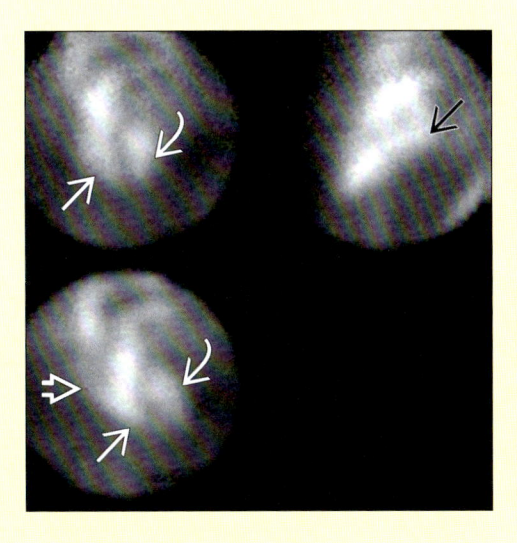

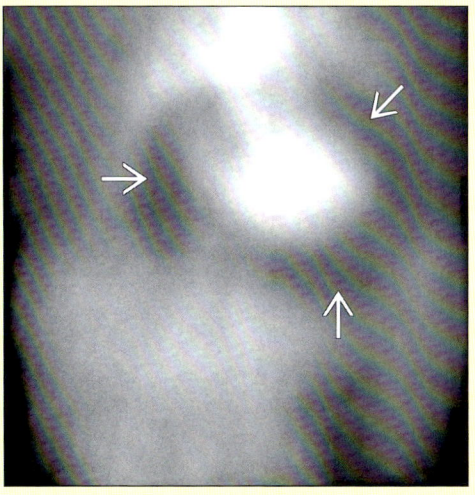

(Left) RNV/MUGA in multiple views shows normal configuration of LA ➡, LV ➡, RA ➧, and RV ➡.
(Right) Anterior RNV/MUGA shows photopenic region ➡ surrounding entire heart in patient with large pericardial effusion.

CARDIOMYOPATHY

Coronal FDG PET demonstrates thickening of left ventricular wall ⊳ and increased endocardial uptake ⇗, consistent with chronic subendocardial ischemia secondary to hypertrophic cardiomyopathy. See next.

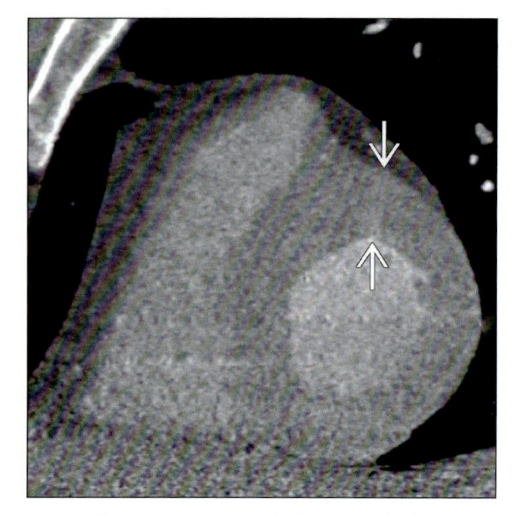

CECT shows concentric thickening of the heart, consistent with hypertrophic cardiomyopathy. Wall thickness ➡ in this case is 1.8 cm.

TERMINOLOGY

Definitions
- Cardiomyopathy: Any disease of myocardium
- Congestive heart failure (CHF): Inadequate circulation causing tissue congestion

IMAGING FINDINGS

General Features
- Best diagnostic clue
  - **Non-ischemic dilated cardiomyopathy (NIDC)**
    - Multi-chamber enlargement, diffuse hypokinesis
    - May show patchy fixed perfusion defects or normal perfusion
    - May occasionally increase left ventricular ejection fraction (LVEF) with exercise
  - **Ischemic dilated cardiomyopathy (IDC)**
    - Stress-induced wall motion abnormalities & drop in LVEF
    - Focal or regional wall motion abnormalities; may also appear similar to NIDC
    - Isolated LV enlargement
    - Focal fixed/reversible perfusion defects
  - **Hypertrophic cardiomyopathy (HC)**
    - Concentric or asymmetric wall thickening (especially septal)
    - Normal to ↑ LVEF
    - ± Abnormal diastolic parameters, patchy perfusion at rest
  - **Restrictive cardiomyopathy (RC)**
    - Abnormal diastolic parameters
    - LVEF variable
    - Diffuse heart uptake on bone scan (hypercalcemia, amyloidosis, heavy metal)

Nuclear Medicine Findings
- Myocardial perfusion scintigraphy (MPS)
  - Ischemia
    - Stress-induced (reversible) perfusion defects
  - Transmural infarction
    - "Fixed" (non-reversible) segmental defects
    - 25% of infarcted regions by MPS may contain viable myocardium: Viability study (FDG PET, Tl-201, MR)
  - Non-transmural infarction
    - Diminished but not absent perfusion, hypokinesis

DDx: Pericardial Disease, Mimics of Cardiomyopathy

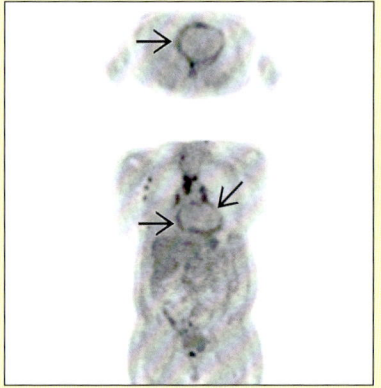

Pericardial Metastases (FDG PET)

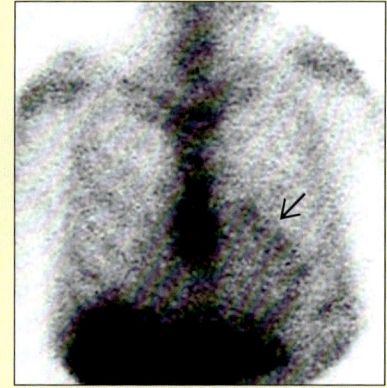

Pericarditis (Ga-67)

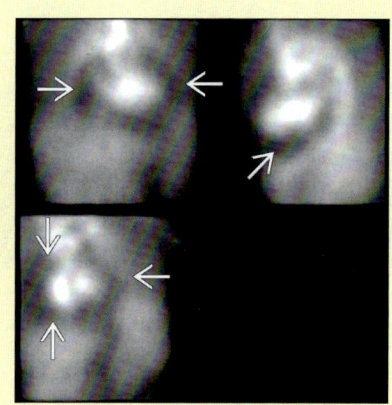

Pericardial Effusion (RNV)

CARDIOMYOPATHY

Key Facts

Imaging Findings
- **Non-ischemic dilated cardiomyopathy (NIDC)**
- Multi-chamber enlargement, diffuse hypokinesis
- May occasionally increase left ventricular ejection fraction (LVEF) with exercise
- **Ischemic dilated cardiomyopathy (IDC)**
- Stress-induced wall motion abnormalities & drop in LVEF
- Isolated LV enlargement
- Focal fixed/reversible perfusion defects
- Concentric or asymmetric wall thickening (especially septal)
- Normal to ↑ LVEF
- **Restrictive cardiomyopathy (RC)**
- Abnormal diastolic parameters
- LVEF variable
- Diffuse heart uptake on bone scan (hypercalcemia, amyloidosis, heavy metal)

Top Differential Diagnoses
- Constrictive Pericardial Disease
- Background Artifacts
- Region of Interest Issues

Diagnostic Checklist
- Technique duplication on serial MUGAs critical
- Prefer Tl-201 > FDG PET for viability testing in patients with type II diabetes mellitus
- Diastolic parameters on RNV to distinguish pericardial constriction from RC
- Gate both rest and stress MPS images to detect apparent volume changes with stress

---

- Hibernating (severely ischemic) myocardium may mimic
  - Fixed perfusion defects
    - Occasionally seen with cardiomyopathy
  - Patchy reversible/fixed defects
    - Diabetes mellitus, small vessel disease
- Radionuclide ventriculography (RNV) = multigated acquisition (MUGA)
  - Focal wall motion abnormality favors ischemic > non-ischemic: But not consistent
  - Chemotherapy-induced cardiomyopathy: Many agents cause, doxorubicin most significant
    - Baseline LVEF < 45%: May be ineligible for chemotherapy
    - May require stopping drug: ↓ LVEF by > 10% units from baseline; ↓ LVEF to < 30% when baseline 30-50%; ↓ LVEF to < 50% when baseline normal
- Abnormal diastolic function: Best assessed with RNV, best used to distinguish pericardial constriction from RC or normal heart
  - Peak LV filling rates
    - Pericardial constriction: 4.23-7.32 EDVs/sec
    - Normal: 2.62-4.45 EDVs/sec
  - First 1/3-1/2 diastolic filling fractions: Constrictive pericarditis > normal > restrictive cardiomyopathy
  - Time to peak filling
    - Pericardial constriction: 110 ± 14 ms
    - RC: 195 ± 45 ms
    - Normal: 173 ± 32 ms
  - Percent atrial contribution to ventricular filling
    - Pericardial constriction: 21 ± 6%
    - RC: 45 ± 17%
    - Normal: 24 ± 9%
  - HC: Abnormal diastolic filling in ~ 20%, may improve with therapy
- PET
  - Rb-82, N-13 ammonia perfusion
    - Stress-induced perfusion defects in ischemia
    - Fixed stress/rest defects in infarction
  - F-18 FDG
    - Diffuse uptake in all chambers in NIDC
    - Uptake in viable myocardium
- Tl-201
  - Stress/rest determinations of ischemia/infarction
  - 24 h imaging for viability

Imaging Recommendations
- Best imaging tool
  - Ventricular morphology: MR
  - Perfusion abnormalities: MPS, PET (Rb-82, [N-13]NH3 PET, Gd-enhanced MR perfusion (gaining acceptance)
  - Coronary artery lesions: Conventional angiography, CTA
  - Valvular assessment: Echocardiography, MR
  - Ventricular function: MUGA, MR, echocardiography
  - Viability: Tl-201 (24 h imaging), FDG PET, MR
  - Diastolic parameters: MUGA, echocardiography, MR
- Protocol advice
  - RNV/MUGA
    - Diastolic parameters: 32-frame acquisition recommended (conventional MUGA typically 16-20 frame)
    - Consistency in ventricular & background regions of interest critical to serial determinations
  - MPS: Gate both rest and stress images to detect apparent volume changes
  - Viability testing: Tl-201 preferred over FDG PET for insulin-resistant diabetes; FDG uptake insulin dependent

DIFFERENTIAL DIAGNOSIS

Constrictive Pericardial Disease
- Thickened or calcified pericardium
- Many causes: Idiopathic, infection, neoplastic, post-surgical, connective tissue disease, trauma, radiation, renal failure, infiltrative, post-MI

Background Artifacts
- Poor RBC tagging ⇒ alters background activity ⇒ inconsistent LVEF calculation
- Background over region with too many counts (e.g., spleen) ⇒ LVEF artificially high

CARDIOMYOPATHY

- Background over region with too few counts (e.g., stomach) ⇒ LVEF artificially low

Region of Interest Issues
- Inconsistent regions of interest on serial MUGAs ⇒ artifactual changes in LVEF

PATHOLOGY

General Features
- Genetics
  - HC: Autosomal dominant with incomplete penetrance
  - Idiopathic dilated cardiomyopathy: Family history positive in ~ 20% of patients; autosomal dominant
  - Arrhythmogenic right ventricular dysplasia (ARVD): Mutations on chromosomes 1 & 14
- Etiology
  - IDC: Atherosclerosis (coronary artery disease), microvascular disease (diabetes)
  - NIDC: Nutritional deficiency, valvular heart disease, anemia, stress, viral, alcohol, idiopathic, cocaine, high output state, chemotherapy
  - HC: Hypertension, aortic stenosis, hypercalcemia, asymmetric septal hypertrophy, genetic abnormality (disordered muscle growth)
  - RC: Amyloid, idiopathic myocardial fibrosis (e.g., heart transplant), sarcoid, hemochromatosis, radiation fibrosis, tumor, endocardial disease
  - Diastolic dysfunction: Idiopathic, post-cardiac surgery, amyloidosis, radiation therapy, hypertension, ischemic cardiac disease
- Epidemiology
  - Dilated cardiomyopathy
    - Prevalence 35 per 100,000
    - Incidence 5-8 cases per 100,000 population per year
  - Chemotherapy-induced cardiomyopathy
    - Cumulative doxorubicin of ≤ 300 mg/m^2 → 2% CHF rate
    - Cumulative dose ≥ 550 mg/m^2 → > 20% CHF rate

Gross Pathologic & Surgical Features
- Patchy involvement of myocardium common: Decreases sensitivity of biopsy
- HC: Plaques in upper interventricular septum, thickening of anterior mitral leaf

Microscopic Features
- RC: Fine interstitial fibrosis
- HC: Myofibrillar disarray, disorganized muscle bundles with whorling & interstitial fibrosis

CLINICAL ISSUES

Presentation
- Most common signs/symptoms
  - Chest pain
  - CHF signs/symptoms (e.g., dyspnea, lower extremity swelling)
- Other signs/symptoms: Abnormal ECG (e.g., anterior Q waves, intraventricular conduction abnormalities, arrhythmias)

Demographics
- Age: 3% to 5% of elderly have CHF
- Gender: M > F

Natural History & Prognosis
- Dilated cardiomyopathy: 50% of deaths sudden (arrhythmias)
- Hypertensive heart failure: 25-30% survival at 5 y
- Chemotherapeutic: Late toxicity can occur > 10 y after drug

Treatment
- Prevention
  - Reduce risk factors: Hypertension, hyperlipidemia, inactivity, obesity, smoking, hyperglycemia
  - Prevent exacerbations: Limit salt, alcohol intake
  - Limit cumulative doxorubicin < 550 mg/m^2; epirubicin < 900 mg/m^2
- Medical: ACE inhibitors, beta blockers, diuretics, vasodilators, digoxin, antiarrhythmics, antithrombogenics
- Interventional: Implantable defibrillator, cardiac resynchronization; myectomy/myotomy for hypertrophic myopathy

DIAGNOSTIC CHECKLIST

Image Interpretation Pearls
- Technique duplication on serial MUGAs critical
- Prefer Tl-201 > FDG PET for viability testing in patients with type II diabetes mellitus
- Diastolic parameters on RNV to distinguish pericardial constriction from RC
  - 32-frame acquisition
- Gate both rest and stress MPS images to detect apparent volume changes with stress

SELECTED REFERENCES

1. Knaapen P et al: Regional heterogeneity of resting perfusion in hypertrophic cardiomyopathy is related to delayed contrast enhancement but not to systolic function: a PET and MRI study. J Nucl Cardiol. 13(5):660-7, 2006
2. Panjrath GS et al: Monitoring chemotherapy-induced cardiotoxicity: Role of cardiac nuclear imaging. J Nucl Cardiol. 13(3):415-426, 2006
3. Bax JJ: Assessment of myocardial viability in ischemic cardiomyopathy. Heart Lung Circ. 14 Suppl 2:S8-13, 2005
4. Le Guludec D et al: Imaging inflammatory cardiomyopathies. J Nucl Cardiol. 12(6):731-9, 2005
5. Wachtell K et al: Change in diastolic left ventricular filling after one year of antihypertensive treatment: The Losartan Intervention For Endpoint Reduction in Hypertension (LIFE) Study. Circulation. 105(9):1071-6, 2002
6. Aroney CN et al: Differentiation of restrictive cardiomyopathy from pericardial constriction: assessment of diastolic function by radionuclide angiography. J Am Coll Cardiol. 13(5):1007-14, 1989

CARDIOMYOPATHY

IMAGE GALLERY

Typical

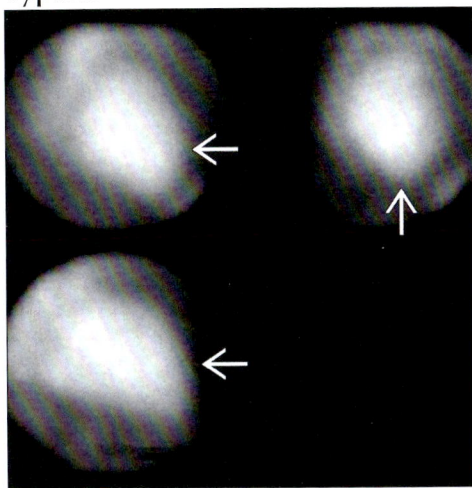

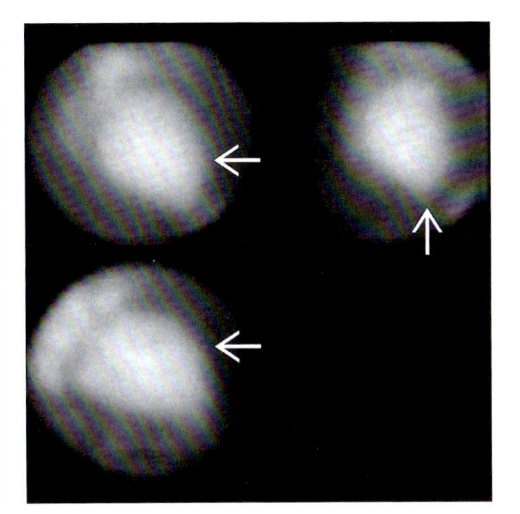

(Left) Multi-plane end-diastolic RNV shows isolated, massive enlargement of left ventricle ➡. See next image. *(Right)* Multi-plane end-systolic RNV in same patient at left shows isolated, massive enlargement of left ventricle ➡ with little change from end-diastolic images. This patient had previous occlusion of left main coronary artery, resulting in ischemic cardiomyopathy.

Typical

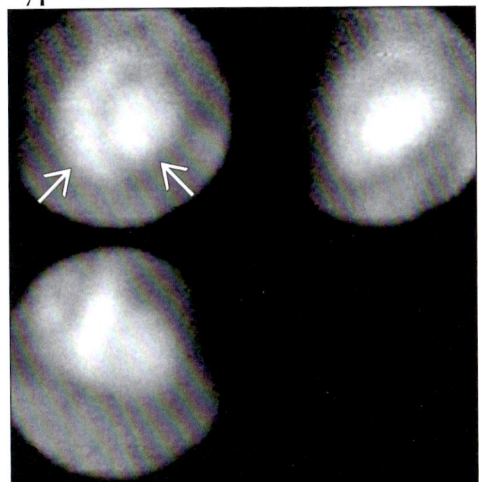

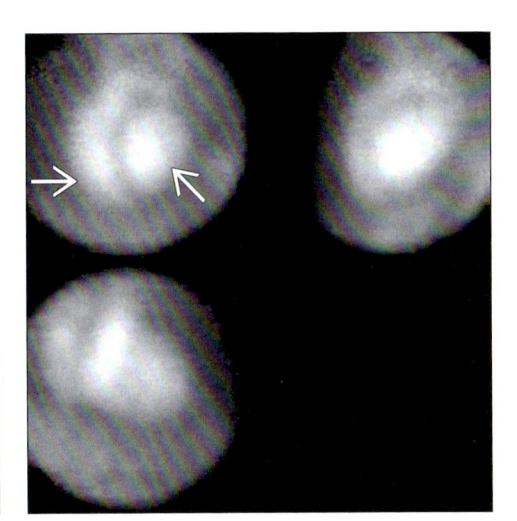

(Left) Multi-plane end-diastolic RNV shows diffuse biventricular enlargement ➡. See next image. *(Right)* Multi-plane end-systolic RNV in same patient at left shows biventricular enlargement ➡, diffuse hypokinesis, & little change from end-diastolic images in patient with idiopathic dilated cardiomyopathy.

Typical

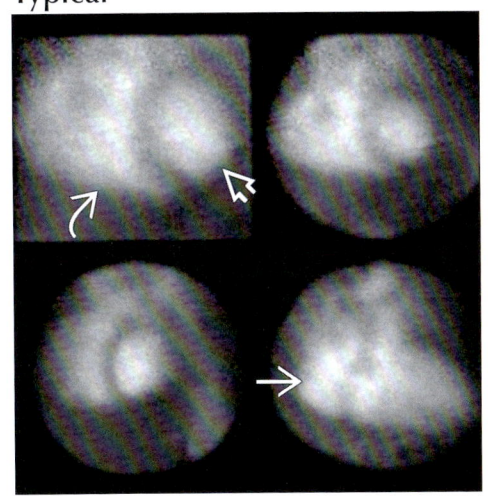

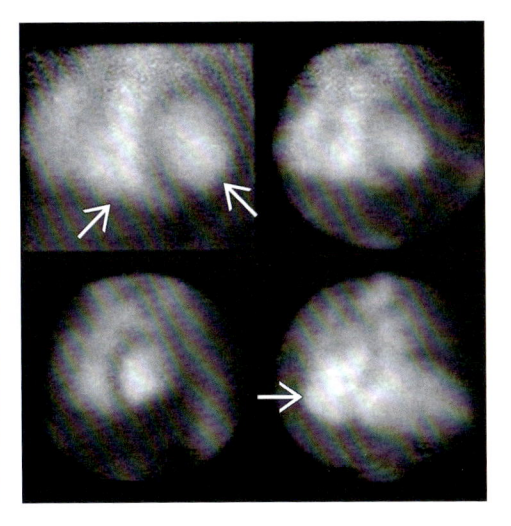

(Left) Multi-plane end-diastolic RNV shows marked enlargement of right atrium ➡, right ventricle ➡, and left ventricle ➡. See next image. *(Right)* Multi-plane end-systolic RNV in same patient at left shows marked multichamber enlargement ➡, diffuse hypokinesis & little change in ventricular volumes compared to end-diastolic images in patient with viral-induced cardiomyopathy.

CARDIOMYOPATHY

Variant

(Left) Multi-plane end-diastolic RNV shows marked enlargement of right atrium ➡ and left atrium ➡. See next image. (Right) Multi-plane end-systolic RNV in same patient at left shows marked enlargement of right atrium ➡ and left atrium ➡, slightly increased LVEF (70%) due to severe tricuspid and mitral insufficiency.

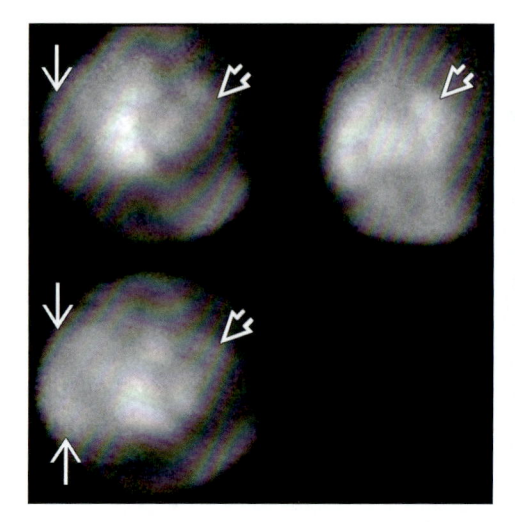

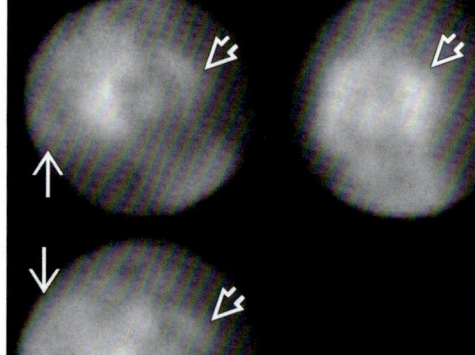

Variant

(Left) LAO RNV shows massive enlargement of right ventricle ➡ and pulmonary outflow tract ➡ in patient with chronic pulmonary embolism. See next image. (Right) Sagittal CECT shows right ventricular hypertrophy ➡ with dilation of pulmonary outflow tract ➡ due to severe pulmonary hypertension.

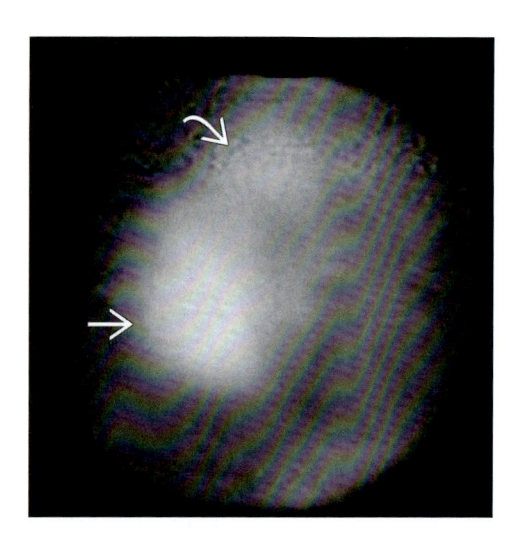

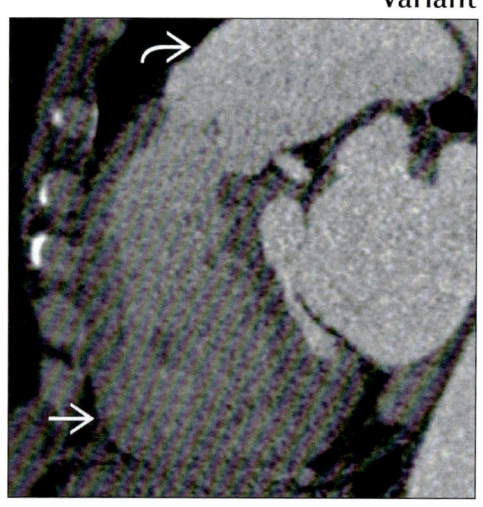

Typical

(Left) Myocardial perfusion scintigraphy shows ischemic cardiomyopathy with a dilated left ventricle, an inferior wall infarction ➡, and apical ischemia ➡. (Right) End-diastole ➡ and end-systole ➡ LAO RNV frames after two cycles of doxorubicin shows mild left ventricular enlargement and low LVEF (38%). Pre-chemo LVEF was 60%. Doxorubicin was not continued.

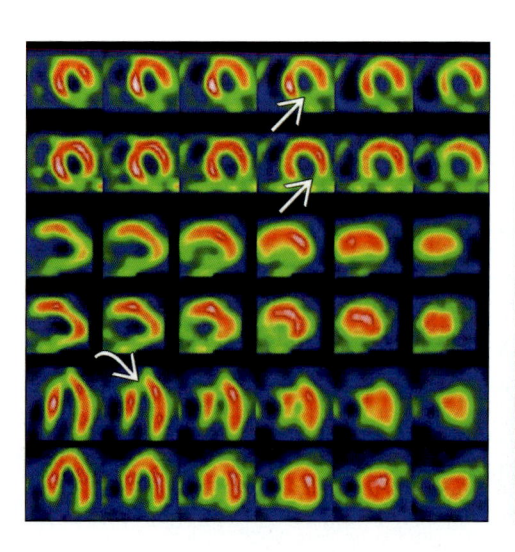

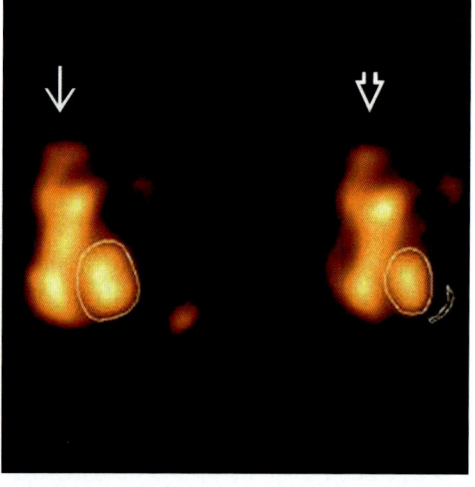

CARDIOMYOPATHY

Variant

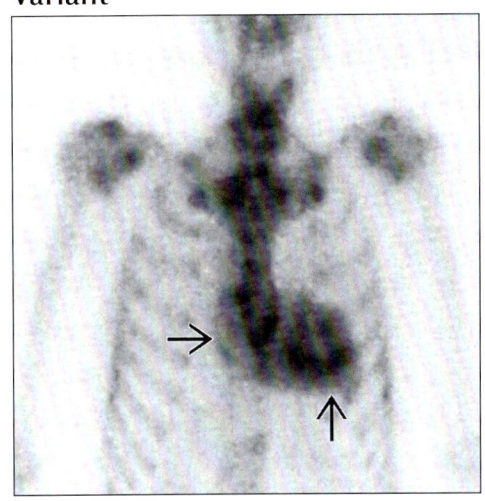

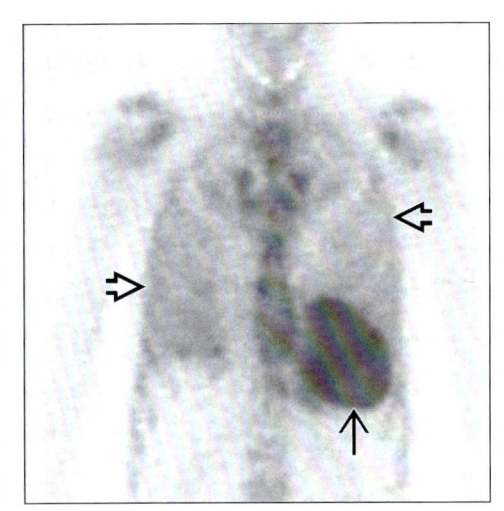

(Left) Anterior planar Tc-99m MDP bone scan shows diffuse uptake in both chambers of the heart ➡ in patient with restrictive cardiomyopathy due to amyloidosis. *(Right)* Anterior planar Tc-99m MDP bone scan shows uptake in heart ➡ and in lungs ▷ in patient with cardiomyopathy due to hypercalcemia (secondary hyperparathyroidism).

Typical

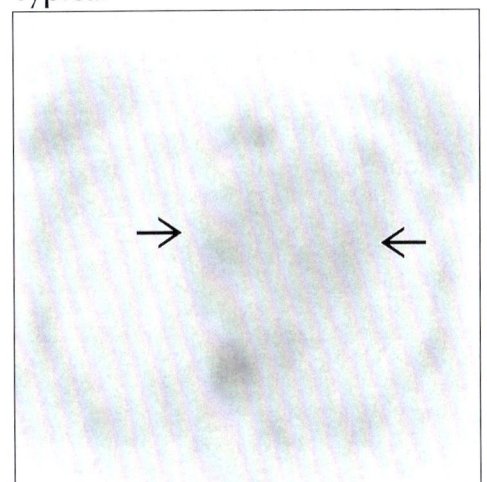

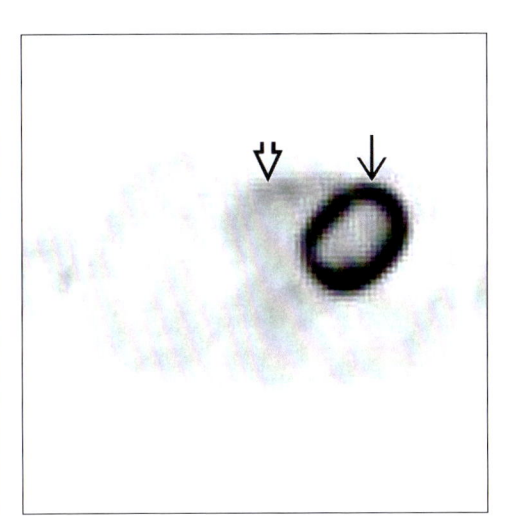

(Left) Axial FDG PET in patient after 12 h of fasting shows minimal blood pool ➡. Absence of myocardial activity is due to low-insulin state. *(Right)* Axial FDG PET in non-fasting patient shows uptake in left ventricle ➡, but little RV activity ▷. This is a normal pattern when insulin is present.

Variant

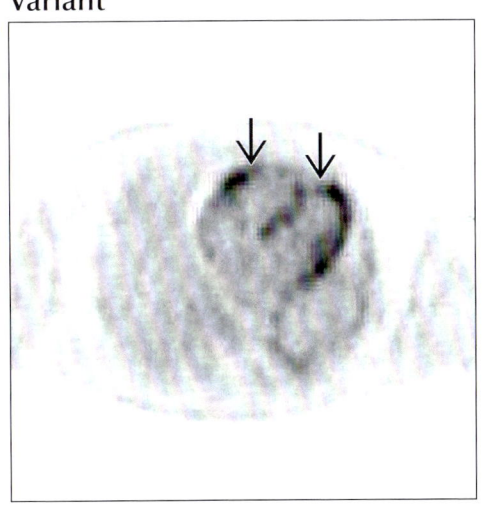

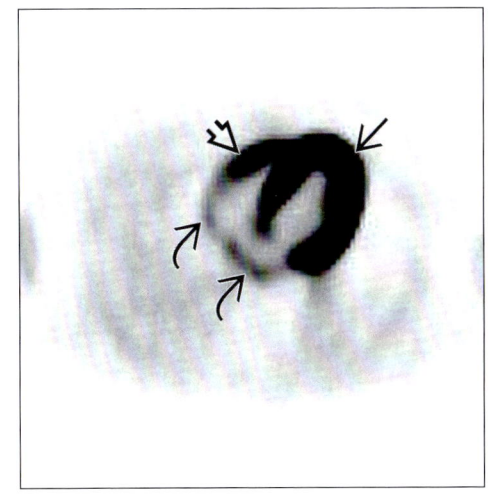

(Left) Axial FDG PET in non-fasting patient with type II diabetes mellitus shows very poor, patchy uptake in both ventricles ➡. This is a typical pattern with insulin resistance due to type II diabetes. *(Right)* Axial FDG PET in fasting patient with non-ischemic cardiomyopathy shows diffuse uptake in right ▷ and left ➡ ventricles, as well as both atria ➡. Typical pattern in non-ischemic cardiomyopathy, possibly from impaired fatty acid utilization.

VALVULAR HEART DISEASE

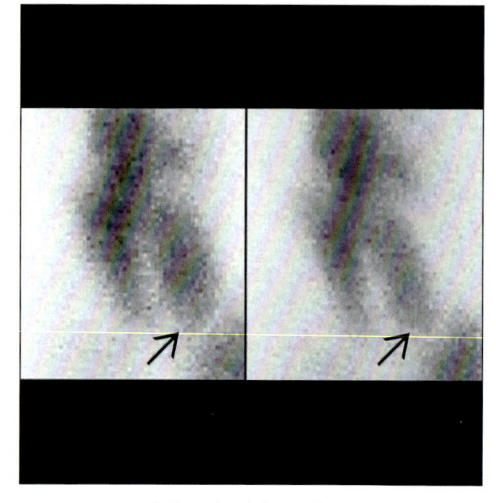

Severe AR: End-diastole (left) and end-systole (right) images from RNV show "wind-sock" elongated LV with bulbous, dyskinetic apex, which mimics apical aneurysm.

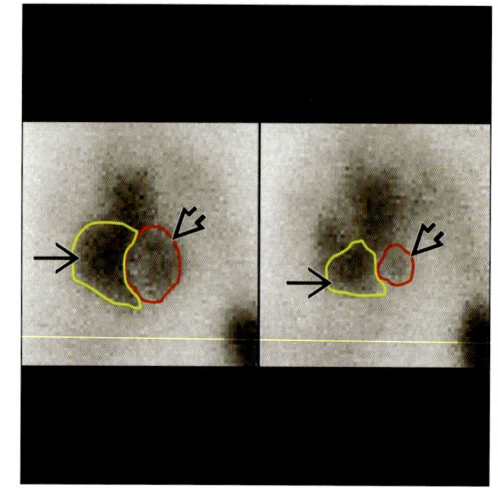

End-diastole (left) and end-systole (right) images from RNV show regions of interest for measuring LV and RV stroke volumes.

TERMINOLOGY

Abbreviations and Synonyms
- Synonyms for radionuclide ventriculography (RNV): Multigated acquisition (MUGA), equilibrium radionuclide angiography (ERNA)
- Myocardial perfusion scintigraphy (MPS)
- Functional parameters: Ejection fraction (EF), stroke volume (SV), stroke volume index (SVI)
- Aortic regurgitation/stenosis (AR, AS)
- Pulmonic regurgitation/stenosis (PR, PS)
- Mitral regurgitation/stenosis (MR, MS),
- Tricuspid regurgitation/stenosis (TR, TS) pulmonic regurgitation (PR)
- Chambers: Left ventricle (LV), right ventricle (RV), left atrium (LA), right atrium (RA)
- Increased chamber volume: LA, RA or ventricular enlargement/dilatation (LAE, RAE, LVE, RVE)
- Increased wall thickness: Left ventricular hypertrophy (LVH), right ventricular hypertrophy (RVH)
- End-diastole (ED), end-systole (ES)

Definitions
- Valvular stenosis: Narrowing of valve resulting in elevated systolic pressure and chamber hypertrophy
- Valvular regurgitation: Valvular insufficiency resulting in backflow during diastole; chamber dilation
- Valvular heart disease: Stenosis, regurgitation/insufficiency, or failure of any one or more of four heart valves

IMAGING FINDINGS

General Features
- Best diagnostic clue
  - Echocardiography: 1st line in valvular disease
    - Characteristic findings in valvular anatomy/area, gradients, directional blood flow, chamber size and function
- Location
  - May affect any or all cardiac chambers
  - AS: Concentric LVH
  - AR: Eccentric occurring with concentric cardiac hypertrophy
  - MS: RVE

DDx: LV Aneurysms Mimic Valvular Regurgitation

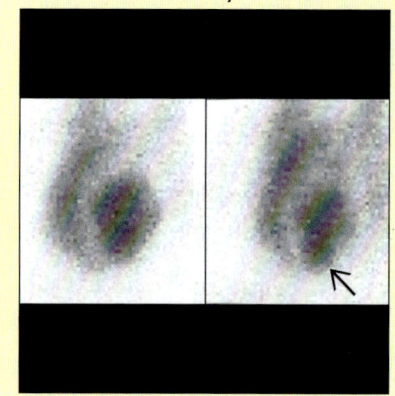

Apical Aneurysm: Mimics AR

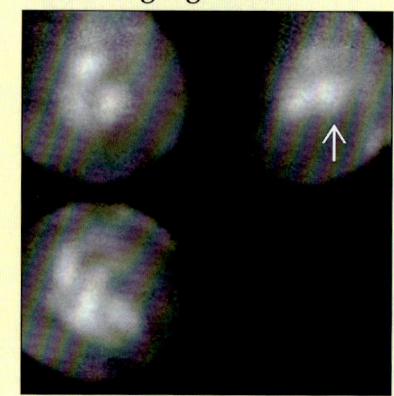

Post LV Aneurysm (ED): Mimics LAE

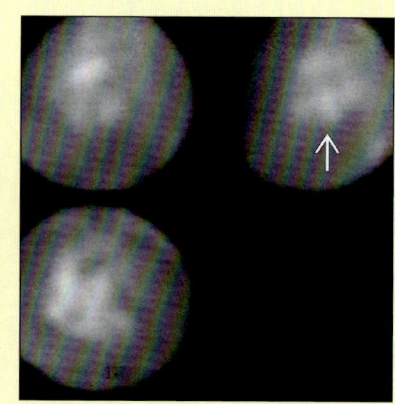

Post LV Aneurysm (ES): Mimics LAE

VALVULAR HEART DISEASE

Key Facts

Terminology
- Valvular stenosis: Narrowing of valve resulting in elevated systolic pressure and chamber hypertrophy
- Valvular regurgitation: Valvular insufficiency resulting in backflow during diastole; chamber dilation

Imaging Findings
- LVEF normal: 50-60% by RNV
- AR and MR: LVEF usually ↑ (> 65%) unless concurrent ventricular failure
- Stress-induced ↓ in EF more sensitive for valvular-induced ventricular failure than resting EF: Also seen with ischemia
- Stroke volume (SV): ED-ES; measurement of regurgitant index from LV and RV
- Normal SVI (LVSV/RVSV) = 1
- Because of contribution of RA to RV counts, normal SVI range is 1-1.7
- SVI > 1.7 suggests AR or MR
- SVI < 1 suggests PR or TR
- SVI: More accurate in detecting than in quantifying degree of regurgitation
- SVI: Inaccurate when ventricular failure present
- Echocardiography: 1st line modality for valvular anatomy/area, gradients, blood flow

Top Differential Diagnoses
- Myocardial Wall Thickening
- Left Ventricular Aneurysms
- Ventricular Failure
- Pulmonary Artery Hypertension (PAH)

  ○ MR: LAE, eccentric cardiac hypertrophy

Nuclear Medicine Findings
- RNV
  ○ Chamber dilatation with regurgitation: Ventricular volume measurements less accurate than CT, MR, echocardiography
    ▪ MPS: Artifactually decreases volume measurements with small heart, obesity, tachycardia, motion
    ▪ RNV: Attenuation confounds determinations of ventricular volumes
  ○ Myocardial wall hypertrophy (stenosis): Nuclear techniques often inaccurate for wall thickness
  ○ MPS: Also allows assessment of ischemia
- Ventricular ejection fraction (EF): (ED-ES)/ES; measurement of contraction of LV and RV
  ○ LVEF normal: 50-60% by RNV
    ▪ LVEF measurements: LAO projection by RNV; Δ volumes on gated MPS
  ○ RVEF normal: 55-65% by (equilibrium) RNV due to technical problems, not physiology
    ▪ First-pass technique more accurate for RVEF: Gated or rapid dynamic imaging
  ○ AR and MR: LVEF usually ↑ (> 65%) unless concurrent ventricular failure
  ○ Stress-induced ↓ in EF more sensitive for valvular-induced ventricular failure than resting EF: Also seen with ischemia
- Stroke volume (SV): ED-ES; measurement of regurgitant index from LV and RV
  ○ Stroke volume index (SVI): LVSV/RVSV
    ▪ SVI: Measured on LAO projection on RNV; regions of interest (ROI) around LV and RV for end-systole, end-diastole
    ▪ Normal SVI (LVSV/RVSV) = 1
    ▪ Because of contribution of RA to RV counts, normal SVI range is 1-1.7
    ▪ SVI > 1.7 suggests AR or MR
    ▪ SVI < 1 suggests PR or TR
    ▪ SVI: More accurate in detecting than in quantifying degree of regurgitation
    ▪ SVI: Inaccurate when ventricular failure present

Imaging Recommendations
- Best imaging tool
  ○ Echocardiography: 1st line modality for valvular anatomy/area, gradients, blood flow
    ▪ Transesophageal echocardiography: Defines mechanism of mitral regurgitation, excludes LA thrombus
    ▪ Stress echo: Stress-induced changes more significant than at rest in many patients
  ○ MR: Improved techniques, equipment increasing role in valvular disease
    ▪ Severity of regurgitant, stenotic lesions: Combination of cine gradient echo MR, steady-state free precession, cine-phase contrast
    ▪ Dynamic MR = standard of reference in evaluation of ventricular function: Critical in timing valve replacement
  ○ Fast/cine cardiac CT: Allows detailed visualization of cardiac valves, calcification, vegetations, chamber anatomy, wall motion
  ○ RNV: Excellent for serial measurements of LVEF, SVI, but largely replaced by other modalities for valvular disease
- Protocol advice
  ○ Radionuclide ventriculography (RNV)
    ▪ In-vitro labeling results in a higher tagging efficiency of red blood cells
    ▪ Withdraw and re-inject blood using a 21-gauge or larger bore catheter to minimize cell destruction
    ▪ Image with a caudal tilt in LAO view, minimum frames/cycle = 16

DIFFERENTIAL DIAGNOSIS

Myocardial Wall Thickening
- Systemic hypertension: Concentric LV hypertrophy mimics that of AS

Left Ventricular Aneurysms
- Posterior wall aneurysm mimics enlargement of left atrium due to MR

VALVULAR HEART DISEASE

- Apical aneurysm mimics dilatation of apex due to AR

Ventricular Failure
- May mask valvular regurgitation as identified by SVI

Pulmonary Artery Hypertension (PAH)
- May result in RAE: Mimic TR

PATHOLOGY

General Features
- Genetics: Death from valvular diseases appears familial, suggesting genetic link
- Etiology
  - AR
    - Aortic root dilation: Idiopathic in > 80% of cases; also secondary to aging and hypertension
    - Inflammatory retraction of valve cusps: Endocarditis, rheumatic fever, collagen vascular disease
    - Fenfluramine/dexfenfluramine
  - AS: Congenital anomalies, bicuspid aortic valve, rheumatic fever, age-related calcification
  - PR: Dilated cardiomyopathy, pulmonary hypertension
  - PS: Congenital
  - MR: Myxomatous degeneration, papillary muscle dysfunction, ruptured chordae tendinea, rheumatic fever, fenfluramine/dexfenfluramine
  - MS: Rheumatic fever
  - TR: Pulmonary hypertension, RV outflow obstruction, infective endocarditis, papillary muscle dysfunction, blunt trauma, Ebstein anomaly
  - TS: Rheumatic fever, usually associated with a dominant MS
- Epidemiology
  - Primary cause of death: 20,000/yr in US
  - Contributing cause of death: 42,000/yr in US
  - Aortic valve disease: 63% of valvular deaths
  - Mitral valve disease: 14% of valvular deaths

Gross Pathologic & Surgical Features
- Concentric hypertrophy from early aortic stenosis; later, ventricular dilation and failure occurs
- Eccentric hypertrophy from regurgitant fraction in aortic insufficiency

CLINICAL ISSUES

Presentation
- Most common signs/symptoms
  - Decrease in exercise tolerance due to congestive heart failure (CHF)
  - Peripheral edema from CHF
  - Dyspnea from pulmonary edema
  - Neurologic deficits from embolic events
  - Fever from endocarditis
  - Syncope from AS
- Other signs/symptoms: Cardiac murmurs, abnormal electrocardiogram, cardiomegaly, pulmonary congestion

Demographics
- Age: Bimodal: Congenital defects in pediatric population; acquired disease in elderly
- Gender
  - Valvular disease of particular concern in pregnancy
    - Blood volume increase → acute CHF

Natural History & Prognosis
- Prognosis highly dependent upon LVEF
- RNV: Accurate, reproducible measurement of LVEF; guides therapy

Treatment
- Treatment goal: Maintain ventricular function, LVEF
- Pharmacologic: ACE inhibitors, antiarrhythmics, antibiotic prophylaxis, anticoagulants, beta blockers, diuretics
- Surgical: Valvuloplasty, repair, replacement
- Lifestyle: Reasonably active lifestyle should be maintained

DIAGNOSTIC CHECKLIST

Consider
- AR and MR: LVEF usually ↑ (> 65%) unless concurrent ventricular failure
- Calculate SVI when LVEF > 65% (AR or MR may be present)
- Stress-induced ↓ in EF more sensitive for valvular-induced ventricular failure than resting EF: Also seen with ischemia
- MPS: Artifactually decreases volume measurements with small heart, obesity, tachycardia, motion
- RNV: Attenuation confounds determinations of ventricular volumes

SELECTED REFERENCES

1. Cannistra AJ: Adult valvular heart disease: a practical approach. Prim Care. 32(4):1109-14, ix, 2005
2. El-Maghraby TA et al: Clinical relevance of left ventricular volumes and function assessed by gated SPECT in paediatric patients. Int J Cardiovasc Imaging. 20(2):127-34, 2004
3. Horne BD et al: Evidence for a heritable component in death resulting from aortic and mitral valve diseases. Circulation. 110(19):3143-8, 2004
4. Patsilinakos SP et al: Adenosine stress myocardial perfusion tomographic imaging in patients with significant aortic stenosis. J Nucl Cardiol. 11(1):20-5, 2004
5. Carabello B: Pathophysiology of valvular heart disease: implications for nuclear imaging. J Nucl Cardiol. 9(1):104-13, 2002
6. Shipton B et al: Valvular heart disease: review and update. Am Fam Physician. 63(11):2201-8, 2001
7. Shi R et al: The value of 99mTc-MIBI myocardial perfusion spect imaging in detecting coronary artery disease in patients with valvular disease before operation. Chin Med Sci J. 15(1):64-6, 2000
8. Nicod P et al: Radionuclide techniques for valvular regurgitant index: comparison in patients with normal and depressed ventricular function. J Nucl Med. 23(9):763-9, 1982

VALVULAR HEART DISEASE

IMAGE GALLERY

Typical

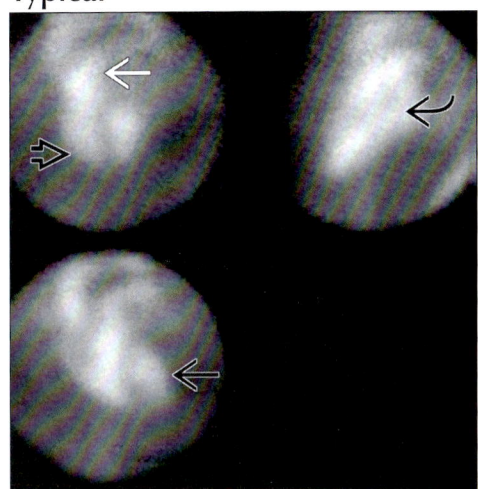

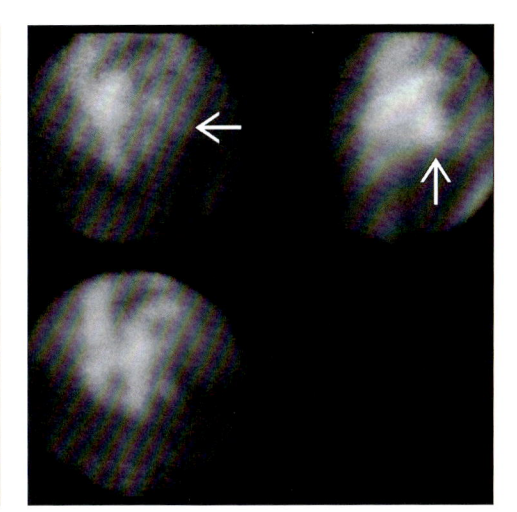

(Left) Multi-projection end-diastole frames from RNV shows normal configuration of 4 chambers of the heart: Right atrium ➡, right ventricle ➡, left atrium ➡, left ventricle ➡. (Right) Multi-projection end-systole frames from RNV shows enlargement of the left atrium ➡ due to mitral valve disease.

Typical

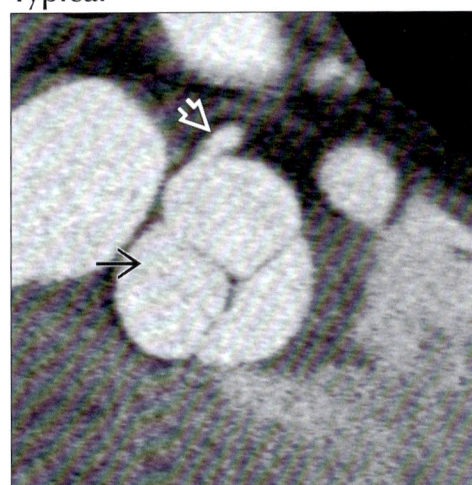

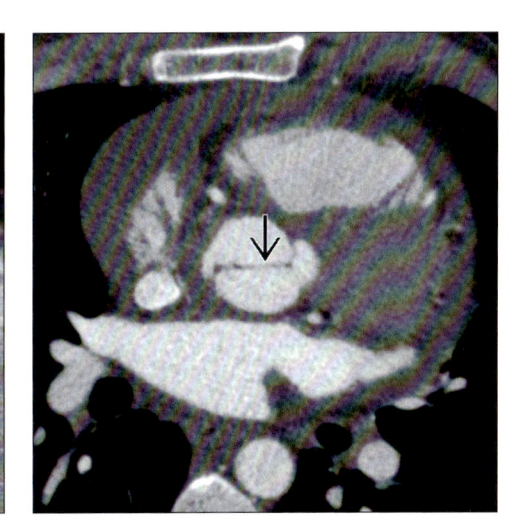

(Left) Axial CECT shows a normal three-leaflet aortic valve ➡. Note the left main coronary artery ➡, with its origin off the left aortic valve cusp. (Right) Axial CECT shows a two-leaflet (bicuspid) aortic valve ➡, a congenital defect that can cause aortic stenosis.

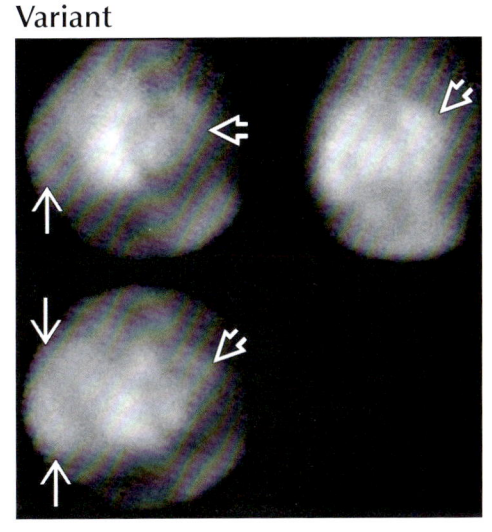

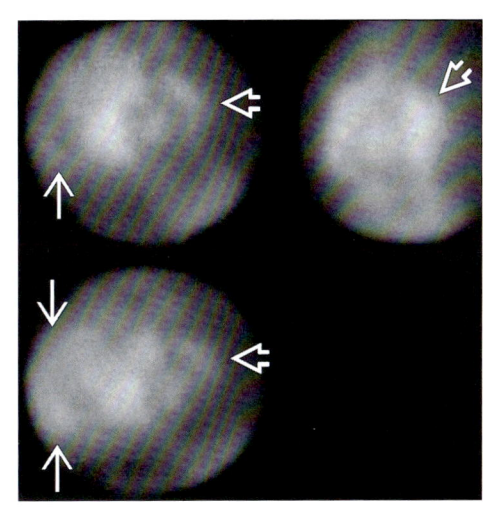

Variant

(Left) Multi-projection end-diastole frames from RNV show massive enlargement of right ➡ and left atria ➡. See next image. (Right) Multi-projection end-systole frames from RNV in same patient at left accentuate massive enlargement of right ➡ and left atria ➡ in patient with severe TR and MR 2° to rheumatic heart disease.

MYOCARDIAL ISCHEMIA

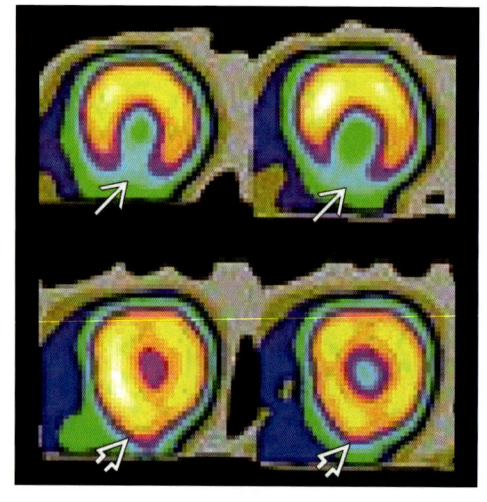

Short axis Rb-82 PET perfusion shows inferior perfusion defect on stress ➡, which is not evident on rest images ➡. This is consistent with inferior wall ischemia.

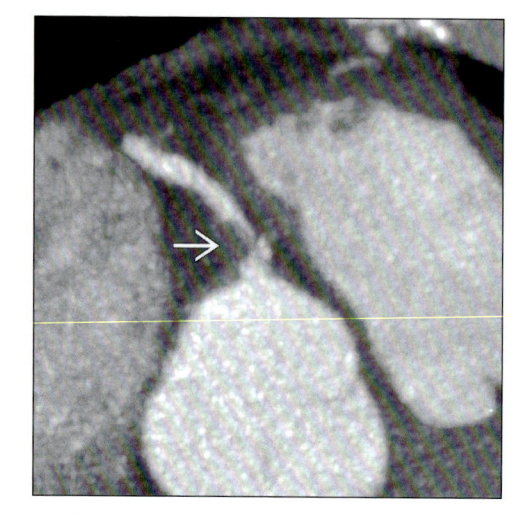

Axial CECT of same patient as left shows soft plaque ➡ in proximal right coronary artery causing > 90% stenosis. (Courtesy C. Newton, MD, FACC).

TERMINOLOGY

Abbreviations and Synonyms
- Ischemic heart disease (IHD); coronary artery disease (CAD)

Definitions
- Ischemia: Inadequate oxygen supply to an organ

IMAGING FINDINGS

General Features
- Best diagnostic clue
  - Reversible myocardial perfusion defect
    - < 5% of myocardium: Low risk (~ 1% annualized risk of hard cardiac event)
    - 5-10% of myocardium: Intermediate risk (~ 1-3% annualized risk of hard cardiac event)
    - > 10% of myocardium: High risk (> 3% annualized risk of hard cardiac event)
  - Transient ischemic dilatation (TID): High-risk variable; predictor of serious cardiac event
- Size
  - Regional ischemia (single or double vessel disease)
  - Diffuse (triple vessel or left main disease)

Nuclear Medicine Findings
- Myocardial perfusion scintigraphy (MPS)
  - Reversible perfusion defect, worse on stress: Ischemia
  - Fixed perfusion defect with associated wall motion abnormalities: Infarction
- TID: Multivessel or left main disease, subendocardial ischemia: Decreased subendocardial perfusion and apparent dilation
- Decreased ventricular function post-stress compared to rest: Ventricular stunning due to extensive ischemia; more commonly when imaged at time of stress, e.g., Tl-201, Rb-82
- Tc-99m agents (tetrofosmin, sestamibi): No redistribution for several hours
- Tl-201: Rapid redistribution (minutes); lung-heart ratio of > 0.5 is poor prognostic sign (stress-induced ventricular dysfunction)
- PET perfusion imaging: Quantification of absolute myocardial blood flow

DDx: Non-Ischemic Abnormalities on Myocardial Perfusion Scintigraphy

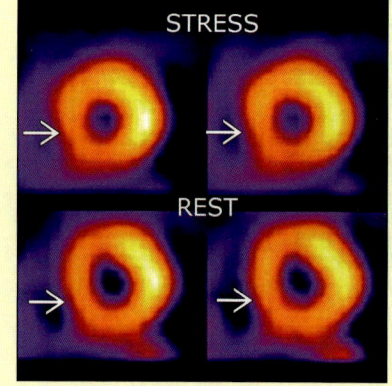

LBBB: Septal ↓

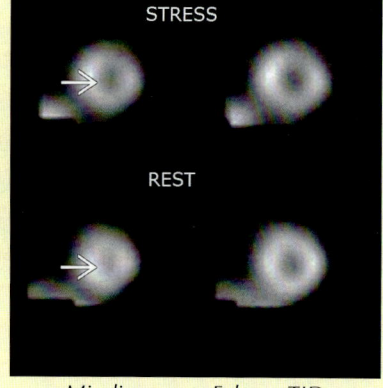

Misalignment: False + TID

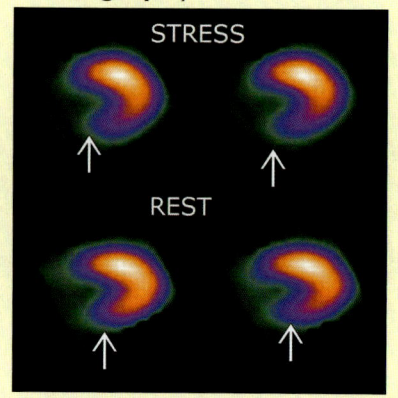

Soft Tissue Attenuation: Diaphragm

MYOCARDIAL ISCHEMIA

Key Facts

Imaging Findings
- Reversible perfusion defect, worse on stress: Ischemia
- Fixed perfusion defect with associated wall motion abnormalities: Infarction
- TID: Multivessel or left main disease, subendocardial ischemia: Decreased subendocardial perfusion and apparent dilation
- Decreased ventricular function post-stress compared to rest: Ventricular stunning due to extensive ischemia; more commonly when imaged at time of stress, e.g., Tl-201, Rb-82
- Tc-99m agents (tetrofosmin, sestamibi): No redistribution for several hours
- Tl-201: Rapid redistribution (minutes); lung-heart ratio of > 0.5 is poor prognostic sign (stress-induced ventricular dysfunction)
- PET perfusion imaging: Quantification of absolute myocardial blood flow

Top Differential Diagnoses
- Artifacts
- Microvascular Coronary Disease
- Balanced Ischemia
- Left Bundle Branch Block

Clinical Issues
- Age: 1:2 men, 1:3 women > age 40 have CAD
- Gender: Average age of first heart attack: 65.8 y in men and 70.4 y in women
- Annual mortality: 2-3% in patients with recent onset exertional angina
- Untreated unstable angina: 30% risk of hard cardiac event ≤ 3 months

Imaging Recommendations
- Best imaging tool
  - MPS: Moderate risk factors (optimize post-test probability of CAD)
  - Angiography, CT angiography: High-risk patients
- Protocol advice
  - Patient preparation: Withhold cardiac meds if no known CAD; may scan on meds to evaluate efficacy of drugs
  - For MPS, quality control critical: Center of rotation, patient motion, detector uniformity, energy and tomographic uniformity
  - Tc-99m sestamibi, tetrofosmin
    - Rest: 8-15 mCi (300-550 MBq); image 30-45 min post-injection
    - Stress, 1-day protocol: 25-35 mCi (925-1295 MBq); image 15 min after exercise, 45 min after vasodilator stress
    - Stress, 2-day protocol: 8-15 mCi (300-550 MBq); image 15 min after exercise, 45 min after vasodilator stress
    - SPECT imaging optimal; planar if patient morbidly obese
  - Tl-201
    - Stress: 3-3.5 mCi (111-129 MBq), image immediately
    - Redistribution: Image ~ 4 h after stress [0.5-1 mCi (19-37 MB)] may be given 15 min prior to imaging
  - Combination Tl-201 (inject 15 min prior to stress), Tc-99m agent (stress injection)
    - Dual isotope imaging; rapid throughput; cannot compare ventricular volumes
  - Imaging: Gate both rest and stress studies to evaluate ventricular volumes
  - Planar vs SPECT imaging: Sensitivity similar to SPECT but ↓ specificity
  - Image processing: Use standard filters (e.g., Butterworth 0.16 frequency and order of 10); set intensity levels independently for each acquisition
  - Scan interpretation: View images in continuous color scale
  - Quantitative, semiquantitative programs: Polar map, bullseye, washout (planar), quantitative SPECT comparing perfusion to gender-matched normals
- Stress protocols: Severe complications ~ 5 of 10,000 patients in hospital setting
  - Exercise: Treadmill
    - Target heart rate (HR): 85% of predicted maximum [(220 - age) x 0.85]
    - Contraindications: Severe aortic stenosis, left bundle branch block (LBBB), severe hypertension, unstable or recent severe cardiac event
  - Pharmacologic stress: Vasodilators
    - Dipyridamole: 0.142 mg/kg/min x 4 min
    - Adenosine: 140 µg/kg/min x 6 min
    - Side effects: Headache, dyspnea, nausea, hypotension, anxiety, arrhythmias; Rx: 75-225 mg aminophylline IV usually reverses
    - Contraindications: Pulmonary disease; 2nd or 3rd degree AV block (without pacemaker); caffeine within 12 h; unstable or recent cardiac event
  - Pharmacologic stress: Chronotrope/inotrope
    - Dobutamine: 5 µg/kg/min increasing to 10, 20, 30 and 40 µg/kg/min at 3 minute intervals, as required, to achieve target heart rate
    - Atropine: 0.5 to 1.0 mg IV in 0.1-0.2 mg increments if HR suboptimal with dobutamine
    - Side effects: Arrhythmias, nausea, nervousness; atropine causes difficult urination; Rx: stop dobutamine, give beta blockers
    - Contraindications: Same as for exercise
- PET perfusion scanning: Separate rest, stress injections
  - Rb-82: Generator produced; T½ = 75 sec; typical total dose = 60 mCi (2220 MBq)
  - N-13 ammonia: Cyclotron produced; T½ = 10 min; typical dose = 20 mCi (740 MBq)
  - PET advantages over SPECT: Routine attenuation correction; ↑ resolution; ↑ contrast (higher photon flux); ↓ patient radiation; accuracy for CAD: ~ 95% (PET) vs. ~ 85% (SPECT); high throughput
  - PET disadvantages: Exercise stress difficult; Rb-82 generators expensive; N-13 ammonia labor intensive (cyclotron); reimbursement similar to SPECT

MYOCARDIAL ISCHEMIA

- Reporting findings
  - Raw images: Artifacts (if any), extracardiac activity, lung-heart ratio (Tl-201), overall scan quality
  - Perfusion images: Fixed or reversible perfusion defects; extent and severity of defects; TID; appearance of right ventricle (Tl-201)
  - Functional images: Wall motion, wall thickening, ejection fraction, left ventricular volumes
  - Type and adequacy of stress
- Reporting conclusions
  - Perfusion images: Positive or negative for inducible ischemia (reversibility, severity, extent), presence of myocardial infarction
  - Gated images: Wall motion, LVEF, LV end diastolic volume, differences between stress & rest
  - Other: Extracardiac findings, limitations of study, ECG findings
- Imaging evaluation of acute chest pain
  - High-risk patient: Angiography
  - Low-risk patient: MPS, cardiac CTA

DIFFERENTIAL DIAGNOSIS

Artifacts
- Attenuation: False + defects in inferior wall (diaphragm), anterolateral wall (breast)
- Cardiac creep: False + inferior wall defect; heart moves superior as patient relaxes
- Patient motion: Horizontal (hurricane sign), vertical (inferior & anterior defects)
- Overlapping bowel activity: False - due to photon scatter; false (+) due to ramp artifact
- Image misalignment: False + or - TID

Microvascular Coronary Disease
- Diabetes mellitus: Patchy defects

Balanced Ischemia
- Triple vessel disease may appear normal on SPECT

Left Bundle Branch Block
- LBBB: False + reversible septal defects (also see with ↑ RV pressures) with exercise, dobutamine

PATHOLOGY

General Features
- Genetics: Family history: Significant if first cardiac event occurs < age 55 in close male relative or < age 65 in close female relative
- Etiology
  - Obstructive CAD most common etiology
  - 90% of patients with ischemia have > 75% stenosis in at least one vessel
- Epidemiology: CAD leading cause of death worldwide

Gross Pathologic & Surgical Features
- Fatty streaks → fibrous cap → plaque rupture → thrombus formation
- Calcified plaques: More stable, less likely to rupture

Microscopic Features
- Acute obstruction (platelet aggregation); vasospasm; inflammation

CLINICAL ISSUES

Presentation
- Most common signs/symptoms
  - Typical angina: Substernal chest pain, exacerbated by stress, relieved by rest or nitroglycerin
  - Often vague symptoms or asymptomatic: Women, diabetes mellitus
  - No prior symptoms: 50% of men and 64% of women with sudden CAD death
- Other signs/symptoms: Dyspnea: Common presenting symptom of myocardial ischemia

Demographics
- Age: 1:2 men, 1:3 women > age 40 have CAD
- Gender: Average age of first heart attack: 65.8 y in men and 70.4 y in women

Natural History & Prognosis
- Annual mortality: 2-3% in patients with recent onset exertional angina
- Untreated unstable angina: 30% risk of hard cardiac event ≤ 3 months

Treatment
- Medical: Lifestyle modification; antiplatelet, lipid-lowering, antihypertensive drugs
- Interventional: Revascularization most effective when myocardial ischemia affects > 10% of myocardium

DIAGNOSTIC CHECKLIST

Consider
- False (-): Suboptimal stress, caffeine consumption prior to vasodilator, balanced ischemia
- False (+): Artifacts, microvascular disease, LBBB and exercise/dobutamine stress
- Extracardiac uptake: Cancer, infection, thyroid abnormalities
- Planar cardiac imaging in morbidly obese patients: Sensitivity similar to SPECT

SELECTED REFERENCES

1. Berman DS et al: Roles of nuclear cardiology, cardiac computed tomography, and cardiac magnetic resonance: assessment of patients with suspected coronary artery disease. J Nucl Med. 47(1):74-82, 2006
2. Berman DS et al: Roles of nuclear cardiology, cardiac computed tomography, and cardiac magnetic resonance: Noninvasive risk stratification and a conceptual framework for the selection of noninvasive imaging tests in patients with known or suspected coronary artery disease. J Nucl Med. 47(7):1107-18, 2006
3. Machac J: Cardiac positron emission tomography imaging. Semin Nucl Med. 35(1):17-36, 2005
4. Takalkar A et al: PET in cardiology. Radiol Clin North Am. 43(1):107-19, xi, 2005

MYOCARDIAL ISCHEMIA

IMAGE GALLERY

Typical

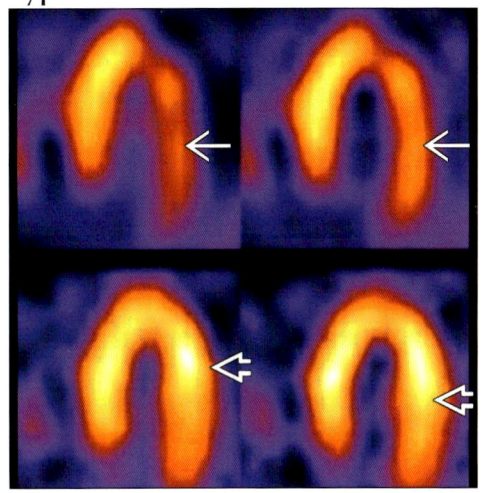

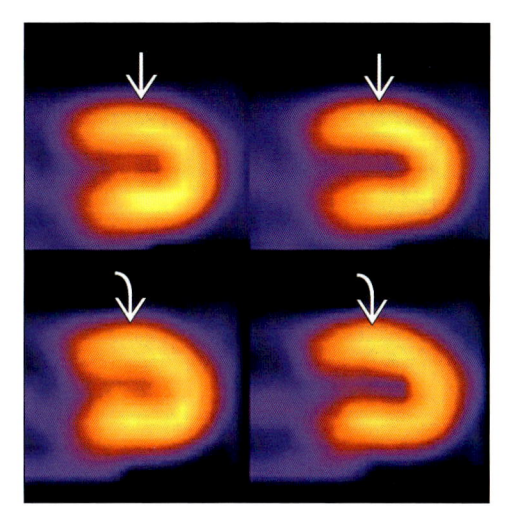

(Left) Long axis horizontal MPS shows perfusion defect ➡ in lateral wall on stress that is not evident on rest ➡, consistent with ischemia. See next image. *(Right)* Vertical long axis MPS shows normal perfusion at stress ➡ and rest ➡ using Tc-99m tetrofosmin.

Typical

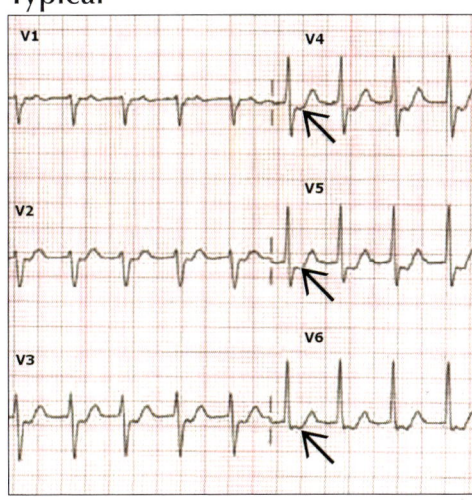

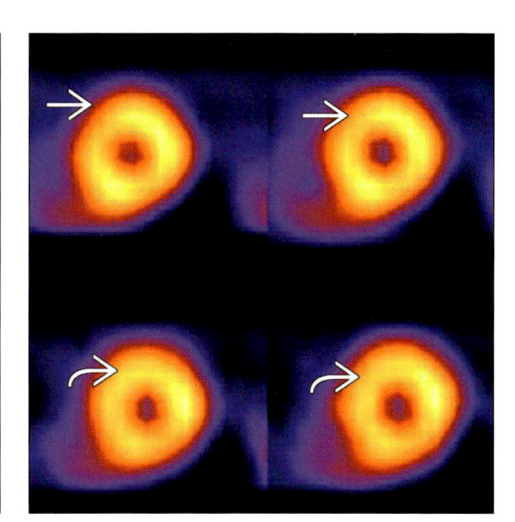

(Left) Stress ECG in same patient at left shows ST depression in lateral leads ➡, consistent with lateral wall ischemia. *(Right)* Short axis MPS shows normal perfusion at stress ➡ and rest ➡ using Tc-99m tetrofosmin.

Typical

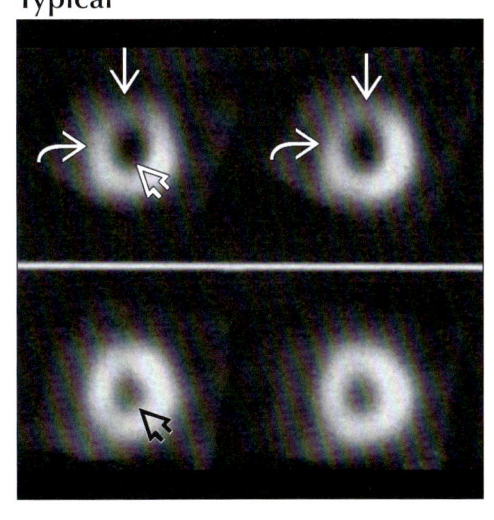

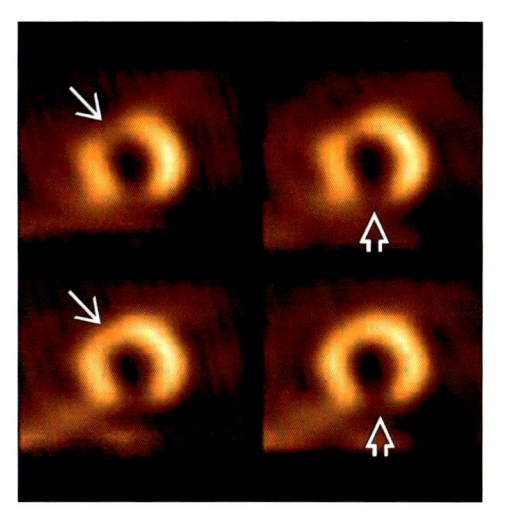

(Left) Short axis MPS shows transient ischemic dilation of ventricular cavity ➡ when compared with rest ➡. There is ↓ perfusion in anterior wall ➡ and septum ➡, consistent with high-risk ischemia. (Courtesy F. Mishkin, MD). *(Right)* Short axis MPS shows reversible anterior and anterior septal defects ➡ and fixed inferior wall defects ➡, consistent with anterior ischemia & inferior infarct.

MYOCARDIAL ISCHEMIA

(Left) Myocardial perfusion imaging QPS surface rendering shows decreased perfusion in anterior wall ➡ on stress, less apparent on rest ➡. The reversible region is evident on lower panel images ➡. The fixed inferior wall defect is also evident ➡. **(Right)** QPS polar segments show quantitative stress ➡ and rest ➡ perfusion. Note apical and anterior reversibility ➡, indicating ischemia. Inferior myocardial infarction also evident ➡.

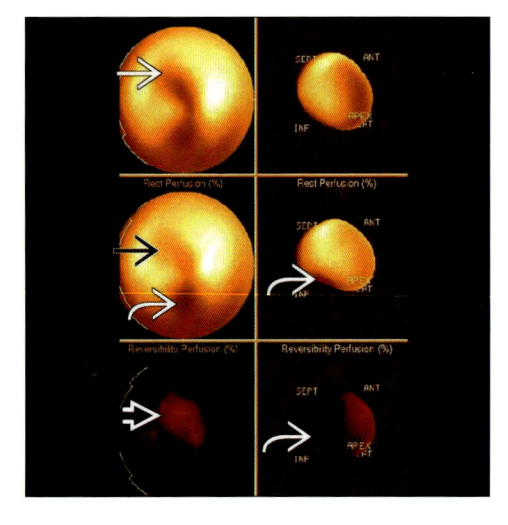

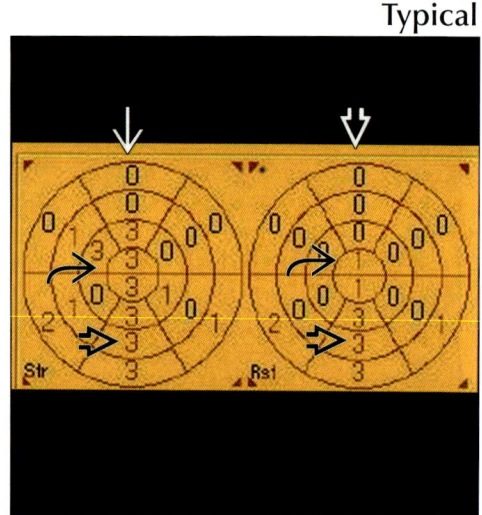

(Left) Myocardial perfusion imaging Horizontal long axis Tl-201 MPS shows apical redistribution ➡ when compared to stress ➡, consistent with ischemia. Incomplete redistribution may indicate apical thinning, non-transmural scarring, severe ischemia. **(Right)** Short axis MPS shows fixed anterolateral defect ➡ that appears worse on lower-count rest images ➡. Gated images shows normal wall motion, indicating breast attenuation.

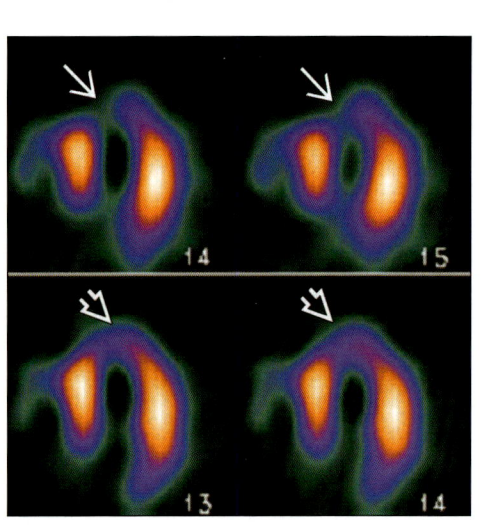

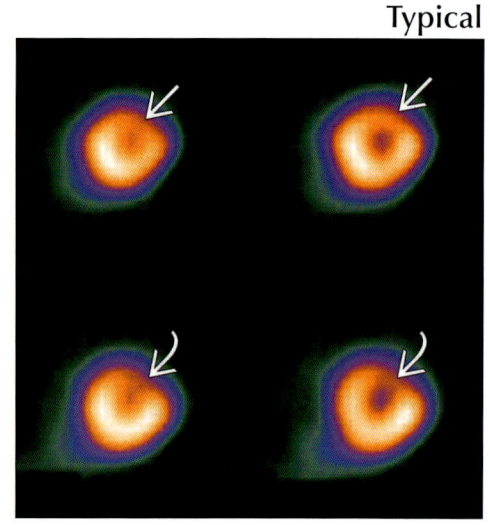

(Left) Short axis MPS shows ↑ tracer in lateral wall ➡ consistent with normal ventricular papillary muscle. This can also be seen with hypertrophic myocardium. **(Right)** Horizontal long axis MPS shows adjacent GI activity ➡ on stress performed with Tc-99m tetrofosmin. Resting images performed with Tl-201 show no GI activity ➡. Tl-201 produces less bowel and liver uptake.

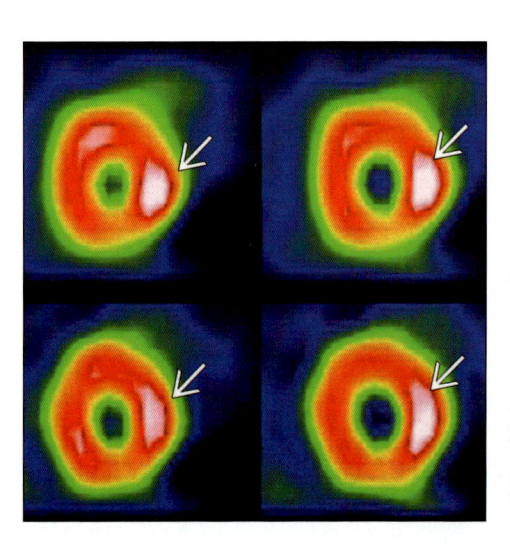

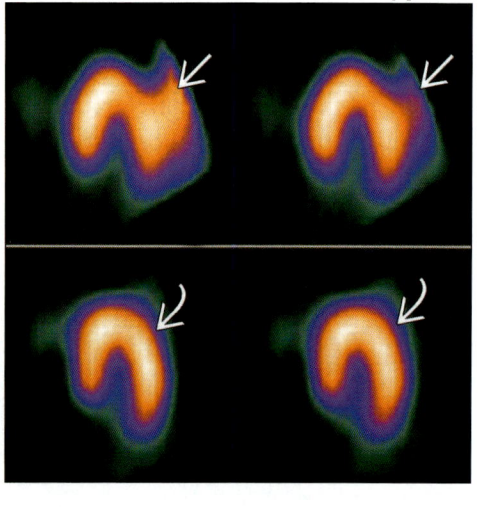

MYOCARDIAL ISCHEMIA

Typical

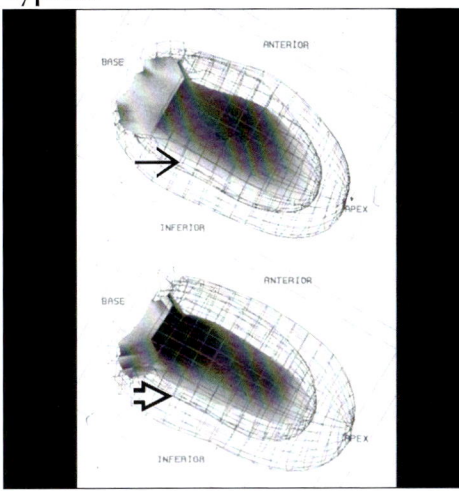

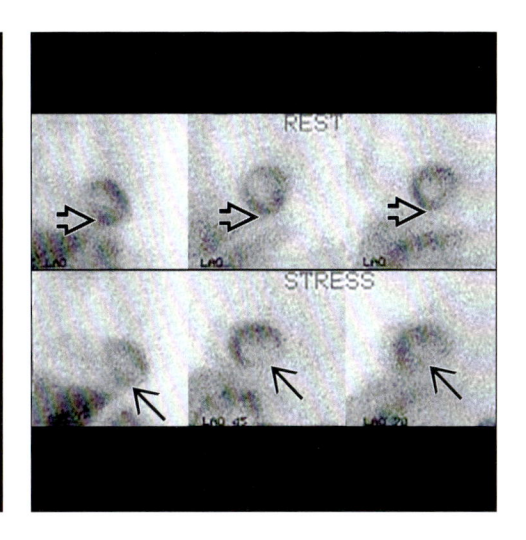

(Left) Three dimensional MPS shows ventricular dilation at stress ➔ compared with rest ⇨, indicative of high-risk coronary artery disease. (Right) Planar stress Tl-201 MPS shows reversible perfusion defect in inferior wall ➔ not seen on rest ⇨, consistent with ischemia.

Variant

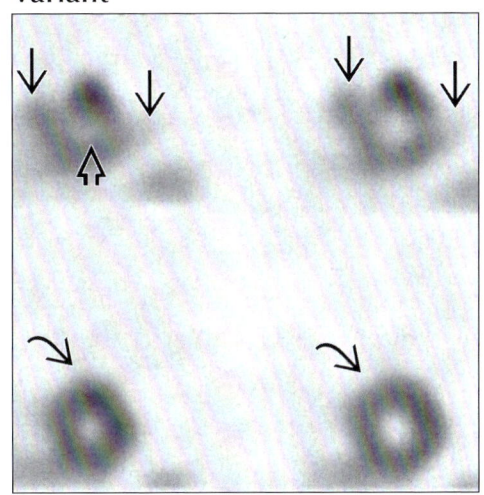

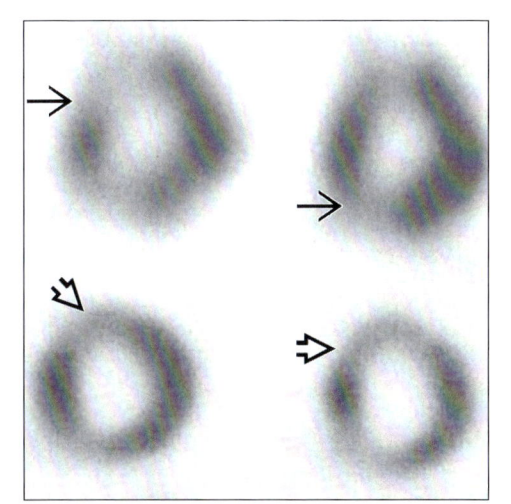

(Left) Short axis MPS at stress shows hurricane sign ➔ and obliteration of ventricular cavity ⇨, consistent with lateral patient motion. Rest images ➔ are normal. (Right) Short axis MPS shows patchy uptake at stress ➔ throughout ventricle with "spreading" of counts, consistent with low counts due to extravasation of tracer. Repeat injection resulted in good-quality images ⇨.

Other

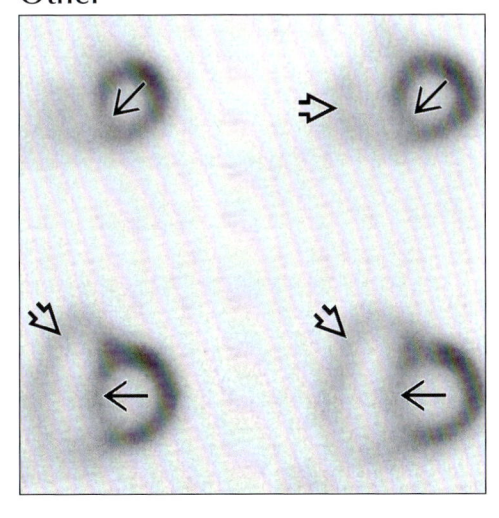

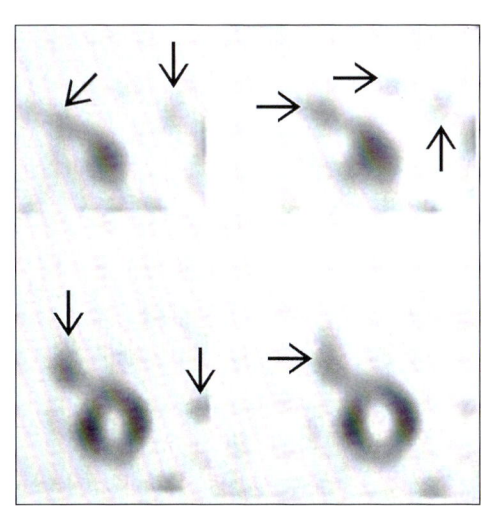

(Left) Short axis MPS in patient with pulmonary artery hypertension and RV enlargement ⇨ shows ↓ septal counts ➔ (usually worse on stress than rest) due to ↑ RV pressures, septal compression. Finding also seen with LBBB. (Right) Short axis MPS shows multiple foci of extracardiac activity ➔ in patient with renal cell carcinoma metastatic to lungs. Both Tc-99m agents and Tl-201 show avidity for many tumors.

MYOCARDIAL VIABILITY

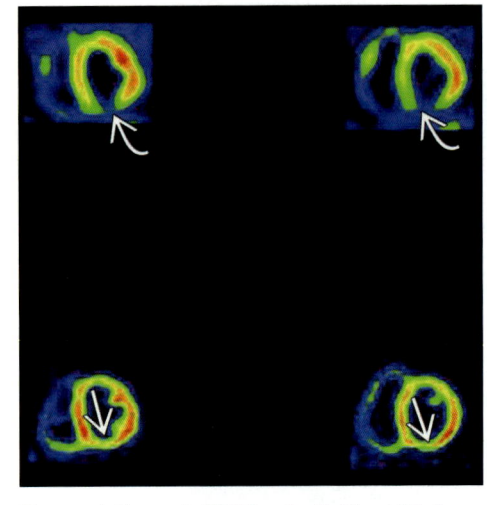

Top panel: Short axis SPECT resting Tc-99m MPS shows absent activity in inferior wall ➔, consistent with infarction. Lower panel: Comparable FDG PET images demonstrate uptake ➔, thus viability.

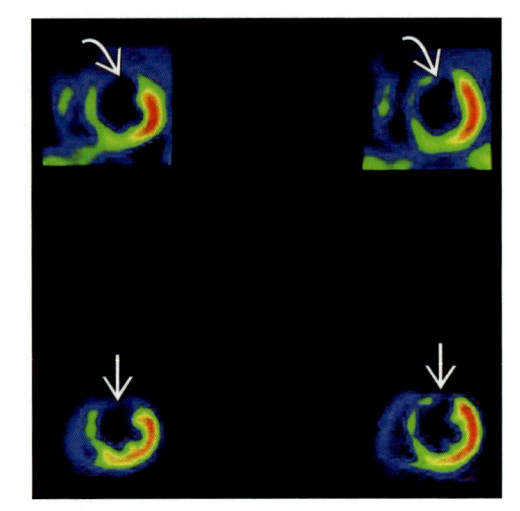

Top panel: Short axis SPECT resting Tc-99m MPS shows absent activity in anterior wall ➔, consistent with infarction. Lower panel: FDG PET images demonstrate lack of uptake ➔, confirming non-viability.

TERMINOLOGY

Abbreviations and Synonyms
- Myocardial hibernation, myocardial stunning

Definitions
- Myocardial viability testing: To identify ongoing metabolic function in regions of suspected myocardial infarction (MI)
- Hibernating myocardium: Adaptation of left ventricular dysfunction secondary to chronic ischemia
- Stunned myocardium: Left ventricular dysfunction after transient severe ischemia

IMAGING FINDINGS

General Features
- Best diagnostic clue
  - CE MR: Non-viability indicated by decreased initial perfusion, wall motion abnormality, delayed contrast-enhancement
  - Tl-201: Non-viability indicated by absent uptake on 24 hour imaging
  - F-18 fluorodeoxyglucose (FDG) PET: Non-viability indicated by absent uptake in presence of elevated insulin levels
- Morphology: Myocardial viability requires: Sarcolemmal membrane integrity, preserved metabolic activity, adequate myocardial perfusion

Nuclear Medicine Findings
- Conventional Tc-99m, Tl-201 myocardial perfusion scans (MPS): Viability is present in 25% of regions called "infarcted", and 50% of patients with "infarcted" segments
  - More definitive viability study indicated where MI suspected by MPS and surgery/revascularization may be beneficial
- Myocardial uptake of Tl-201 indicates myocardial perfusion and sarcolemmal membrane integrity
- FDG uptake indicates preserved glucose metabolism; may be increased in presence of ischemia (forced anaerobic metabolism)

Imaging Recommendations
- Best imaging tool
  - F-18 FDG PET at rest is gold standard for viability testing

DDx: False (+) and (-) Viability Studies

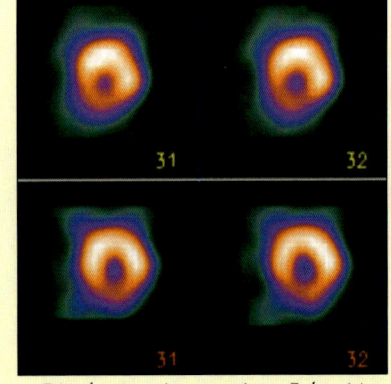

Diaphragm Attenuation: False 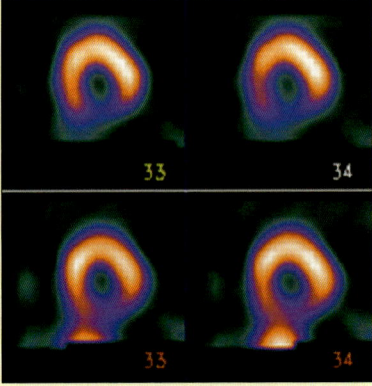 (-) *Overlapping Bowel: False 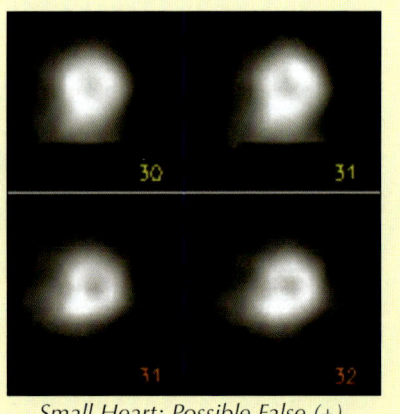 (+)* *Small Heart: Possible False (+)*

MYOCARDIAL VIABILITY

Key Facts

Imaging Findings
- F-18 FDG PET at rest is gold standard for viability testing
- CE MR: Increasingly preferred over nuclear techniques because of availability; reader confidence, reimbursement
- CE-MR: Also evaluates scar burden, coronary perfusion, and contractile reserve
- Rest-redistribution, 24 h delayed Tl-201 myocardial SPECT provides comparable results to PET imaging when the LVEF > 25%
- Choice of study for viability dictated by availability: Good correlation between CE MR, FDG PET, 24 h Tl-201

Top Differential Diagnoses
- Severe type-II diabetes: Absent FDG myocardial uptake despite insulin; Tl-201 preferred
- Attenuation artifacts cause apparent defects in uptake: Diaphragm, breasts, soft tissue
- Poor count statistics due to obesity, insufficient imaging time, use of Tl-201, incorrect isotope peaking
- Reconstruction alignment errors
- Movement during imaging
- Inadequate time for redistribution on Tl-201 imaging (image at both 4 and 24 h after injection)
- Overlapping bowel activity masking inferior wall defects
- Partial volume effect in small hearts masks defects in tracer uptake

---

    - Reimbursement requires previous conventional myocardial perfusion scan suggestive of infarction
  ○ CE MR: Increasingly preferred over nuclear techniques because of availability; reader confidence, reimbursement
    - CE-MR: Also evaluates scar burden, coronary perfusion, and contractile reserve
  ○ Rest-redistribution, 24 h delayed Tl-201 myocardial SPECT provides comparable results to PET imaging when the LVEF > 25%
  ○ Choice of study for viability dictated by availability: Good correlation between CE MR, FDG PET, 24 h Tl-201
  ○ Nitrate enhanced rest SPECT with Tc-99m sestamibi, Tc-99m tetrofosmin: Less well studied; may be comparable to Tl-201 rest/24 h imaging
- Protocol advice
  ○ Long imaging times recommended to enhance counting statistics on Tl-201 rest imaging
  ○ When the 4 hour delayed Tl-201 image shows absent uptake, a 24 hour delayed image indicated to increase sensitivity
  ○ FDG PET
    - Obtain rest myocardial perfusion scan prior to FDG PET scan
    - Fast 6-12 hours prior to FDG PET
    - Glucose load (25-100 mg) or euglycemic hyperinsulinemic clamp to switch primary myocardial energy substrate from free fatty acids to glucose
    - Inject 10 mCi of F-18 FDG at 45-90 min after glucose load, with blood sugar is < 150 mg/dL
    - Imaging performed at 30-60 minutes after FDG injection
- Correlative imaging features
  ○ Echocardiography: Viable myocardium shows improved wall motion with low dose dobutamine infusion (5-7.5 μg/kg/min); subsequent deterioration of wall motion on high infusion rates (> 20 μg/kg/min)
- Alternative nuclear medicine techniques
  ○ FDG SPECT: Concordance with FDG PET is about 92%; image quality similar to 24 h Tl-201
  ○ I-123 BMIPP SPECT: Measures fatty acid metabolism; used in combination with perfusion and glucose metabolism imaging

DIFFERENTIAL DIAGNOSIS

False-Negative Scan
- Severe type-II diabetes: Absent FDG myocardial uptake despite insulin; Tl-201 preferred
- Attenuation artifacts cause apparent defects in uptake: Diaphragm, breasts, soft tissue
- Poor count statistics due to obesity, insufficient imaging time, use of Tl-201, incorrect isotope peaking
- Reconstruction alignment errors
- Movement during imaging
- Inadequate time for redistribution on Tl-201 imaging (image at both 4 and 24 h after injection)

False-Positive Scan
- Overlapping bowel activity masking inferior wall defects
- Partial volume effect in small hearts masks defects in tracer uptake

PATHOLOGY

General Features
- Genetics
  ○ Family history is significant and independent predictor of coronary artery disease
  ○ Family history considered positive when evidence of coronary artery disease in a parent or sibling before 60 yrs of age
- Etiology: Chronically decreased myocardial perfusion
- Epidemiology
  ○ 400,000 new cases of heart failure a year in the U.S.
  ○ Prevalence approximately 2%

MYOCARDIAL VIABILITY

Gross Pathologic & Surgical Features
- Loss of contractile function
- Myocardial wall thinning in areas of mixed scar and viable tissue

Microscopic Features
- Loss of myocyte contractile material
- Accumulation of glycogen in the cytosol
- Cellular ATP is maintained without the buildup of lactate
- Similar features found in the fetal heart
  - Dedifferentiation may be a normal adaptive response to chronic ischemia
  - Myocytes become glucose dependent, similar to that found in the fetal heart

CLINICAL ISSUES

Presentation
- Most common signs/symptoms
  - Anginal chest pain
  - Shortness of breath
  - Peripheral swelling
  - Fatigue
- Other signs/symptoms: Patients with viable myocardium often asymptomatic: Imaging plays vital role in evaluation for possible myocardial viability

Demographics
- Age
  - Men > 45 years
  - Women > 55 years
  - Younger individuals: Typically have significant comorbid factors: Obesity, diabetics, amphetamine abuse
- Gender: M = F

Natural History & Prognosis
- Patients with viable myocardium: Benefit from revascularization; if untreated, risk of cardiac death or nonfatal MI is increased
- Patients with non-viable myocardium: Increased morbidity and mortality with revascularization
- Viability testing most important in patients with heart failure
  - 50% of patients with heart failure: Death within 5 years
  - Revascularization: Decreases morbidity and mortality where viable myocardium is present

Treatment
- Revascularization should be considered in patients with residual viable myocardium after MI

DIAGNOSTIC CHECKLIST

Consider
- Use of multiple tracers (e.g., FDG and Tl-201) increases accuracy of viability assessment

Image Interpretation Pearls
- Tl-201 preferred over FDG PET in severe type-II diabetes: Lack of FDG uptake due to insulin resistance
- Planar imaging helpful when using Tl-201 in large patients
- False-negative Tl-201 scans often due to inadequate count statistics or imaging too early after tracer injection

SELECTED REFERENCES

1. Rahimtoola SH et al: Hibernating myocardium: another piece of the puzzle falls into place. J Am Coll Cardiol. 47(5):978-80, 2006
2. Slart RH et al: Imaging techniques in nuclear cardiology for the assessment of myocardial viability. Int J Cardiovasc Imaging. 22(1):63-80, 2006
3. Unlu M et al: Cardiac MRI in ischemic heart disease with severe coronary artery stenosis. Acad Radiol. 13(11):1387-93, 2006
4. Canty JM Jr et al: Hibernating myocardium. J Nucl Cardiol. 12(1):104-19, 2005
5. Hunt SA et al: ACC/AHA 2005 Guideline Update for the Diagnosis and Management of Chronic Heart Failure in the Adult: a report of the American College of Cardiology/American Heart Association Task Force on Practice Guidelines (Writing Committee to Update the 2001 Guidelines for the Evaluation and Management of Heart Failure): developed in collaboration with the American College of Chest Physicians and the International Society for Heart and Lung Transplantation: endorsed by the Heart Rhythm Society. Circulation. 112(12):e154-235, 2005
6. Tamaki N et al: SPET in cardiology. Diagnosis, prognosis, and management of patients with coronary artery disease. Q J Nucl Med Mol Imaging. 49(2):193-203, 2005
7. Lim ET et al: Should we be screening for myocardial hibernation in heart failure? J Nucl Cardiol. 11(2):114-7, 2004
8. Jessup M et al: Heart failure. N Engl J Med. 348(20):2007-18, 2003
9. Sloof GW et al: Nuclear imaging is more sensitive for the detection of viable myocardium than dobutamine echocardiography. Nucl Med Commun. 24(4):375-81, 2003
10. Beanlands R et al: Myocardial viability. In: Positron Emission Tomography. Philadelphia, Lippincott Williams & Wilkins. 334-50, 2002
11. Camici PG et al: Repetitive stunning, hibernation, and heart failure: contribution of PET to establishing a link. Am J Physiol Heart Circ Physiol. 280(3):H929-36, 2001
12. Visser FC: Imaging of cardiac metabolism using radiolabelled glucose, fatty acids and acetate. Coron Artery Dis. 12 Suppl 1:S12-8, 2001
13. Auerbach MA et al: Prevalence of myocardial viability as detected by positron emission tomography in patients with ischemic cardiomyopathy. Circulation. 99(22):2921-6, 1999
14. Di Carli MF: Predicting improved function after myocardial revascularization. Curr Opin Cardiol. 13(6):415-24, 1998
15. Sambuceti G et al: Perfusion-contraction mismatch during inotropic stimulation in hibernating myocardium. J Nucl Med. 39(3):396-402, 1998
16. Wijns W et al: Hibernating myocardium. N Engl J Med. 339(3):173-81, 1998
17. Afridi I et al: Dobutamine echocardiography in myocardial hibernation. Optimal dose and accuracy in predicting recovery of ventricular function after coronary angioplasty. Circulation. 91(3):663-70, 1995

MYOCARDIAL VIABILITY

IMAGE GALLERY

Typical

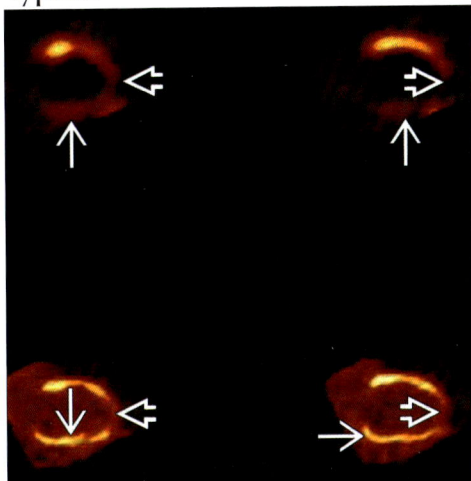

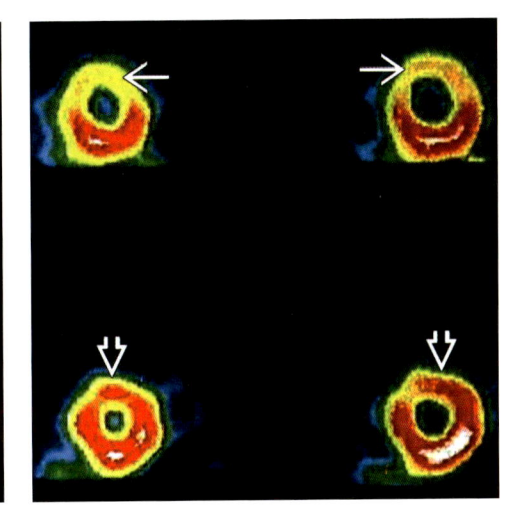

(Left) Top panel: Short axis resting Tc-99m MPS shows severely decreased activity in apex ➡, inferior wall ➡. Lower panel: Comparable FDG PET images demonstrate non-viable apex ➡, viable inferior wall ➡. *(Right)* Top panel: Short axis 4 h Tl-201 scan shows severely decreased uptake in anterior wall ➡, suggesting infarction. Lower panel: Comparable 24 h images show redistribution ➡, confirming viability.

Typical

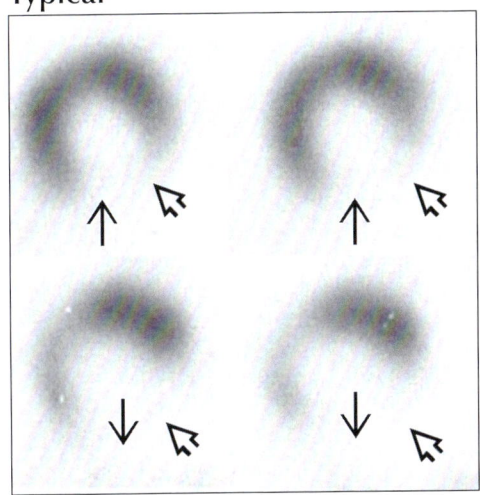

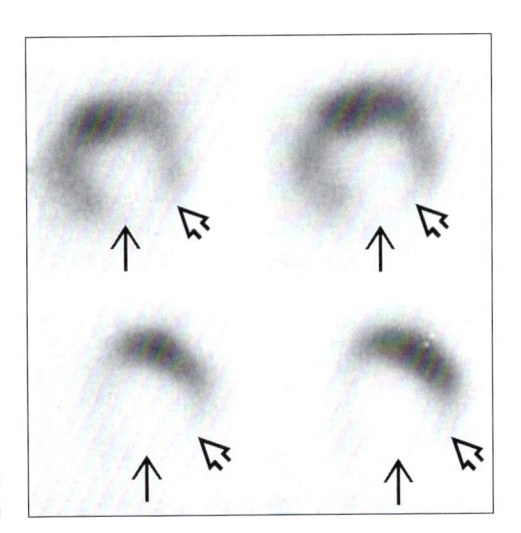

(Left) Short axis images from 4 h Tl-201 scan shows absent uptake in inferior ➡ and inferolateral ➡ walls, consistent with infarction. See next image. *(Right)* Same case as previous image. Short axis images from 24 h Tl-201 scan persistent absence of uptake in inferior ➡ and inferolateral ➡ walls, confirming non-viability.

Typical

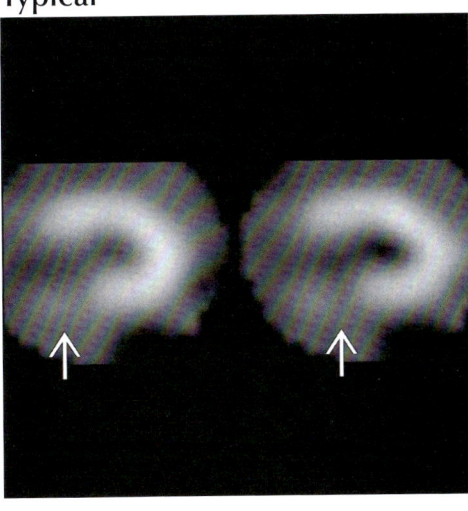

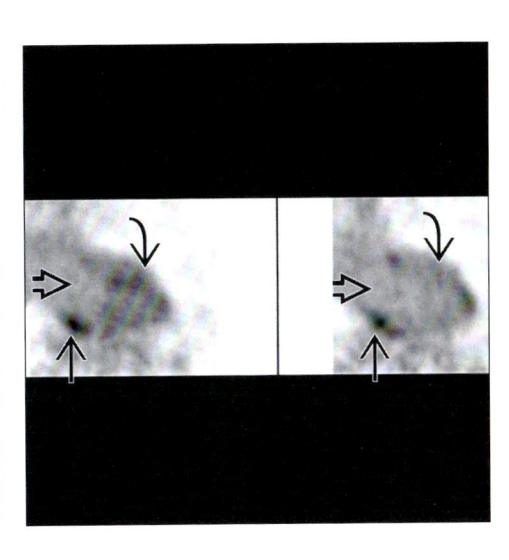

(Left) Vertical long axis images from resting Tc-99m sestamibi scan show severely decreased activity in proximal inferior wall ➡, consistent with infarction. Patient had severe type II diabetes and chest pain. See next image. *(Right)* Comparable vertical long axis FDG PET images (same as previous image) show poor, patchy uptake in myocardium ➡ and high blood pool ➡, typical of type II diabetes. Proximal inferior wall ➡ is viable.

MYOCARDIAL INFARCTION

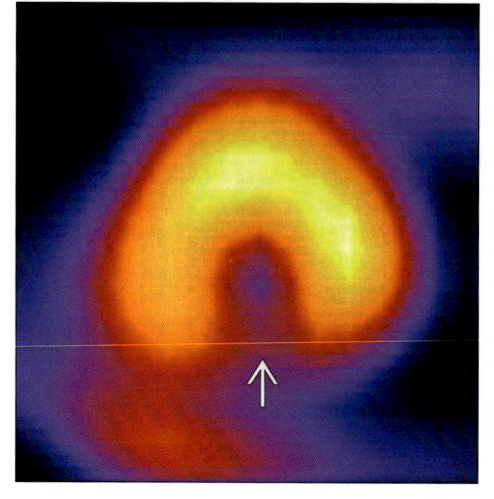

Short axis MPI shows inferior wall perfusion defect ➡ at rest, consistent with inferior myocardial infarction.

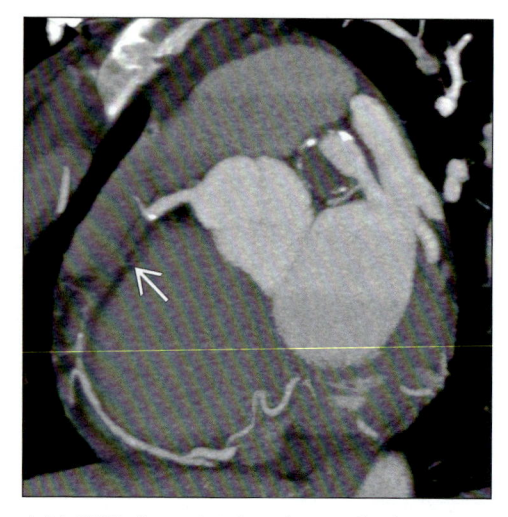

Axial CECT shows 100% occlusion of right coronary artery ➡, the vascular territory supplying inferior myocardial wall. (Courtesy C. Newton, MD).

TERMINOLOGY

Abbreviations and Synonyms
- Myocardial infarction (MI); acute myocardial infarction (AMI)

Definitions
- MI: Irreversible myocardial cell death and necrosis

IMAGING FINDINGS

General Features
- Best diagnostic clue
  - Myocardial perfusion imaging (MPI)
    - Fixed perfusion defect on rest-stress MPI images
- Location
  - Anterior/septal wall: Left anterior descending (LAD) artery
  - Lateral wall: Circumflex artery
  - Inferior wall: Posterior descending artery (PDA)
    - From right coronary artery (RCA) in 85% (right dominant)
    - From continuation of circumflex in 15% (left dominant)
  - Apex: Usually from LAD, but variable or in part from PDA in many

Imaging Recommendations
- Best imaging tool
  - Coronary angiography: Best option for high risk patients with acute coronary syndrome
    - Direct visualization of occluded vessel(s)
    - Diagnosis with potential for immediate percutaneous revascularization
  - Multislice CT angiography (CTA): Best option for low risk patients with acute coronary syndrome
    - Immediate result in acute chest pain setting
    - Direct visualization of occluded vessel(s), thinned myocardium
    - Concomitant calcium scoring
    - Similar in sensitivity to MPI
  - MPI: Equivalent to CTA in low risk patients with acute coronary syndrome
    - Stress-rest MPI: Sensitive noninvasive test to determine prognosis (MI extent, ischemia, left ventricular ejection fraction)

DDx: Artifacts that Mimic Myocardial Infarction

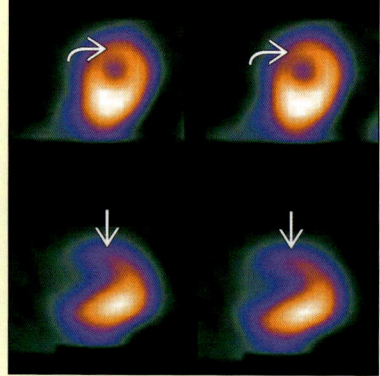

Breast Attenuation 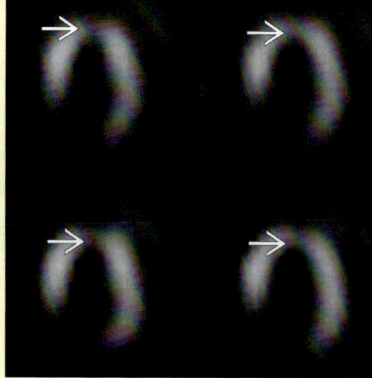 | *Normal Apical Thinning* 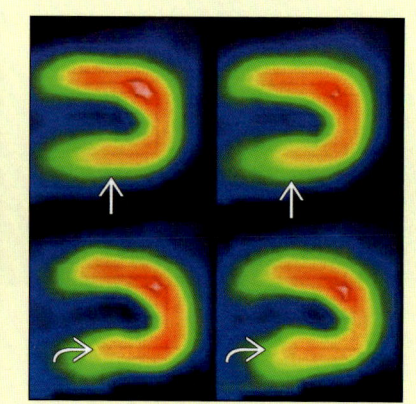 | *Diaphragmatic Attenuation*

MYOCARDIAL INFARCTION

Key Facts

Terminology
- MI: Irreversible myocardial cell death and necrosis

Imaging Findings
- Coronary angiography: Best option for high risk patients with acute coronary syndrome
- Direct visualization of occluded vessel(s)
- Diagnosis with potential for immediate percutaneous revascularization
- Multislice CT angiography (CTA): Best option for low risk patients with acute coronary syndrome
- Immediate result in acute chest pain setting
- Direct visualization of occluded vessel(s), thinned myocardium
- Concomitant calcium scoring
- MPI: Equivalent to CTA in low risk patients with acute coronary syndrome
- When evaluating AMI, attempt to inject Tc-99m perfusion tracer within 2 hours of pain episode: May image later
- Choice of multidetector CTA vs. MPI in acute coronary artery syndrome: Dictated by availability, patient size, renal function

Top Differential Diagnoses
- Artifact
- Vasospastic disease (Prinzmetal angina)
- Microvascular disease (e.g., diabetes mellitus, syndrome X)
- Stress-rest MPI "overcalls" MI in 25% of regions and 50% of patients with fixed defects: Shown viable by 24 hr Tl-201, CEMR, FDG

- AMI: Perfusion defect on Tc-99m sestamibi or Tc-99m tetrofosmin SPECT
- Chronic MI: Perfusion defect on resting Tl-201, Tc-99m sestamibi, Tc-99m tetrofosmin MPI
- Rest MPI: Diagnosis/risk assessment in patients with acute coronary syndrome, nondiagnostic electrocardiogram (ECG), negative cardiac enzymes
- Protocol advice
  - When evaluating AMI, attempt to inject Tc-99m perfusion tracer within 2 hours of pain episode: May image later
  - Choice of multidetector CTA vs. MPI in acute coronary artery syndrome: Dictated by availability, patient size, renal function
- Other nuclear medicine imaging options
  - Radionuclide angiography
    - Regional and global LV function
  - Other nuclear medicine studies
    - Rubidium-82 or N-13 ammonia PET perfusion: Absent activity
    - Tc-99m pyrophosphate (PYP): Binds intracellular calcium; ↑ activity 24-48 hours after MI; false (+) extremely rare
- CE MR
  - Assessment of myocardial viability in setting of known or suspected MI
  - Early contrast-enhancement of affected myocardial segment in AMI
  - Delayed contrast-enhancement in scar
  - Wall motion/thickness assessment
  - Dobutamine stress assessment of ischemic changes
- Echocardiography
  - MI = myocardial wall hypokinesis, akinesis, dyskinesis, thinned myocardium

DIFFERENTIAL DIAGNOSIS

Artifact
- Left ventricular hypertrophy: Relative lateral wall defect (fixed)
- Soft tissue attenuation of photons: Breast, diaphragm
- Motion artifact (vertical, horizontal)
- SPECT: Misaligned center of rotation
- Normal apical thinning
- Photopenic defect in inferior wall due to adjacent bowel, liver activity (reconstruction artifact)
- Scatter of photons into inferior wall due to adjacent bowel, liver activity

Other Vascular Disease
- Vasospastic disease (Prinzmetal angina)
- Microvascular disease (e.g., diabetes mellitus, syndrome X)

Myocardial Hibernation
- Myocardium with little/no perfusion, but viable due to anaerobic glycolysis
- Stress-rest MPI "overcalls" MI in 25% of regions and 50% of patients with fixed defects: Shown viable by 24 hr Tl-201, CEMR, FDG

PATHOLOGY

General Features
- Genetics
  - PIA2 polymorphic allele (prothrombotic genetic factor); ↑ risk of premature MI
  - ALOX5AP encoding 5-lipoxygenase activating protein (FLAP); ↑ leukotrienes ⇒ arterial wall inflammation ⇒ ↑ risk of MI
- Etiology
  - Ruptured coronary artery plaque disrupts myocardial blood supply
    - Myocardial necrosis begins in 20-30 minutes, spreading from sub- to epicardium
  - Distribution
    - Left anterior descending artery (40%)
    - Right coronary artery (27%)
    - Circumflex artery (11%)
    - Other: Obtuse marginal, diagonal branches (22%)
  - Risk factors
    - Hyperlipidemia

MYOCARDIAL INFARCTION

- Diabetes mellitus
- Hypertension
- Obesity
- Cigarette smoking
- Family history
- Epidemiology
  - Lifetime incidence of CAD > 35 yrs exceeds 25%
  - US: > 1 million MIs per year
  - Worldwide: 12 million MIs per year
- Associated abnormalities: Transmural MI: ST segment elevation on ECG typical, although not necessary

Gross Pathologic & Surgical Features
- Coronary plaque
  - Stable: Thick, calcified cap with small fatty core
  - Unstable: Thin, calcified cap with large fatty core

Microscopic Features
- Eosinophilic coagulative necrosis ⇒ granulation tissue ⇒ fibrous scar

Staging, Grading or Classification Criteria
- Q-wave MI: Transmural, ~ 100% arterial occlusion
- Non-Q-wave MI: Nontransmural, up to 50% of culprit vessels patent

CLINICAL ISSUES

Presentation
- Most common signs/symptoms
  - Heavy, substernal chest pain
  - Tombstones: ST elevation on ECG
- Other signs/symptoms
  - Nausea (M < F)
  - Dyspnea (M < F)
  - Diaphoresis (M > F)
  - Pain radiating to neck, jaw, arms, or back
  - Asymptomatic: 25% of MIs (diabetic, elderly)

Demographics
- Age
  - Men: Usually > 45 yrs old
  - Women: Usually > 55 yrs old
  - < 45 yrs: MI usually due to cigarettes, cocaine, methamphetamine, diabetes
- Gender
  - M > F in patients 40-70 yrs old
  - M = F in patients > 70 yrs old

Natural History & Prognosis
- Death within 1 year in up to 50% of patients
  - 50% of deaths occur in first few hrs of MI
  - Anterior MI: Highest risk
  - Lateral MI: Intermediate risk
  - Inferior/posterior MI: Lowest risk
- MI caused by left main coronary occlusion can ⇒ death within minutes ("widow-maker")

Treatment
- Acute
  - Medical: Oxygen, aspirin, beta blockers, nitrates, thrombolytics
  - Revascularization: Cardiac catheterization-based intervention or bypass surgery
- Long term therapy
  - Medical therapy for damaged myocardium
    - Beta blockers
    - ACE inhibitors
  - Anti-platelet medication
    - Aspirin
    - Clopidogrel bisulfate
  - Risk factor reduction
    - Antihypertensive medications
    - Exercise
    - Cholesterol-lowering drugs
    - Cigarette cessation
- Therapeutic response
  - Monitor with stress-rest MPI
  - BMIPP fatty acid imaging: Altered myocardial metabolism due to intermittent ischemia

DIAGNOSTIC CHECKLIST

Consider
- Diagnostic standard for AMI
  - 2x normal elevation of cardiac enzymes
  - ECG changes usually present, highly variable
  - ± Chest pain
- Diagnostic standard for chronic MI
  - MPI: Fixed perfusion defect
  - MPI, CT, MR, echocardiography, cardiac angiography: Hypokinesis, akinesis, dyskinesis in myocardial segment
  - ECG: Q waves

Image Interpretation Pearls
- Septal hypokinesis common in absence of MI, especially after coronary artery bypass graft surgery
- Review raw images to identify artifacts, extracardiac radiotracer uptake (breast cancer, lymphoma, lung, infection)
- Increased activity in bowel or liver can cause artifactual increased or decreased activity in inferior wall
- In first few days after MI, necrotic area infiltrates with red blood cells: May cause false-negative perfusion scan

SELECTED REFERENCES

1. Barnett K et al: Noninvasive imaging techniques to aid in the triage of patients with suspected acute coronary syndrome: a review. Emerg Med Clin North Am. 23(4):977-98, 2005
2. Mowatt G et al: Systematic review of the prognostic effectiveness of SPECT myocardial perfusion scintigraphy in patients with suspected or known coronary artery disease and following myocardial infarction. Nucl Med Commun. 26(3):217-29, 2005
3. Klocke FJ et al: ACC/AHA/ASNC guidelines for the clinical use of cardiac radionuclide imaging--executive summary: a report of the American College of Cardiology/American Heart Association Task Force on Practice Guidelines (ACC/AHA/ASNC Committee to Revise the 1995 Guidelines for the Clinical Use of Cardiac Radionuclide Imaging). J Am Coll Cardiol. 42(7):1318-33, 2003
4. Heston TF et al: Gender bias in acute myocardial infarction. Am J Cardiol. 79(6):844, 1997

MYOCARDIAL INFARCTION

IMAGE GALLERY

Typical

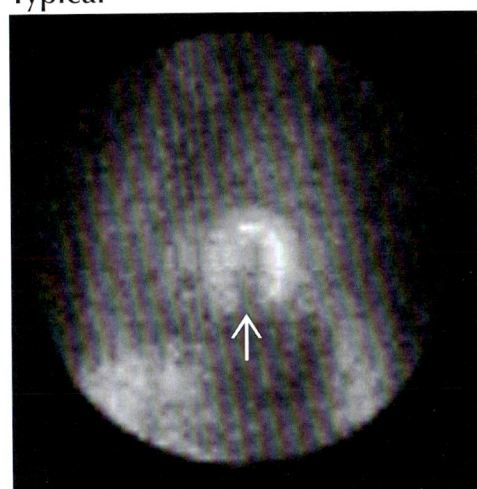

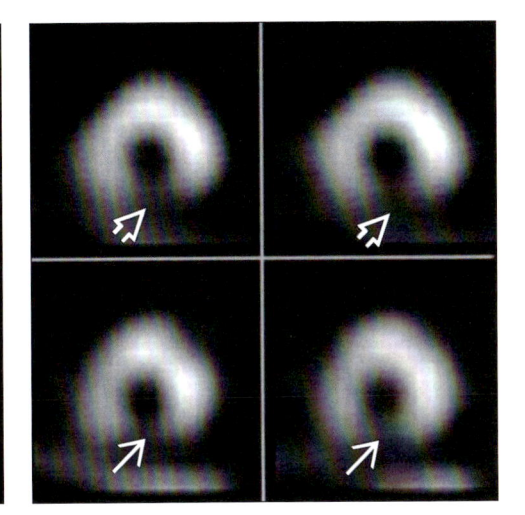

(Left) Left lateral planar MPI shows resting perfusion defect ➡ in inferoapical wall, consistent with myocardial infarction. Planar images can be obtained in patients too obese for imaging tables. *(Right)* Short axis MPI shows decreased activity in inferior wall on rest ➡, more pronounced on stress images ➡, signifying myocardial infarction with peri-infarct ischemia.

Typical

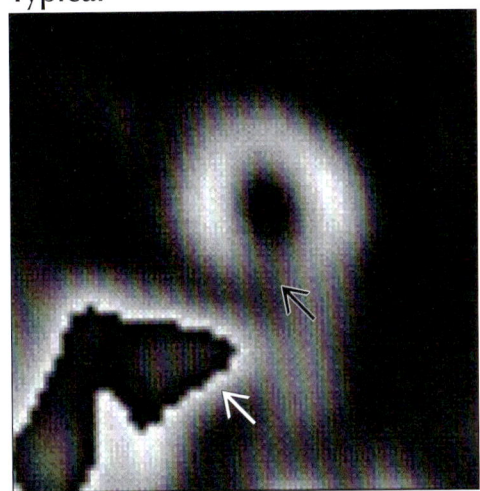

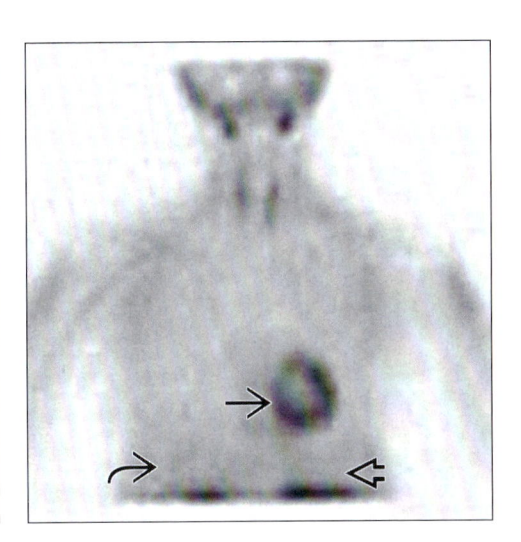

(Left) Short axis MPI shows ↓ activity in inferior wall ➡ due to artifact caused by adjacent extracardiac activity ➡. (Courtesy Washington University School of Medicine). See next image. *(Right)* Anterior MPI at 90 minutes shows retained activity in myocardium ➡. Note tracer washout from liver ➡ and bowel ➡. If bowel or liver activity is adjacent to inferior wall, prone or delayed imaging can decrease artifact.

Typical

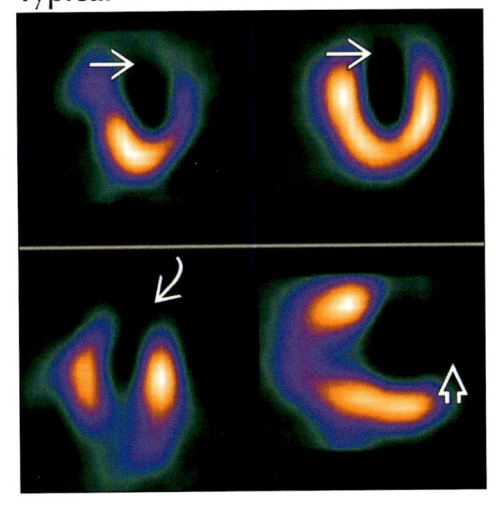

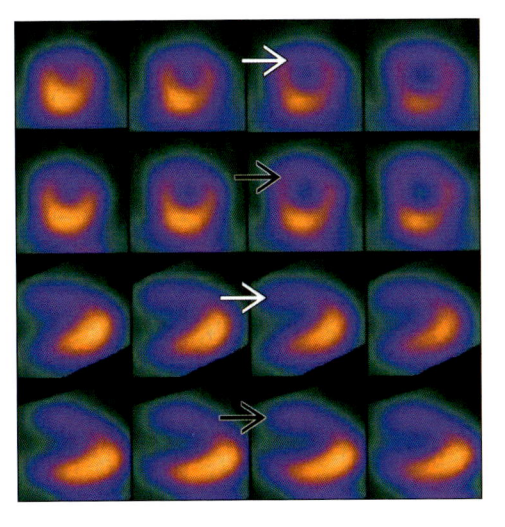

(Left) MPI shows large anteroapical defect on short axis ➡, vertical long axis ➡, and horizontal long axis ➡ views. *(Right)* MPI shows decreased activity ➡ on rest in anterior wall that becomes more pronounced on stress images ➡ in patient with Prinzmetal angina. No coronary artery disease was present on catheterization.

MYOCARDIAL INFARCTION

Typical

(Left) LAO MUGA end-diastole frame in patient with history of apical infarct ➔. See next 2 images. *(Right)* LAO MUGA end-systole frame shows probable dyskinesis of cardiac apex ➔, suspicious for aneurysm.

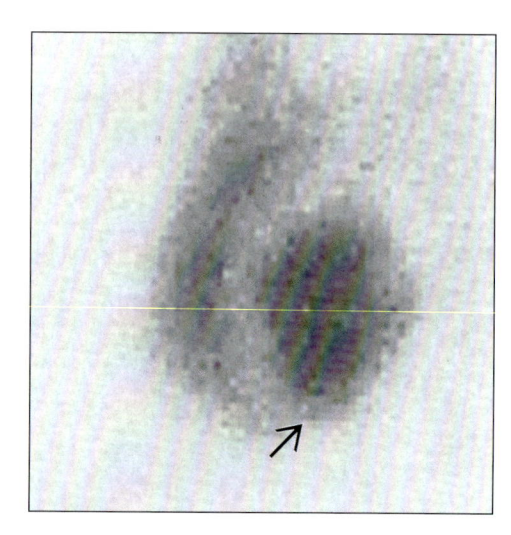

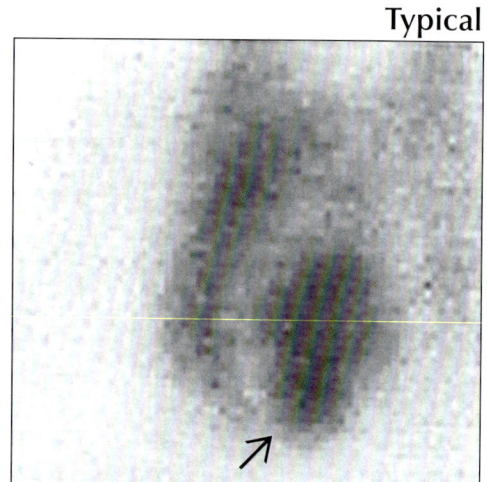

Variant

(Left) Phase image confirms complete out-of-phase focus in cardiac apex ➔, consistent with apical aneurysm. *(Right)* LAO planar Tc-99m PYP scan shows donut sign ➔ of peripheral increased activity with central photopenia, consistent with large anteroapical infarct with central necrosis. This finding is associated with high risk of ventricular rupture.

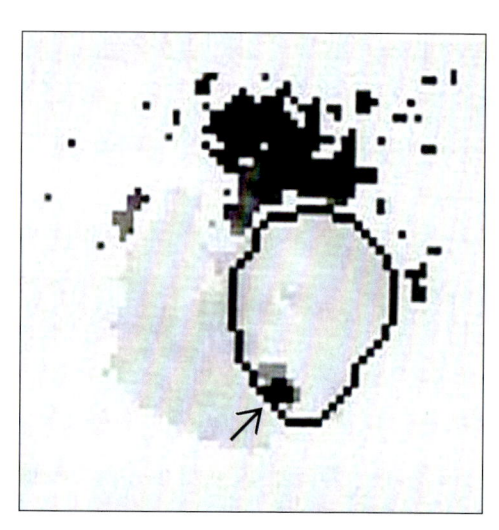

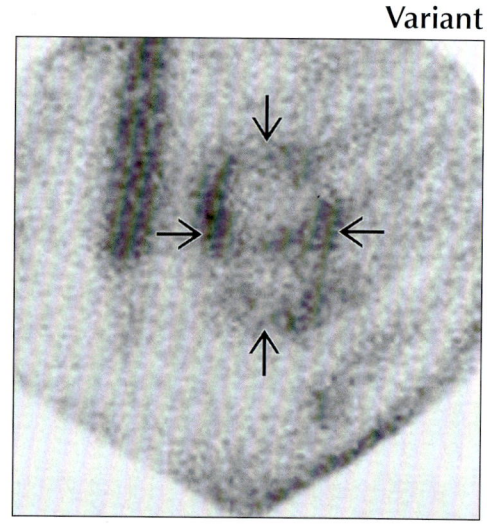

Typical

(Left) Anterior planar Tc-99m PYP scan shows focal ovoid region of uptake to left of sternum ➔ consistent with acute myocardial infarction. See next. *(Right)* Left lateral planar Tc-99m PYP scan confirms focus of activity ➔ correspond to anterior wall. Finding is consistent with acute myocardial infarction.

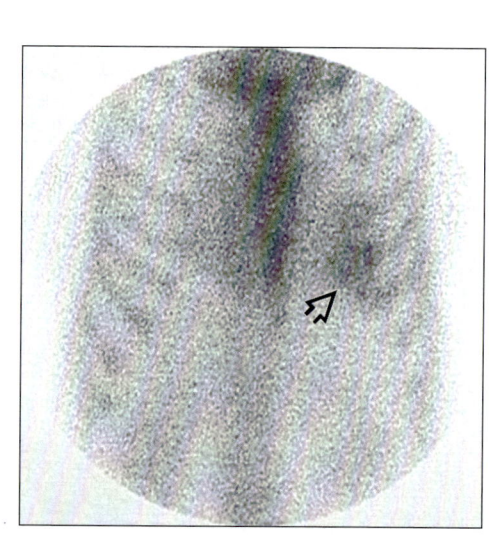

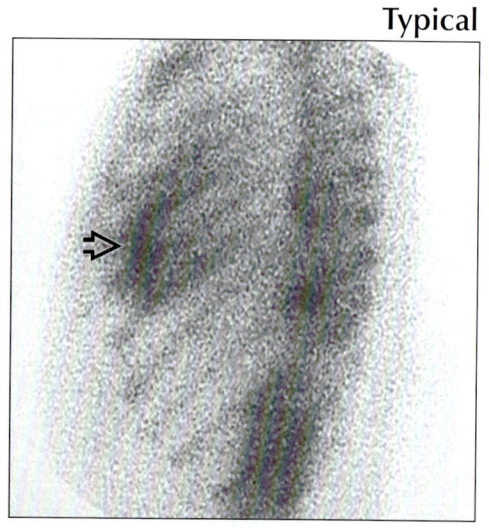

MYOCARDIAL INFARCTION

Typical

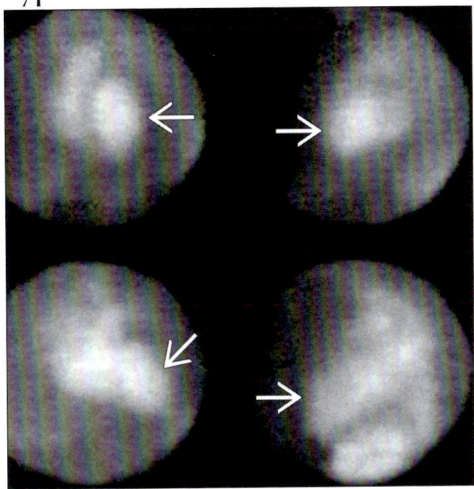

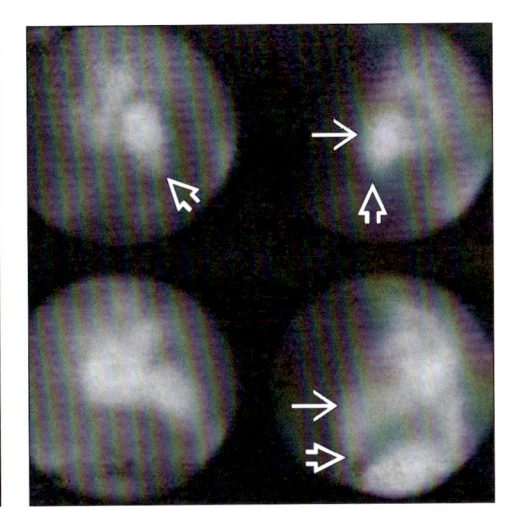

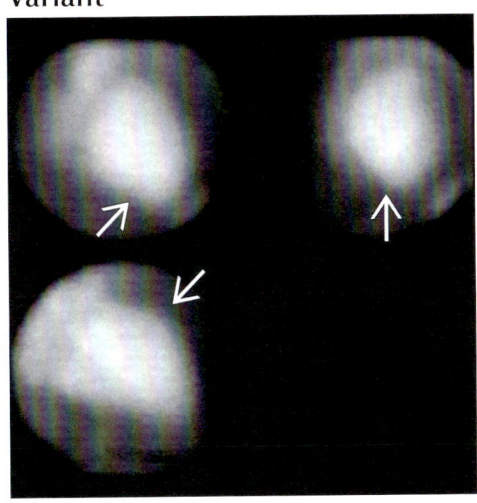

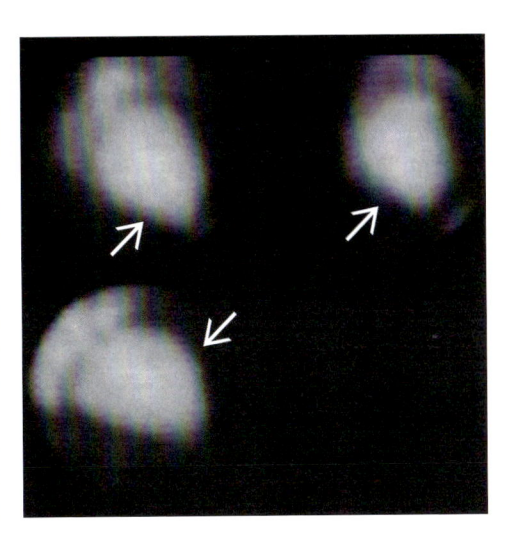

(Left) Multi-plane end-diastole MUGA frames show enlarged left ventricle ➡. See next. *(Right)* Multi-plane end-systole MUGA frames show enlarged left ventricle with akinesis of anterior wall ➡ and dyskinesis of apex ➡, consistent with large anteroapical infarct with apical aneurysm.

Variant

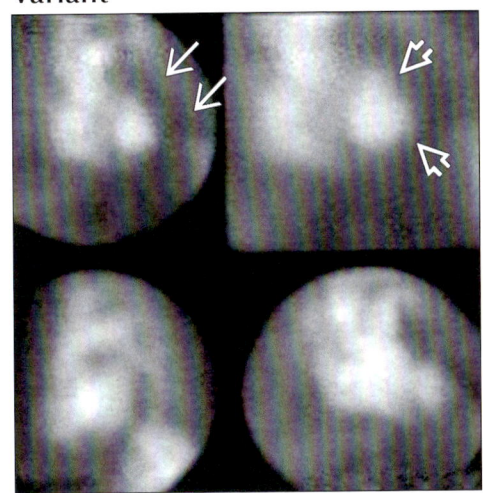

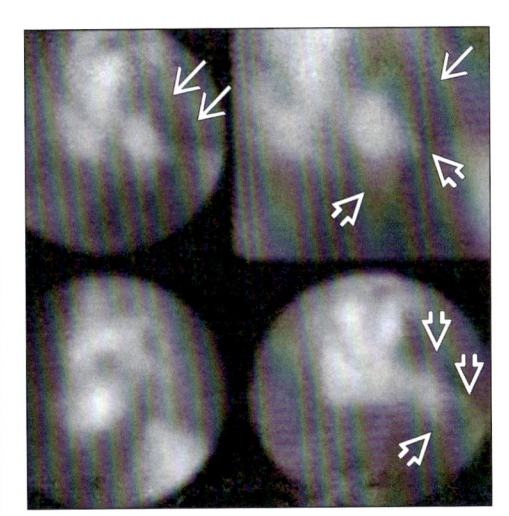

(Left) Multi-plane end-diastole MUGA frames show photopenic region around heart ➡ with irregular LV configuration ➡ in a patient with previous aneurysmectomy. See next. *(Right)* Multi-plane end-systole MUGA frames show multiple finger-like extensions ➡ (surgically-proven pseudoaneurysms). Photopenia around heart ➡ is clot in pericardium.

Variant

(Left) Multi-plane end-diastole MUGA frames show huge left ventricle ➡. See next. *(Right)* Multi-plane end-systole MUGA frames show little wall motion in huge left ventricle ➡, due to left main coronary artery infarction with left dominant circulation.

CARDIAC TRANSPLANT

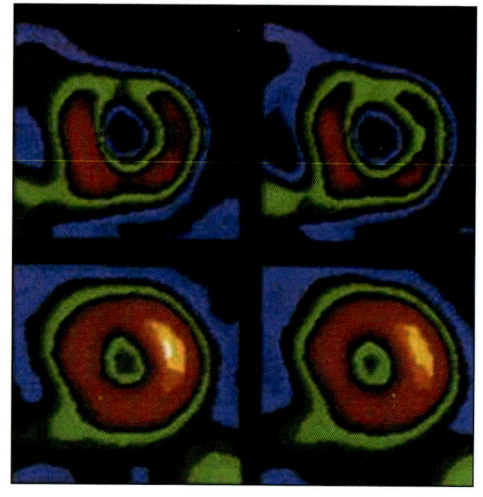

Axial stress (top) and rest (bottom) MPS in heart transplant patient shows severe, diffuse ischemia and transient ischemic dilatation. Diffuse coronary disease confirmed at angiography.

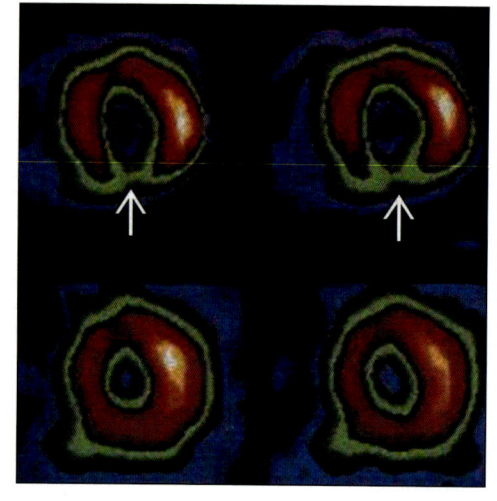

Axial stress (top) and rest (bottom) MPS in patient with cardiac transplantation x 6 years, no symptoms. Inferior wall ischemia ➡ required stenting of RCA lesion.

TERMINOLOGY

Abbreviations and Synonyms
- Cardiac transplantation, heart-lung transplant, transplant evaluation, cardiac allograft, cardiac replacement
- United Network for Organ Sharing (UNOS)
- Multigated acquisition (MUGA) = radionuclide ventriculography

Definitions
- Cardiac allograft vasculopathy (CAV): Diffuse narrowing and occlusion of transplanted coronary arteries

IMAGING FINDINGS

General Features
- Best diagnostic clue
  - Pretransplant evaluation
    - Myocardial uptake of F-18 FDG or Tl-201 indicates myocardial viability: May respond to revascularization
    - Severely decreased left ventricular ejection fraction
    - Decreased myocardial uptake of metaiodobenzylguanidine (MIBG): Heart-to-mediastinal ratio of < 1.7 indicates severe congestive failure; poor response to antiadrenergics, better candidate for transplantation (investigational)
  - Transplant rejection: Worsening ventricular function on MUGA, echo, gated SPECT, MR
    - ↓: In serial measurements of L or R ventricular ejection fraction, peak ejection rate
    - ↑: In L or R end diastolic volumes, time to peak ejection rate
  - Transplant rejection: Investigational techniques to identify cell death
    - ↑ Myocardial uptake of In-111 antimyosin antibodies: Heart-to-lung ratio of ≥ 1.55 indicates disordered cell death (necrosis)
    - ↑ Myocardial uptake of Tc-99m annexin: Programmed cell death (apoptosis)
  - Transplant rejection: CAV
    - Perfusion defects on gated SPECT or PET perfusion scintigraphy

DDx: MUGA Findings in Various States of Transplant Rejection

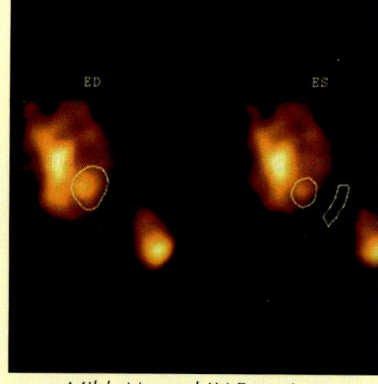

Mild: Normal LV Function 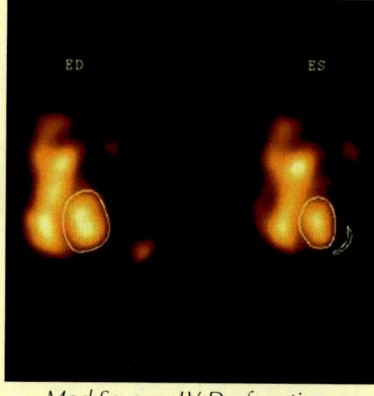 *Mod-Severe: LV Dysfunction* 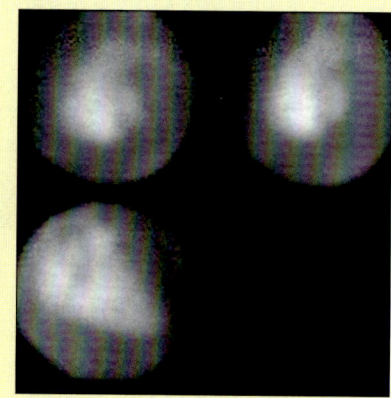 *Chronic: Small Noncompliant LV*

CARDIAC TRANSPLANT

Key Facts

Terminology
- Cardiac allograft vasculopathy (CAV): Diffuse narrowing and occlusion of transplanted coronary arteries

Imaging Findings
- Normal stress myocardial perfusion scintigraphy at 1 year post transplantation best predictor of long-term survival
- Acute rejection: Focal wall motion abnormalities, drop in ejection fraction seen only with moderate-severe rejection
- Chronic rejection: Small, non-compliant ventricle (abnormal diastolic parameters on MUGA), may also see as transplant "ages"
- Stress myocardial perfusion imaging to detect cardiac allograft vasculopathy: Affects long-term survival
- Cardiac computed tomography angiography (CTA) may be superior to conventional angiography in detecting CAV

Pathology
- Allograft vascular disease: Primary cause of late cardiac failure/death in heart transplant recipients
- Bronchiolitis obliterans syndrome: Common cause of death in heart-lung recipients

Clinical Issues
- Heart-lung transplant recipients are relatively spared from allograft coronary artery disease compared to heart transplant recipients
- Chest pain may be absent due to cardiac denervation
- ~ 80% survival at year 1; ~ 70% survival at year 5; ~ 20% survival at 15-20 years

---

- Decrease in absolute myocardial blood flow on PET perfusion scintigraphy
  ○ Long-term survival and complications
    ▪ Normal stress myocardial perfusion scintigraphy at 1 year post transplantation best predictor of long-term survival
    ▪ Dual-energy X-ray absorptiometry best test to monitor for development of osteoporosis, a common complication following organ transplantation
- Location
  ○ Endocardial biopsy takes a small sample from the right ventricle only
    ▪ Limited sensitivity for transplant rejection
  ○ Nuclear cardiac imaging: Increases sensitivity by evaluating both right and left ventricular function

Imaging Recommendations
- Best imaging tool
  ○ Pretransplant evaluation
    ▪ Myocardial viability: F-18 FDG PET (preferred) or rest-redistribution Tl-201 (acceptable)
    ▪ Ventricular function assessment: MUGA, gated SPECT, echocardiography, MR
    ▪ Sympathetic innervation: I-123 MIBG
  ○ Transplant rejection
    ▪ Myocyte death: In-111 antimyosin antibodies (necrosis, inflammation), Tc-99m annexin (apoptosis)
    ▪ CAV: PET myocardial perfusion imaging able to assess both regional perfusion defects and also quantify absolute myocardial blood flow; gated SPECT able to assess regional perfusion defects but poorly detects a global decrease in myocardial blood flow
    ▪ Worsening ventricular function: MUGA, gated SPECT, echocardiography, MR
    ▪ Acute rejection: Focal wall motion abnormalities, drop in ejection fraction seen only with moderate-severe rejection
    ▪ Chronic rejection: Small, non-compliant ventricle (abnormal diastolic parameters on MUGA), may also see as transplant "ages"
  ○ Long-term survival
    ▪ Stress myocardial perfusion imaging to detect cardiac allograft vasculopathy: Affects long-term survival
    ▪ Cardiac computed tomography angiography (CTA) may be superior to conventional angiography in detecting CAV
- Protocol advice
  ○ Exercise MUGA may increase sensitivity for detecting rejection compared to a rest only
  ○ Serial testing to detect early changes in perfusion, function

DIFFERENTIAL DIAGNOSIS

Pretransplantation: End Stage Cardiomyopathy
- Primary pulmonary hypertension
- Severe pulmonary disease
- Hypothyroidism
- Recurrent pulmonary embolism

Transplant Rejection: Clinical Mimics
- Musculoskeletal chest wall pain
- Peptic ulcer disease
- Depression, anxiety
- Medication side effects

PATHOLOGY

General Features
- Genetics: Most recipients Caucasian: Possible bias secondary to insurance coverage; genetic predisposition unproven
- Etiology
  ○ Cardiac failure prior to transplantation: Idiopathic cardiomyopathy (54%); ischemic cardiomyopathy (45%); congenital heart disease; valvular heart disease
  ○ Transplant rejection

CARDIAC TRANSPLANT

- Rejection initiated by invasion of inflammatory cells into the heart, causing myocardial damage
- Rejection results in the initiation of apoptosis
○ Death after transplantation
  - Allograft vascular disease: Primary cause of late cardiac failure/death in heart transplant recipients
  - Bronchiolitis obliterans syndrome: Common cause of death in heart-lung recipients
- Epidemiology: Nearly 2x as many patients on the waiting list than available organ donors
- Associated abnormalities
  ○ Denervation results in upregulation of β-adrenergic receptors during the early post-transplantation period (~ first 6 months)
  ○ Overall, no upregulation present late after transplantation, however, ratio of β2/β1 receptors increases

Microscopic Features
- Myocardial cell damage surrounded by lymphomononuclear cell infiltrate

CLINICAL ISSUES

Presentation
- Most common signs/symptoms
  ○ Early or mild transplant rejection: Shortness of breath, fever, flu-like symptoms, fatigue, persistent resting tachycardia, normal ventricular function
  ○ Severe transplant rejection: Hypotension, tachycardia, peripheral cyanosis, decreased heart sounds on auscultation
  ○ Transplant complications
    - Infections (secondary to chronic immunosuppression): Fever may or may not be present; leukocytosis may or may not be present; pain at site of infection may be decreased due to suppression of a normal inflammatory response
    - Heart-lung transplant recipients are relatively spared from allograft coronary artery disease compared to heart transplant recipients
    - Osteoporosis: Typically asymptomatic prior to fracture; back pain secondary to compression fractures
  ○ Normal signs and symptoms in recipients
    - Chest pain may be absent due to cardiac denervation
    - Decreased exercise tolerance secondary to loss of vasomotor tone
    - Increased resting heart rate
    - Decreased elevation of heart rate with stress
    - Depression

Demographics
- Age: Upper age limit for the recipient is ~ 65 y of age: 1/2 of recipients 50-65 y
- Gender: Male predominance

Natural History & Prognosis
- ~ 80% survival at year 1; ~ 70% survival at year 5; ~ 20% survival at 15-20 years

Treatment
- Increased surveillance for patients with rising In-111 antimyosin antibody uptake during the first 3 months
- Immunosuppression; steroids for acute rejection
- No smoking, stay active, blood pressure control, lipid lowering

DIAGNOSTIC CHECKLIST

Consider
- Mild rejection: Normal ventricular function
- Transplant ischemia: Often silent
- Chronic rejection: Abnormal diastolic function, small, non-compliant ventricle

SELECTED REFERENCES

1. Iyengar S et al: Detection of coronary artery disease in orthotopic heart transplant recipients with 64-detector row computed tomography angiography. J Heart Lung Transplant. 25(11):1363-6, 2006
2. Yap KS et al: Evaluation of sympathetic re-innervation in heterotopic cardiac transplants by iodine-123-metaiodobenzylguanidine (I-123-MIBG) imaging. J Heart Lung Transplant. 25(8):977-80, 2006
3. Hacker M et al: Dobutamine myocardial scintigraphy for the prediction of cardiac events after heart transplantation. Nucl Med Commun. 26(7):607-12, 2005
4. Khaw BA: Antibodies for molecular imaging in the cardiovascular system. J Nucl Cardiol. 12(5):591-604, 2005
5. Streeter RP et al: Stability of right and left ventricular ejection fractions and volumes after heart transplantation. J Heart Lung Transplant. 24(7):815-8, 2005
6. Bax JJ et al: Heart and lung transplantation. In: Diagnostic Nuclear Medicine. 4th ed. Philadelphia, Lippincott Williams & Wilkins, 2003
7. Dae MW: MIBG imaging. In: Nuclear Cardiac Imaging. 3rd ed. Oxford, Oxford University Press, 2003
8. Narula J et al: Development of newer radiotracers for evaluation of myocardial and vascular disorders. In: Nuclear Cardiac Imaging. 3rd ed. Oxford, Oxford University Press, 2003
9. Shirani J et al: Relation of thallium uptake to morphologic features of chronic ischemic heart disease: evidence for myocardial remodeling in noninfarcted myocardium. J Am Coll Cardiol. 38(1):84-90, 2001
10. Elhendy A et al: Accuracy of dobutamine tetrofosmin myocardial perfusion imaging for the noninvasive diagnosis of transplant coronary artery stenosis. J Heart Lung Transplant. 19(4):360-6, 2000
11. Ballester M et al: Noninvasive detection of acute heart rejection: the quest for the perfect test. J Nucl Cardiol. 4(3):249-55, 1997
12. Verhoeven PP et al: Prognostic value of noninvasive testing one year after orthotopic cardiac transplantation. J Am Coll Cardiol. 28(1):183-9, 1996
13. Kemkes BM et al: Noninvasive methods of rejection diagnosis after heart transplantation. J Heart Lung Transplant. 11(4 Pt 2):S221-31, 1992
14. Follansbee WP et al: Changes in left ventricular systolic function that accompany rejection of the transplanted heart: a serial radionuclide assessment of fifty-three consecutive cases. Am Heart J. 121(2 Pt 1):548-56, 1991

CARDIAC TRANSPLANT

IMAGE GALLERY

Typical

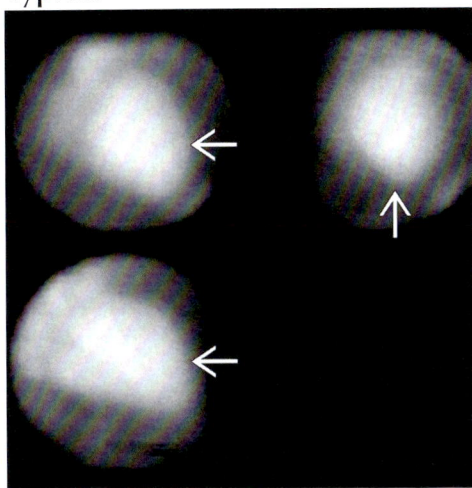

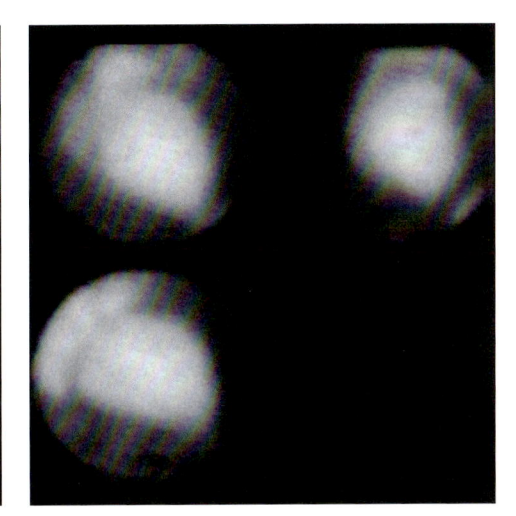

(Left) Resting MUGA, end diastole views, show massive dilatation of the left ventricle ➡ in patient with past history of left main coronary artery occlusion. See next image. *(Right)* Resting MUGA, end systole views show minimal change in appearance of left ventricle. LV ejection fraction = 15%. Patient subsequently received a heart transplant.

Typical

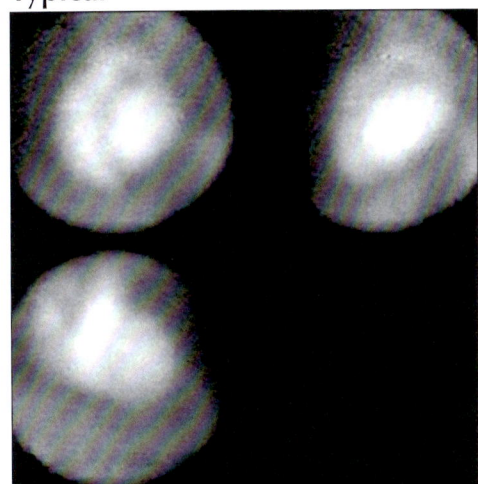

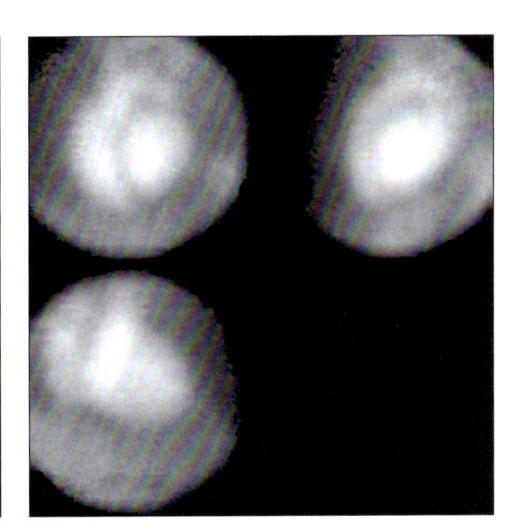

(Left) Resting MUGA, end diastole views show biventricular enlargement in patient with history of idiopathic dilated cardiomyopathy. See next image. *(Right)* Resting MUGA, end systole views show little change in size of either ventricle, global severe hypokinesis. LVEF = 5%. Patient subsequently received heart transplant.

Typical

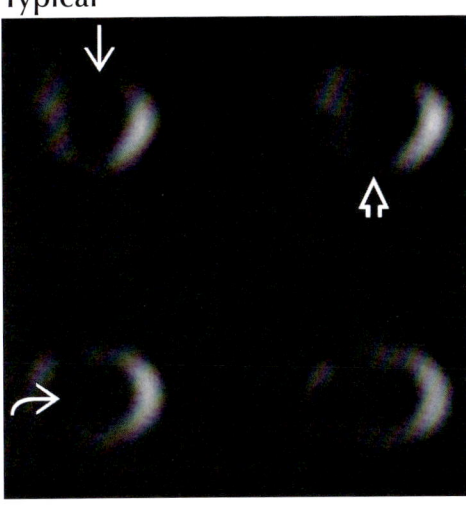

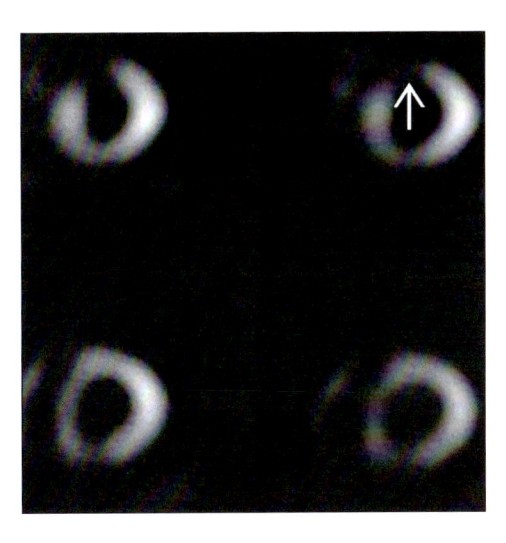

(Left) Pretransplant evaluation in patient with severe ventricular dysfunction: Axial stress MPS shows near absent perfusion to anterior ➡ septal ➡, and inferior ➡ walls. See next image. *(Right)* Axial rest MPS shows improved perfusion to anterior, septal and inferior walls, consistent with ischemia, as well as distal anterior infarct ➡. Revascularized with improved function.

LEFT-TO-RIGHT INTRACARDIAC SHUNTS

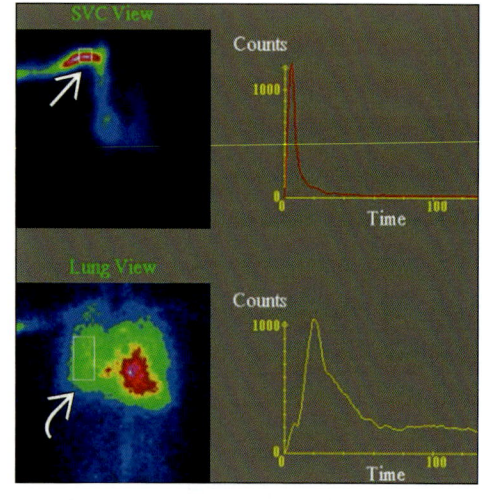

Raw data acquisition of a left-to-right intracardiac shunt analysis. Images show ROI over superior vena cava (SVC) ➡ and lung ➢. Note compact tracer bolus seen the in SVC graph.

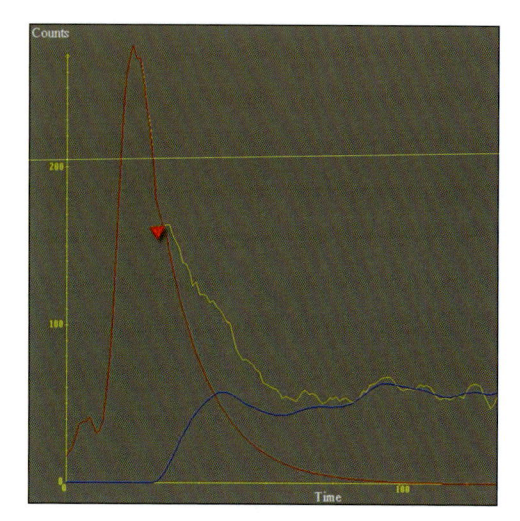

Gamma variate analysis of same patient as previous image shows measured lung activity (yellow) and fitted curve (red). Area under blue curve quantifies the shunt. (Courtesy F. Mishkin, MD).

TERMINOLOGY

Abbreviations and Synonyms
- Pulmonary blood flow (Qp), systemic blood flow (Qs)

Definitions
- Abnormal flow from systemic to pulmonary circulation typically due to cardiac septal defect

IMAGING FINDINGS

General Features
- Best diagnostic clue: Interatrial or interventricular septal defect with left-to-right flow on echocardiography or cine MR
- Location: Defect most commonly involves the interatrial or interventricular septum
- Size: Variable

Nuclear Medicine Findings
- Tracer injected IV as bolus has abnormal circulation kinetics through lungs with an early recirculation curve (may not be apparent on visual inspection)
  - Presence and degree of recirculation calculated by gamma variate function analysis
    - Qp/Qs ratio greater than 1.2:1 significant

CT Findings
- Direct visualization of septal defect can be incidental finding on CECT of chest

MR Findings
- Cardiac gated cine-MR shows defect, characterizes velocity and flow direction

Other Modality Findings
- Cardiac catheterization to evaluate differential oxygen saturation and calculate Qp/Qs ratio

Echocardiographic Findings
- Echo with Doppler shows defect, characterizes velocity and flow direction

Imaging Recommendations
- Best imaging tool: Echocardiography is preferred modality for primary evaluation
- Protocol advice

DDx: Right-to-Left Shunts with Other Imaging Modalities

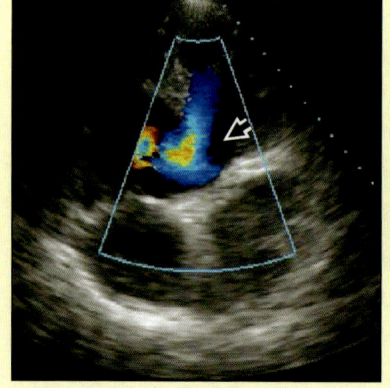

VSD on Doppler Echo

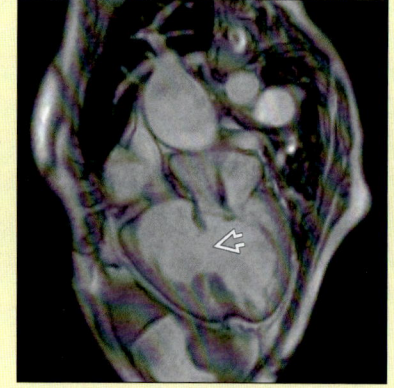

VSD on Cardiac MR

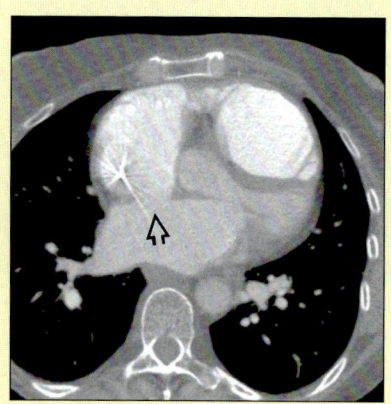

ASD on Contrast CT

LEFT-TO-RIGHT INTRACARDIAC SHUNTS

Key Facts

Terminology
- Abnormal flow from systemic to pulmonary circulation typically due to cardiac septal defect

Imaging Findings
- Best diagnostic clue: Interatrial or interventricular septal defect with left-to-right flow on echocardiography or cine MR
- Tracer injected IV as bolus has abnormal circulation kinetics through lungs with an early recirculation curve (may not be apparent on visual inspection)
- Presence and degree of recirculation calculated by gamma variate function analysis
- Qp/Qs ratio greater than 1.2:1 significant
- Compact bolus of radionuclide activity is required for accurate quantitation

○ Tc-99m pertechnetate most common tracer but other Tc-99m compounds can be used
○ Compact bolus of radionuclide activity is required for accurate quantitation
- Valsalva such as crying must be avoided
- High specific activity dose reduces volume of tracer dose
- Jugular injection site preferred over arm
- If arm must be injected, basilic vein preferred as it flows directly to central circulation

DIFFERENTIAL DIAGNOSIS

Extracardiac Left-to-Right Shunts
- Patent ductus arteriosus, extracardiac arteriovenous malformation, various congenital cardiac anomalies

PATHOLOGY

General Features
- Associated abnormalities
  ○ Other congenital cardiac anomalies
  ○ Situs anomalies of abdominal viscera (e.g., right-sided stomach)
  ○ Asplenia
  ○ Polysplenia

CLINICAL ISSUES

Presentation
- Most common signs/symptoms: Range from asymptomatic to pulmonary hypertension

Natural History & Prognosis
- Depends on severity of shunt
  ○ Eisenmenger syndrome: Left-to-right shunt leading to pulmonary vascular disease and increased pulmonary vascular resistance ultimately causing a net reversal of shunt flow (right-to-left)

Treatment
- Surgical closure of septal defect if clinically indicated

DIAGNOSTIC CHECKLIST

Image Interpretation Pearls
- Valvular regurgitant lesions contraindicate NM study

SELECTED REFERENCES

1. Eterovic D et al: Gated versus first-pass radioangiography in the evaluation of left-to-right shunts. Clin Nucl Med. 20(6):534-7, 1995
2. Port SC: Recent advances in first-pass radionuclide angiography. Cardiol Clin. 12(2):359-72, 1994
3. Madsen MT et al: An improved method for the quantification of left-to-right cardiac shunts. J Nucl Med. 32(9):1808-12, 1991

IMAGE GALLERY

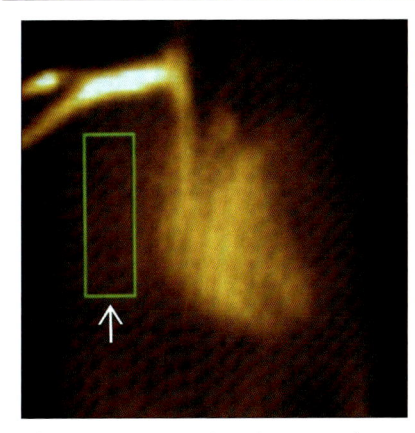

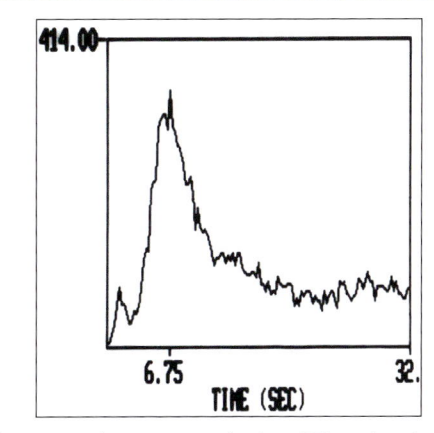

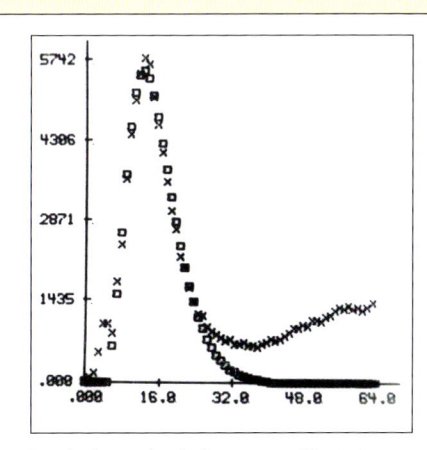

(Left) Anterior intracardiac shunt scan shows the region of interest over the lung ➡ used to determine the lung circulation curve. *(Center)* Time/activity curve for the lung is used for gamma variate calculation and Qp/Qs analysis. *(Right)* Lung recirculation curve (crosses) is fitted to the calculated curve (squares) showing no early recirculation of tracer into the pulmonary circulation.

RIGHT-TO-LEFT INTRACARDIAC SHUNTS

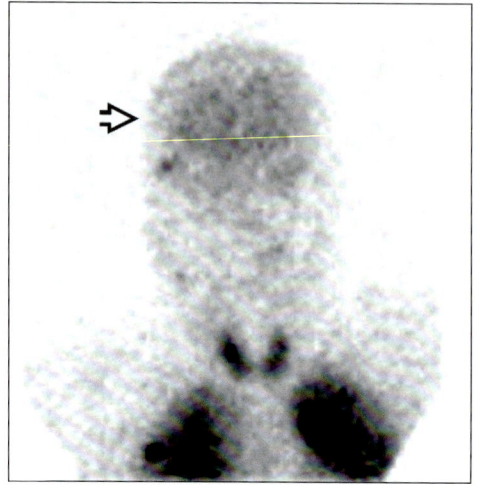

Anterior intracardiac shunt scan shows a disproportional amount of brain uptake ⇨ seen in this patient with a pulmonary to systemic shunt.

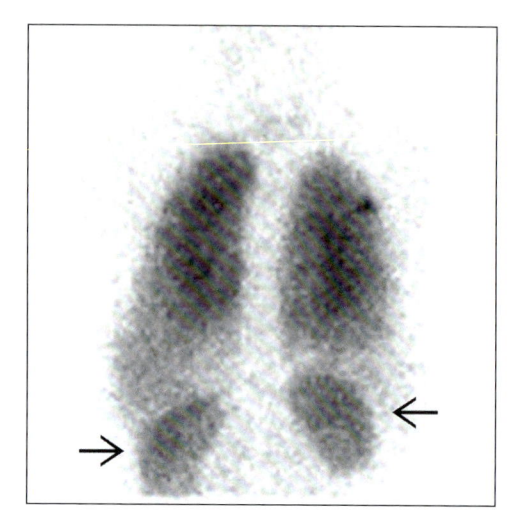

Posterior intracardiac shunt scan shows increased renal uptake ⇨ in the same patient as previous image. Greater than 95% of MAA should be trapped by the pulmonary capillary bed in normal patients.

TERMINOLOGY

Definitions
- Abnormal flow from pulmonary to systemic circulation bypassing the pulmonary capillary bed

IMAGING FINDINGS

General Features
- Best diagnostic clue: Septal defect showing right-to-left flow on echocardiography or cine-MRI
- Location: Defect most commonly involves the interatrial or interventricular septum
- Size: Variable

Nuclear Medicine Findings
- Macroaggregated albumin (MAA) injected intravenously is trapped by first capillary bed encountered, normally lungs
  - If right-to-left shunt is present, particles crossing the shunt bypass lungs and are trapped mostly in brain and renal capillaries with amount of activity proportional to size of shunt
    - Right to left shunt % = (total body counts - lung counts)/total body counts x 100
    - Normal physiologic shunting can be up to 5% of injected dose
- Early systemic appearance of tracer on nuclear angiogram is less sensitive and not quantitative
- Right-to-left shunt can be incidental finding on any study using MAA

CT Findings
- Direct visualization of septal defect is generally incidental finding on CECT

MR Findings
- Cardiac gated cine-MRI visualizes defect and characterizes flow direction and velocity

Echocardiographic Findings
- Echo with Doppler visualizes defect and characterizes flow direction and velocity

Imaging Recommendations
- Best imaging tool: Echocardiography is the primary imaging modality for initial evaluation
- Protocol advice

DDx: Additional Examples of Right-to-Left Shunt

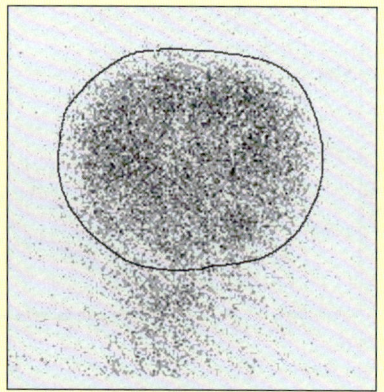

```
Tc-99m MAA

Total Lung Cts   = 12156.50
Total Brain Cts  = 15922.75
Total Kidney Cts = 17756.00

Percent of Total
Lung   = 27 %
Brain  = 35 %
Kidney = 39 %
```

Large Shunt (Brain) 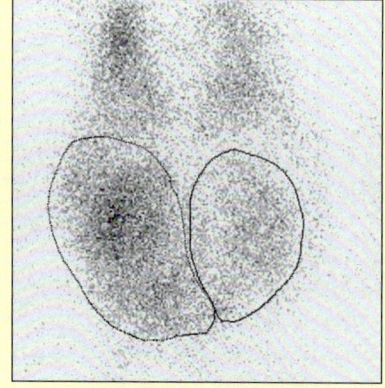 *Large Shunt (Abdomen)* 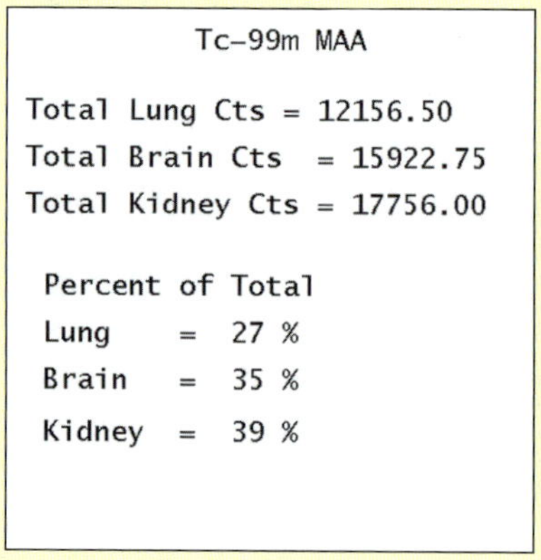 *Shunt Calculation*

RIGHT-TO-LEFT INTRACARDIAC SHUNTS

Key Facts

Terminology
- Abnormal flow from pulmonary to systemic circulation bypassing the pulmonary capillary bed

Imaging Findings
- Best diagnostic clue: Septal defect showing right-to-left flow on echocardiography or cine-MRI
- Location: Defect most commonly involves the interatrial or interventricular septum

- Best imaging tool: Echocardiography is the primary imaging modality for initial evaluation
- Reduce particles from typical lung scan dose of 700,000 to 80,000-100,000 for safety
- On serial studies, inject same extremity: Can affect measured shunt size

Diagnostic Checklist
- NM imaging findings not specific for shunt location

○ Reduce particles from typical lung scan dose of 700,000 to 80,000-100,000 for safety
○ On serial studies, inject same extremity: Can affect measured shunt size
○ After Blalock Taussig procedure, half of patients will have upper lobe lung reduced perfusion with an arm injection ipsilateral to the side of the surgery which usually corrects on a subsequent lower extremity injection

DIFFERENTIAL DIAGNOSIS

Possible Causes of Systemic Visualization of MAA
- Tetralogy of Fallot, VSD or ASD with Eisenmenger physiology, intrapulmonary shunts, hepatopulmonary syndrome, other congenital heart defects

PATHOLOGY

General Features
- Associated abnormalities: Defects can be isolated or associated with other congenital cardiac anomalies

CLINICAL ISSUES

Presentation
- Most common signs/symptoms: Variable ranging from asymptomatic to paradoxical emboli and heart failure

Natural History & Prognosis
- Depends on severity of shunt

Treatment
- Surgical closure if clinically indicated

DIAGNOSTIC CHECKLIST

Image Interpretation Pearls
- NM imaging findings not specific for shunt location
- When performing MAA lung scan on patient with history of congenital heart disease consider imaging brain and kidneys

SELECTED REFERENCES

1. Lu G et al: Tc-99m MAA total-body imaging to detect intrapulmonary right-to-left shunts and to evaluate the therapeutic effect in pulmonary arteriovenous shunts. Clin Nucl Med. 21(3):197-202, 1996
2. Hurwitz RA et al: Role of radionuclide shunt studies in management of infants and children. Clin Nucl Med. 11(11):781-5, 1986
3. Treves S et al: Radionuclide evaluation of circulatory shunts. Cardiol Clin. 1(3):427-39, 1983

IMAGE GALLERY

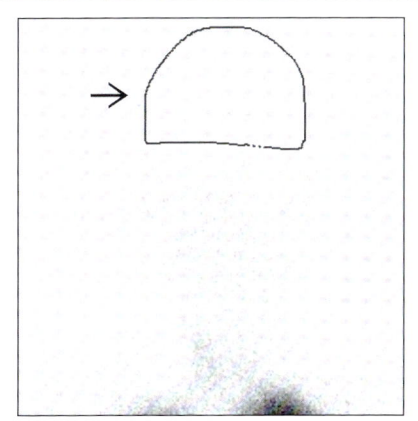

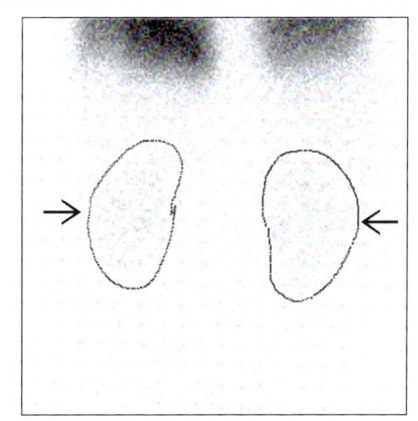

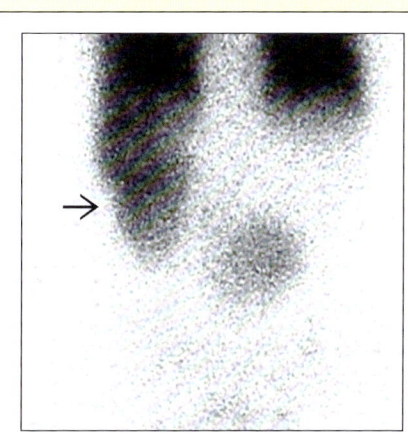

(Left) Anterior intracardiac shunt scan shows a brain region of interest ➔ which contains virtually no activity consistent with a normal right-to-left shunt study in a patient post shunt repair. *(Center)* Posterior intracardiac shunt scan shows renal regions of interest ➔ in the same patient as previous image consistent with no residual right-to-left shunt. *(Right)* Posterior V/Q scan shows marked renal uptake ➔ (the right kidney is ectopic) due to an atrial septal defect with bidirectional shunting.

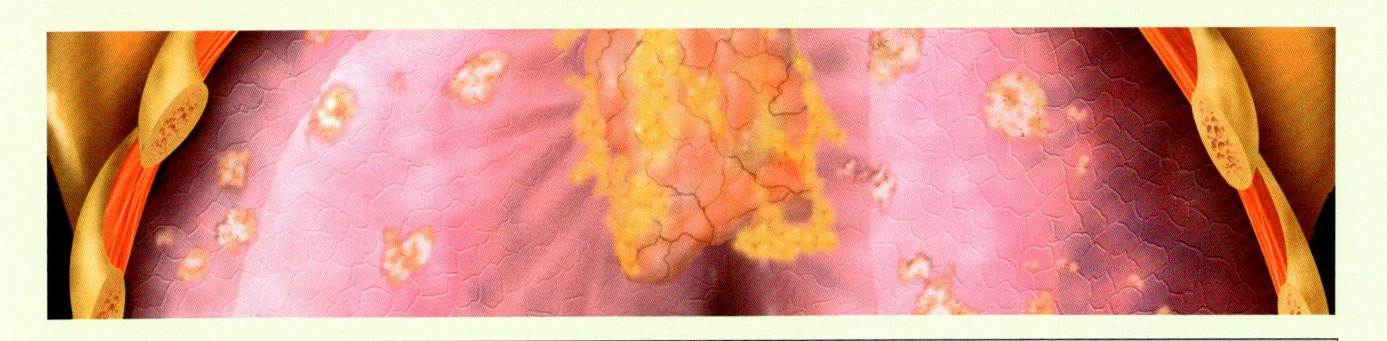

SECTION 4: Chest and Mediastinum

Introduction and Overview
V/Q Scan Overview   4-2

Lung Ventillation & Perfusion Abnormalities
V/Q, Pulmonary Embolism   4-6
V/Q, Quantitative   4-10

Lung Infection & Inflammation
Pneumocystis Carinii Pneumonia   4-16
Interstitial Lung Disease   4-20
Granulomatous Disease   4-24

Lung Cancer
Solitary Pulmonary Nodule   4-28
Non-Small Cell Lung Cancer   4-32
Metastases, Lungs & Mediastinum   4-38

Pleura
Pleural Disease, Malignant & Inflammatory   4-42

Mediastinum
Thymic Evaluation   4-46
Pericardial Disease, Malignant & Inflammatory   4-50

V/Q SCAN OVERVIEW

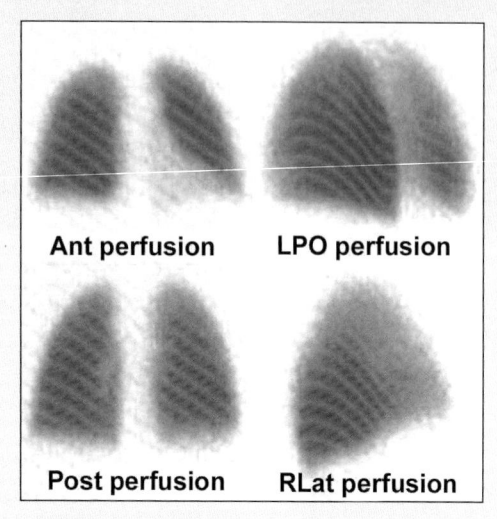

Multiple planar Tc-99m MAA Q images show homogeneous symmetrical distribution throughout both lungs. No segmental or subsegmental defects present. Interpretation: Normal (acute PE < 4%). Dx: No PE.

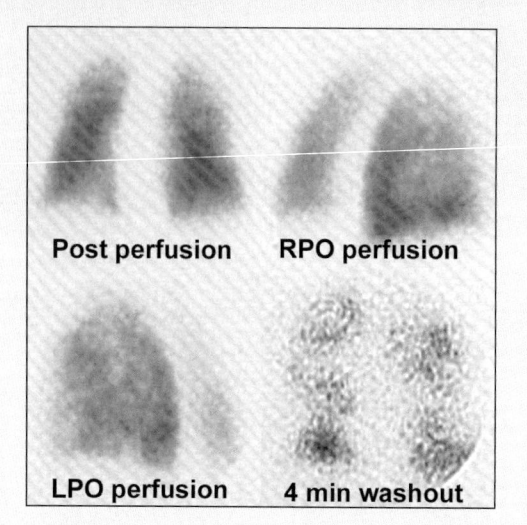

3 multiplanar Q images show small perfusion defects throughout both lungs. Interpretation: Low probability for acute PE (< 20%), regardless of V or CXR. Xe-133 retention suggests air trapping. Dx: Emphysema.

TERMINOLOGY

Abbreviations
- Prospective Investigation of Pulmonary Embolism Diagnosis (PIOPED) study
- Ventilation (V), perfusion (Q), V/Q scan (radionuclide ventilation and perfusion scan)
- Pulmonary embolism (PE)

Definitions
- V/Q scan: Scintigraphic diagnostic imaging test to assess pulmonary perfusion and ventilation, to determine likelihood of PE or quantification of regional and relative lung function
- V/Q mismatch: Perfusion defect with normal regional ventilation
- V/Q match: Ventilation and perfusion defects of same size and location

RADIOPHARMACEUTICALS

Perfusion
- Tc-99m macroaggregated albumin (MAA)
  - Tc-99m physical characteristics: 6 hour half-life, 140 keV, IT decay
  - Administration: 1-5 mCi (40-150 MBq); intravenous injection
  - Pediatric dose: 0.02-0.08 mCi/kg with minimum of 0.2 mCi (7-8 MBq)
  - Particle number: 200,000-700,000; < 300,000 for children, right to left shunt, severe pulmonary hypertension
  - Dosimetry
    - Target organ: Lung [(.067 mGy/MBq), (0.25 rad/mCi)]
    - Effective dose: 0.012 mSv/MBq (0.044 rem/mCi)
    - Pediatric dosimetry: Lung [(0.21 mGy/MBq), (0.78 rad/mCi)]; effective dose [(0.038 mSv/MBq), (0.14 rem/mCi)]

Ventilation
- Xe-133 gas
  - Xe-133 physical characteristics: 5.2 day half-life, 81 keV, beta decay
  - Administration: 5-20 mCi (200-750 MBq); inhaled via mouthpiece or facemask
  - Alternate route of administration: Xe-133 in saline, intravenous injection
  - Dosimetry
    - Target organ: Lung [(0.0011 mGy/MBq), (0.0041 rad/mCi)]
    - Effective dose: 0.0008 mSv/MBq (0.0030 rem/mCi)
    - Pediatric dosimetry: Lung [(0.21 mGy/MBq), (0.014 rad/mCi)]; effective dose [(0.0027 mSv/MBq), (0.01 rem/mCi)]
- Tc-99m DTPA aerosol
  - Tc-99m physical characteristics: 6 hour half-life, 140 keV, IT decay
  - Administration: 25-35 mCi (900-1300 MBq), from which patient receives ~ 0.5-1.0 mCi (20-40 MBq) to lungs; inhaled from nebulizer
  - Dosimetry
    - Target organ: Bladder [(0.047 mGy/MBq), (0.17 rad/mCi)]
    - Effective dose: 0.0070 mSv/MBq (0.026 rem/mCi)
    - Pediatric dosimetry: Bladder [(0.12 mGy/MBq), (0.44 rad/mCi)]; effective dose [(0.020 mSv/MBq), (0.074 rem/mCi)]
- Kr-81m gas: Rarely used because of cost and availability of Rb-81 generator

V/Q SCAN TECHNIQUE

Chest X-ray or Chest CT
- To exclude obvious causes of symptomatology
- Required for interpretation of V/Q scan
- Should be obtained prior to V/Q scan
- PA and lateral CXR preferred over portable AP
- If stable symptoms: CXR within 24 hour of V/Q scan is adequate
- If changing symptoms: CXR within 1 hour of V/Q scan is recommended

V/Q SCAN OVERVIEW

Interpretative Criteria

High Probability (HP): ≥ 80% Acute PE
- ≥ 2 large V/Q mismatched segments or arithmetic equivalent, regionally clear CXR/CT
- 2 large V/Q mismatches are borderline for acute PE (80% probability)
  - May categorize as either IP or HP

Intermediate Probability (IP): 20-79% Acute PE
- 1 moderate to 2 large V/Q mismatched defects, regionally clear CXR
- Moderate or large matched defect(s) with corresponding CXR opacity (same size as Q defect)
- CXR or CT opacity appreciably smaller than Q defect can be counted as mismatched
- Pattern not categorized as either LP or HP

Low Probability (LP): < 20% Acute PE
- Small Q defects (regardless of number); non-segmental Q defects
- VQ matching defects, CXR regionally clear
- Single moderate-to-large VQ match, CXR clear: 20% chance of PE (can be either IP or LP)
- Q defect substantially smaller than corresponding radiographic opacity
- Matched VQ defect with matching CXR or CT opacity stable in size > 10 days

Normal or Near-Normal Q: < 5% Probability of Acute PE
- Classified by Q pattern, regardless of V or CXR

Perfusion Scan (Q)
- Can be done before or after ventilation scan: If Tc-99m aerosol used for V, count rate for second study must exceed first by 3-4 fold
- If Q done first, with normal or low probability defects, V need not be done
- Prior to injection: Have patient cough and take several deep breaths
- Patient supine or near supine for injection
- Used well-flushed IV site; do not draw blood into syringe or IV site prior to injection (will cause clumping and hot spots in lungs)
- Inject in IV site close to skin (MAA sticks to tubing)
- Inject slowly over 3-5 breath cycles, flush well
- Imaging upright (sitting) preferred
- Projections: Anterior, posterior, R/L lateral, R/L anterior/posterior obliques
- High resolution collimator, 256 x 256 matrix
- Minimum 500,000 count ID posterior image, then same time for remaining images, typically 2-4 min
- Ventilation scan (V)
  - Tc-99m aerosol
    - Administered through mouthpiece with nose occluded, during tidal breathing
    - 300,000-500,000 count image in posterior projection, then for same time in other projections
    - High resolution collimator, upright imaging preferred
    - Advantage: Can view lungs in multiple projections for better correlation between V and Q defects
    - Disadvantage: Aerosol deposition altered by turbulent flow, central deposition degrades images
  - Xe-133 gas
    - Low energy collimator
    - Inhale through mouthpiece, nose clamped, preferably upright
    - Preferably image posteriorly, upright (if possible)
    - Alternative position: Do Q scan first, then position for optimal delineation of Q defect
    - Deep breath hold image for 15 sec image, 3-5 minute rebreathing (equilibrium) image, then serial 1 minute washout images x 5
  - Kr-81m: Breath continuously from generator until reaches single breath distribution, medium energy collimator

Information to be Obtained Prior to V/Q Scan
- Pregnancy status: Less dose to fetus from CTA than V/Q scan
- Issues requiring reduction in particle number: Severe pulmonary hypertension, right to left shunt, pediatric patient
- Pertinent clinical information
  - Symptoms: Chest pain, dyspnea, hemoptysis, pleuritic chest pain, leg/arm swelling/redness
  - Clinical history: Prior PE, cancer, recent surgery, trauma, pulmonary disease, IV drug abuse, antecedent illness, oral contraceptives, pregnancy, congestive failure (CHF), current anticoagulant therapy/status
  - Physical exam: Vital signs, hypoxia, evidence of right heart failure (increased P2 heart sound, right axis deviation on ECG, increased jugular waves)
  - Results of correlative radiography (CXR, CT)
    - Suggestive of PE: Normal radiograph, pleural effusion, peripheral wedge-shaped focal lung opacity, enlarged azygous vein or central pulmonary arteries, pulmonary artery cutoff, pulmonary oligemia
    - Suggestive of other causes: Consolidation with air-bronchograms (pneumonia), cardiomegaly with diffuse pulmonary edema (CHF), emphysema with worsened hyperinflation, atelectasis, bibasilar infiltrates (aspiration), masses
  - Results of other tests for deep venous thrombosis, PE
  - Other: Availability of vascular access, ability to follow instructions, ability to lay supine, ability to sit up, ability to hold breath for 15 seconds

V/Q SCAN OVERVIEW

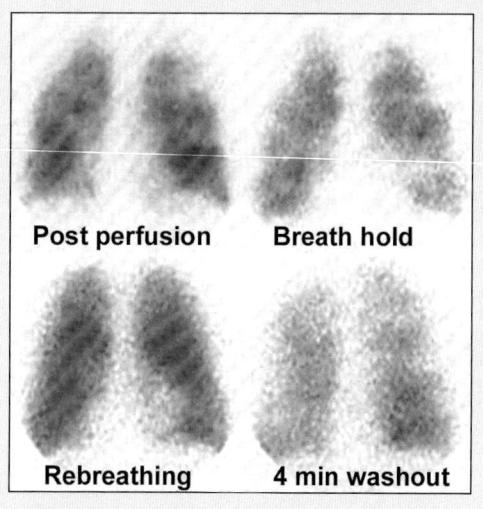

Posterior Tc-99m MAA Q image and 3 Xe-133 V images demonstrate extensive V/Q matching defects. CXR was normal. Interpretation: Low probability of acute PE (< 20%). Dx: Severe emphysema.

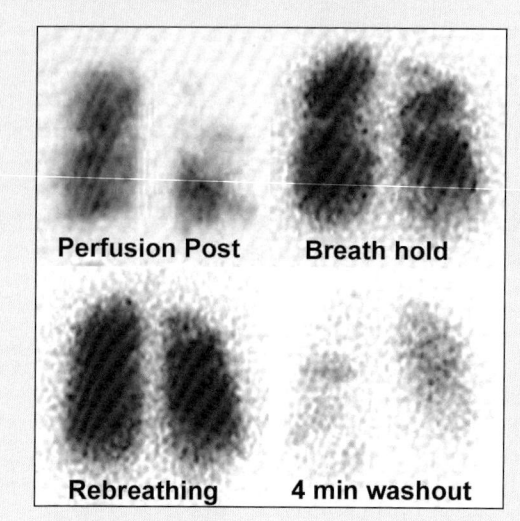

Posterior Tc-99m MAA Q image and 3 Xe-133 V images demonstrate extensive matching V/Q defects. CXR normal. Interpretation: Low probability of acute PE (< 20%). Dx: 14 year old female with asthma.

INTERPRETATION: MODIFIED PIOPED

Perfusion Defects
- Large: > 75% of a bronchopulmonary segment
- Moderate: 25-75% of a bronchopulmonary segment
- Small: < 25% of a bronchopulmonary segment
- Non-segmental: Defects due to extrapulmonary structures or failing to correspond to bronchopulmonary anatomy
  - Examples: Defects due to hilar structures, heart, aorta, extrapleural masses, chest wall deformity, spine, scapula, pleural effusion

High Probability (HP): ≥ 80% Chance of Acute PE
- ≥ 2 large V/Q mismatched segments or arithmetic equivalent, regionally clear CXR
  - Arithmetic equivalent: 2 moderate = 1 large defect
    - Note: Small defects are not additive
- 2 large V/Q mismatches: Borderline for acute PE (80% probability); categorized as either IP or HP

Intermediate Probability (IP): 20-79% Probability of Acute PE
- 1 moderate to 2 large V/Q mismatched defects, regionally clear CXR
- Moderate or large matched defects with corresponding CXR opacity (same size as Q defect)
- CXR or CT opacity appreciably smaller than Q defect can be counted as mismatched
- Pattern not categorized as either LP or HP
- Single moderate-large V/Q match, clear CXR: 20% chance of PE: Can be either LP or IP
- Experienced reader may Gestalt probability within IP range

Low Probability (LP): < 20% Probability of Acute PE
- Small Q defects (regardless of number): V or CXR/CT findings irrelevant
- VQ matching defects, CXR regionally clear
- Non-segmental Q defects
- Single moderate-to-large VQ match, clear CXR: 20% chance of PE: Can be either IP or LP
- Q defect substantially smaller than corresponding radiographic opacity
- Matched VQ defect with matching CXR or CT opacity stable in size > 10 d

Normal to Near-Normal: < 5% Chance of Acute PE
- Defined by perfusion, not ventilation pattern

Ventilation Defects
- Tc99m aerosol: Defect sizes graded as for perfusion imaging
- Xe-133
  - Defects defined either on breath hold, equilibrium or washout images
  - Retention beyond 3-4 minutes washout: Abnormal and implies air trapping
  - Hypoventilation: Diffuse mild retention beyond 3-4 minutes

RELATED REFERENCES

1. Freitas JE et al: Modified PIOPED criteria used in clinical practice. J Nucl Med. 36(9):1573-8, 1995
2. Worsley DF et al: Comprehensive analysis of the results of the PIOPED Study. Prospective Investigation of Pulmonary Embolism Diagnosis Study. J Nucl Med. 36(12):2380-7, 1995
3. Sostman HD et al: Evaluation of revised criteria for ventilation-perfusion scintigraphy in patients with suspected pulmonary embolism. Radiology. 193(1):103-7, 1994
4. Gottschalk A et al: Ventilation-perfusion scintigraphy in the PIOPED study. Part I. Data collection and tabulation. J Nucl Med. 34(7):1109-18, 1993
5. Gottschalk A et al: Ventilation-perfusion scintigraphy in the PIOPED study. Part II. Evaluation of the scintigraphic criteria and interpretations. J Nucl Med. 34(7):1119-26, 1993

V/Q SCAN OVERVIEW

IMAGE GALLERY

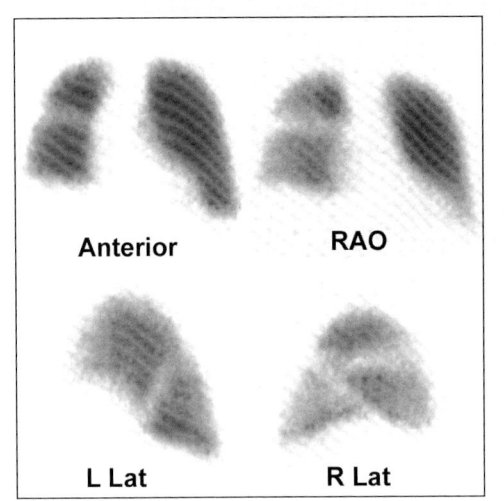

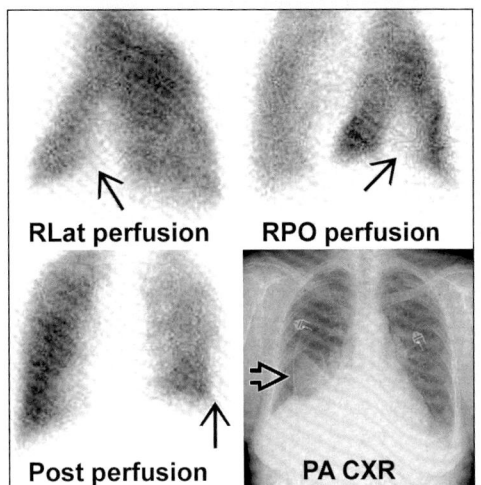

(Left) Multiplanar Tc-99m MAA Q images show widening of all fissures (all defects are non-segmental) without additional defects. CXR: Pleural fluid loculated in all fissures. Interpretation: Low probability for acute PE (< 20%). Dx: Pleural effusions. *(Right)* Multiplanar Q images & PA CXR show single large Q ➔ defect right lung, with corresponding opacity ➔ on CXR. Interpretation: Intermediate probability of acute PE (20-79%). Actual DX: Pneumonia.

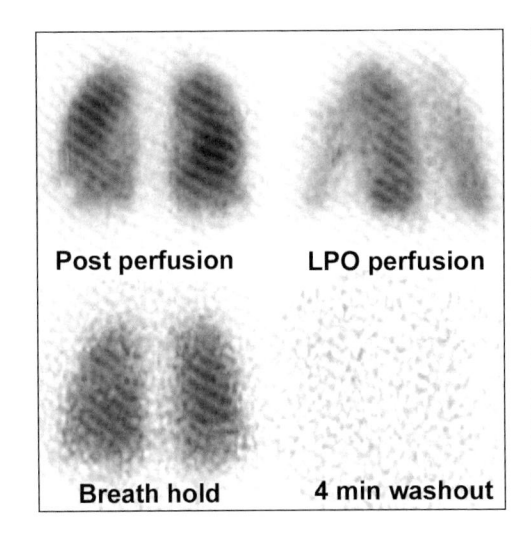

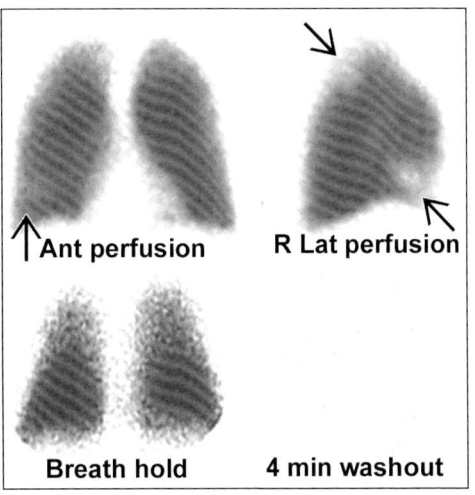

(Left) Tc-99m MAA Q images with corresponding V images show single large V/Q mismatched defect in left lateral base. CXR was regionally clear. Interpretation: Intermediate probability of acute PE (20-79%). *(Right)* Tc-99m MAA Q images with corresponding V images show 2 large V/Q mismatches ➔ in right lung. CXR was regionally clear. Interpretation: High probability of acute PE (borderline at 80%).

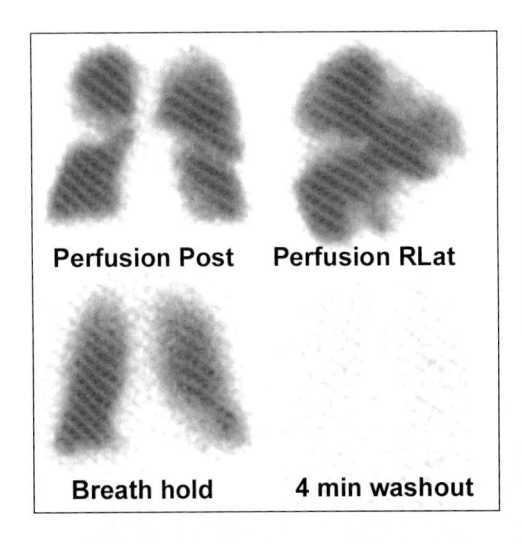

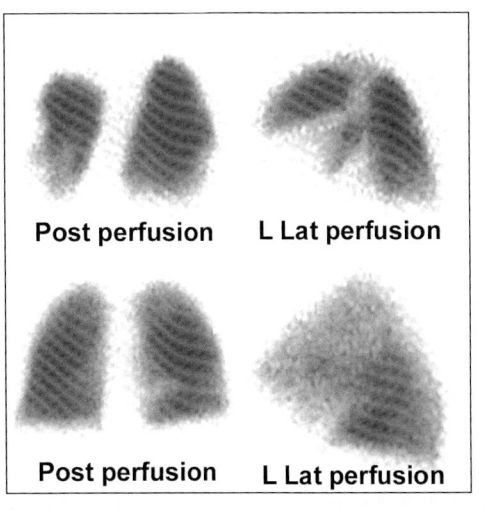

(Left) Multiplanar Tc-99m MAA Q images with corresponding V images show many moderate and large V/Q mismatches in both lungs. CXR was regionally clear. Interpretation: High probability of acute PE (≥ 80%). *(Right)* Upper panel: Multiplanar perfusion images from high probability V/Q scan (V, CXR were normal). Lower panel: Repeat exam 1 week later. Q defects can resolve in < 1 week in normal young patients.

V/Q, PULMONARY EMBOLISM

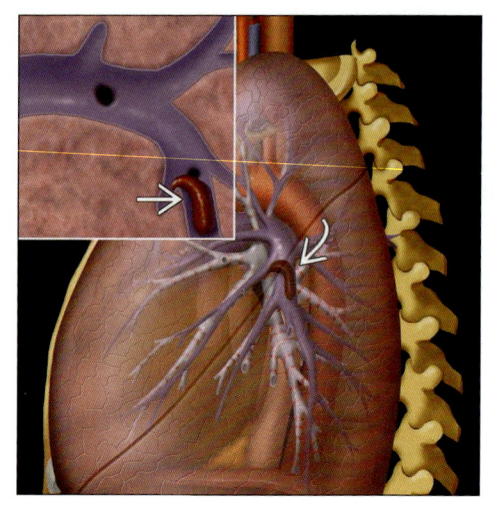

Graphic demonstrates intraluminal thrombus ➤ in the left interlobar pulmonary artery ➤.

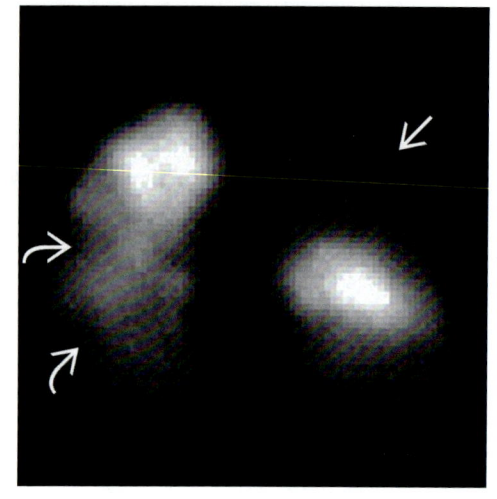

Posterior perfusion lung scan shows several large, segmental perfusion defects in the right ➤ and left ➤ lungs in a patient with acute PE.

TERMINOLOGY

Abbreviations and Synonyms
- Pulmonary embolism (PE)
- Ventilation perfusion scan (V/Q scan)

Definitions
- Venous thromboembolism lodges in pulmonary arterial system

IMAGING FINDINGS

General Features
- Best diagnostic clue: Peripheral, wedge-shaped segmental or subsegmental lung perfusion defects with normal ventilation on V/Q scan
- Location: Lower lobes > upper lobes
- Size
  o Typically at least 2 large segmental perfusion defects
    ▪ Large: > 75% of a segment
    ▪ Moderate: 26-74% of a segment
    ▪ Small: < 25% of a segment
  o V/Q detects > 95% of emboli which completely occlude pulmonary arterioles > 2 mm
- Morphology
  o Wedge shaped
  o Apex of wedge directed toward pulmonary hila
  o At lung periphery: Pleural-based, includes fissures
- Number
  o Usually ≥ 2 pulmonary segments involved in PE

Nuclear Medicine Findings
- V/Q Scan
  o Ventilation imaging combined with perfusion imaging improves specificity of PE diagnosis
  o PE: Key finding is V/Q mismatch (abnormal Q, normal V) with clear radiograph (in that region)
  o Ventilation scan (V) abnormalities
    ▪ Abnormal ventilation and perfusion: Parenchymal lung disease [tumor, infection, chronic obstructive pulmonary disease (COPD), asthma]
    ▪ Ventilation abnormalities larger than perfusion abnormalities (reverse mismatch): Airway obstruction, mucous plugging, airspace disease, pneumonia
  o Perfusion scan (Q)

DDx: Other Causes of V/Q Mismatch

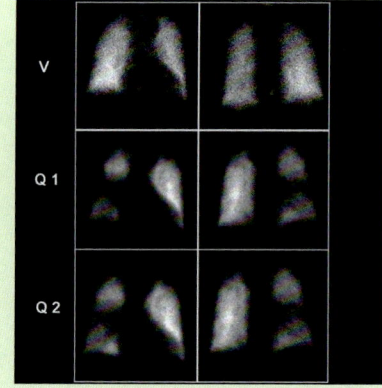

Chronic PE 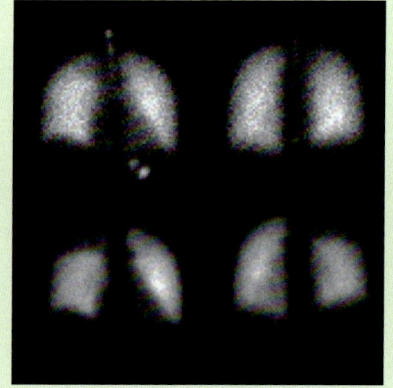 | *Vasculitis* 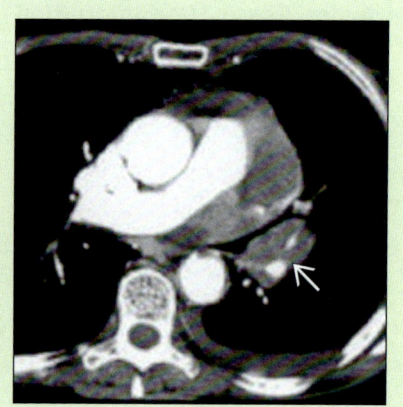 | *Lung Cancer*

V/Q, PULMONARY EMBOLISM

Key Facts

Imaging Findings
- Location: Lower lobes > upper lobes
- V/Q detects > 95% of emboli which completely occlude pulmonary arterioles > 2 mm
- Most patients with acute PE have radiographically normal chest
- Chest X-ray (CXR): To exclude clinical mimics of PE; adjunct to interpretation of V/Q scan
- CTA: Usually first-line PE examination in clinical practice today
- CTA: 83% sensitivity; 96% specificity for PE
- High probability: ≥ 80% likelihood of acute PE
- High probability: At least 2 large (or arithmetic equivalent) mismatched segmental perfusion defects
- Intermediate probability: 20-79% chance of acute PE
- Intermediate probability: At least 1 moderate, but less than 2 large (or arithmetic equivalent), mismatched segmental perfusion defects
- Intermediate probability: Matched V/Q defects with clear chest radiograph
- Intermediate probability: Patterns difficult to categorize as either low or high probability
- Low probability: ≤ 20% likelihood of acute PE
- Low probability: Matched perfusion and ventilation defects with normal chest radiograph (some areas of normal perfusion present)
- Low probability: Small perfusion defects
- Low probability: Nonsegmental perfusion defects (cardiomegaly, enlarged vasculature, overlying structures): Likely normal perfusion

---

    - High sensitivity: Identifying decreased/absent pulmonary perfusion
    - Low specificity: Virtually all parenchymal lung diseases cause decreased perfusion
    - Provides estimate of pulmonary clot burden, hemodynamic effects
  - Usually second-line examination used in clinical practice today (CTA #1)
    - Most often used in patients with CT contraindications
    - Preferred study for morbidly obese patients
    - V/Q imaging can be easily and safely performed in patients with orthopnea, renal insufficiency, contrast allergies
    - False negatives: Partially occluded vessel; low clot burden; subacute clot (retracted)
  - High probability: ≥ 80% likelihood of acute PE
    - High probability: At least 2 large (or arithmetic equivalent) mismatched segmental perfusion defects
    - Moderate or large perfusion defects substantially larger than CXR abnormality (V normal): Can count as mismatched
    - Arithmetic equivalent: 2 moderate = 1 large (note: Small defects do not add up to either moderate or large)
  - Intermediate probability: 20-79% chance of acute PE
    - Intermediate probability: At least 1 moderate, but less than 2 large (or arithmetic equivalent), mismatched segmental perfusion defects
    - Intermediate probability: Matched V/Q defects with clear chest radiograph
    - Intermediate probability: Patterns difficult to categorize as either low or high probability
  - Low probability: ≤ 20% likelihood of acute PE
    - Low probability: Matched perfusion and ventilation defects with normal chest radiograph (some areas of normal perfusion present)
    - Low probability: Perfusion defect with substantially larger abnormality on chest radiograph
    - Low probability: Small perfusion defects
    - Low probability: Nonsegmental perfusion defects (cardiomegaly, enlarged vasculature, overlying structures): Likely normal perfusion
  - Normal (virtually excludes acute PE)
    - No perfusion defects on lung scan

Radiographic Findings
- Most patients with acute PE have radiographically normal chest
- Chest X-ray (CXR): To exclude clinical mimics of PE; adjunct to interpretation of V/Q scan
- Atelectasis or opacity in affected segment
  - Most common positive radiographic finding in patients with PE
  - Also most common finding in patients in whom PE excluded

CT Findings
- CTA
  - Direct visualization of thromboembolism in pulmonary arteries
    - Partial or complete intraluminal filling defect(s) in pulmonary arteries
    - Abrupt pulmonary artery vessel cutoff
  - CTA: Usually first-line PE examination in clinical practice today
    - CTA: 83% sensitivity; 96% specificity for PE
    - Negative predictive value close to 100%
    - Detects asymptomatic PE in 1-3% of patients
    - Higher interobserver agreement than with V/Q
    - May provide etiology of alternate diagnosis if PE excluded
    - CTA is more likely to provide a definite diagnosis in patients with significant CXR abnormalities
  - Technical issues
    - Technically inadequate studies occur in 2-4% of patients
  - Contraindications
    - Iodinated contrast allergy
    - Acute renal failure, renal insufficiency; end-stage renal disease patients on chronic dialysis OK
    - Morbid obesity (table weight restrictions)
    - Claustrophobia

V/Q, PULMONARY EMBOLISM

Imaging Recommendations
- Best imaging tool
  - V/Q scan indicated in patients with
    - Acute renal failure, renal insufficiency
    - Morbid obesity
    - Orthopnea
    - Iodinated contrast allergies
    - Inconclusive CTA
    - Claustrophobia
  - CTA
    - Most common PE examination used in clinical practice today
- Protocol advice: Pregnant women: CTA with abdominal lead shield gives lower dose to fetus than VQ scan

DIFFERENTIAL DIAGNOSIS

Chronic or Unresolved PE
- Often indistinguishable from acute PE without prior scan
- Other patterns include heterogeneous perfusion
- CT: Vascular pruning, mosaic attenuation

Pulmonary Vascular Abnormalities
- Unilateral decrease/absent perfusion in pulmonary artery
  - Extrinsic compression: Tumor, adenopathy
  - Intrinsic vascular obliteration: Vasculitis, pulmonary artery tumor
  - Congenital
    - Pulmonary artery agenesis, hypoplasia

Non-Thromboembolic Intraluminal Occlusions
- Tumor
- Foreign body
- Septic emboli

PATHOLOGY

General Features
- Genetics: Protein C deficiency, protein S deficiency, antithrombin III deficiency, hyperhomocysteinemia, factor V Leiden
- Epidemiology: Incidence of deep venous thromboembolism (DVT) approximately 1:1,000/year

CLINICAL ISSUES

Presentation
- Most common signs/symptoms
  - 97% of patients with PE
    - Dyspnea, tachypnea or pleuritic chest pain present
  - Increased risk with
    - Stasis: Immobilization, recent surgery (< 3 months), trauma, obesity
    - Hypercoagulability: Genetic factors, cancer, cigarette smoking, pregnancy, systemic inflammatory conditions
- Other signs/symptoms
  - Positive D-dimer: High sensitivity, low specificity for venous thromboembolism
  - Hemodynamic instability
  - Acute pulmonary hypertension

Demographics
- Age: Increased risk with age
- Gender
  - M = F for risk factors, clinical signs, symptoms and prevalence
  - Mortality: M > F (hazard ratio 7:1)

Natural History & Prognosis
- Overall mortality among treated patients is 2.5-8%
  - Mortality highest with hemodynamic instability, acute pulmonary hypertension
- Survival beyond first hour following PE requires highly effective treatment
- Resolution depends on: Pulmonary clot burden, type/timing of therapy, cardiopulmonary status, age
- Clot burden at 7-10 days after anticoagulant therapy = good predictor of clot resolution
- 75-80% perfusion defects resolve by 3 months following initiation of anticoagulation

Treatment
- Anticoagulation with heparin, warfarin: Prevent further thromboembolism
- Thrombolytic therapy: Decrease clot burden in lungs
- Venous filters: When thromboembolism occurs despite medical management

DIAGNOSTIC CHECKLIST

Image Interpretation Pearls
- Normal V/Q scan excludes clinically significant PE
- Low probability V/Q and low clinical likelihood of disease do not require further study or treatment
- Low probability V/Q scan with intermediate/high clinical likelihood of PE: Venous Dopplers, CTA
- Intermediate V/Q scan: Venous Doppler ultrasound to evaluate for DVT
- High probability V/Q with low clinical likelihood of PE require further study (CTA, angiography)
- High probability V/Q with high clinical likelihood of PE requires treatment; no further test necessary

SELECTED REFERENCES
1. Stein PD et al: Multidetector computed tomography for acute pulmonary embolism. N Engl J Med. 354(22):2317-27, 2006
2. Wells PS et al: Diagnosis of pulmonary embolism: when is imaging needed? Clin Chest Med. 24(1):13-28, 2003
3. Worsley DF et al: Radionuclide imaging of acute pulmonary embolism. Semin Nucl Med. 33(4):259-78, 2003
4. Freitas JE et al: Modified PIOPED criteria used in clinical practice. J Nucl Med. 36(9):1573-8, 1995
5. Sostman HD et al: Evaluation of revised criteria for ventilation-perfusion scintigraphy in patients with suspected pulmonary embolism. Radiology. 193(1):103-7, 1994

V/Q, PULMONARY EMBOLISM

IMAGE GALLERY

Typical

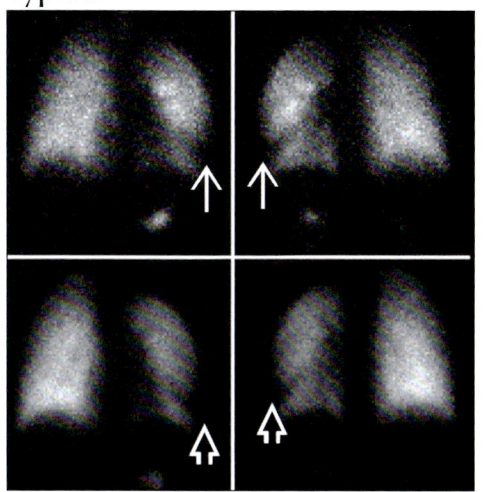

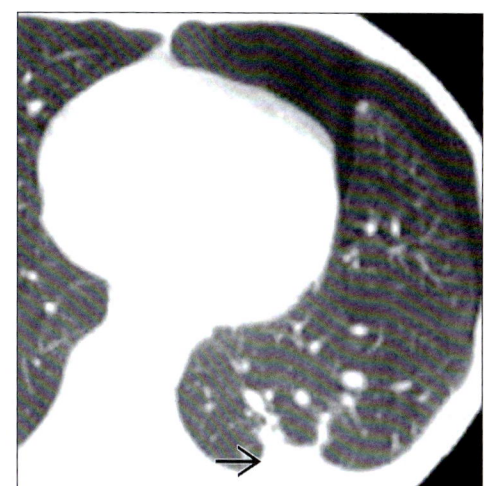

(Left) Anterior and posterior Tc-99m aerosol ventilation shows peripheral ventilation defect ➡ in left lung (upper panels). Perfusion images show matching moderate defect ➡ in left lung (lower panels). Same patient as next image. *(Right)* Axial NECT shows left pneumothorax and focal opacity ➡ in posterior lower lobe, corresponding to V and Q defect. Interpretation: Intermediate probability for acute PE.

Typical

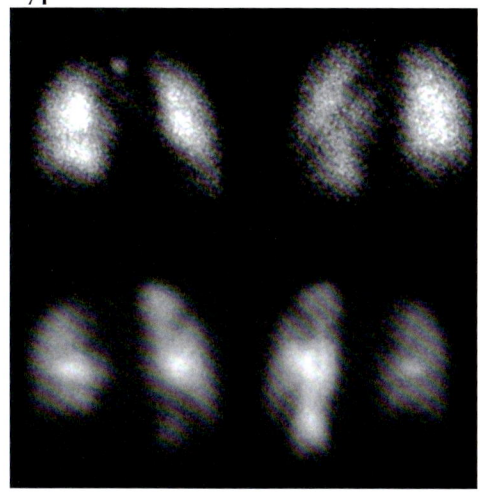

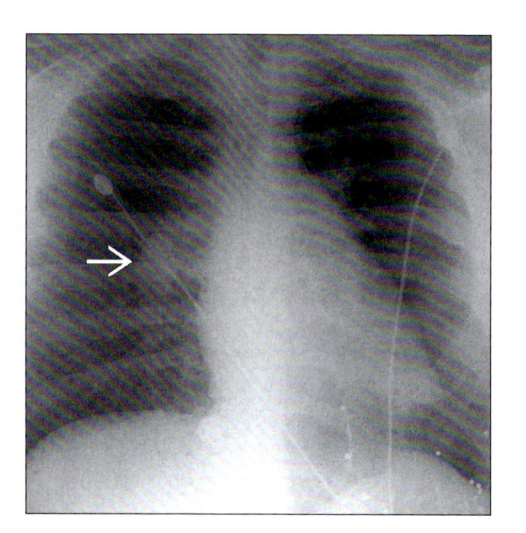

(Left) Anterior and posterior ventilation (top row) and perfusion (bottom row) images show generalized V/Q mismatch within the entire right lung and multiple segmental regions of V/Q mismatch within the left lung. Same patient as next image. *(Right)* Anteroposterior radiograph shows corresponding hyperlucency within the right hemithorax and an enlarged right pulmonary artery ➡. Interpretation: High probability for acute PE.

Typical

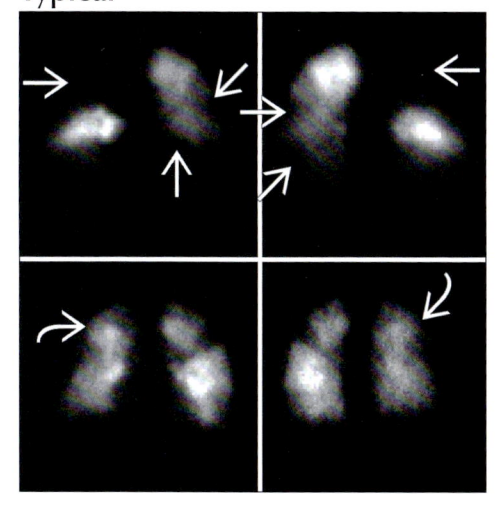

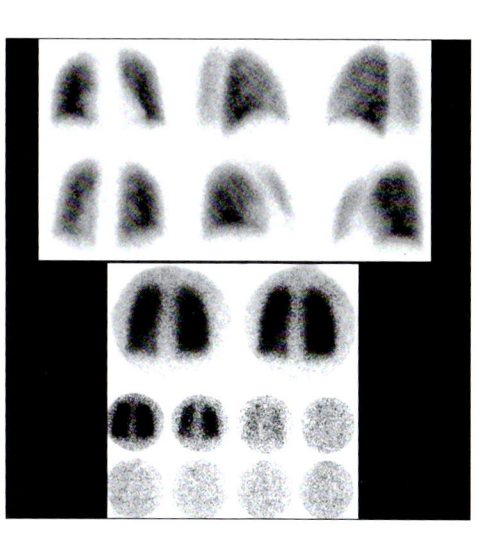

(Left) Anterior and posterior perfusion images show multiple segmental perfusion defects ➡ in patient with acute PE (upper panels). Three months later, images show improved pulmonary perfusion ➡ (lower panels). *(Right)* Upper panel: Normal 6 view perfusion lung scan (anterior, LPO, RPO, posterior, RAO and LAO). Lower panel: Normal posterior Xe-133 ventilation images (breath hold, equilibrium and washout).

V/Q, QUANTITATIVE

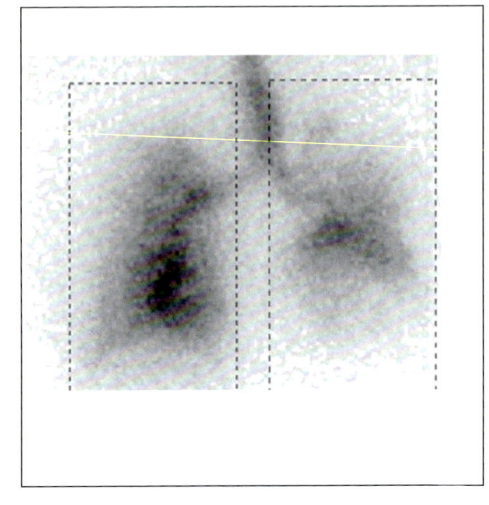

Posterior initial single breath ventilation image in transplant patient (right lung is native). L/R scintigraphic inspiratory volume ratio is 63/37 (L/R). Same patient as next image.

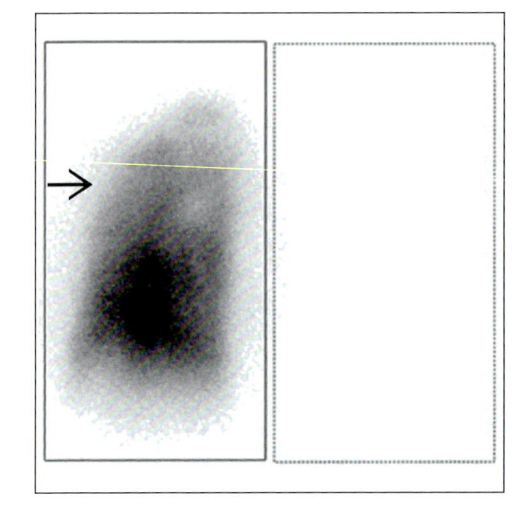

Posterior perfusion image. L/R perfusion ratio is 98/2. Most of the perfusion is to the transplanted lung ➔, despite ventilation to the native right lung. No rejection. Same patient as previous image.

TERMINOLOGY

Abbreviations and Synonyms
- Quantitative perfusion/ventilation (QVQ)
- Ventilation (V); perfusion (Q)

Definitions
- Quantitative comparison of global and regional pulmonary ventilation and perfusion using radioisotopic methods

IMAGING FINDINGS

General Features
- Best diagnostic clue
  - Congenital heart disease (CHD)
    - Asymmetry of lung Q, evaluate response to intervention
    - Brain and kidney uptake of macro-aggregated albumin (MAA) with right-to-left (R-L) shunt
  - Pre- and post-lung transplant evaluation
    - Identify most diseased lung prior to transplant
    - Serve as baseline post-transplant
    - Serially assessment of subtle compromise (rejection, infection)
  - Evaluation prior to lobectomy or partial pneumonectomy (tumor, bullae)
    - Prediction of post-operative lung function, surgical candidacy
  - Early lung inflammation/irritation: Enhanced rate of clearance of radiolabeled aerosol
- Location: V and Q defects correspond to location of airway (V) or vascular (Q) compromise
- Morphology
  - V and Q defects can be diffuse, regional or focal
  - V defects may appear as slow or absent initial uptake (gas, aerosol) and/or retention on washout (gas)

Nuclear Medicine Findings
- Pre-lung transplant
  - QVQ to identify lung with worst function (for transplantation)
- Post-lung transplant
  - Expect improved V and Q in transplanted lung
  - Early rejection: Subtle discordance between V and Q in transplanted lung

DDx: Other Causes of Abnormal Tc-99m Perfusion Scans

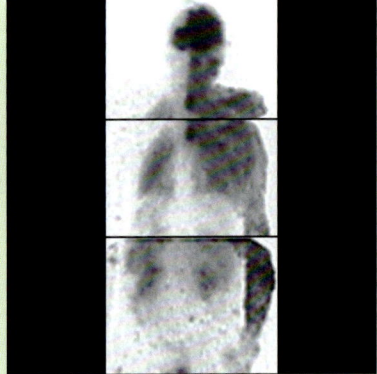

Brachiocephalic Vein/Artery Fistula

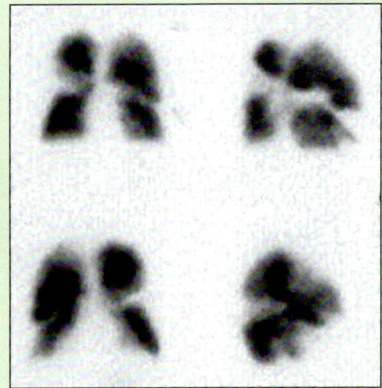

Pulmonary Embolism

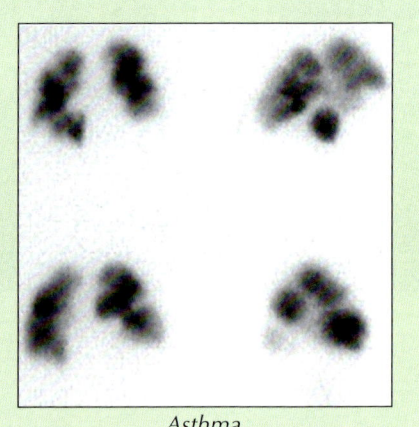

Asthma

V/Q, QUANTITATIVE

Key Facts

Imaging Findings
- QVQ to identify lung with worst function (for transplantation)
- Expect improved V and Q in transplanted lung
- Early rejection: Subtle discordance between V and Q in transplanted lung
- Trend toward further discordance on serial scans with transplant rejection
- Enhanced clearance of aerosolized particles increased in infection/inflammation
- To calculate post-operative FEV_1, multiply predicted % post-operative retained Q to pre-operative FEV_1
- Predicted post-operative FEV_1 < 0.8-1.5 L/min, undue dyspnea on exertion (DOE), or evidence of interstitial lung disease: May preclude resection
- Evaluate R-L shunt: Post atrial window, conduit or baffle to re-direct flow
- Percent MAA in brain and kidneys should be < 5% total body
- Evaluate effect of interventional procedures (e.g., dilating or stenting right or left pulmonary artery)

Top Differential Diagnoses
- Pulmonary Embolism
- Central Tumor
- Pneumonia
- Asthma

Diagnostic Checklist
- Transplant, pneumonectomy: Communication with surgical team paramount for optimal study

---

- Trend toward further discordance on serial scans with transplant rejection
- Ventilation usually declines faster than perfusion in rejection
- On single study: Discordance of ≥ 20% likely significant
- On serial studies: Relative change of ≥ 10% likely significant
- Infection/inflammation
  - VQ defects usually matched, focal
  - Enhanced clearance of aerosolized particles increased in infection/inflammation
    - Mechanism: Increased epithelial permeability
- Predict pneumonectomy: Quantitative Q applied to pre-operative pulmonary function tests (PFTs)
  - To calculate post-operative FEV_1, multiply predicted % post-operative retained Q to pre-operative FEV_1
    - Calculate percent Q to be retained following lung resection
    - Predicted post-operative FEV_1 > 2 L/min (> 80% normal), absence of dyspnea on exertion and interstitial lung disease: Correlates with decreased post-operative complications
    - Predicted post-operative FEV_1 < 0.8-1.5 L/min, undue dyspnea on exertion (DOE), or evidence of interstitial lung disease: May preclude resection
- Congenital heart disease (CHD)
  - Evaluate R-L shunt: Post atrial window, conduit or baffle to re-direct flow
    - Percent MAA in brain and kidneys should be < 5% total body
    - Higher risk of septic emboli or clots in brain or body with R-L shunt, bypasses pulmonary capillary "sieve"
  - Determine relative and regional lung perfusion
    - Evaluate effect of interventional procedures (e.g., dilating or stenting right or left pulmonary artery)
    - Note: Baffle or shunting procedures can selectively direct venous return to specific portion of lung depending on site/side of injection

Radiographic Findings
- Correlate QVQ with plain radiograph/CT
- Define anatomy, location of pleural effusions, mass lesions, infiltrates, postsurgical changes

Angiographic Findings
- MRA, CTA, contrast angiography: In CHD to define initial anatomy; evaluate success of intervention (shunt, baffle, stent, etc.)

Other Modality Findings
- Echocardiography: Cardiac anatomy, relative pressure data, shunt, valvular, blood flow

Imaging Recommendations
- Best imaging tool
  - Pre-operative lung transplant
    - Quant V/Q scan: Relative lung function (V & Q)
    - CECT: Presurgical anatomical detail
  - Post-operative lung transplant
    - Quant V/Q: Early assessment of rejection
    - HRCT: Air trapping, infiltrate, evaluate anatomy
  - CHD
    - Quantitative Q: Evaluate extent of R-L shunt with whole body images
    - First-pass (Q) images often needed on initial CHD studies if complex surgery (baffles, conduits)
    - QVQ: Evaluate relative/regional lung perfusion after pulmonary stent
  - Pre-pneumonectomy
    - Pre-operative QVQ to predict post-operative FEV_1
- Protocol advice
  - Ventilation scan
    - Xenon-133 gas 148-740 MBq (4-20 mCi)
    - Air trapping: Serial images taken after patient breathing room air (abnormal if delayed washout > 3-4 minutes)
    - Scintigraphic inspiratory volume ratio: 15-second image of gas delivery to lungs in single breath, each lung measured separately, expressed as relative percent of total (R/L)

V/Q, QUANTITATIVE

- Scintigraphic vital capacity ratio: 15-second image breath hold counts both with maximum inspiration and expiration (may require measuring on different breaths), each lung measured separately, expressed as [(Linsp - Lexp)/Linsp]/[(Rinsp - Rexp)/Rinsp]
  o Perfusion scan
    - Tc-99m macro-aggregated albumin (MAA) 111-185 MBq (3-5 mCi) IV; image ant, post, both laterals
  o CHD evaluation
    - R-L shunt: [(brain+kidneys)/(brain+kidneys+lungs)] > 5%
    - Ensure venous return from injection site (leg, right arm, left arm) does not significantly bypass lung: Foot injection may be best
  o Quantitative Q: Used to predict post-operative FEV_1 after pneumonectomy/lobectomy
    - Perform initial pulmonary function tests (PFTs) for FEV_1
    - Geometric mean calculation for % MAA perfusion of R & L lungs from anterior & posterior image region of interests (ROIs) of Q scan
    - Percent contributed by each lobe: Calculated from ROIs around individual lobes on lateral images, applied to single lung percent perfusion
    - Calculate % total lung perfusion contributed by each lobe
    - Calculate predicted post-operative FEV_1: Pre-operative FEV_1 x [1 - (% total Q to be removed)]
    - Significant discordance between V and Q invalidates predictive value of Q for post-operative lung function
  o Post-transplant: Similar protocols required for serial studies to distinguish subtle functional degradation
  o Aerosol lung clearance: Identify active lung infection/inflammation
    - 4 minute inhalation of 900-1200 MBq (25-35 mCi) Tc-99m DTPA or carbon dust aerosol (delivering about 20-40 MBq to lung); dynamic study: 1 minute images x 30
    - T-½ in healthy lung: Average 60 min (> 40 is normal); T-½ in smoker's lung: Average 21 min; T-½ in areas of pneumocystis pneumonia: Average 4 min

DIFFERENTIAL DIAGNOSIS

Pulmonary Embolism
- Acute PE: Multiple large, moderate Q defects, normal V, clear chest

Central Tumor
- Either V, Q, or both may be completely abolished by tumor compression of airway, pulmonary arteries

Pneumonia
- Matching V and Q defects with matching area of consolidation or airspace disease

Asthma
- Reversible matched V and Q defects, usually with radiograph/CT

PATHOLOGY

General Features
- Etiology: Wide variety of etiologies

CLINICAL ISSUES

Presentation
- Most common signs/symptoms: Shortness of breath, dyspnea on exertion

DIAGNOSTIC CHECKLIST

Consider
- Transplant, pneumonectomy: Communication with surgical team paramount for optimal study
- CHD: Communication with cardiologist, cardiothoracic surgeon required for optimal study

Image Interpretation Pearls
- "Hot spots" in lungs usually due to mixing tracer with blood prior to injection (in syringe or line): Leads to Tc-99m MAA clumping

SELECTED REFERENCES

1. Petersson J et al: Physiological evaluation of a new quantitative SPECT method measuring regional ventilation and perfusion. J Appl Physiol. 96(3):1127-36, 2004
2. Piai DB et al: The use of SPECT in preoperative assessment of patients with lung cancer. Eur Respir J. 24(2):258-62, 2004
3. Beckles MA et al: The physiologic evaluation of patients with lung cancer being considered for resectional surgery. Chest. 123(1 Suppl):105S-114S, 2003
4. Chenuel B et al: Effect of exercise on lung-perfusion scanning in patients with bronchogenic carcinoma. Eur Respir J. 20(3):710-6, 2002
5. Fratz S et al: More accurate quantification of pulmonary blood flow by magnetic resonance imaging than by lung perfusion scintigraphy in patients with fontan circulation. Circulation. 106(12):1510-3, 2002
6. Hunsaker AR et al: Lung volume reduction surgery for emphysema: correlation of CT and V/Q imaging with physiologic mechanisms of improvement in lung function. Radiology. 222(2):491-8, 2002
7. Kreck TC et al: Determination of regional ventilation and perfusion in the lung using xenon and computed tomography. J Appl Physiol. 91(4):1741-9, 2001
8. Gierada DS et al: Patient selection for lung volume reduction surgery: An objective model based on prior clinical decisions and quantitative CT analysis. Chest. 117(4):991-8, 2000
9. Hardoff R et al: The prognostic value of perfusion lung scintigraphy in patients who underwent single-lung transplantation for emphysema and pulmonary fibrosis. J Nucl Med. 41(11):1771-6, 2000
10. Reilly JJ Jr: Evidence-based preoperative evaluation of candidates for thoracotomy. Chest. 116(6 Suppl):474S-476S, 1999
11. Chacon RA et al: Comparison of the functional results of single lung transplantation for pulmonary fibrosis and chronic airway obstruction. Thorax. 53(1):43-9, 1998

V/Q, QUANTITATIVE

IMAGE GALLERY

Typical

Typical

Typical

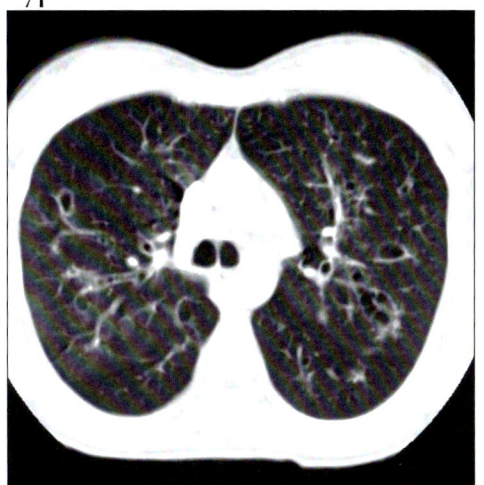

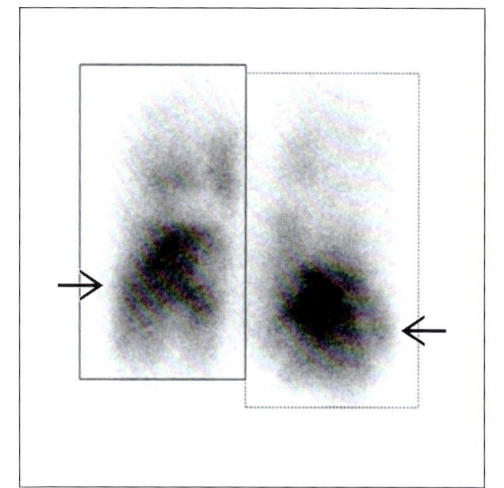

(Left) Axial NECT of the chest shows typical cystic/bronchiectatic changes of cystic fibrosis. Same patient as next two images. *(Right)* Posterior planar perfusion image in patient with cystic fibrosis shows basal predominant perfusion ➡. L/R perfusion ratio is 55/45.

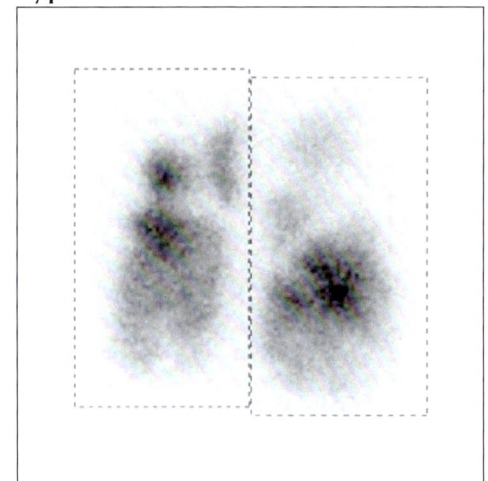

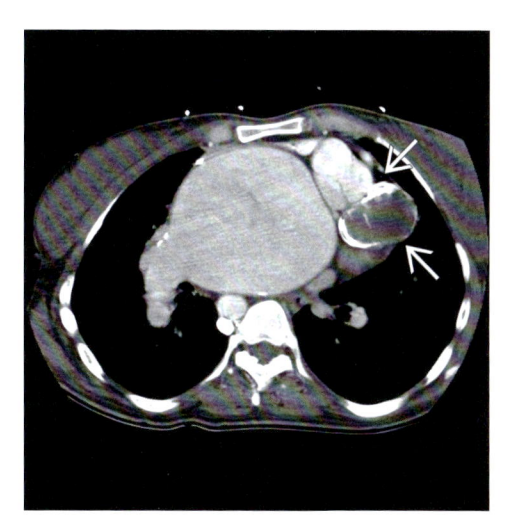

(Left) Posterior breath hold ventilation image in patient with cystic fibrosis shows patchy areas of ventilatory absence, corresponding to areas of diminished perfusion. *(Right)* CECT through atrial level in patient with CHD shows very enlarged atrium and vascular conduit ➡. Same patient as next two images.

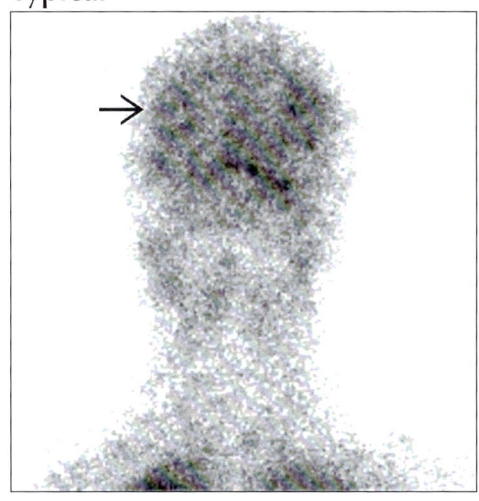

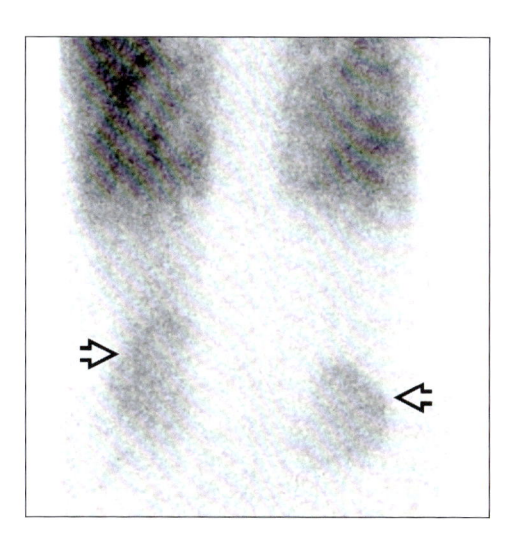

(Left) Tc-99m MAA perfusion scan in patient with CHD and a vascular conduit. Posterior view of base of head shows particle in brain ➡. R-L shunt was calculated at 16%. *(Right)* Posterior Tc-99m MAA perfusion scan in patient with CHD and vascular conduit. Posterior view of abdomen shows particles in kidneys ➡. R-L shunt was calculated at 16%. Anterior and posterior images with geometric mean measurements may be used.

V/Q, QUANTITATIVE

(Left) Anterior perfusion flow in a patient with left pulmonary artery stenosis shows reduced perfusion to left lung ➡. Same patient as next image. **(Right)** Anterior perfusion imaging confirms marked flow discrepancy. L/R perfusion ratio is 17/83. No shunt R-L shunt is identified.

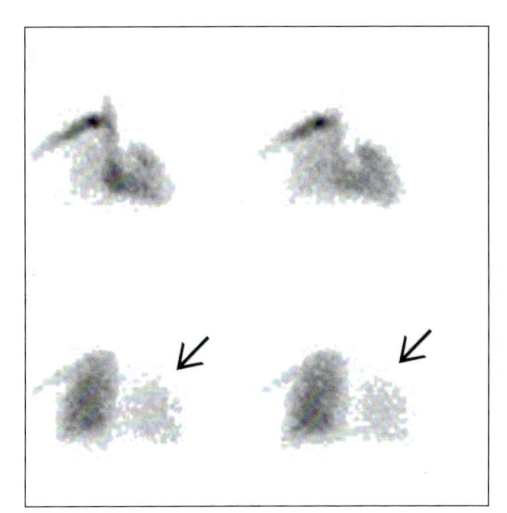

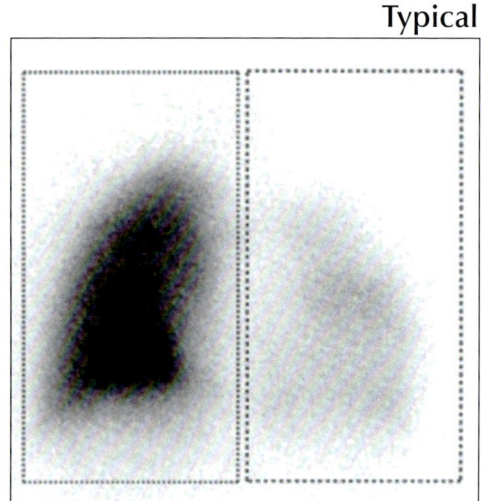

Typical

(Left) Perfusion flow images in patient with severe right pulmonary stenosis. Tc-99m MAA injected in right antecubital vein is directed strongly to the left lung ➡. Same patient as next image. **(Right)** Multi perfusion images in same patient as previous. Perfusion L/R ratio 96/4. Study was repeated with left arm injection with less L/R discrepancy. Variant anatomy can alter perfusion based on site of injection.

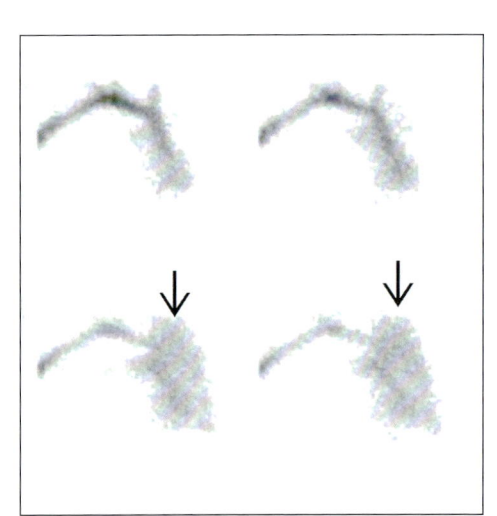

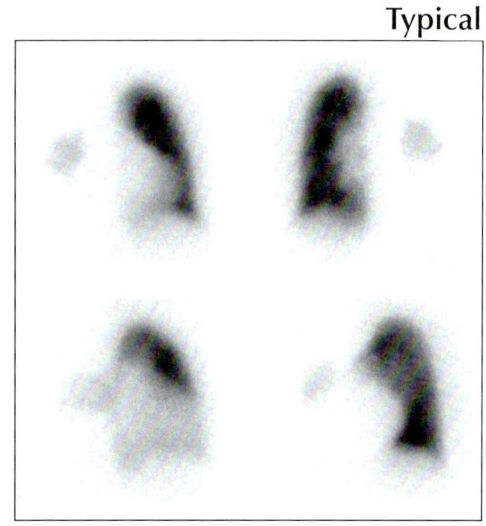

Typical

(Left) Axial NECT of the chest shows bilateral lower lobe emphysema and fibrosis in patient being evaluated for lung transplant. Same patient as next image. **(Right)** Planar perfusion images shows bibasilar decreased perfusion (L/R 47/53). Ventilation was concordant (scintigraphic vital capacity L/R 44/56), with basal slow wash-in and wash-out.

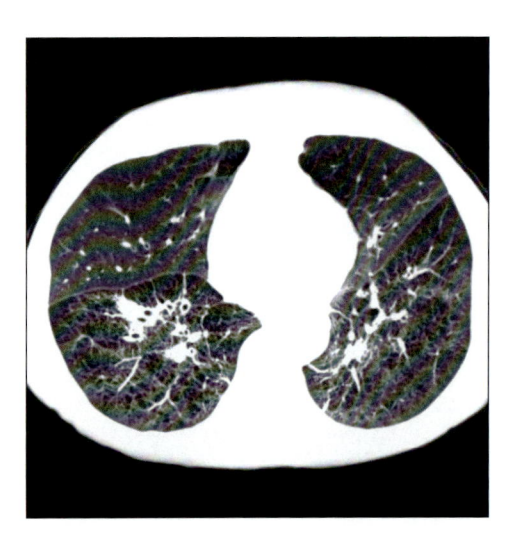

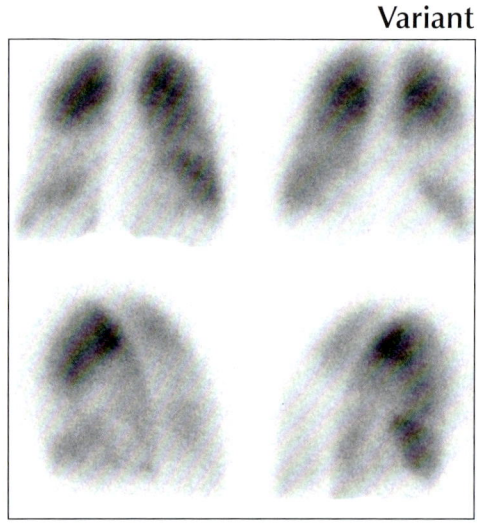

Variant

V/Q, QUANTITATIVE

Typical

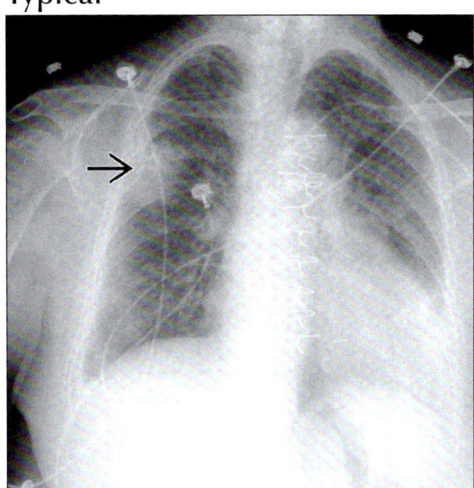

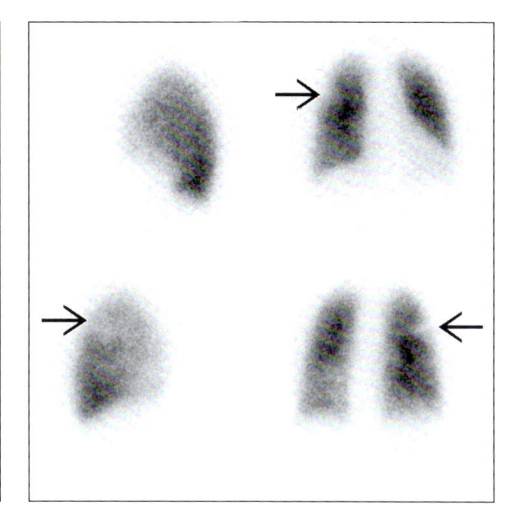

(Left) AP plain radiograph of the chest shows right lung mass ➔. Right upper and middle lobectomy was planned. Same patient as next two images. *(Right)* Multi perfusion images show L/R ratio of 44/56 in patient with right upper lobe malignancy ➔. Ventilation was concordant.

Typical

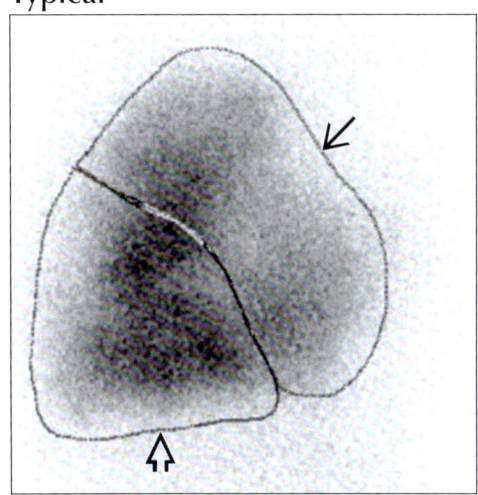

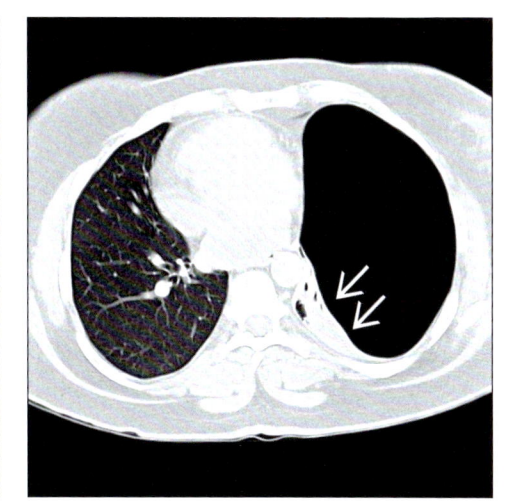

(Left) Right lateral Q image shows technique for separation of upper/middle ➔ from lower ⇨ lobe. Upper and mid to lower perfusion ratio of 40/60. Predicted post-operative FEV1 was adequate at 1.6. Contribution of opposite lung is minimal. *(Right)* Axial CT of the chest shows large bulla, compressive atelectasis of the left lung ➔. Same patient as next two images.

Typical

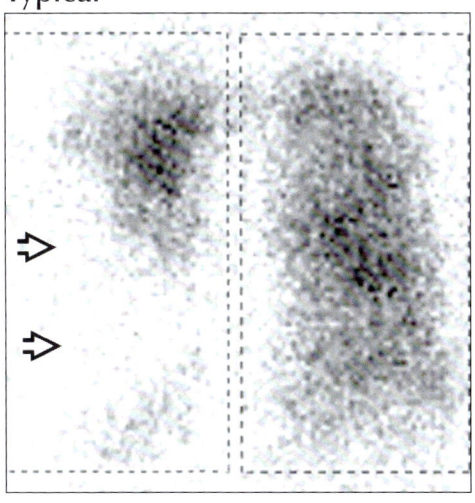

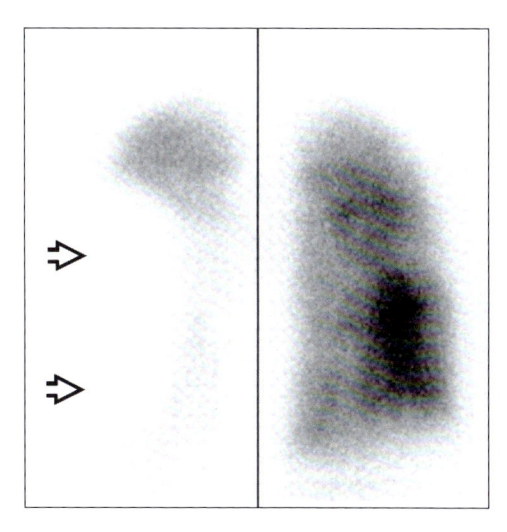

(Left) Posterior first breath image in patient with COPD shows absent ventilation in large bulla ⇨. Scintigraphic inspiratory volume ratio is 33/67 (L/R), scintigraphic vital capacity ratio is 25/75 (L/R). *(Right)* Posterior perfusion scan shows large perfusion defect in mid and lower left lung ⇨, corresponding to ventilation defect. L/R perfusion ratio is 19/81. Same patient as previous two images.

PNEUMOCYSTIS CARINII PNEUMONIA

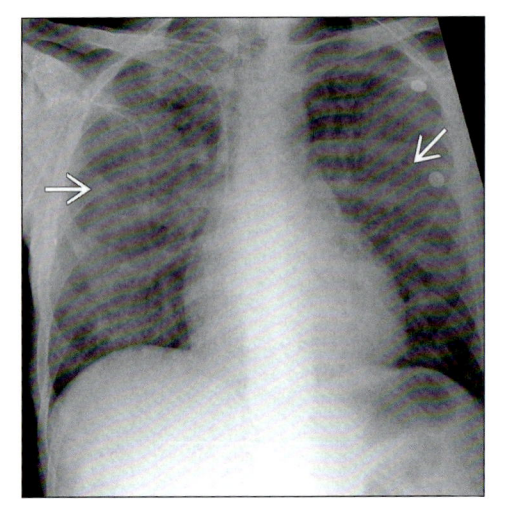

Anterior chest radiograph shows diffuse hazy infiltrates ➡ bilaterally in patient with PCP.

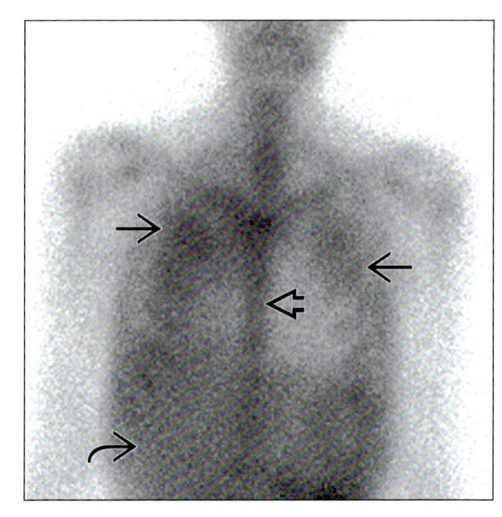

Anterior Ga-67 scintigraphy in same patient as left shows diffuse pulmonary activity ➡ equal to or greater than liver ➚ or sternum ⮕.

TERMINOLOGY

Abbreviations and Synonyms
- Pneumocystis carinii pneumonia (PCP)

Definitions
- Opportunistic pulmonary fungus that causes alveolitis
  - Most common in immunocompromised

IMAGING FINDINGS

General Features
- Best diagnostic clue
  - Ga-67 scintigraphy: Diffuse, bilateral pulmonary activity in immunocompromised patient with cough, fever and X-ray infiltrates
  - Partially treated PCP: Focal Ga-67 activity, often upper lung zones

Nuclear Medicine Findings
- Increased activity in lungs may be present with several radiopharmaceutical capable of detecting alveolitis
  - Ga-67 citrate, Tl-201, F-18 FDG PET
  - Tc-99m or In-111 WBC's poorly sensitive for PCP
- Ga-67 scintigraphy at 48 hours post injection
  - Activity may be focal or diffuse
  - Activity may be dominant in a specific region (i.e., perihilar or upper lobe)
  - Pulmonary activity compared to reference tissue (liver or sternum)
    - 0 (normal): Activity < soft tissue
    - 1+ (equivocal): Activity = soft tissue
    - 2+ (mildly positive): Activity > soft tissue but < liver or sternum
    - 3+ (moderately positive): Activity = liver or sternum
    - 4+ (strongly positive): Activity > liver or sternum
  - Intensity of activity correlates with degree of alveolitis
  - May be strongly positive despite negative chest radiograph
  - Poor prognostic sign: Strongly positive in afebrile subjects with few, no pulmonary symptoms
  - If necessary, biopsy site of highest activity on Ga-67 scintigraphy

DDx: Other Inflammatory Alveolitis (Ga-67)

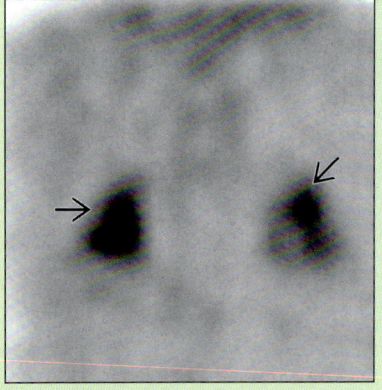

| Aspiration Pneumonia | Granulomatous Pneumonia | Bacterial Pneumonia |

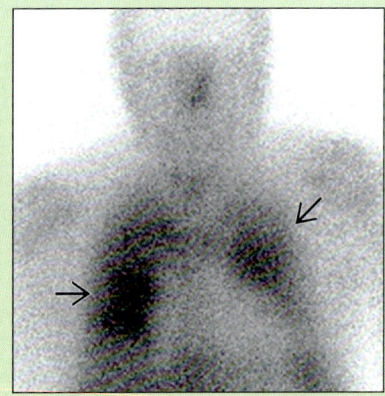

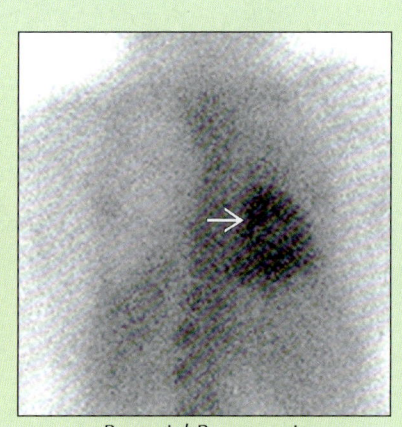

PNEUMOCYSTIS CARINII PNEUMONIA

Key Facts

Terminology
- Opportunistic pulmonary fungus that causes alveolitis
- Most common in immunocompromised

Imaging Findings
- Ga-67 scintigraphy: Diffuse, bilateral pulmonary activity in immunocompromised patient with cough, fever and X-ray infiltrates
- Partially treated PCP: Focal Ga-67 activity, often upper lung zones
- Ga-67 scintigraphy at 48 hours post injection
- 0 (normal): Activity < soft tissue
- 1+ (equivocal): Activity = soft tissue
- 2+ (mildly positive): Activity > soft tissue but < liver or sternum
- 3+ (moderately positive): Activity = liver or sternum
- 4+ (strongly positive): Activity > liver or sternum
- High negative predictive value: Negative Ga-67 scintigraphy excludes active PCP

Top Differential Diagnoses
- Non-Cardiogenic Pulmonary Edema
- Cytomegalovirus Pneumonitis
- Diffuse Pulmonary Hemorrhage Syndromes
- Hypersensitivity Pneumonitis
- Pulmonary Alveolar Proteinosis

Pathology
- Patchy and often extensive areas of consolidated lung tissue
- Cysts common in AIDS, usually in subpleural lung
- Intra-alveolar foamy exudate with fungus seen as bubble-like areas

Radiographic Findings
- Diffuse infiltrates, often ground-glass appearance
- Consolidation may be evident in advanced cases
- If cysts evident, mainly in upper lung zones

CT Findings
- High-resolution CT (HRCT) modality of choice
- Most common: Diffuse, bilateral ground-glass opacities
- Peripheral upper lobe cysts: Can be seen in HIV+
- Consolidation: Late finding in untreated cases

Imaging Recommendations
- Best imaging tool
  - HRCT usually positive in diffuse disease even when chest radiograph negative
  - Ga-67 scintigraphy highly sensitive but not specific for PCP infection
    - Ga-67 scintigraphy positive in virtually every lung infection (except histiocytosis X in adult)
    - High negative predictive value: Negative Ga-67 scintigraphy excludes active PCP
- Protocol advice
  - 5 mCi Ga-67 IV
  - Whole-body anterior and posterior planar images at 48 hours post injection

DIFFERENTIAL DIAGNOSIS

Non-Cardiogenic Pulmonary Edema
- Diffuse ground-glass to consolidative appearance
- Onset rapid, usually < 24 hours
- Fever not characteristic
- Small bilateral pleural effusions common

Cytomegalovirus Pneumonitis
- Most common infection associated with PCP due to immunocompromise
- Bilateral ground-glass opacities, multiple small nodules most common
- HRCT
  - Ground-glass, reticular opacities, multiple small nodules
  - Patchy consolidation less common

Diffuse Pulmonary Hemorrhage Syndromes
- Wegener granulomatosis, Goodpasture syndrome, Churg-Strauss syndrome, connective tissue vasculitis, microscopic polyangiitis, bone marrow transplantation and idiopathic pulmonary hemosiderosis
- Diffuse or extensive bilateral ground-glass and consolidative opacities
- Usually acute onset of dyspnea, often < 24 hours

Hypersensitivity Pneumonitis
- Common causes: Medications or extrinsic allergens
- Dyspnea and non-productive cough: Subacute or chronic onset
- Mild hypoxia, fever not common
- Diffuse ground-glass opacities most common
- HRCT
  - Ill-defined centrilobular nodules
  - Cysts very uncommon
  - Air-trapping common

Pulmonary Alveolar Proteinosis
- Fever and severe hypoxia uncommon
- Symptoms indolent (often over months), except rarely in patients with hematological malignancy
- HRCT
  - Ground-glass with concurrent intralobular and interlobular septal thickening ("crazy paving" pattern)

PATHOLOGY

General Features
- Etiology
  - Impaired T-cell mediated immunity predisposes to PCP
    - AIDS, especially with CD4 < 200
    - Long-term corticosteroid therapy, particularly during taper

PNEUMOCYSTIS CARINII PNEUMONIA

- Organ, bone marrow transplant and chemotherapy
- Congenital immunodeficiency (e.g., thymic aplasia, bare T-cell disease and severe combined immunodeficiency syndrome)
  - Premature infants predisposed
  - Malnourished predisposed
- Epidemiology: Organism can be found in normal lungs
- Associated abnormalities
  - Patients with PCP at risk for other immunosuppressed-related infections or neoplasms
    - Cytomegalovirus
    - Mycobacterium tuberculosis
    - Disseminated mycobacteria avium complex (MAC)
    - Lymphoma
    - Kaposi sarcoma

Gross Pathologic & Surgical Features
- Patchy and often extensive areas of consolidated lung tissue
- Cysts common in AIDS, usually in subpleural lung

Microscopic Features
- Intra-alveolar foamy exudate with fungus seen as bubble-like areas
  - Mild-moderate interstitial pneumonitis
  - Chronic diffuse alveolar damage common
- Giemsa stain useful to demonstrate trophozoites
- Gomori methenamine silver (GMS) stain excellent for detecting cysts
- Cysts, necrotizing granulomas and subpleural emphysematous blebs common
- Non-HIV+: Foamy exudates absent in 50%

CLINICAL ISSUES

Presentation
- Most common signs/symptoms
  - Presenting symptoms variable: Non-productive cough, fever and hypoxia
    - AIDS: Symptoms often subacute, with prodrome of malaise, fever and dyspnea gradually worsening over 2-6 weeks
    - Immunocompromised, HIV-: Symptoms often more rapid, usually presenting over 4-10 days
    - Indolent course with minimal symptoms less common, seen in HIV-
  - Hypoxia very common and important clinical feature, especially evident during minimal exercise
    - Absence of hypoxia should place other potential disease processes above PCP
- Other signs/symptoms
  - Crackles on auscultation
  - 90% have elevated serum lactate dehydrogenase (LDH)
    - Prognostic implications: Rising LDH despite therapy ⇒ poor outcome

Demographics
- Age: Any, depends on risk factors

Natural History & Prognosis
- AIDS
  - Diagnosis often straightforward: High fungal load with minimal inflammation
  - Usually develop PCP with CD4 < 200
  - Thin-walled cysts may develop; predispose to pneumothorax
  - Sputum and/or bronchoalveolar lavage (BAL) often positive
- Non-HIV+ immunocompromised
  - More difficult diagnosis: Lower fungal load, higher inflammatory component
  - Negative sputum and/or BAL may lead physician to consider another diagnosis
    - High clinical suspicion required
    - Transbronchial biopsy may be required

Treatment
- Very good prognosis: Up to 90% cured with appropriate treatment
  - Trimethoprim-sulfamethoxazole or pentamidine IV effective in most
    - Chest radiograph may worsen initially due to pulmonary edema from large amounts of IV fluids administered with antibiotics
  - Severe hypoxia: Early adjunctive treatment with corticosteroids shown to decrease rate of respiratory failure
- Prophylactic therapy for AIDS and chronic corticosteroid therapy
  - Oral trimethoprim-sulfamethoxazole or, if allergic, dapsone

DIAGNOSTIC CHECKLIST

Image Interpretation Pearls
- Entire Ga-67 scintigraphy should be evaluated
  - Ga-67 localizes in other infections, neoplasms (lymphoma)
- WBC scintigraphy insensitive for atypical pulmonary infection

SELECTED REFERENCES

1. Sojan SM et al: Pneumocystis carinii pneumonia on F-18 FDG PET. Clin Nucl Med. 30(11):763-4, 2005
2. Win Z et al: FDG-PET imaging in Pneumocystis carinii pneumonia. Clin Nucl Med. 30(10):690-1, 2005
3. Kroe DM et al: Diagnostic strategies for Pneumocystis carinii pneumonia. Semin Respir Infect. 12(2):70-8, 1997
4. Kramer EL: PCP, AIDS and nuclear medicine. J Nucl Med. 35(6):1034-7, 1994
5. Tumeh SS et al: Ga-67 scintigraphy and computed tomography in the diagnosis of pneumocystis carinii pneumonia in patients with AIDS. A prospective comparison. Clin Nucl Med. 17(5):387-94, 1992
6. Barron TF et al: Pneumocystis carinii pneumonia studied by gallium-67 scanning. Radiology. 154(3):791-3, 1985
7. Levin M et al: Pneumocystis pneumonia: importance of gallium scan for early diagnosis and description of a new immunoperoxidase technique to demonstrate Pneumocystis carinii. Am Rev Respir Dis. 128(1):182-5, 1983

PNEUMOCYSTIS CARINII PNEUMONIA

IMAGE GALLERY

Typical

Typical

Typical

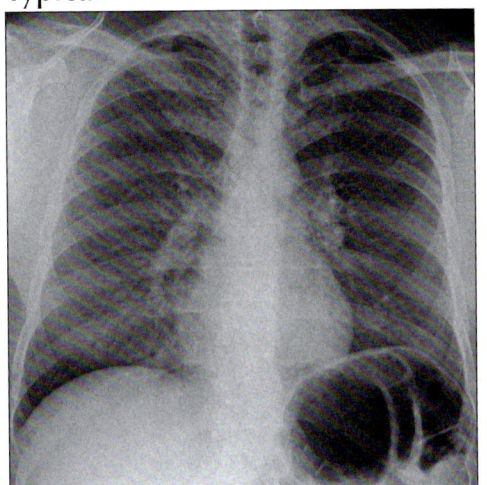

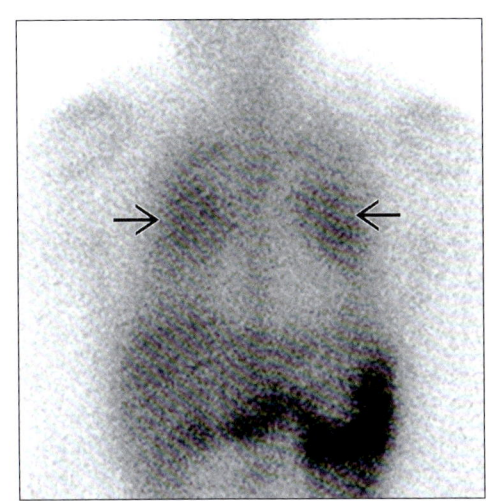

(Left) Anterior chest radiograph in hypoxic patient with acquired immunodeficiency syndrome shows no pulmonary infiltrates that would suggest PCP. (Right) Anterior Ga-67 scintigraphy in same patient as left shows diffuse pulmonary activity ➡ bilaterally, signifying PCP, later proven with biopsy.

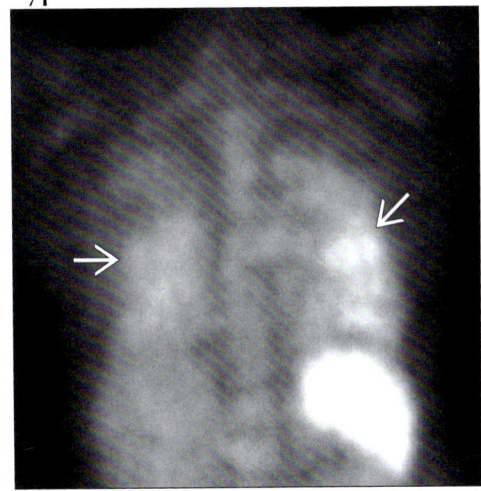

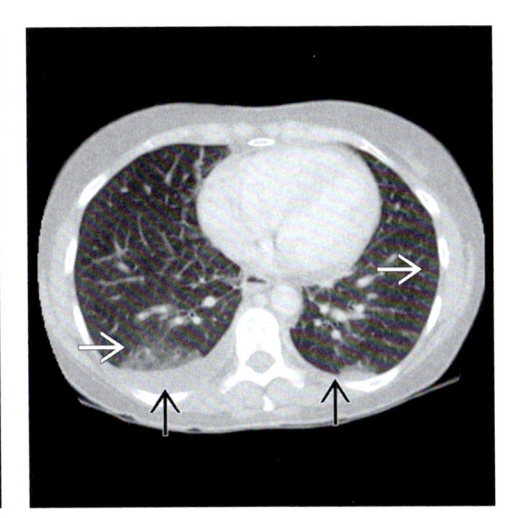

(Left) Coronal FDG PET shows diffusely increased activity ➡ in both lungs in HIV+ patient. (Right) Axial NECT in same patient as previous image shows bilateral ground-glass infiltrates ➡, consistent with PCP infection. Pleural effusions (right > left) ➡ also present.

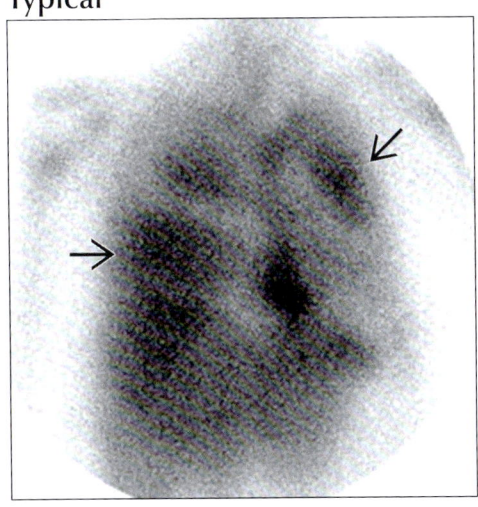

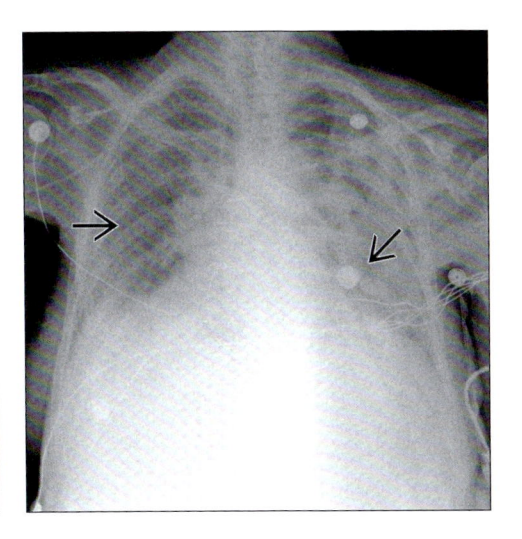

(Left) Anterior labeled leukocyte scintigraphy in HIV+ patient with fever and possible PCP shows increased activity ➡ in both hemithoraces. (Right) Anterior chest radiograph of patient at left shows bilateral diffuse, hazy infiltrates ➡, consistent with PCP. Labeled WBC scan usually poor sensitivity for PCP. Positive scan should suggest complicating bacterial infection or ARDS.

INTERSTITIAL LUNG DISEASE

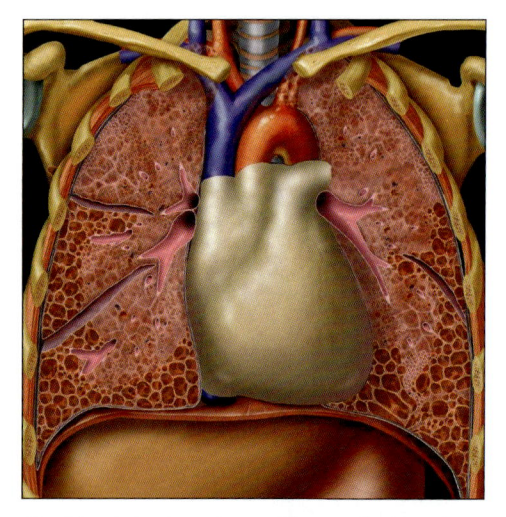

Graphic of the lungs in a mid coronal plane shows bibasilar and subpleural distribution of fibrosis and cysts in idiopathic pulmonary fibrosis.

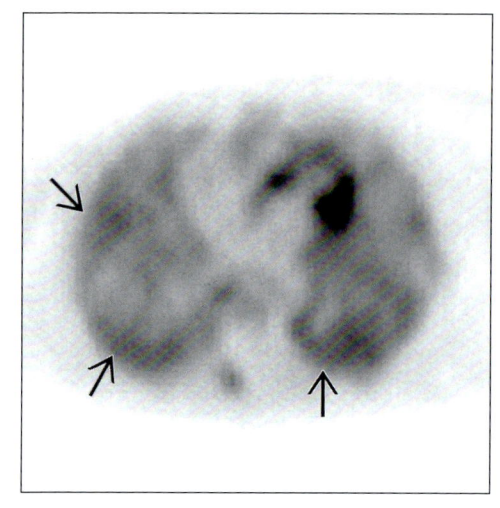

Axial PET shows extensive diffuse bilateral hypermetabolism with accentuation of subpleural regions ➔, confirming active inflammatory component, in a patient with idiopathic pulmonary fibrosis.

TERMINOLOGY

Abbreviations and Synonyms
- Interstitial lung disease (ILD)
- Idiopathic pulmonary fibrosis (IPF)
- Idiopathic interstitial pneumonia (IIP)
- Usual interstitial pneumonia (UIP)
- Desquamative interstitial pneumonia (DIP)
- Bronchiolitis obliterans with organizing pneumonia (BOOP)

Definitions
- Variety of chronic lung disorders caused by known or unknown initial damage, followed by airway inflammation and fibrosis of interstitium

IMAGING FINDINGS

General Features
- Best diagnostic clue
  - HRCT: Nodules, linear and reticular opacities, cystic lesions, ground-glass opacity (GGO), consolidation
  - GGO may indicate inflammatory component
  - Ga-67 scintigraphy, FDG PET: Positive with active disease, useful in assessing response to treatment
- Location: Vary with etiology of ILD
- Size: Nodules typically 1 mm to 1 cm
- Morphology: Highly variable, overlap in patterns with different etiologies of ILD

Nuclear Medicine Findings
- Ga-67 Scintigraphy
  - Positive Ga-67 with all types of active interstitial lung disease except Langerhans cell histiocytosis (histiocytosis X) in adults
  - Ga-67 grading system based on comparison of lung to liver, bone, background
    - Grade I: Less than bone but discernibly above background
    - Grade II: Equal to bone
    - Grade III: Equal to liver
    - Grade IV: Greater than liver
  - Ga-67 uptake decreases with good response to treatment
- FDG PET or PET/CT
  - FDG PET: Positive in active forms of interstitial lung disease

DDx: Mimics of Interstitial Lung Disease

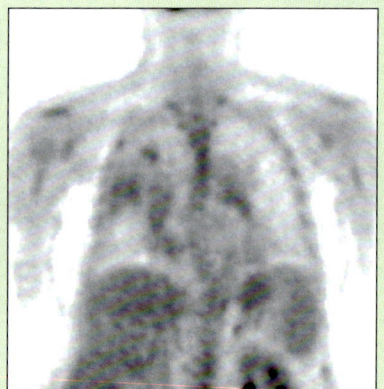

Bacterial Pneumonia (PET)

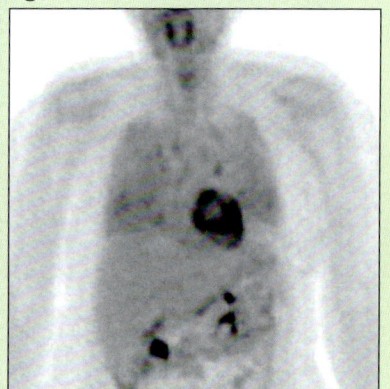

Lymphangitic Metastases (PET)

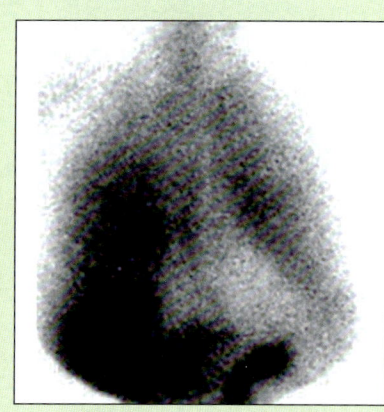

PCP Pneumonia (Ga-67)

INTERSTITIAL LUNG DISEASE

Key Facts

Imaging Findings
- Positive Ga-67 with all types of active interstitial lung disease except Langerhans cell histiocytosis (histiocytosis X) in adults
- Ga-67 grading system based on comparison of lung to liver, bone, background
- Ga-67 uptake decreases with good response to treatment
- FDG PET: Positive in active forms of interstitial lung disease
- Regions of FDG uptake correspond to active or inflammatory areas of disease
- PET useful in assessing response to treatment (FDG uptake should decrease)

- HRCT: Best tool for evaluating pulmonary interstitium, secondary pulmonary lobule, diagnosis and assessment of diffuse disease
- FDG PET or Ga-67: For evaluating active inflammatory component

Top Differential Diagnoses
- Sarcoidosis
- Bronchioloalveolar Carcinoma
- Miliary Tuberculous/Fungal Diseases
- Lymphangitic Carcinomatosis
- Pulmonary Edema

Clinical Issues
- Steroids, smoking cessation, removal of offending antigen or drug

---

- Regions of FDG uptake correspond to active or inflammatory areas of disease
- More false positives with PET due to malignancy than with Ga-67
- PET useful in assessing response to treatment (FDG uptake should decrease)
- IPF: Diffuse FDG uptake in subpleural location, most prominent in bases

Radiographic Findings
- Radiography
  - Plain chest radiograph: Peripheral reticular, linear, nodular lesions, GGO most common findings
  - Radiography normal in 10-15% of symptomatic patients

CT Findings
- HRCT
  - Nodular opacities: Involve both airspace and interstitial, 1 mm to 1 cm in diameter
    - Perilymphatic nodules (subpleural, interlobular septa and fissures, bronchovascular bundles, patchy distribution): Sarcoidosis, lymphangitic carcinomatosis, silicosis
    - Centrilobular nodules (diffuse or patchy): Extrinsic allergic alveolitis, respiratory bronchiolitis, Langerhans cell histiocytosis, bronchioalveolar cell carcinoma
    - Diffuse nodules (random or perivascular): Hematogenous spread of malignancy, miliary tuberculosis, miliary fungal disease
  - Linear and reticular opacities: Interlacing lines suggesting mesh; due to fibrosis, edema and infiltration of interstitium
    - Reticular pattern: Large (thickened interlobular septa), intermediate (honeycomb pattern), fine (thickened intralobular septa)
    - Interlobular septal thickening (smooth): Pulmonary edema, lymphatic carcinomatosis, pulmonary hemorrhage, amyloidosis, alveolar proteinosis
    - Interlobular septal thickening (nodular): Lymphangitic carcinomatosis, sarcoidosis, pneumoconiosis
    - Interlobular septal thickening (irregular): Architectural distortion (interstitial fibrosis, UIP, asbestosis), honeycomb (IPF)
    - Intralobular septal thickening: Irregular linear opacities and fine reticular pattern (UIP, asbestosis, sarcoidosis)
  - Cystic lesions: Thin-walled, circumscribed, air or fluid-filled, fibrous or epithelial wall
    - Cystic pattern: Seen in Histiocytosis X, lymphangioleiomyomatosis, honeycombing
    - Honeycombing: Cystic airspace with thick, definable wall lined with bronchiolar epithelium, bases and subpleural location (idiopathic pulmonary fibrosis)
  - GGO: Hazy increased attenuation with preserved bronchovascular markings
    - Usual context: Active inflammation, microscopic fibrosis
    - May contribute to specific diagnosis in DIP, hypersensitivity pneumonitis, pulmonary alveolar proteinosis
  - Consolidation: Replacement of alveolar air by fluid, cells, or tissue obscuring underlying vascular structures; may be associated with air bronchograms
    - Commonly seen with BOOP, chronic eosinophilic pneumonia, lipoid pneumonia, bronchoalveolar carcinoma, pneumonia

Imaging Recommendations
- Best imaging tool
  - HRCT: Best tool for evaluating pulmonary interstitium, secondary pulmonary lobule, diagnosis and assessment of diffuse disease
  - FDG PET or Ga-67: For evaluating active inflammatory component
- Protocol advice
  - FDG PET: 10-20 mCi IV, 60-90 min uptake interval, PET/CT best for co-registration
  - Ga-67: 5 mCi IV; planar and SPECT of chest 48-72 h post injection

INTERSTITIAL LUNG DISEASE

DIFFERENTIAL DIAGNOSIS

Sarcoidosis
- GGO, micronodules, nodules, beaded vessels and fissures
- Positive on FDG PET and Ga-67

Bronchioloalveolar Carcinoma
- Progressive ground-glass, airspace opacities
- May have low-to-moderate level uptake on FDG PET; not Ga-67 avid

Miliary Tuberculous/Fungal Diseases
- Small nodules (1-2 mm), hematogenous pattern, tree-in-bud appearance
- Positive on both FDG PET and Ga-67 scintigraphy

Lymphangitic Carcinomatosis
- History of carcinoma
- Positive on FDG PET, variable on Ga-67 scintigraphy

Pulmonary Edema
- If not causes by inflammation, not typically positive on FDG PET or Ga-67

PATHOLOGY

General Features
- Etiology
  - Idiopathic: UIP, IPF, acute interstitial pneumonia, nonspecific interstitial pneumonia
  - Drug-induced lung disease: Amiodarone, nitrofurantoin, gold salts, methotrexate, vincristine, fludarabine
  - Radiation toxicity
  - Collagen vascular disorders: Scleroderma, rheumatoid arthritis
  - DIP and respiratory bronchiolitis with interstitial lung disease: Smokers, steroid responsive
  - Asbestosis
  - Langerhans cell histiocytosis (histiocytosis X): Smoking related but unknown cause
  - Healing diffuse alveolar damage
  - Occupational exposures: Silicosis, berylliosis, coal dust, many others
  - Antigens: Many types of hypersensitivity pneumonitis
- Epidemiology: Smoking association: DIP, respiratory bronchiolitis with interstitial lung disease, Langerhans cell histiocytosis
- Associated abnormalities: Variable with etiology in systemic granulomatous diseases, Langerhans cell histiocytosis, collagen vascular diseases, tuberous sclerosis

Gross Pathologic & Surgical Features
- Highly variable with etiology

Microscopic Features
- Highly variable with etiology

CLINICAL ISSUES

Presentation
- Most common signs/symptoms: Shortness of breath, cough, not typically febrile
- Other signs/symptoms: Abnormal pulmonary function tests
- Although history and imaging may suggest cause, biopsy usually required for definitive diagnosis

Demographics
- Age: Variable with etiology
- Gender: Variable with etiology

Natural History & Prognosis
- Variable with etiology

Treatment
- Steroids, smoking cessation, removal of offending antigen or drug

DIAGNOSTIC CHECKLIST

Consider
- FDG PET/CT and Ga-67 scintigraphy to assess active/inflammatory component of ILD

SELECTED REFERENCES

1. Meissner HH et al: Idiopathic pulmonary fibrosis: evaluation with positron emission tomography. Respiration. 73(2):197-202, 2006
2. Grijm K et al: Semiquantitative 67Ga scintigraphy as an indicator of response to and prognosis after corticosteroid treatment in idiopathic interstitial pneumonia. J Nucl Med. 46(9):1421-6, 2005
3. Mura M et al: Inflammatory activity is still present in the advanced stages of idiopathic pulmonary fibrosis. Respirology. 10(5):609-14, 2005
4. Hang LW et al: A pilot trial of quantitative Tc-99m HMPAO and Ga-67 citrate lung scans to detect pulmonary vascular endothelial damage and lung inflammation in patients of collagen vascular diseases with active diffuse infiltrative lung disease. Rheumatol Int. 24(3):153-6, 2004
5. O'Connell M et al: Progressive massive fibrosis secondary to pulmonary silicosis appearance on F-18 fluorodeoxyglucose PET/CT. Clin Nucl Med. 29(11):754-5, 2004
6. Zompatori M et al: Diagnostic imaging of diffuse infiltrative disease of the lung. Respiration. 71(1):4-19, 2004
7. Milman N et al: Fluorodeoxyglucose PET scan in pulmonary sarcoidosis during treatment with inhaled and oral corticosteroids. Respiration. 70(4):408-13, 2003
8. Blum R et al: Role of 18FDG-positron emission tomography scanning in the management of histiocytosis. Leuk Lymphoma. 43(11):2155-7, 2002
9. Nishiyama O et al: Serial high resolution CT findings in nonspecific interstitial pneumonia/fibrosis. J Comput Assist Tomogr. 24:41-6, 2000
10. Baughman RP et al: Radionuclide imaging in interstitial lung disease. Curr Opin Pulm Med. 2(5):376-9, 1996
11. Ramsay SC et al: Quantitative pulmonary gallium scanning in interstitial lung disease. Eur J Nucl Med. 19(2):80-5, 1992

INTERSTITIAL LUNG DISEASE

IMAGE GALLERY

Typical

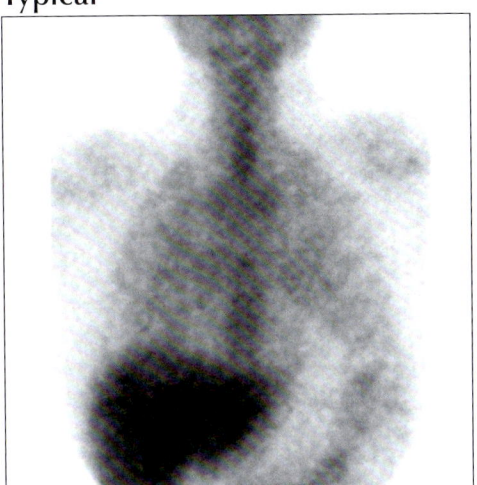

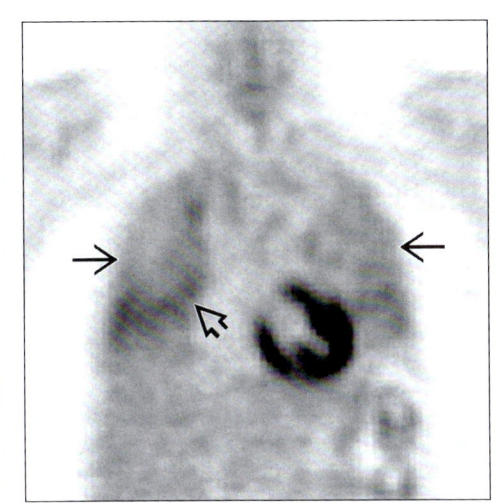

(Left) Anterior planar Ga-67 scan of the chest shows diffuse bilateral lung uptake consistent with active interstitial lung disease. Activity would be classified as grade II (equal to bone). *(Right)* PET shows diffuse uptake throughout both lungs ➔ in a patient with active UIP. Note prominence of subpleural regions ⊳, typical of the diagnosis.

Variant

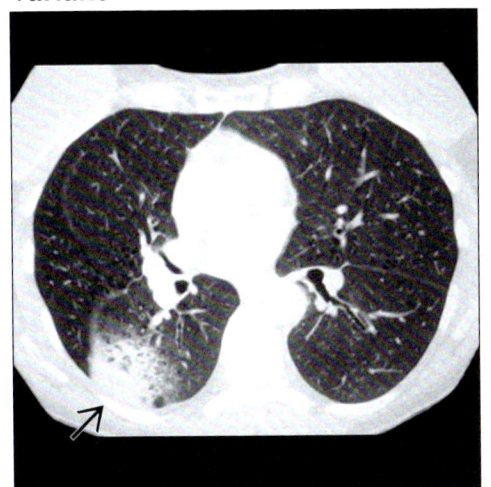

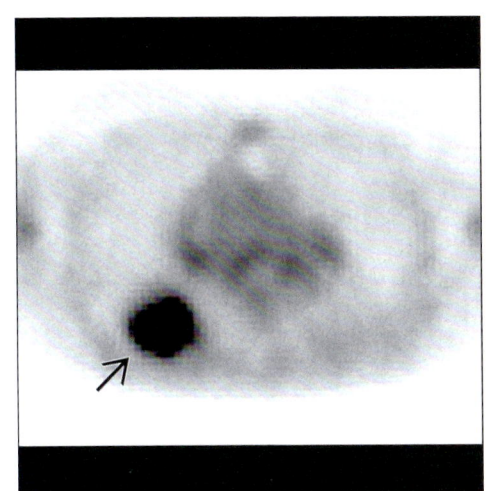

(Left) Axial CT of the chest shows focal area of consolidation in superior segment of right lower lobe ➔, confirmed at biopsy to be BOOP. Same as next image. *(Right)* Focal area of consolidation on CT corresponds to region of intense uptake on FDG PET ➔ in patient with biopsy proven BOOP. Same as previous image.

Variant

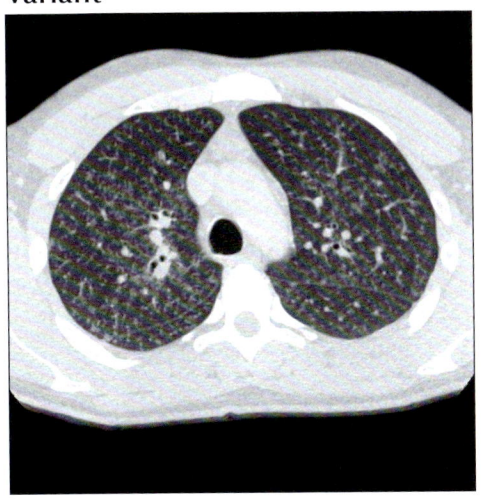

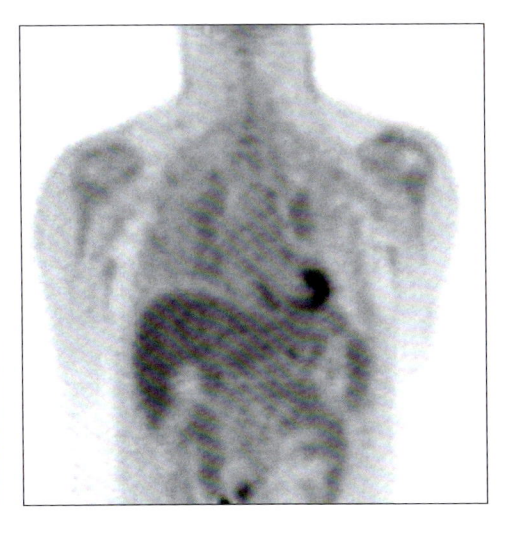

(Left) Axial CT chest shows numerous tiny nodules throughout both lung fields in a patient with drug (bleomycin)-induced pneumonitis. Same as next image. *(Right)* Coronal FDG PET shows diffuse bilateral lung uptake of FDG in patient with proven drug-induced pneumonitis (bleomycin). Same as previous image.

GRANULOMATOUS DISEASE

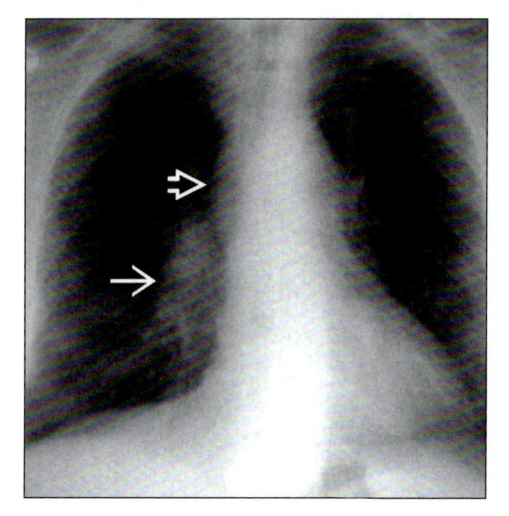

AP plain radiograph of the chest shows bulky bilateral hilar ➔ and mediastinal ➔ lymphadenopathy in a 28 year old male. Same patient as next image. Biopsy confirmed sarcoidosis.

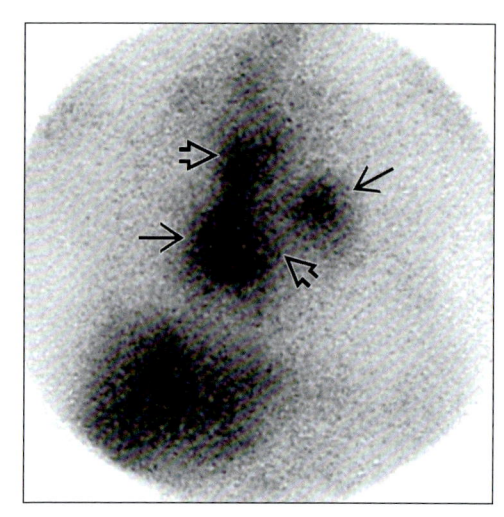

Same as previous. AP planar Ga-67 scan of the chest 72 h post injection demonstrates increased uptake in bulky hilar ➔ and mediastinal ➔ lymph nodes. Biopsy confirmed sarcoidosis.

TERMINOLOGY

Abbreviations and Synonyms
- Tuberculosis (TB), mycobacterium avium complex (MAC), chronic granulomatous disease (CGD)

Definitions
- Granulomatous diseases of either infectious or non-infectious etiology

IMAGING FINDINGS

General Features
- Best diagnostic clue
  - CT, plain film: Symmetrical, balanced hilar and mediastinal adenopathy, upper lobe predilection for nodules
  - Primary TB usually asymmetrical
  - FDG PET, Ga-67: Increased uptake on FDG PET, Ga-67 scan indicates active disease
- Location
  - Any site, varies with etiology
  - Commonly involves hilar/mediastinal lymph nodes and/or lungs (sarcoidosis, silicosis, fungal, mycobacterial)
  - All pulmonary granulomatous nodules: Upper lung predilection
- Size
  - Lymph nodes: Subtle enlargement to bulky "potato"
  - Nodules: Miliary to moderate size
- Morphology
  - Nodular opacities most common
  - Confluent nodules (progressive massive fibrosis), reticulonodular opacities, airspace disease also seen

Nuclear Medicine Findings
- PET
  - Active granulomatous disease is FDG avid
  - Magnitude of FDG uptake cannot distinguish from lung cancer
  - FDG PET patterns suggesting granulomatous disease rather than tumor
    - Symmetrical balanced distribution involving both hila and mediastinum
    - Bilateral upper lobe distribution

DDx: Mimics of Granulomatous Disease

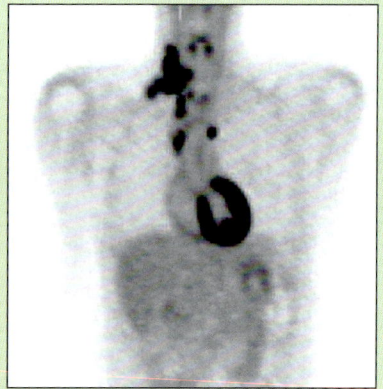

Metastatic Disease 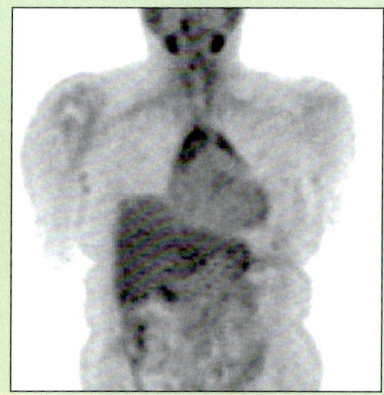 *Normal Thymus* 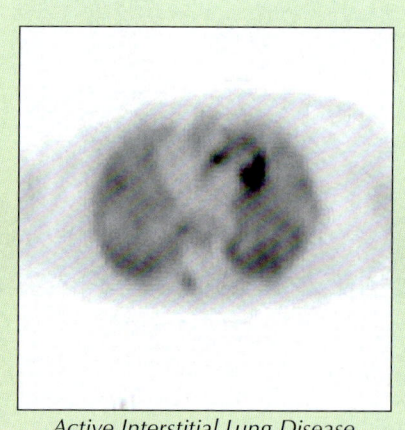 *Active Interstitial Lung Disease*

GRANULOMATOUS DISEASE

Key Facts

Terminology
- Granulomatous diseases of either infectious or non-infectious etiology

Imaging Findings
- Active granulomatous disease is FDG avid
- Magnitude of FDG uptake cannot distinguish from lung cancer
- FDG PET patterns suggesting granulomatous disease rather than tumor
- Symmetrical balanced distribution involving both hila and mediastinum
- Bilateral upper lobe distribution
- Bilateral hilar nodes with absence of intervening mediastinal activity
- Association with calcified nodes (note: Calcified nodes not usually FDG avid)
- Trial of systemic steroids may decreased FDG uptake and help confirm granulomatous disease
- Active granulomatous disease is Ga-67 avid
- Adenocarcinoma, squamous cell carcinoma not typically Ga-67 avid
- Radiography (CT or plain film) usually sufficient for diagnosis and follow-up
- Ga-67, FDG PET may be abnormal with normal chest radiograph

Top Differential Diagnoses
- Non-small cell lung cancer can be primarily hilar/mediastinal, more symmetrical than non-small cell
- Metastatic nodules tend to be dependent, lower lobes
- Metastatic adenopathy tends to be asymmetrical
- Unknown primary found with FDG PET/CT in ~ 45%

        - Bilateral hilar nodes with absence of intervening mediastinal activity
        - Association with calcified nodes (note: Calcified nodes not usually FDG avid)
    - Trial of systemic steroids may decreased FDG uptake and help confirm granulomatous disease
- Ga-67 Scintigraphy
    - Active granulomatous disease is Ga-67 avid
    - Adenocarcinoma, squamous cell carcinoma not typically Ga-67 avid

Radiographic Findings
- Thoracic sarcoidosis
    - Symmetric hilar and mediastinal lymphadenopathy; without or with pulmonary opacities
    - Reticulonodular opacities (90%) predominately upper lung zones
    - Atypical lymphadenopathy: Unilateral hilar, posterior mediastinal
    - Atypical lung disease: Unilateral lung disease, cavitary lung lesions, or pleural effusion
    - Pulmonary fibrosis
        - Upper lobe and superior segment lower lobe predominance
        - Upper lobe cyst formation (honeycombing), traction bronchiectasis with severe disease
    - Large airspace nodules with air bronchograms (alveolar sarcoid)
- Berylliosis, silicosis, coal workers pneumoconiosis
    - Occupational history
    - Similar radiographically to sarcoidosis
- Tuberculosis
    - Primary TB: Lymphadenopathy asymmetric and ipsilateral with the consolidation, pleural effusion
    - Miliary TB: Random nodule distribution, little or no lymphadenopathy
- Fungal (histoplasmosis, coccidiomycosis, cryptococcus)
    - Asymmetric lymphadenopathy
    - Lung nodules diffuse or focal
- Langerhans cell histiocytosis
    - Minimal adenopathy, lacks peribronchial distribution, cysts more common
- Hypersensitivity pneumonitis
    - No adenopathy, lacks peribronchial distribution, mosaic attenuation more common from small airways disease
- Pulmonary Wegener granulomatosis
    - Chronic fluctuating pattern of nodules, fluffy parenchymal opacities
    - Association with other clinical findings (nose, sinuses, kidneys, skin, eyes, joints)

Imaging Recommendations
- Best imaging tool
    - Radiography (CT or plain film) usually sufficient for diagnosis and follow-up
    - Ga-67, FDG PET may be abnormal with normal chest radiograph
    - Ga-67 or FDG PET differentiates active vs. inactive (FDG PET not currently approved by committee on medicare and medicaid services for this purpose)
- Protocol advice
    - CT: NECT first to evaluate nodal calcification pattern; CECT for hilar, mediastinum nodes, liver and spleen nodules; HRCT to define pulmonary parenchymal pattern
    - Ga-67: 5 mCi (185 MBq) IV, planar, SPECT at 72 h
    - FDG PET: 10-15 mCi (370-555 MBq), 60-90 min uptake before scanning

DIFFERENTIAL DIAGNOSIS

Lymphoma
- Lymphoma usually asymetric or predominantly mediastinal nodal enlargement

Primary Lung Cancer
- Non-small cell lung cancer can be primarily hilar/mediastinal, more symmetrical than non-small cell

Metastatic Disease
- Metastatic nodules tend to be dependent, lower lobes
- Metastatic adenopathy tends to be asymmetrical

GRANULOMATOUS DISEASE

- Known primary tumor
- Unknown primary found with FDG PET/CT in ~ 45%

PATHOLOGY

General Features
- General path comments
  - Widespread noncaseating granulomas that resolve or cause fibrosis
  - Exclusion of an alternative etiology
- Etiology
  - Infectious
    - Fungal: Coccidiomycosis, histoplasmosis, blastomycosis, aspergillosis, crytpcoccosis, sporotrichosis
    - Protozoa and metazoa: Leishmaniasis, schistosomiasis, toxoplasmosis
    - Spirochetes: Syphilis
    - Bacteria: Cat scratch fever, lymphogranuloma venereum, mycobacterium tuberculosis, nontuberculous mycobacteria
  - Non-infectious
    - Neoplasms: Carcinomas, sarcomas
    - Foreign substances: Foreign body, berylliosis, silicosis, coal-workers pneumoconiosis, extrinsic allergic alveolitis
    - Immunological defect: Primary biliary cirrhosis, Churg-Strauss allergic granulomatosis, hypogammaglobulinemia, Wegener granulomatous, giant cell arteritis
    - Congenital: Chronic granulomatous disease of childhood
    - Collagen disease: Lupus erythematosus
    - Idiopathic: Crohn disease, Langerhans cell histiocytosis, relapsing panniculitis, sarcoidosis, Whipple disease, lymphomatoid granulomatosis
    - Other: Chemotherapy, radiotherapy, granulomatous lesions of unknown significance (GLUS)
- Epidemiology
  - Infectious causes: Endemic regions, immunocompromised patients
  - Sarcoidosis shows geographic predilection: Swedish, Danish, Japanese
    - Constitutional symptoms more frequent in African-Americans and Asian-Indians

Gross Pathologic & Surgical Features
- Enlarged lymph nodes
- Granulomas caseating (mycobacterial), non-caseating (non-mycobacterial)
- Calcifications centrally, peripherally (egg-shell)

Microscopic Features
- Granulomas with rim of lymphocytes and fibroblasts, +/- central caseating necrosis
- Perilymphatic interstitial distribution of granulomas

CLINICAL ISSUES

Presentation
- Most common signs/symptoms
  - Wide range of organ specific symptoms and signs
  - Systemic symptoms common: Fatigue, malaise, weight loss, fever, night sweats
  - Asymptomatic: 50% (sarcoidosis)
- Other signs/symptoms
  - Multiorgan disorder: Symptoms from skin, muscle, bone, joint, neurologic, eye, cardiac, renal, genital, gastrointestinal involvement
  - Sarcoidosis: Increased angiotensin-converting enzyme level, hypercalcemia

Demographics
- Age
  - Childhood to late middle age
  - Sarcoidosis: Usually 20-40, onset rare > age 65
- Ethnicity: Sarcoidosis: Predilection in African-American females (most severe disease)

Natural History & Prognosis
- Highly variable between and within etiologies

Treatment
- Steroids, immunosuppression, treatment of infectious etiologies

DIAGNOSTIC CHECKLIST

Image Interpretation Pearls
- Upper lobe small nodules: Differential diagnosis includes all granulomatous diseases
- FDG PET: Granulomatous if balanced symmetrical metabolically active hilar nodes with smaller or absent intervening mediastinal nodes

SELECTED REFERENCES

1. Koyama T et al: Radiologic manifestations of sarcoidosis in various organs. Radiographics. 24(1):87-104, 2004
2. Barrington SF et al: Limitations of PET for imaging lymphoma. Eur J Nucl Med Mol Imaging. 30 Suppl 1:S117-27, 2003
3. Higashi K et al: Value of whole-body FDG PET in management of lung cancer. Ann Nucl Med. 17(1):1-14, 2003
4. Slart RH et al: Clinical value of gallium-67 scintigraphy in assessment of disease activity in Wegener's granulomatosis. Ann Rheum Dis. 62(7):659-62, 2003
5. Alavi A et al: Positron emission tomography imaging in nonmalignant thoracic disorders. Semin Nucl Med. 32(4):293-321, 2002
6. Gungor T et al: Diagnostic and therapeutic impact of whole body positron emission tomography using fluorine-18-fluoro-2-deoxy-D-glucose in children with chronic granulomatous disease. Arch Dis Child. 85(4):341-5, 2001
7. Goo JM et al: Pulmonary tuberculoma evaluated by means of FDG PET: findings in 10 cases. Radiology. 216(1):117-21, 2000
8. Yamada Y et al: Fluorine-18-fluorodeoxyglucose and carbon-11-methionine evaluation of lymphadenopathy in sarcoidosis. J Nucl Med. 39(7):1160-6, 1998
9. Kapala GB et al: Ga-67 chest imaging. Chronic granulomatous disease. Clin Nucl Med. 8(12):632, 1983
10. Rohatgi PK et al: Quantitative gallium scanning in pulmonary sarcoidosis. Respiration. 44(4):304-13, 1983

GRANULOMATOUS DISEASE

IMAGE GALLERY

Typical

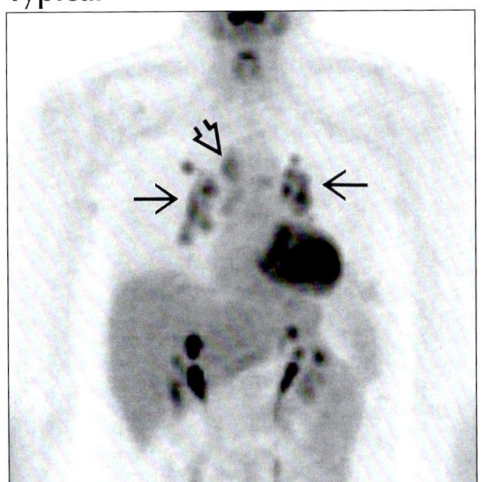

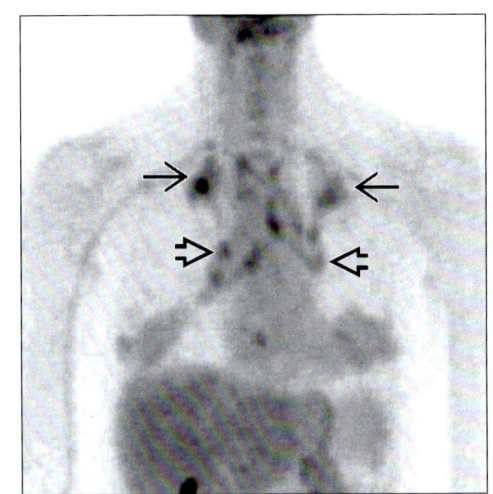

(Left) AP maximum intensity projection (MIP) FDG PET image shows symmetrical hypermetabolic hilar ➡ lymph nodes; fewer mediastinal ➡ nodes (mostly right paratracheal), typical of sarcoidosis. *(Right)* AP maximum intensity projection (MIP) FDG PET image shows bilateral apical focal hypermetabolism ➡, bilateral hilar ➡ and mediastinal hypermetabolic lymph nodes in patient with reactivated TB.

Variant

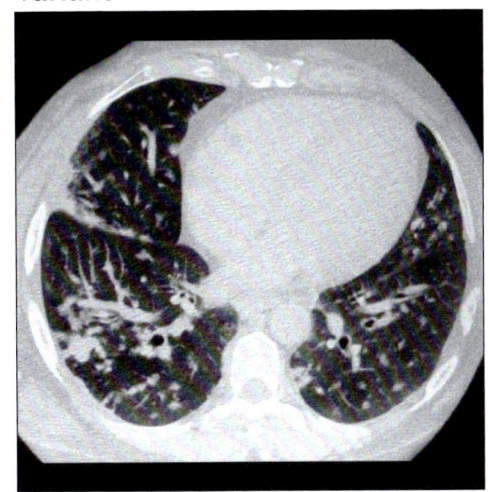

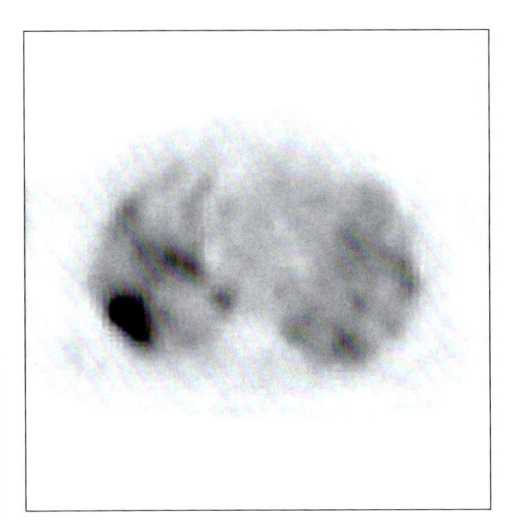

(Left) Transaxial CT shows bilateral nodular opacities, septal and peribronchial thickening. Biopsy confirmed sarcoidosis. Same patient as next image. *(Right)* Transaxial FDG PET shows patchy and focal hypermetabolism throughout both lungs in patient with active sarcoidosis. Same as patient as previous image.

Variant

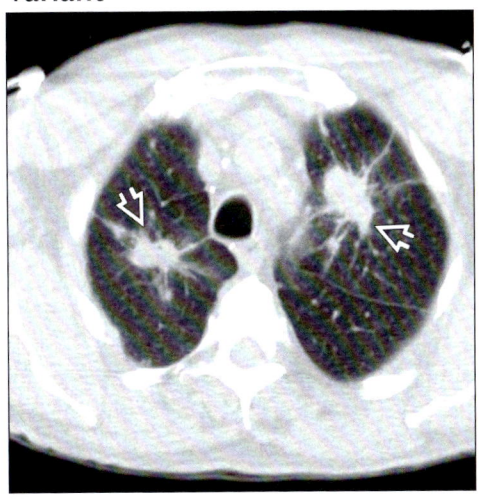

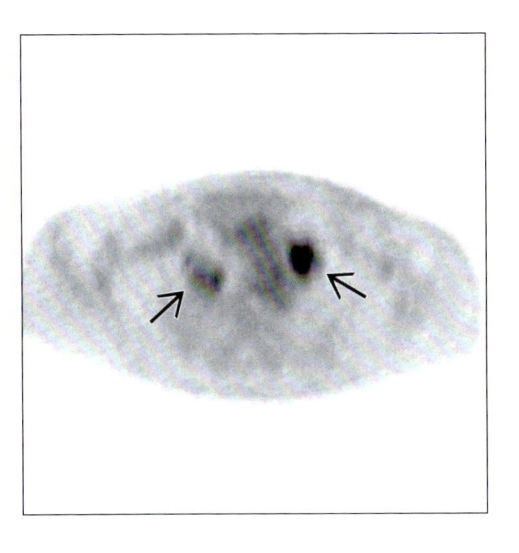

(Left) Transaxial CT shows bilateral apical spiculated masses ➡ in retired coal miner. Confirmed progressive massive fibrosis. Same patient as next image. *(Right)* Transaxial FDG PET shows focal hypermetabolism in bilateral apical masses ➡ in retired coal miner. Confirmed progressive massive fibrosis. Same patient as previous image.

SOLITARY PULMONARY NODULE

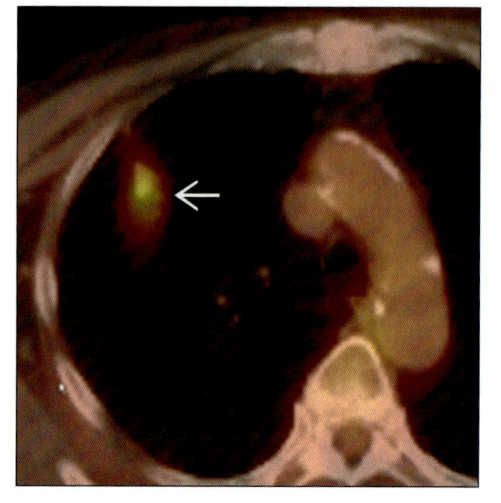

Axial PET shows SPN with focally increased FDG activity most prominent posterolaterally ➡. This observation guided the subsequent percutaneous CT-guided biopsy. See next image.

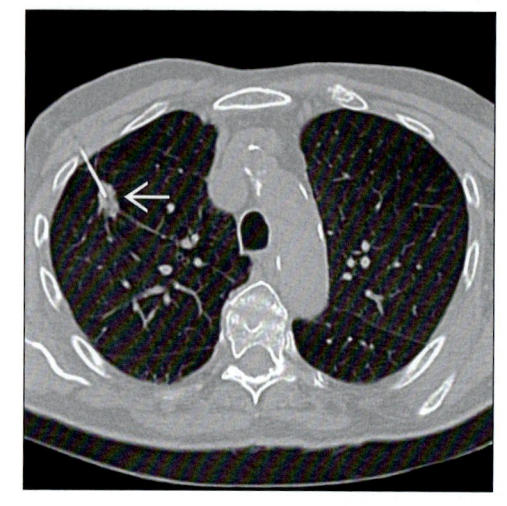

Axial NECT of same patient as previous image shows guided fine needle aspiration of the spiculated nodule ➡. Biopsy was diagnostic for adenocarcinoma.

TERMINOLOGY

Abbreviations and Synonyms
- Solitary pulmonary nodule (SPN)

Definitions
- Focal pulmonary parenchymal opacity < 3 cm in size

IMAGING FINDINGS

General Features
- Best diagnostic clue
  - Most likely malignant
    - SPN with higher SUV (≥ 2.5): As predictive of malignancy; confirmation of growth by CT
    - Also concerning for malignancy: Any detectable FDG activity higher than background for SPN < 1.5 cm; FDG activity > mediastinal blood pool
    - Risk of malignancy highest when SUV > 2.5 and nodule spiculated
  - Most likely benign
    - Smooth border and negative PET more likely benign but requires CT follow-up
- Location
  - SPN may occur anywhere within lung
  - 2/3 of primary lung CA occurs in upper lobes
  - Metastatic SPN more common in outer 1/3 of lower lobes
- Size
  - Nodule < 30 mm, mass > 30 mm
  - Likelihood of malignancy related to size; > 85% if > 20 mm in diameter
  - Growth
    - 26% increase in diameter = one doubling in volume; time to 26% increase in diameter = one doubling time
    - Most cancer doubling times ~ 30-200 day range
    - Nodule dimension stability: > 2 years highly suggestive of benignity
    - Increase in size < 30 days with infection, infarction, lymphoma, fast-growing metastases
- Morphology
  - Margin characteristics
    - Benign lesions: Well-circumscribed, smooth borders
    - Malignant nodules: Ill-defined, irregular, lobulated, spiculated borders

DDx: Solitary Pulmonary Nodule

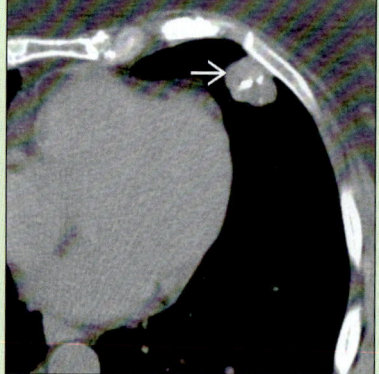

Hamartoma

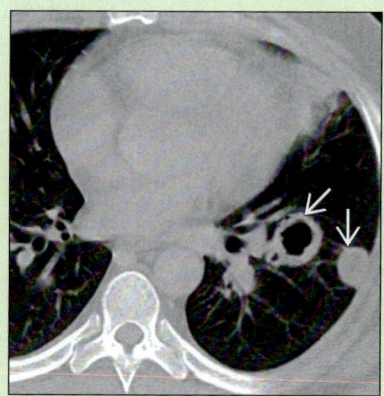

Wegener Granulomatosis

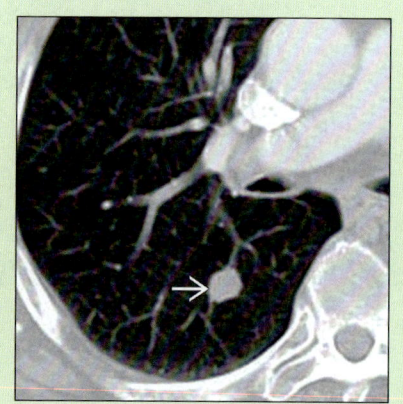

Leiomyosarcoma Metastasis

SOLITARY PULMONARY NODULE

Key Facts

Imaging Findings
- SPN with higher SUV (≥ 2.5): As predictive of malignancy; confirmation of growth by CT
- Also concerning for malignancy: Any detectable FDG activity higher than background for SPN < 1.5 cm; FDG activity > mediastinal blood pool
- Risk of malignancy highest when SUV > 2.5 and nodule spiculated
- Smooth border and negative PET more likely benign but requires CT follow-up
- Series with SPNs ≥ 10 mm: PET sensitivity 95-98% and specificity 73-85%

Pathology
- Age: Risk of malignancy 3% at 35-39 yrs, 15% at 40-49 yrs, 43% at 50-59 yrs, > 50% at 60+ yrs

- History of smoking, malignancy, TB, pulmonary mycosis
- Travel to regions endemic to mycosis
- Occupational risk factors for malignancy (asbestos, radon, nickel, chromium, vinyl chloride, polycyclic hydrocarbons)

Clinical Issues
- Most SPNs asymptomatic, incidental finding

Diagnostic Checklist
- Continued CT follow-up in PET-negative SPN
- If nodule has features of BAC, a negative PET does not rule out malignancy
- For small nodules (< 1.5 cm), any FDG activity higher than background or mediastinal blood pool = concerning for malignancy

---

- Not unusual for malignant lesion to have smooth contour (e.g., carcinoid)
- 90% of spiculated nodules are malignant
- 20% of smoothly/sharply marginated nodules malignant
- Density characteristics
  - Calcified nodule: More likely to be benign
  - Approximately 10% of malignant nodules demonstrate calcification (usually stippled, peripheral/eccentric)
  - Most ground-glass opacities (GGO) are inflammatory; bronchoalveolar carcinoma (BAC) may be entirely GGO
  - Fat or water density indicates benign etiology
  - Lung cancer enhances more prominently than benign pathology
- Air bronchograms
  - "Air bronchogram" sign in 25-65% of cancers, much less common in benign lesion
- Pseudocavitation
  - More commonly found in malignancy (e.g., BAC)
- Cavitation
  - 10% of malignancies; 80% of cavitary lung cancers = squamous cell carcinoma
  - 85% of cavities with wall thickness > 15 mm are malignant; 95% of cavities with wall thickness < 5 mm are benign
- Air-fluid level
  - Air-fluid level in cavitary nodule suggests benign lesion, particularly abscess
- Satellite nodules
  - Small nodules adjacent dominant nodule, suggest benign, likely granulomatous, lesion

Nuclear Medicine Findings
- PET
  - SPN detectability is dependent on nodule size, metabolic activity
  - Metabolism quantified by standardized uptake value (SUV)
    - SUV > 2.5 suggested as marker of malignancy; but significant overlap between benign and malignant
    - In general, the higher the SUV, the more likely the nodule will be malignant
  - False-positive PET
    - Non-malignant metabolically active conditions (e.g., infection, granuloma, inflammation, hamartoma)
  - False-negative PET
    - Tumors with low metabolic rates (BAC, carcinoid), tumors < 15 mm, "stunned" tumors following therapy, high serum glucose levels during PET
  - Sensitivity & specificity of PET in SPN
    - Depends on many factors: Patient selection, region, referral bias, criteria for positive or negative study, instrumentation
    - Series with SPNs ≥ 10 mm: PET sensitivity 95-98% and specificity 73-85%
  - Prognosis
    - PET staging may be more accurate than pathology in predicting survival or recurrence
    - Staging with PET ⇒ excellent prognostic information; even with stage I on PET, a high SUV (> 5-10) in primary nodule = poor prognosis
  - Other radiopharmaceuticals are not as sensitive as FDG PET (Ga-67, Tc-99m MIBI, Tl-201, Tc-99m depreotide)

Radiographic Findings
- Chest X-ray (CXR) relatively insensitive in detecting noncalcified nodules < 1 cm
- Screening studies in adults: 1-2 SPN per 1,000 CXRs

CT Findings
- Better detection & characterization of margin, density, calcification pattern than CXR

Angiographic Findings
- Vascular malformations detectable (e.g., arteriovenous malformation, hereditary hemorrhagic telangiectasia/Osler-Weber-Rendu syndrome)

Imaging Recommendations
- Best imaging tool: PET/CT superior to CT or PET alone for overall accuracy

SOLITARY PULMONARY NODULE

DIFFERENTIAL DIAGNOSIS

Malignant Lesions
- Usually strongly FDG positive
  - Primary lung cancer: Bronchogenic carcinoma; small cell, large cell, adenocarcinoma, & squamous cell carcinoma
  - Metastatic disease: Most non-mucinous adenocarcinoma, sarcoma, lymphoma, melanoma, lymphoma
- Variable to low FDG uptake
  - Primary lung cancer: Carcinoid, bronchoalveolar carcinoma
  - Metastatic disease: Highly mucinous adenocarcinoma, testicular, renal cell, prostate, hepatocellular carcinoma

Benign Lesions
- Usually FDG positive
  - Inflammation/infection
    - Infectious [tuberculosis (TB), fungal] and non-infectious (rheumatoid, Wegener, sarcoid) granulomatous disease
    - Bacterial infection
    - Inhalation (silicosis, lipoid pneumonia)
  - Other
    - Bronchiolitis obliterans organizing pneumonia
    - Pulmonary infarction
    - Round atelectasis
    - Lymph node
    - Mucoid impaction
    - Soft tissue tumor
- Usually FDG negative
  - Inactive granulomatous disease, bronchogenic cyst, hamartoma, pleural plaque
  - Other: Lipoma, fibroma, AVM, pulmonary varix, congenital cystic adenomatoid malformation

PATHOLOGY

General Features
- Epidemiology
  - 150,000 SPNs detected annually in US
    - Malignancy incidence range 10-70%; depends on population under study (e.g., age, smoking status, referral pattern, study location)
  - Important features in patient history
    - Age: Risk of malignancy 3% at 35-39 yrs, 15% at 40-49 yrs, 43% at 50-59 yrs, > 50% at 60+ yrs
    - History of smoking, malignancy, TB, pulmonary mycosis
    - Travel to regions endemic to mycosis
    - Occupational risk factors for malignancy (asbestos, radon, nickel, chromium, vinyl chloride, polycyclic hydrocarbons)

CLINICAL ISSUES

Presentation
- Most common signs/symptoms
  - Most SPNs asymptomatic, incidental finding
  - SPN in setting of another primary (breast, head & neck, colon, etc.) is most often a primary bronchogenic carcinoma

Natural History & Prognosis
- Low-risk population
  - If no risk factors, clinical history, prior images, or concerning imaging features to suggest high-risk patient
  - Current recommendations are to prove stability over 2-yr period with follow-up imaging
- High-risk population
  - Depends on clinical scenario
  - Management may include
    - Interval CT follow-up
    - Percutaneous biopsy, bronchoscopic/transesophageal biopsy
    - Bronchoscopic washings
    - Video-assisted thoracoscopic surgery
    - Resection of nodule

DIAGNOSTIC CHECKLIST

Consider
- Continued CT follow-up in PET-negative SPN
- If nodule has features of BAC, a negative PET does not rule out malignancy
- For small nodules (< 1.5 cm), any FDG activity higher than background or mediastinal blood pool = concerning for malignancy

SELECTED REFERENCES

1. Lejeune C et al: Use of a decision analysis model to assess the medicoeconomic implications of FDG PET imaging in diagnosing a solitary pulmonary nodule. Eur J Health Econ. 2005
2. Mavi A et al: Fluorodeoxyglucose-PET in characterizing solitary pulmonary nodules, assessing pleural diseases, and the initial staging, restaging, therapy planning, and monitoring response of lung cancer. Radiol Clin North Am. 43(1):1-21, ix, 2005
3. Drosten R: CT-Guided thoracic interventions in "Multidetector-row CT of the Thorax", Schoepf UJ: Springer-Verlag. 23-452, 2004
4. Fischer BM et al: Positron emission tomography of incidentally detected small pulmonary nodules. Nucl Med Commun. 25(1):3-9, 2004
5. Comber LA et al: Solitary pulmonary nodules: impact of quantitative contrast-enhanced CT on the cost-effectiveness of FDG-PET. Clin Radiol. 58(9):706-11, 2003
6. Hickeson M et al: Use of a corrected standardized uptake value based on the lesion size on CT permits accurate characterization of lung nodules on FDG-PET. Eur J Nucl Med Mol Imaging. 29(12):1639-47, 2002
7. Erasmus JJ et al: Solitary pulmonary nodules: Part I. Morphologic evaluation for differentiation of benign and malignant lesions. Radiographics. 20(1):43-58, 2000
8. Erasmus JJ et al: Solitary pulmonary nodules: Part II. Evaluation of the indeterminate nodule. Radiographics. 20(1):59-66, 2000
9. Lowe VJ et al: Prospective investigation of positron emission tomography in lung nodules. J Clin Oncol. 16(3):1075-84, 1998

SOLITARY PULMONARY NODULE

IMAGE GALLERY

Typical

Typical

Typical

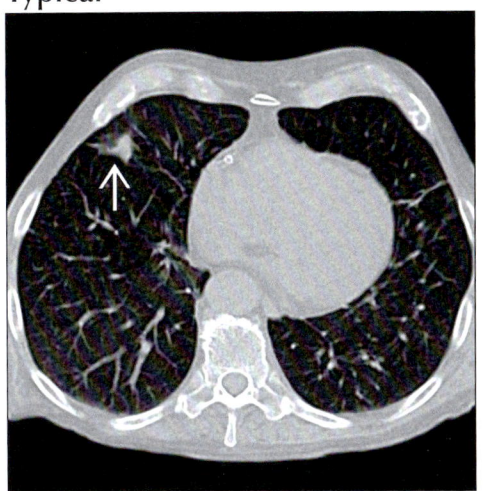

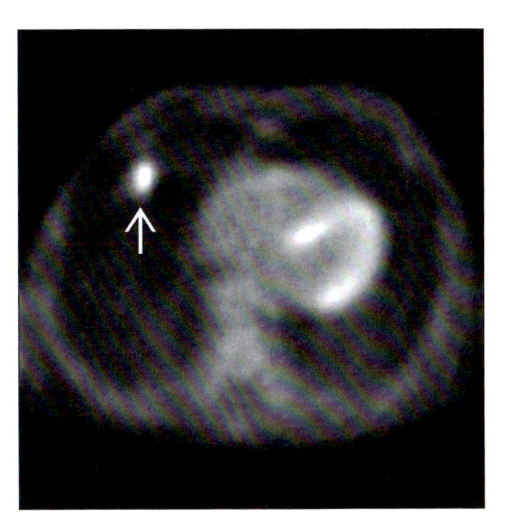

(Left) Axial NECT in patient with significant smoking history shows a spiculated SPN ➡. See next image. *(Right)* Axial PET of same patient as previous image shows increased FDG activity in the SPN ➡. This was pathologically proven non-small cell lung carcinoma.

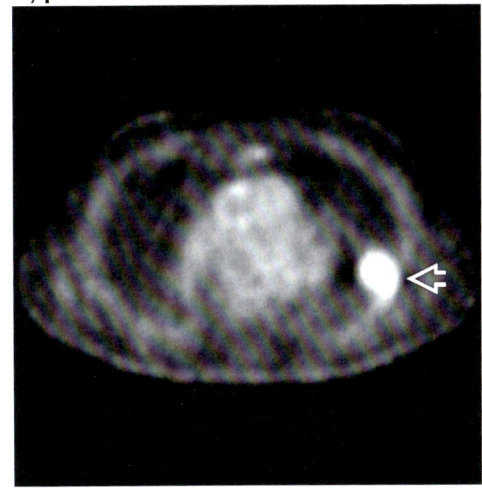

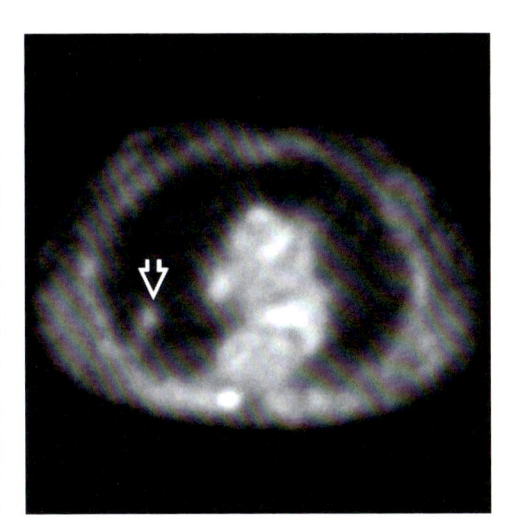

(Left) Axial PET shows increased FDG activity in a left lung lesion ➡. Upon biopsy, this was a granulomatous pneumonia. *(Right)* Axial PET shows mildly increased FDG activity in a right upper lobe nodule ➡. Upon biopsy, this was an organizing pneumonia.

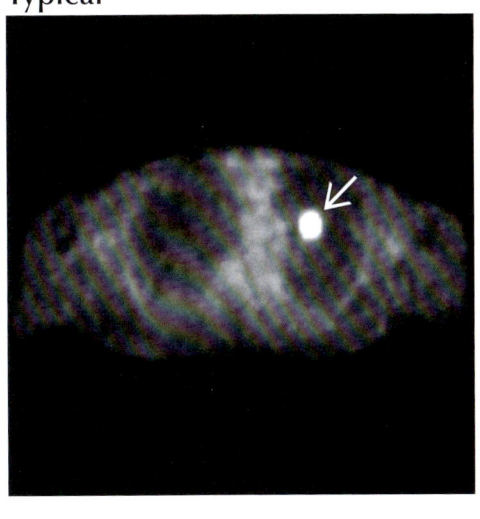

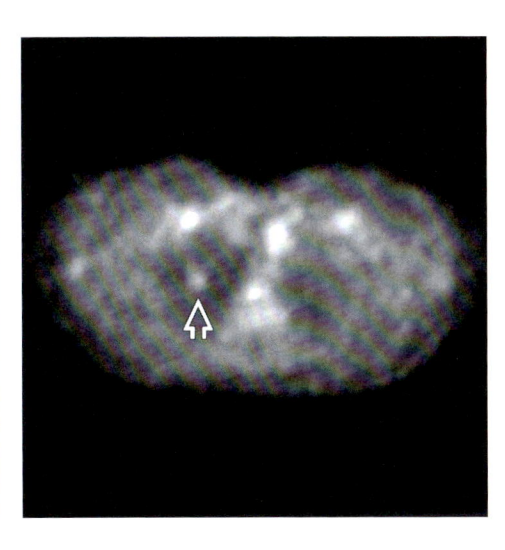

(Left) Axial PET shows increased FDG activity in a left upper lobe lesion ➡, confirmed cytologically to represent large cell lung carcinoma. *(Right)* Axial PET shows mildly increased FDG activity in a right upper lobe nodule ➡. Biopsy demonstrated bronchoalveolar carcinoma, which commonly shows low-grade FDG activity.

NON-SMALL CELL LUNG CANCER

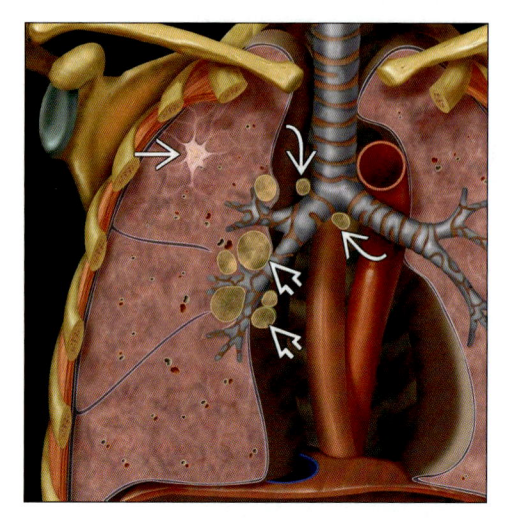

Graphic illustrates appearance of spiculated lesion in RUL, pathologically enlarged lymph node in ipsilateral hilum and mediastinum.

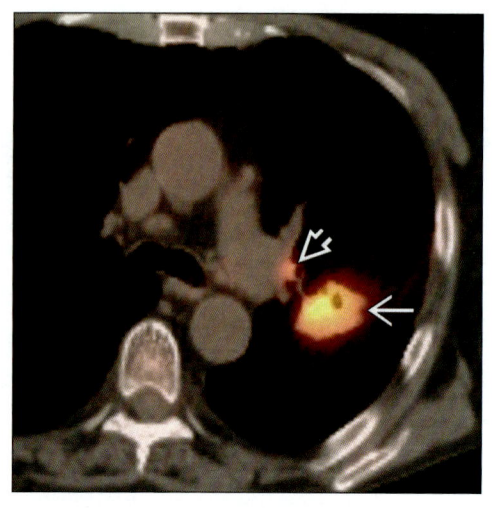

Axial fused PET CT shows left lung mass (NSCLC) and ipsilateral unenlarged, but definitively FDG avid, left hilar lymph node consistent with tumor spread.

TERMINOLOGY

Abbreviations and Synonyms
- Non-small cell lung cancer (NSCLC), bronchogenic carcinoma (CA), adenocarcinoma (adenoCA), squamous cell carcinoma (SCCA), large cell carcinoma (LCCA), bronchoalveolar carcinoma (BAC)

Definitions
- Group of primary lung neoplasms arising from secretory cells (glandular features)

IMAGING FINDINGS

General Features
- Best diagnostic clue: Spiculated pulmonary nodule in a smoker; hilar and mediastinal lymphadenopathy
- Location
  - Central: Typical of SCCA
  - Upper lobe, peripheral: Typical of adenoCA
- Size
  - Average size at detection is approx; 25 mm by CXR
  - CT or screening detected lesion is usually 8-15 mm
- Morphology
  - Borders: Spiculated, lobulated, smooth
  - Density: Solid, mixed solid/ground-glass, less often pure ground-glass without soft tissue component
    - Cavitation more common with SCCA
    - Ground-glass is associated with adenoCA and BAC

Nuclear Medicine Findings
- V/Q Scan
  - Consider pulmonary embolus (PE) in every patient (including oncology patients) with a pleural effusion
  - Quantitative V/Q for prediction of post-operative pulmonary function
- PET
  - PET/CT has revolutionized initial and post therapy evaluation and management of NSCLC
  - PET/CT can predict prognosis, assess Rx response, influence Rx plans by demonstrating occult disease
  - FDG PET may be more accurate than pathology in predicting survival or recurrence
  - SPN > 10 mm: PET 95-98% sensitive, 73-85% specific
  - FDG PET criteria for malignancy: Activity > mediastinal background, max SUV ≥ 2.5, any appreciable activity in lesion < 1-1.5 cm

DDx: Non-Small Cell Lung Cancer

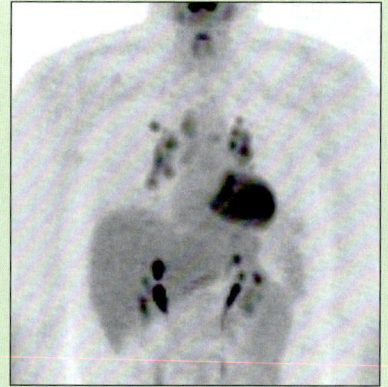

Granulomatous Disease 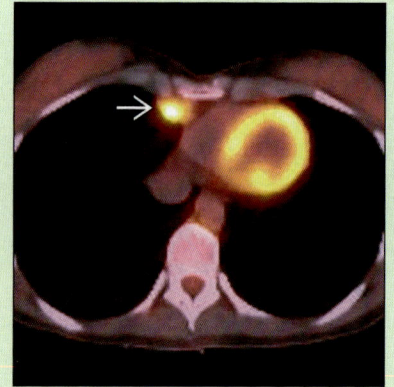 | *Lymphoma* 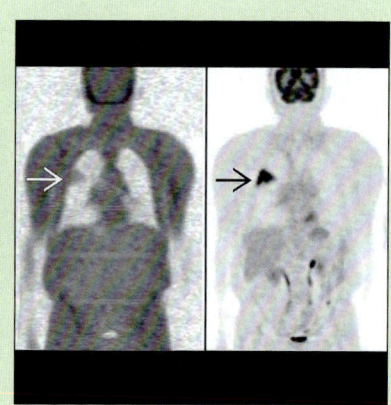 | *Infarct*

NON-SMALL CELL LUNG CANCER

Key Facts

Imaging Findings
- Best diagnostic clue: Spiculated pulmonary nodule in a smoker; hilar and mediastinal lymphadenopathy
- MR is used to evaluate brachial plexus invasion by superior sulcus (Pancoast) tumor
- PET/CT has revolutionized initial and post therapy evaluation and management of NSCLC
- PET/CT can predict prognosis, assess Rx response, influence Rx plans by demonstrating occult disease
- FDG PET may be more accurate than pathology in predicting survival or recurrence
- SPN > 10 mm: PET 95-98% sensitive, 73-85% specific
- FDG PET avoids nontherapeutic thoracotomy in 20% by detecting previously occult distant disease

Pathology
- General path comments: Sputum cytology for central tumors: False in 40%
- > 85% smoke; 50% in former smokers
- Environmental: Asbestos, radon, passive smoking
- Epidemiology: In US: 170,000 new cases/year; 150,000 deaths/year (most common CA death)

Clinical Issues
- Majority are diagnosed with advanced stage disease

Diagnostic Checklist
- Suspicious CT morphology: Biopsy even with negative PET
- Suspicious on FDG PET: Biopsy/remove without required followed growth on CT

- Positive FDG PET has same predictive value of malignancy as nodule growth on CT
  - Partial volume effects on SUV: Lower measured maximum SUV in nodules < 2.5 cm measure
  - Apply recovery coefficient to correct max SUV in smaller nodules: Recommended for quantitative determinations
  - False (+) PET: Non-malignant metabolically active conditions (active inflammation, infectious, granulomatous disease)
  - False (-) PET: Tumor with low metabolic rate (low grade adenoCA, BAC, carcinoid), tumor < 10 mm, "stunned" tumor post therapy, high serum glucose (competition)
  - Prognostic information from FDG PET: Max SUV > 5 suggests aggressive neoplasm, poorer prognosis
  - Response to treatment: Compare max SUV before and ≥ 3 cycles of chemoradiation: > 60% reduction = good response
  - FDG PET avoids nontherapeutic thoracotomy in 20% by detecting previously occult distant disease
  - Negative FDG PET: Does not exclude microscopic disease; does not preclude mediastinal/hilar surgical staging
  - FDG PET/CT increasingly used in simulations for radiation treatment planning

Radiographic Findings
- Radiography
  - Peripheral lesion 1-10 cm: Nodules < 1 cm are rarely detected by conventional radiography
  - Central tumor with hilar or mediastinal lymph node enlargement
  - Rib or spine destruction with chest wall invasion

CT Findings
- NECT
  - Usually adequate for evaluation of primary tumor, hilar and mediastinal lymph node enlargement
  - Advantage: No nephrotoxicity/contrast reaction, adrenal nodule evaluation (adenoma vs. metastasis)
  - Disadvantage: Difficult detecting enlarged hilar lymph nodes, vascular invasion, liver lesions
  - Peripheral lesions
    - Cavitation more frequent in squamous histology
    - Peripheral adenoCA may be solid, mixed solid and ground-glass, or ground-glass
  - Metastases in non-tumor lobe, multiple, bilateral
  - HRCT to evaluate for lymphangitic carcinomatosis
- CECT
  - Increased conspicuity for small endobronchial lesion
  - Bronchial obstruction with lobar collapse or post-obstructive pneumonitis
  - Size criteria for lymph node pathology: > 0.5 mm hilar, > 10 mm mediastinal lymph node short axis
  - Demonstrates pleural metastases in pleural effusion

MR Findings
- Slightly more sensitive than CT for chest wall invasion
- MR is used to evaluate brachial plexus invasion by superior sulcus (Pancoast) tumor

Imaging Recommendations
- Best imaging tool
  - CT characterizes the pattern and extent of disease: Readily available, widespread expertise
  - Whole body PET/CT is superior to CT or PET alone: Prognosis, staging
  - MR to evaluate the brain, brachial plexus invasion in superior sulcus (Pancoast) tumors
- Protocol advice
  - CT thorax is incomplete if the adrenal glands are not completely imaged
  - Screening CT studies should be performed without contrast and with the lowest possible mAs
  - FDG PET: Serum glucose < 150 ng/dl; 90 minute uptake interval

DIFFERENTIAL DIAGNOSIS

Pulmonary Infarct, Infection
- FDG uptake as great as with lung cancer

Granulomatous Disease
- Multiple upper lobe nodules, calcified nodes

NON-SMALL CELL LUNG CANCER

- Balanced, symmetrical FDG avid hilar and mediastinal nodes

Mediastinal Mass
- Consider small cell lung cancer, lymphoma (both "hot" on PET)

Hamartoma
- Typically low FDG activity, popcorn calcification

PATHOLOGY

General Features
- General path comments: Sputum cytology for central tumors: False in 40%
- Genetics: AdenoCA: 30% ras oncogene mutation; worse prognosis
- Etiology
  - \> 85% smoke; 50% in former smokers
  - Environmental: Asbestos, radon, passive smoking
- Epidemiology: In US: 170,000 new cases/year; 150,000 deaths/year (most common CA death)
- Associated abnormalities: COPD, emphysema

Gross Pathologic & Surgical Features
- AdenoCA (may have BAC features); SCCA (cavitate); LCCA (> 4 cm at diagnosis)

Microscopic Features
- AdenoCA: Forms glands, mucus production
- SCCA: Irregular nuclei, large nucleoli, intercellular bridging, + keratin stain
- LCCA: Difficult to identify, may have neuroendocrine features

Staging, Grading or Classification Criteria
- Primary lesion (T): Tx: Tumor cannot be assessed, + sputum/washings; T0: No evidence of primary tumor; Tis: Carcinoma in situ; T1: < 3 cm, completely surrounded by lung; no main bronchi invasion; T2: > 3 cm, involving main bronchus > 2 cm from the carina, visceral pleura; atelectasis/pneumonitis extending to hila; T3: Invading chest wall, diaphragm, mediastinal pleura, parietal pericardium, main bronchus < 2 cm from the carina; total atelectasis of whole lung; T4: Invading the mediastinal structures, vertebrae, carina; separate tumor nodules in same lobe; malignant pleural effusion
- Mediastinal and hilar lymph nodes (N): N1: Hilar lymph nodes at vessel branch point; N2: Ipsilateral to primary tumor (subcarinal lymph node is ipsilateral); N3: Contralateral lymph node, supraclavicular fossa
- Metastases (M): Mx: Metastases cannot be assessed; M0: No distant metastases; M1: Distant metastases, including separate tumor in different lobe
- SCCA limited stage: One lung, ipsilateral lymph nodes
- SCCA extensive stage: Contralateral lung, lymph nodes, distant organs, malignant pleural effusion
- Stages: O(TisN0M0); 1A(T1N0M0); IB(T2N0M0); IIA(T1N1M0); IIB[(T2N1M0),(T3N0M0)]; IIIA[(T1-3N2M0),(T3N1M0]; IIIB[(any T,N3M0), (T4,any N,M0)]; IV(any T,any N,M1)

CLINICAL ISSUES

Presentation
- Most common signs/symptoms: 10% asymptomatic; symptoms with advanced disease
- Other signs/symptoms: Pain, recurrent pneumonia in same lobe, constitutional symptoms, paraneoplastic syndrome

Demographics
- Age: > 50 years
- Gender: M > F = 2:1; mortality higher in males, increasing in females
- Ethnicity: African-American: Caucasian males = 2:1

Natural History & Prognosis
- Majority are diagnosed with advanced stage disease
- AdenoCA: Per stage, worse prognosis than SCCA (except T1N0)

Treatment
- Stage 1 & 2: Surgery, then adjuvant chemo in selected
- Stage 3A: Neoadjuvant chemoradiation, then surgery in selected; stage 3B: Chemoradiation, then surgery in selected T4N0
- Stage 4: Chemotherapy, palliative radiation in selected; solitary brain mets: Resection of brain met and primary if possible
- Radiation or RFA: Symptomatic non-operable lesions

DIAGNOSTIC CHECKLIST

Consider
- Suspicious CT morphology: Biopsy even with negative PET
- Suspicious on FDG PET: Biopsy/remove without required followed growth on CT

SELECTED REFERENCES

1. Bruzzi JF et al: PET/CT Imaging of Lung Cancer. J Thorac Imaging. 21(2):123-36, 2006
2. Pottgen C et al: Value of 18F-fluoro-2-deoxy-D-glucose-positron emission tomography/computed tomography in non-small-cell lung cancer for prediction of pathologic response and times to relapse after neoadjuvant chemoradiotherapy. Clin Cancer Res. 12(1):97-106, 2006
3. Hoekstra CJ et al: Prognostic relevance of response evaluation using [18F]-2-fluoro-2-deoxy-D-glucose positron emission tomography in patients with locally advanced non-small-cell lung cancer. J Clin Oncol. 23(33):8362-70, 2005
4. Ravenel JG: Lung cancer staging. Semin Roentgenol. 39(3):373-85, 2004
5. Vansteenkiste J et al: Positron-emission tomography in prognostic and therapeutic assessment of lung cancer: systematic review. Lancet Oncol. 5(9):531-40, 2004
6. Pastorino U et al: Fluorodeoxyglucose positron emission tomography improves preoperative staging of resectable lung metastasis. J Thorac Cardiovasc Surg. 126(6):1906-10, 2003

NON-SMALL CELL LUNG CANCER

IMAGE GALLERY

Typical

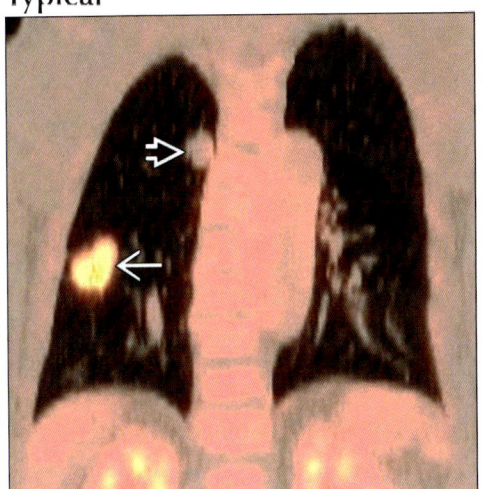

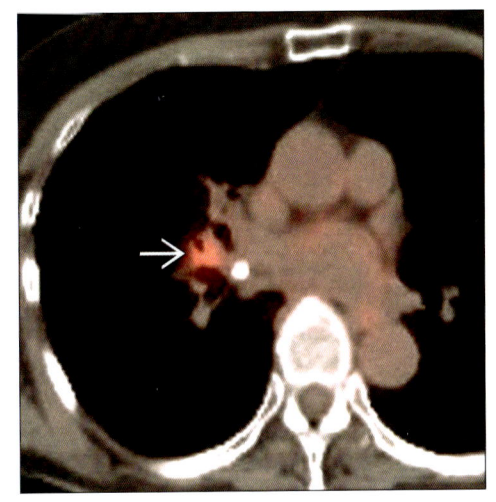

(Left) Coronal PET/CT fusion image shows prominently FDG avid RLL mass ➡ (NSCLC) and non FDG avid RUL hamartoma ➡. (Right) Axial PET/CT shows tumor recurrence ➡ in right paramediastinal radiation field. Post radiation lung fibrosis remains hypermetabolic indefinitely. Focal elevated avidity may indicate recurrence.

Typical

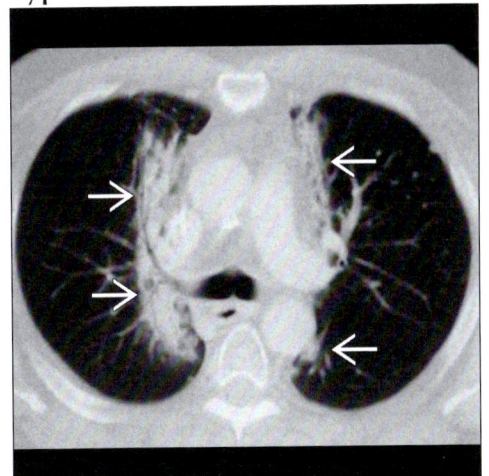

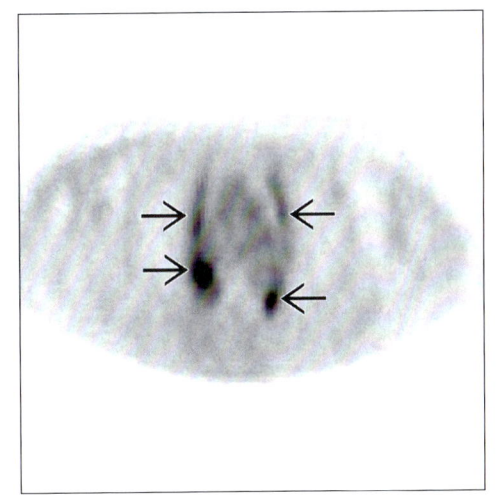

(Left) Axial NECT following mediastinal radiation shows fibrotic changes within radiation field ➡, which can remain FDG avid indefinitely. Same patient as next image. (Right) Axial FDG PET shows extensive hypermetabolism in region of post-radiation fibrosis ➡, a finding that can persist indefinitely. Same patient as previous image.

Typical

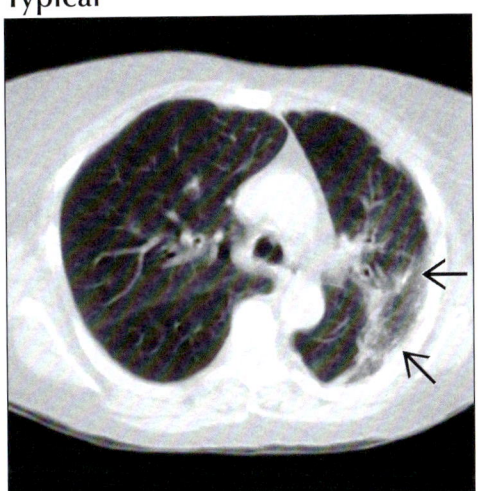

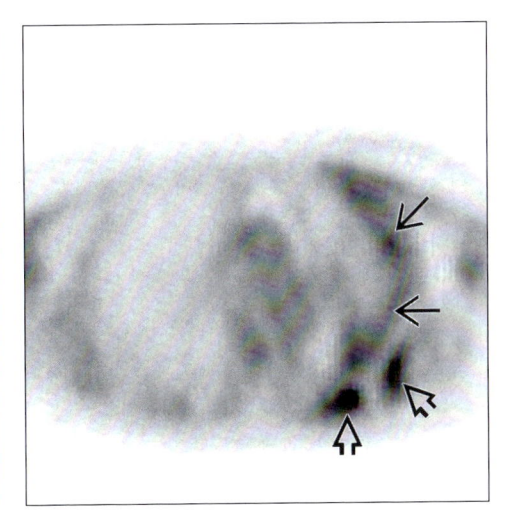

(Left) Axial CT shows scarring and pleural thickening ➡ after partial pneumonectomy for NSCLC. Architectural distortion and tissue thickening make evaluation for local recurrence difficult by CT. Same patient as next image. (Right) Axial FDG PET shows diffuse hypermetabolic pleural rind ➡ following partial pneumonectomy, which can persist indefinitely. Also note uptake in chest wall due to post-thoracotomy inflammation ➡.

NON-SMALL CELL LUNG CANCER

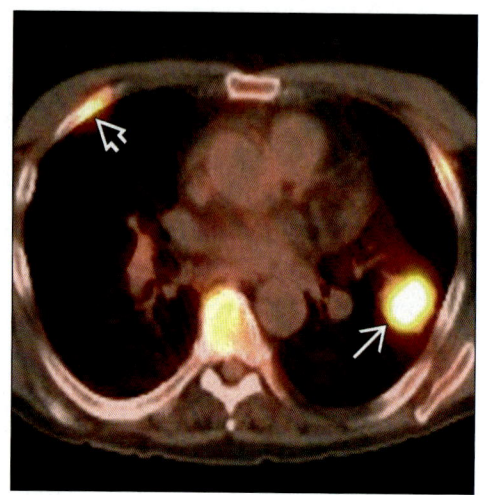

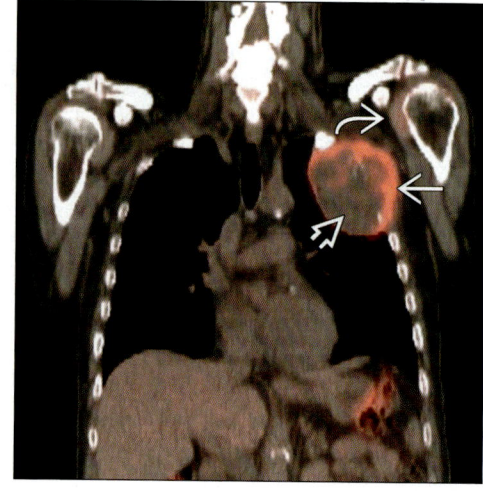

(Left) Axial fused FDG PET/CT shows LLL NSCLC ➡ and also demonstrates a clinically occult right anterolateral rib ➡ and vertebral body metastases, which upgrades staging.
(Right) Coronal fused PET/CT shows NSCLC invading chest wall. Note prominent peripheral FDG avid viable tumor ➡, central absence of metabolism ➡ representing necrosis, and mildly FDG avid left shoulder arthritic effusion ➡.

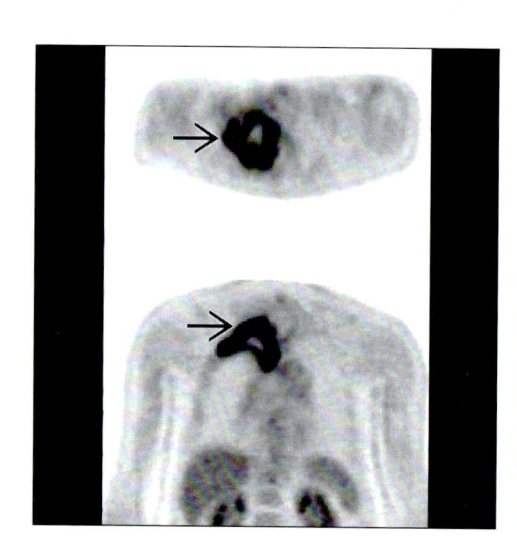

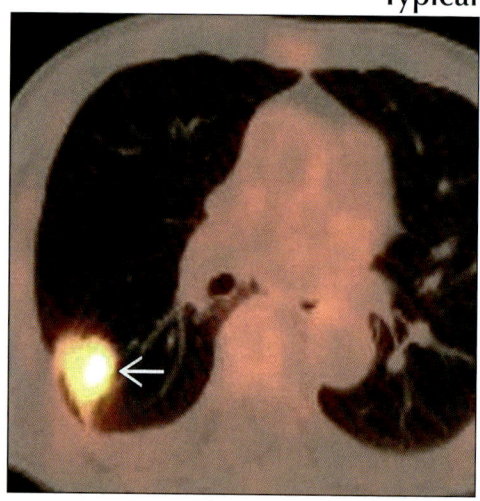

(Left) FDG PET shows hypermetabolic mass in right superior sulcus ➡. Patient presented with Horner syndrome and pain due to biopsy proven Pancoast tumor. (Right) Axial fused PET/CT shows prominently hypermetabolism in RLL mass ➡, biopsy-proven NSCLC.

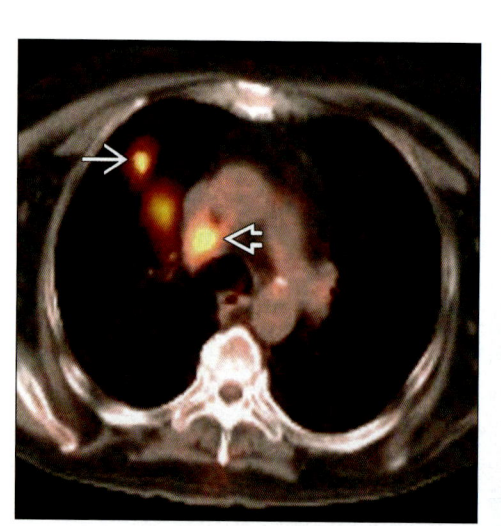

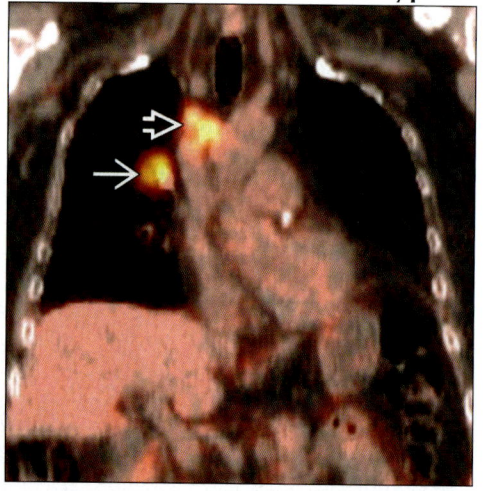

(Left) Axial fused FDG PET/CT shows prominently FDG avid RUL NSCLC ➡ with ipsilateral mediastinal hypermetabolic lymph nodes ➡ consistent with tumor involvement. Same patient as next image. (Right) Coronal fused FDG PET/CT shows prominently FDG avid ipsilateral hilar ➡ and mediastinal ➡ lymph nodes. Same patient as previous image.

NON-SMALL CELL LUNG CANCER

Typical

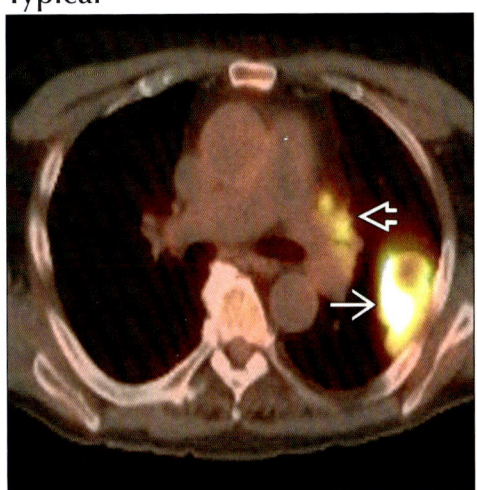

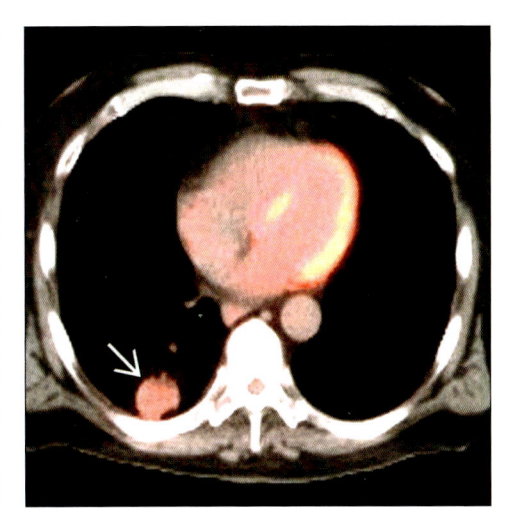

(Left) Axial fused FDG PET/CT image shows markedly hypermetabolic LLL NSCLC ⇨, as well as left hilar lymph nodal involvement ⇨. *(Right)* Axial fused FDG PET/CT shows moderately FDG avid RLL mass ⇨ pathologically shown to be a moderately well differentiated NSCLC.

Variant

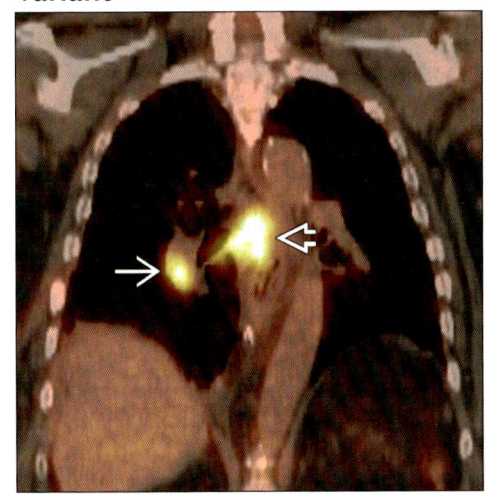

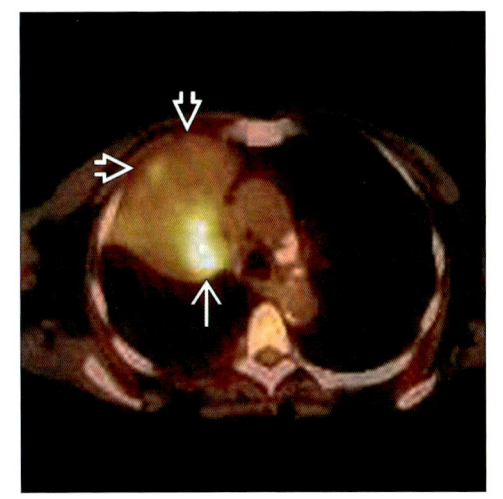

(Left) Coronal fused FDG PET/CT shows right perihilar primary NSCLC ⇨ with prominently FDG avid ipsilateral and subcarinal mediastinal involved lymph nodes ⇨. *(Right)* Axial fused FDG PET/CT demonstrates medial hypermetabolic mass ⇨, a NSCLC, producing post-obstructive pneumonia and consolidation of the right upper lobe ⇨.

Variant

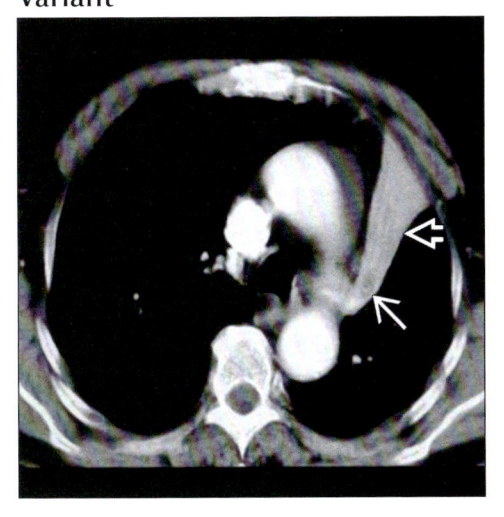

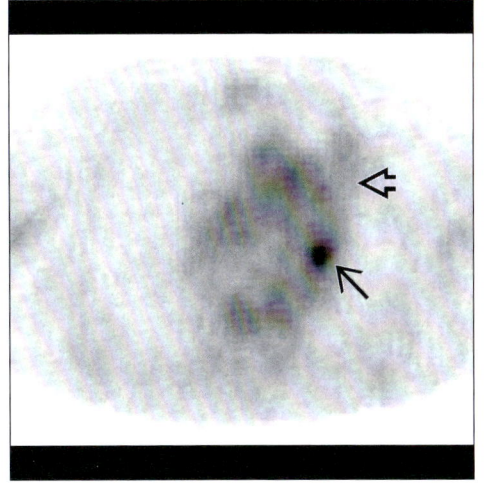

(Left) Axial CECT shows focal mass ⇨ at central apex of atelectatic lung ⇨, proved at bronchoscopy to be an endobronchial SCCA. Same patient as next image. *(Right)* Axial FDG PET demonstrated focal hypermetabolism at site of small endobronchial mass ⇨ producing post-obstructive collapse of LUL ⇨, faint in FDG activity. Same patient as previous image.

METASTASES, LUNGS & MEDIASTINUM

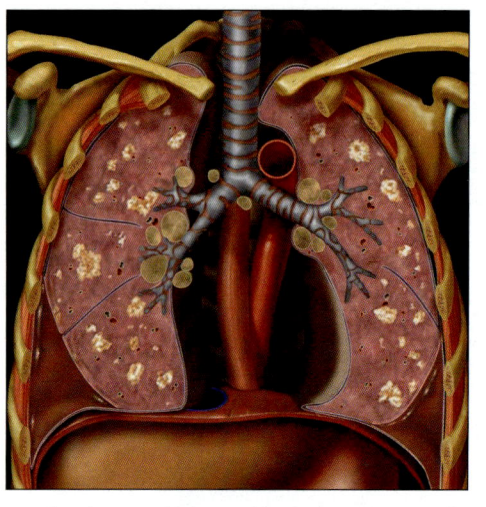

Graphic shows multiple, variably sized metastases to the lung with hilar and mediastinal lymphadenopathy.

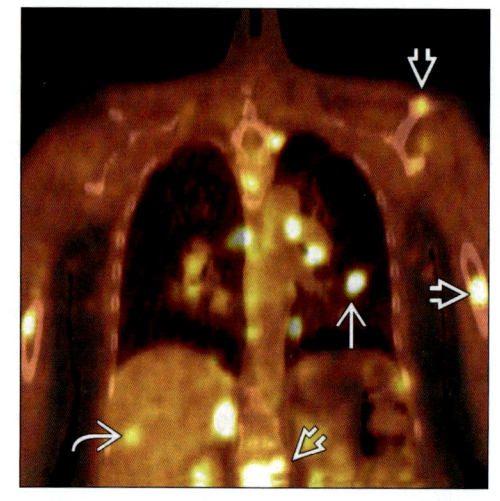

Coronal fused FDG PET/CT demonstrates hypermetabolism in numerous pulmonary ➡, mediastinal, hilar, skeletal ➡, and liver ➡ metastases in a patient with breast cancer.

TERMINOLOGY

Definitions
- Spread of malignancy from the primary site to the lungs and/or mediastinum

IMAGING FINDINGS

General Features
- Best diagnostic clue: Multiple, variable sized, pulmonary parenchymal nodules, enlarged mediastinal lymph nodes, masses
- Location
  o Lymphangitic metastases: Focal, commonly spare an entire lobe
  o Hematogenous metastases: Bases and periphery (regions of greater blood flow) of lungs

Nuclear Medicine Findings
- PET
  o Many metastatic lesions to the lungs are FDG avid
  o FDG PET may be more accurate than pathology in predicting survival or recurrence
  - Staging with FDG PET offers prognostic information: SUV (> 5) suggests prominent metabolism, aggressive neoplasm and a poor prognosis
  o False positive FDG PET: Primary lung malignancy, and virtually any infectious, active inflammatory, or active granulomatous (infectious or non-infectious) process
  o False negative FDG PET: Low grade lung cancers (BAC, carcinoid), tumors < 15 mm, "stunned" tumor during/immediately following therapy, high glucose levels (competition with FDG uptake)
  o False negative FDG PET: Mets from variably FDG avid extrathoracic malignancies (e.g., renal cell carcinoma, hepatoma, testicular carcinoma, mucinous adenocarcinomas)
  o Metastatic disease of unknown primary: FDG PET identifies primary site in ~ 45% of cases
  o Misregistration common between lung nodules and site of PET uptake: Breathing on PET, inspiratory breath hold on CT
- Bone Scan
  o May see uptake in large pulmonary mets on bone scan

DDx: Mimics of Metastases to Lungs and Mediastinum

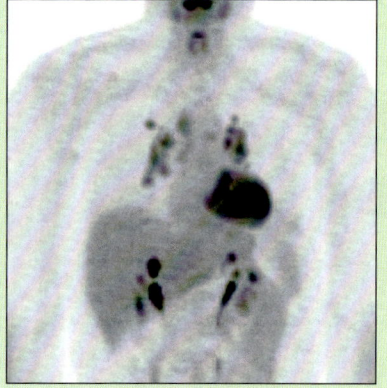

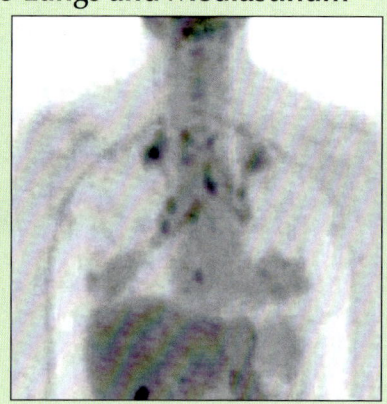

Sarcoidosis | *Reactivated TB* | *Normal Thymus*

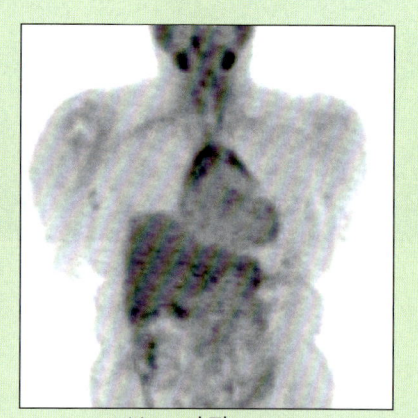

METASTASES, LUNGS & MEDIASTINUM

Key Facts

Imaging Findings
- Lower lobe predominance: Gravity, higher blood flow
- Solitary metastasis: Renal, colon, breast, sarcoma, melanoma
- Miliary pattern: Thyroid, melanoma, renal, ovarian, pancreatic
- Ossifying/calcifying tumors: Osteogenic sarcoma, chondrosarcoma, thyroid (may be confused with benign granulomas)
- May see uptake in large pulmonary mets on bone scan
- More intense uptake on bone scan in osteosarcoma and other calcifying/ossifying tumors
- Staging with FDG PET offers prognostic information: SUV (> 5) suggests prominent metabolism, aggressive neoplasm and a poor prognosis
- Ga-67 avid tumors: Melanoma, lymphoma, hepatocellular carcinoma, testicular cancers, others variable
- Limitation of Ga-67 scan: Many tumors are not Ga-67 avid (e.g., most adenocarcinomas, Kaposi sarcoma)
- PET/CT superior to CT or PET alone: Information about primary malignancy; sensitive in detecting additional sites

Top Differential Diagnoses
- Multiple Benign Pulmonary Nodules
- Endobronchial Carcinoma
- Interstitial Lung Disease and Lymphangitis
- Chronic Consolidation vs. Post-Obstructive Pneumonitis
- Pulmonary Embolus

- More intense uptake on bone scan in osteosarcoma and other calcifying/ossifying tumors
- Ga-67 Scintigraphy
  - Ga-67 avid tumors: Melanoma, lymphoma, hepatocellular carcinoma, testicular cancers, others variable
  - Limitation of Ga-67 scan: Many tumors are not Ga-67 avid (e.g., most adenocarcinomas, Kaposi sarcoma)
  - Practical size limit for detection on Ga-67: ≥ 2 cm
- Other nuclear medicine modalities that may identify metastatic lesions
  - Tl-201, Tc-99m sestamibi or tetrofosmin: Breast cancer, lymphoma, sarcoma, thyroid
  - In-111 octreotide and I-123, I-131 MIBG: Neuroendocrine tumors
  - I123 and 1 scans: Well-differentiated thyroid cancer; reports of uptake in many other tumors
  - Labeled monoclonal antibodies: Occasional identification of metastatic sites (prostate, ovarian, colorectal)

Radiographic Findings
- Radiography
  - Vascular pattern: Hematogenous spread
    - Sharply-defined, variable-sized round pulmonary nodules; ill-defined margins with hemorrhagic metastases (choriocarcinoma, renal, melanoma)
    - Lower lobe predominance: Gravity, higher blood flow
    - Peripheral predominance: 80% within 2 cm of pleura
    - Solitary metastasis: Renal, colon, breast, sarcoma, melanoma
    - Cavitation: Squamous or sarcoma cell types
    - Miliary pattern: Thyroid, melanoma, renal, ovarian, pancreatic
    - Ossifying/calcifying tumors: Osteogenic sarcoma, chondrosarcoma, thyroid (may be confused with benign granulomas)
    - Occasionally associated with spontaneous pneumothorax, esp. sarcoma cell type
  - Lymphangitic pattern: Lymphangitic spread
    - Asymmetric nodular interstitial thickening, often spares a lobe; associated small pleural effusion, hilar or mediastinal lymph node enlargement
  - Endobronchial pattern: Bronchogenic seeding within the airways or hematogenous dissemination to airway wall
    - Atelectasis of lobe or lung or segment: Post-obstructive pneumonitis may be segmental, lobar, or entire lung
    - Seen with bronchioloalveolar cell carcinoma (BAC), basal cell carcinoma of head and neck, breast, renal, sarcoma
  - Pleural pattern: Lymphangitic or hematogenous spread
    - Discrete pleural nodule or mass; pleural effusion may be massive, free-flowing or loculated
  - Consolidative pattern: Hematogenous spread
    - Lipidic growth similar to BAC; peripheral consolidation; air-bronchograms; mimics pneumonia
    - Peripheral consolidation with air-bronchograms; mimics pneumonia
  - Pulmonary embolus pattern: Hematogenous spread
    - Beaded enlarged vessels: Mass conforms to vascular shape, pulmonary infarcts
  - Mediastinal disease: Hematogenous or lymphangitic spread, direct invasion
    - Common with genitourinary, head and neck, melanoma, breast cancers

CT Findings
- CECT
  - Mirrors CXR findings: Metastases predominate in the outer 1/3 of the mid and lower lung zones
  - Beaded dilated vessels and lymphatics for endovascular extension and lymphangitis respectively
- HRCT
  - Hematogenous nodules may have visible feeding artery ("cherry stem")

METASTASES, LUNGS & MEDIASTINUM

- Lymphangitic mets: Centrilobular peribronchial thickening, beaded peripheral interlobular septa (clusters of tumor cell proliferation)
- Hemorrhagic metastasis halo sign (solid central nodule surrounded by ground-glass opacity)

Imaging Recommendations
- Best imaging tool
  - CT characterizes the pattern and extent of disease; readily available, widespread expertise
  - PET/CT superior to CT or PET alone: Information about primary malignancy; sensitive in detecting additional sites

DIFFERENTIAL DIAGNOSIS

Multiple Benign Pulmonary Nodules
- Arteriovenous malformations (AVM): Minimal or no FDG activity
- Granulomas: Benign patterns of calcification, associated with calcified hilar/mediastinal nodal, liver and spleen granulomas
  - Ossifying primary tumor metastases may be confused for granulomas
  - Completely calcified granulomas are not FDG avid; ossifying mets are FDG avid
- Wegener granulomatosis: Cavitating nodules (FDG avid), association with subglottic stenosis
- Sarcoidosis: Typically, nodules predominantly upper lobe; hilar/mediastinal nodes balanced, symmetrical

Endobronchial Carcinoma
- Smoking history, more common than endobronchial metastasis, FDG avid, depending on size

Interstitial Lung Disease and Lymphangitis
- Active interstitial lung disease is typically Ga-67 and FDG avid
- Nodules, septal thickening are frequent mimics of hematogenous, lymphangitic metastases

Chronic Consolidation vs. Post-Obstructive Pneumonitis
- Bronchoalveolar cell carcinoma: < FDG uptake than pneumonitis or post-obstructive pneumonia
- Chronic organizing pneumonia (COP, BOOP): FDG avid

Pulmonary Embolus
- Both acute thrombus and infarct can show FDG uptake
- Transient, acute symptoms, will not distend the vessel, single or multiple, central or peripheral
- Pulmonary artery sarcoma: Central location in main pulmonary artery, solitary lesion
- Tumor thrombus: FDG avid

PATHOLOGY

General Features
- Etiology
  - Metastatic models
    - Mechanical model: Metastases filtered out by draining organ, often lung
    - Environmental model: Metastases flourish in favorable medium
- Epidemiology
  - Vascular pattern: Lung, breast, GI carcinomas, sarcomas
  - Lymphangitic pattern: Adenocarcinomas
  - Pleural pattern: Adenocarcinoma, esp. lung, breast
  - Consolidative pattern: GI carcinoma, lymphoma
  - PE pattern: Hepatoma, breast, renal cell, choriocarcinoma, angiosarcoma
  - Bronchogenic pattern: BAC, basal cell, head and neck carcinoma
  - Mediastinal spread: Nasopharyngeal, GU, breast, melanoma
- Associated abnormalities: Lytic or sclerotic skeletal metastases are common

Gross Pathologic & Surgical Features
- Lipidic growth: No architectural distortion, tumor grows on lung scaffolding (BAC)
- Hilic growth: Architectural distortion, tumor expands and displaces lung (mets)

Microscopic Features
- Important in aiding diagnosis of the primary tumor

Staging, Grading or Classification Criteria
- Regarded as stage IV M1 for most tumor staging

CLINICAL ISSUES

Presentation
- Most common signs/symptoms: Related to disease load, location, invasion compression

Natural History & Prognosis
- Generally poor prognosis
- Germ cell metastases may evolve into benign teratomas (may grow)

Treatment
- Generally palliative radiation or chemotherapy
- Surgical resection: Osteosarcoma, solitary, slow growing mets
- Radiofrequency ablation, catheter delivered chemoembolization

DIAGNOSTIC CHECKLIST

Consider
- Mets if radiographic chest abnormality, cancer history

SELECTED REFERENCES
1. Seo JB et al: Atypical pulmonary metastases: spectrum of radiologic findings. Radiographics. 21:403-17, 2001

METASTASES, LUNGS & MEDIASTINUM

IMAGE GALLERY

Typical

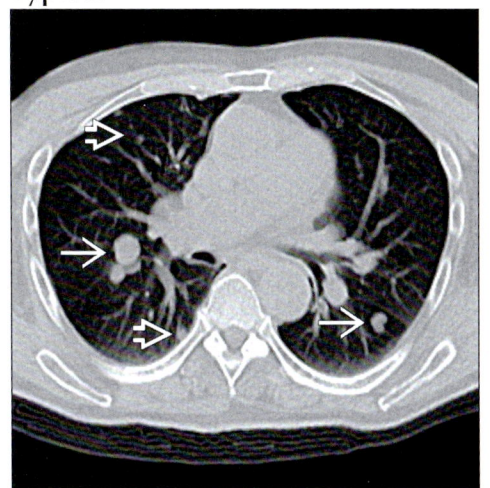

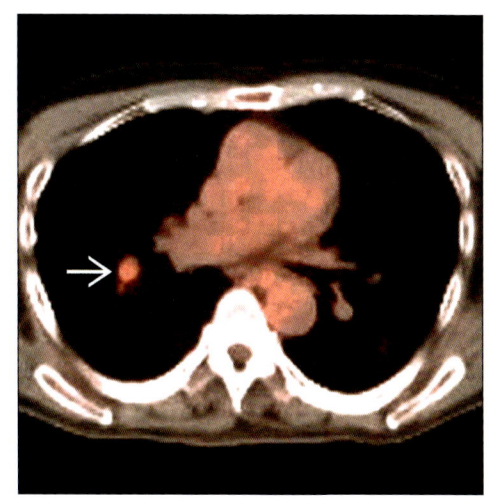

(Left) Axial NECT shows numerous melanoma metastases to the lungs ➡. Smaller lesions ➡ are below the limits of PET detectability. Same patient as next image. *(Right)* Axial CT/PET shows melanoma metastases to the lungs ➡. Smaller lesions seen on CT are beneath the limits of PET detectability. Same patient as previous image.

Variant

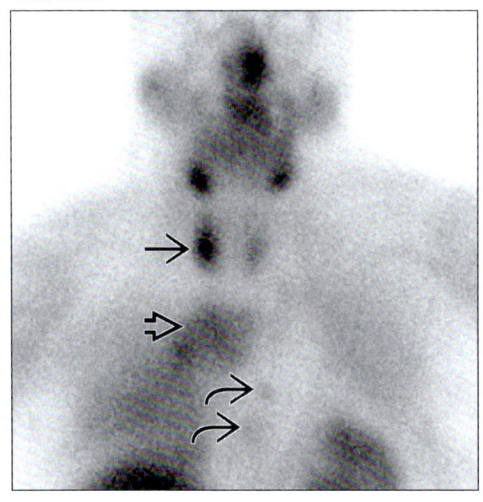

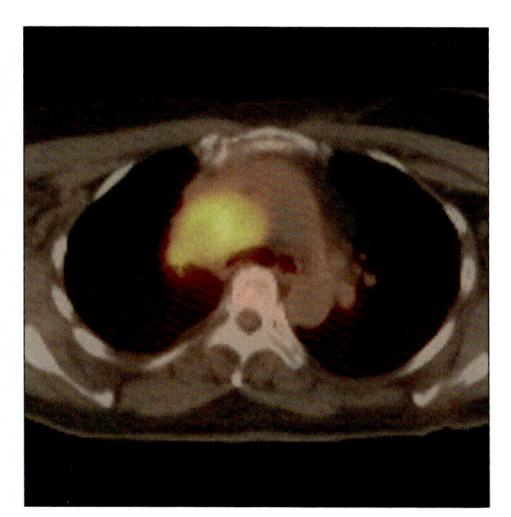

(Left) Anterior Tc-99m sestamibi scan performed for parathyroid adenoma ➡ demonstrates uptake in metastatic mediastinal mass ➡ and nodes ➡ due to breast cancer. Same patient as next image. *(Right)* Axial fused FDG PET/CT confirms hypermetabolic mediastinal mass (due to breast cancer) metastasis, also positive on Tc-99m sestamibi scan. Same patient as previous image.

Variant

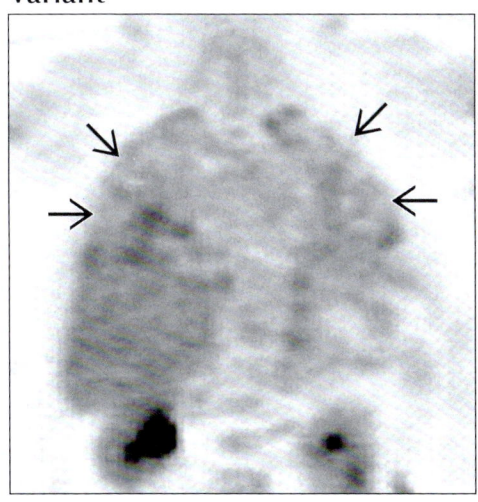

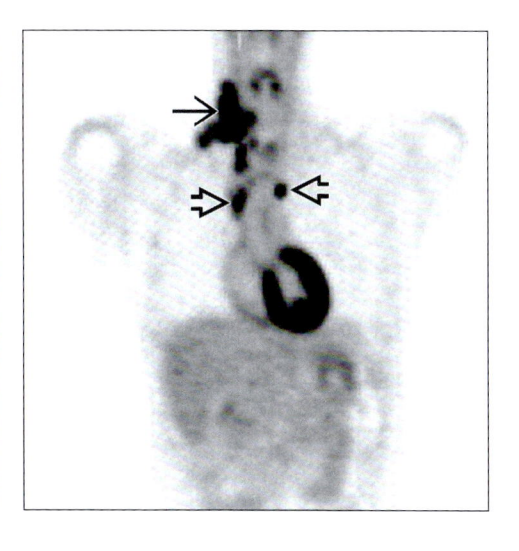

(Left) Coronal FDG PET of chest shows diffuse bilateral patchy pulmonary uptake ➡ in patient with diffuse lymphangitic metastases. Diffuse lung uptake in cancer patients is metastases in ~ 50%. *(Right)* Anterior MIP FDG PET in a patient with a history of ovarian cancer, a rising serum CA-125, and a negative abdomen CT. Hypermetabolic metastases are shown in the mediastinum ➡ and right neck ➡.

PLEURAL DISEASE, MALIGNANT & INFLAMMATORY

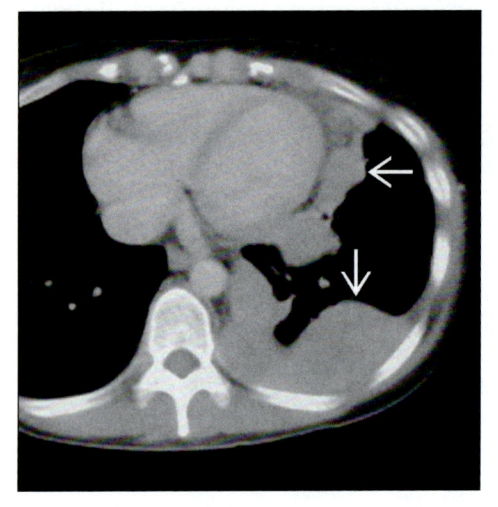

Axial CECT shows malignant thymoma metastatic to left pleura. CECT shows multiple enhancing left pleural lesions ➔. Same patient as next image.

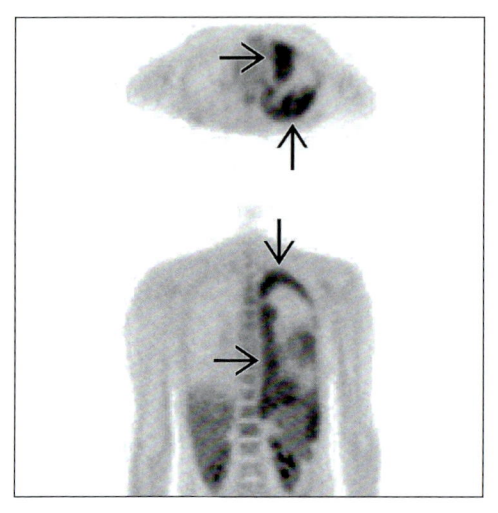

Same patient as previous image. Axial and coronal FDG PET shows hypermetabolic malignant thymoma metastases to left pleura ➔.

TERMINOLOGY

Definitions
- Accumulation of fluid/abnormal tissue in pleural space

IMAGING FINDINGS

General Features
- Morphology: Fluid: Free flowing or loculated, transudate or exudate, fibrinous, hemorrhagic or chylous

Nuclear Medicine Findings
- V/Q Scan: Pulmonary embolism (PE): Consider with a pleural effusion
- PET
  - FDG-avid pleura/effusion suggests neoplasm in setting of known extrapleural malignancy
  - Nodular pleural foci of FDG uptake further supports malignancy
  - FDG-avid pleural fluid: Also with inflammatory, infectious etiologies
  - Absence of FDG uptake does not exclude malignant effusion
- Bone Scan
  - Uptake on bone scan on delayed images: Exudative effusion, leaky capillaries
  - More intense uptake in ossifying pleural metastases (e.g., osteosarcoma)
  - Often best seen on posterior images (layering of fluid)
- Ga-67 Scintigraphy
  - Positive in infected pleural effusion/empyema
  - Ga-67 uptake: Common with melanoma, lymphomatous pleural seeding
  - No Ga-67 uptake in many tumors (e.g., most adenocarcinomas)

Radiographic Findings
- Radiography
  - Decubitus images: Free flowing vs. loculated fluid
  - Air-fluid level: Bronchopleural fistula, Boerhaave syndrome, trauma, empyema

CT Findings
- Pleural fluid: Low (water) to high (soft tissue, calcium, talc), homogeneous or heterogeneous attenuation

DDx: Pleural Thickening Months Following Left Partial Pneumonectomy

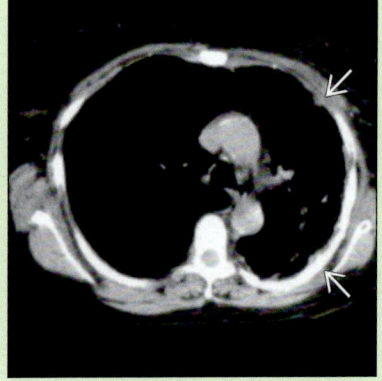

CECT Soft Tissues

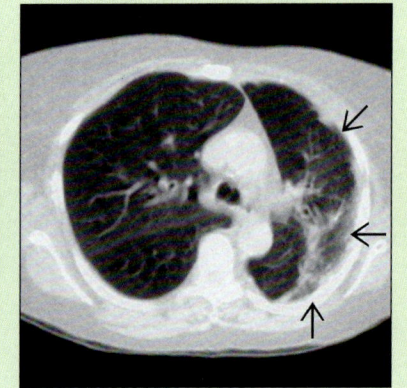

CECT Lung Windows

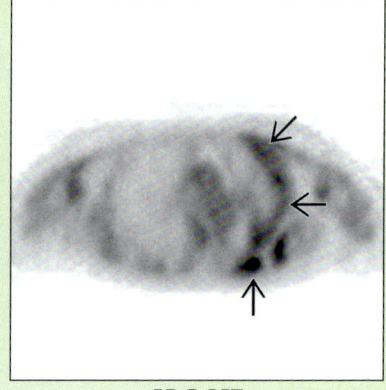

FDG PET

PLEURAL DISEASE, MALIGNANT & INFLAMMATORY

Key Facts

Terminology
- Accumulation of fluid/abnormal tissue in pleural space

Imaging Findings
- Morphology: Fluid: Free flowing or loculated, transudate or exudate, fibrinous, hemorrhagic or chylous
- Decubitus images: Free flowing vs. loculated fluid
- Air-fluid level: Bronchopleural fistula, Boerhaave syndrome, trauma, empyema
- Uptake on bone scan on delayed images: Exudative effusion, leaky capillaries
- FDG-avid pleura/effusion suggests neoplasm in setting of known extrapleural malignancy
- Nodular pleural foci of FDG uptake further supports malignancy
- FDG-avid pleural fluid: Also with inflammatory, infectious etiologies
- Absence of FDG uptake does not exclude malignant effusion
- Positive in infected pleural effusion/empyema
- Ga-67 uptake: Common with melanoma, lymphomatous pleural seeding
- No Ga-67 uptake in many tumors (e.g., most adenocarcinomas)
- Best imaging tool: CECT for anatomic information; US/CT to guide biopsy, drainage

Clinical Issues
- Thoracentesis if exudate suspected
- Important to differentiate empyema (Rx early chest tube drainage) from lung abscess (Rx antibiotics)

- CECT may not differentiate between transudate, exudate and chylous effusion
- Fluid-fluid level: Dependent layering of high attenuation contents suggests hemorrhage
- Loculated effusion: Lenticular configuration, smooth margins, homogeneous attenuation, compressive atelectasis
- High attenuation fluid, thick pleural rind, nodularity, loculation, septations
- Pleura
  - Malignant pleural disease: CT may not differentiate between benign and malignant effusion
    - Pleural thickening suggesting neoplasia: > 1 cm, nodular, mediastinal pleura, circumferentially encasing
    - Mesothelioma: Encased small lung, nodular pleural thickening extends into fissures
  - Empyema: Parietal and visceral enhancement (split pleura sign), elliptical, smooth inner margin, distinct lesion:lung interface
- Lung: Abscess, tumor, bronchopleural fistula, PE
  - Abscess: Round, thick wall, indistinct lesion:lung interface, no mass effect
- Extrapleural fat: Thickening in empyema, stranding/infiltration with infection or tumor
- Mediastinum: Lymphadenopathy, mediastinitis (fat induration), esophageal perforation
- Chest wall involvement: Extension of tumor or infection (empyema necessitans)
- Subdiaphragmatic: Associated subphrenic or liver abscess, tumor, pancreatitis

Fluoroscopic Findings
- Esophagram
  - Esophageal perforation may be demonstrated
  - Lateral displacement away from pleural effusion

Ultrasonographic Findings
- Grayscale Ultrasound
  - Can detect < 50 mL; 100% sensitive for > 100 mL
  - Exudate: Echogenic or anechoic, loculated, septate, pleural thickening
  - Look for subdiaphragmatic inflammatory cause
  - Guide percutaneous thoracentesis or drainage

Imaging Recommendations
- Best imaging tool: CECT for anatomic information; US/CT to guide biopsy, drainage
- Protocol advice: CT: IV contrast to show tumor, pleura enhancement (split pleura sign)

DIFFERENTIAL DIAGNOSIS

Fibrothorax
- Pleural thickening, no fluid, minimal FDG uptake

Solid Primary or Metastatic Tumor to the Pleura, without Effusion
- Focal uptake on FDG PET; enhancing on CECT

Post Pneumonectomy Pleural Thickening
- Mild-moderate uptake on FDG PET (persists for months)

Benign Asbestos Related Pleural Disease
- Minimal uptake on FDG PET

Pleurodesis
- Marked FDG uptake: Persists

PATHOLOGY

General Features
- General path comments: Exudate: Pleural fluid:serum protein > 0.5, pleural fluid:serum LDH > 0.6, pleural fluid LDH > 2/3 of upper limit for serum LDH
- Etiology
  - Passive effusion (transudate): Increased capillary pressure, decreased plasma oncotic pressure (Starling law)
  - Pleural inflammation (pleurisy): Increased pleural surface permeability, accumulation of pleural fluid and/or lymphatic obstruction
  - Neoplastic: Metastases (lung, breast, lymphoma, ovary, gastric), mesothelioma, lymphoma

PLEURAL DISEASE, MALIGNANT & INFLAMMATORY

- Infective: Parapneumonic effusion, bacterial, mycoplasma, viral, TB, fungal, parasitic
- Trauma: Hemothorax, aggressive resuscitation
- Chylothorax: Thoracic duct injury, traumatic or neoplastic (lymphoma)
- Following cardiac surgery or myocardial infarction (Dressler syndrome)
- PE: Exudate in 75%, suggests pulmonary infarction
- Uremic pleuritis
- Collagen vascular disease: Rheumatoid arthritis (RA), systemic lupus erythematosus (SLE)
- Drug induced: Nitrofurantoin, dantrolene, isoniazid, IL-2, bromocriptine, amiodarone, hydralazine, procainamide, phenytoin, chlorpromazine
- GI diseases: Perforated esophagus, pancreatic disease, subdiaphragmatic abscess
- Benign asbestos effusion
- Meigs syndrome: Ovarian fibroma, ascites, pleural effusion
- Yellow nail syndrome: Rhinosinusitis, pleural effusion, bronchiectasis, lymphedema, yellow nails
- Epidemiology: In US, pleural effusion affects 1.3 million/year; internationally > incidence where TB is endemic

Microscopic Features
- Parapneumonic effusion, neutrophils and bacteria; mycotic pleurisy, granulomas
- Chylothorax: High lipid content (neutral fat, fatty acids), low cholesterol, sudanophilic fat droplets; triglyceride level > 110 mg/dL
- Cholesterol effusion: Cholesterol crystals, up to 1 gm/dL; low neutral fat and fatty acids
- Immunohistochemistry and electron microscopy to differentiate mesothelioma (sarcomatoid, epithelioid) from adenocarcinoma

CLINICAL ISSUES

Presentation
- Most common signs/symptoms: Fever, dyspnea, pain
- Other signs/symptoms
  - Dullness to percussion, ↓ breath sounds, tactile fremitus, egophony, pleural rub, mediastinal shift
  - Post cardiac injury (Dressler syndrome)
    - In weeks following MI, cardiac surgery, blunt trauma, pacemaker implantation, angioplasty
    - Fever, pleuropericarditis, unilateral or bilateral small to moderate effusions, lung opacities
  - Clues to etiology: Anasarca, skin changes of chronic liver disease, distended neck veins, S3 gallop, clubbing, breast nodule, intra-abdominal mass
- Clinical Profile
  - Thoracentesis if exudate suspected
    - Fluid for chemistry, bacteriology, cytology
    - Removing < 1000 mL relieves dyspnea
    - Empyema: pH < 7.0, glucose < 40 mg/dL
    - Low glucose < 60 m/dL: TB, malignancy, RA, empyema, hemothorax, SLE
  - Pleural fluid characteristics
    - Blood-tinged: Metastases, mesothelioma, benign asbestos effusion, PE, TB, pancreatitis
    - Bloody: Trauma, anticoagulation, iatrogenic, metastases, uremia
    - Milky: Chylous
    - Brown: Amebic abscess
    - Black: Aspergillus
    - Yellow-green: RA
    - Golden, iridescent: Chronic chylothorax, TB, rheumatoid
    - Putrid odor: Anaerobic infection
  - Important to differentiate empyema (Rx early chest tube drainage) from lung abscess (Rx antibiotics)
  - CT or US-guided pleural biopsy; core sample for mesothelioma, lymphoma; FNA for metastasis
  - Open biopsy or video-assisted thoracic surgery may be needed to establish etiology

Demographics
- Gender
  - Male predominance: RA, pancreatitis, mesothelioma
  - Female predominance: 2/3 of malignant pleural effusions (breast and gynecologic malignancies), yellow nail syndrome, SLE

Natural History & Prognosis
- Malignant pleural effusion, life expectancy 3-6 months
- Benign asbestos effusion 5 to > 30 yrs after exposure

Treatment
- Depends on etiology
  - Antibiotics, thoracentesis, tube thoracostomy, pleurodesis, chemotherapy, surgery, steroids

DIAGNOSTIC CHECKLIST

Image Interpretation Pearls
- Diffusely ↑ activity in pleural effusion on FDG PET suggests infection/inflammation or malignancy
- Nodular, focal ↑ activity on FDG PET with associated pleural effusion strongly suggests malignancy
- Lack of ↑ activity on FDG PET in pleural effusion does not rule out malignant effusion

SELECTED REFERENCES

1. Shim SS et al: Integrated PET/CT and the dry pleural dissemination of peripheral adenocarcinoma of the lung: diagnostic implications. J Comput Assist Tomogr. 30(1):70-6, 2006
2. Toaff JS et al: Differentiation between malignant and benign pleural effusion in patients with extra-pleural primary malignancies: assessment with positron emission tomography-computed tomography. Invest Radiol. 40(4):204-9, 2005
3. Kuhlman JE et al: PET scan-CT correlation: what the chest radiologist needs to know. Curr Probl Diagn Radiol. 33(4):171-88, 2004
4. Melloni B et al: Assessment of 18F-fluorodeoxyglucose dual-head gamma camera in asbestos lung diseases. Eur Respir J. 24(5):814-21, 2004
5. Alavi A et al: Positron emission tomography imaging in nonmalignant thoracic disorders. Semin Nucl Med. 32(4):293-321, 2002
6. Kuhlman JE et al: Complex disease of the pleural space: radiographic and CT evaluation. Radiographics. 17(1):63-79, 1997

PLEURAL DISEASE, MALIGNANT & INFLAMMATORY

IMAGE GALLERY

Typical

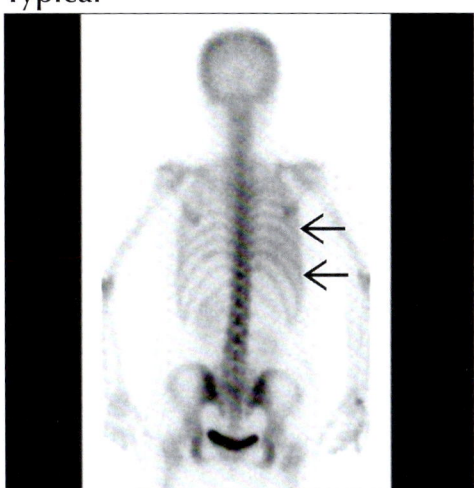

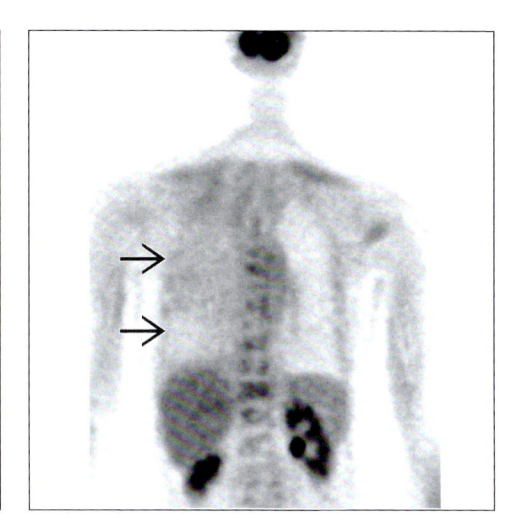

(Left) Posterior bone scan shows mild diffuse uptake ➡ indicative of right malignant pleural effusion. Uptake often better seen on posterior images due to dependent layering. *(Right)* Coronal FDG PET scan shows diffuse hypermetabolism in a malignant right pleural effusion ➡.

Typical

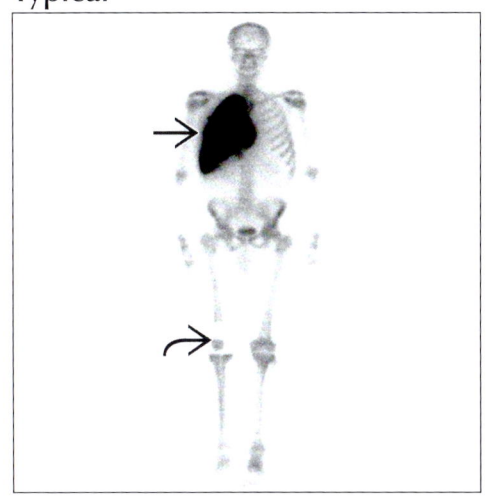

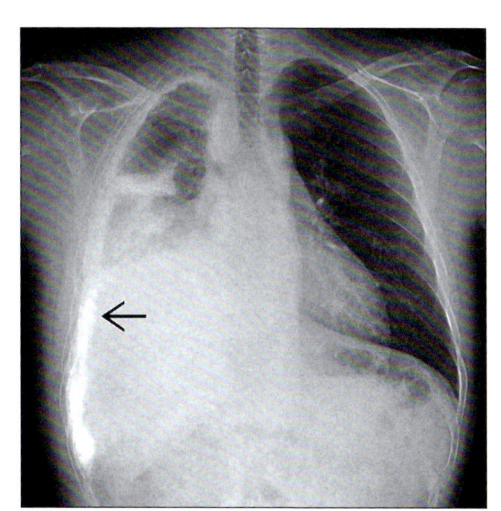

(Left) Anterior bone scan of a 23 year old male with right femur osteosarcoma. Note knee prosthesis ➡. Right hemithorax uptake ➡ due to pleural metastases. Same patient as next two images. *(Right)* Radiography shows prominently calcified right pleural lesions ➡ in metastatic osteosarcoma. Calcification conforms to pattern of uptake on bone scan.

Typical

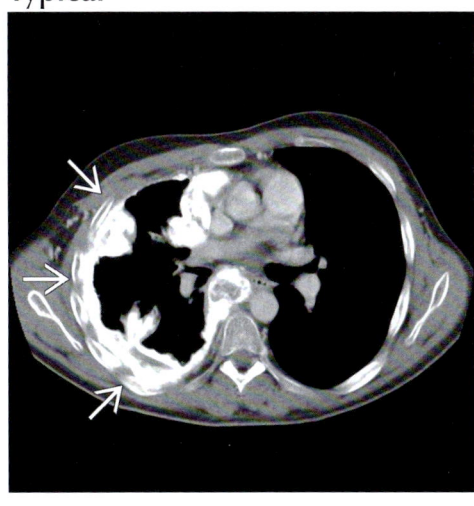

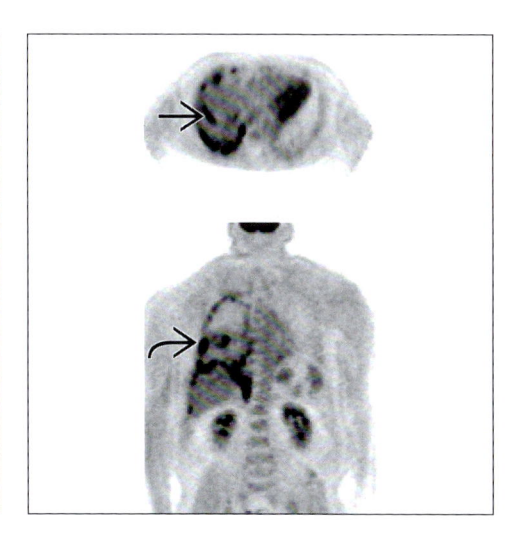

(Left) Axial CECT shows prominently calcifying metastases ➡ corresponding to sites of uptake on bone scan in patient with osteosarcoma metastatic to right pleura. *(Right)* Axial and coronal FDG PET images show FDG avid right pleural lesions due to malignant mesothelioma. Note right inferior lung encasement and extension into major ➡ and minor ➡ fissures.

THYMIC EVALUATION

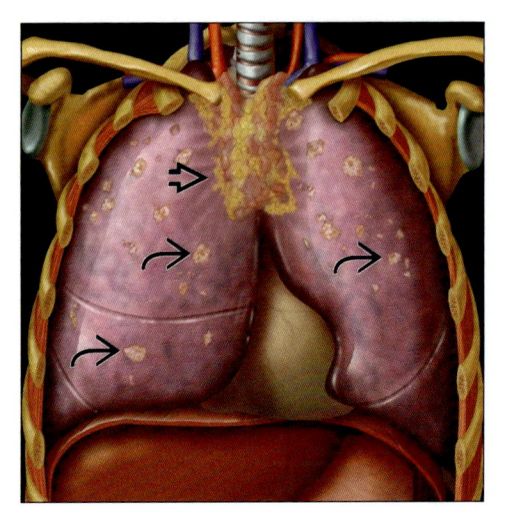

Coronal graphic shows thymic carcinoma in superior anterior mediastinum with multiple bilateral pleural metastases.

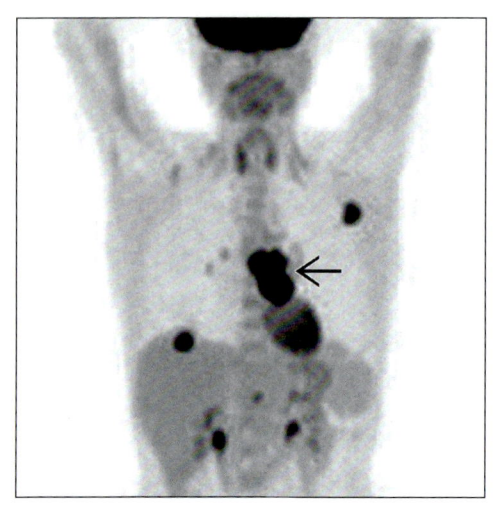

Anterior MIP FDG PET shows hypermetabolic mediastinal mass (thymic carcinoma) with metastases to liver, bone, lung and axilla.

TERMINOLOGY

Definitions
- Thymus: Bilobed ductless gland, contributes to T-cell immune response in early life

IMAGING FINDINGS

General Features
- Best diagnostic clue: CECT: Pathology suggested by convex borders, enlarged for age, focal mass, pleural nodules
- Location
  - Anterior superior mediastinum
  - Originates from the 3rd and 4th pharyngeal pouches
  - Ectopic thymic tissue may extend into neck
- Size: Age-dependent size variation; infancy 10-15 g, puberty ~ 40 g, fat-replaced involuted gland in adult
- Morphology
  - Bilobed ductless organ with cortex and medulla
  - Differentiating normal thymus from neoplasm is made, in part, on basis of morphology
    - < 5 years: Quadrilateral, straight or convex borders
    - 5-15 years: Triangular, straight or concave borders

Nuclear Medicine Findings
- PET
  - Increased FDG activity: Seen in wide range of thymic conditions, both benign and malignant
  - Normal thymic FDG activity: Children and young adults, may persist into 30s
  - Thymic hyperplasia
    - Mild FDG activity (SUV < 4) with associated soft tissue mass; seen in patients < 40 years old
    - Thymic neoplasms: FDG activity in neoplasm typically > hyperplasia, but significant overlap
  - "Thymic rebound": Seen following chemotherapy, even without thymic activity on pre-chemotherapy PET
    - Increased activity of thymic medullary epithelial cells, regeneration of lymphocytes during recovery from chemotherapy
    - "Thymic rebound" usually regressed within 3-6 months, but may persistent longer
  - Thymoma: Spectrum from benign to malignant
    - Thymomas (benign and invasive/malignant) show moderate FDG avidity

DDx: Mimics of Thymic Pathology

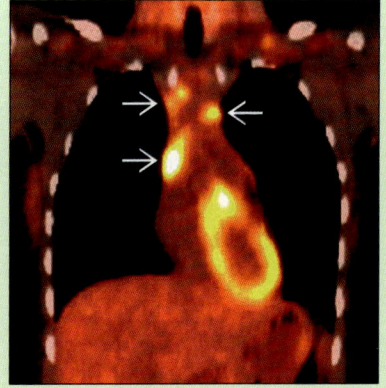

Lymphoma

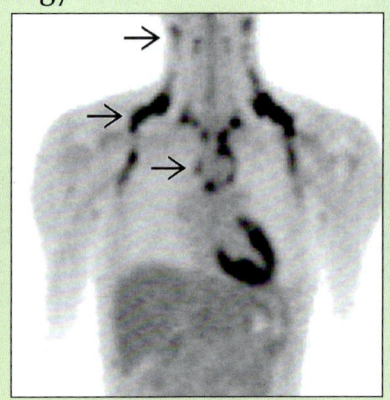

Hypermetabolic Brown Fat

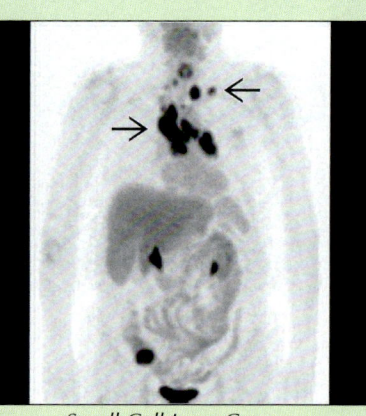

Small Cell Lung Cancer

THYMIC EVALUATION

Key Facts

Imaging Findings
- "Thymic rebound": Seen following chemotherapy, even without thymic activity on pre-chemotherapy PET
- Thymomas (benign and invasive/malignant) show moderate FDG avidity
- Cannot distinguish benign from malignant thymoma based on FDG activity
- Thymic rebound following chemotherapy is commonly Ga-67 avid - may persist for ≥ 1 year
- I-131 total body scans for thyroid cancer: Thymic uptake is normal finding, may mimic mediastinal metastases
- In-111 octreotide scan: Define receptor status and extent of disease in malignant thymoma
- CECT: Convex borders, enlarged for age, focal mass, pleural nodules suggest pathology

Top Differential Diagnoses
- Hypermetabolic Brown Fat
- Primary Thymic Neoplasms
- Metastases
- Substernal Thyroid
- Germ Cell Tumors
- Lymphoma

Diagnostic Checklist
- Hypermetabolic brown adipose tissue can occur in mediastinum
- Hyperplasia and thymic rebound can occur as late as 30s and 40s

---

- Cannot distinguish benign from malignant thymoma based on FDG activity
○ Myasthenia gravis (MG): 30-40% of thymoma patients
  - Exacerbations may occur in the premenstrual period and during, or shortly, after pregnancy
  - Lambert-Eaton myasthenic syndrome (LEMS): Thymus is usually normal on CT, PET imaging
○ Graves disease: Symmetric thymic hyperplasia, skeletal muscle ↑ FDG avidity (thymus not always FDG avid)
  - Thymic thyrotropin receptor acts as an autoantigen possibly involved in the development of Graves disease
○ Systemic lupus erythematosus (SLE)
  - ↑ FDG activity in thymus in active SLE; ↑ FDG uptake in lymph nodes in active and inactive SLE
○ Rosai-Dorfman disease
  - Massive, painless, bilateral cervical lymph node pathology in 90%; extranodal disease in 43%
  - Moderate to prominent ↑ thymic FDG uptake
○ Lymphomatous infiltration: Common site for many types of lymphoma
- Ga-67 Scintigraphy
  ○ Ga-67 avid tumors include lymphoma, thymic CA, melanoma, HCC, sarcoma, testicular
  ○ Thymic rebound following chemotherapy is commonly Ga-67 avid - may persist for ≥ 1 year
- I-131 scintigraphy
  ○ I-131 total body scans for thyroid cancer: Thymic uptake is normal finding, may mimic mediastinal metastases
- In-111 octreotide (pentetreotide): Somatostatin analogue
  ○ In-111 octreotide uptake in carcinoid, including (rare) thymic carcinoid, now known as primary neuroendocrine tumor of the thymus
  ○ In-111 octreotide scan: Define receptor status and extent of disease in malignant thymoma

Imaging Recommendations
- Best imaging tool
  ○ CECT: Initial evaluation, post therapy follow-up
  ○ FDG PET/CT: Pre and post therapy evaluation
- Correlative imaging features
  ○ CECT: Convex borders, enlarged for age, focal mass, pleural nodules suggest pathology

DIFFERENTIAL DIAGNOSIS

Hypermetabolic Brown Fat
- FDG uptake in (brown) adipose tissue: Can occur in superior mediastinum

Thymic Cysts
- Thymic cysts are common (3rd branchial pouch)
- Not all simple appearing thymic cysts are benign; cysts may form near a thymic neoplasm

Thymolipoma
- May be large; not FDG-avid

Primary Thymic Neoplasms
- Thymic carcinoma: Aggressive cytology (in contrast with malignant thymoma), rare, propensity for pleural and distant metastases, usually ↑↑ FDG avidity (SUV > 5)
  ○ Thymoma (invasive or noninvasive): All cytologically similar and benign, mild-moderate FDG activity (SUV < 5)
- Thymic carcinoid: Often aggressive, with extrathoracic metastases in 30-40% at diagnosis
  ○ Consider in patient with Cushing syndrome (ectopic ACTH) and a thymic tumor (occurs in 30% of patients with thymic carcinoid)
  ○ Associations: Paraneoplastic syndromes, multiple endocrine neoplasia (MEN I or II)

Metastases
- Lymph node metastases typically have known primary
- Metastasis from an occult 1° malignancy unlikely to manifest as solitary large thymic tumor

Substernal Thyroid
- Marked enhancement, calcification, cyst formation, low FDG activity

THYMIC EVALUATION

Germ Cell Tumors
- Thymus is a classic site of extragonadal primary germ cell tumor: Commonly seminoma, teratoma
- 75% are teratomas: Calcification, cyst formation, or fat attenuation
- Seminoma and rare malignant nonseminomatous germ cell tumors: Rare in women
- Alpha fetoprotein (αFP) and β-HCG may aid DX
- FDG activity highly variable, often low

Lymphoma
- Most common anterior mediastinal malignancy
- Typically marked FDG activity (Mantle cell may be lower)

PATHOLOGY

General Features
- Epidemiology: Most common anterior mediastinal tumor: 20-25% of all mediastinal tumors, 50% of anterior mediastinal tumors
- Associated abnormalities
  - 30-40% thymomas: MG symptoms
  - Other thymoma associations: Red cell aplasia, dermatomyositis, systemic lupus erythematous, Cushing syndrome, and the syndrome of inappropriate antidiuretic hormone secretion

Gross Pathologic & Surgical Features
- Large in neonates, larger during puberty, involutes after puberty, replaced by fat > 30 years

Microscopic Features
- No clear histologic distinction between benign and malignant thymomas: Originate in epithelial cells of thymus
- Thymic tissue: Cortex (lymphocytes) and medulla (lymphocytopenic), basic structural unit a stellate epithelial cell; keratinizing squamous pearls, or Hassall corpuscles

CLINICAL ISSUES

Presentation
- Most common signs/symptoms: Incidental mass ± ↑ FDG activity
- Other signs/symptoms
  - For lung cancer: Clinical symptoms of LEMS precede detection of the underlying disease
  - Consider thymic carcinoid in patient with Cushing syndrome (ectopic ACTH) and a thymic tumor (occurs in 30% of patients with thymic carcinoid)

Demographics
- Age
  - Thymoma: 4th-5th decade, M = F
  - Thymic carcinoma: 5th, 6th decade
  - Rebound thymic hyperplasia: Post chemotherapy, particularly in younger patients (generally < 40 years)
  - MG: All ages, sometimes in association with thymic CA, thyrotoxicosis, RA or SLE

Treatment
- No therapy: Thymic rebound
- Surgery: Thymic neoplasm, MG
- Chemotherapy ± radiation therapy: Thymic neoplasm

DIAGNOSTIC CHECKLIST

Consider
- Hypermetabolic brown adipose tissue can occur in mediastinum
- Cannot distinguish benign from malignant thymoma by histology or magnitude of FDG activity
- Hyperplasia and thymic rebound can occur as late as 30s and 40s

SELECTED REFERENCES

1. Godart V et al: Intense 18-fluorodeoxyglucose uptake by the thymus on PET scan does not necessarily herald recurrence of thyroid carcinoma. J Endocrinol Invest. 28(11):1024-8, 2005
2. Gorospe L et al: Whole-body PET/CT: spectrum of physiological variants, artifacts and interpretative pitfalls in cancer patients. Nucl Med Commun. 26(8):671-87, 2005
3. Kaste SC et al: 18F-FDG-avid sites mimicking active disease in pediatric Hodgkin's. Pediatr Radiol. 35(2):141-54, 2005
4. Markou A et al: [18F]fluoro-2-deoxy-D-glucose ([18F]FDG) positron emission tomography imaging of thymic carcinoid tumor presenting with recurrent Cushing's syndrome. Eur J Endocrinol. 152(4):521-5, 2005
5. Chen YK et al: Elevated 18F-FDG uptake in skeletal muscles and thymus: a clue for the diagnosis of Graves' disease. Nucl Med Commun. 25(2):115-21, 2004
6. Ferdinand B et al: Spectrum of thymic uptake at 18F-FDG PET. Radiographics. 24(6):1611-6, 2004
7. Lim R et al: FDG PET of Rosai-Dorfman disease of the thymus. AJR Am J Roentgenol. 182(2):514, 2004
8. Nowak M et al: A pilot study of the use of 2-[18F]-fluoro-2-deoxy-D-glucose-positron emission tomography to assess the distribution of activated lymphocytes in patients with systemic lupus erythematosus. Arthritis Rheum. 50(4):1233-8, 2004
9. Yeung HW et al: Patterns of (18)F-FDG uptake in adipose tissue and muscle: a potential source of false-positives for PET. J Nucl Med. 44(11):1789-96, 2003
10. Alavi A et al: Positron emission tomography imaging in nonmalignant thoracic disorders. Semin Nucl Med. 32(4):293-321, 2002
11. Santana L et al: Best cases from the AFIP: thymoma. Radiographics. 22 Spec No:S95-S102, 2002
12. Brink I et al: Increased metabolic activity in the thymus gland studied with 18F-FDG PET: age dependency and frequency after chemotherapy. J Nucl Med. 42(4):591-5, 2001
13. Nakahara T et al: FDG uptake in the morphologically normal thymus: comparison of FDG positron emission tomography and CT. Br J Radiol. 74(885):821-4, 2001
14. Shreve PD et al: Pitfalls in oncologic diagnosis with FDG PET imaging: physiologic and benign variants. Radiographics. 19(1):61-77; quiz 150-1, 1999
15. Kubota K et al: PET imaging of primary mediastinal tumours. Br J Cancer. 73(7):882-6, 1996

THYMIC EVALUATION

IMAGE GALLERY

Typical

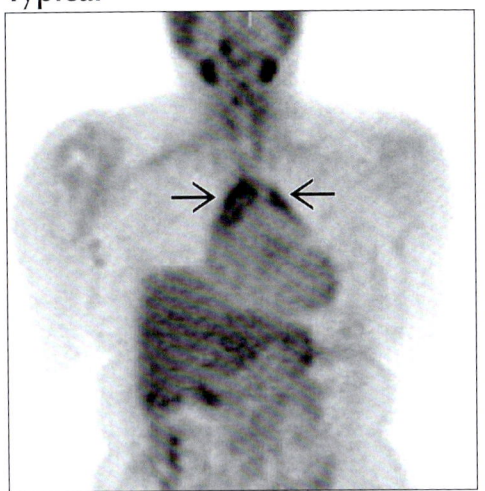

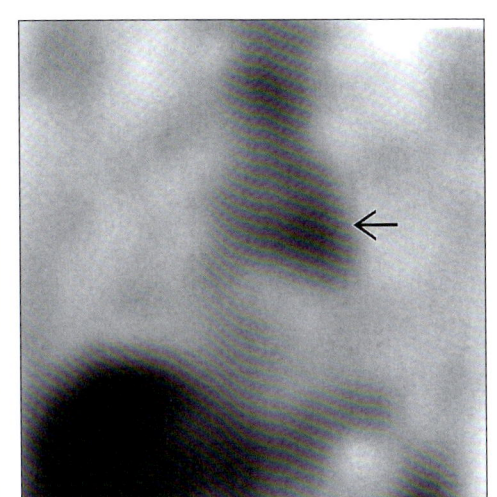

(Left) Coronal FDG PET following chemotherapy shows typical thymic rebound ➔: Moderate uptake in a typical chevron-shaped configuration. *(Right)* Coronal Ga-67 SPECT image of chest post chemotherapy for lymphoma shows typical thymic rebound ➔, with sail-like configuration and moderate Ga-67 avidity.

Variant

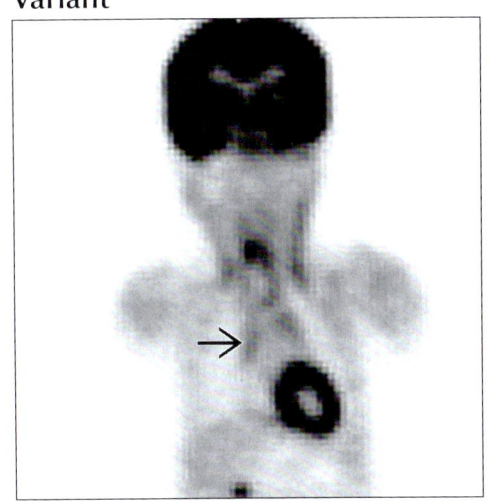

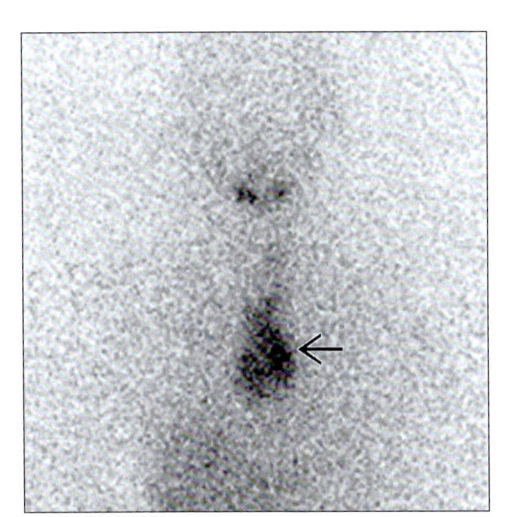

(Left) Coronal FDG PET in pediatric patient shows typical superior mediastinal uptake within normal thymus ➔. *(Right)* Anterior planar I-131 scan in 15 year old patient undergoing surveillance for previously treated thyroid cancer shows I-131 activity ➔ in normal thymic tissue.

Typical

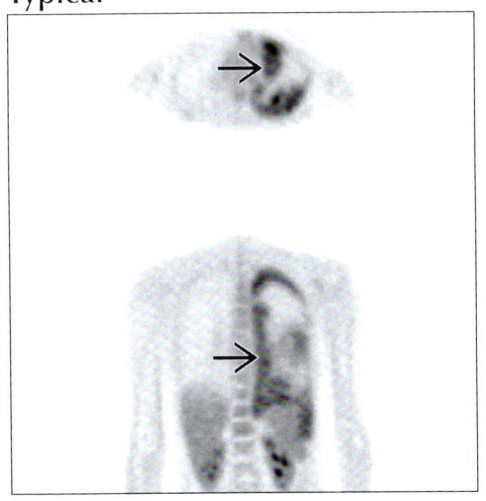

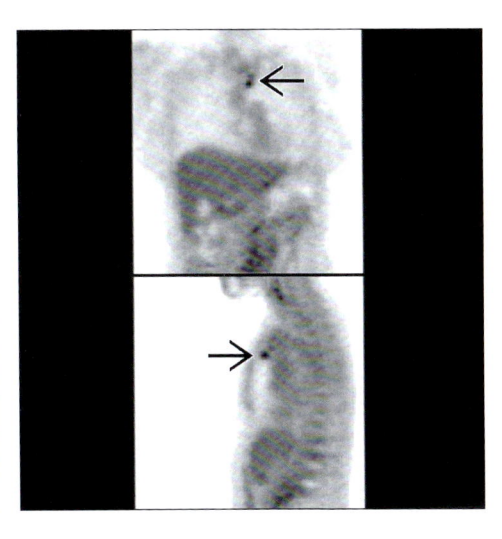

(Left) Axial (top) and coronal (bottom) PET shows increased activity in pleural metastases ➔ in patient with thymic carcinoma. *(Right)* Coronal (top) and sagittal (bottom) PET in middle-aged woman with myasthenia gravis shows activity in two small anterior mediastinal thymomas ➔.

PERICARDIAL DISEASE, MALIGNANT & INFLAMMATORY

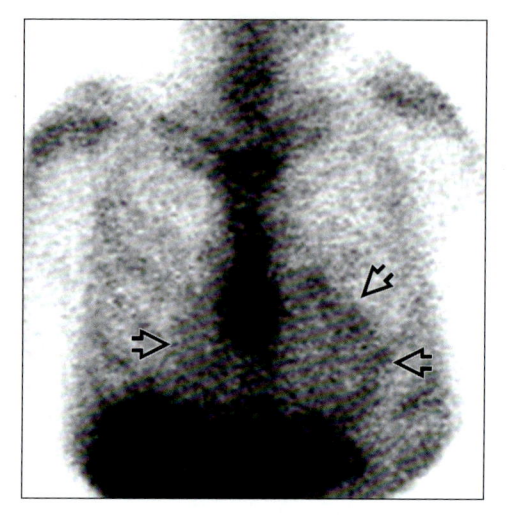

Anterior Ga-67 scintigraphy shows uptake around the heart in a patient with viral pericarditis. Same patient as next image.

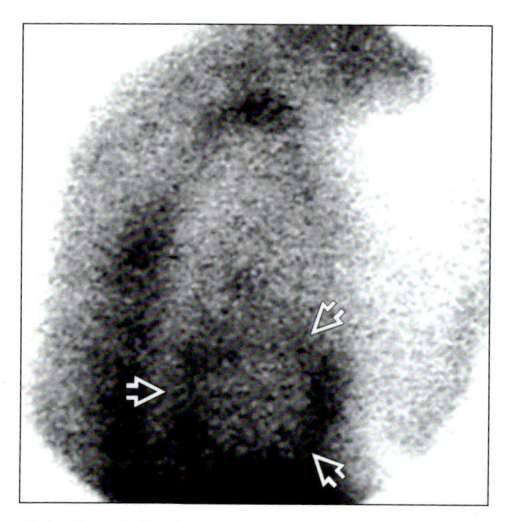

Right lateral Ga-67 scintigraphy in same patient as previous image shows uptake around heart due to viral pericarditis.

TERMINOLOGY

Definitions
- Increased volume and/or abnormal character of fluid in pericardial space

IMAGING FINDINGS

General Features
- Best diagnostic clue
  - Enlarging, globular cardiac silhouette on CXR
  - Increased dimensions of pericardial space: Small effusion < 1 cm, large effusion > 1 cm in diameter
- Size
  - Pericardial space normally contains 15-50 cc of fluid
    - Originates from visceral pericardium as an ultrafiltrate of plasma
  - Total protein levels are low; but, concentration of albumin is increased (low molecular weight)
- Morphology
  - Elevated volume of pericardial fluid
  - Pericardium may be thickened, enhance, demonstrate calcification, nodules/masses, fibrinous strands

Nuclear Medicine Findings
- PET
  - FDG uptake in effusion or pericardium suggests neoplasm in patient with known extrapericardial malignancy
  - Absence of FDG uptake does not exclude malignant pericardial effusion
  - Hypermetabolic pericardial fluid on FDG PET often seen with inflammation/infection
- Bone Scan
  - Bone scan: Increased uptake in fluid on delayed images in exudative effusions
  - More intense uptake in malignant pericardial involvement due to osteosarcoma and calcifying tumors (rare)
- Ga-67 Scintigraphy
  - Ga-67: Pericardium better evaluated on anterior images
  - Ga-67 uptake: Infected pericardial effusion/empyema, viral pericarditis

DDx: Benign Pericardial Effusion

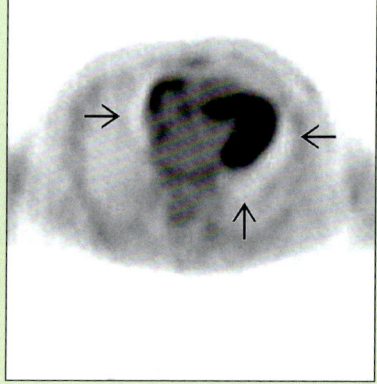

Axial FDG PET

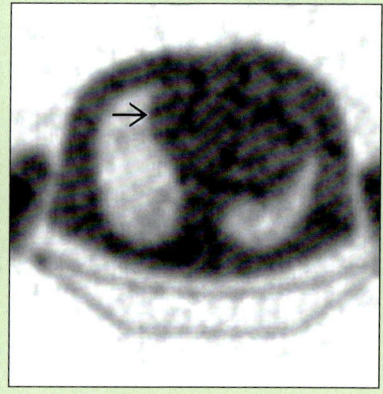

Transmission PET

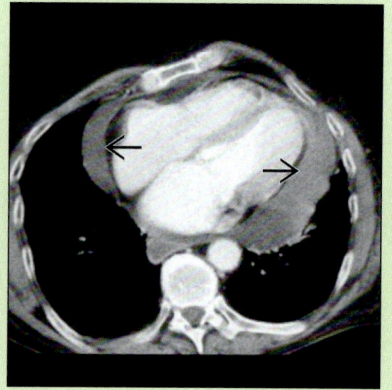

Axial CECT

PERICARDIAL DISEASE, MALIGNANT & INFLAMMATORY

Key Facts

Terminology
- Increased volume and/or abnormal character of fluid in pericardial space

Imaging Findings
- Bone scan: Increased uptake in fluid on delayed images in exudative effusions
- FDG uptake in effusion or pericardium suggests neoplasm in patient with known extrapericardial malignancy
- Absence of FDG uptake does not exclude malignant pericardial effusion
- Hypermetabolic pericardial fluid on FDG PET often seen with inflammation/infection
- Ga-67: Pericardium better evaluated on anterior images
- Ga-67 uptake: Infected pericardial effusion/empyema, viral pericarditis
- Ga-67 uptake in malignant pericardial effusion: Most common with melanoma, lymphoma, sarcoma
- Little or no Ga-67 uptake in malignant effusion due to many tumors (e.g. most adenocarcinomas)
- MUGA (radionuclide ventriculography): Photopenic defect around heart on all projections
- Best imaging tool: ECHO best for detection; MR, CT/PET for characterization
- Protocol advice: Fused PET/CT allows both anatomic and functional information

Top Differential Diagnoses
- Medial Pleural Effusion/Thickening
- Pericardial Thickening/Mass
- Myocardial Thickening

  ○ Ga-67 uptake in malignant pericardial effusion: Most common with melanoma, lymphoma, sarcoma
  ○ Little or no Ga-67 uptake in malignant effusion due to many tumors (e.g. most adenocarcinomas)
- MUGA (radionuclide ventriculography): Photopenic defect around heart on all projections

Radiographic Findings
- Radiography unreliable in suggesting or refuting pericardial effusion diagnosis
- Enlarged cardiac silhouette (water-bottle heart)
- Pericardial fat stripe ("Oreo cookie" sign)
- Coexisting pleural effusion in 33%
- CXR advantage: Identifying pericardial calcifications and may suggest diagnosis of large pericardial effusion at low cost and radiation dose

CT Findings
- CT may detect as little as 50 cc of fluid; potentially determine composition of fluid
- Fewer false-positives than with echocardiography

Non-Vascular Interventions
- Pericardiocentesis: Contrast ECHO using agitated saline may be used to exclude needle placement within ventricular cavity when bloody fluid aspirated
  ○ Balloon pericardotomy: Fluoroscopic or CT-guided placement of catheter in pericardial space; then balloon inflation creating channel to pleural space, allowing drainage of fluid
- Pericardial sclerosis: Reported success ~ 90% at 30 days
- Pericardioscopy

MR Findings
- MR may detect as little as 30 cc of fluid
- MR differentiates hemorrhagic from nonhemorrhagic effusions
- More difficult to perform than CT acutely

Fluoroscopic Findings
- Utilized during interventional/therapeutic procedures (e.g., balloon pericardiotomy)

Ultrasonographic Findings
- Screening for pericardial and pleural effusion: Should be routine in US of abdomen

Echocardiographic Findings
- Echocardiography (ECHO) and transesophageal echocardiography (TEE) gold standard for noninvasive diagnosis
- TEE: Useful in demonstrating small & characterizing loculated effusions
- Early effusions: Accumulate posteriorly (expandable posterolateral pericardium)
- Severe cases may be accompanied by diastolic collapse of RA and RV (and in hypovolemic patients left coronary artery and left ventricle)
- Large effusions: Characterized by excessive motion within pericardial sac

Imaging Recommendations
- Best imaging tool: ECHO best for detection; MR, CT/PET for characterization
- Protocol advice: Fused PET/CT allows both anatomic and functional information

DIFFERENTIAL DIAGNOSIS

Medial Pleural Effusion/Thickening
- CECT with coronal reformatting may better define anatomy

Pericardial Thickening/Mass
- Enhancement on CECT; uptake on FDG PET depends on etiology

Myocardial Thickening
- Most problematical with NECT

PATHOLOGY

General Features
- Etiology

PERICARDIAL DISEASE, MALIGNANT & INFLAMMATORY

- o Idiopathic
- o Hydropericardium: Congestive heart failure, valvular disease
- o Neoplastic: Malignant, nonmalignant (not all cancer-associated effusions are malignant)
  - Mediastinal lymphoma, Hodgkin disease and metastatic breast cancer may cause transient effusions with no long-term sequelae
- o Infectious: Bacterial, viral, fungal, parasitic, tuberculosis, HIV related
- o Autoimmune, connective tissue disorders: Systemic lupus erythematosus, rheumatoid arthritis, systemic sclerosis, vasculitides
- o Other: Trauma, uremia, drugs, postpericardiotomy syndrome, chylopericardium, myxedema, radiation
- Epidemiology
  - o Pericardial effusion in 3-4% of autopsies; higher with certain diseases
  - o 21% of cancer patients have pericardial metastases: Mostly lung, breast, leukemia/lymphoma
  - o Asymptomatic effusion in 41-87% with HIV, +/- AIDS; moderate to severe effusion in 13%

Gross Pathologic & Surgical Features
- Serous, purulent, hemorrhagic, fibrinous, malignant lesions

Microscopic Features
- Purulent, hemorrhagic, fibrinous, malignant cells

CLINICAL ISSUES

Presentation
- Most common signs/symptoms
  - o Small pericardial effusions often are asymptomatic
  - o Time course to development impacts symptoms
    - Rapid accumulation of as little as 80 cc of pericardial fluid may cause elevated intrapericardial pressure
    - Slowly developing effusions can grow to 2 liters without symptoms
- Other signs/symptoms
  - o Cardiovascular: Chest pain, pressure, discomfort, light-headedness, syncope, palpitations, cyanosis
    - Beck triad: Hypotension, jugular venous distension, muffled heart sounds
    - Pulsus paradoxus, pericardial friction rub, widened pulse pressure, tachycardia, hepatojugular reflux, weakened peripheral pulses, edema
  - o Respiratory: Cough, dyspnea, hoarseness, tachypnea, ↓ breath sounds (pleural effusions), Ewart sign (dullness to percussion beneath left scapula due to lung compression from pericardial effusion)
  - o Gastrointestinal: Hiccough, hepatosplenomegaly
  - o Neurologic: Anxiety, confusion

Demographics
- Age: Observed in all age groups: Mean 4th or 5th decades, earlier with HIV

Natural History & Prognosis
- Depends on etiology and comorbid condition(s)
- Idiopathic effusions are well tolerated in most; up to 50% with large, chronic effusions are asymptomatic during long-term follow-up
- Pericardial effusion is primary or contributory cause of death in 86% of cancer patients with symptomatic effusions
- Survival rate in HIV with symptomatic pericardial effusion: 36% at 6 months, 19% at 1 year

Treatment
- Medical therapy: Determine etiology, IV resuscitation, chemotherapy, corticosteroids and NSAIDs
- Surgical therapy: Subxiphoid pericardial window, VATS, thoracotomy, median sternotomy

DIAGNOSTIC CHECKLIST

Image Interpretation Pearls
- FDG PET: Hypermetabolic activity suggest infection/inflammation or malignancy
- FDG PET: Lack of hypermetabolic activity in pericardial effusion does not exclude malignant effusion
- MUGA: Photopenic defect around heart on all projections = pericardial effusion

SELECTED REFERENCES

1. Bhargava P et al: FDG PET in Primary Effusion Lymphoma (PEL) of the Pericardium. Clin Nucl Med. 31(1):18-19, 2006
2. Marta MJ et al: Constrictive tuberculous pericarditis: case report and review of the literature. Rev Port Cardiol. 22(3):391-405, 2003
3. Patel AD et al: Detection of pericardial effusion during Tc-99m sestamibi cardiac imaging. J Nucl Cardiol. 10(1):102-4, 2003
4. Sidley JA et al: Percutaneous balloon pericardiotomy as a treatment for recurrent pericardial effusion in 6 dogs. J Vet Intern Med. 16(5):541-6, 2002
5. Silva-Cardoso J et al: Pericardial involvement in human immunodeficiency virus infection. Chest. 115(2):418-22, 1999
6. Flores RM et al: Video-assisted thoracic surgery pericardial resection for effusive disease. Chest Surg Clin N Am. 8(4):835-51, 1998
7. Herzog E et al: Diagnosis of pericardial effusion and its effects on ventricular function using gated Tc-99m sestamibi perfusion SPECT. Clin Nucl Med. 23(6):361-4, 1998
8. Nugue O et al: Pericardioscopy in the etiologic diagnosis of pericardial effusion in 141 consecutive patients. Circulation. 94(7):1635-41, 1996
9. Prvulovich EM et al: Gallium-67 imaging of pericardial lymphoma in AIDS. J Nucl Med. 37(6):995-6, 1996
10. Weisse AB et al: Contrast echocardiography as an adjunct in hemorrhagic or complicated pericardiocentesis. Am Heart J. 131(4):822-5, 1996
11. Chong HH et al: Pericardial effusion and tamponade: evaluation, imaging modalities, and management. Compr Ther. 21(7):378-85, 1995
12. Heidenreich PA et al: Pericardial effusion in AIDS. Incidence and survival. Circulation. 92(11):3229-34, 1995
13. Rokey R et al: Assessment of experimental pericardial effusion using nuclear magnetic resonance imaging techniques. Am Heart J. 121(4 Pt 1):1161-9, 1991

PERICARDIAL DISEASE, MALIGNANT & INFLAMMATORY

IMAGE GALLERY

Other

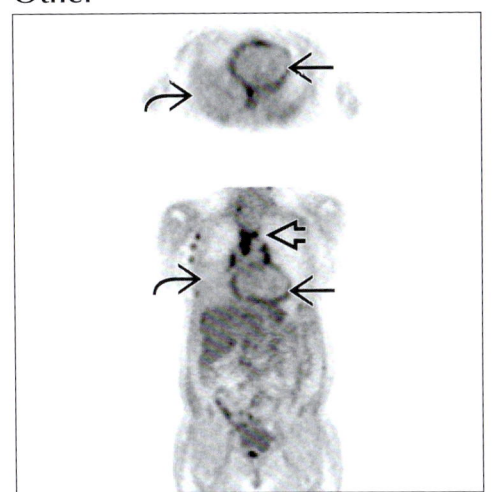

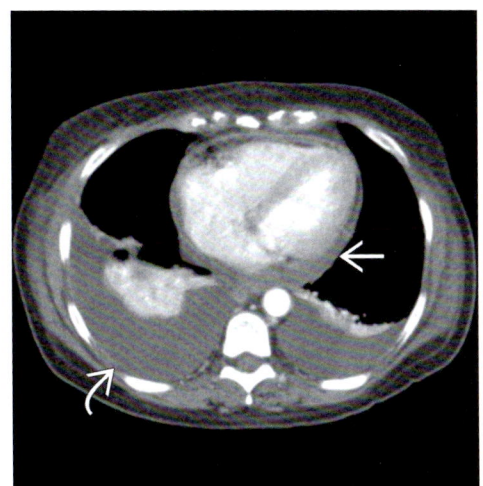

(Left) Axial and coronal FDG PET shows hypermetabolism in pericardium ➔, mediastinal lymph nodes ➔ and pleural effusion ➔, all consistent with metastatic involvement. Same patient as next image. *(Right)* Axial CECT in same patient as previous image shows pericardial ➔ and bilateral pleural ➔ effusions due to metastatic involvement.

Other

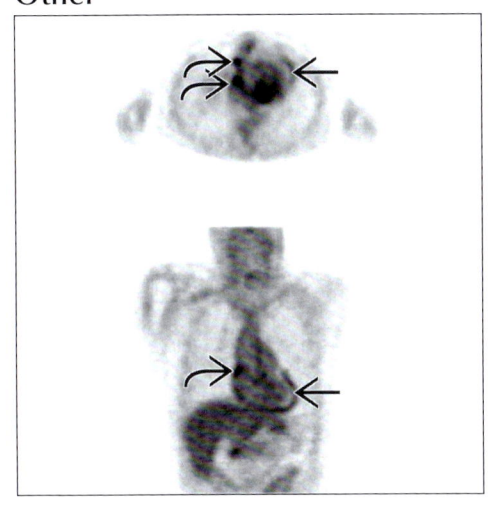

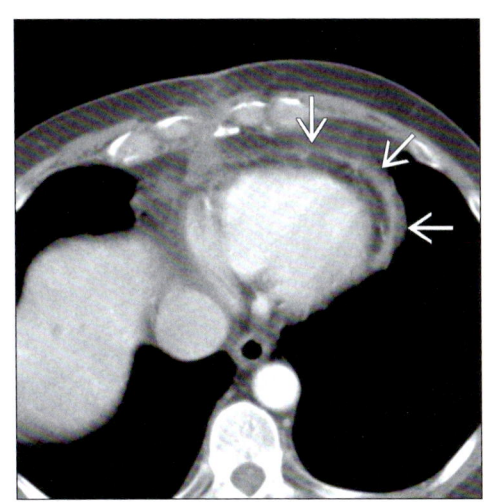

(Left) Axial and coronal FDG PET shows hypermetabolic rim around the heart ➔ due to breast cancer metastases to the pericardium. Note nodular component ➔. Same patient as next image. *(Right)* Axial CECT in same patient as previous image shows nodular pericardial thickening/effusion ➔ due to metastatic breast cancer.

Other

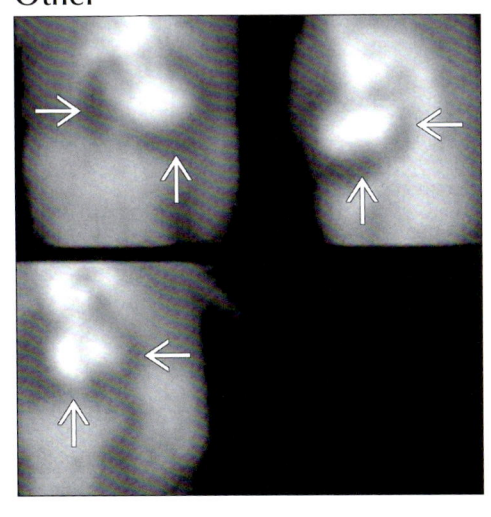

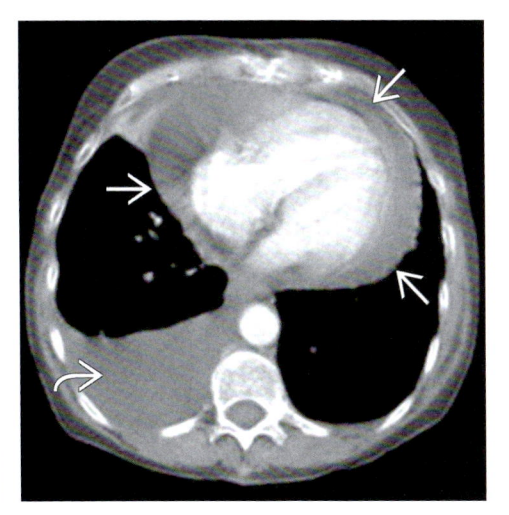

(Left) Planar MUGA (radionuclide ventriculogram) images show a large photopenic region around the heart ➔ due to a large malignant effusion. Same patient as next image. *(Right)* Axial CECT in same patient as previous image shows a large pericardial effusion ➔ and right pleural effusion ➔ due to metastatic breast cancer.

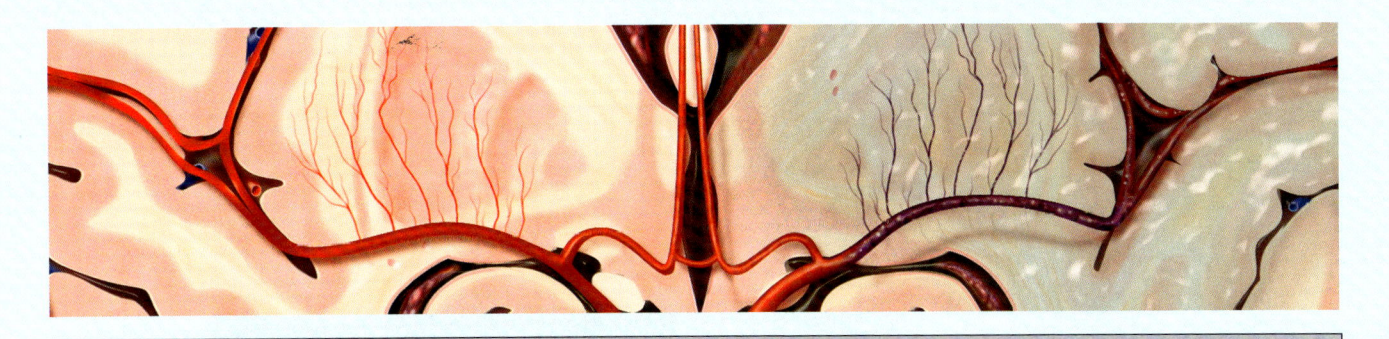

SECTION 5: CNS

Introduction and Overview
Brain Imaging Overview 5-2

Vascular Assessment
Brain Death 5-4
Cerebral Vascular Occlusion 5-10
Blood Brain Barrier Disruption 5-14

Seizure Assessment
Seizure Evaluation 5-16

Dementia & Neurodegenerative
Alzheimer Disease 5-22
Dementia & Neurodegenerative, Other 5-26

Neurooncology
Gliomas & Astrocytomas 5-32
Primary CNS Lymphoma 5-36
Metastases, Brain 5-40
Radiation Necrosis vs. Recurrent Tumor 5-44

CSF Imaging
CSF Leak 5-50
Ventricular Shunt Dysfunction 5-54
Normal Pressure Hydrocephalus 5-58

Miscellaneous
Heterotopic Gray Matter 5-64
Brain Infection & Inflammation 5-70
Psychiatry, Drug Addiction & Forensics 5-74

BRAIN IMAGING OVERVIEW

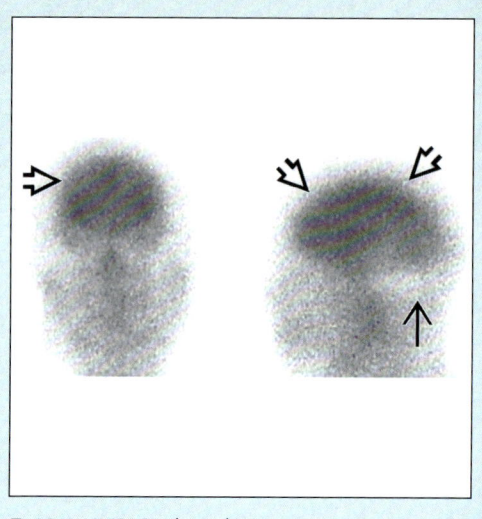

Tc-99m HMPAO planar brain scan in a patient with clinical brain death shows absence of perfusion to the posterior fossa ➔, intact perfusion to supratentorial brain ➔.

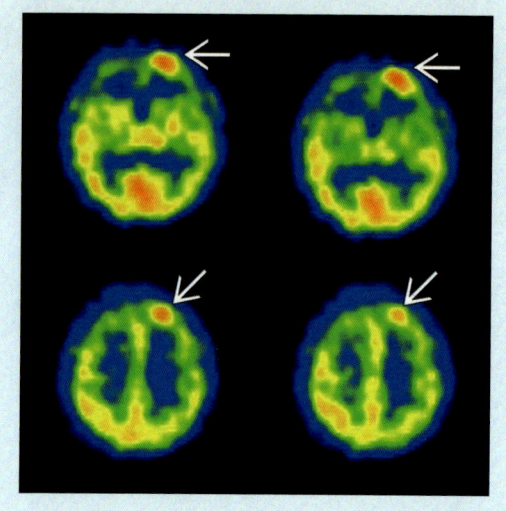

Multi-axial Tc-99m ECD SPECT images of the brain in patient injected at onset of seizure (ictal SPECT). Images show increased uptake in seizure focus in left frontal lobe ➔.

KEY RADIOPHARMACEUTICALS

Tc-99m Hexamethylpropylene Amine Oxime (HMPAO, Exametazime, Ceretec)
- Dose: 370-1110 MBq (10-30 mCi)
- Adult dosimetry
  - Target organ (kidneys): 0.034 mGy/MBq (0.126 rad/mCi)
  - Effective dose: 0.0093 mSv/MBq (0.034 rem/mCi)
- Pediatric dosimetry
  - Target organ (thyroid): 0.14 mGy/MBq (0.52 rad/mCi)
  - Effective dose: 0.026 mSv/MBq (0.096 rem/mCi)
- Tc-99m pertechnetate should be freshly eluted (< 2 hours old)
- Available in unstabilized and stabilized forms
  - Unstabilized: Should be injected no more than 10 minutes pre and 30 minutes post reconstitution
  - Stabilized (preferred): Should be injected no more than 10 minutes pre and 4 hours post reconstitution
- Time from injection to imaging: ≥ 90 minutes for best result; excessive delay (> 4 hours) to be avoided
- Inject and uptake at rest, eyes open, low light, low noise

Tc-99m Ethyl Cysteinate Dimer, Bicisate (ECD, Neurolite)
- Dose: 370-1110 MBq (10-30 mCi) IV
- Adult dosimetry
  - Target organ (bladder wall): 0.073 mGy/MBq (0.27 rad/mCi)
  - Effective dose: 0.011 mSv/MBq (0.042 rem/mCi)
- Pediatric dosimetry
  - Target organ (bladder wall): 0.083 mGy/MBq (0.31 rad/mCi)
  - Effective dose: 0.023 mSv/MBq (0.085 rem/mCi)
- Tc-99m pertechnetate should be freshly eluted (< 2 hours old)
- Time from injection to imaging: ≥ 45 minutes for best result; excessive delay (> 4 hours) to be avoided
- Inject and uptake at rest, eyes open, low light, low noise

F-18 Fluorodeoxyglucose (FDG)
- Dose: ~ 10 mCi (370 MBq) IV
- Adult dosimetry
  - Target organ (heart wall): 2.78 mGy/MBq (0.278 rad/mCi)
  - Effective dose: 0.592 mSv/MBq (0.059 rem/mCi)
- Time from injection to imaging: 30-45 minutes
- Inject and uptake at rest, eyes open, low light, low noise

APPLICATIONS

"Conventional" Brain Scan
- Purpose: Rarely indicated
  - Historically used to identify regions of focal blood brain barrier (BBB) disruption
  - Current applications to confirm adequacy of therapeutic disruption of BBB
- Radiopharmaceuticals: Tracers rapidly excreted but excluded by blood brain barrier
  - Tc-99m glucohepatate
  - Tc-99m pertechnetate
  - Tc-99m diethylenetriamine pentaacetic acid (DTPA)

Brain Death Determination
- Purpose: To assess cerebral blood flow (CBF) in patients clinically suspected as brain dead
  - Facilitate familial acceptance of withdrawal of life support
  - Expedite organ harvest for transplantation
- Patient preparation: High levels of barbiturates can decrease CBF
- Radiopharmaceuticals
  - Non-brain binding agents: Typically Tc-99m DTPA (diethylamine pentaacetic acid), glucoheptanate, or pertechnetate
    - Generally considered inferior to brain binding agents: Cannot assess posterior circulation; often non-diagnostic when poor bolus or severely reduced cardiac output
  - Brain binding agents now preferred (HMPAO, ECD)

BRAIN IMAGING OVERVIEW

Primary Indications for Radionuclide Brain Imaging

Brain Death
- Brain binding agents now preferred (HMPAO, ECD) over non-brain binding agents (Tc-99m DTPA, pertechnetate, glucoheptanate)
  - Flow study not critical; allows assessment of posterior circulation

SPECT: Many indications, reimbursed
- Cerebrovascular insufficiency
- Dementia
- Epilepsy monitoring (especially ictal)
- Assessment of brain injury

FDG PET
- Likely superior to SPECT for many applications
- Only few reimbursed indications at this time
  - Epilepsy (interictal), AD vs. frontotemporal dementia (many pre-conditions)
  - Primary brain tumors (if enrolled in NOPR)

- Flow study not critical
- Allows visualization of relative and global CBF

Brain SPECT
- Likely inferior to FDG PET for most applications, but significant reimbursement and cost limitations make FDG less available
- Purposes: Multiple
  - Evaluation of dementia
  - Cerebrovascular insufficiency
    - Baseline and Diamox-challenged SPECT for clinically significant vascular insufficiency
    - In conjunction with Wada test to assess adequacy of collateral flow prior to vascular sacrifice
    - Evaluation of acute stroke
  - Epilepsy monitoring
    - Preferred method for ictal studies
  - Assessment of brain injury
    - Prognostic significance in acute setting
    - Use in forensics and personal-injury litigation is controversial

Brain FDG PET
- Currently only few indications approved for reimbursement by Centers for Medicare and Medicaid Services (CMS)
  - Epilepsy monitoring (interictal)
  - To distinguish Alzheimer disease (AD) from frontotemporal dementia (many criteria must first be met)
  - Evaluation of dementia in conjunction with a CMS approved clinical trial
  - Evaluation of primary brain tumors if entered into National Oncologic PET Registry (NOPR)
- Promising results for many other non-reimbursed indications

RELATED REFERENCES

1. Knowlton RC: The role of FDG-PET, ictal SPECT, and MEG in the epilepsy surgery evaluation. Epilepsy Behav. 8(1):91-101, 2006
2. Wang SX et al: FDG-PET on irradiated brain tumor: ten years' summary. Acta Radiol. 47(1):85-90, 2006
3. Lascola C: Molecular imaging in Alzheimer's disease. Neuroimaging Clin N Am. 15(4):827-35, x-xi, 2005
4. Pakrasi S et al: Emission tomography in dementia. Nucl Med Commun. 26(3):189-96, 2005
5. Giammarile F et al: High and low grade oligodendrogliomas (ODG): correlation of amino-acid and glucose uptakes using PET and histological classifications. J Neurooncol. 68(3):263-74, 2004
6. Benard F et al: Imaging gliomas with positron emission tomography and single-photon emission computed tomography. Semin Nucl Med. 33(2):148-62, 2003
7. Conrad GR et al: Scintigraphy as a confirmatory test of brain death. Semin Nucl Med. 33(4):312-23, 2003
8. Lee JK et al: Usefulness of semiquantitative FDG-PET in the prediction of brain tumor treatment response to gamma knife radiosurgery. J Comput Assist Tomogr. 27(4):525-9, 2003
9. Padma MV et al: Prediction of pathology and survival by FDG PET in gliomas. J Neurooncol. 64(3):227-37, 2003
10. Roelcke U et al: Operated low grade astrocytomas: a long term PET study on the effect of radiotherapy. J Neurol Neurosurg Psychiatry. 66(5):644-7, 1999

IMAGE GALLERY

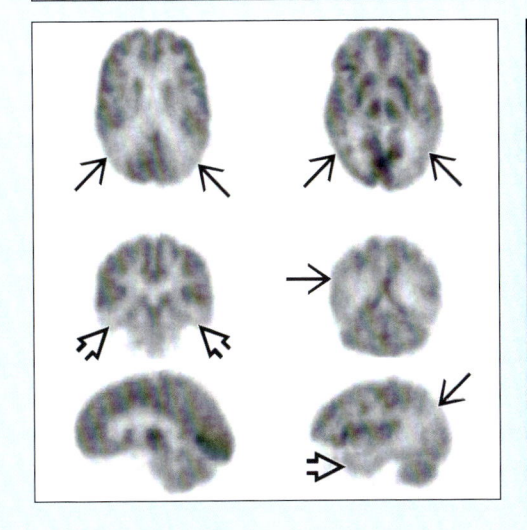

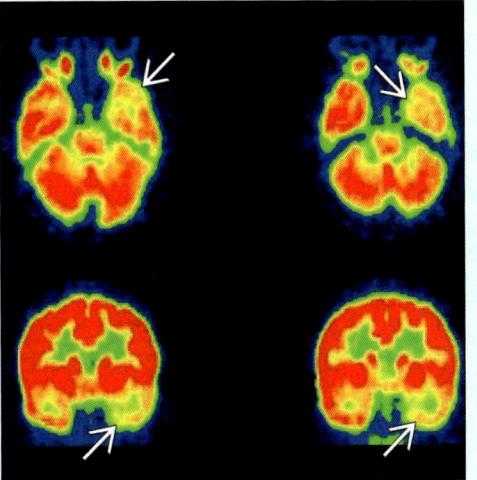

(Left) Axial (top panel), coronal (middle panel) and sagittal (lower panel) FDG PET images of the brain in a demented patient shows typical pattern of Alzheimer dementia: Decreased temporal ⇒ and parietal uptake ➡. *(Right)* Axial (top panel) and coronal (lower panel) FDG PET images of the brain in a patient with partial complex seizures (interictal injection) show hypometabolism in seizure focus in left medial and anterior temporal lobe ➡.

BRAIN DEATH

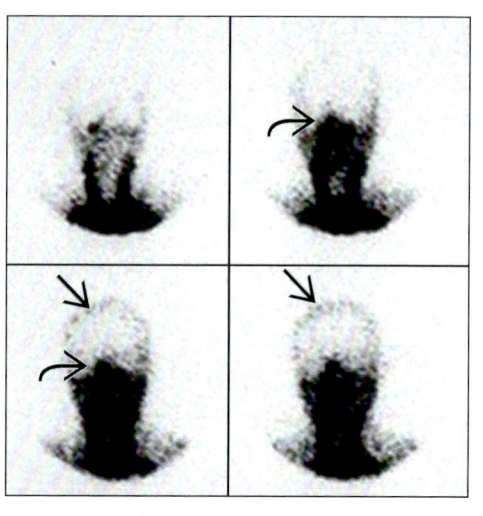

Tc-99m pertechnetate angiographic phase shows absence of "trident sign" with shunting of blood to scalp ("empty light bulb sign") and to central face ("hot nose sign").

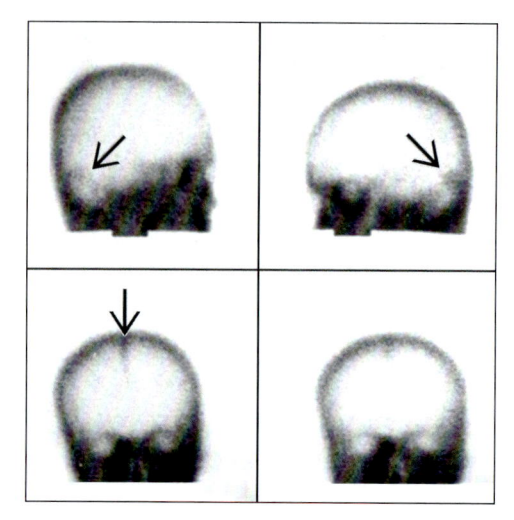

Same patient as left. Despite lack of cerebral blood flow, venous sinuses are visualized. This can be seen in brain death due to centrally draining scalp perforator vessels.

TERMINOLOGY

Abbreviations and Synonyms
- Brain death (BD)

Definitions
- Complete, irreversible cessation of brain function
- Medical determination of death has serious legal ramifications
  - Includes status for organ donation
  - Often has forensic implications
- Legal definition (as based from Draft form of Uniform Determination of Death Act, on which most states have modelled their definition
  - An individual who (is dead) has sustained either
    - (1) Irreversible cessation of circulatory and respiratory functions
    - (2) Irreversible cessation of all functions of the entire brain, including the brain stem
  - A determination of death must be made in accordance with accepted medical standards

IMAGING FINDINGS

General Features
- Best diagnostic clue
  - Absence of uptake lipophyllic brain tracer [Tc-99m HMPAO (Ceretec), ECD (Neurolite, bicisate)] = brain death
    - Lipophyllic tracers: Do not require bolus technique
    - Lipophyllic tracers: Allow assessment of cerebrum & cerebellum/brainstem
  - Absence of brain perfusion on CBF scan (Tc-99m DTPA or Tc-99m pertechnetate) = brain death
    - Limited in that requires good bolus technique and adequate cardiac output
    - Limited in that only allows assessment of anterior circulation (anterior and middle cerebral arteries)
- Location: In many states, must assess CBF to both supra- and infratentorial brain (brainstem, cerebellum)
- Imaging may confirm but does not substitute for clinical criteria

DDx: Other Findings on Brain Death Scan

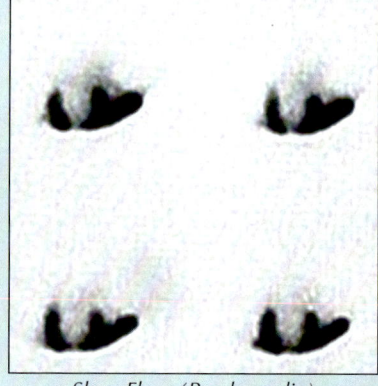

Slow Flow (Bradycardia) 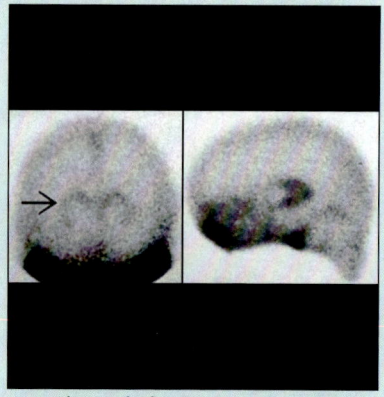 | *Choroid Plexus (Tc-99m O 4-)* 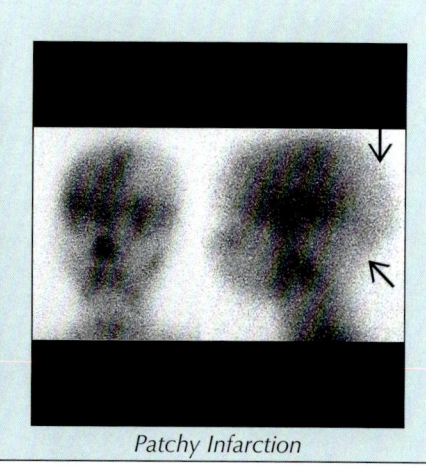 | *Patchy Infarction*

BRAIN DEATH

Key Facts

Terminology
- Complete, irreversible cessation of brain function
- Medical determination of death has serious legal ramifications
- An individual who (is dead) has sustained either
- (1) Irreversible cessation of circulatory and respiratory functions
- (2) Irreversible cessation of all functions of the entire brain, including the brain stem
- A determination of death must be made in accordance with accepted medical standards

Imaging Findings
- Absence of uptake lipophyllic brain tracer [Tc-99m HMPAO (Ceretec), ECD (Neurolite, bicisate)] = brain death
- Lipophyllic tracers: Do not require bolus technique
- Lipophyllic tracers: Allow assessment of cerebrum & cerebellum/brainstem
- Absence of brain perfusion on CBF scan (Tc-99m DTPA or Tc-99m pertechnetate) = brain death
- Imaging may confirm but does not substitute for clinical criteria
- Best imaging tool: Scintigraphy using lipophyllic tracers (consider bedside imaging if available) + EEG

Top Differential Diagnoses
- Diffuse Cerebral Edema
- Technical Difficulty
- Massive Cerebral Infarction

Clinical Issues
- Remember: BD is primarily clinical diagnosis, legal criteria vary

Nuclear Medicine Findings
- Lipophyllic radionuclide brain tracers: Tc-99m exametazime (HMPAO), Tc-99m ethyl cysteinate dimer (ECD) (bicisate)
  - Normal
    - Uptake in all portions of brain
  - Brain injury but not brain dead
    - Patchy areas of absent or diminished uptake
    - May provide prognostic information despite lack of brain death
  - Brain death
    - Absence of uptake in all portions of brain
- Cerebral blood flow (CBF) scan (Tc-99m DTPA, pertechnetate, may not meet legal requirements of brain stem or posterior fossa assessment)
  - Normal
    - Angiographic phase: Early arterial visualization of both anterior (seen together) and middle cerebral arteries - "trident sign"
    - Blood pool phase: Visualization of venous sinuses, but not brain
  - Brain damaged but not brain death
    - Angiographic phase: May see asymmetrical flow or incomplete trident
    - Blood pool phase: May see uptake in epidural hematoma, choroid plexus (pertechnetate) or areas of blood brain barrier breakdown
  - Brain death
    - Angiographic phase: Absence of trident, "empty light bulb sign", "hot nose sign" due to shunting to ECA
    - Blood pool phase: May visualize venous sinuses from centrally draining scalp perforators

CT Findings
- CTA: No intravascular enhancement
- NECT
  - Diffuse cerebral edema (GM/WM borders effaced)
    - "Reversal sign" (density of cerebellum >> cerebral hemispheres)
  - Gyri swollen, ventricles/cisterns compressed
- CECT: No enhancement of intracranial arteries or veins

Angiographic Findings
- Conventional
  - No intracranial flow
  - Contrast stasis (ECA fills, supraclinoid ICA does not)

MR Findings
- T1WI
  - Hypointense, GM/WM differentiation lost
  - Complete central brain herniation
- T2WI: Cortex hyperintense, gyri swollen
- DWI
  - Hemispheric high signal, severe apparent diffusion coefficient (ADC) drop
  - Diffusion anisotropy diminishes between 1-12 hours after BD
- MRA: No intracranial flow demonstrated

Other Modality Findings
- EEG isoelectric

Ultrasonographic Findings
- Orbital Doppler
  - Absence/reversal of end-diastolic flow in ophthalmic, central retinal arteries
  - Markedly increased arterial resistive indices
- Transcranial Doppler
  - Global circulatory arrest
  - Oscillating "to and fro" signal
  - Caution: 20% have ICA flow demonstrated despite cerebral circulatory arrest

Imaging Recommendations
- Best imaging tool: Scintigraphy using lipophyllic tracers (consider bedside imaging if available) + EEG
- Protocol advice
  - Tc-99m lipophyllic tracers (trade names: Ceretec, ECD, Neurolite)
    - Venous injection of 10-30 mCi Tc-99m lipophyllic brain tracer

BRAIN DEATH

- Anterior and lateral planar views may be acquired within 10-20 minutes of injection (SPECT usually not required)
- Chin slightly "tucked" on lateral view to allow visualization of posterior fossa
- If not yet brain dead, may repeat exam with 2x dose in 6 h
- Quality control on tracer important since inadequate preparation may result in agent that fails to show uptake in brain
  - Tc-99m DTPA or pertechnetate
    - Large bore, small volume rapid venous injection 15-20 mCi Tc-99m DTPA or pertechnetate
    - May repeat in 6 hours if necessary

DIFFERENTIAL DIAGNOSIS

Diffuse Cerebral Edema
- From reversible causes: Drug overdose, status epilepticus
  - Clinically can mimic BD

Technical Difficulty
- Missed bolus
- Dissection, vasospasm (catheter angiography)
- Poor binding of metabolic agent (HMPAO, ECD) with Tc-99m (quality control should detect in advance of study)
- Not an issue with current radionuclide studies

Massive Cerebral Infarction
- "Malignant" MCA infarct can mimic BD

PATHOLOGY

General Features
- General path comments: BD is anatomically, physiologically complex
- Etiology
  - Severe cell swelling ↑ intracranial pressure (ICP)
  - Markedly elevated ICP decreases cerebral blood flow
  - If ICP > end-diastolic pressure in cerebral arteries, diastolic reversal occurs
  - If ICP > systolic pressure, blood flow ceases
  - Complete and irreversible loss of brain function
  - Brainstem level responses and spinal reflexes sequentially fade out
- Epidemiology
  - Trauma: Could be accidental, criminal (battered child or assault), or combination
  - Vascular (stroke, hypoxia/anoxia)
  - Neoplastic (with mixtures of the above as natural or iatrogenic progression)
  - Infectious

Gross Pathologic & Surgical Features
- Markedly swollen brain with severely compressed sulci
- Bilateral descending transtentorial herniation
  - Downwards displacement of diencephalon
  - "Grooving" of temporal lobes by tentorial incisura

CLINICAL ISSUES

Presentation
- Most common signs/symptoms
  - Profound coma (GCS = 3) "known cause"
  - Reversible causes of coma must be excluded!
- Clinical Profile
  - Clinical diagnosis of BD highly reliable if examiners are experienced, use established criteria
  - Remember: BD is primarily clinical diagnosis, legal criteria vary

Natural History & Prognosis
- Ancillary studies [absent brainstem auditory evoked responses (BAER), "isoelectric" cortical EEG, no intracranial flow on imaging studies], and neurologic exam help confirm clinical diagnosis

DIAGNOSTIC CHECKLIST

Consider
- Prior to study
  - Quality control on HMPAO and ECD are important, as poor tag negates study
  - Focused history, including head trauma, surgery, possibility of hypothermia or drug overdose, and review of anatomic imaging
  - Support (respiratory and monitoring) personnel in place
- Cerebral blood flow agents (pertechnetate, DTPA)
  - Successful anterior (posterior occasionally) flow sequence critical; consider viewing dynamically
  - 5-30 minute delayed posterior (anterior) plus lateral
- Lipophyllic tracers (Ceretec, Neurolite, ECD)
  - Flow sequence not critical
  - Planar anterior (posterior) and lateral at 10-20 minutes or longer
  - SPECT may be helpful but usually not necessary

SELECTED REFERENCES

1. Booth CM et al: Is this patient dead, vegetative, or severely neurologically impaired? Assessing outcome for comatose survivors of cardiac arrest. JAMA 291(7):870-9, 2004
2. Dosemeci L et al: Utility of transcranial doppler ultrasonography for confirmatory diagnosis of brain death: two sides of the coin. Transplantation. 77(1):71-5, 2004
3. Belber CJ: Brain death documentation: analysis and issues. Neurosurgery. 53(4):1009; author reply 1009, 2003
4. Conrad GR et al: Scintigraphy as a confirmatory test of brain death. Semin Nucl Med. 33(4):312-23, 2003
5. Donohoe KJ et al: Procedure guideline for brain death scintigraphy. J Nucl Med. 44(5):846-51, 2003
6. Harding JW et al: Outcomes of patients referred for confirmation of brain death by 99mTc-exametazime scintigraphy. Intensive Care Med. 29(4):539-43, 2003
7. Shih LC et al: Perfusion-weighted magnetic resonance imaging thresholds identifying core, irreversibly infarcted tissue. Stroke. 34(6):1425-30, 2003
8. Flowers WM Jr et al: Accuracy of clinical evaluation in the determination of brain death. South Med J. 93(2):203-6, 2000
9. Haupt WF et al: European brain death codes: a comparison of national guidelines. J Neurol. 246(6):432-7, 1999

BRAIN DEATH

IMAGE GALLERY

Other

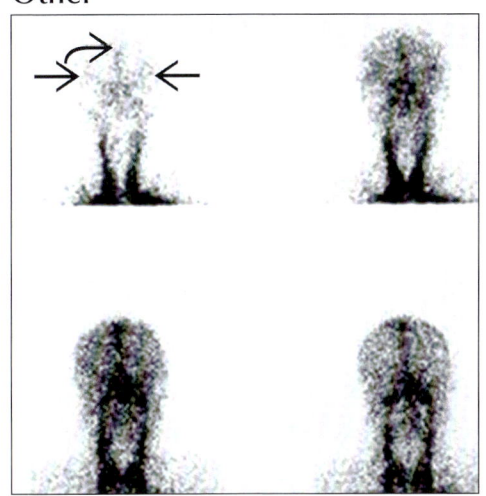

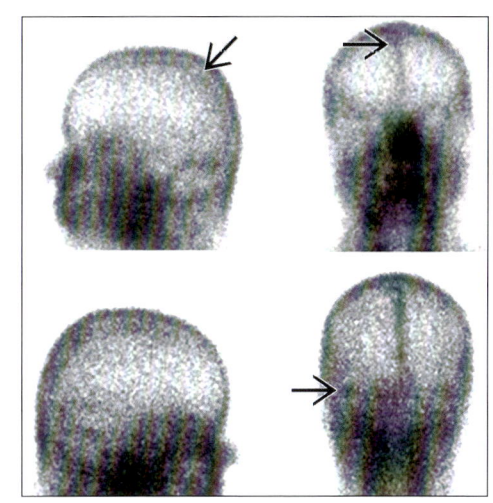

(Left) Normal CBF scan in the angiographic phase. Second image demonstrates normal "trident sign" consisting of middle cerebrals ➡ and paired anterior cerebral ➡ arteries. *(Right)* Normal study in same patient as left. Blood pool images show normal venous sinus activity ➡. No activity in brain itself (this is normal).

Variant

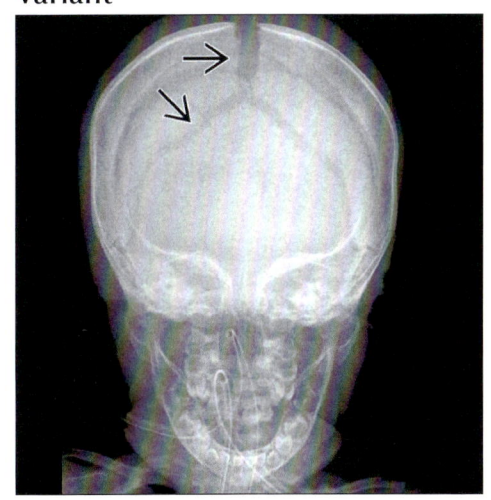

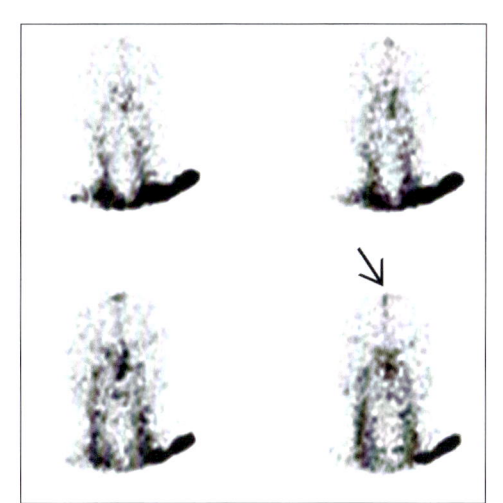

(Left) AP plain skull radiograph shows widely patent sutures ➡ in this young individual, giving the cranium considerable flexibility. Same patient as next image. *(Right)* Late angiographic images show venous sinus activity ➡, which may mimic arterial flow. Early angiographic images in this patient showed no CBF.

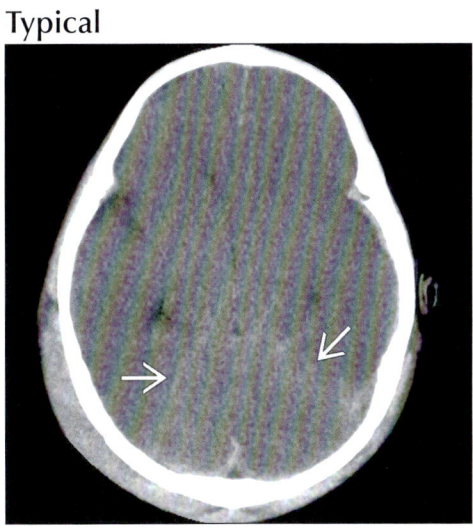

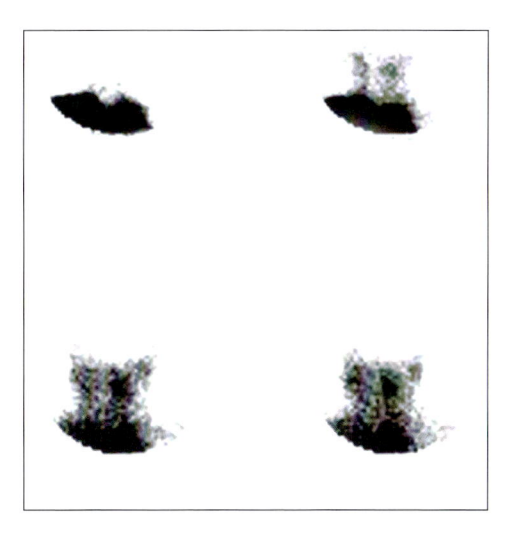

Typical

(Left) NECT at the level of the tentorium cerebelli shows high density (blood) ➡ along the tentorium. *(Right)* Anterior angiographic sequence (pertechnetate) shows lack of flow in the upper brain. Free blood caused brain swelling, cutting off flow, leading to brain death.

BRAIN DEATH

(Left) Brain death with very poor cardiac output. Angiographic phase of CBF scan (Tc-99m pertechnetate) is non-diagnostic due to lack of adequate bolus. **(Right)** Blood pool phase of CBF scan (Tc-99m pertechnetate) in same patient as previous and next. No definite venous sinus activity suggests (but does not confirm) brain death.

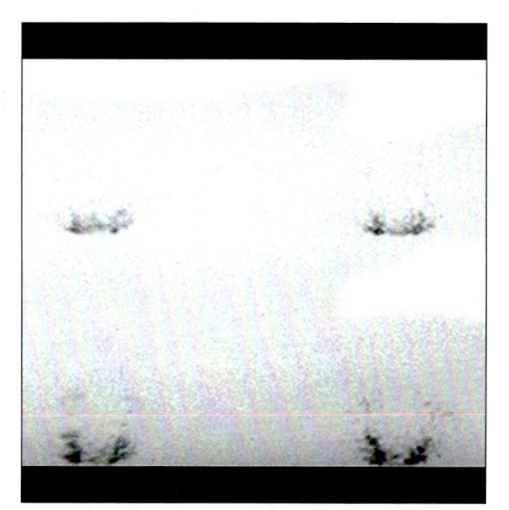

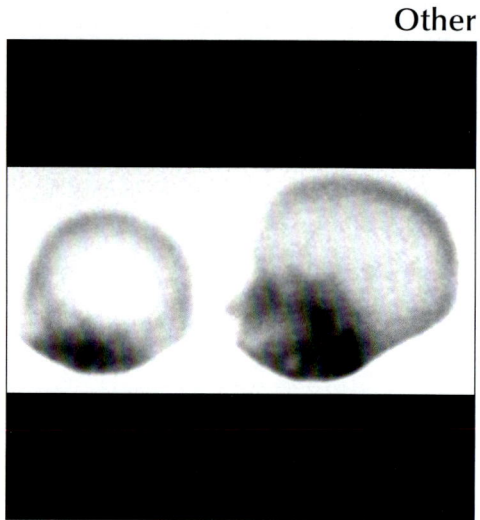

(Left) Repeat scan with Tc-99m HMPAO in same patient as previous image. Extensive salivary activity but no brain uptake. Brain death confirmed. See next image for normal comparison. **(Right)** Normal Tc-99m lipophyllic (HMPAO, ECD) brain scan shows uptake in all portions of the brain, including brain stem and cerebellum.

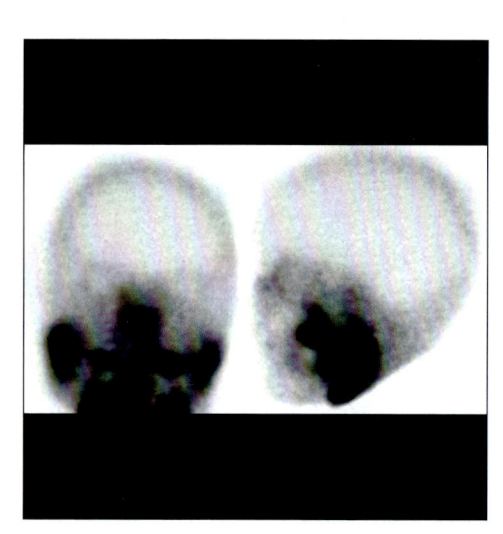

(Left) Anterior Tc-99m HMPAO brain scan. Absence of left hemispheric activity, subfalcine herniation ➡, poor uptake in right cerebral hemisphere. Not brain dead but prognosis dire. **(Right)** Tc-99m HMPAO brain scan. Motorcycle helmet vs. overhanging tree limb. Avulsed vertebral arteries. No brain stem or cerebellar activity ➡. Not legally brain dead but prognosis is dire.

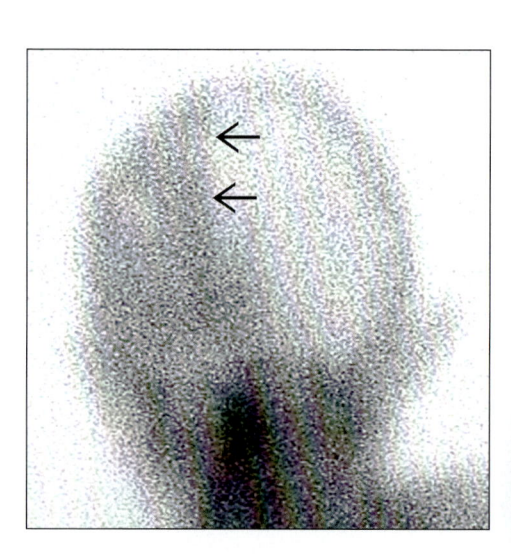

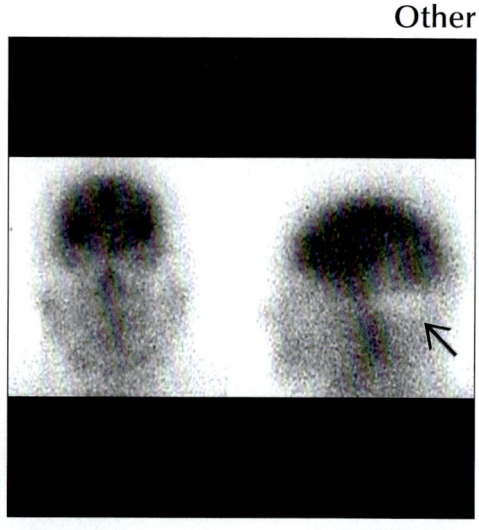

BRAIN DEATH

Other

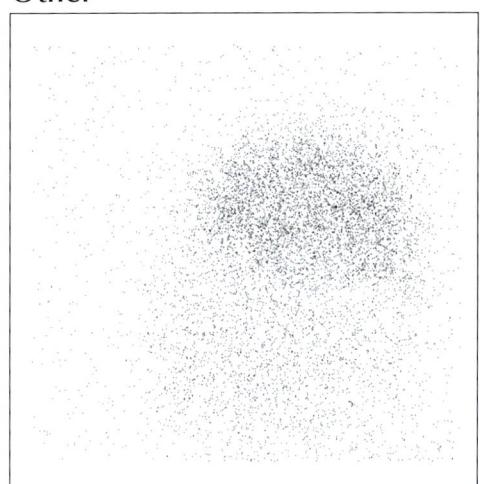

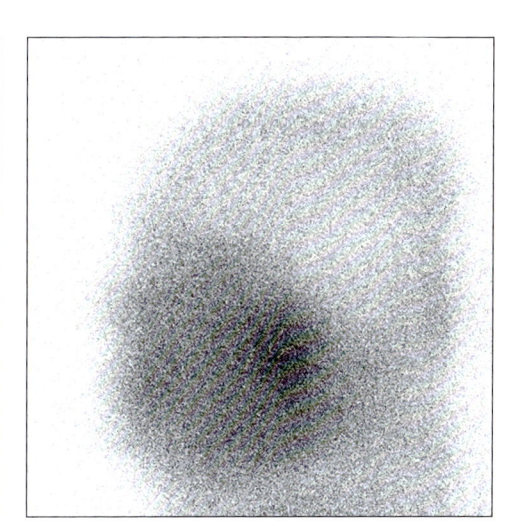

(Left) Lateral Tc-99m HMPAO brain scan shows very faint brain activity, the residua of a Tc-99m HMPAO brain scan performed 24 h earlier (with diffuse brain uptake). *(Right)* Same patient as left following reinjection of Tc-99m HMPAO) has progressed to brain death (the counts on pre-injection lateral over the brain were only 2% of the counts on this study).

Other

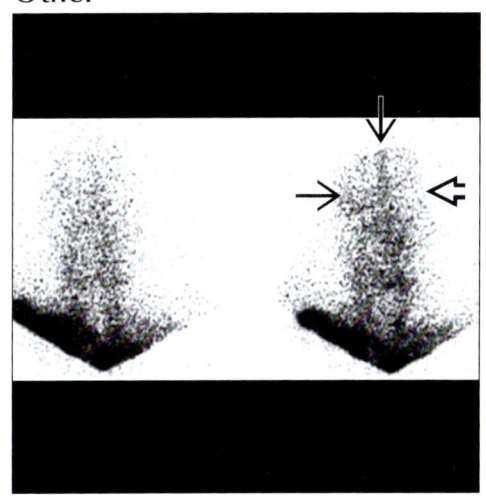

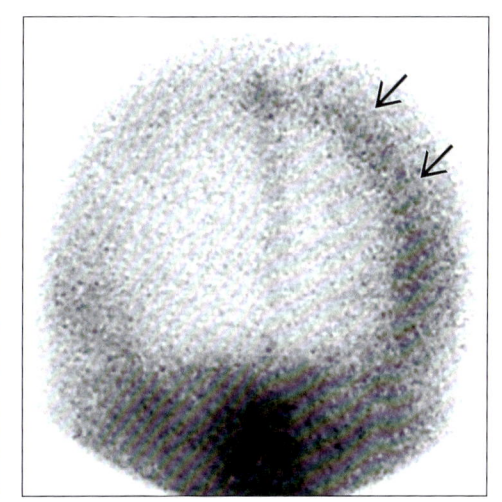

(Left) CBF scan (Tc-99m pertechnetate), angiographic phase shows absence of flow to left middle cerebral artery ⇨, but intact right and anterior cerebral arteries →. *(Right)* CBF scan (Tc-99m pertechnetate). Anterior delayed blood pool image demonstrates diffuse activity in over left cerebral hemisphere →. Patient had large left subdural hematoma.

Other

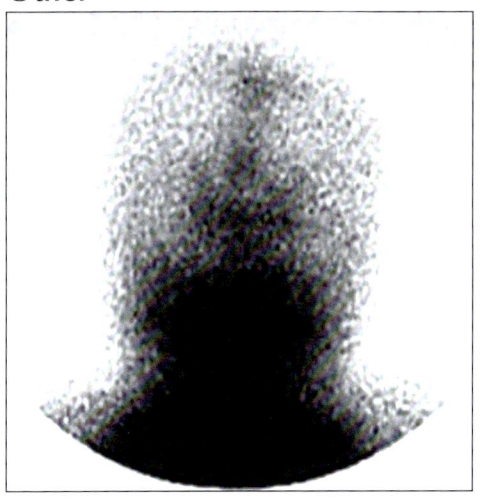

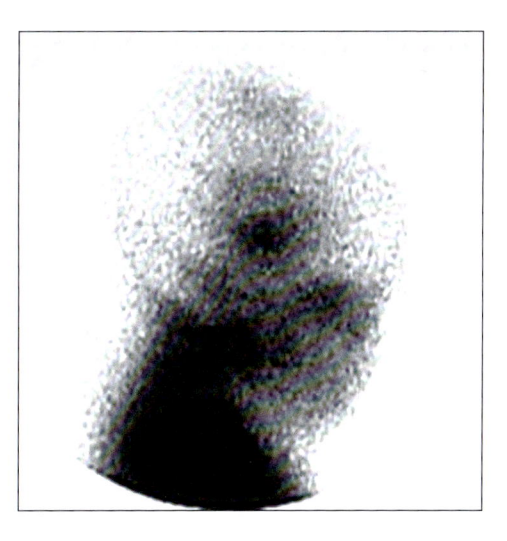

(Left) Anterior view of Tc-99m HMPAO brain scan in clinically, but not legally brain dead child; shows activity in interhemispheric and deep brain structures (basal ganglia, brain stem). *(Right)* Lateral view of Tc-99m HMPAO brain scan in same patient as left shows activity in interhemispheric (motor cortex region), and deep brain structures (basal ganglia, brain stem). Not legally brain dead but prognostically dire.

CEREBRAL VASCULAR OCCLUSION

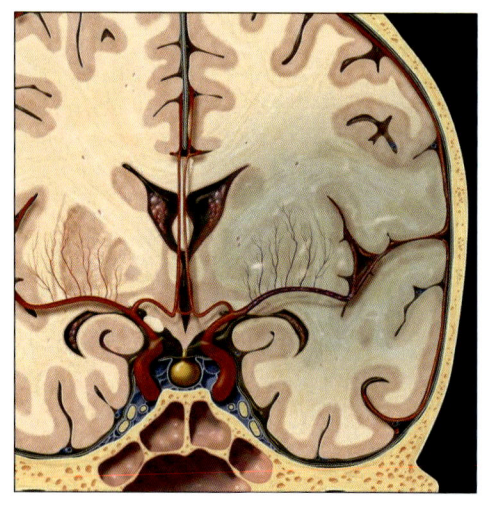

Coronal graphic illustrates left M1 occlusion. Such proximal occlusion will affect the entire MCA territory, including the deep nuclei, which are perfused by lenticulostriate arteries.

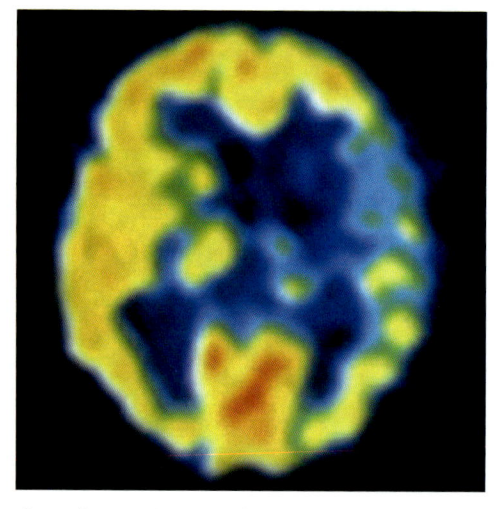

Coronal HMPAO SPECT shows decreased perfusion in the left MCA territory in a patient with acute stroke x 8 h. Small amount of residual perfusion may warrant revascularization, despite subacute presentation.

TERMINOLOGY

Abbreviations and Synonyms
- Stroke: Lay term for sudden onset neurologic symptoms
- Cerebrovascular accident (CVA)
- Transient ischemia attack (TIA)

Definitions
- Decrease or interruption of blood supply to any portion of the brain

IMAGING FINDINGS

General Features
- Best diagnostic clue: Acute infarction: Diffusion restriction with correlating ADC (apparent diffusion coefficient)
- Location: One or more vascular territories, watershed regions
- Size: Dependent on extent of compromise and collateral flow
- Morphology
  - Gray matter: Peripheral, wedge-shaped
  - White matter: Variable shapes

Nuclear Medicine Findings
- Cerebral infarction in problem or equivocal cases: ECD or HMPAO SPECT
  - Assessment of penumbra at risk for extension of infarction: Decreased perfusion surrounding region of infarction
  - Assessment of subacute infarction: Small amounts of perfusion in regions of suspected infarction may support salvage procedure
- Post interventional assessment: ECD or HMPAO SPECT
  - Spasm or post-interventional vascular compromise: Decreased uptake
  - Prediction of hyperperfusion syndrome following ECA-ICA and other bypass: Increased uptake
- Assessment of functional vascular reserve: ECD or HMPAO SPECT with Diamox challenge
  - Diamox (acetazolamide): Carbonic anhydrase inhibitor, results in increased pCO2, increased CBF with normal vessels, failure to increase with stenosis
  - Increased sensitivity over non-Diamox SPECT for detection of ischemic regions of clinical significance

DDx: Mimics of Stroke

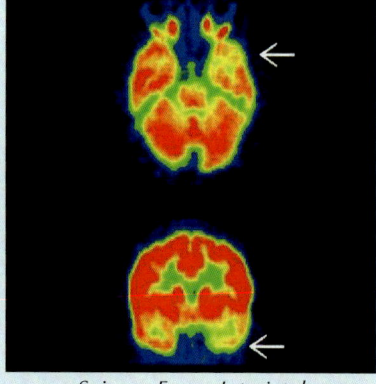

Seizure Focus Interictal

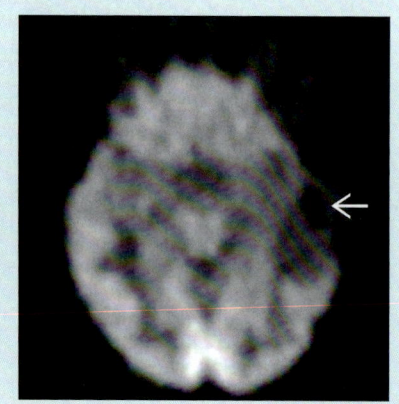

Brain Radiation

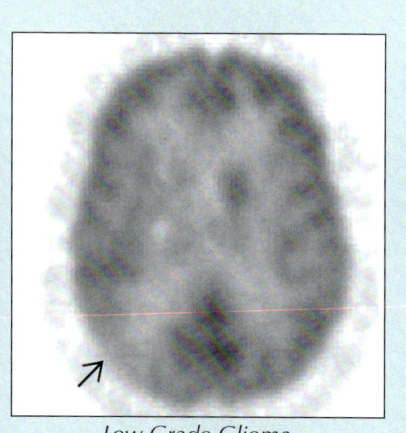

Low Grade Glioma

CEREBRAL VASCULAR OCCLUSION

Key Facts

Imaging Findings
- NECT: Hemorrhagic vs. ischemic, hyperintense clotted vessel
- MR: CE with PWI, DWI
- Acute infarction: Diffusion restriction with correlating ADC map
- Subacute infarction: Gyral edema and enhancement +/- hemorrhagic transformation
- Chronic infarction: Volume loss with marginal gliosis
- Cerebral infarction in problem or equivocal cases: ECD or HMPAO SPECT
- Post interventional assessment: ECD or HMPAO SPECT
- Assessment of functional vascular reserve: ECD or HMPAO SPECT with Diamox challenge
- Preoperative assessment prior to carotid sacrifice: Balloon occlusion test (BOT) with SPECT

Top Differential Diagnoses
- Embolic
- Neoplasm
- Cerebritis
- Cerebral Contusion
- Venous Infarct

Clinical Issues
- "Time is brain" - IV rTPA window is < 3 h; IA rTPA is < 6 h
- Patient selection is most important
- Symptom onset < 6 h
- No hemorrhage by CT
- < 1/3 MCA territory hypodensity

- Preoperative assessment prior to carotid sacrifice: Balloon occlusion test (BOT) with SPECT
  ○ Decreased uptake on SPECT following BOT (> 15% decreased compared to contralateral side)
- Additional nuclear medicine imaging options
  ○ Xe-133 SPECT, XeCT and O-15 H2O PET: Assessment of regional cerebral blood flow
    ▪ Gold standard methods for quantifying (PET) or comparing (SPECT, CT) regional cerebral flood flow
  ○ Tc-99m diethylenetriaminepentaacetic acid (DTPA) SPECT: Assessment of blood brain barrier disruption (BBBD)
    ▪ Magnitude of disruption (> 2.5 times opposite normal side) correlates with lack of functional recovery

CT Findings
- NECT: Hemorrhagic vs. ischemic, hyperintense clotted vessel

MR Findings
- MR: CE with PWI, DWI
  ○ Acute infarction: Diffusion restriction with correlating ADC map
  ○ Subacute infarction: Gyral edema and enhancement +/- hemorrhagic transformation
  ○ Chronic infarction: Volume loss with marginal gliosis

Imaging Recommendations
- Best imaging tool
  ○ CEMR with DWI, PWI for acute/chronic cerebral vascular occlusive disease
  ○ MRA or contrast angiography for vascular anatomy
  ○ SPECT for problem solving in equivocal cases
- Protocol advice
  ○ ECD, HMPAO SPECT
    ▪ Place butterfly and allow to rest until no further discomfort
    ▪ Inject with 20-30 mCi ECD or HMPAO
    ▪ Wait 1 h before imaging (although can image after 10 minutes if critical)
    ▪ Decrease sensory input and motor activity for first 30 minutes after injection
    ▪ Diamox challenge: 1 g IV, wait 30 min before injecting tracer
  ○ Balloon occlusion test (BOT)
    ▪ With balloon inflated, injection 20-30 mCi ECD or HMPAO peripherally
    ▪ Ideally, allow balloon occlusion for 15 minutes prior to injection (if patient asymptomatic) to allow collateral vascular dilation
    ▪ Ideally, leave balloon inflated for 10-15 minutes after injection of tracer (if patient asymptomatic) to allow localization of tracer
    ▪ If abnormal, consider baseline study

DIFFERENTIAL DIAGNOSIS

Embolic
- Clot from left ventricle: Atrial fibrillation, poor ventricular function
- Clot from venous circulation through right-to-left shunt
- Clot discharged from unstable plaque

Neoplasm
- Enhancing mass rather than gyral enhancement
- Lack of regression on follow-up imaging

Cerebritis
- Early: Edema, enhancement, non-vascular territory, different clinical presentation
- Late: Gyriform ring enhancing patterns, volume loss, gliosis

Cerebral Contusion
- Lack of vascular territory

Venous Infarct
- Non-arterial territory, hypercoagulable state

CEREBRAL VASCULAR OCCLUSION

PATHOLOGY

General Features
- Genetics
  - Some genetic diseases predispose to stroke
    - Sickle cell disease, familial hyperlipidemia, familial hypercoagulable diseases, familial causes of aneurysms (adult polycystic kidney disease, many connective tissue diseases)
- Etiology
  - Vascular occlusive
    - Critical narrowing: Due to atherosclerosis, vasculitis, spasm, compression, dissection, thrombosis on unstable plaque
  - Embolic
    - Clot from heart or unstable plaque most common
  - Hemorrhagic
    - Causal factors: Hypertension, trauma, infarction from any cause, aneurysms, anticoagulant therapy
- Epidemiology
  - Stroke: Second most common cause of death worldwide
  - Number 1 cause of mortality in US
- Associated abnormalities: Cardiac disease, prothrombotic states

Gross Pathologic & Surgical Features
- Acute infarction: Pale, swollen brain, GM/WM boundary "smudging"
- Subacute infarction: Mass effect, frank hemorrhage, necrosis
- Chronic infarction: Liquefaction and cyst formation

Microscopic Features
- After 4 h: Eosinophilic neurons with pyknotic nuclei
- 15-24 h: Neutrophil invasion, necrotic nuclei ("eosinophil ghosts")
- 2-3 days: Blood derived phagocytes enter
- 1 week: Reactive astrocytosis, increased capillary density
- Late: Fluid-filled cavity lines with astrocytes

CLINICAL ISSUES

Presentation
- Most common signs/symptoms: Focal neurologic deficit
- Other signs/symptoms: Weakness, aphasia, decreased mental status

Demographics
- Age
  - Usually older adults
  - Younger patient: Consider underlying or genetic disease (sickle cell disease, Moyamoya, neurofibromatosis I, cardiac origin, drugs)
- Gender: M = F

Natural History & Prognosis
- Clinical presentation is confusing in 15-20% of strokes
- Malignant stroke (coma, death) in up to 10% of stroke patients

Treatment
- "Time is brain" - IV rTPA window is < 3 h; IA rTPA is < 6 h
- Patient selection is most important
  - Symptom onset < 6 h
  - No hemorrhage by CT
  - < 1/3 MCA territory hypodensity

DIAGNOSTIC CHECKLIST

Consider
- DWI with all MRs

Image Interpretation Pearls
- DWI positive for acute stroke only if ADC correlates
- SPECT can be useful for equivocal cases, penumbra imaging, presentation > 6 h

SELECTED REFERENCES

1. Hori M et al: The magnetic resonance Matas test: Feasibility and comparison with the conventional intraarterial balloon test occlusion with SPECT perfusion imaging. J Magn Reson Imaging. 21(6):709-14, 2005
2. Lampl Y et al: Prognostic significance of blood brain barrier permeability in acute hemorrhagic stroke. Cerebrovasc Dis. 20(6):433-7, 2005
3. Maulaz A et al: Selecting patients for early stroke treatment with penumbra images. Cerebrovasc Dis. 20 Suppl 2:19-24, 2005
4. Sitburana O et al: Magnetic resonance imaging: implication in acute ischemic stroke management. Curr Atheroscler Rep. 7(4):305-12, 2005
5. Ueda T et al: Single-photon emission CT imaging in acute stroke. Neuroimaging Clin N Am. 15(3):543-51, x, 2005
6. Mahagne MH et al: Voxel-based mapping of cortical ischemic damage using Tc 99m L,L-ethyl cysteinate dimer SPECT in acute stroke. J Neuroimaging. 14(1):23-32, 2004
7. Latchaw RE et al: Guidelines and recommendations for perfusion imaging in cerebral ischemia: A scientific statement for healthcare professionals by the writing group on perfusion imaging, from the Council on Cardiovascular Radiology of the American Heart Association. Stroke. 34(4):1084-104, 2003
8. Rudd JH et al: Imaging atherosclerotic plaque inflammation with [18F]-fluorodeoxyglucose positron emission tomography. Circulation. 105(23):2708-11, 2002
9. Sugawara Y et al: Usefulness of brain SPECT to evaluate brain tolerance and hemodynamic changes during temporary balloon occlusion test and after permanent carotid occlusion. J Nucl Med. 43(12):1616-23, 2002
10. Yamamoto Y et al: Preliminary results of Tc-99m ECD SPECT to evaluate cerebral collateral circulation during balloon test occlusion. Clin Nucl Med. 27(9):633-7, 2002
11. Ozgur HT et al: Correlation of cerebrovascular reserve as measured by acetazolamide-challenged SPECT with angiographic flow patterns and intra- or extracranial arterial stenosis. AJNR Am J Neuroradiol. 22(5):928-36, 2001
12. Baird AE et al: Sensitivity and specificity of 99mTc-HMPAO SPECT cerebral perfusion measurements during the first 48 hours for the localization of cerebral infarction. Stroke. 28(5):976-80, 1997

CEREBRAL VASCULAR OCCLUSION

IMAGE GALLERY

Typical

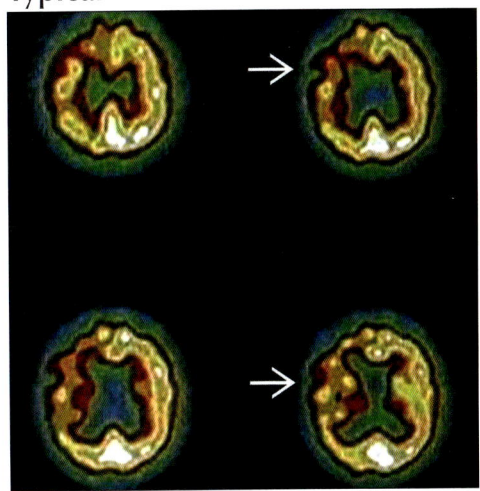

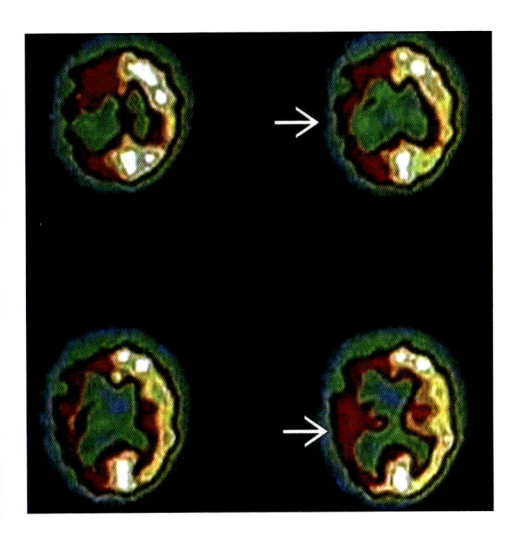

(Left) Axial HMPAO SPECT shows mild decreased perfusion in right cerebral hemisphere ➡ in patient with known right carotid occlusion. This is a baseline study. See next. *(Right)* Repeat SPECT with Diamox challenge in same patient as left shows lack of functional vascular reserve on right ➡, indicative of brain-at-risk (improved sensitivity over baseline study).

Typical

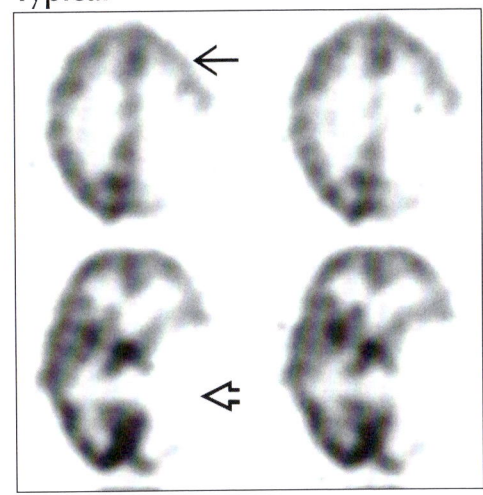

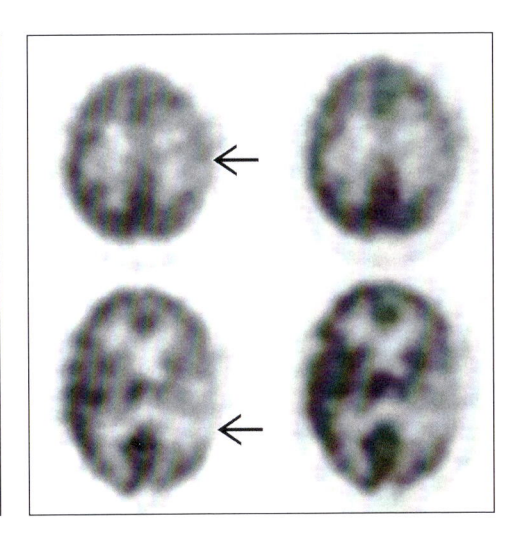

(Left) Axial HMPAO SPECT in conjunction with balloon occlusion of left ICA test to assess collateral adequacy. Good collateral flow from ACA territory ➡ but poor collateral to PCA, MCA territory ⇨. See baseline next. *(Right)* Baseline HMPAO SPECT (same patient as previous) shows some baseline decrease in the compromised territory ➡, likely due to mass effect from base of skull tumor.

Typical

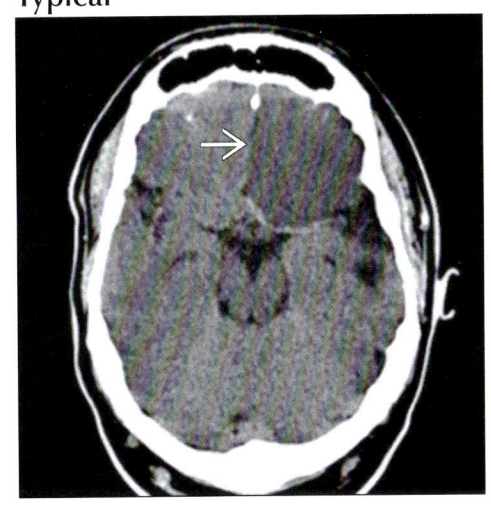

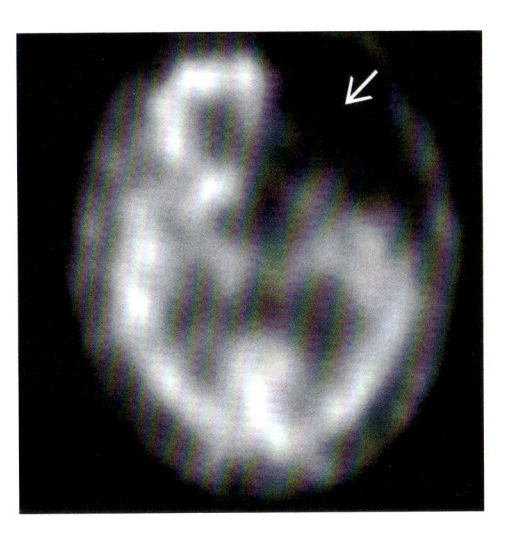

(Left) Axial NECT in 30 year old male with traumatic dissection of left ICA. Hypoattenuating left frontal lobe ➡ suggests infarcted brain. See next. *(Right)* Axial HMPAO SPECT in same patient as previous image confirms complete infarction ➡ of left frontal lobe, but intact perfusion to temporal and parietal lobes, suggesting collateral perfusion from left PCA.

BLOOD BRAIN BARRIER DISRUPTION

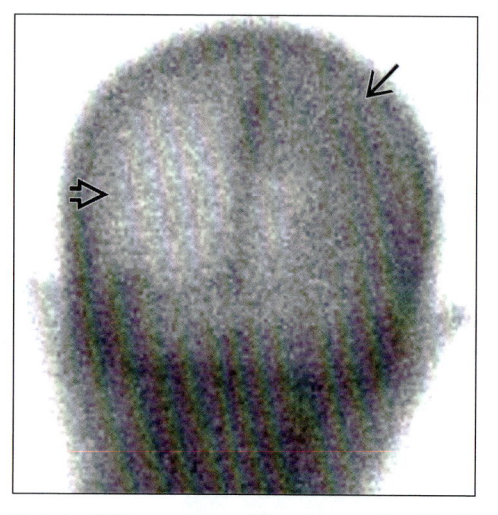

Posterior BBB scan shows diffuse, increased activity in right cortex ➔ after therapeutic right internal carotid BBBD in patient with CNS lymphoma. Compare to activity in normal left cortex ⇨.

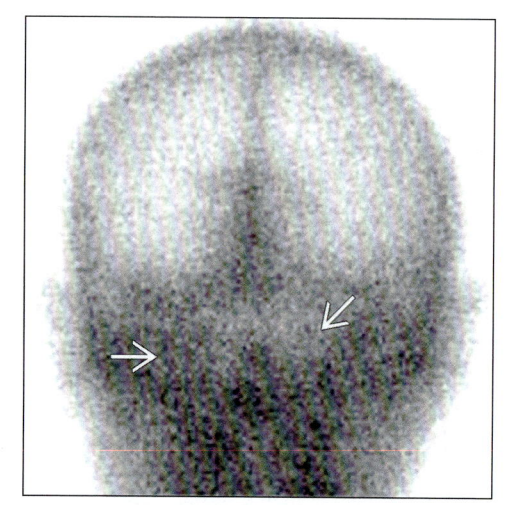

Posterior BBB scan shows diffuse, irregular activity ➔ in cerebellum after therapeutic vertebral artery BBBD in patient with cerebellar metastasis.

TERMINOLOGY

Abbreviations and Synonyms
- Blood brain barrier (BBB) disruption (BBBD)
- Therapeutic BBBD

Definitions
- Temporarily circumvent BBB, allowing local delivery of palliative chemotherapy to CNS neoplasm
  - Intra-arterial hyperosmolar mannitol into right/left internal carotid (R/LIC), vertebral arteries to chemically disrupt basement membrane
  - Chemotherapeutic agents instilled immediately following BBBD (5-20 minutes)
  - Palliative treatment of CNS neoplasms: Lymphoma, primitive neuroectodermal tumor, metastases
  - Experimental: Performed ~ 9 sites worldwide

IMAGING FINDINGS

General Features
- Best diagnostic clue
  - Irregular, increased activity at BBBD on Tc-99m glucoheptonate (GH) scan
  - Activity can diffuse over cerebral artery distribution

Nuclear Medicine Findings
- BBB Scan
  - 925 MBq (25 mCi) Tc-99m glucoheptonate IV
  - GH leaks across basement membrane of BBB
  - Quantification of BBBD
    - Subjective: Excellent > moderate > fair > nil
    - Ratio calculation: Anterior and middle circulation ratio for R/LIC, cerebellar fossa and posterior circulation ratio for vertebrobasilar

Imaging Recommendations
- Best imaging tool
  - Tc-99m GH BBB scan
    - First choice in patient who cannot undergo CECT: Contrast allergy, hardware artifacts, seizure
  - CECT (most common)
    - IV isosmotic non-ionic iodine contrast
    - Low seizure risk
    - Subjective quantification of BBBD
- Protocol advice

DDx: Blood Brain Barrier Disruption

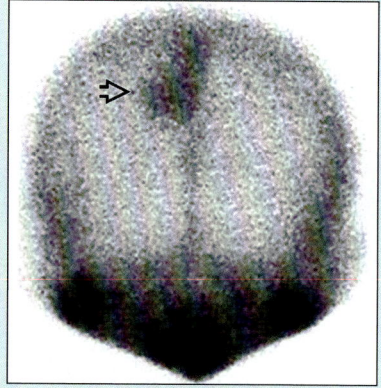

Post-Traumatic

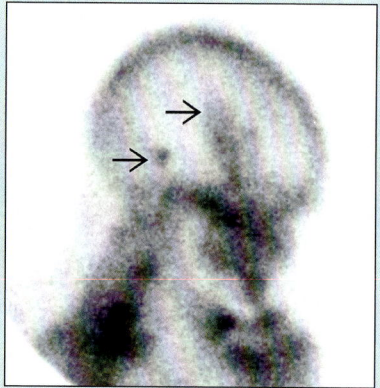

CNS Metastases

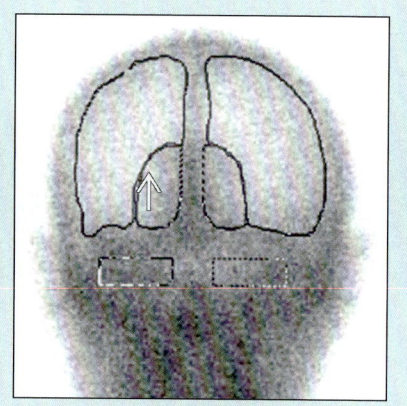

Normal BBB

BLOOD BRAIN BARRIER DISRUPTION

Key Facts

Terminology
- Therapeutic BBBD
- Temporarily circumvent BBB, allowing local delivery of palliative chemotherapy to CNS neoplasm

Imaging Findings
- Irregular, increased activity at BBBD on Tc-99m glucoheptonate (GH) scan
- Activity can diffuse over cerebral artery distribution
- 925 MBq (25 mCi) Tc-99m glucoheptonate IV

- GH leaks across basement membrane of BBB
- First choice in patient who cannot undergo CECT: Contrast allergy, hardware artifacts, seizure

Diagnostic Checklist
- Compare therapeutic BBBD to baseline BBB scan
- Incidental detection of BBBD: Radiotracers administered for other indications (bone scan, thyroid scan) can show BBBD

- Baseline: Identify preprocedure BBBD (CNS neoplasm, trauma, CVA)
- Post-BBBD: Identify extent of therapeutic BBBD
  - GH IV 1-2 minutes post BBBD and chemotherapy
  - Image 60-120 minutes post BBBD
- Imaging recommendations
  - BBBD ⇒ severe headache: Smooth, gentle transport and imaging procedures required
  - Monitor patient for complications post R/LIC, vertebral catheterization (bleeding, CVA)
  - Vertex: Flexible lead shield around neck ("Elizabethan collar") to block body counts
  - Posterior: Tuck chin (moves sigmoid and straight sinus activity from cerebellum)
- Correlative imaging features
  - CECT: Enhancement at BBBD

CLINICAL ISSUES

Presentation
- Most common signs/symptoms: Headache, seizure
- Other signs/symptoms: ↓ Mental status, ototoxicity

DIAGNOSTIC CHECKLIST

Image Interpretation Pearls
- Compare therapeutic BBBD to baseline BBB scan
- Incidental detection of BBBD: Radiotracers administered for other indications (bone scan, thyroid scan) can show BBBD
  - Tc-99m MDP localizes in BBBD, BBB calcification
  - Tc-99m pertechnetate localizes in BBBD

DIFFERENTIAL DIAGNOSIS

Medical
- Hypertension
- Infection/inflammation
- Cerebrovascular accident
- CNS malignancy

Injury
- Trauma
- ↑ Intracranial pressure

Iatrogenic
- Radiation therapy

SELECTED REFERENCES
1. Roman-Goldstein S et al: Osmotic blood-brain barrier disruption: CT and radionuclide imaging. AJNR Am J Neuroradiol. 15(3):581-90, 1994
2. Neuwelt EA et al: Osmotic blood-brain barrier modification: clinical documentation by enhanced CT scanning and/or radionuclide brain scanning. AJR Am J Roentgenol. 141(4):829-35, 1983
3. Neuwelt EA et al: Osmotic blood-brain barrier disruption. Computerized tomographic monitoring of chemotherapeutic agent delivery. J Clin Invest. 64(2):684-8, 1979

IMAGE GALLERY

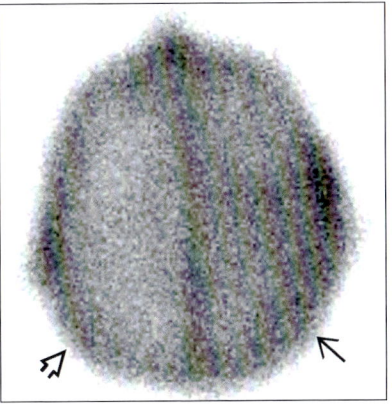

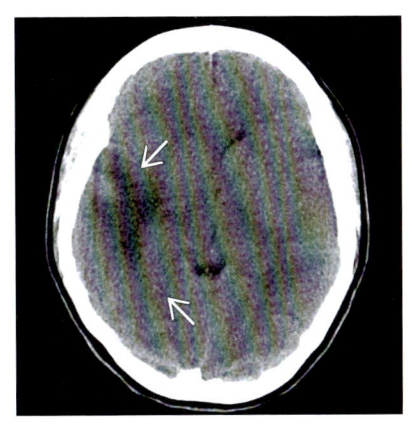

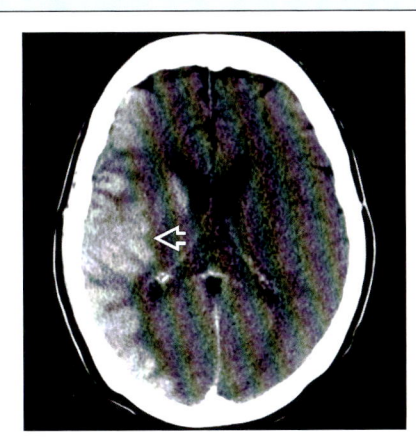

(Left) Vertex BBB scan shows diffuse, irregular activity in right cortex due to right internal carotid BBBD ➡ in patient who underwent therapeutic BBBD for CNS lymphoma. Compare to activity in left cortex ➡, with no BBBD. (Center) Axial CECT shows marked right temporal and deep white matter hypodensity ➡ in patient with CNS lymphoma. (Right) Axial CECT shows diffuse enhancement ➡ after therapeutic right internal carotid artery BBBD.

SEIZURE EVALUATION

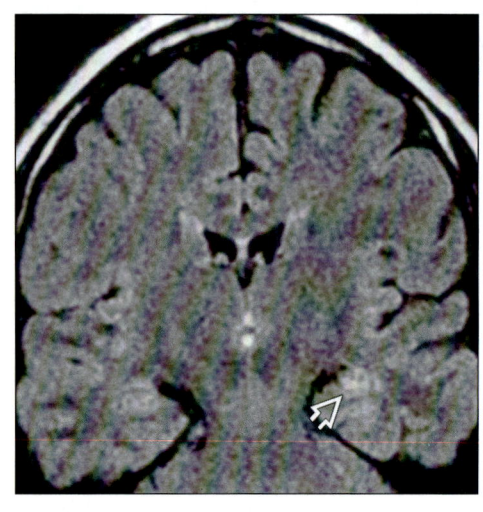

Coronal T2WI MR shows abnormal hyperintensity in the left hippocampus ➔ in a patient with TLE. Findings are characteristic for MTS.

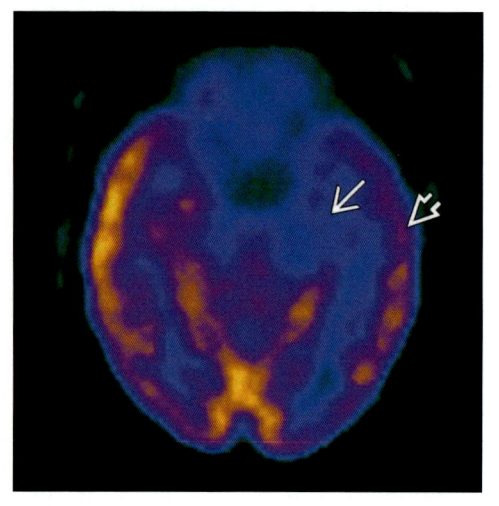

Axial interictal FDG PET, optimized for temporal lobe viewing, shows decreased mesial temporal ➔ and lateral temporal ➔ activity. FDG PET and MR consistent with left TLE and MTS.

TERMINOLOGY

Abbreviations and Synonyms
- Temporal lobe epilepsy (TLE), mesial temporal sclerosis (MTS)

Definitions
- Seizure: Hypersynchronous cortical neuron discharges
- Refractory seizure: Seizure not controlled by antiepileptic drugs
- Epilepsy: Disorder characterized by at least 2 unprovoked seizures
- Seizure classifications
  - Generalized: Diffuse, bilateral epileptiform on EEG; unable to localize
  - Partial onset: Focal origin from gray matter, often temporal lobe (TLE); may remain partial or become generalized
  - Unclassified: Cannot classify as partial or generalized

IMAGING FINDINGS

General Features
- Best diagnostic clue
  - Hypometabolism of mesial temporal lobe on interictal FDG-PET in TLE with lateralization on non-invasive EEG
  - T2WI MR demonstrating increased signal of the hippocampus as well as atrophy identifies hippocampal sclerosis
- Location: Mesial temporal lobe; bilateral findings in 20% of cases

Nuclear Medicine Findings
- Ictal SPECT imaging
  - Focal increase on ictal SPECT at epileptogenic zone if rapid injection (20-30 sec) from seizure onset
  - Variable pattern with poor localization if late injection (switching phenomenon)
  - Lipophilic radiopharmaceuticals for SPECT
    - Hexamethyl propylene amine oxime (HMPAO)
    - Ethylene cystine dimer (ECD) sodium bicisate
  - Advantages

DDx: Hypometabolic Foci in Non-Epileptic Subjects

Stroke

Lewy Body Disease

Alzheimer's with Infarct

SEIZURE EVALUATION

Key Facts

Imaging Findings
- Hypometabolism of mesial temporal lobe on interictal FDG-PET in TLE with lateralization on non-invasive EEG
- T2WI MR demonstrating increased signal of the hippocampus as well as atrophy identifies hippocampal sclerosis
- Location: Mesial temporal lobe; bilateral findings in 20% of cases
- Focal increase on ictal SPECT at epileptogenic zone if rapid injection (20-30 sec) from seizure onset
- FDG PET excellent in TLE (80-96% accuracy for interictal PET)

Top Differential Diagnoses
- Status Epilepticus
- Low Grade Astrocytoma
- Cortical Dysplasia

Pathology
- MTS associated with second lesion in 15%
- Decrease in hippocampal neurons and gliosis

Clinical Issues
- EEG often helpful for localization (60-90%)
- Intracranial EEG (subdural or depth electrodes) may be indicated if noninvasive studies discordant

Diagnostic Checklist
- T2 hyperintensity and atrophy of hippocampus most sensitive signs of MTS
- Relative decrease in affected temporal lobe with FDG PET

- High accuracy (85-90% in TLE; 60-90% in extra temporal lobe epilepsy) relative to other imaging modalities, including MR and MRS
- More accurate than interictal PET in extra temporal epilepsy
- Decision-making test if EEG, MR, and PET are equivocal or discordant
- Improved accuracy if subtraction and coregistration techniques are used
  - Disadvantages
    - Requires highly trained personnel and dedicated facility for monitoring
    - Supervised anti-seizure medication withdrawal
    - Patients with infrequent seizures are problematic
    - Injection within 20-30 seconds of seizure onset
- Interictal SPECT imaging
  - Accuracy is less than ictal SPECT or interictal PET
  - May be helpful when ictal SPECT is equivocal (late injection or rapid propagation)
  - Digital subtraction of interictal SPECT from ictal SPECT may improve accuracy by increasing the activation signal
  - Digital processing may improve accuracy
    - Subtraction ictal SPECT co-registered to MR (SISCOM)
    - Comparing relative perfusion on ictal or interictal SPECT to a normal database
- FDG PET
  - FDG PET excellent in TLE (80-96% accuracy for interictal PET)
  - Poor localization in extratemporal epilepsy (50-80% accuracy for interictal PET)
  - Not generally useful in ictal localization due to slow accumulation and short half life
  - Digital processing may improve accuracy
    - Three dimensional stereotactic surface projection (3D-SSP) to locate region of hypometabolism as compared to a normal data base (z score > 3 standard deviations from the mean are significant)

CT Findings
- NECT: Typically normal, insensitive to MTS

Angiographic Findings
- Wada testing, neuropsychological testing after intracarotid Amytal injection, may be performed prior to seizure surgery to assess feasibility of surgery

MR Findings
- T2WI
  - Hyperintense signal in the hippocampus
  - Atrophy of hippocampus

Imaging Recommendations
- Best imaging tool
  - High resolution MR for diagnosis
  - FDG PET if TLE is suspected and potential for surgery
  - Ictal SPECT for extratemporal epilepsy, or if unable to localize with MR and/or FDG PET after EEG
- Protocol advice
  - Injection within 30 seconds following seizure onset (ictal SPECT)
  - Temporal lobe and oblique processing and display (SPECT and PET)
  - EEG monitoring of interictal studies (SPECT and PET)

DIFFERENTIAL DIAGNOSIS

Status Epilepticus
- MR, ictal SPECT for focus location

Low Grade Astrocytoma
- FDG PET often negative

Cortical Dysplasia
- MR for evaluation

Choroidal Fissure Cyst
- Patients asymptomatic
- MR for diagnosis

Hippocampal Sulcus Remnant
- Patients asymptomatic

SEIZURE EVALUATION

- MR for diagnosis

Dysembryoplastic Neuroepithelial Tumor (DNET)
- MR for evaluation
- Patients with partial complex seizures

Cavernous Malformation
- MR for evaluation

PATHOLOGY

General Features
- General path comments
  - MTS is primary cause of complex partial seizures
  - MTS associated with second lesion in 15%
  - Hippocampus has complex anatomy
    - Ammon horn, dentate gyrus, hippocampal sulcus, fimbria, alveus, subiculum, parahippocampal gyrus, collateral sulcus
  - Ammon horn, cornu ammonis (CA), contains 4 zones of granular cells: CA1, CA2, CA3, CA4
    - CA1 most susceptible to ischemia
    - CA4 is also susceptible to ischemia
- Genetics: Familial cases of TLE reported
- Etiology
  - Controversial, may be acquired or developmental
    - Acquired: Shown to be related to changes after prolonged febrile seizures, status epilepticus, complicated delivery, and ischemia
    - Developmental: 2nd developmental lesion in 15%
  - Likely that MTS represents a common outcome of both acquired and developmental processes
  - Multiple seizures in early childhood are associated with hippocampal atrophy
- Epidemiology
  - MTS accounts for majority of patients undergoing temporal lobe surgery
  - Cortical dysplasia is most common dual pathology

Gross Pathologic & Surgical Features
- Atrophy of mesial temporal lobe
  - Hippocampal body (88%)
  - Hippocampal tail (61%)
  - Hippocampal head (51%)
  - Amygdala (12%)
- No hemorrhage or necrosis

Microscopic Features
- Decrease in hippocampal neurons and gliosis
- CA1, CA4, and CA3 are most affected
- May involve entire cornu ammonis and dentate gyrus
- Chronic astrogliosis with a fine fibrillary background containing bland nuclei of astrocytes and few remaining neurons

CLINICAL ISSUES

Presentation
- Most common signs/symptoms
  - Partial complex seizures
  - Other signs/symptoms
    - May progress to tonic-clonic seizures
- Clinical Profile
  - EEG often helpful for localization (60-90%)
  - Intracranial EEG (subdural or depth electrodes) may be indicated if noninvasive studies discordant
  - Patients often have remote history of childhood febrile seizures, medically intractable seizures

Demographics
- Age: Disease of childhood, young adults
- Gender: No gender predominance

Natural History & Prognosis
- Anterior temporal lobectomy successful in 70-95% patients with MR findings of MTS
- If MR is normal, success of anterior temporal lobectomy is 40-55%
- If amygdala involved, decreased success of surgery, approximately 50%

Treatment
- Medical treatment successful in only 25%
- Anterior temporal lobe resection for medically intractable disease
  - Resection includes anterior temporal lobe, majority of hippocampus, variable portions of amygdala
- Surgical removal of MTS is approximately 90% effective in seizure control

DIAGNOSTIC CHECKLIST

Consider
- MTS is most common cause of partial complex seizures
- Imaging findings of MTS may occasionally be found in normal, seizure-free, patients

Image Interpretation Pearls
- T2 hyperintensity and atrophy of hippocampus most sensitive signs of MTS
- Relative decrease in affected temporal lobe with FDG PET

SELECTED REFERENCES

1. Kuzniecky RI et al: Neuroimaging of epilepsy. Semin Neurol. 22(3):279-88, 2002
2. Jack CR Jr et al: Mesial temporal sclerosis: diagnosis with fluid-attenuated inversion-recovery versus spin-echo MR imaging. Radiology. 199(2):367-73, 1996
3. Ho SS et al: Parietal lobe epilepsy: clinical features and seizure localization by ictal SPECT. Neurology. 44(12):2277-84, 1994
4. Spencer SS: The relative contributions of MRI, SPECT, and PET imaging in epilepsy. Epilepsia. 35 Suppl 6:S72-89, 1994
5. Radtke RA et al: Temporal lobe hypometabolism on PET: predictor of seizure control after temporal lobectomy. Neurology. 43(6):1088-92, 1993
6. Marks DA et al: Localization of extratemporal epileptic foci during ictal single photon emission computed tomography. Ann Neurol. 31(3):250-5, 1992
7. Theodore WH et al: Pathology of temporal lobe foci: correlation with CT, MRI, and PET. Neurology. 40(5):797-803, 1990
8. Editorial. PET and SPECT in epilepsy. Lancet. 1:135-7, 1989

SEIZURE EVALUATION

IMAGE GALLERY

Typical

Typical

Typical

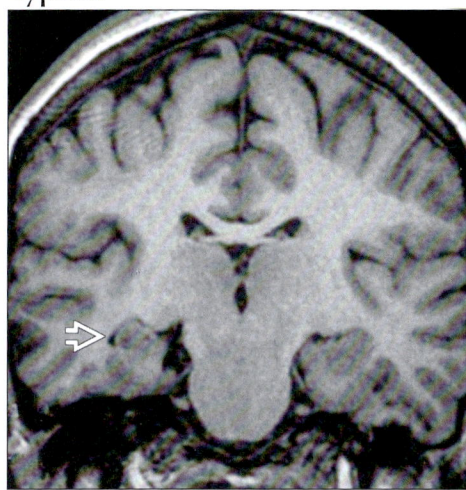

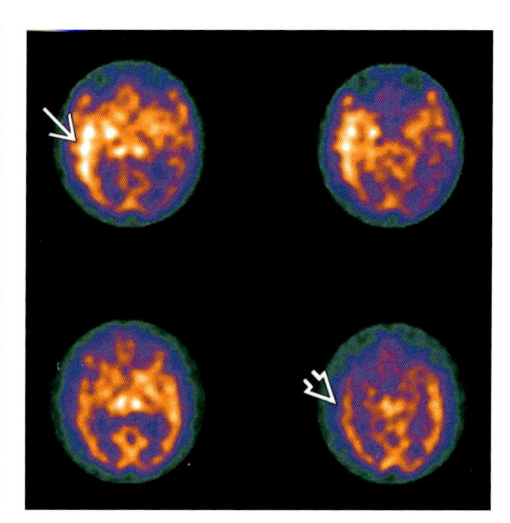

(Left) Coronal T1WI MR shows right hippocampal atrophy ➡ in patient with TLE. (Right) Upper: Ictal SPECT with Tc-99m HMPAO demonstrates right temporal perfusion increase ➡. Lower: Interictal SPECT with hypoperfusion of right temporal lobe ➡.

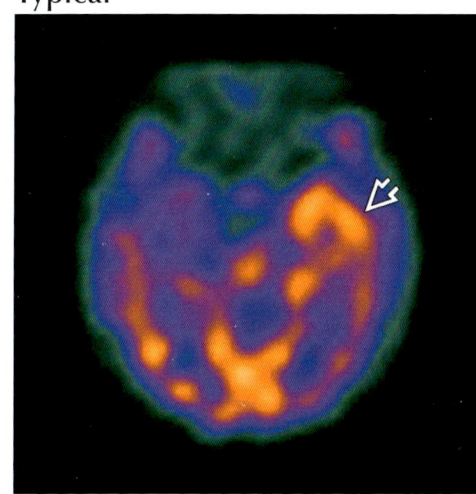

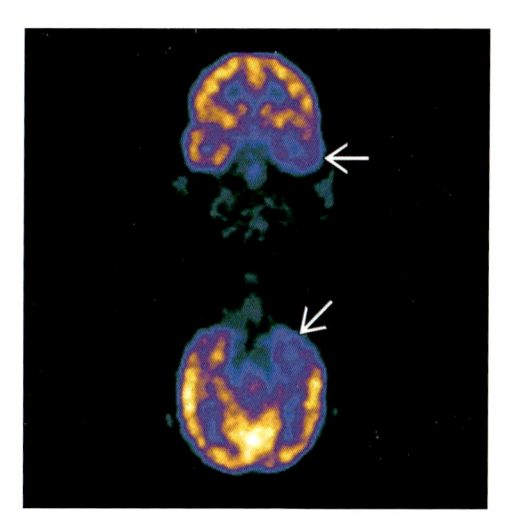

(Left) Axial ictal SPECT in patient with TLE and MTS of the left temporal lobe shows left temporal hyperperfusion ➡. (Right) Coronal and axial FDG PET on same patient shows hypometabolism of the left temporal lobe ➡ on interictal study.

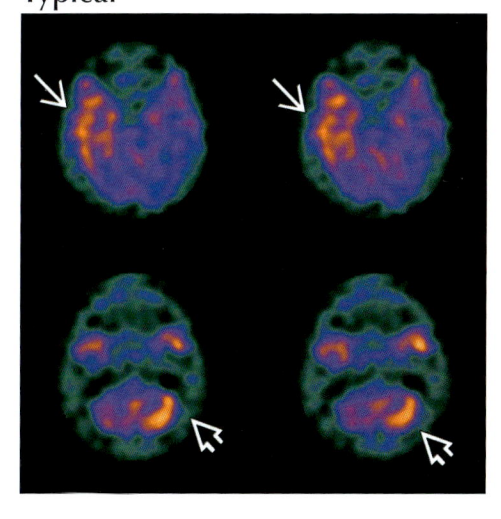

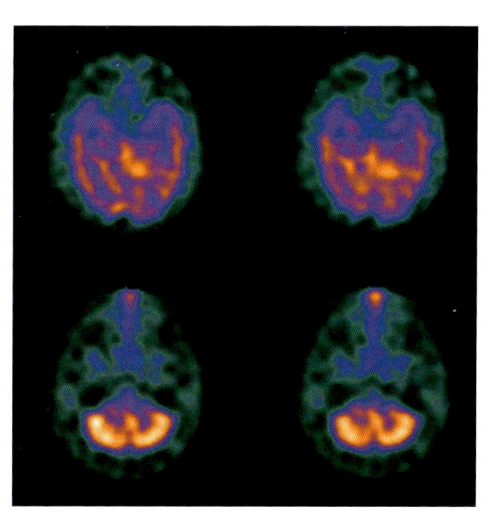

(Left) Ictal SPECT shows right temporal lobe hyperperfusion ➡ in patient with TLE. Note the crossed cerebellar increase ➡ often seen with ictal SPECT on opposite side of epileptogenic focus. (Right) Interictal SPECT (in same patient as left) with normalization of ictal SPECT findings.

SEIZURE EVALUATION

(Left) Axial ictal SPECT shows increased perfusion to the left temporal lobe ➡ in patient with TLE. (Right) Inferior view of dual threshold 3D surface rendered SPECT (in the same patient as left) shows epileptogenic focus ➡.

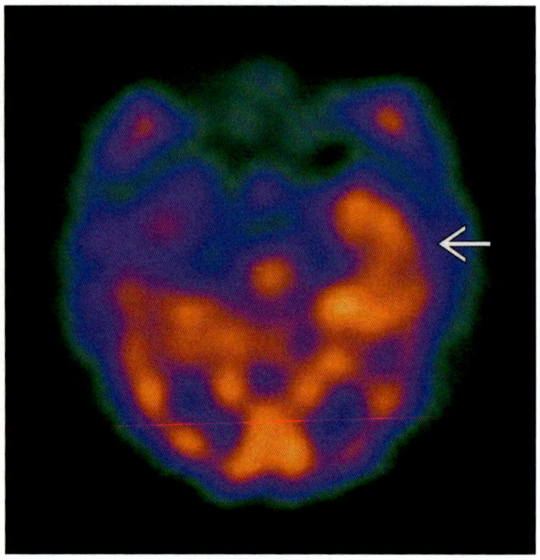

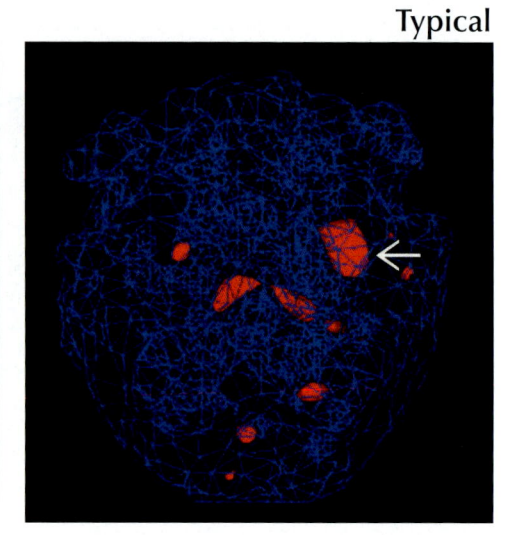

Typical

(Left) Axial ictal SPECT from upper brain (top) and mid brain through basal ganglia (bottom). Note prior surgery of right frontal and temporal regions and persistent multifocal hyperperfused regions ➡. Pattern associated with poor prognosis. (Right) Axial interictal SPECT (in same patient as left) shows normalization of ictal findings.

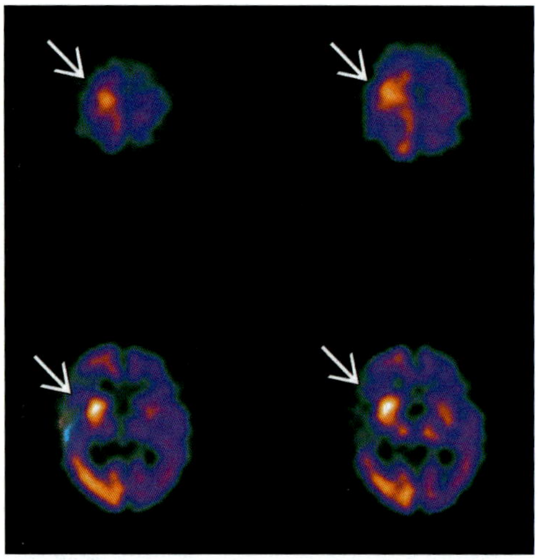

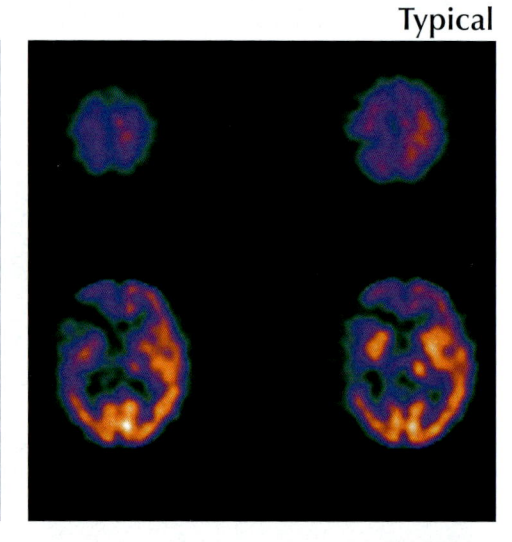

Typical

(Left) Axial ictal SPECT with data transformation to MR image. Note right frontal cortex localization ➡. (Right) Three dimensional stereotactic surface projection (3D-SSP) in same patient as left (Courtesy D. Eliashiv, MD).

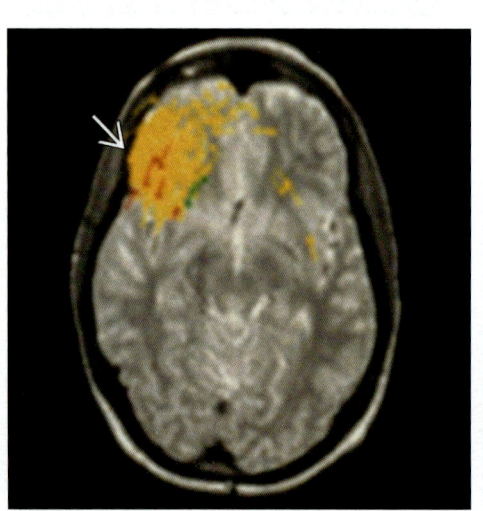

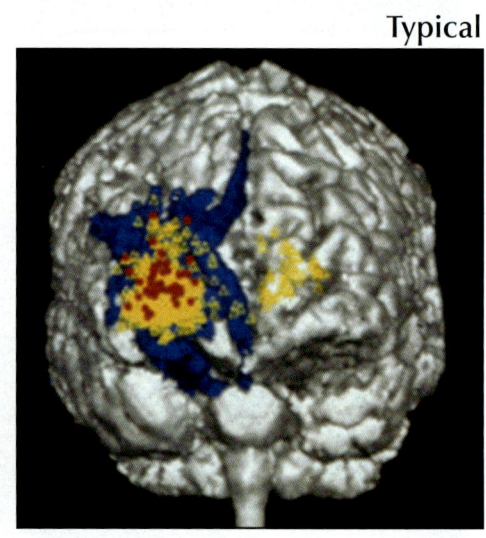

Typical

SEIZURE EVALUATION

Typical

Typical

Typical

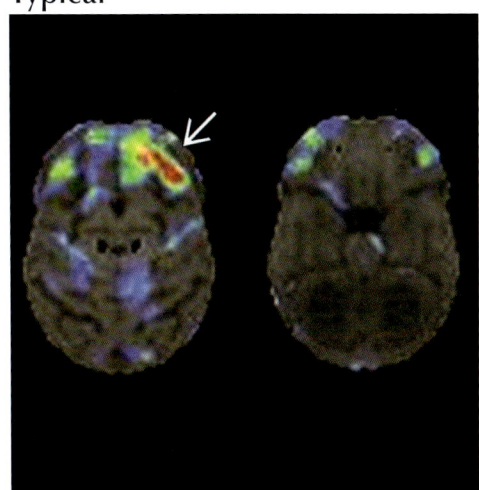

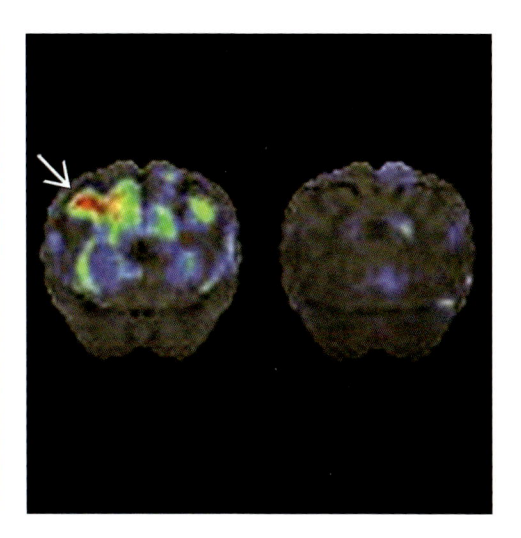

(Left) 3D-SSP ictal SPECT localizing ictal focus to superior right frontal cortex ➡. Superior and inferior surface views are shown. (Right) 3D-SSP in same patient as left shows anterior and posterior projections of localizing ictal focus ➡ (Courtesy S. Minoshima, MD).

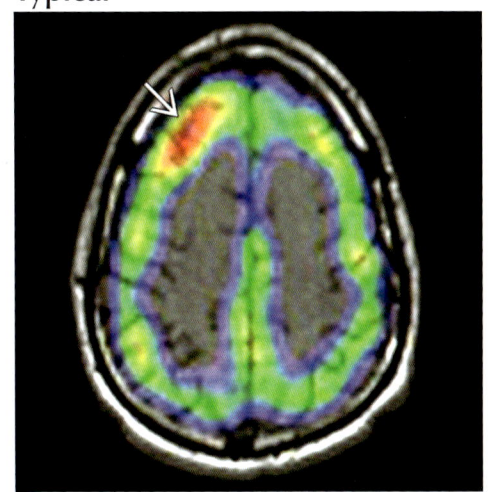

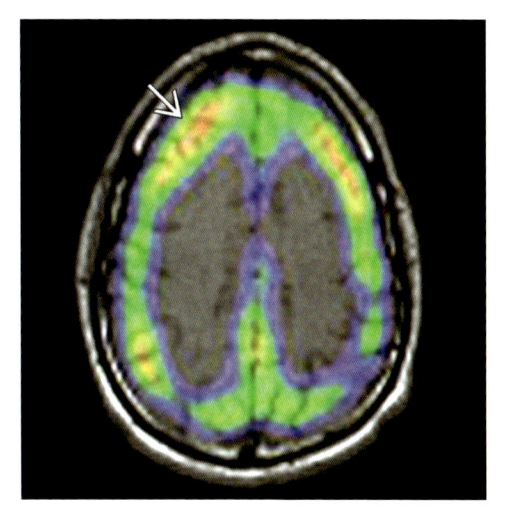

(Left) Axial ictal SPECT fused to MR shows right frontal epileptogenic focus ➡. (Right) Adjacent axial slice in same patient as left shows focus ➡ less clearly due to narrow cortical focus.

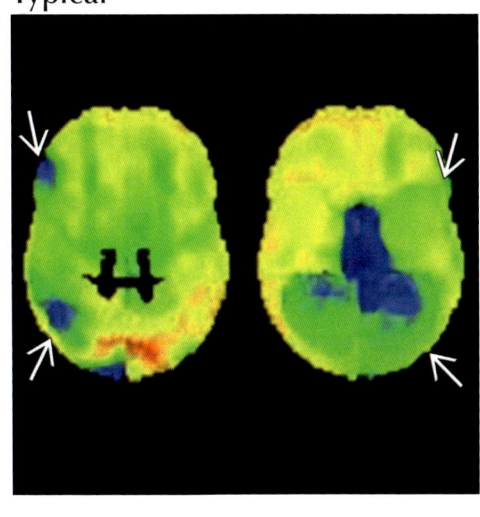

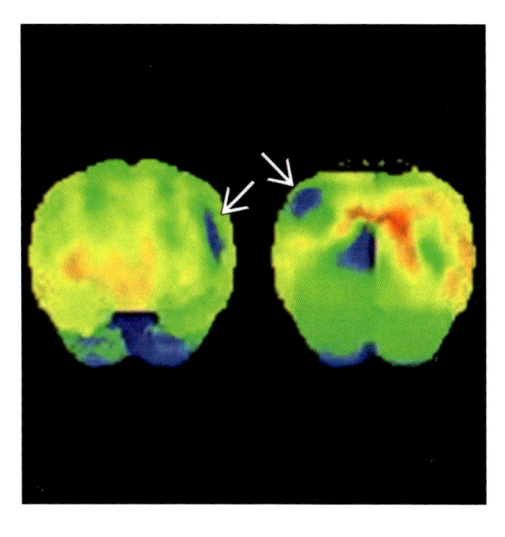

(Left) Superior and inferior views of C11 Flumazenil PET (benzodiazepine receptor antagonist). 3D-SSP images in patient with TLE. Reduced binding to benzodiazepine receptors in left temporal and parietal regions correspond to the epileptogenic zone ➡. (Right) Anterior and posterior projections in same patient as left show epileptogenic zone ➡ in the right temporal and parietal regions (Courtesy S. Minoshima, MD).

ALZHEIMER DISEASE

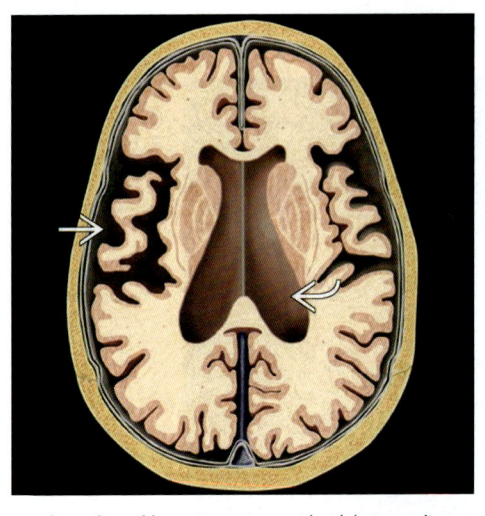

Axial graphic of brain in patient with Alzheimer disease shows temporal-parietal atrophy ➡ and ventricular enlargement ➡.

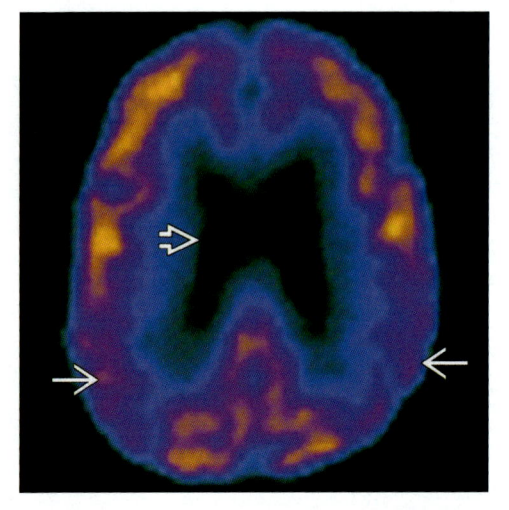

Axial FDG PET of brain in elderly patient with AD shows reduced metabolism in the parietal/posterior temporal regions ➡ and ventricular enlargement ➡.

TERMINOLOGY

Abbreviations and Synonyms
- Alzheimer disease (AD)
- Dementia of the Alzheimer type (DAT)
- Mild cognitive impairment (MCI)

Definitions
- Progressive neurodegenerative disease of brain of unknown etiology, likely related to amyloid cascade with β-amyloid and tau protein deposition ⇒ neuronal, glial cell death

IMAGING FINDINGS

General Features
- Best diagnostic clue
  - Parietal, posterior temporal lobes: Relative reduction in metabolism (FDG PET) or perfusion (SPECT)
  - Volume loss in parietal, temporal lobes on CT/MR: Nonspecific for AD
  - Hippocampal and entorhinal cortex volume loss on MR improves specificity
  - Serial studies show progression
  - Early AD: Highest sensitivity (80%) and specificity with FDG PET

Nuclear Medicine Findings
- PET and SPECT
  - Early AD
    - Relative reduction in activity in parietal, temporal lobes and posterior cingulate gyri
    - Usually symmetric, asymmetry not unusual
  - Early and advanced AD
    - Sparing of sensory motor cortex, basal ganglia, thalamus, primary visual cortex
  - Advanced AD
    - Progression of findings present in early AD
    - Usually symmetric
    - Frontal lobe reduction
    - Moderate to severe atrophy
  - FDG PET sensitivity for possible/probable AD > SPECT (80% vs. 65%)
  - FDG PET accuracy for possible/probable AD: 15-20% greater than SPECT
  - Accuracy of diagnosis with FDG PET or SPECT > clinical assessment, especially in early AD

DDx: Non-Alzheimer Dementia

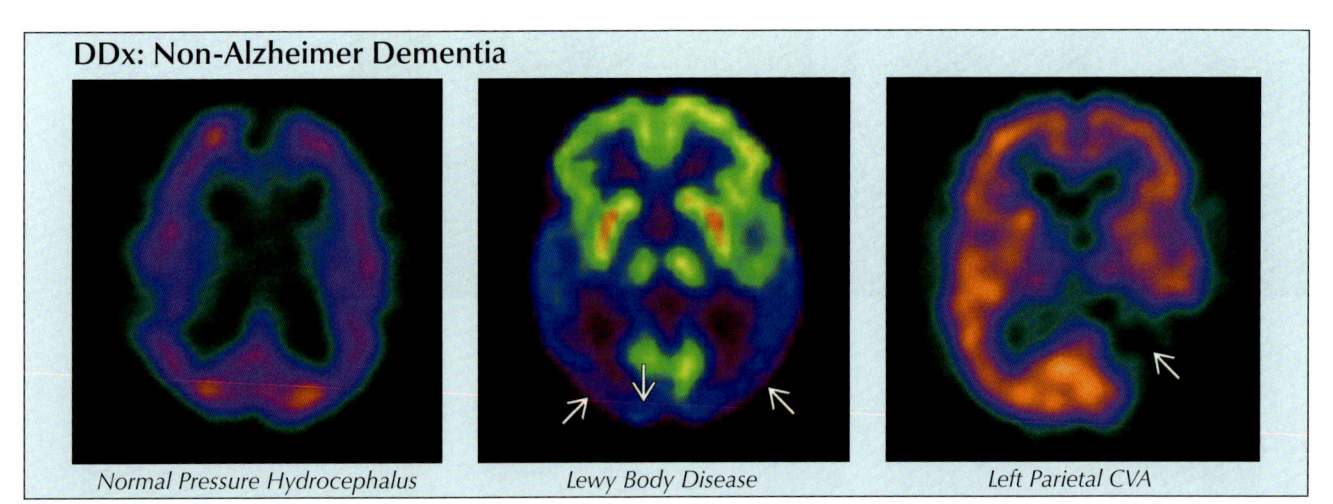

Normal Pressure Hydrocephalus | *Lewy Body Disease* | *Left Parietal CVA*

ALZHEIMER DISEASE

Key Facts

Terminology
- Progressive neurodegenerative disease of brain of unknown etiology, likely related to amyloid cascade with β-amyloid and tau protein deposition ⇒ neuronal, glial cell death

Imaging Findings
- Parietal, posterior temporal lobes: Relative reduction in metabolism (FDG PET) or perfusion (SPECT)
- Accuracy of diagnosis with FDG PET or SPECT > clinical assessment, especially in early AD
- Severity of findings on FDG PET or SPECT: Parallel or often precede clinical dementia, degree of cognitive impairment
- Probability of AD low if no progression on FDG PET or SPECT within 12-18 months

Top Differential Diagnoses
- Vascular Dementia
- Lewy Body Disease
- Frontotemporal Dementia
- Creutzfeldt-Jakob Disease
- Progressive Supranuclear Palsy
- Corticobasal Degeneration
- Reversible Dementias

Diagnostic Checklist
- Parietal/temporal with occipital involvement on FDG PET or SPECT likely Lewy body disease, not AD
- Hippocampal atrophy on MR with biparietal defects on FDG PET or SPECT predicts AD
- Basal ganglia defects along with classic AD findings on FDG PET or SPECT suggests vascular disease also contributing to dementia

---

  ○ Severity of findings on FDG PET or SPECT: Parallel or often precede clinical dementia, degree of cognitive impairment
  ○ Probability of AD low if no progression on FDG PET or SPECT within 12-18 months

CT Findings
- NECT
  ○ ↑ Perihippocampal fissures due to atrophy of hippocampus and parahippocampal gyrus
  ○ Temporal & parietal lobe volume loss

MR Findings
- T1WI, T2WI
  ○ Entorhinal cortex, hippocampal volume loss
- MR volumetric analysis of hippocampi and parahippocampal gyri may help distinguish patients with mild cognitive impairment (at risk for proceeding to AD) from normal elderly subjects

Imaging Recommendations
- Best imaging tool
  ○ FDG PET
    ▪ Differentiate AD from other causes of memory impairment in MCI patients
    ▪ Differentiate AD from other dementias when exact cause uncertain
- Protocol advice
  ○ Patient preparation critical
    ▪ IV in place for 10-15 min prior to injection
    ▪ Inject in dimly lit room with only background noise allowed
    ▪ Image 45-60 min post injection
  ○ 10 mCi (370 MBq) F-18 FDG IV
  ○ 20-25 mCi (740-925 MBq) Tc-99m HMPAO; 20-25 mCi (740-925 MBq) Tc-99m ECD
- Confirm findings with MR
  ○ Hippocampus and entorhinal atrophy
  ○ Evaluate ventricular size and presence/absence of vascular disease
- Research PET radiotracers
  ○ 11C-PIB (congo red analog); F-18 FDDNP (thioflavin analog)
    ▪ Both bind to β-amyloid marker

DIFFERENTIAL DIAGNOSIS

Vascular Dementia
- Cerebrovascular accident (CVA) in large, small vessels

Lewy Body Disease
- Findings similar to AD, especially parietal and posterior temporal
- Occipital involvement usually present ; ± visual hallucinations

Frontotemporal Dementia
- Pick disease
- Non-Pick disease frontotemporal (tau protein pathology)
- Reduction in activity in frontal lobes, anterior temporal lobes predominate
  ○ Advanced disease may be difficult to separate from advanced AD

Creutzfeldt-Jakob Disease
- Mad cow disease (prion disorder)
- Rapidly progressive cortical destruction
- May involve any region of cortex

Progressive Supranuclear Palsy
- Primarily frontal lobe with involvement of basal ganglia

Corticobasal Degeneration
- Frontal/parietal asymmetric defects with basal ganglia involvement

Reversible Dementias
- Normal pressure hydrocephalus: Enlarged ventricles, cortical hypoperfusion and metabolism due to compression
- Subdural fluid collections
- Depression
- Hypothyroidism
- Mass lesions

ALZHEIMER DISEASE

- Infection
- Autoimmune disorders

PATHOLOGY

General Features
- General path comments: Degenerative process starts in medial temporal lobes ⇒ parahippocampal gyri ⇒ temporal and frontal lobes ⇒ motor and visual cortex
- Genetics
  - Most cases spontaneous; 5-10% familial
  - Early-onset, familial, autosomal dominant AD
    - Mutations in amyloid precursor protein gene on chromosome 21
  - Aggressive AD often associated with apolipoprotein E (ApoE) ϵ4 allele on chromosome 19
- Etiology
  - β-amyloid precursor protein has pivotal role in AD
  - Neurofibrillary tangles (NTs) and senile plaques
    - Abnormal protein deposition: β-amyloid in senile/neuritic plaques, tau in NTs
  - Amyloid and tau deposited along course of cortical memory pathways cause neuronal damage
  - Senile plaques extraneuronal, promote attack by microglia ("inflammatory cascade")
- Epidemiology: AD most common cause of cerebral atrophy and neurodegenerative dementia in elderly

Gross Pathologic & Surgical Features
- Shrunken gyri, widened sulci

Microscopic Features
- Neuritic plaques (NPs), NTs in hippocampus, neocortical/some subcortical areas
- Amyloid angiopathy (β-amyloid major component of NPs and blood vessels in AD)
- Disruption/loss of axonal membranes, myelin

Staging, Grading or Classification Criteria
- Transentorhinal stage = clinically asymptomatic: NTs develop in parahippocampal gyrus
- Limbic stage = MCI: NTs dramatically increase, begin to develop in hippocampus
- Neocortical stage = severe dementia: NTs in temporal and parietal cortex, eventually spread to entire cortex

CLINICAL ISSUES

Presentation
- Most common signs/symptoms
  - Initial symptom = memory impairment
  - Major dysfunction in memory and cognition
  - Personality changes
- Clinical Profile
  - Clinical subtypes
    - MCI: Early, mild memory impairment; no deficits in cognitive domains other than memory
    - Possible AD: Dementia features in presence of second disease that could cause memory deficit but not likely cause
    - Probable AD: Memory deficits on neuropsychological testing, progressive worsening of memory and ≥ 2 cognitive functions
- Primarily disease of old age; autosomal dominant AD as early as 4th decade
- Visual variant of AD: Impaired visuospatial skills without memory complaints

Demographics
- Age
  - Prevalence increases with age
  - 50% of population > 80 years have dementia
  - 70% of all dementias due to AD
- Gender: M:F = 1:2

Natural History & Prognosis
- Progressive impairment of intellectual functions
- MCI conversion to AD is 10-15% per year

Treatment
- Cholinesterase inhibitors (not curative)
- Amyloid vaccine under investigation

DIAGNOSTIC CHECKLIST

Image Interpretation Pearls
- Parietal/temporal with occipital involvement on FDG PET or SPECT likely Lewy body disease, not AD
- Hippocampal atrophy on MR with biparietal defects on FDG PET or SPECT predicts AD
- Basal ganglia defects along with classic AD findings on FDG PET or SPECT suggests vascular disease also contributing to dementia

SELECTED REFERENCES

1. Norfray JF et al: Alzheimer's disease: neuropathologic findings and recent advances in imaging. AJR Am J Roentgenol. 182(1):3-13, 2004
2. Sair HI et al: In vivo amyloid imaging in Alzheimer's disease. Neuroradiology. 46(2):93-104, 2004
3. Silverman DH: Brain 18F-FDG PET in the diagnosis of neurodegenerative dementias: comparison with perfusion SPECT and with clinical evaluations lacking nuclear imaging. J Nucl Med. 45(4):594-607, 2004
4. Chetelat G et al: Mild cognitive impairment: Can FDG-PET predict who is to rapidly convert to Alzheimer's disease? Neurology. 60(8):1374-7, 2003
5. Drzezga A et al: Cerebral metabolic changes accompanying conversion of mild cognitive impairment into Alzheimer's disease: a PET follow-up study. Eur J Nucl Med Mol Imaging. 30(8):1104-13, 2003
6. Devous MD Sr: Functional brain imaging in the dementias: role in early detection, differential diagnosis, and longitudinal studies. Eur J Nucl Med Mol Imaging. 29(12):1685-96, 2002
7. Herholz K et al: Direct comparison of spatially normalized PET and SPECT scans in Alzheimer's disease. J Nucl Med. 43(1):21-6, 2002
8. Silverman DH et al: Added clinical benefit of incorporating 2-deoxy-2-[18F]fluoro-D-glucose with positron emission tomography into the clinical evaluation of patients with cognitive impairment. Mol Imaging Biol. 4(4):283-93, 2002

ALZHEIMER DISEASE

IMAGE GALLERY

Typical

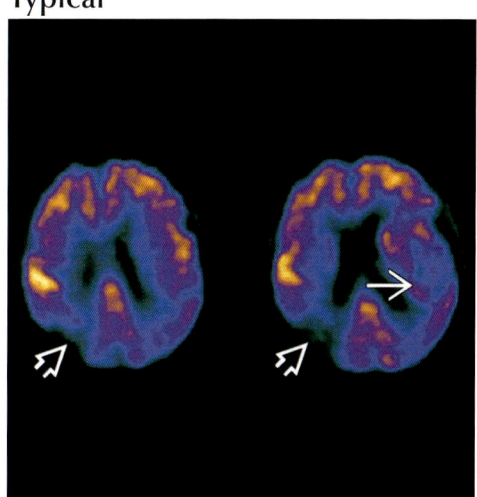

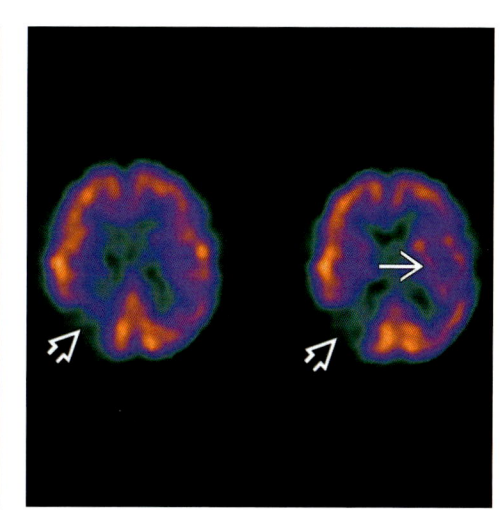

(Left) Axial FDG PET of brain in patient with AD shows concomitant right parietal stroke ➡ in addition to decreased activity in left parietotemporal lobes ➡. *(Right)* Axial slices of Tc-99m ECD SPECT scan in same patient as left. Note right parietal stroke ➡. Findings in temporoparietal regions ➡ are more subtle than on FDG PET.

Typical

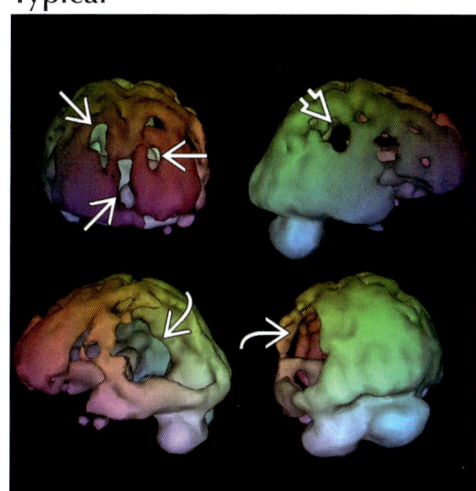

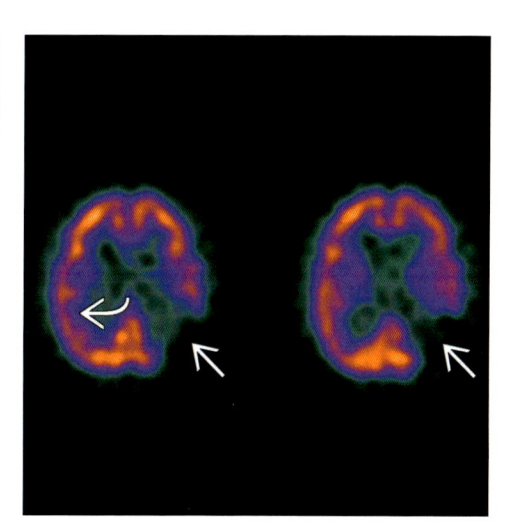

(Left) Tc-99m ECD surface-rendered SPECT images in patient with early AD shows left parietal stroke ➡ and mild defect in right parietal cortex ➡. Additionally, mild atrophic/degenerative changes noted in frontal lobes ➡. *(Right)* Axial Tc-99m ECD SPECT in same patient as left. Note mild perfusion defect in right parietal cortex ➡ corresponding to that on surface-rendered images. Left parietal stroke also evident ➡.

Typical

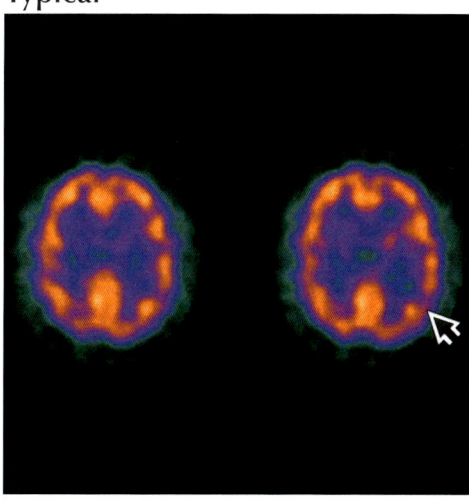

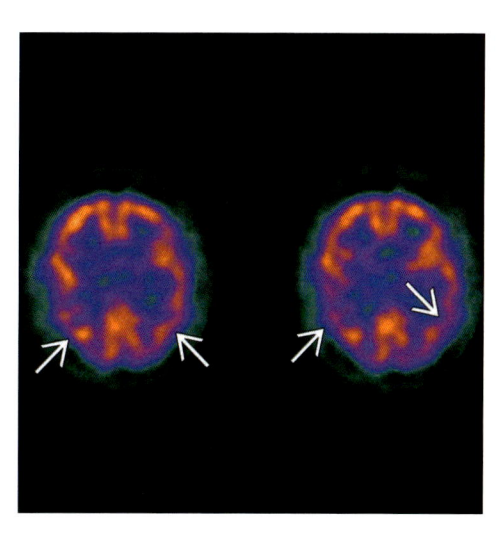

(Left) Axial SPECT of brain in patient with mild cognitive impairment. Note mild reduction in parietal perfusion on left ➡. *(Right)* Axial SPECT of brain in same patient at left 22 months later. Note marked reduction in parietal perfusion bilaterally ➡, signifying progression to AD.

DEMENTIA & NEURODEGENERATIVE, OTHER

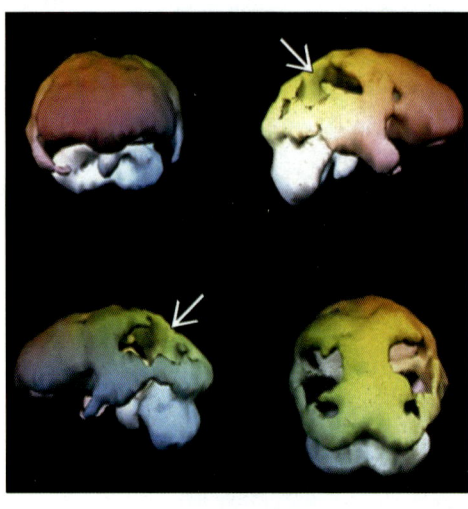

Alzheimer dementia. Note parietal and posterior temporal reductions ➡ and sparing of occipital and frontal lobes.

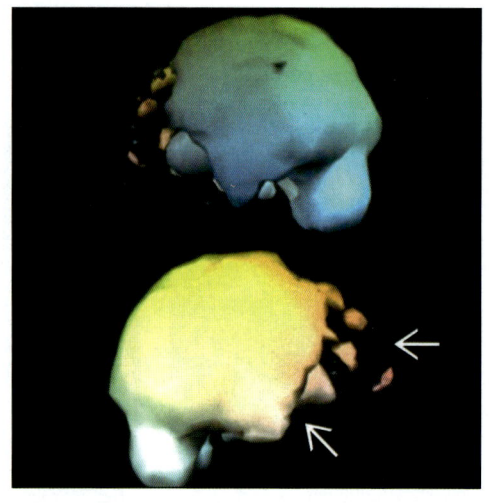

Frontotemporal dementia. Note frontal and anterior temporal reductions ➡ and sparing of parietal, posterior temporal, and occipital regions.

TERMINOLOGY

Abbreviations and Synonyms
- Lewy body disease (LBD); frontotemporal dementia (FTD) or Pick disease; Creutzfeldt-Jakob disease (CJD); progressive supranuclear palsy (PSP); corticobasal degeneration (CBD); vascular dementia (VaD), multi-infarct dementia (MID); normal pressure hydrocephalus (NPH); post-traumatic dementia (PDT); Huntington disease (HD); multiple system atrophy (MSA)

Definitions
- Decline in memory, intellectual and cognitive function caused by damage to, or progressive degeneration of, neuronal and glial cells
- Characterized by amnestic and combination of personality, behavioral, or motor disturbances

IMAGING FINDINGS

General Features
- Best diagnostic clue
  - LBD: Generalized decreased cortical perfusion (SPECT) and metabolism (FDG PET) mainly parietal and posterior temporal
    - LBD similar to Alzheimer dementia (AD); greater occipital lobe involvement
  - FTD: Frontal and temporal lobe hypometabolism or hypoperfusion on FDG PET or SPECT; parietal lobe involvement in advanced cases
  - CJD: Characteristic features on MR include "hockey stick" sign in putamen and head of caudate nucleus, "pulvinar" sign in bilateral pulvinar thalamic nuclei; FDG PET and perfusion SPECT demonstrate cortical and striatal defects that correlate with pathologic sites
  - PSP: Hypometabolic/hypoperfusion pattern primarily of frontal lobe, caudate and putamen
  - CBD: Asymmetric reductions in frontal/parietal lobes and basal ganglia
  - VaD/MID: Cortical and striatal lesions on CT or MR, including white matter; acetazolamide perfusion SPECT may worsen from baseline (reduced cerebrovascular reserve)

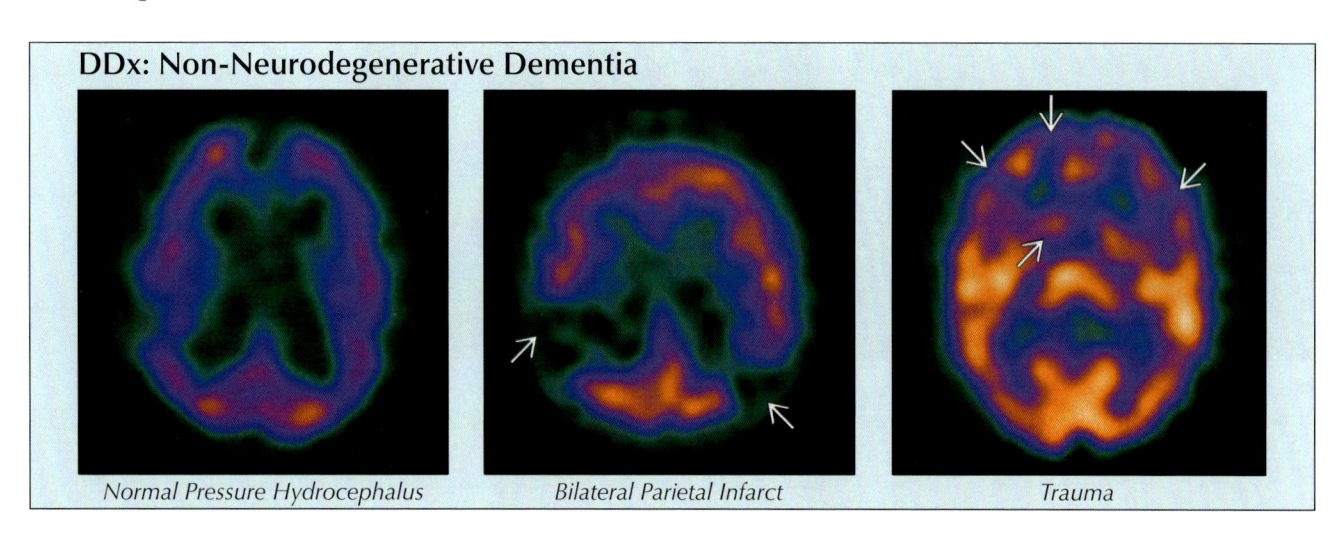

DDx: Non-Neurodegenerative Dementia

Normal Pressure Hydrocephalus

Bilateral Parietal Infarct

Trauma

DEMENTIA & NEURODEGENERATIVE, OTHER

Key Facts

Terminology
- Lewy body disease (LBD); frontotemporal dementia (FTD) or Pick disease; Creutzfeldt-Jakob disease (CJD); progressive supranuclear palsy (PSP); corticobasal degeneration (CBD); vascular dementia (VaD), multi-infarct dementia (MID); normal pressure hydrocephalus (NPH); post-traumatic dementia (PDT); Huntington disease (HD); multiple system atrophy (MSA)

Imaging Findings
- LBD: Generalized decreased cortical perfusion (SPECT) and metabolism (FDG PET) mainly parietal and posterior temporal
- LBD similar to Alzheimer dementia (AD); greater occipital lobe involvement
- FTD: Frontal and temporal lobe hypometabolism or hypoperfusion on FDG PET or SPECT; parietal lobe involvement in advanced cases
- CJD: Characteristic features on MR include "hockey stick" sign in putamen and head of caudate nucleus, "pulvinar" sign in bilateral pulvinar thalamic nuclei; FDG PET and perfusion SPECT demonstrate cortical and striatal defects that correlate with pathologic sites
- PSP: Hypometabolic/hypoperfusion pattern primarily of frontal lobe, caudate and putamen
- CBD: Asymmetric reductions in frontal/parietal lobes and basal ganglia
- VaD/MID: Cortical and striatal lesions on CT or MR, including white matter; acetazolamide perfusion SPECT may worsen from baseline (reduced cerebrovascular reserve)

Nuclear Medicine Findings
- FDG PET and SPECT (functional brain imaging)
  - High sensitivity for identifying neurodegenerative abnormalities (PET > SPECT)
  - Moderate specificity for subcategorizing dementias
    - Superior to clinical assessment and cross-sectional imaging alone
    - Specificity ~ 75% for functional brain imaging in diagnosing AD
  - Can help differentiate between AD and non-Alzheimer dementias
    - Occipital lobe involvement usually present in LBD but not AD
    - Decreased activity of frontal and anterior temporal lobes distinguish FTD from AD (hypometabolic pattern initially seen in posterior temporal and parietal lobes)
    - Variable asymmetric cortical reduction seen in VaD/MID usually distinct from parietal/temporal lobe pattern seen in AD; MR confirmation and/or cerebrovascular reserve testing helpful
    - PSP: Global hypometabolism with relative selectivity in frontal lobe; decreased regional cerebral blood flow in caudate and putamen
    - "Swiss cheese" pattern seen with drug abuse dementia
  - Functional brain imaging useful in differentiating neurodegenerative from other dementias
    - Psychiatric dementia usually normal functional brain study; severe depression may have frontal lobe reduction
    - NPH demonstrates major reduction in periventricular/ventricular regions; In-111 DTPA cysternography useful in confirming diagnosis and determining shunt candidate
    - Normal pattern on functional brain imaging seen in hypothyroid dementia

MR Findings
- T1WI, T2WI
  - LBD: Superior to CT in identifying hippocampal atrophy
  - CJD: Preferred imaging test; "hockey stick", "pulvinar" signs
  - VaD: White matter lesions (not seen in LBD)
  - FTD: T2 hyperintense frontotemporal white matter
  - PSP: Midbrain atrophy (not seen in CBD), both with eye movement disturbance
  - MSA: "Hot cross bun" sign (T2 hyperintensity cruciform pontine), atrophy of pons, cerebellum, cortex

Imaging Recommendations
- Best imaging tool
  - Functional brain imaging (PET > SPECT) for LBD, FTD, HD, PSP; MR may be helpful
  - MR for CJD, MSA, VaD/MID; SPECT/PET may be helpful
- Protocol advice: Minimal stimulation (resting) protocol for FDG PET or SPECT (acetazolamide SPECT for cerebrovascular reserve is exception)

DIFFERENTIAL DIAGNOSIS

Alzheimer Disease
- Reduced activity in parietal, posterior temporal and posterior cingulate regions early, frontal lobes late
- Hippocampal atrophy on MR

Normal Pressure Hydrocephalus
- Dilated ventricles on CT or MR
- Metabolic or perfusion reductions in lateral cortex (frontal and parietal), separation of caudate heads
- Reduced activity in periventricular white matter and ventricular regions > expected for age

Huntington Disease
- Major reduction in basal ganglia metabolism and perfusion (worse in caudate)
- Cortical reductions (late)

Post-Traumatic Dementia
- Pattern of abnormality on functional imaging variable: Depends on severity, directional forces at injury
- Chronic subdural may cause significant asymmetry

DEMENTIA & NEURODEGENERATIVE, OTHER

- Deceleration injury may cause anterior frontal and temporal tip reductions
- Atrophic pattern may occur; worse with increasing severity of injury
- Focal reduction correlates with encephalomalacia and other cortical abnormalities on CT or MR
- Basal ganglia, thalamic abnormalities may be present

Drug Related Dementia
- Cocaine and amphetamine abuse: Random small focal defects throughout the brain
  - "Swiss cheese" pattern on FDG PET and SPECT
- Alcohol abuse: May demonstrate frontal lobe decrease

Autoimmune Dementia
- Vasculitis pattern in systemic lupus; frontal watershed abnormalities
- Small cortical defects mainly frontal lobe

PATHOLOGY

General Features
- Lewy body disease
  - Generalized protein folding disorder of brain; inclusion bodies (α-synuclein) in abnormal regions
  - 2nd most common neurodegenerative dementia; nearly 30% of AD subjects have LBD
- Frontotemporal dementia (Pick disease)
  - Tau protein abnormality in grey and white matter, mainly frontal and temporal lobes
  - Gliosis and neuronal degeneration at times with Pick inclusion bodies in swollen neurons
  - 25-40% of FTD is familial; 3rd most common neurodegenerative dementia
- Creutzfeldt-Jakob disease
  - Definitive diagnosis by biopsy
  - Laboratory demonstration of prion protein in CSF
  - Prion (protein-like particle with no DNA or RNA) capable of causing a spongiform encephalopathy
  - Marked loss of neurons with astrocytosis and gliosis
  - Most common form is sporadic; less common is new variant form acquired by ingestion of infected beef products or iatrogenic, usually human pituitary tissue derivatives or rarely CNS surgical procedures
- Vascular dementia
  - Common findings of vascular based lesions in patients with AD
  - Vascular dementia may have genetic link to AD
    - Apolipoprotein (ApoE) involved in lipid metabolism, encoded on chromosome 19 by epsilon 4 allele: Increases probability of AD or VaD by 400% vs. non-carriers
    - VaD due to multiple small infarctions
    - MID often due to large emboli with MR correlates
    - 2nd most common dementia in elderly behind AD and often a contributing factor in AD
    - Myelin and axonal loss with astrocytosis

CLINICAL ISSUES

Presentation
- Lewy body disease
  - Visual and auditory hallucinations
  - Progressive dementia with fluctuating cognitive function, including memory and attention span
- Vascular dementia
  - Transient motor or cognitive symptoms; neurologic findings depend on involved sites
  - Depression more common, more severe than other dementias; progression rate is variable
- Frontotemporal dementia
  - Usual presentation is memory loss with behavioral and language change
  - Clinical presentation depends on distribution of pathologic involvement
- Creutzfeldt-Jakob disease
  - Rapidly progressing signs and symptoms: Dementia, pyramidal and extrapyramidal
  - Cerebellar related signs and/or rapid cognitive decline are seen in most subjects
  - Additional findings dependent on location of pathology
  - Psychiatric symptoms common; spinal cord involvement may occur
  - No effective treatment, death within months of onset

DIAGNOSTIC CHECKLIST

Image Interpretation Pearls
- FDG PET or perfusion SPECT
  - Temporal-parietal reductions with normal occipital metabolism and perfusion likely AD
  - Temporal-parietal with occipital reduction suggests LBD; global reduction later stage
  - Frontal-temporal reduction greater than normal age-related decline seen in FTD
  - Moderate to severe cortical and/or basal ganglia hypometabolic regions in rapidly progressive dementia suggests CJD
    - Similar pattern for CBD, MR with "hockey stick" sign in CJD
  - Major reduction in ventricular and periventricular activity with lateral parietal and frontal reductions indicates NPH

SELECTED REFERENCES

1. Galariotis V et al: Frontotemporal dementia--part III. Clinical diagnosis and treatment. Ideggyogy Sz. 58(9-10):292-7, 2005
2. Pakrasi S et al: Emission tomography in dementia. Nucl Med Commun. 26(3):189-96, 2005
3. Minoshima S et al: Alzheimer's disease versus dementia with Lewy bodies: cerebral metabolic distinction with autopsy confirmation. Ann Neurol. 50(3):358-65, 2001
4. Hoffman JM et al: FDG PET imaging in patients with pathologically verified dementia. J Nucl Med. 41(11):1920-8, 2000
5. Goldman S et al: Positron emission tomography and histopathology in Creutzfeldt-Jakob disease. Neurology. 43(9):1828-30, 1993

DEMENTIA & NEURODEGENERATIVE, OTHER

IMAGE GALLERY

Typical

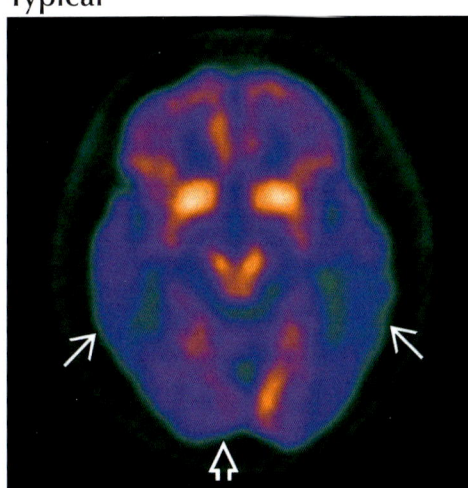

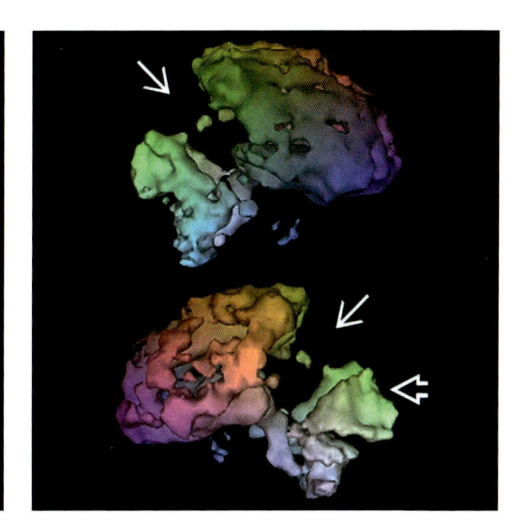

(Left) Axial FDG PET in patient with Lewy body disease. Note parietal and posterior temporal reduction similar to AD ➔, but occipital cortex is also involved ➔. (Right) Surface rendered Tc-99m ECD SPECTs in same patient as previous image demonstrate severe reductions of parietal, temporal ➔, and occipital cortex ➔.

Typical

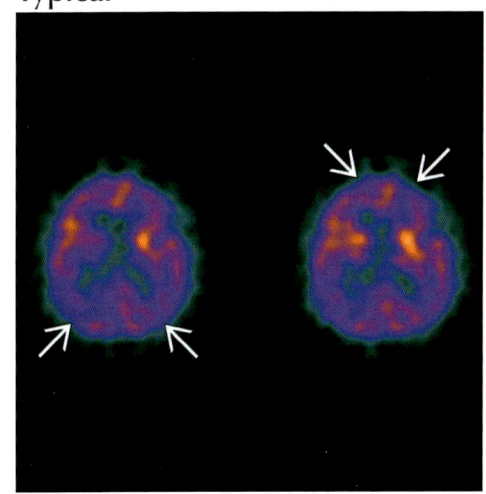

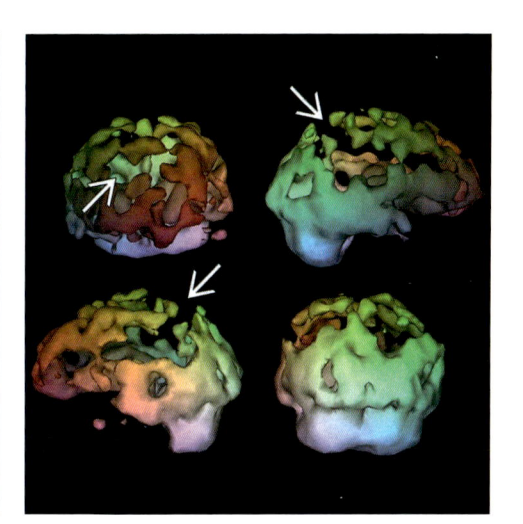

(Left) Axial FDG PET in autopsy-proven CJD. Note multiple cortical defects ➔. (Right) Surface rendered Tc-99m ECD SPECT shows pattern similar to AD ➔, however clinical course was that of a rapid progressive dementia ending in death within 12 months of onset.

Typical

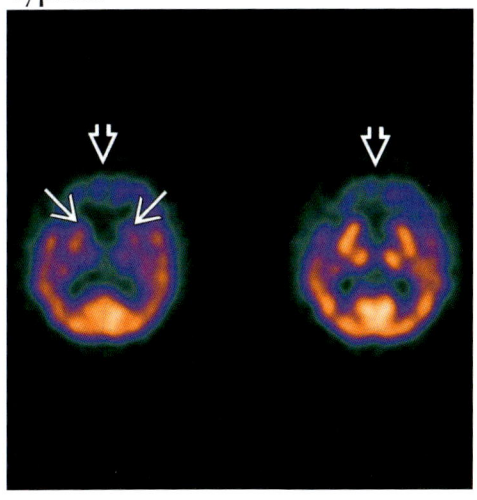

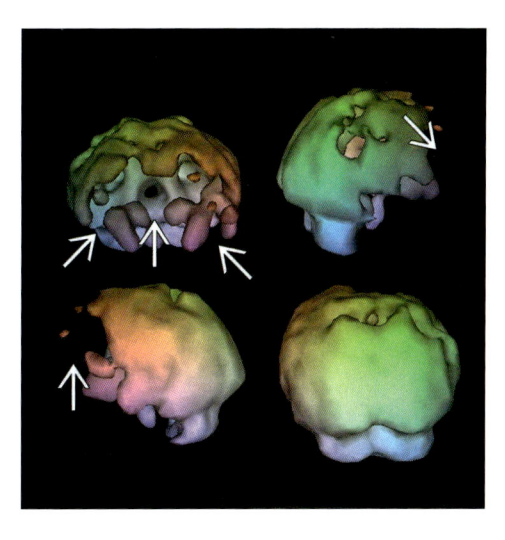

(Left) Axial Tc-99m ECD SPECT in patient with clinical PSP presentation. Note severe frontal lobe decrease ➔ and mild reduction in caudate heads ➔. (Right) Surface rendered Tc-99m ECD SPECT demonstrating severe frontal decrease relative to parietal and occipital cortex ➔.

DEMENTIA & NEURODEGENERATIVE, OTHER

(Left) Axial Tc-99m ECD SPECT (baseline) in patient with early FTD. Note frontal atrophy and mild reduction in perfusion ➡. Same patient as next 3 images. (Right) Axial Tc-99m ECD SPECT in same patient as previous image (18 months post-baseline) demonstrates significant decrease of frontal lobe activity from baseline study ➡, consistent with worsening dementia.

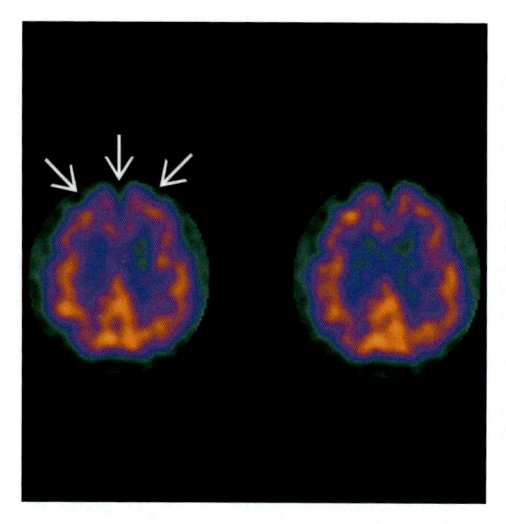

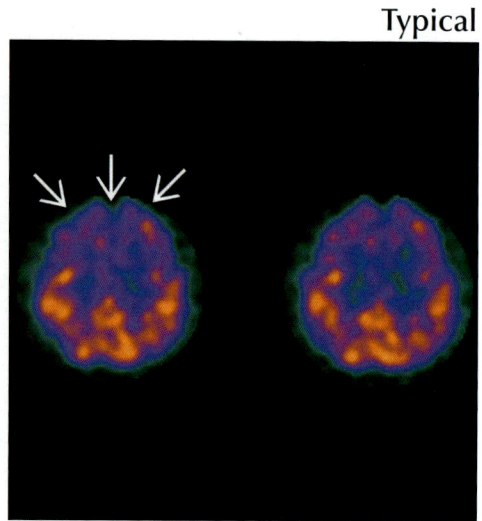

(Left) Surface rendered Tc-99m ECD SPECT of same patient as previous image (baseline) demonstrating mild frontal lobe findings ➡. (Right) Surface rendered Tc-99m ECD SPECT 18 months post-baseline demonstrates worsening ➡.

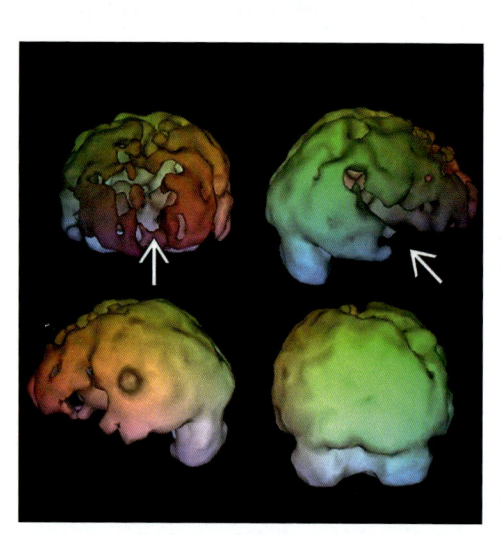

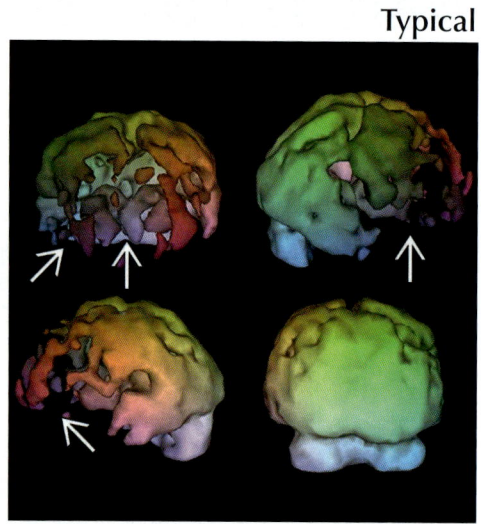

(Left) Axial FDG PET in patient with Huntington disease with mild dementia. Note severe reduction in basal ganglia ➡. (Right) Surface rendered Tc-99m ECD SPECT in same patient. Note mild frontal ➡ and parietal reductions ➡.

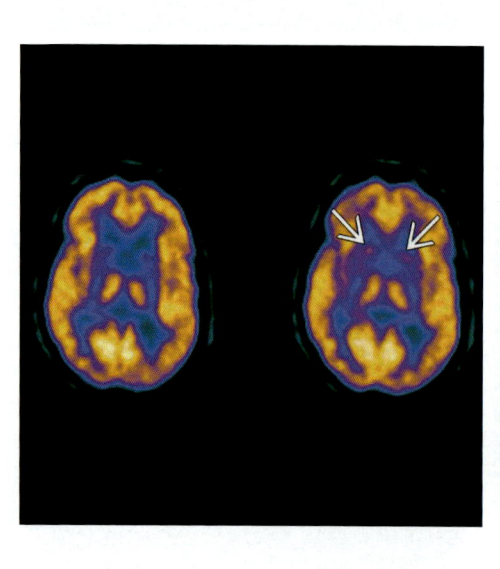

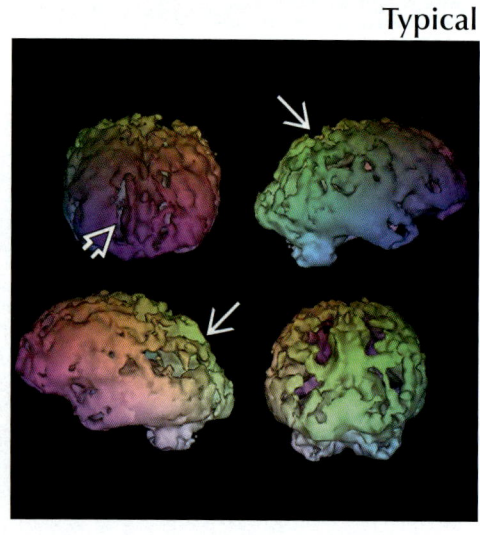

DEMENTIA & NEURODEGENERATIVE, OTHER

Typical

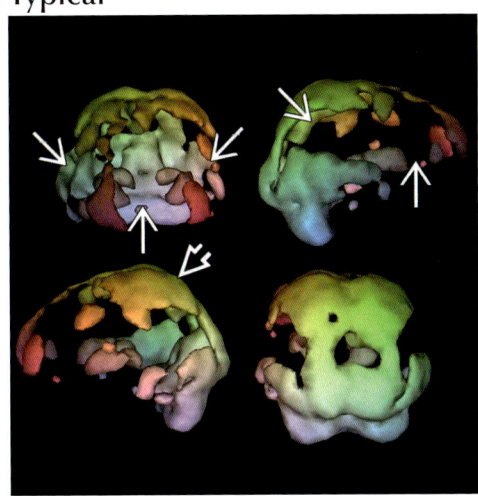

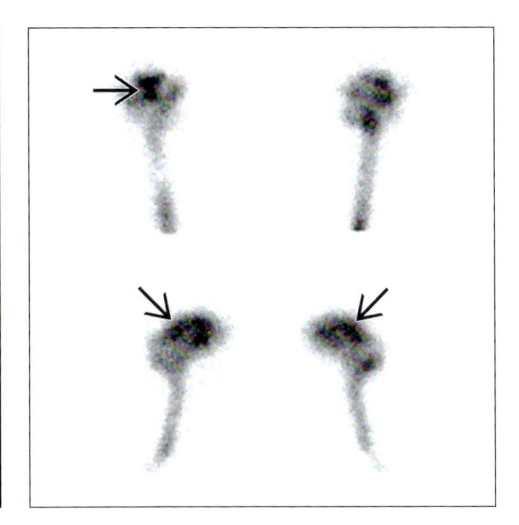

(Left) Surface rendered Tc-99m ECD SPECT in patient with NPH. Note severe frontal and parietal defects ➡ with preservation of vertex ➡. Same patient as next image. *(Right)* In-111 DTPA cysternogram (24 hour) in same patient as previous image. Note abnormal ventricular activity ➡.

Typical

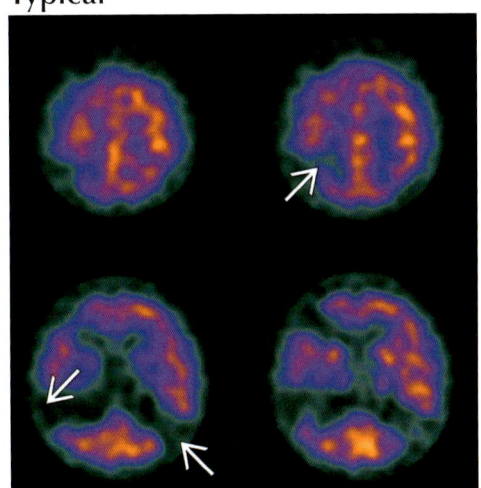

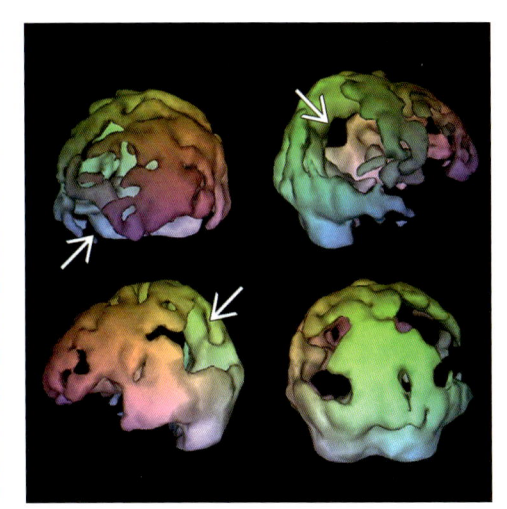

(Left) Axial Tc-99m ECD SPECT in patient with MID. Note multiple infarcts of the frontal & parietal cortex ➡. Same patient as next image. *(Right)* Surface rendered Tc-99m ECD SPECT in same patient as previous image. Note asymmetric cortical findings ➡.

Typical

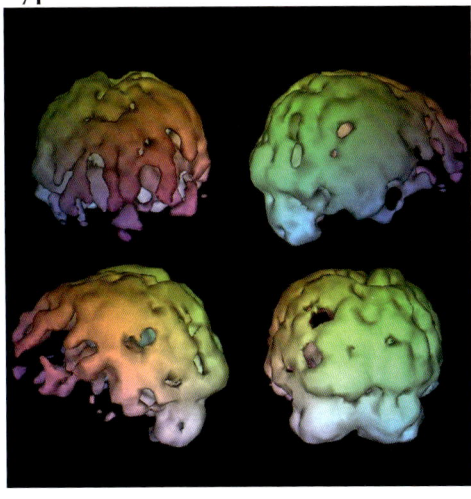

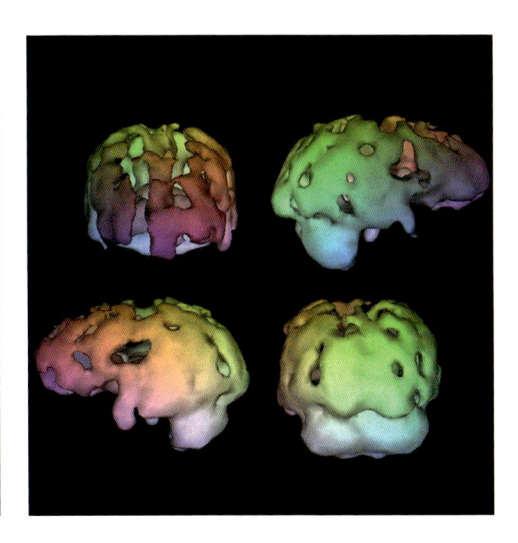

(Left) Surface rendered Tc-99m ECD SPECT in patient with history of cocaine abuse and early dementia. Note diffuse cortical findings. *(Right)* Surface rendered Tc-99m ECD SPECT in patient with history of methamphetamine abuse and early dementia.

GLIOMAS & ASTROCYTOMAS

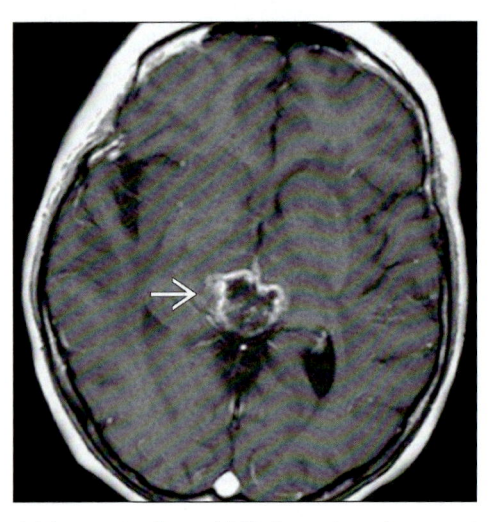

Axial contrast-enhanced MR shows ring-enhancement and central necrosis ➡ following radiation therapy. The differential diagnosis includes radiation necrosis vs. tumor. See next image.

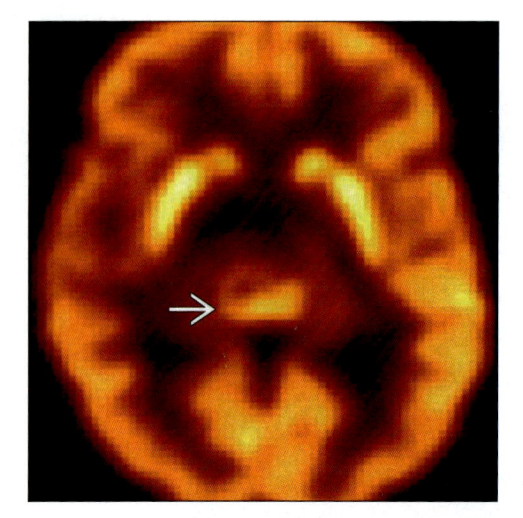

Axial PET shows focal intense FDG uptake ➡ correlating to the enhancing lesion on MR in the previous image following radiation therapy compatible with residual/recurrent tumor.

TERMINOLOGY

Abbreviations and Synonyms
- Low grade gliomas (LGG), astrocytomas, glioblastoma multiforme (GBM)

Definitions
- Imaging of neoplasms of glial or astrocyte origin
- World Health Organization (WHO) grade I: Most benign
  - Example: Pilocytic astrocytoma
- WHO grade II: Benign to semi benign
  - Example: Astrocytoma and oligoastrocytoma
- WHO grade III: Semi benign to malignant
  - Example: Astrocytoma
- WHO grade IV: Malignant
  - Example: GBM
  - Two types, primary (de novo) and secondary (degeneration from lower grade tumors)

IMAGING FINDINGS

General Features
- Best diagnostic clue
  - MR shows variable amounts of enhancement, with most low grade gliomas showing little if any enhancement, high grade tumors with extensive enhancement
  - MRS shows abnormal choline: Creatine (Cho/Cr) ratio and decreased N-acetylaspartate (NAA)
  - FDG PET shows little activity in low grade gliomas and increasing amounts of FDG uptake in higher grade tumors
- Location
  - Intra-axial location
  - 2/3 supratentorial and 1/3 infratentorial for low grade gliomas
  - Most anaplastic astrocytomas and GBMs are hemispheric
- Size: Variable, from a few millimeters to several centimeters; smaller tumors < 6 mm often not visualized by FDG PET
- Morphology: Variably sized intra-axial tumor +/- enhancement with surrounding vasogenic edema

DDx: PET Performed for Abnormal Enhancing MR

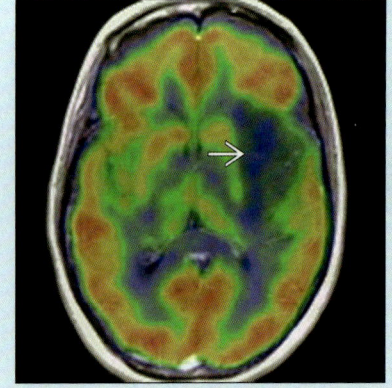

Low Grade Glioma 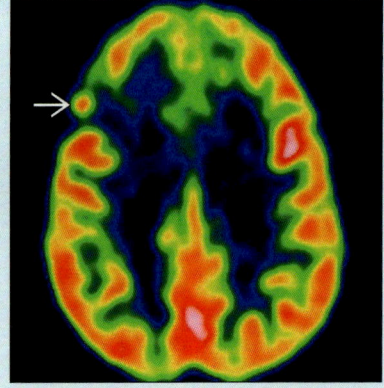 — *Glioblastoma Multiforme* 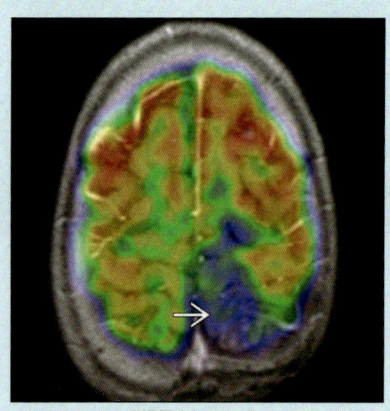 — *XRT Necrosis*

GLIOMAS & ASTROCYTOMAS

Key Facts

Terminology
- Low grade gliomas (LGG), astrocytomas, glioblastoma multiforme (GBM)
- Imaging of neoplasms of glial or astrocyte origin

Imaging Findings
- MR shows variable amounts of enhancement, with most low grade gliomas showing little if any enhancement, high grade tumors with extensive enhancement
- FDG PET shows little activity in low grade gliomas and increasing amounts of FDG uptake in higher grade tumors
- MR: Most primary CNS tumors will show some enhancement except low grade gliomas (grade I-II); usually accompanied by vasogenic edema

Clinical Issues
- FDG PET has 75-88% sensitivity and 81% specificity for detecting recurrent tumor as opposed to radiation necrosis

Diagnostic Checklist
- Initial imaging evaluation should include MR with contrast +/- FDG PET
- Primary roles for FDG PET are tumor grading, prognosis and differentiating recurrent tumor from radiation necrosis
- Low grade gliomas may only have mildly increased FDG uptake compared to normal white matter
- Areas of intense FDG uptake in a patient with a low grade glioma likely represent tumor transformation to higher grade (i.e., GBM)

Nuclear Medicine Findings
- Metabolic activity in primary glial and astrocytic tumors correlates with tumor grade and prognosis
- Low grade gliomas show mild FDG uptake, generally more than normal white matter; much less than normal cortex
- Higher grade tumors have increasing FDG activity, with GBM being very FDG-avid; as much or more than normal cortex

CT Findings
- NECT: Ill-defined mass occasionally with calcifications (up to 20% in LGG, rare in anaplastic and GBM)
- CECT
  - Low grade gliomas should have no enhancement
  - GBM will typically enhance and may have necrosis centrally

MR Findings
- FLAIR: Typically will show a larger area of involvement representing edema
- T1 C+: No enhancement with low grade and variable amounts of enhancement, mass effect and central necrosis with GBM
- MRS: Elevated Cho/Cr ratio and decreased NAA

Imaging Recommendations
- Best imaging tool
  - MR: Primary tumor usually demonstrates enhancement
  - MR: FLAIR images show extent of vasogenic edema
  - MR: Shows mass effect, hemorrhage, necrosis and signs of increased intracranial pressure
  - FDG PET: Increased uptake in higher grade gliomas & astrocytomas, pilocytic astrocytomas
- Protocol advice
  - Minimize auditory and visual stimulation during FDG uptake phase
  - Dynamic acquisition
- Additional nuclear medicine imaging options
  - SPECT
- Other PET tracers for neurooncology (investigational)
  - C11-Methionine: Amino acid transport
  - C11-Tyrosine: Amino acid transport
  - C11-Choline: Membrane synthesis, proliferation
  - F-18 Fluorothymidine: Proliferation
- Correlative imaging features
  - CT: Variable appearance, difficult to see without contrast unless large
  - MR: Most primary CNS tumors will show some enhancement except low grade gliomas (grade I-II); usually accompanied by vasogenic edema

DIFFERENTIAL DIAGNOSIS

Metastases
- Primary can not be differentiated from a metastatic lesion by imaging; whole body FDG PET can help identify primary lesion if outside the brain

Abscess
- Usually can not be differentiated by imaging; usually have other infectious symptoms such as fever and elevated white blood cell count

Infarct
- Little or no FDG uptake

Multiple Sclerosis (MS)
- Tumefactive MS can look similar to an intracranial neoplasm

Radiation Necrosis
- PET negative in most cases, whereas tumor tends to have increased levels of FDG uptake

PATHOLOGY

General Features
- Genetics: Loss, mutation or hypermethylation of tumor suppressor gene TP53
- Etiology: Variable
- Epidemiology

GLIOMAS & ASTROCYTOMAS

- Gliomas: Incidence is 6-8/100,000, with 50% being malignant subtypes
- GBM: 3-4/100,000, approximately 50% of all gliomas are GBM
- Younger patients tend to have lower grade gliomas with grade increasing in older age groups

Microscopic Features
- Grade depends on degree of cellularity, cellular pleomorphism, mitotic figures, necrosis and vascular proliferation

CLINICAL ISSUES

Presentation
- Most common signs/symptoms: Various neurologic symptoms including headaches, seizures or visual disturbances
- Other signs/symptoms: Other symptoms related to mass effect or hemorrhage

Demographics
- Age
  - Low grade gliomas typically occur in younger patients
  - Higher grade tumors typically occur in older patients
- Gender: Males and females equally affected

Natural History & Prognosis
- Overall prognosis poor, 5 year survival 30% for all astrocytomas; worse with increasing age; worse for GBM 2% 5 year survival
- Spread along tracts, along surfaces and across the meninges
- Some GBMs may arise from lower grade tumors; PET often helpful if baseline shows tumor has no or low FDG activity and follow-up shows intense uptake

Treatment
- Combination of primary surgical resection with chemoradiation
- FDG PET has 75-88% sensitivity and 81% specificity for detecting recurrent tumor as opposed to radiation necrosis

DIAGNOSTIC CHECKLIST

Consider
- Initial imaging evaluation should include MR with contrast +/- FDG PET
- Primary roles for FDG PET are tumor grading, prognosis and differentiating recurrent tumor from radiation necrosis

Image Interpretation Pearls
- Low grade gliomas may only have mildly increased FDG uptake compared to normal white matter
- Small lesions < 1 cm may not be seen due to the large amount of FDG activity in normal brain and partial volume averaging
- Areas of intense FDG uptake in a patient with a low grade glioma likely represent tumor transformation to higher grade (i.e., GBM)
- FDG PET generally very good for differentiating radiation necrosis from recurrent tumor
- Areas of decreased FDG activity can be seen following radiotherapy

SELECTED REFERENCES

1. Chen W et al: Imaging proliferation in brain tumors with 18F-FLT PET: comparison with 18F-FDG. J Nucl Med. 46(6):945-52, 2005
2. Kim S et al: 11C-methionine PET as a prognostic marker in patients with glioma: comparison with 18F-FDG PET. Eur J Nucl Med Mol Imaging. 32(1):52-9, 2005
3. Henze M et al: PET and SPECT for detection of tumor progression in irradiated low-grade astrocytoma: a receiver-operating-characteristic analysis. J Nucl Med. 45(4):579-86, 2004
4. Pardo FS et al: Correlation of FDG-PET interpretation with survival in a cohort of glioma patients. Anticancer Res. 24(4):2359-65, 2004
5. Lee JK et al: Usefulness of semiquantitative FDG-PET in the prediction of brain tumor treatment response to gamma knife radiosurgery. J Comput Assist Tomogr. 27(4):525-9, 2003
6. Padma MV et al: Prediction of pathology and survival by FDG PET in gliomas. J Neurooncol. 64(3):227-37, 2003
7. Tralins KS et al: Volumetric analysis of 18F-FDG PET in glioblastoma multiforme: prognostic information and possible role in definition of target volumes in radiation dose escalation. J Nucl Med. 43(12):1667-73, 2002
8. Mirzaei S et al: Diagnosis of recurrent astrocytoma with fludeoxyglucose F18 PET scanning. N Engl J Med. 344(26):2030-1, 2001
9. De Witte O et al: FDG-PET as a prognostic factor in high-grade astrocytoma. J Neurooncol. 49(2):157-63, 2000
10. Bruehlmeier M et al: Effect of radiotherapy on brain glucose metabolism in patients operated on for low grade astrocytoma. J Neurol Neurosurg Psychiatry. 66(5):648-53, 1999
11. Gross MW et al: The value of F-18-fluorodeoxyglucose PET for the 3-D radiation treatment planning of malignant gliomas. Int J Radiat Oncol Biol Phys. 41(5):989-95, 1998
12. Kaschten B et al: Preoperative evaluation of 54 gliomas by PET with fluorine-18-fluorodeoxyglucose and/or carbon-11-methionine. J Nucl Med. 39(5):778-85, 1998
13. Sfakianakis G: Preoperative grading of gangliogliomas using FDG PET and Tl-201 SPECT: comments from a nuclear medicine view. AJNR Am J Neuroradiol. 19(5):811, 1998
14. Barker FG 2nd et al: 18-Fluorodeoxyglucose uptake and survival of patients with suspected recurrent malignant glioma. Cancer. 79(1):115-26, 1997
15. Deshmukh A et al: Impact of fluorodeoxyglucose positron emission tomography on the clinical management of patients with glioma. Clin Nucl Med. 21(9):720-5, 1996
16. Ogawa T et al: Clinical positron emission tomography for brain tumors: comparison of fludeoxyglucose F 18 and L-methyl-11C-methionine. AJNR Am J Neuroradiol. 17(2):345-53, 1996

GLIOMAS & ASTROCYTOMAS

IMAGE GALLERY

Typical

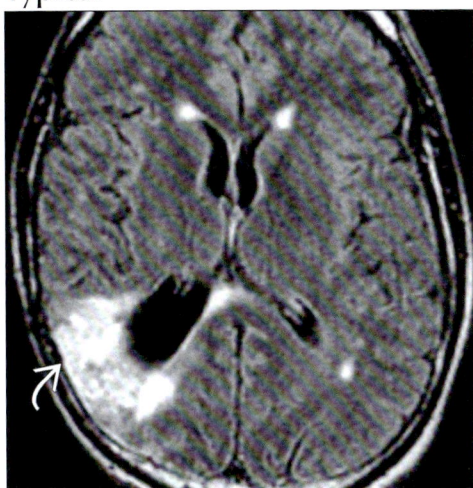

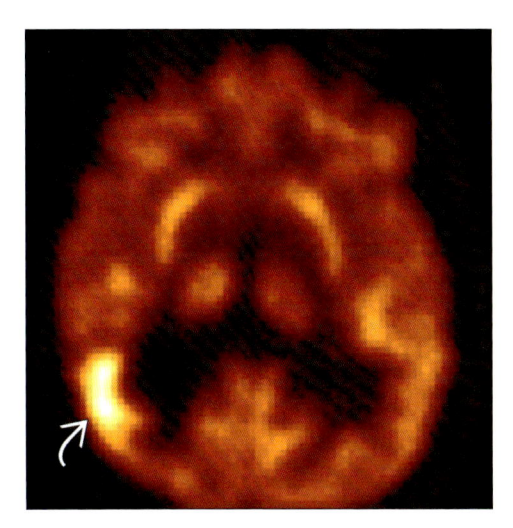

(Left) Axial FLAIR MR shows abnormal signal ➔ in a patient with a GBM treated with gamma knife. Differential includes radiation necrosis vs. recurrent tumor. MR spectroscopy was equivocal. *(Right)* Axial PET shows intense FDG activity ➔ in the area of signal abnormality on the previous image compatible with residual/recurrent tumor rather than radiation necrosis.

Typical

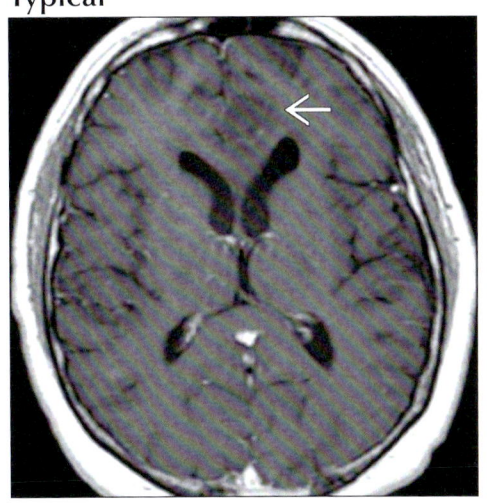

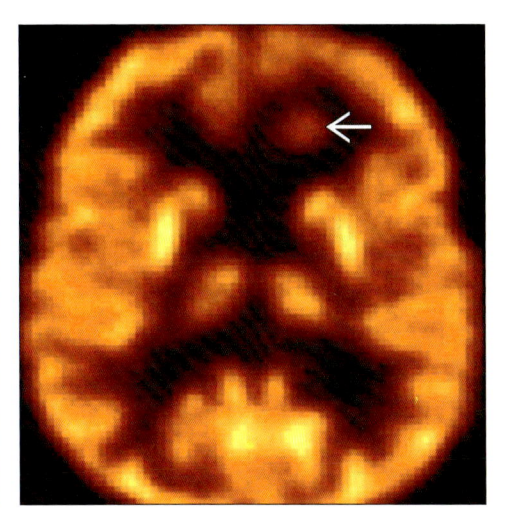

(Left) Axial post-gadolinium T1 weighted MR shows a left frontal lesion ➔ with minimal posterior enhancement following radiation treatment for a WHO grade III lesion equivocal for residual tumor. *(Right)* Axial PET shows moderate FDG activity ➔ correlating to the lesion on MR (previous image). Compared to normal white matter, the FDG uptake is fairly intense, compatible with low grade tumor.

Variant

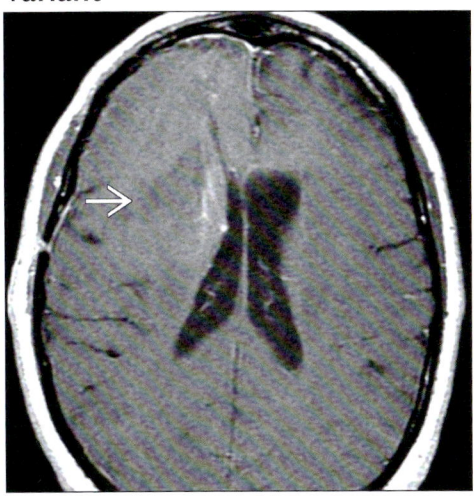

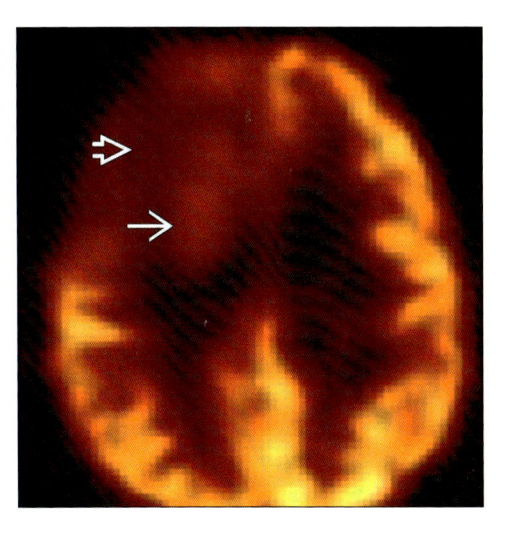

(Left) Axial T1 post-contrast MR shows a right frontal mass ➔ with mass effect on the right lateral ventricle but no significant enhancement in this patient with a WHO grade 1 glioma after radiotherapy (XRT). *(Right)* Axial PET shows diffuse hypometabolism in the right frontal lobe ➔ compatible with post XRT changes plus mild FDG uptake in the right frontal tumor ➔ compatible with residual low grade tumor.

PRIMARY CNS LYMPHOMA

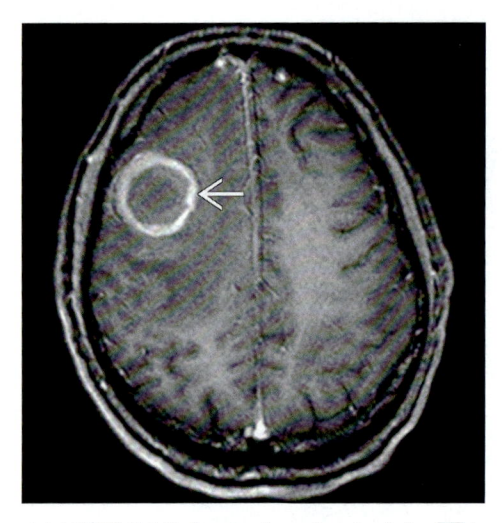

Axial CE T1WI MR shows a ring-enhancing lesion ➔ in right frontal lobe. In this HIV+ patient, the differential diagnosis is opportunistic infection with toxoplasmosis vs. primary CNS lymphoma.

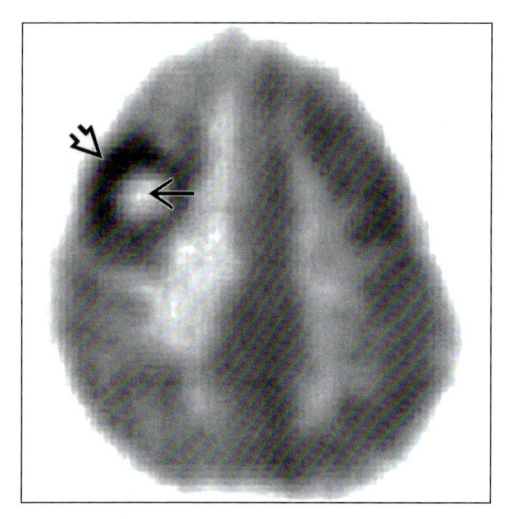

Axial PET shows focal ring of increased activity ➔ with central photopenia ➔ in right frontal lobe, consistent with primary CNS lymphoma. Biopsy proved non-Hodgkin lymphoma, large B-cell type.

TERMINOLOGY

Abbreviations and Synonyms
- Primary CNS lymphoma (PCNSL)
- Lymphoma

Definitions
- Malignant neoplasm composed of B lymphocytes

IMAGING FINDINGS

General Features
- Best diagnostic clue
  - Hypermetabolic lesion(s) in basal ganglia, periventricular white matter on F-18 FDG PET
  - Peripheral ring of increased activity surrounding photopenic core in HIV+ = central necrosis
- Location
  - 90% supratentorial, often gray-white junction
  - Deep gray nuclei commonly affected
  - Often involve, cross corpus callosum
- Morphology: Well-circumscribed mass > infiltrative
- Number: Single or multiple

Nuclear Medicine Findings
- F-18 FDG PET
  - Evaluate immunocompromised patients with ring-enhancing lesion(s) on MR
  - Differentiate lymphoma from opportunistic infection/inflammation (e.g., toxoplasmosis) with 80-95% specificity
  - Increased activity = lymphoma (SUV usually > 3.5)
  - Low, mild activity = infection/inflammation
  - Improved resolution (6-10 mm) over single photon radiotracers
- Tl-201 SPECT
  - Sensitive for lesions ≥ 2 cm
  - Initial and delayed images (3-4 hours)
    - Lymphoma: Tl-201 activity increases with time
    - Infection/inflammation: Tl-201 activity decreases with time
  - Toxoplasma IgG titer + SPECT findings improves diagnostic accuracy
- Ga-67 SPECT
  - Malignant lesions concentrate Ga-67 and Tl-201
  - Infectious/inflammatory lesions usually take up Ga-67, but not Tl-201

DDx: Primary CNS Lymphoma

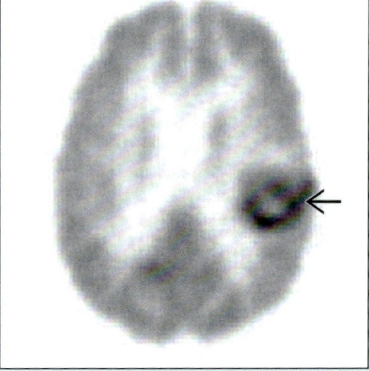

Abscess

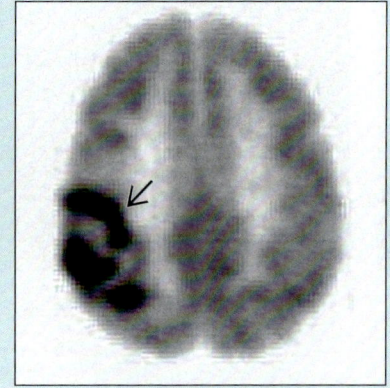

High Grade Glioma

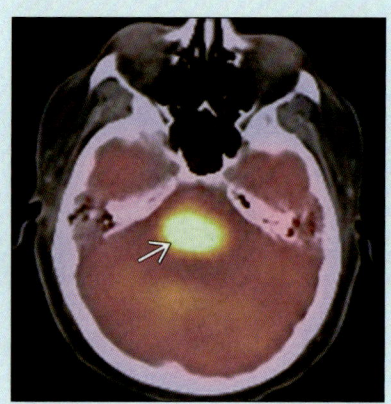

Myelitis

PRIMARY CNS LYMPHOMA

Key Facts

Terminology
- Malignant neoplasm composed of B lymphocytes

Imaging Findings
- Hypermetabolic lesion(s) in basal ganglia, periventricular white matter on F-18 FDG PET
- Evaluate immunocompromised patients with ring-enhancing lesion(s) on MR
- Differentiate lymphoma from opportunistic infection/inflammation (e.g., toxoplasmosis) with 80-95% specificity
- Increased activity = lymphoma (SUV usually > 3.5)
- Improved resolution (6-10 mm) over single photon radiotracers
- Guide stereotactic biopsy
- Monitor treatment response
- Computer coregistration of F-18 FDG PET and CE MR usually required

Top Differential Diagnoses
- Toxoplasmosis
- Other Primary CNS Malignancy (e.g., Glioblastoma Multiforme)
- Brain Metastases
- Abscess
- Progressive Multifocal Leukoencephalopathy
- Myelitis, Demyelination Disorder

Diagnostic Checklist
- Corticosteroid treatment may decrease F-18 FDG activity on PET
- Coregistration of F-18 FDG PET with CE MR increases sensitivity and specificity of PET findings

MR Findings
- T1 C+
  - Immunocompetent: Strong, homogeneous enhancement
  - Immunocompromised: Peripheral enhancement with central necrosis or homogeneous enhancement

Imaging Recommendations
- Best imaging tool
  - F-18 FDG PET
    - Evaluate immunocompromised patients with ring-enhancing lesion(s) on MR to distinguish lymphoma from opportunistic infection
    - Guide stereotactic biopsy
    - Monitor treatment response
- Protocol advice
  - Computer coregistration of F-18 FDG PET and CE MR usually required
    - Small lesions: Increase sensitivity of FDG PET findings
    - Multiple lesions
    - Increase specificity: Distinguish activity in regions of peripheral enhancement vs. surrounding edema/inflammation

DIFFERENTIAL DIAGNOSIS

Toxoplasmosis
- Critical differential diagnosis for immunocompromised patients
- Empiric toxoplasma therapy required if in differential

Other Primary CNS Malignancy (e.g., Glioblastoma Multiforme)
- F-18 FDG PET
  - Higher SUV = higher tumor grade
  - Central photopenia in necrotic tumors
  - SUV may correlate with tumor grade better than enhancement on CE MR
- 201-Tl
  - Increased activity in malignancy on early and delayed imaging

Brain Metastases
- F-18 FDG PET: Uptake depends on metabolic activity of primary
- Multiple lesions common
- Primary tumor often known

Abscess
- F-18 FDG PET: No hypermetabolic activity (+/- surrounding activity in associated inflammation)

Progressive Multifocal Leukoencephalopathy
- F-18 FDG PET: Lesions may be hypermetabolic
- 201-Tl, Ga-67: No increased activity

Myelitis, Demyelination Disorder
- F-18 FDG PET
  - Foci of active demyelination may be hypermetabolic
  - Regional cortical activity may be reduced in patients with multiple sclerosis

PATHOLOGY

General Features
- General path comments
  - CNS is a site of "extranodal lymphoma" since CNS does not have lymphoid tissue or lymphatic circulation
  - Immunocompetent: 98% B cell, non-Hodgkin lymphoma; rarely T-cell, Burkitt lymphoma, large cell anaplastic types
  - Immunocompromised: 70-90% high grade; 20% intermediate grade
- Etiology
  - Inherited or acquired immunodeficiency predisposes
  - EBV in immunocompromised
- Epidemiology
  - Incidence increasing
    - Immunocompetent: 4-7% of newly diagnosed primary CNS malignancies (up from 0.5-1.5% pre-1975)

PRIMARY CNS LYMPHOMA

- Immunocompromised: 2-6% of AIDS patients
- Associated abnormalities
  - Can be preceded by flu-like and/or gastrointestinal illness
  - Demyelinating disorder (+/- Lyme disease)
  - PCNSL is an AIDS-defining condition

Gross Pathologic & Surgical Features
- Single or multiple masses in cerebral hemispheres
- Well-circumscribed mass > infiltrative
- HIV+: Often central necrosis, hemorrhage

Microscopic Features
- Several subtypes: Nearly 50% large cell subtype
- High nuclear/cytoplasmic ratio
- Angiocentric: Surrounds, infiltrates vessels and perivascular spaces

CLINICAL ISSUES

Presentation
- Most common signs/symptoms
  - Altered mental status
  - Focal neurological deficits
- Other signs/symptoms
  - Headache
  - Seizure
  - Cognitive/neuropsychiatric disturbance
- Clinical Profile
  - CSF
    - Elevated protein
    - Decreased glucose
    - Cytology typically negative for lymphoma

Demographics
- Age
  - Immunocompetent
    - 45-70 years (mean 60)
  - Immunocompromised
    - AIDS: Mean 39 years
    - Organ transplant recipients: Mean 37 years
    - Inherited immunodeficiency: Mean 10 years
- Gender: Male predominance (1.4-2:1)

Natural History & Prognosis
- Poor prognosis: Median survival 17-45 months; 2-6 months in AIDS
- Favorable prognostic factors
  - Single lesion
  - No meningeal involvement
  - Immunocompetent
  - Age < 60 years
- Often dramatic, short-lived response to steroids and radiation therapy

Treatment
- Corticosteroids
  - Reduce associated inflammation, edema, mass effect
  - Improves clinical symptoms
- Radiation therapy
  - Stereotactic: Single, sometimes multiple lesions
  - Whole brain: Single and multiple lesions
- Chemotherapy
  - Blood brain barrier disruption may enhance efficacy
- Empiric toxoplasma medication
  - Initial treatment in immunocompromised patients pre-biopsy for pathological differentiation between PCNSL and toxoplasmosis

DIAGNOSTIC CHECKLIST

Consider
- Corticosteroid treatment may decrease F-18 FDG activity on PET

Image Interpretation Pearls
- Coregistration of F-18 FDG PET with CE MR increases sensitivity and specificity of PET findings

SELECTED REFERENCES

1. Young RJ et al: Lesion size determines accuracy of thallium-201 brain single-photon emission tomography in differentiating between intracranial malignancy and infection in AIDS patients. AJNR Am J Neuroradiol. 26(8):1973-9, 2005
2. Von Schulthess GK: Clinical Molecular Anatomic Imaging: PET, PET/CT, and SPECT/CT. Rev ed. Philadelphia, Lippincott Williams & Wilkins.172, 2003
3. Plasswilm L et al: Primary central nervous system (CNS) lymphoma in immunocompetent patients. Ann Hematol. 81(8): 415-23, 2002
4. Bataille B et al: Primary intracerebral malignant lymphoma: report of 248 cases. J Neurosurgery. 92:261-6, 2000
5. Paulus W et al: Malignant lymphomas. Pathology & Genetics of Tumours of the Nervous System. IARC Press. 198-203, 2000
6. Schlegel U et al: Primary CNS lymphoma: clinical presentation, pathological classification, molecular pathogenesis and treatment. J Neurol Sci. 181(1-2): 1-12, 2000
7. Skiest DJ et al: SPECT thallium-201 combined with Toxoplasma serology for the presumptive diagnosis of focal central nervous system mass lesions in patients with AIDS. J Infect. 40(3):274-81, 2000
8. DeAngelis LM: Primary CNS lymphoma: treatment with combined chemotherapy and radiotherapy. J Neurooncol. 43(3): 249-57, 1999
9. Iranzo A et al: Absence of thallium-201 brain uptake in progressive multifocal leukoencephalopathy in AIDS patients. Acta Neurol Scand. 100(2):102-5, 1999
10. Lee VW et al: Intracranial mass lesions: sequential thallium and gallium scintigraphy in patients with AIDS. Radiology. 211(2):507-12, 1999
11. Bakshi R et al: High-resolution fluorodeoxyglucose positron emission tomography shows both global and regional cerebral hypometabolism in multiple sclerosis. J Neuroimaging. 8(4):228-34, 1998
12. Koeller KK et al: Primary central nervous system lymphoma: radiologic-pathologic correlation. Radiographics. 17(6): 1497-526, 1997
13. Heald AE et al: Differentiation of central nervous system lesions in AIDS patients using positron emission tomography (PET). Int J STD AIDS. 7(5):337-46, 1996
14. Villringer K et al: Differential diagnosis of CNS lesions in AIDS patients by FDG-PET. J Comput Assist Tomogr. 19(4):532-6, 1995
15. Hoffman JM et al: FDG-PET in differentiating lymphoma from nonmalignant central nervous system lesions in patients with AIDS. J Nucl Med. 34(4):567-75, 1993

PRIMARY CNS LYMPHOMA

IMAGE GALLERY

Typical

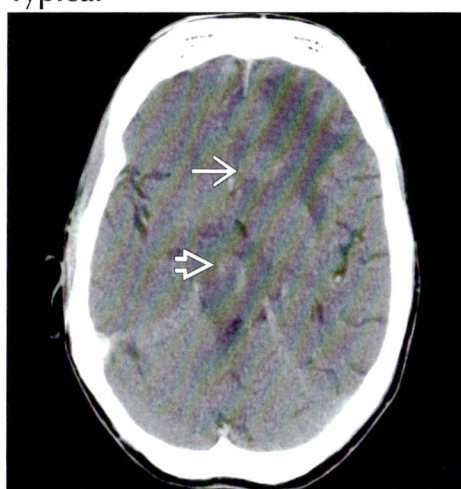

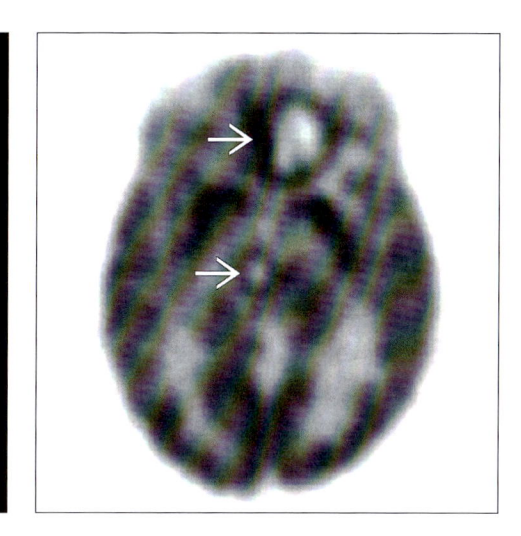

(Left) Axial NECT shows lesions in the left frontal lobe ➡ and brainstem ➡ with iso/hyperdense rim and surrounding vasogenic edema in an HIV+ patient. *(Right)* Axial PET in same patient as left shows two peripherally hypermetabolic lesions (left frontal lobe and brainstem) ➡, consistent with primary CNS lymphoma.

Typical

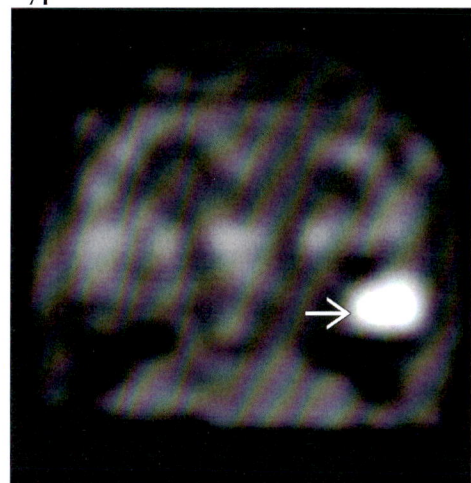

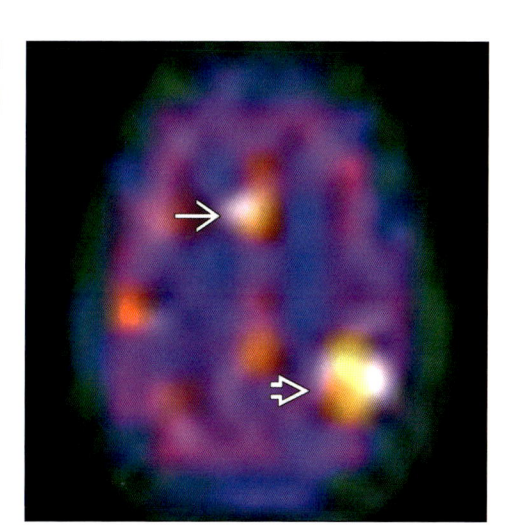

(Left) Coronal PET shows hypermetabolic focus of CNS lymphoma in left temporal lobe ➡. *(Right)* Axial PET shows focal hypermetabolic lesions in right frontal ➡ and left parietal ➡ lobes, signifying primary CNS lymphoma with intracranial metastasis.

Typical

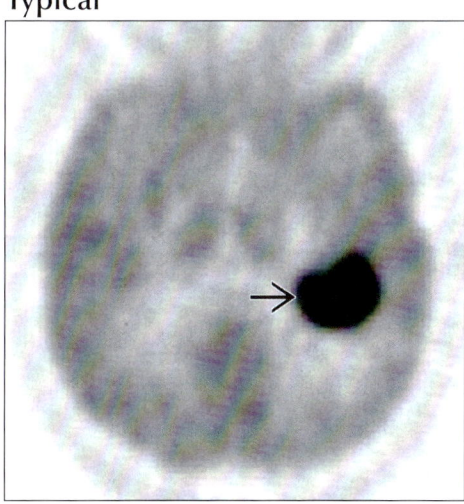

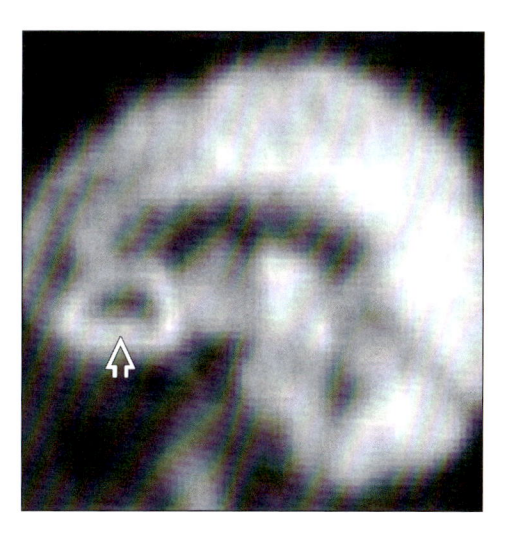

(Left) Axial PET shows primary CNS lymphoma in left temporoparietal region ➡. *(Right)* Sagittal PET shows hypermetabolic ring surrounding central photopenia in frontal lobe ➡ lesion. Central necrosis often present in HIV+ patients with primary CNS lymphoma.

METASTASES, BRAIN

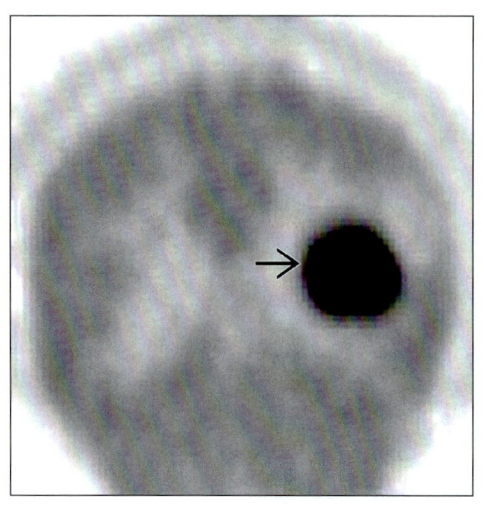

Coronal PET shows hypermetabolic left cerebral metastasis in patient with primary colorectal cancer.

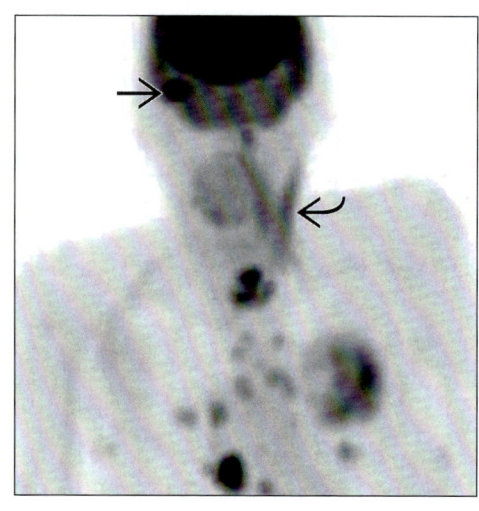

3D PET shows right cerebellar metastasis in patient with head-and-neck cancer. Note post-radiation change in neck and lung/mediastinal metastases.

TERMINOLOGY

Abbreviations and Synonyms
- Central nervous system (CNS) metastases

Definitions
- Secondary tumors in brain or spinal cord originating from primary extracranial or CNS malignancy

IMAGING FINDINGS

General Features
- Best diagnostic clue: Focal hypermetabolic activity in the brain or spinal cord
- Location
  - Classic
    - Cerebral hemispheres (80%)
    - Cerebellum (15%)
    - Basal ganglia (3%)
  - Less common
    - Choroid plexus
    - Ventricular ependyma
    - Pituitary gland
    - Pineal gland
    - Leptomeninges
  - Uncommon
    - Diffusely infiltrating tumors (carcinomatous encephalitis)
    - Perivascular
    - Perineural
  - Rare
    - Brainstem
- Size: Microscopic to several cm
- Morphology
  - Usually discrete, spherical
  - Infiltrating
  - Along vascular or neural structures
- Number
  - One (50%)
  - Two (20%)
  - ≥ Three (30%)

Nuclear Medicine Findings
- PET
  - FDG PET
    - Activity in CNS metastases depends on tumor histology

DDx: CNS Lesions on PET

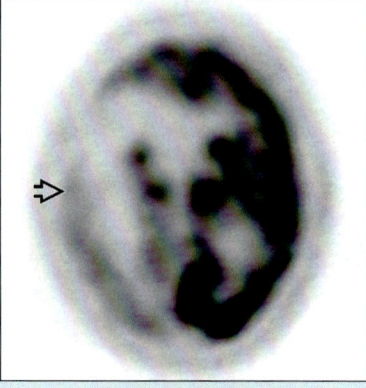

Cerebrovascular Accident

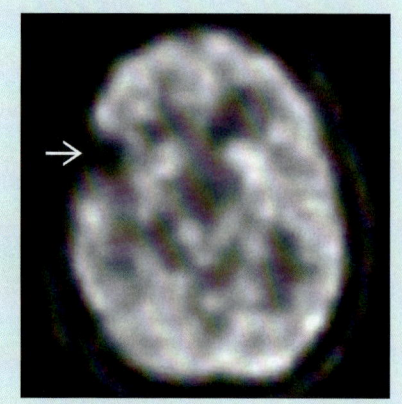

Resection Cavity

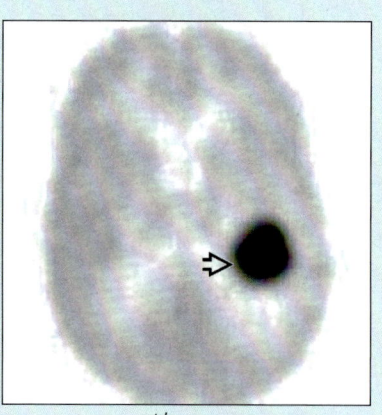

Abscess

METASTASES, BRAIN

Key Facts

Imaging Findings
- Classically hypermetabolic on FDG PET: Lung, breast, colorectal, head and neck, melanoma, thyroid
- Classically hypometabolic on FDG PET: Mucinous adenocarcinoma, renal cell carcinoma
- Variable uptake on FDG PET: Gliomas, lymphoma
- Can detect ≈ 1.5 cm metastases
- Cannot rule out small metastases with PET (CEMR gold standard)
- Normal brain metabolism of FDG (glucose) can hide small metastases
- To increase sensitivity, re-window image to make normal brain activity less intense
- Review three-dimensional and tomographic images

Top Differential Diagnoses
- Abscess
- Cerebrovascular Accident
- Primary Brain Tumor
- Meningioma
- Post-Treatment Effects
- Epilepsy

Pathology
- Number of patients with CNS metastases diagnosed annually: 100,000-500,000
- Metastases account for ≈ 50% of cerebral tumors
- 25% of cancer patients have CNS metastases at autopsy
- 90% of patients with CNS metastases have metastases in other organs

---

- Classically hypermetabolic on FDG PET: Lung, breast, colorectal, head and neck, melanoma, thyroid
- Classically hypometabolic on FDG PET: Mucinous adenocarcinoma, renal cell carcinoma
- Variable uptake on FDG PET: Gliomas, lymphoma
- Central hypometabolism suggests necrosis
- SPECT
  - Tl-201, Tc-99m sestamibi, Tc-99m tetrofosmin
  - Focal increased activity suggests metastasis

CT Findings
- NECT
  - Iso- or hypodense mass
  - Peritumoral edema: None to striking
  - Intracranial hemorrhage (ICH) variable
- CECT
  - Enhancement patterns
    - Intense
    - Punctate
    - Nodular
    - Ring enhancement

MR Findings
- T1WI
  - Iso- or hypointense mass
  - Metastases with intrinsically short T1 may be hyperintense (e.g., melanoma)
  - ICH: Atypical evolution compared to nonneoplastic etiology
- T2WI
  - Usually hyperintense
  - May mimic vascular disease if metastases scattered
- FLAIR
  - Usually moderately hyperintense
  - Hyperintense peritumoral edema
- T1 C+
  - Enhancement patterns
    - Usually intense
    - Uniform
    - Punctate
    - Solid
    - Ring enhancement
  - Delayed sequences can show additional lesions
- MRS
  - Strong Cho peak at long TE
  - No Cho elevation in peritumoral edema characteristic
  - Lipid or lipid/lac present with necrosis
  - No Cr peak in 80-85%

Imaging Recommendations
- Best imaging tool
  - FDG PET
    - Improved resolution over SPECT
    - Can detect ≈ 1.5 cm metastases
    - Cannot rule out small metastases with PET (CEMR gold standard)
- Protocol advice
  - Normal brain metabolism of FDG (glucose) can hide small metastases
  - To increase sensitivity, re-window image to make normal brain activity less intense
  - Review three-dimensional and tomographic images

DIFFERENTIAL DIAGNOSIS

Abscess
- Usually hypermetabolic
- Central hypometabolism signifies necrosis

Cerebrovascular Accident
- Hyper- or hypometabolic

Primary Brain Tumor
- Anaplastic astrocytoma/oligodendroglioma, glioblastoma multiforme (GBM)
- Lymphoma

Meningioma
- Hypometabolic

Post-Treatment Effects
- Hypermetabolic activity acutely (surgery, radiotherapy)
- Hypometabolic regions correspond to treated tumor

METASTASES, BRAIN

Epilepsy
- Seizure activity after FDG injection can cause focal hypermetabolic activity

PATHOLOGY

General Features
- Etiology
  - Hematogenous spread
    - Lung, breast, melanoma most common
    - Receptor-mediated attachment of circulating tumor cells in CNS
    - 10% unknown source
  - Local extension
    - Extension to dura from calvarium
    - Through skull base or via foramina, fissures
    - Perineural
    - Perivascular
    - Cerebrospinal fluid
  - Regional metastasis from CNS primary (e.g., GBM, lymphoma)
- Epidemiology
  - Number of patients with CNS metastases diagnosed annually: 100,000-500,000
  - Metastases account for ≈ 50% of cerebral tumors
  - 25% of cancer patients have CNS metastases at autopsy
- Associated abnormalities
  - Extracranial metastases
    - 90% of patients with CNS metastases have metastases in other organs

Gross Pathologic & Surgical Features
- Round, confluent tan or gray-white mass
- Edema
- Local mass effect
- Hemorrhage (common in melanoma, choriocarcinoma, lung and renal cell carcinomas)

Microscopic Features
- Usually similar to primary
- Usually displaces brain parenchyma
- Necrosis common
- Neovascularity common
- Marked mitotic figures

CLINICAL ISSUES

Presentation
- Most common signs/symptoms
  - Neurological
    - Headache
    - Seizure
    - Mental status changes: Confusion, obtundation
    - Ataxia
    - Nausea and vomiting
    - Vision problems
    - Papilledema
  - 10% of patients with CNS metastases asymptomatic

Demographics
- Age
  - Incidence increases with age
    - Rare in children (skull/dura more common site than parenchyma)
    - Peak prevalence over 65 years
- Gender: Slight male predominance

Natural History & Prognosis
- Progressive increase in size and number of metastases
- No treatment: Approximate 1 month survival
- With treatment: Median survival improved, but < 1 year

Treatment
- Medical management
  - Corticosteroids: Diminish effects of edema
  - Anticonvulsants: Seizure prophylaxis
  - Hyperosmolar agents: Decrease intracranial pressure
- Whole brain external beam radiotherapy
  - Prolong survival, improve neurological function
- Stereotactic radiotherapy (masses < 3 cm)
  - Prolong survival, minimally invasive, symptom palliation slower than with surgery
- Surgical resection
  - Prolong survival, symptom palliation, histopathologic tissue sample

SELECTED REFERENCES

1. Barker FG 2nd: Surgical and radiosurgical management of brain metastases. Surg Clin North Am. 85(2):329-45, 2005
2. Young RJ et al: Neuroimaging of metastatic brain disease. Neurosurgery. 57(5 Suppl):S10-23; discusssion S1-4, 2005
3. Gajewicz W et al: The use of proton MRS in the differential diagnosis of brain tumors and tumor-like processes. Med Sci Monit. 9(9):MT97-105, 2003
4. Kremer S et al: Dynamic contrast-enhanced MRI: differentiating melanoma and renal carcinoma metastases from high-grade astrocytomas and other metastases. Neuroradiology. 45(1):44-9, 2003
5. Lassman AB et al: Brain metastases. Neurol Clin. 21(1):1-23, vii, 2003
6. Miller KD et al: Occult central nervous system involvement in patients with metastatic breast cancer: prevalence, predictive factors and impact on overall survival. Ann Oncol. 14(7):1072-7, 2003
7. Rohren EM et al: Screening for cerebral metastases with FDG PET in patients undergoing whole-body staging of non-central nervous system malignancy. Radiology. 226(1):181-7, 2003
8. Yamamoto Y et al: 99mTc-MIBI and 201Tl SPET in the detection of recurrent brain tumours after radiation therapy. Nucl Med Commun. 23(12):1183-90, 2002
9. Yamamoto AJ et al: Detection of cranial metastases by F-18 FDG positron emission tomography. Clin Nucl Med. 26(5):402-4, 2001
10. Choi JY et al: Brain tumor imaging with 99mTc-tetrofosmin: comparison with 201Tl, 99mTc-MIBI, and 18F-fluorodeoxyglucose. J Neurooncol. 46(1):63-70, 2000
11. Ericson K et al: Positron emission tomography using 18F-fluorodeoxyglucose in patients with stereotactically irradiated brain metastases. Stereotact Funct Neurosurg. 66 Suppl 1:214-24, 1996

METASTASES, BRAIN

IMAGE GALLERY

Typical

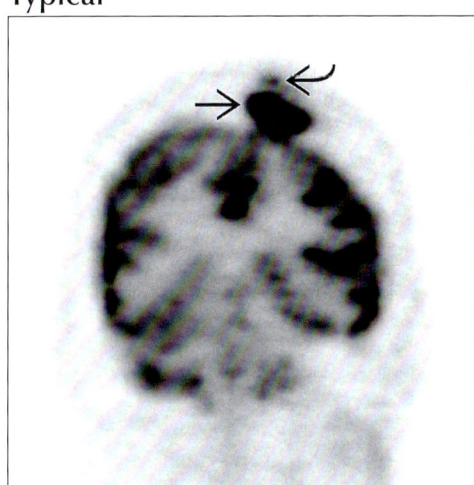

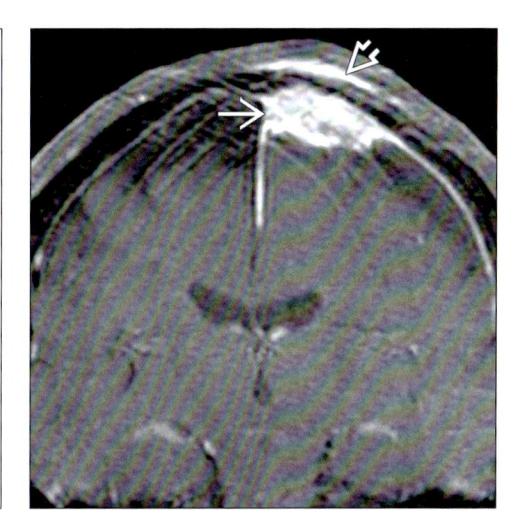

(Left) Coronal PET shows hypermetabolic melanoma metastasis extending from left cerebral hemisphere ➡. Adjacent hypermetabolic focus ➡ suggests extension of metastasis to skull. *(Right)* Coronal CE T1WI MR of patient at left shows enhancement of a soft tissue mass ➡. Calvarial enhancement confirms metastatic involvement ➡.

Typical

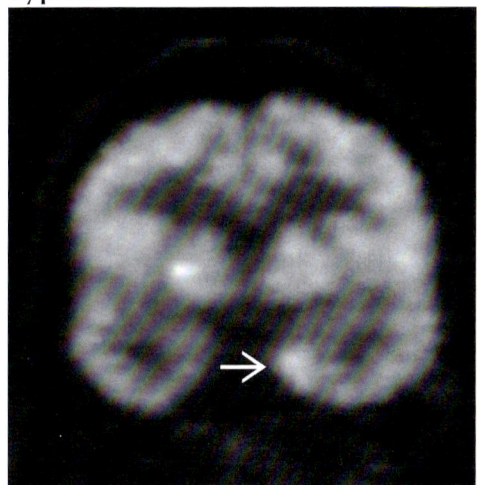

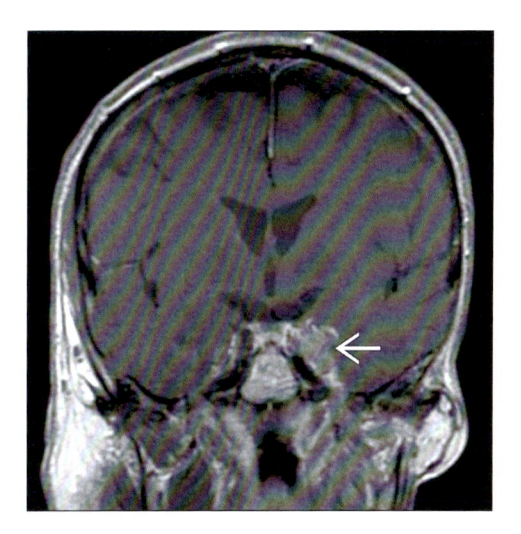

(Left) Coronal PET shows focal hypermetabolic activity in perineural spread of head and neck carcinoma ➡. *(Right)* Coronal CE T1WI MR of patient at left shows enhancement in the region of the cavernous sinus ➡, signifying perineural spread and corresponding to focal hypermetabolic activity on PET.

Typical

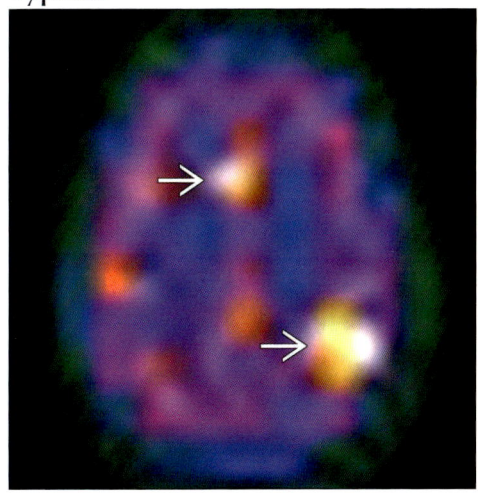

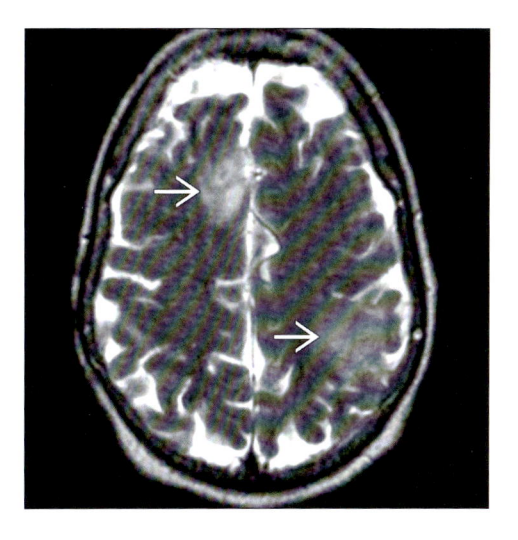

(Left) Axial PET shows two focal hypermetabolic lesions ➡ in patient with primary CNS lymphoma that metastasized throughout brain. *(Right)* Axial T2WI MR of patient at left shows two focal enhancing masses ➡, corresponding to focal hypermetabolic activity on PET.

RADIATION NECROSIS VS. RECURRENT TUMOR

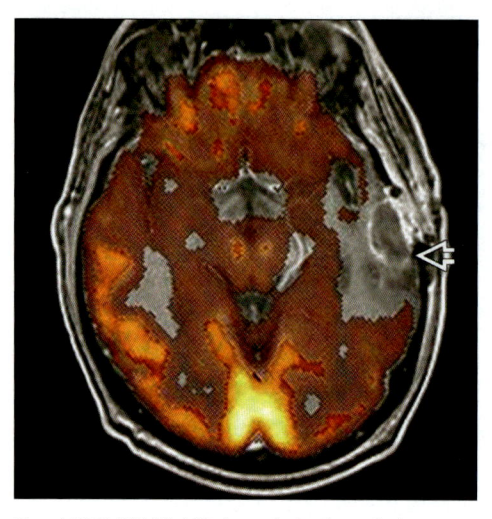

Fused FDG PET/T1 MR shows lack of metabolic activity in region of enhancement at site of XRT consistent with radiation necrosis ⇨. Same patient as next image.

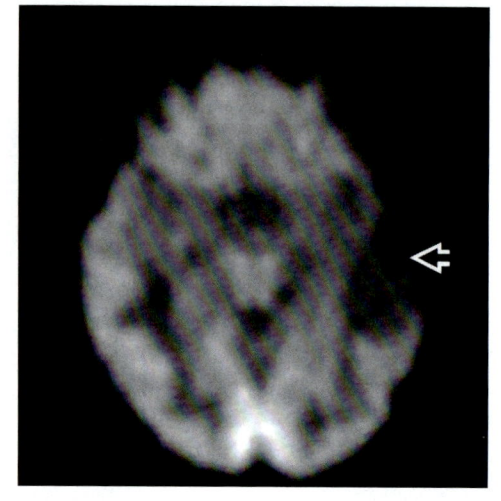

FDG PET in same patient as previous image shows lack of metabolic activity in region of enhancement on MR ⇨ following XRT, consistent with radiation necrosis.

TERMINOLOGY

Abbreviations and Synonyms
- Radiation-induced injury, external radiation (XRT) changes, chemotherapy effects, treatment-related changes

Definitions
- Includes edema, arteritis, leukoencephalopathy, mineralizing microangiopathy, necrotizing leukoencephalopathy, posterior reversible encephalopathy syndrome (PRES), radiation injury, radiation-induced tumors
- Radiation-induced injury may be divided into acute, early delayed injury, late delayed injury

IMAGING FINDINGS

General Features
- Best diagnostic clue
  - Multivoxel MRS: Characteristic patterns in recurrent tumor, radiation necrosis
  - FDG PET: Tendency for increased metabolism in recurrent tumor, low in radiation necrosis
    - However, FDG PET currently not typically reimbursed for radiation necrosis vs. recurrent brain tumor
  - CEMR, CECT: Irregular enhancing lesions for both radiation necrosis, recurrent tumor
- Location
  - Radiation injury occurs in radiation port
    - Periventricular WM especially susceptible
    - Subcortical U-fibers and corpus callosum spared
  - Metastases typically multiple
    - Gray matter (GM) and white matter (WM) junctions vulnerable
  - Recurrent glioma can be anywhere, usually spatially related to primary site
    - Can spread along subcortical U-fibers and corpus callosum
- Size
  - Edema, mass effect often greater than size of radiation necrosis
  - Glioma often greater in size than imaging findings

DDx: Metabolic Abnormalities on FDG PET Brain Scans

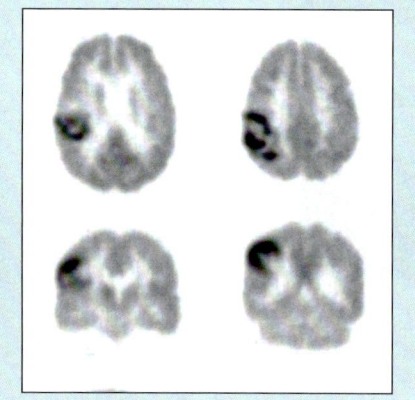

High Grade Right Glioma

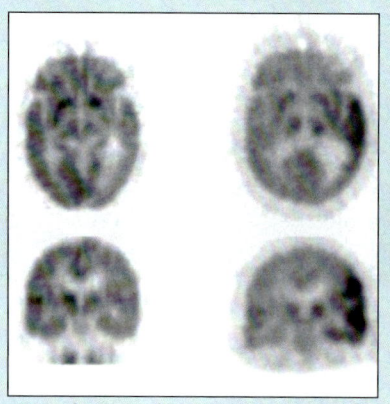

Cerebritis Early (Right), Late (Left)

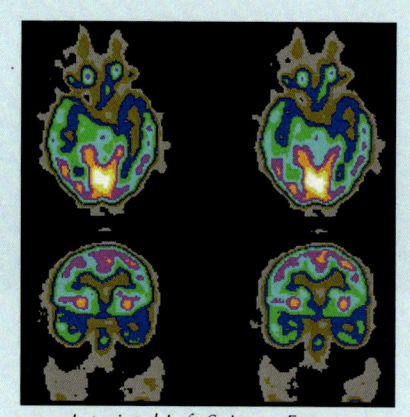

Interictal Left Seizure Focus

RADIATION NECROSIS VS. RECURRENT TUMOR

Key Facts

Terminology
- Includes edema, arteritis, leukoencephalopathy, mineralizing microangiopathy, necrotizing leukoencephalopathy, posterior reversible encephalopathy syndrome (PRES), radiation injury, radiation-induced tumors

Imaging Findings
- Multivoxel MRS: Characteristic patterns in recurrent tumor, radiation necrosis
- FDG PET: Tendency for increased metabolism in recurrent tumor, low in radiation necrosis
- However, FDG PET currently not typically reimbursed for radiation necrosis vs. recurrent brain tumor

Top Differential Diagnoses
- Abscess
- Multiple Sclerosis
- Vascular Dementia
- Progressive Multifocal Leukoencephalopathy

Pathology
- XRT: Spectrum from edema to cavitating WM necrosis; demyelination; coagulation necrosis: Favors WM

Diagnostic Checklist
- Distinguishing residual/recurrent neoplasm from XRT necrosis difficult using morphology alone
- MRS, FDG PET, Tl-201 or Tc-99m sestamibi SPECT all options for recurrent tumor from radiation necrosis

Nuclear Medicine Findings
- FDG PET: Radiation necrosis
  - FDG PET has 75-88% sensitivity, 81% specificity for distinction of radiation necrosis vs. recurrent tumor
  - If < metabolism than contralateral white matter, can suggest radiation necrosis
  - Radiation necrosis, especially after gamma knife, can show inflammatory hypermetabolism on FDG PET
    - Whole brain XRT inflammation resolves by 2-3 months; gamma knife may persist indefinitely
- FDG PET: Recurrent tumor
  - Increased uptake on FDG PET (> contralateral WM) suggestive of recurrent tumor
  - Lower grade gliomas usually poorly FDG avid
    - Conversion to higher grade glioma suggested by hypermetabolism
  - Small tumors < 6 mm may be undetectable by FDG PET
  - Metastases and gliomas not distinguishable by FDG PET but may allow search for primary elsewhere
- Thallium 201 or Tc-99m Sestamibi SPECT
  - Radiation necrosis typically decreased uptake
  - Recurrent glioma typically increased uptake
  - Reimbursed but probably inferior to FDG PET and MRS

CT Findings
- NECT
  - Acute XRT: Confluent WM low density edema
  - Delayed XRT: Focal/multiple WM low density
  - Leukoencephalopathy: Symmetric WM hypodensity
  - Mineralizing microangiopathy: Basal ganglia (BG) and subcortical WM Ca++, atrophy
  - Necrotizing leukoencephalopathy: Extensive areas of WM necrosis, posterior Ca++
  - PRES: Subcortical WM edema, posterior circulation

Angiographic Findings
- Radiation induced vasculopathy: Progressive narrowing of supraclinoid ICA and proximal anterior circulation vessels; may develop moyamoya pattern

MR Findings
- T1WI
  - Acute XRT: Periventricular WM hypointense edema
  - Delayed XRT: Focal or multiple WM hypointensities
  - Leukoencephalopathy: Diffuse, symmetric WM hypointensity; spares subcortical U-fibers
  - Mineralizing microangiopathy: Putamen hyperintensity, atrophy
  - Necrotizing diffuse leukoencephalopathy: Extensive areas of WM necrosis
  - PRES: Symmetric posterior WM hypointensity
  - Radiation-induced cryptic vascular malformations: Blood products
- T2WI
  - Acute XRT: Periventricular WM hyperintense edema
  - Early delayed XRT: Focal or multiple hyperintense WM lesions with edema, demyelination
    - Spares subcortical U-fibers and corpus callosum
  - Late delayed XRT: Diffuse WM injury or necrosis
    - Hyperintense WM lesion(s), +/- hypointense rim
    - Mass effect and edema
  - Leukoencephalopathy: Diffuse, symmetric involvement of central and periventricular WM, relative sparing of subcortical U-fibers
  - Mineralizing microangiopathy: Decreased signal
  - Necrotizing leukoencephalopathy: Extensive WM necrosis
  - PRES: Confluent, symmetric hyperintensity in subcortical WM, +/- cortex, posterior circulation
  - Radiation-induced cryptic vascular malformations: Blood products
- T2* GRE: Radiation-induced cryptic vascular malformations: "Blooming" related to blood products
- T1 C+
  - Acute XRT: No enhancement
  - Early delayed XRT: +/- Patchy enhancement
  - Late delayed XRT: Enhancement often resembles residual/recurrent tumor about resection cavity
  - Necrotizing leukoencephalopathy: Marked enhancement, may ring-enhance
  - PRES: +/- Enhancement
- MRS

RADIATION NECROSIS VS. RECURRENT TUMOR

- Radiation necrosis: Markedly reduced metabolites [choline (Cho), creatine (Cr) and N-acetylaspartate (NAA), +/- lactate/lipid peaks
- Recurrent tumor: Depends on tumor grade, typically elevated Cho/Cr, reduced NAA in high grade gliomas

Imaging Recommendations
- Best imaging tool
  - CEMR with multivoxel MRS
  - FDG PET, Tl-201 or sestamibi SPECT if question of XRT vs. recurrent neoplasm
- Protocol advice: Wait at least 2-3 months after XRT for FDG PET

DIFFERENTIAL DIAGNOSIS

Abscess
- Ring-enhancing mass, thinner margin along ventricle; T2 hypointense rim; diffusion restriction characteristic

Multiple Sclerosis
- Often incomplete "horseshoe-shaped" enhancement, open towards cortex; often lacks mass effect; other lesions in typical locations; young patients

Vascular Dementia
- Large and small infarcts, WM disease, typically older patients

Progressive Multifocal Leukoencephalopathy
- WM T2 hyperintensity; involves subcortical U-fibers; may cross corpus callosum; nonenhancing typical; immunosuppressed patients

Vasculitis
- Multiple small WM areas of T2 hyperintensity; gray matter involvement; enhancement may be seen

Foreign Body Reaction
- Can mimic tumor recurrence, radiation necrosis

PATHOLOGY

General Features
- General path comments
  - Acute: Mild and reversible, vasogenic edema
  - Early delayed injury: Edema & demyelination
  - Late delayed injury: More severe, irreversible
  - Most XRT injury is delayed (months/years)
  - Second neoplasms: Meningiomas (70%), gliomas (20%), sarcomas (10%); tend to be more aggressive
- Etiology
  - Radiation-induced vascular injury: Permeability alterations, endothelial and basement membrane damage, accelerated atherosclerosis, telangiectasia formation
  - Radiation-induced neurotoxicity: Glial and WM damage (sensitivity of oligodendrocytes >> neurons)
  - Mineralizing microangiopathy: Common with chemotherapy & XRT, appears ≥ 2 years after XRT
  - Necrotizing leukoencephalopathy: Combined XRT and chemotherapy, progressive disease
  - PRES: Related to elevated blood pressure which exceeds autoregulatory capacity of brain vasculature
- Epidemiology: Overall incidence of radionecrosis 5-24%; second neoplasms: 3-12%

Gross Pathologic & Surgical Features
- Radiation necrosis
  - XRT: Spectrum from edema to cavitating WM necrosis; demyelination; coagulation necrosis: Favors WM

Microscopic Features
- Acute XRT injury: WM edema from capillary damage
- Early delayed injury: Vasogenic edema, demyelination, leukocyte infiltration, gliosis
- Late delayed injury: WM necrosis, demyelination, astrocytosis, vasculopathy, Ca++, thrombosis

CLINICAL ISSUES

Presentation
- Most common signs/symptoms: Highly variable
- Radiation injury to the brain is divided into 3 groups
  - Acute injury: 1-6 weeks after or during treatment
  - Early delayed injury: 3 weeks to several months
  - Late delayed injury: Months to years after treatment

Natural History & Prognosis
- Younger patient at time of treatment: Worse prognosis
- Radiation necrosis is a dynamic pathophysiological process; often progressive, irreversible

Treatment
- Biopsy if imaging does not resolve tumor vs. radionecrosis
- Surgery if mass effect, edema
- Acute radiation injury may respond to steroids

DIAGNOSTIC CHECKLIST

Consider
- Distinguishing residual/recurrent neoplasm from XRT necrosis difficult using morphology alone

Image Interpretation Pearls
- MRS, FDG PET, Tl-201 or Tc-99m sestamibi SPECT all options for recurrent tumor from radiation necrosis

SELECTED REFERENCES
1. Chernov M et al: Differentiation of the radiation-induced necrosis and tumor recurrence after gamma knife radiosurgery for brain metastases: importance of multi-voxel proton MRS. Minim Invasive Neurosurg. 48(4):228-34, 2005
2. Hustinx R et al: PET imaging for differentiating recurrent brain tumor from radiation necrosis. Radiol Clin North Am. 43(1):35-47, 2005
3. Siepmann DB et al: Tl-201 SPECT and F-18 FDG PET for assessment of glioma recurrence versus radiation necrosis. Clin Nucl Med. 30(3):199-200, 2005
4. Benard F et al: Imaging gliomas with positron emission tomography and single-photon emission computed tomography. Semin Nucl Med. 33(2):148-62, 2003

RADIATION NECROSIS VS. RECURRENT TUMOR

IMAGE GALLERY

Variant

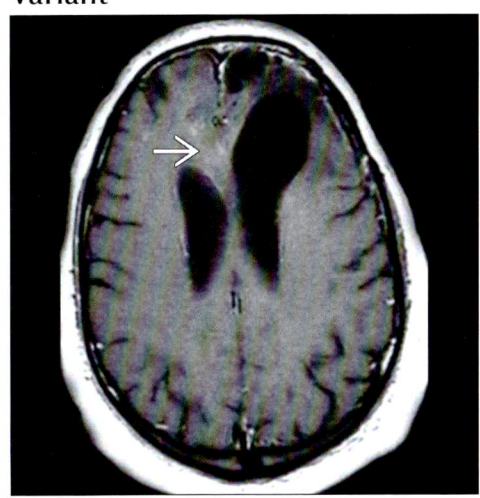

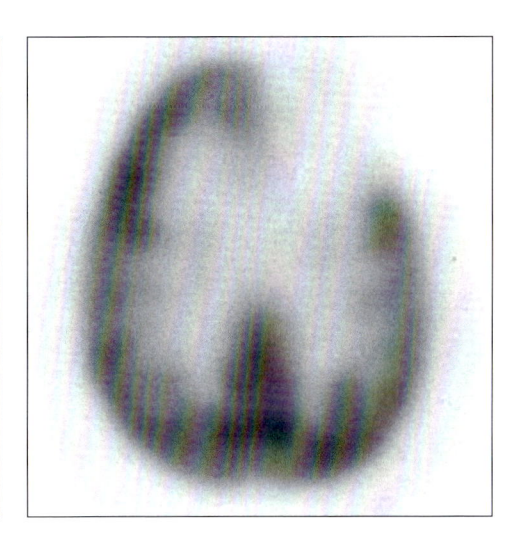

(Left) Axial T1 CEMR demonstrates partial enhancement in region of apparent gliosis ➡ in corpus callosum near surgical defect following XRT. See next image. *(Right)* Axial FDG PET in same patient as previous image. Lack of metabolic activity in area of concern on MR is suggestive of post XRT gliosis, not recurrent tumor.

Typical

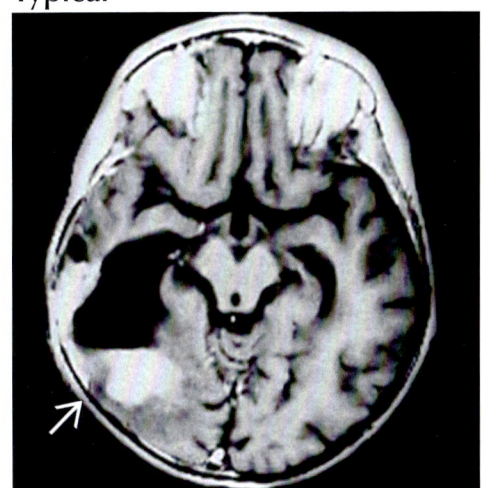

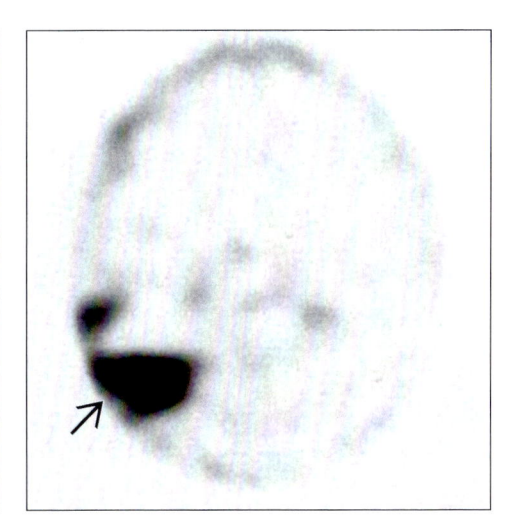

(Left) Axial T1 CEMR shows enhancement at margin of surgical cavity following XRT for GBM ➡. See next image. *(Right)* Tl-201 SPECT in same patient as previous image shows intense uptake at site of enhancement, consistent with recurrent GBM ➡.

Typical

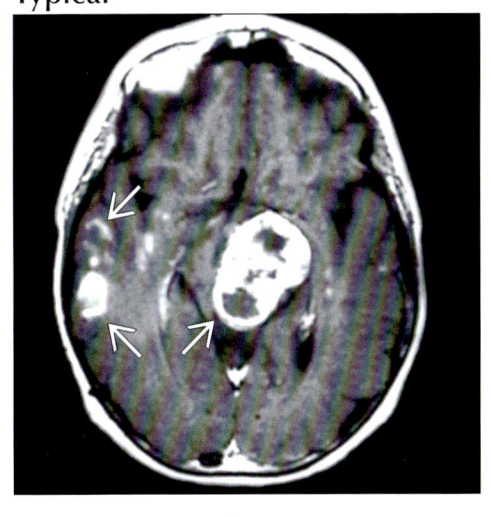

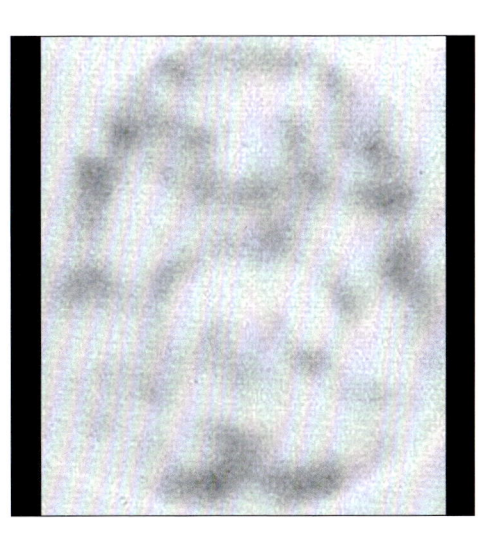

(Left) T1 CEMR shows areas of enhancement/necrosis following whole brain and stereotactic XRT for medulloblastoma ➡. See next image. *(Right)* Tl-201 SPECT in same patient as previous image demonstrates no abnormal uptake at site of enhancement. Findings consistent with radiation necrosis.

RADIATION NECROSIS VS. RECURRENT TUMOR

(Left) Axial T1 CEMR shows enhancing ring ➡ post surgery, XRT. See next image. *(Right)* Axial PET shows focal hypermetabolism ➡ at site of enhancing lesion consistent with recurrent tumor. Same patient as previous image.

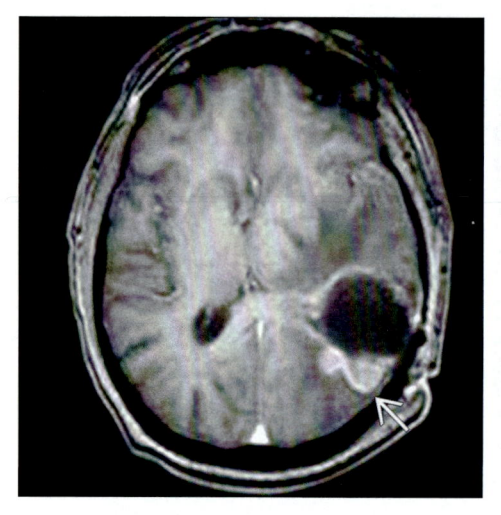

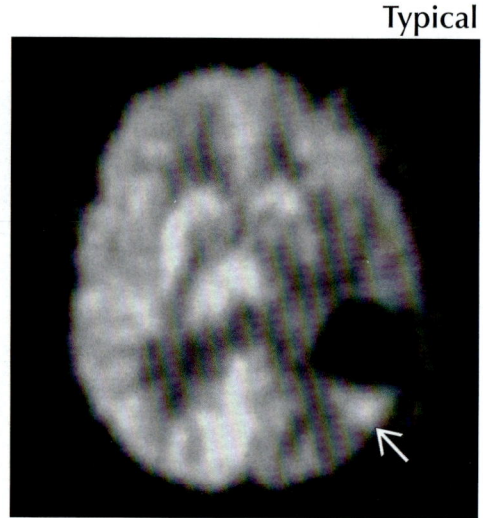

(Left) Axial T2 MR shows edema in large region of temporal lobe ➡, previously radiated. See next image. *(Right)* FDG PET in same patient shows hypermetabolism along posterior margin of region of edema ➡. Directed biopsy demonstrated recurrent glioma. Hypometabolic region is radiation necrosis ➡.

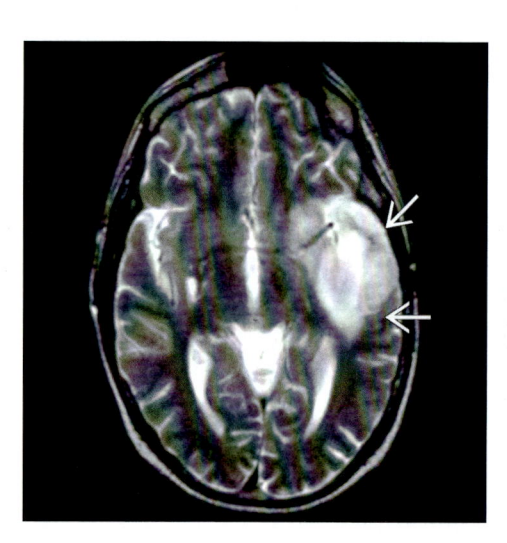

(Left) Axial T1 CEMR demonstrates ring of enhancement with central necrosis following XRT for glioma ➡. See next image. *(Right)* FDG PET in same patient as previous image shows absent metabolism in same region as enhancement, ➡ consistent with radiation necrosis.

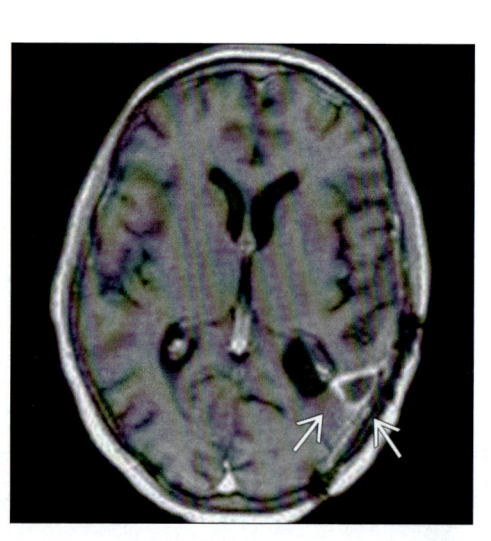

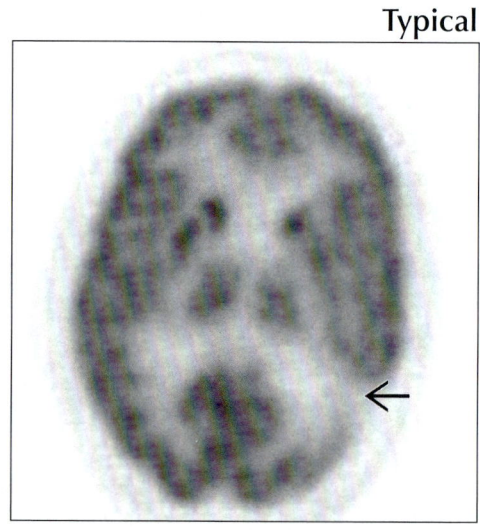

RADIATION NECROSIS VS. RECURRENT TUMOR

Typical

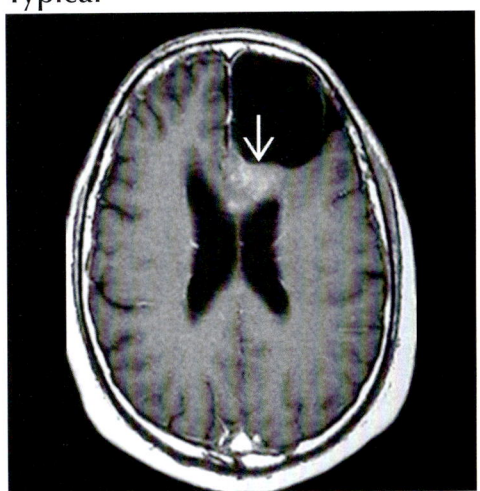

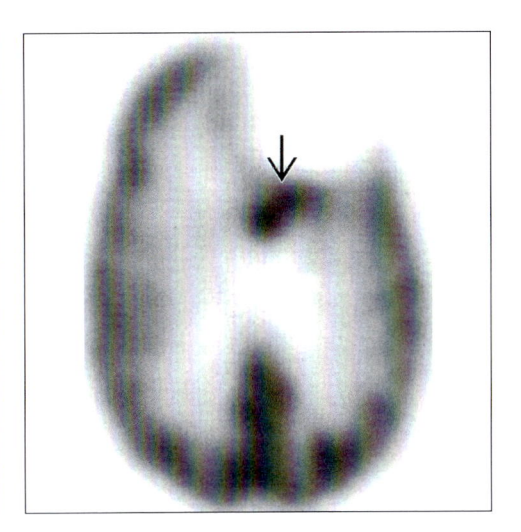

(Left) Axial T1 CEMR shows region enhancement near surgical cavity post XRT ➔. See next image. *(Right)* FDG PET in same patient as previous image shows focal hypermetabolism ➔ at site of enhancement and apparent gliosis consistent with recurrent glioma.

Variant

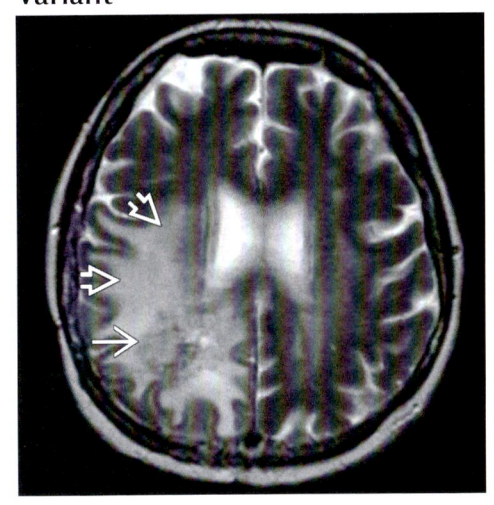

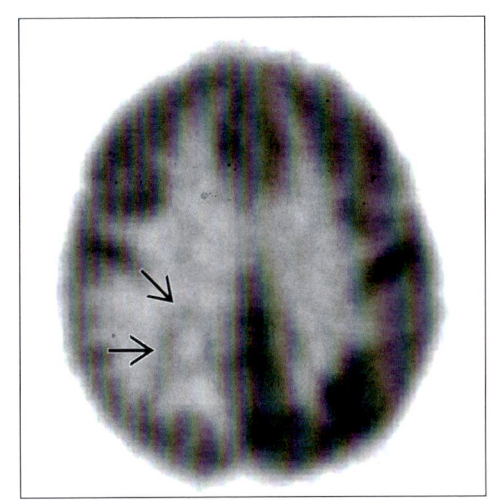

(Left) Axial T2 MR following XRT shows nodular region ➔ in large area of edema ➔ following XRT. Same patient as next 3 images. *(Right)* Axial FDG PET in same patient as previous image shows subtle ring-like metabolism ➔ suspicious, but not diagnostic, for recurrent tumor. See next 2 images.

Typical

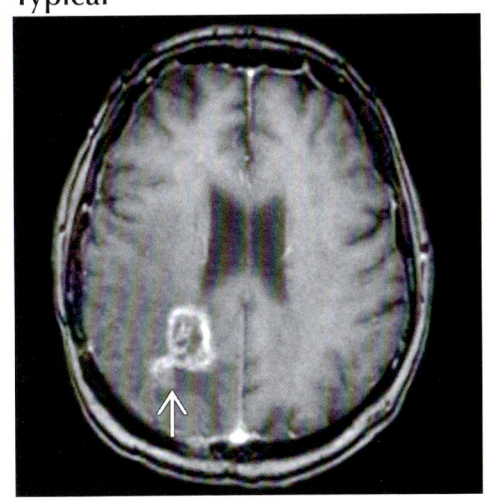

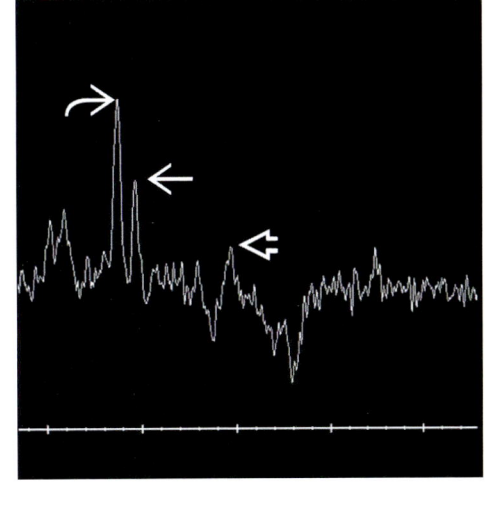

(Left) Axial T1 CEMR with localizer for MRS shows irregular, nodular ring-like enhancement ➔ with adjacent edema. *(Right)* MRS pattern (elevated Cho ➔/Cr ➔ ratio, and reduced NAA ➔) is suggestive of recurrent glioma, confirmed by biopsy.

CSF LEAK

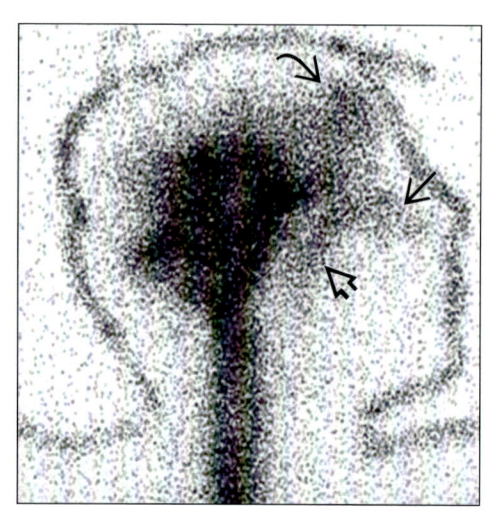

Tc-99m DTPA cisternogram. Right lateral with surface anatomy drawn with point source. Cribriform plate leak results in activity in frontal sinus ⇗, nose ⇒, and nasopharynx ⊳.

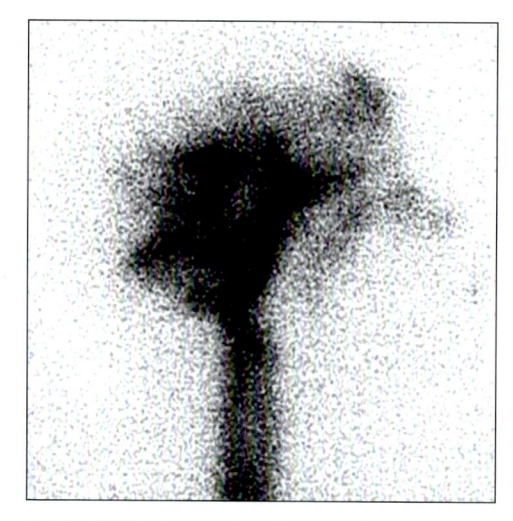

Tc-99m DTPA cisternogram of same patient as previous image but without surface anatomy map. Cribriform plate leak results in activity in frontal sinus, nose, and nasopharynx.

TERMINOLOGY

Abbreviations and Synonyms
- Cerebrospinal fluid (CSF) rhinorrhea, CSF otorrhea, CSF fistula, pseudomeningocele
- Spontaneous intracranial hypotension (SIH), intracranial hypotension (IH)
- Cerebrospinal fluid hypovolemia

Definitions
- Spontaneous, iatrogenic or post traumatic escape of CSF from the normal CSF space

IMAGING FINDINGS

General Features
- Best diagnostic clue: Visualization of CSF outside of its expected location
- Location: Nose, nasopharynx, paranasal sinuses, temporal bone or ear, along spinal canal
- Size: Varies from very small to large

Nuclear Medicine Findings
- Activity seen outside the expected location of CSF
- Activity in nose or ear packs significantly higher than level in a concurrent blood sample
  - Nose or ear pack counts are much more sensitive than imaging
    - Pack counts are considered positive if more than double blood counts, but in positive studies are often several orders of magnitude hotter than blood
  - If pack counts are positive there is a leak despite negative images

CT Findings
- NECT
  - Dilated epidural veins, arachnoid diverticula/meningocele
  - Direct visualization of CSF collection
  - May see inner ear anomalies in congenital leaks
  - May see fractures with post traumatic leaks
- CECT
  - May see enhancing epidural veins
  - Myelography or CT myelography
    - May visualize the actual leak

DDx: Other Leak Examples

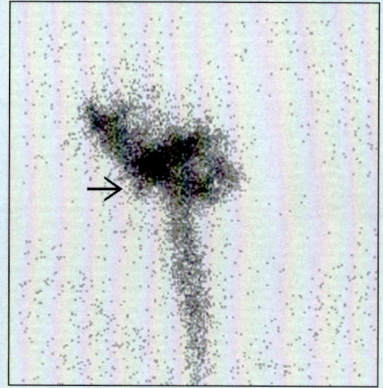

Nasopharynx Leak

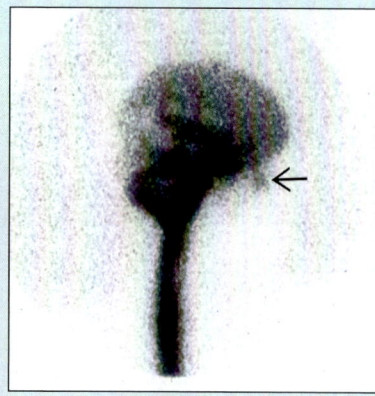

Nasopharynx Leak

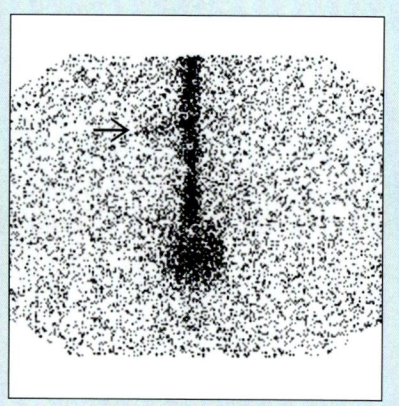

Lumbar Spine Leak

CSF LEAK

Key Facts

Terminology
- Cerebrospinal fluid (CSF) rhinorrhea, CSF otorrhea, CSF fistula, pseudomeningocele
- Spontaneous, iatrogenic or post traumatic escape of CSF from the normal CSF space

Imaging Findings
- Best diagnostic clue: Visualization of CSF outside of its expected location
- Location: Nose, nasopharynx, paranasal sinuses, temporal bone or ear, along spinal canal
- Activity seen outside the expected location of CSF
- Activity in nose or ear packs significantly higher than level in a concurrent blood sample
- Nose or ear pack counts are much more sensitive than imaging

- Pack counts are considered positive if more than double blood counts, but in positive studies are often several orders of magnitude hotter than blood
- CSF is labeled with In-111 DTPA about 500 microcuries by intrathecal injection (2-5 mCi Tc-99m DTPA for overpressure technique)
- Tracer injection must be done carefully to avoid leakage of tracer out of injection site
- Mixing tracer with metrizamide prior to injection will cause metrizamide to act as transport vehicle, bringing tracer to potential leak site sooner for intracranial level leaks and facilitating combined nuclear and CT imaging
- Packs should not be removed if possible until tracer is seen on images bathing area of clinical concern

---

- CT myelography more sensitive than myelography alone

MR Findings
- T1WI: May see abnormal fluid collection
- T2WI: May see congenital anomalies or abnormal fluid collections

Imaging Recommendations
- Best imaging tool
  - CSF imaging
    - CSF is labeled with In-111 DTPA about 500 microcuries by intrathecal injection (2-5 mCi Tc-99m DTPA for overpressure technique)
    - Tracer injection must be done carefully to avoid leakage of tracer out of injection site
    - Penetrate dura with needle bevel parallel to longitudinal plane of dural fibers
    - Keep patient Trendelenburg for five minutes after tracer injection before removing the needle
    - Mixing tracer with metrizamide prior to injection will cause metrizamide to act as transport vehicle, bringing tracer to potential leak site sooner for intracranial level leaks and facilitating combined nuclear and CT imaging
  - CSF counting
    - Nose is packed and packs removed and counted
    - Packs should not be removed if possible until tracer is seen on images bathing area of clinical concern
    - A simultaneous blood sample should be drawn when nasal pledgets are removed to compare pledget count levels with blood levels of tracer
    - Pledget counts should classically be at least 1.5-2x blood levels to call positive, but in practice leaks often have orders of magnitude more counts than blood in positive studies
- Protocol advice
  - Tracer can be injected with normal pressure or CSF overpressure (injection of artificial CSF or Elliott's B solution)
    - Normal pressure technique: Leaked tracer appears more slowly; place pledgets after tracer reaches basal cisterns if possible
    - Overpressure technique: Leaked tracer appears quickly; place pledgets prior to tracer injection; imaging started earlier
    - Overpressure technique generally requires neurosurgeon, infusion pump, manometer (transient headache common)
    - Overpressure technique: Stop infusion if pressure > 500 cc H_2O, or headache
  - Imaging protocol
    - Tracer can be injected alone or mixed with CT contrast for combined CT imaging and aid in gravity flow
    - External radioactive markers or a flood source aid anatomic orientation
    - Tracer monitored by preliminary images until bathes the area of clinical concern, at which time images obtained
    - Nuclear tomography (SPECT) may increase imaging sensitivity
    - With overpressure technique imaging can be completed in less than one hour
    - With normal pressure technique, imaging should start at 1-2 hours and continue until 6-8 hours or longer if necessary
    - Early and continuous imaging for spinal leaks
  - Pledgets should be placed under direct visualization by ENT surgeon with consistent protocol
    - Six nasal pledgets, three on each side at anterior, middle, and posterior locations or near superior meatus, middle meatus, and near cribriform plate
    - Pledgets should be clearly labeled
    - Ear pledgets should be placed if CSF otorrhea suspected
    - Pledgets removal does not require an ENT specialist but should be removed anterior, then middle, then posterior to avoid contaminating one pledget with another

CSF LEAK

- Venous blood sample drawn immediately before or after pledget removal, red cells sedimented by centrifugation, 100 μl of serum counted in gamma well counter, along with pledgets (each in separate tube)
- Remove excess nasal mucous from surface of pledget prior to weighing and counting
- Weigh pledgets before placement and before counting to establish fluid volume (1 g = 1)
- Abnormal result: Counts in pledget > 1.5 times counts in equal volume serum

DIFFERENTIAL DIAGNOSIS

Artifact
- Patient moving head during imaging session
- Contamination on surface of patient

PATHOLOGY

General Features
- Genetics: 20% of spontaneous CSF leaks have minor skeletal features of Marfan syndrome
- Etiology
  - Basilar skull fracture, paranasal sinus fracture
  - Spontaneous, congenital, idiopathic
  - Complication of skull, sinus, or pituitary surgery
  - Complication of lumbar puncture
  - Post infectious
  - Vigorous exercise or violent coughing, rupture of arachnoid diverticulum
- Associated abnormalities
  - Subdural hematoma
  - Marfan syndrome
  - Spina bifida

Gross Pathologic & Surgical Features
- The abnormal fluid collection and the associated abnormality or defect

Microscopic Features
- Thickened dura with fibrosis and dilated thin walled vessels

CLINICAL ISSUES

Presentation
- Most common signs/symptoms
  - CSF rhinorrhea or otorrhea
  - Headaches affected by postural maneuvers
  - Lumbar puncture demonstrates low CSF pressure
- Other signs/symptoms
  - Lab tests of leaking fluid identify as CSF
  - Symptoms of meningitis, recurrent meningitis, encephalopathy
  - Conductive hearing loss
  - Cranial nerve palsies
  - Visual disturbances
- Clinical Profile: Onset of postural headache after surgery, trauma or lumbar puncture

Demographics
- Age: Peak age 30-40 years
- Gender: Female to male 2:1 for spontaneous CSF leaks

Natural History & Prognosis
- Most leaks will resolve spontaneously within several months
- Some leaks will persist including persistent headaches
- Continued symptoms, CSF hypotension, meningitis without repair of those that persist
- Prognosis is excellent, although deaths have been reported

Treatment
- Conservative treatment with fluid replacement and bed rest
- Autologous blood patch
- Epidural saline infusion
- Surgical repair of a defect

DIAGNOSTIC CHECKLIST

Consider
- Combining tracer with CT contrast and utilizing both nuclear imaging and CT cisternography

SELECTED REFERENCES

1. Yilmazlar S et al: Cerebrospinal fluid leakage complicating skull base fractures: analysis of 81 cases. Neurosurg Rev. 29(1):64-71, 2006
2. Kerr JT et al: Cerebrospinal fluid rhinorrhea: diagnosis and management. Otolaryngol Clin North Am. 38(4):597-611, 2005
3. Schlosser RJ et al: Nasal cerebrospinal fluid leaks: critical review and surgical considerations. Laryngoscope. 114(2):255-65, 2004
4. Payne RJ et al: Role of computed tomographic cisternography in the management of cerebrospinal fluid rhinorrhea. J Otolaryngol. 32(2):93-100, 2003
5. Rice DH: Cerebrospinal fluid rhinorrhea: diagnosis and treatment. Curr Opin Otolaryngol Head Neck Surg. 11(1):19-22, 2003
6. Stern RH et al: Scintigraphic cerebral spinal fluid leak study in a child with recurrent meningitis after resection of a frontal meningocele. Clin Nucl Med. 20(2):136-9, 1995
7. Lewis DH et al: Benefit of tomography in the scintigraphic localization of cerebrospinal fluid leak. J Nucl Med. 32(11):2149-51, 1991
8. Zu'bi SM et al: Intestinal activity visualized on radionuclide cisternography in patients with cerebrospinal fluid leak. J Nucl Med. 32(1):151-3, 1991
9. Primeau M et al: Spinal cerebrospinal fluid leak demonstrated by radioisotopic cisternography. Clin Nucl Med. 13(10):701-3, 1988
10. Curnes JT et al: CSF rhinorrhea: detection and localization using overpressure cisternography with Tc-99m-DTPA. Radiology. 154(3):795-9, 1985
11. Glaubitt D et al: Detection and quantitation of intermittent CSF rhinorrhea during prolonged cisternography with 111In-DTPA. AJNR Am J Neuroradiol. 4(3):560-3, 1983
12. Colletti PM et al: Posttraumatic lumbar cerebrospinal fluid leak: detection by retrograde in-111-DTPA myeloscintigraphy. Clin Nucl Med. 6(9):403-4, 1981

CSF LEAK

IMAGE GALLERY

Typical

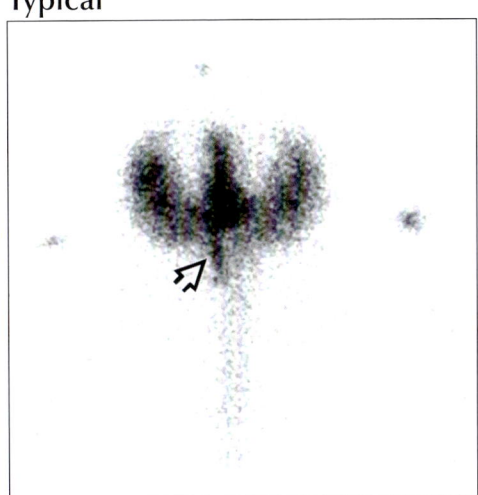

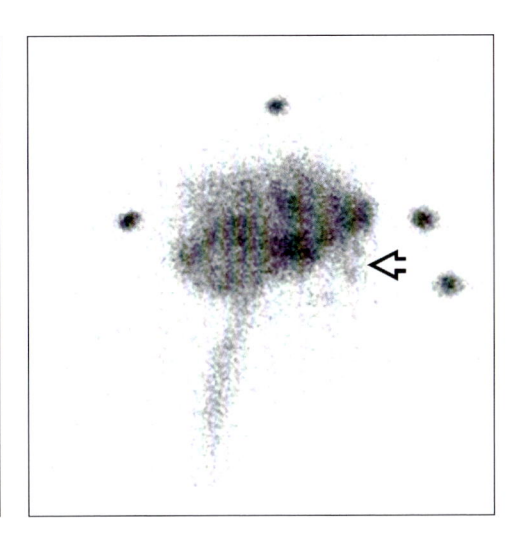

(Left) Anterior CSF leak Evaluation-Radionuclide shows tracer extending below the skull base ⇨ into the right nasopharynx in this patient post sinus surgery. *(Right)* Right lateral CSF leak Evaluation-Radionuclide in the same patient as left shows the abnormal activity ⇨ below the skull base. Pledget counts were 500 times plasma.

Variant

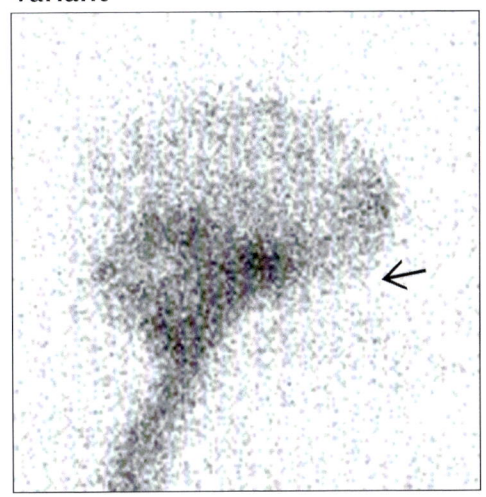

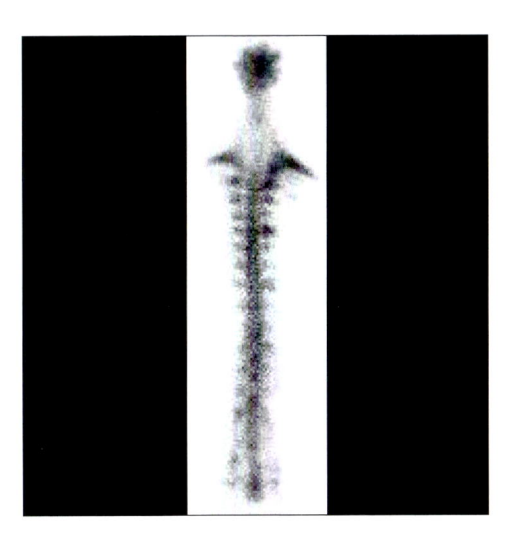

(Left) Right lateral CSF leak Evaluation-Radionuclide shows no activity below the level of the skull base ⇨ despite pledget counts 200 times greater than plasma. This is not uncommon. *(Right)* Posterior Tc-99m DTPA cisternogram in patient with thoracolumbar dural tear and low CSF pressure shows extent of subarachnoid and extradural space. Site of such tears is difficult to find.

Typical

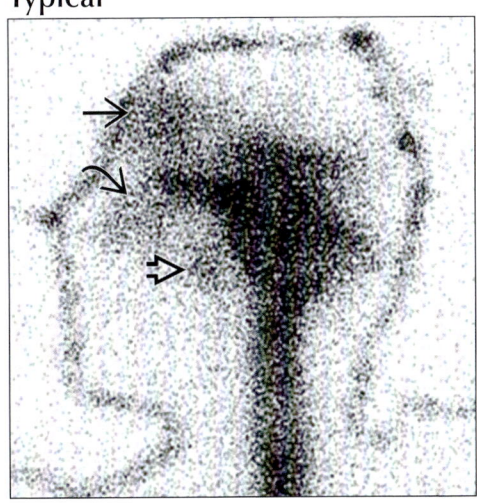

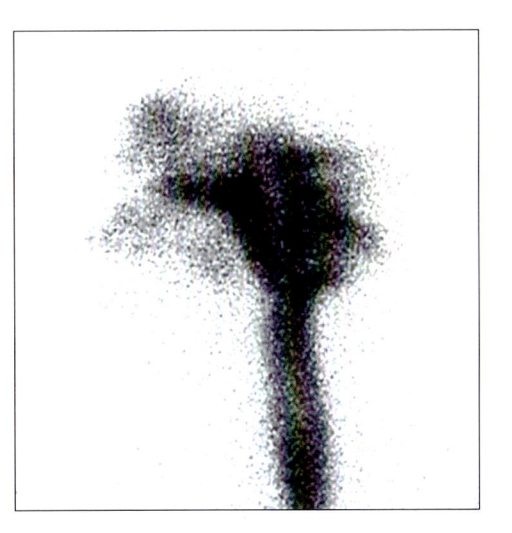

(Left) Left lateral Tc-99m DTPA overpressure CSF study with surface anatomy: Leak from posterior fontal sinus results in activity in frontal sinus ⇨, nose ⇨ and pharynx ⇨. See next image. *(Right)* Left lateral CSF leak Evaluation-Radionuclide of the same patient as previous image but without surface map.

VENTRICULAR SHUNT DYSFUNCTION

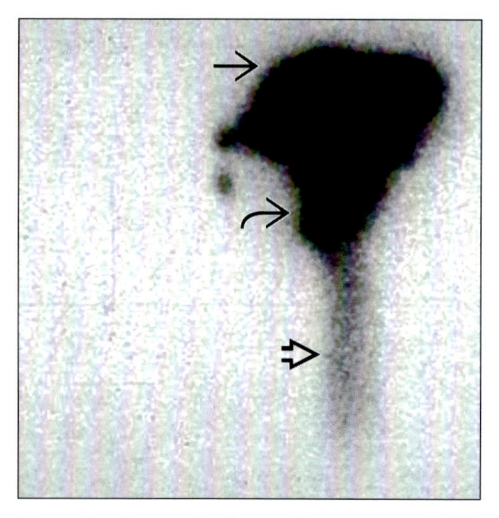

Ventricular shunt study shows reflux into ventricle ➔, basal cistern ➔ and subarachnoid space of spinal cord ➔. Tube was never visualized, consistent with shunt dysfunction.

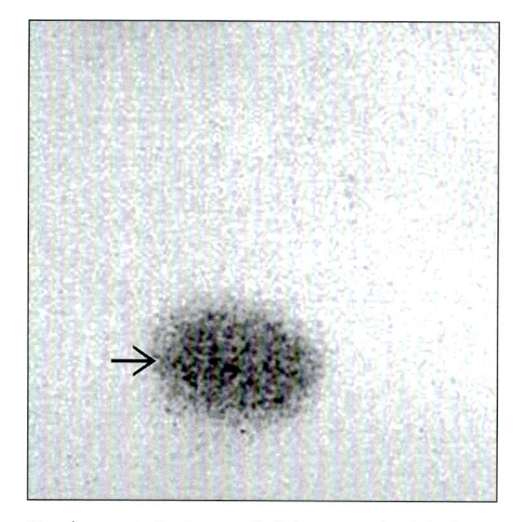

Two-hour anterior image of abdomen and pelvis shows focal collection in urinary bladder ➔, signifying systemic absorption of Tc-99m DTPA and renal excretion.

TERMINOLOGY

Abbreviations and Synonyms
- Cerebrospinal fluid (CSF) diversionary shunt
  - Ventriculoperitoneal (VP)
  - Lumbar peritoneal (LP), lumbar pleural
  - Ventriculopleural (VPL)
  - Ventriculoatrial (VA)

Definitions
- CSF diversionary shunt
  - Decreases amount of CSF in hydrocephalic ventricles/subarachnoid space and deposits into systemic circulation
  - Tube extends from ventricles/subarachnoid space into body cavity, vascular space

IMAGING FINDINGS

General Features
- Best diagnostic clue
  - No radiotracer flow through tube into body cavity
  - No radiotracer reflux into ventricles or subarachnoid space (proximal tube site)
- Location
  - Proximal end of tube
    - Obstructive hydrocephalus: Usually in lateral ventricle
    - Communicating (normal pressure) hydrocephalus: Lateral ventricle, extraventricular subarachnoid space
  - Middle of tube
    - Traverses the neck, thorax and abdomen, depending on distal site
  - Distal end of tube
    - Peritoneal space
    - Pleural space
    - Rarely: Central venous system (e.g., right atrium)

Nuclear Medicine Findings
- Normal
  - Radiotracer reflux from reservoir to ventricles and/or subarachnoid space
  - Visualization of radiotracer in tube
  - Radiotracer disperses in distal cavity
    - Pleural space

DDx: Patent Ventriculoperitoneal Shunt

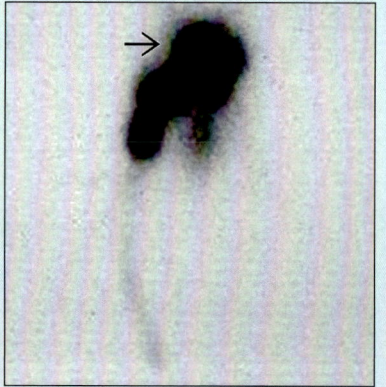

| Ventricular Reflux | Thoracolumbar Tube | Peritoneal Dispersion |

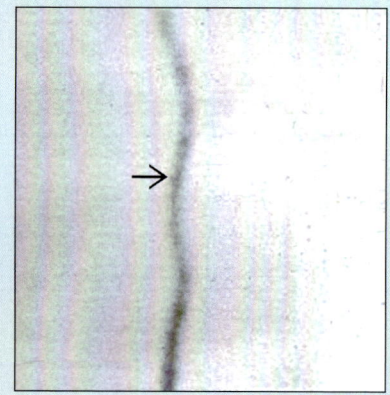

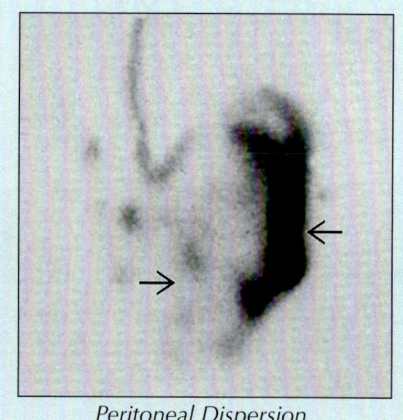

VENTRICULAR SHUNT DYSFUNCTION

Key Facts

Imaging Findings
- Lack of radiotracer reflux into ventricle/subarachnoid space: Blocked proximal tube from ventricle/subarachnoid space to reservoir
- Nonvisualization of distal tube: Distal tube blocked (may not see exact site of blockage)
- Collection or tracking in subcutaneous tissue around tube: Tube broken
- Radiotracer confinement in small space at tube tip: Obstruction due to loculation at/around tube end
- Best imaging tool: Radionuclide CSF shunt patency study
- Radiographs required to define reservoir position, tube course, identify breaks in tube
- Position patient supine over/near gamma camera for immediate imaging of reservoir/head
- Inject 1 mCi Tc-99m DTPA in 0.1 mL sterile (non-bacteriostatic) water or saline into reservoir
- Flush: 0.3 mL sterile (non-bacteriostatic) water/saline
- Release tube compression when reflux into ventricle evident on immediate imaging
- With patient supine, image anterior abdomen/pelvis

Diagnostic Checklist
- Important: Ensure proper reservoir access and needle placement by imaging injection site
- Compress tube to confirm proximal tube patency
- Demonstrate dispersion of tracer into distal cavity
- Post-void image: Bladder activity easily confused with peritoneal dispersion
- Loculation: Attempt dispersion of radiotracer with lateral decubitus
- Increase image intensity to visualize tube

  - Peritoneal space
  - Visualization of kidneys, urinary bladder signifies systemic absorption
- Abnormal
  - Focal accumulation in tissue around reservoir
    - Failure to insert needle into shunt reservoir, radiopharmaceutical infiltration
    - Increased blood pool, kidney, urinary bladder activity
    - Lack of ventricle visualization, subarachnoid space, proximal or distal tubing, distal body cavity
  - Lack of radiotracer reflux into ventricle/subarachnoid space: Blocked proximal tube from ventricle/subarachnoid space to reservoir
    - Activity in distal tube and dispersion in body cavity may be normal
  - Nonvisualization of distal tube: Distal tube blocked (may not see exact site of blockage)
    - Proximal tube and ventricular reflux may be normal
    - No radiotracer dispersion in body cavity
    - Often increased radiotracer in subarachnoid space around brain and spinal cord
  - Collection or tracking in subcutaneous tissue around tube: Tube broken
    - Radiotracer distribution assumes significantly wider diameter than tube
  - Radiotracer confinement in small space at tube tip: Obstruction due to loculation at/around tube end

Imaging Recommendations
- Best imaging tool: Radionuclide CSF shunt patency study
- Protocol advice
  - Preliminary
    - Radiographs required to define reservoir position, tube course, identify breaks in tube
  - Injection technique
    - Position patient supine over/near gamma camera for immediate imaging of reservoir/head
    - Reservoir site shaved, sterile prep and drape
    - Using aseptic technique, access reservoir (or tube if no reservoir) with 25-g needle
    - Point needle tip cephalad: Maximizes reflux into ventricles/subarachnoid space
    - Compress tube distal to reservoir or injection site: Maximizes reflux into ventricle
    - Inject 1 mCi Tc-99m DTPA in 0.1 mL sterile (non-bacteriostatic) water or saline into reservoir
    - Flush: 0.3 mL sterile (non-bacteriostatic) water/saline
    - Release tube compression when reflux into ventricle evident on immediate imaging
    - Some reservoirs can be pumped to facilitate antegrade CSF flow
  - Imaging technique
    - Initial images of injection site/head: Ensure needle in reservoir and proximal tube patent
    - After initial images, patient may get up and move around to facilitate distal flow into body cavity
    - With patient supine, image anterior abdomen/pelvis
    - Lateral decubitus: May be necessary to confirm lack of fluid loculation in distal body cavity
    - Post-void image: Distinguish pelvic pooling in body cavity from radiotracer in urinary bladder
- Correlative imaging features
  - Radiograph
    - Locate reservoir
    - Evaluate tube for defects
  - Head MR, CT
    - Hydrocephalus (↑ ventricle size)
    - Subependymal CSF leak
  - Abdominal CT, ultrasound
    - Loculated fluid collection around distal tube tip

DIFFERENTIAL DIAGNOSIS

No Reflux into Ventricle
- VPL shunt
  - Radiotracer pulled from ventricle into pleural space due to negative pressure during respiration
- Ventricular reflux may not be seen with VA shunt

VENTRICULAR SHUNT DYSFUNCTION

- Ventricular reflux may not occur even when all portions of shunt patent

Radiotracer Tracking Outside of Tube
- Due to tube breakage with CSF leaking/tracking through tract surrounding tube
- May mimic activity inside tube, but with wider diameter

Bladder Activity
- May mimic peritoneal dispersion of radiotracer
- Seen with functional and dysfunctional shunts
  - Radiotracer absorbed from subarachnoid space with renal excretion

PATHOLOGY

General Features
- Etiology
  - Tube break
  - Tube blockage
    - Normal cellular debris
    - Infection
  - Tube disconnection at reservoir
  - Loculation at/around tube tip

CLINICAL ISSUES

Presentation
- Most common signs/symptoms
  - Increasing headache
  - Mental status changes
  - Ataxia
  - Incontinence
  - Ventriculomegaly without symptoms: May not require shunting
- Other signs/symptoms
  - Fever, elevated white blood cell count (infection)
  - Fluctuant mass around tube (if broken)

Treatment
- Blocked or broken tube
  - Tube replacement
- Infection
  - Tube removal
  - Placement of new shunt at another site
  - IV antibiotics
- Tube disconnected at reservoir
  - Reconnect/replace tube
- Loculation at tube tip
  - Reposition tube in body cavity

DIAGNOSTIC CHECKLIST

Image Interpretation Pearls
- Important: Ensure proper reservoir access and needle placement by imaging injection site
- Compress tube to confirm proximal tube patency
- Demonstrate dispersion of tracer into distal cavity
  - Post-void image: Bladder activity easily confused with peritoneal dispersion
- Loculation: Attempt dispersion of radiotracer with lateral decubitus
- Increase image intensity to visualize tube

SELECTED REFERENCES

1. Gnanalingham KK et al: Isolated diastasis of cranial sutures: unusual presentation of a blocked shunt in an infant. Childs Nerv Syst. 21(10):936-8, 2005
2. Kumar R et al: Shunt revision in hydrocephalus. Indian J Pediatr. 72(10):843-7, 2005
3. Mangano FT et al: Early programmable valve malfunctions in pediatric hydrocephalus. J Neurosurg. 103(6 Suppl):501-7, 2005
4. Arnell K et al: Distal catheter obstruction from non-infectious cause in ventriculo-peritoneal shunted children. Eur J Pediatr Surg. 14(4):245-9, 2004
5. Owen R et al: Delayed external ventriculoperitoneal shunt infection. J Ky Med Assoc. 102(8):349-52, 2004
6. Yadav YR et al: Lumboperitoneal shunts: review of 409 cases. Neurol India. 52(2):188-90, 2004
7. Tomes DJ et al: Stretching and breaking characteristics of cerebrospinal fluid shunt tubing. J Neurosurg. 98(3):578-83, 2003
8. Acharya R et al: Laparoscopic management of abdominal complications in ventriculoperitoneal shunt surgery. J Laparoendosc Adv Surg Tech A. 11(3):167-70, 2001
9. Gilkes CE et al: Pressure compensation in shunt-dependent hydrocephalus with CSF shunt malfunction. Childs Nerv Syst. 17(1-2):52-7, 2001
10. Kazan S et al: Proof of the patent subcutaneous fibrous tract in children with V-P shunt malfunction. Childs Nerv Syst. 16(6):351-6, 2000
11. Sood S et al: Evaluation of shunt malfunction using shunt site reservoir. Pediatr Neurosurg. 32(4):180-6, 2000
12. Zemack G et al: Seven years of clinical experience with the programmable Codman Hakim valve: a retrospective study of 583 patients. J Neurosurg. 92(6):941-8, 2000
13. Gilkes CE et al: A classification of CSF shunt malfunction. Eur J Pediatr Surg. 9 Suppl 1:19-22, 1999
14. Zingale A et al: Infections and re-infections in long-term external ventricular drainage. A variation upon a theme. J Neurosurg Sci. 43(2):125-32; discussion 133, 1999
15. Williams MA et al: Evaluation of shunt function in patients who are never better, or better than worse after shunt surgery for NPH. Acta Neurochir Suppl. 71:368-70, 1998
16. Caldarelli M et al: Shunt complications in the first postoperative year in children with meningomyelocele. Childs Nerv Syst. 12(12):748-54, 1996
17. Piatt JH Jr: Pumping the shunt revisited. A longitudinal study. Pediatr Neurosurg. 25(2):73-6; discussion 76-7, 1996
18. Vanaclocha V et al: Shunt malfunction in relation to shunt infection. Acta Neurochir (Wien). 138(7):829-34, 1996
19. Lundar T: Shunt removal or replacement based on intraventricular infusion tests. Childs Nerv Syst. 10(5):337-9, 1994
20. Kontny U et al: CSF shunt infections in children. Infection. 21(2):89-92, 1993
21. Walters BC: Cerebrospinal fluid shunt infection. Neurosurg Clin N Am. 3(2):387-401, 1992
22. Jamjoom AH et al: Misleading clinical syndromes of CSF shunt malfunction. Br J Neurosurg. 2(3):391-4, 1988
23. Graham P et al: Evaluation of CSF shunt patency by means of technetium-99m DTPA. J Neurosurg. 57(2):262-6, 1982
24. Di Chiro G et al: Evaluation of surgical and spontaneous cerebrospinal fluid shunts by isotope scanning. J Neurosurg. 24(4):743-8, 1966

VENTRICULAR SHUNT DYSFUNCTION

IMAGE GALLERY

Typical

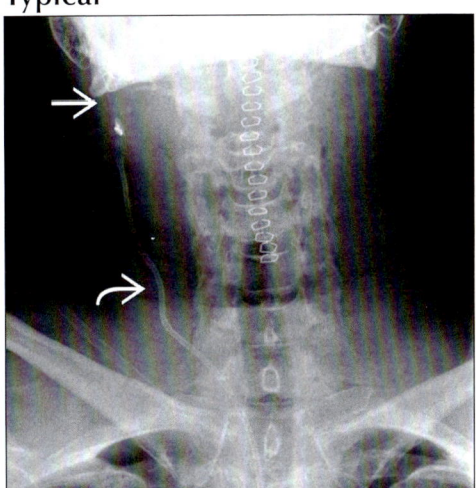

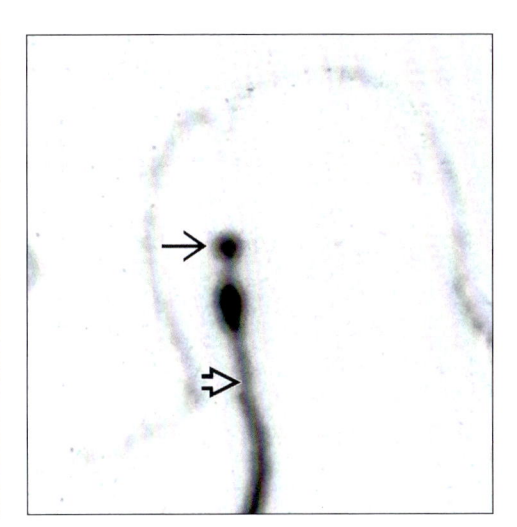

(Left) Anterior radiograph of neck shows reservoir ➡, which is not radiopaque and not to be confused with disconnected tube. Tube ➡ is radiopaque. *(Right)* Right lateral ventricular shunt study of patient with ventriculopleural shunt shows radiotracer in reservoir ➡ and tube ➡. No radiotracer reflux into ventricle is normal due to negative pleural pressure with respiration.

Typical

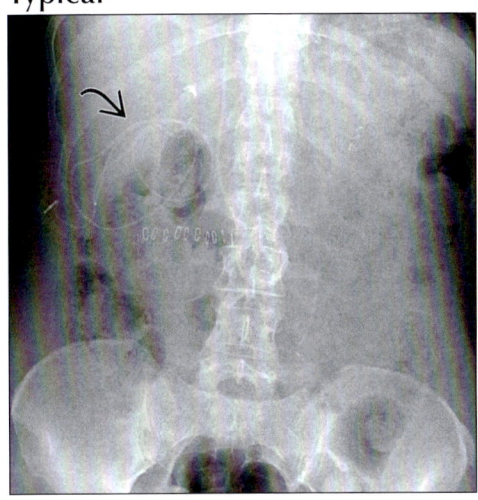

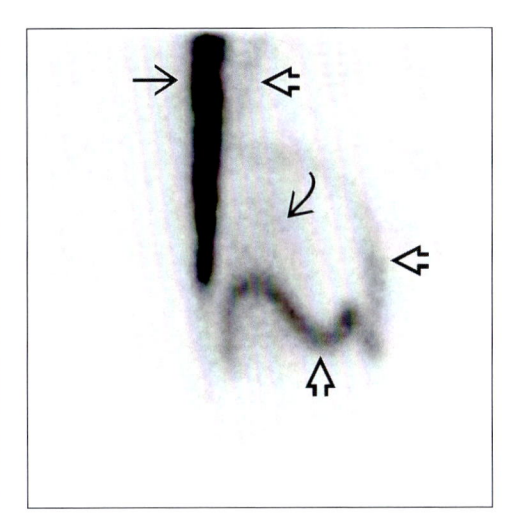

(Left) Anterior radiograph shows distal tube coiled over right upper quadrant ➡. The distal tip is in right pleural space, signifying a ventriculopleural shunt. *(Right)* Right lateral ventricular shunt study over thorax in patient at left shows subarachnoid space ➡, shunt tube ➡, and dispersion into pleural space ➡.

Typical

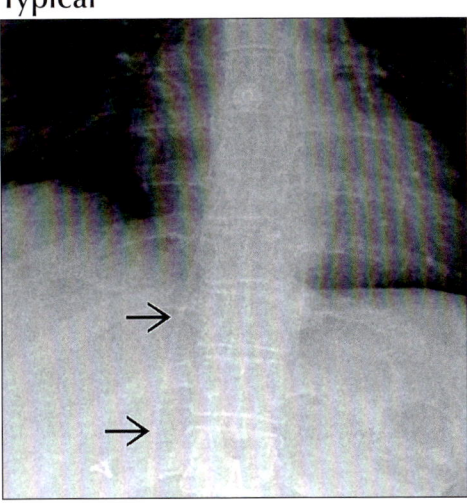

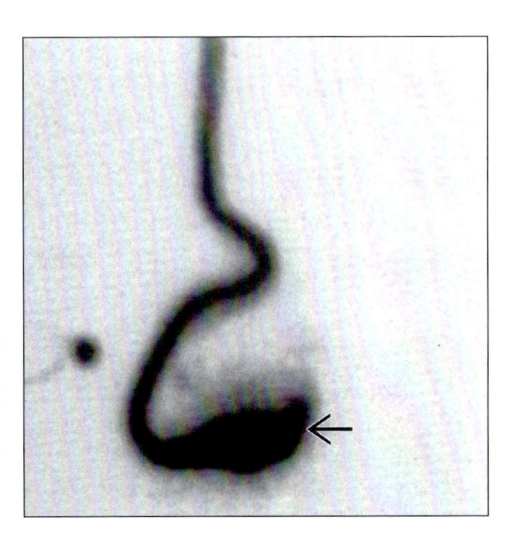

(Left) Anterior radiograph shows intact shunt tube in thorax and upper abdomen ➡ in patient with ventriculoperitoneal shunt. *(Right)* Anterior ventricular shunt study in patient at left shows fluid collection at distal tube tip ➡ which did not disperse freely into abdomen and pelvis. This signifies loculated CSF collection in abdomen.

NORMAL PRESSURE HYDROCEPHALUS

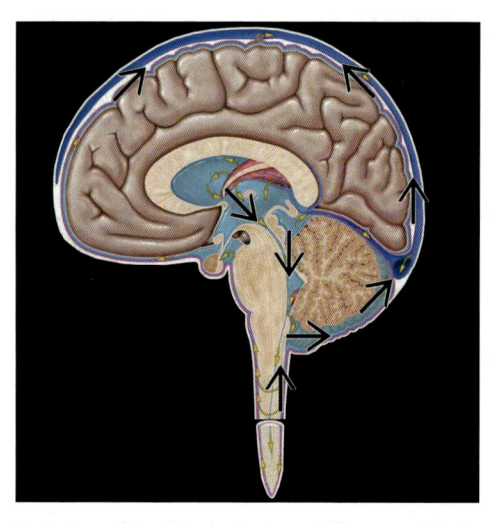

Sagittal graphic of the brain shows CSF spaces (blue). ➡ show direction of flow of CSF to top of brain where absorbed into venous system by arachnoid granulations.

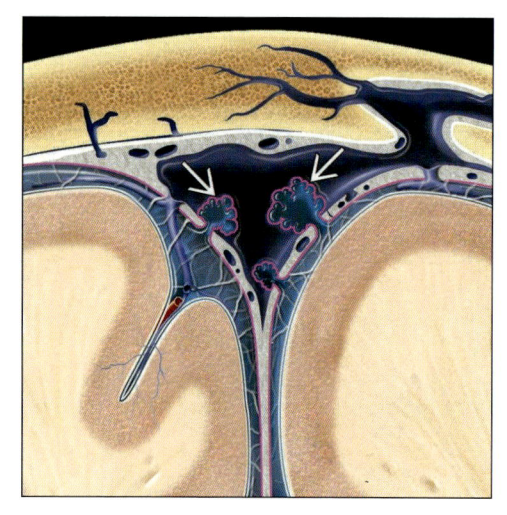

Coronal graphic shows CSF (light blue) is absorbed by arachnoid granulations ➡ and enters venous blood.

TERMINOLOGY

Abbreviations and Synonyms
- Normal pressure hydrocephalus (NPH)
- Radionuclide cisternography (RNC)

Definitions
- Ventriculomegaly with normal cerebrospinal fluid (CSF) pressure, altered CSF dynamics

IMAGING FINDINGS

General Features
- Best diagnostic clue
  - Prominent ventricular activity at 24 h on In-111 DTPA cisternography is best indicator of NPH
  - "Flow void" in aqueduct on MR indicates NPH (vs. high obstructive hydrocephalus)
  - NHP: 50% correlation with improvement after shunt
- Morphology
  - Ventriculomegaly is prominent in all 3 horns of lateral ventricles and 3rd ventricle, with relative sparing of 4th ventricle
  - CT and MR: Ventricles and Sylvian fissures symmetrically dilated out of proportion to sulcal enlargement
  - Normal hippocampus (which distinguishes NPH from atrophy)
- Diagnostic challenge = identify shunt-responsive NPH

Nuclear Medicine Findings
- In-111 DTPA radionuclide cisternography (RNC)
  - Normal immediate RNC images: Rapidly ascent to head
  - Normal 1-2 h RNC images: Ascends to basal cisterns
  - Normal 4-6 h RNC images: Reaches Sylvian & suprasellar cisterns, ventricular penetration
  - Normal 24 h RNC images: No ventricular activity on planar images (may be faint on SPECT); flow over convexities to top of head
  - Normal 48 h RNC images: Homogeneous distribution of tracer around brain
  - NPH: Prominent ventricular activity at 24 h and beyond
  - NPH: Flow to top of head may be normal or slow

CT Findings
- NECT

DDx: "Christmas Tree" Appearance Following Epidural or "Split" Injection of Tracer

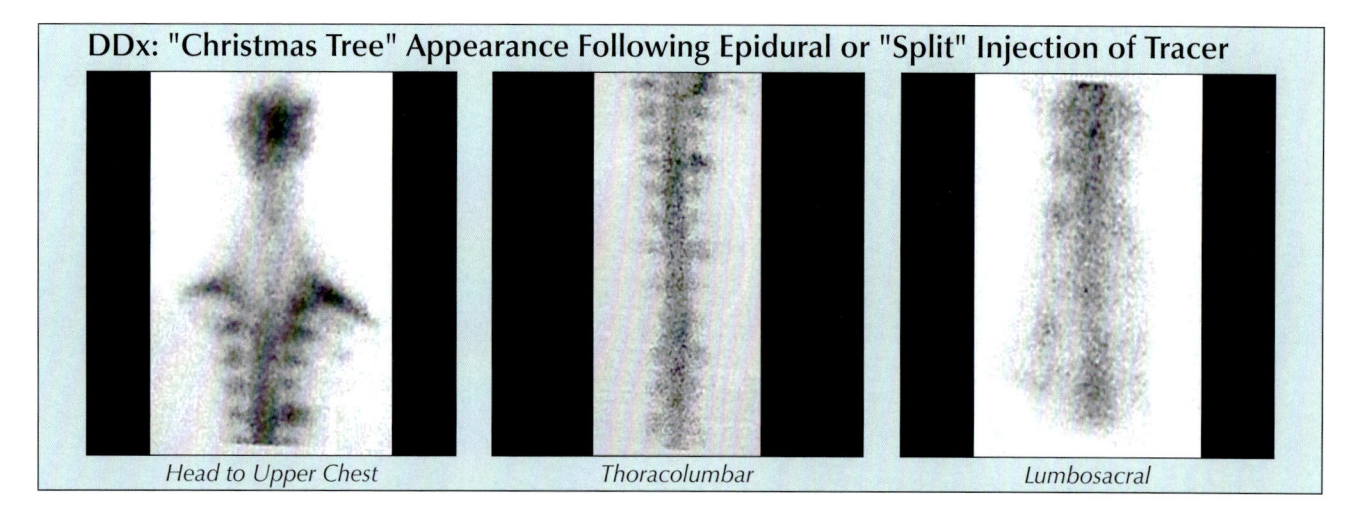

Head to Upper Chest | *Thoracolumbar* | *Lumbosacral*

NORMAL PRESSURE HYDROCEPHALUS

Key Facts

Terminology
- Normal pressure hydrocephalus (NPH)
- Radionuclide cisternography (RNC)

Imaging Findings
- Prominent ventricular activity at 24 h on In-111 DTPA cisternography is best indicator of NPH
- "Flow void" in aqueduct on MR indicates NPH (vs. high obstructive hydrocephalus)
- NHP: 50% correlation with improvement after shunt
- Normal immediate RNC images: Rapidly ascent to head
- Normal 1-2 h RNC images: Ascends to basal cisterns
- Normal 4-6 h RNC images: Reaches Sylvian & suprasellar cisterns, ventricular penetration
- Normal 24 h RNC images: No ventricular activity on planar images (may be faint on SPECT); flow over convexities to top of head
- Normal 48 h RNC images: Homogeneous distribution of tracer around brain
- NPH: Prominent ventricular activity at 24 h and beyond
- NPH: Flow to top of head may be normal or slow

Clinical Issues
- Heterogeneous triad (10% of NPH): Dementia, gait apraxia, urinary incontinence

Diagnostic Checklist
- Whether ventricular dilation is solely due to atrophy
- Prominent ventricular activity at 24 h is single diagnostic feature of NPH on RNC

- Ventriculomegaly with rounded frontal horns, out of proportion to sulcal atrophy (ventriculosulcal disproportion)
- Frontal and occipital periventricular hypodensities (representing transependymal CSF flow)
- Corpus callosal thinning (nonspecific)

MR Findings
- T1WI
  - Lateral ventricles enlarge
  - +/- Aqueductal "flow void"
- T2WI
  - Regions of moving CSF demonstrate no signal
  - Periventricular high signal, primarily anterior to frontal horns or posterior to occipital horns (transependymal CSF flow)
  - 50-60% have periventricular and deep white matter lesions
    - Correlates with poor outcome after shunting, but should not exclude patients from surgery
- MRS
  - Proton chemical shift imaging (^{1}H-CSI): Lactate peaks in lateral ventricles in NPH patients, but not in patients with other types of dementia
    - Reflects ischemic changes in periventricular regions despite normal CSF pressure in patients with NPH
    - May be key factor in differentiating NPH from other dementias
    - May be useful as follow-up study after continuous spinal drainage
- Hypointense or absent signal in proximal 4th ventricle on T2WI, PD, FLAIR, with surrounding CSF appearing hyperintense
- Dilatation of optic and infundibular recesses of anterior 3rd ventricle and downward displacement of hypothalamus
- Corpus callosum bowed upwards (may be impinged by falx)
- Aqueductal "flow void" sign
  - Reflects increased CSF velocity through aqueduct
  - May be reduced if flow-compensation, FSE techniques used
- Cortical and subcortical lacunar infarctions (basal ganglia, internal capsule)

Other Modality Findings
- CSF flow studies to detect increased velocity ("hyperdynamic" flow)
  - Cardiac-gated 2D-FISP
  - Aqueduct stroke volume > 42 mL reported to correlate with good response to shunt
  - Some patients with normal CSF flow values also improve
- ICP monitoring: Wave amplitude > 9 mm Hg correlates with post-shunt cognitive improvement

Imaging Recommendations
- Best imaging tool
  - In-111 DTPA radionuclide cisternography
  - MR with CSF flow study also acceptable
- Protocol advice
  - In-111 DTPA radionuclide cisternography
    - 500 µCi In-111 DTPA injected sterilely via lumbar puncture
    - Immediate imaging to confirm intrathecal placement, ascending activity
    - 4, 24 and 48 h planar images of head: Anterior, posterior, both laterals and vertex (image over top of head)
    - 24 h SPECT images of head if ventricular activity equivocal
  - MR
    - T1WI, T2WI with CSF flow study

DIFFERENTIAL DIAGNOSIS

Normal Aging Brain
- Thin periventricular high signal rim without white matter hyperintensities ("successfully aging brain")

Alzheimer Dementia
- Dementia out of proportion to gait disturbance
- Large parahippocampal fissures, small hippocampi, sulcal enlargement

NORMAL PRESSURE HYDROCEPHALUS

Multi-Infarct Dementia (MID)
- Multiple infarcts on imaging

Subcortical Arteriosclerotic Encephalopathy (Binswanger Disease)
- Continuous, irreversible ischemic degeneration of periventricular and deep white matter
- MR shows extensive periventricular and deep white matter hyperintensities, enlarged ventricles

PATHOLOGY

General Features
- General path comments: Pathogenesis of NPH poorly understood
- Etiology
  - 50% idiopathic
  - 50% other (e.g., subarachnoid hemorrhage, meningitis, neurosurgery, or head trauma)
  - Age-related changes in CSF formation/absorption include increased resistance to CSF outflow
  - Dysfunctional CSF dynamics
    - Reduced absorption through arachnoid villi
    - Compensatory CSF flow into periventricular white matter
    - Transcapillary CSF resorption
  - NPH: Reduced CBF, altered CSF resorption without increased CSF pressure
    - Brain expands in systole, causes CSF displacement
    - Loss of parenchymal compliance, altered viscoelastic properties of ventricular wall
    - Increased interstitial fluid
    - Pulsations directed toward ventricles, "water hammer effect"
- Epidemiology: Accounts for approximately 0.5-5% of dementias

Gross Pathologic & Surgical Features
- Enlarged ventricles, normal CSF pressure
- Periventricular white matter is stretched and dysfunctional due to inadequate perfusion, without actually being infarcted

Microscopic Features
- Arachnoid fibrosis in 50%
- Periventricular tissue: Disruption of ependyma; edema, neuronal degeneration, gliosis
- Cerebral parenchyma
  - Almost 50% show no significant parenchymal pathology
  - 20% have changes of Alzheimer dementia
  - 10% have arteriosclerosis, ischemic changes

CLINICAL ISSUES

Presentation
- Most common signs/symptoms
  - Heterogeneous triad (10% of NPH): Dementia, gait apraxia, urinary incontinence
  - Symptom severity is related to CSF levels of neurofilament protein, a marker of neuronal degeneration
- Clinical Profile: Reversible cause of dementia

Demographics
- Age
  - Most common in patients > 60 y
  - Idiopathic form of NPH tends to present in elderly
  - Patients with chronic communicating hydrocephalus due to prior known insult tend to present at an earlier age
- Gender: M > F
- Ethnicity: No racial predilection

Natural History & Prognosis
- Natural course: Continuing cognitive and motor decline, akinetic mutism, and eventual death
- Potentially reversible cause of dementia when shunted
- Some patients worsen after shunting

Treatment
- Predictors of positive response to shunting
  - Absence of central atrophy or ischemia
  - Gait apraxia as dominant clinical symptom
  - Prominent CSF flow void
  - Known history of intracranial infection or bleeding (nonidiopathic NPH)
- After shunt surgery
  - Variable outcome: 1/3 of patients improve, 1/3 display arrest of symptom progression, and 1/3 continue to deteriorate

DIAGNOSTIC CHECKLIST

Consider
- Whether ventricular dilation is solely due to atrophy

Image Interpretation Pearls
- Prominent ventricular activity at 24 h is single diagnostic feature of NPH on RNC

SELECTED REFERENCES

1. Czosnyka M et al: Age dependence of cerebrospinal pressure-volume compensation in patients with hydrocephalus. J Neurosurg. 94:482-6, 2001
2. Kizu O et al: Proton chemical shift imaging in normal pressure hydrocephalus. Am J Neuroradiol. 22:1659-64, 2001
3. Tullberg M et al: Normal pressure hydrocephalus: vascular white matter changes on MR images must not exclude patients from shunt surgery. Am J Neuroradiol. 22:1665-73, 2001
4. Parkkola RK et al: Cerebrospinal fluid flow in patients with dilated ventricles studied with MR imaging. Eur Radiol. 10:1442-6, 2000
5. Bech RA et al: Frontal brain and leptomeningeal biopsy specimens correlated with CSF outflow resistance and B-wave activity in patients suspected of NPH. Neurosurg. 40:497-502, 1997
6. Harbert JC et al: Computed cranial tomography and radionuclide cisternography in hydrocephalus. Semin Nucl Med. 7(2):197-200, 1977

NORMAL PRESSURE HYDROCEPHALUS

IMAGE GALLERY

Other

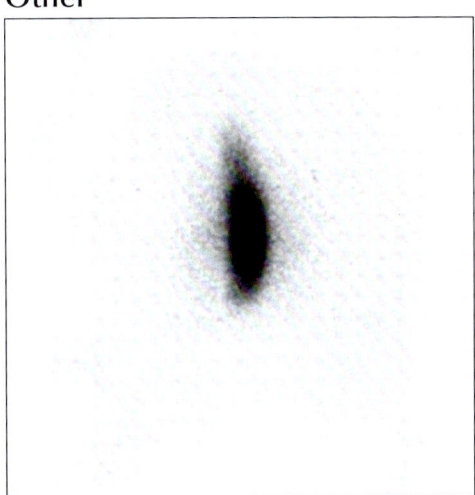

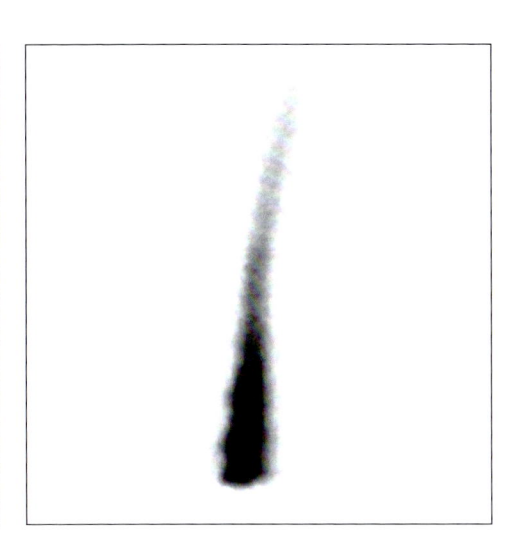

(**Left**) Initial image following LP injection of In-111 DTPA shows little flow of CSF. This was an epidural injection. (**Right**) Normal radionuclide cisternogram. Immediate images following LP introduction of tracer show normal cephalad flow of tracer. This was appropriately injected into the intrathecal space. See next 4 images.

Other

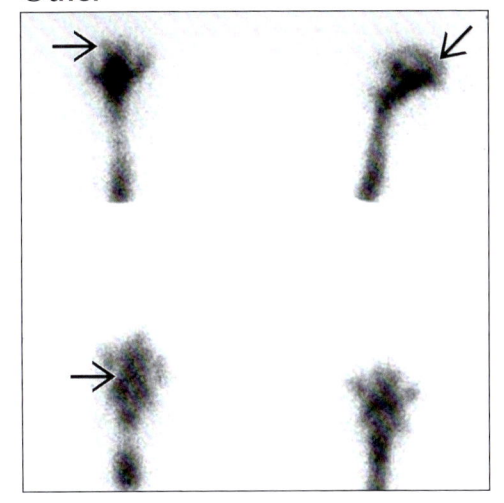

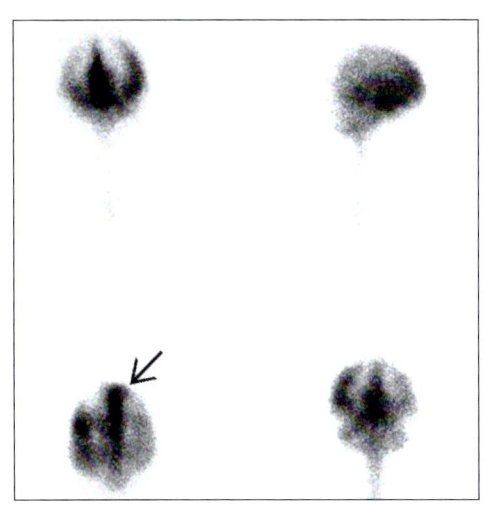

(**Left**) Normal study. 4 h multiplanar images of the head show normal flow to basal, Sylvian and suprasellar cisterns, with faint ventricular activity ➡. See next image. (**Right**) Same patient as left. Normal study. 24 h multiplanar images show flow of tracer over convexities and into interhemispheric fissure ➡. No definite ventricular activity. See next image.

Other

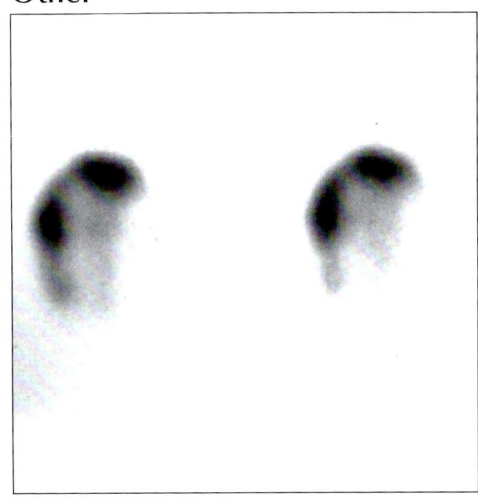

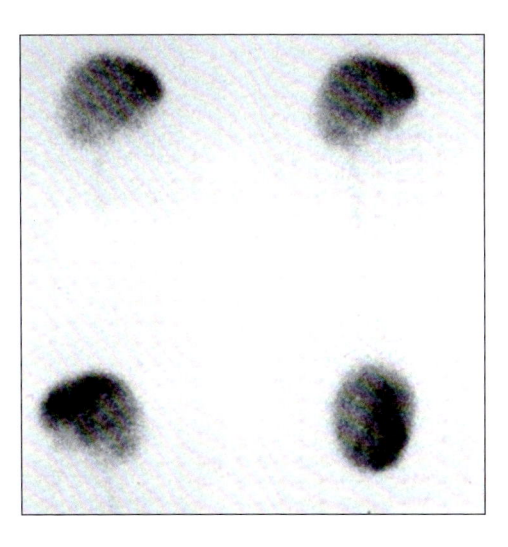

(**Left**) Normal study. 24 h transaxial SPECT images confirm no ventricular activity. Mild asymmetry to flow over convexities is present, and can be normal. See next image. (**Right**) Normal study. 48 h multiplanar images show homogeneous distribution of tracer over brain.

NORMAL PRESSURE HYDROCEPHALUS

(Left) Multiplanar images 4 h after LP injection of In-111 DTPA. Patient with normal pressure hydrocephalus. Normal tracer accumulation in basal, suprasellar, and Sylvian fissures. Normal ventricular penetration. See next 5 image. *(Right)* Normal pressure hydrocephalus. 24 h multiplanar images show tracer in lateral ventricle ⇨, confirmed by vertex and SPECT images following.

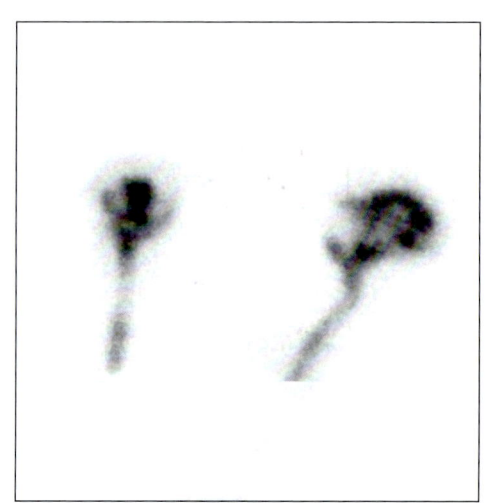

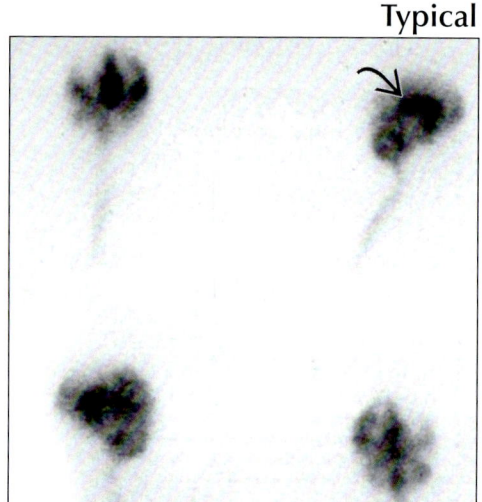

(Left) Planar vertex view (top of head with shielding around shoulders) shows clear activity in lateral ventricles ⇨, confirming diagnosis of normal pressure hydrocephalus. *(Right)* Axial SPECT. Normal pressure hydrocephalus confirmed by visualization of significant ventricular activity at 24 h ⇨.

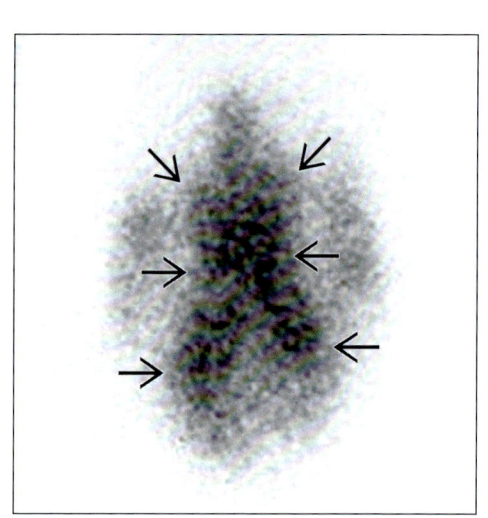

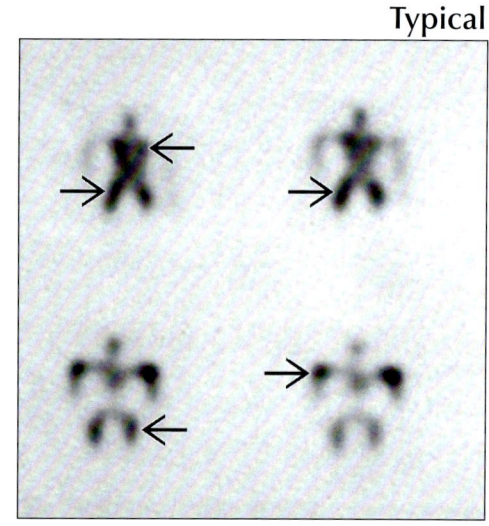

(Left) Additional axial SPECT images. Normal pressure hydrocephalus confirmed by visualization of significant ventricular activity at 24 h ⇨. See next image. *(Right)* 24 h sagittal SPECT clearly demonstrates significant tracer in the lateral ventricle ⇨, confirming normal pressure hydrocephalus.

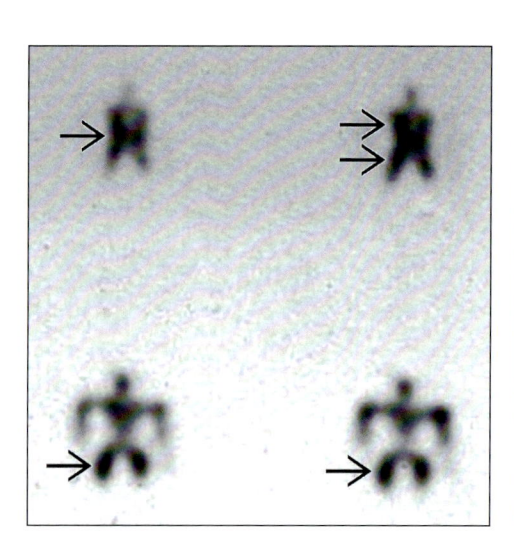

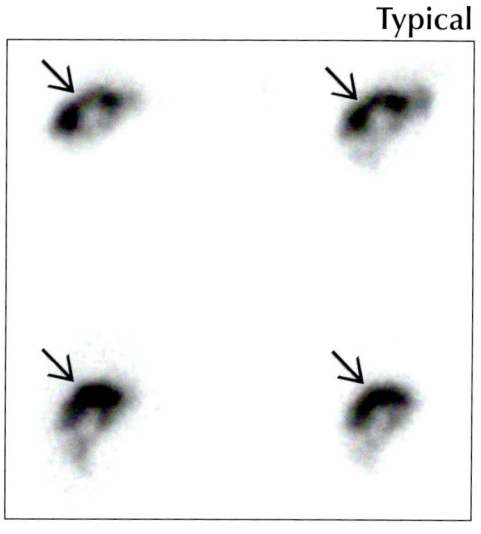

NORMAL PRESSURE HYDROCEPHALUS

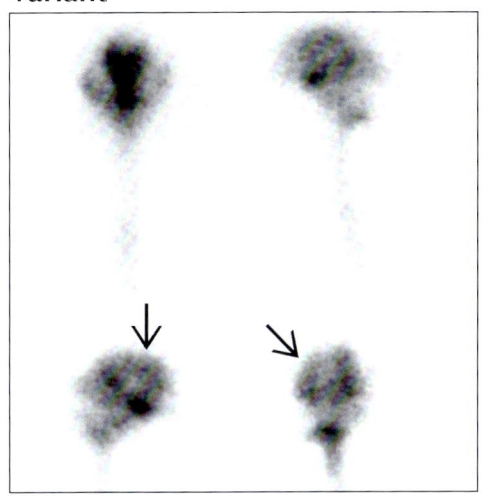

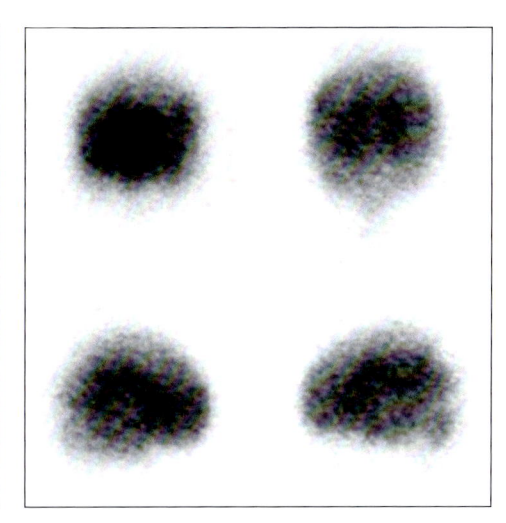

Variant

(Left) Normal pressure hydrocephalus. 4 h multiplanar images show normal uptake in basal, Sylvian and suprasellar cisterns, and in lateral ventricles ⇒. See next 5 images. (Right) Normal pressure hydrocephalus. Lateral ventricle activity is difficult to identify on multiplanar anterior, posterior, and lateral images.

Variant

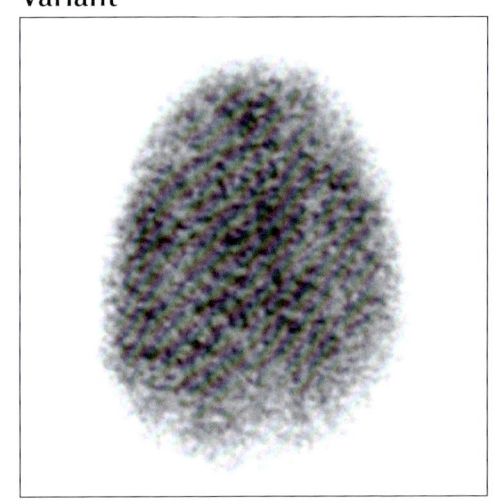

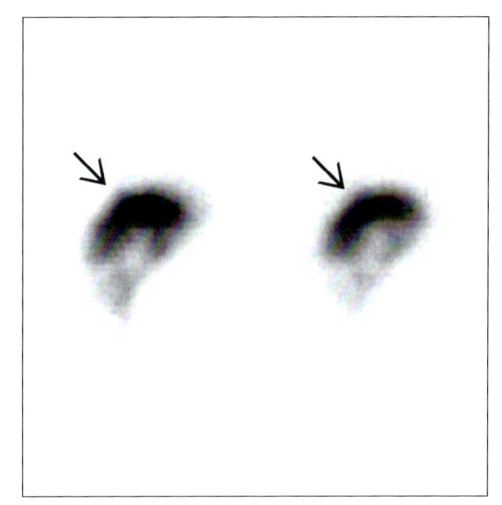

(Left) Normal pressure hydrocephalus. Vertex (top of head) view suggests lateral ventricle activity, obscured by overlying tracer. (Right) 24 h sagittal SPECT demonstrates marked ventricle activity ⇒, confirming presence of normal pressure hydrocephalus.

Variant

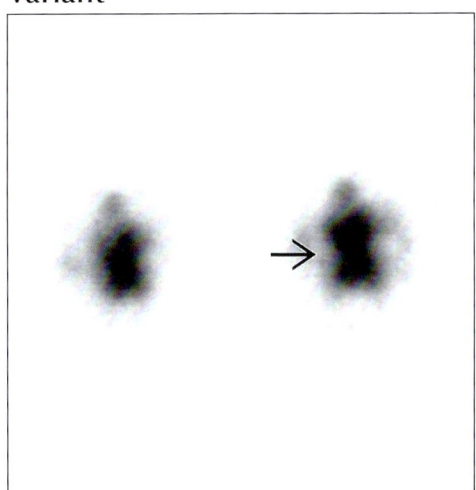

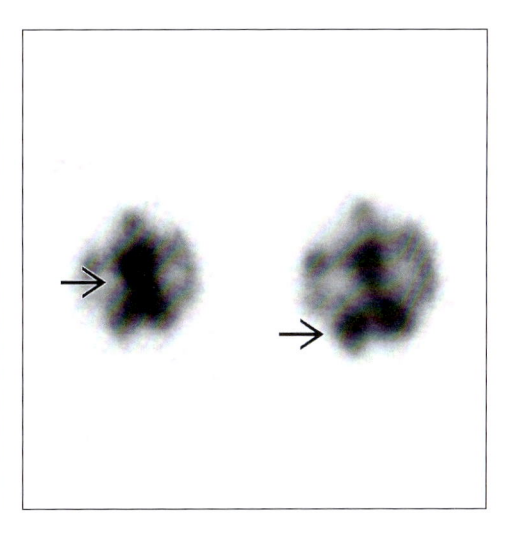

(Left) 24 h axial SPECT demonstrates marked ventricle activity ⇒, confirming presence of normal pressure hydrocephalus. (Right) Additional 24 h axial SPECT images demonstrate marked ventricle activity ⇒, confirming presence of normal pressure hydrocephalus.

HETEROTOPIC GRAY MATTER

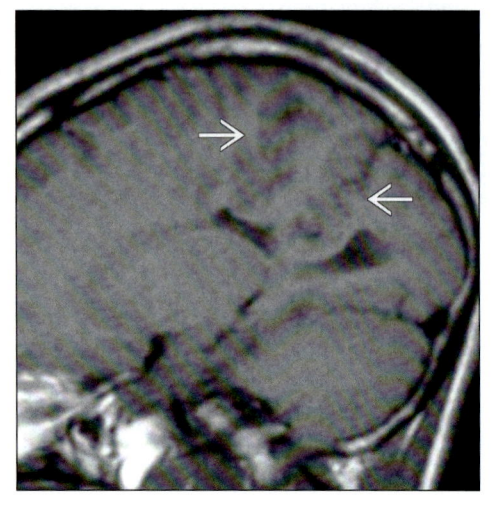

Sagittal T1WI MR demonstrates parietal bands of heterotopic gray matter (HGM) extending into white matter regions ➡. See FDG PET scan at right.

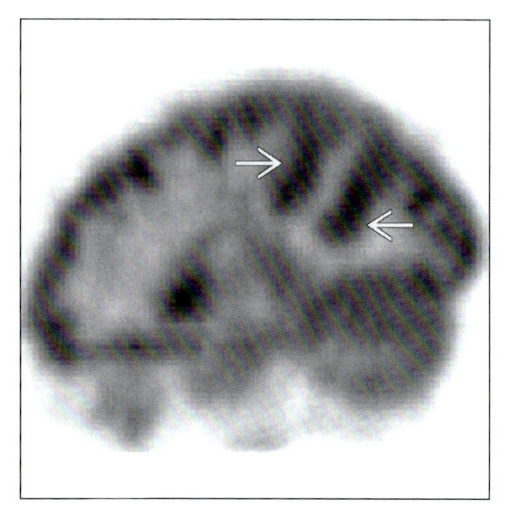

Sagittal FDG PET (same patient as previous image) demonstrates metabolic activity (similar to normal cortex) in parietal bands of heterotopic gray matter ➡.

TERMINOLOGY

Abbreviations and Synonyms
- Heterotopic gray matter (HGM)
- Cerebral ectopia
- Neuronal migration disorder
- Malformations of cortical development

Definitions
- Arrested/disrupted neurons along migration path from periventricular germinal zone to cortex
  - Can be inherited
  - Can be acquired (maternal trauma, infection, or toxin)

IMAGING FINDINGS

General Features
- Best diagnostic clue
  - Nodule or ribbon on MR, isointense with gray matter (GM), "stuck" in wrong place (+/- thin overlying cortex)
  - Identification of seizure focus within HGM: Interictal FDG PET (isocortical metabolism) plus ictal SPECT ("hot") superior to all other modalities
- Location: Can leave "heterotopic" neuronal deposits along migration path
- Size: Diffuse or focal
- Morphology
  - Subependymal heterotopia (most common)
    - GM nodules + focal/multifocal indentation of ventricle
  - Band heterotopia ("double cortex")
    - Thick inner GM band + thin, abnormal cortex (seizure risk)
    - Thin/partial inner band + normal cortex = normal function
  - Lissencephaly type 1
    - Part of agyria, agyria/pachygyria spectrum
    - Thick inner band GM, cell sparse WM zone, thin outer layer GM
    - Shallow Sylvian fissure with "hour-glass" cerebral configuration
  - Lissencephaly type 2 ("cobblestone")
    - Usually occurs with congenital muscular dystrophies

DDx: Mimics of Heterotopic Gray Matter

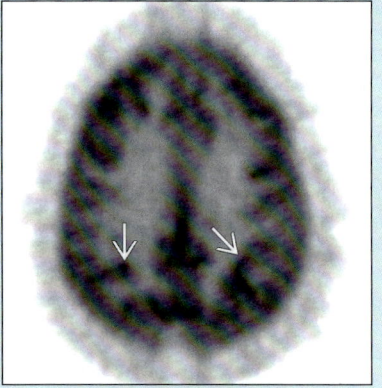

Normal Asymmetry

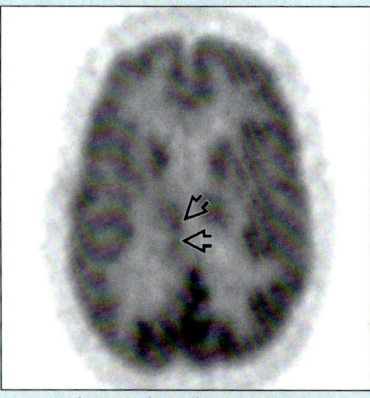

Subependymal Tumor: PET

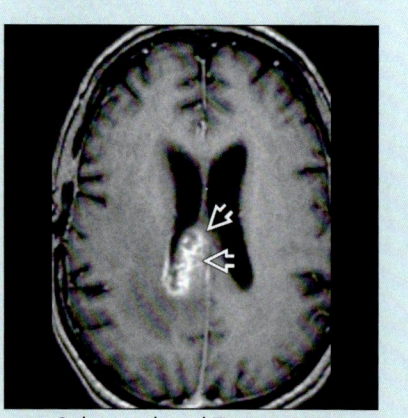

Subependymal Tumor: MR

HETEROTOPIC GRAY MATTER

Key Facts

Imaging Findings
- Nodule or ribbon on MR, isointense with gray matter (GM), "stuck" in wrong place (+/- thin overlying cortex)
- Identification of seizure focus within HGM: Interictal FDG PET (isocortical metabolism) plus ictal SPECT ("hot") superior to all other modalities
- Subependymal heterotopia (most common)
- Band heterotopia ("double cortex")
- Lissencephaly type 1
- Lissencephaly type 2 ("cobblestone")
- Subcortical heterotopia: Large foci have thinned and dysplastic overlying cortex, small foci don't
- FDG uptake in region of HGM usually similar to normal cortex (also slightly greater or slightly less)
- FDG uptake in overlying normal cortex may be decreased
- SPECT
- Tc-99m hexamethylpropyleneamine oxime (HMPAO), bicisate
- Interictal: Uptake similar to normal cortex
- Ictal: Focal increased uptake with spread to overlying cortex

Top Differential Diagnoses
- Normal Gray Matter
- Tumors
- Tuberous Sclerosis
- Zellweger Syndrome (Peroxisomal Disorder)
- Cytomegalovirus

   - Neurons "over migrate" through gaps in external layer of cortex ⇒ "pebbled" surface of brain
   - Associated ocular, cerebellar anomalies common
  ○ Subcortical heterotopia: Large foci have thinned and dysplastic overlying cortex, small foci don't
   - Focal HGM nodules
   - Large nodular HGM (can mimic neoplasm!)
   - Swirling, curvilinear GM mass continuous both with cortex, underlying ventricular surface

Nuclear Medicine Findings
- PET
  ○ FDG uptake in region of HGM usually similar to normal cortex (also slightly greater or slightly less)
  ○ FDG uptake in overlying normal cortex may be decreased
- SPECT
  ○ Tc-99m hexamethylpropyleneamine oxime (HMPAO), bicisate
  ○ Interictal: Uptake similar to normal cortex
  ○ Ictal: Focal increased uptake with spread to overlying cortex

CT Findings
- NECT: Always isodense with GM (extremely rare dysplastic Ca++)
- CECT: No enhancement
- Xenon-CT: ↑ Regional cerebral blood flow (rCBF) during functional testing suggests HGM is functional

MR Findings
- T1WI
  ○ Imaging characteristics match GM
  ○ Margins may be distinct
- T2WI
  ○ Imaging characteristics of GM
  ○ If subcortical, look for continuity with cortex and ventricular surface
- FLAIR: No abnormal signal
- DWI: Eigenvectors (DTI) pass through band heterotopia, connectivity patterns may explain absence of focal neurologic deficits
- MRS: Choline and NAA are variable

Ultrasonographic Findings
- Grayscale Ultrasound: Fetal US and fetal MR have documented subependymal heterotopia

Imaging Recommendations
- MR + thin slice SPGR (surface coil/3D reconstruction) for subtle lesions

DIFFERENTIAL DIAGNOSIS

Normal Gray Matter
- Normal asymmetry, particularly due to non-precise head positioning during imaging
- More problematical with PET than other modalities

Tumors
- Foci of iso-cortical FDG metabolism in lower grade gliomas and some metastases

Tuberous Sclerosis
- Subependymal nodules of tuberous sclerosis may resemble heterotopias
- Subependymal nodules often calcify, may enhance

Zellweger Syndrome (Peroxisomal Disorder)
- Abnormal neuronal migration, hypomyelination

Syndromes Including HGM
- Agenesis CC, Chiari 2 are the most common of these

Cytomegalovirus
- Periventricular calcifications

PATHOLOGY

General Features
- General path comments
  ○ GM nodules/masses in wrong location
  ○ Embryology complicated, process dependent upon multiple molecular mechanisms

HETEROTOPIC GRAY MATTER

- Cell cycle control, cell-cell adhesion, growth factor, neurotransmitter release, interaction with matrix proteins
- Etiology
  - Genetic: Mutations alter molecular reactions at multiple migration points ⇒ migrational arrest ⇒ HGM
  - Acquired: Toxins/infections ⇒ reactive gliosis/macrophage infiltration ⇒ disturbed neuronal migration/cortical positioning
    - CMV-infected cells can fail to migrate ⇒ lissencephaly
    - Toxins (alcohol, XRT) ⇒ slow/abnormal migration
- Epidemiology
  - 17% of neonatal CNS anomalies at autopsy
  - Found in up to 40% of patients with intractable epilepsy

Gross Pathologic & Surgical Features
- Spectrum: Agyria to normal cortex + small ectopic nodules GM
- Persistent fetal leptomeningeal vascularization if severe

Microscopic Features
- Multiple neuronal cell types, immature/dysplastic neurons
  - Excess of excitatory over inhibitory neuronal circuitry
- Neuronal numbers, positioning abnormal

Staging, Grading or Classification Criteria
- Classification by specific location, type, and size of HGM may predict specific gene mutation
  - Nodular/band/curvilinear, anterior/posterior, subcortical, subependymal

CLINICAL ISSUES

Presentation
- Most common signs/symptoms: Cognitive function, age of seizure (Sz) onset/severity depend on location/amount of abnormally positioned GM
- Clinical Profile: Young child with developmental delay and Sz

Demographics
- Age
  - Severe cases present in infancy with Sz & associated malformations
  - Mild cases or simple subcortical nodules can be asymptomatic and only incidental findings on imaging or autopsy
- Gender: Males with X-linked disorders have significantly worse brain malformation and outcome

Natural History & Prognosis
- Variable life span dependent upon extent of malformation
  - Type 2 lissencephaly: Months
  - Focal heterotopias: Can be normal (depends on Sz control)

Treatment
- Surgery reserved for intractable Sz
  - Resect small accessible epileptogenic nodules
  - Corpus callosotomy if bilateral or diffuse unresectable lesions

DIAGNOSTIC CHECKLIST

Consider
- HGM is common and commonly associated with other anomalies

Image Interpretation Pearls
- HGM doesn't enhance and doesn't calcify
- Subcortical HGM can appear mass-like, mimic tumor

SELECTED REFERENCES
1. Conrad GR et al: FDG PET imaging of subependymal gray matter heterotopia. Clin Nucl Med. 30(1):35-6, 2005
2. Hammers A et al: Grey and white matter flumazenil binding in neocortical epilepsy with normal MRI. A PET study of 44 patients. Brain. 126(Pt 6):1300-18, 2003
3. Duncan JS: Epileptogenic networks: cerebral dysplasias and cerebral ectopias. Rev Neurol (Paris). 157(8-9 Pt 1):741-6, 2001
4. Hwang SI et al: Comparative analysis of MR imaging, positron emission tomography, and ictal single-photon emission CT in patients with neocortical epilepsy. AJNR Am J Neuroradiol. 22(5):937-46, 2001
5. Kraemer M et al: Metabolic and electrophysiological alterations in an animal model of neocortical neuronal migration disorder. Neuroreport. 12(9):2001-6, 2001
6. Andermann F: Cortical dysplasias and epilepsy: a review of the architectonic, clinical, and seizure patterns. Adv Neurol. 84:479-96, 2000
7. Barkovich AJ et al: Gray matter heterotopia. Neurology. 55:1603-8, 2000
8. Gressens P: Mechanisms and disturbances of neuronal migration. Pediatric Research. 48:725-30, 2000
9. Morioka T et al: Functional imaging in periventricular nodular heterotopia with the use of FDG-PET and HMPAO-SPECT. Neurosurg Rev. 22(1):41-4, 1999
10. Morioka T et al: Functional imaging in schizencephaly using [18F]fluoro-2-deoxy-D-glucose positron emission tomography (FDG-PET) and single photon emission computed tomography with technetium-99m-hexamethyl-propyleneamine oxime (HMPAO-SPECT). Neurosurg Rev. 22(2-3):99-101, 1999
11. Haase CG et al: Bilateral periventricular nodular heterotopia. PET and MRI of a patient with focal seizures. Clin Nucl Med. 22(2):119-20, 1997
12. Preul MC et al: Function and organization in dysgenic cortex. Case report. J Neurosurg. 87(1):113-21, 1997
13. Calabrese P et al: Left hemispheric neuronal heterotopia: a PET, MRI, EEG, and neuropsychological investigation of a university student. Neurology. 44(2):302-5, 1994
14. De Volder AG et al: Brain glucose utilization in band heterotopia: synaptic activity of "double cortex". Pediatr Neurol. 11(4):290-4, 1994
15. Miura K et al: Magnetic resonance imaging and positron emission tomography of band heterotopia. Brain Dev. 15(4):288-90, 1993

HETEROTOPIC GRAY MATTER

IMAGE GALLERY

Typical

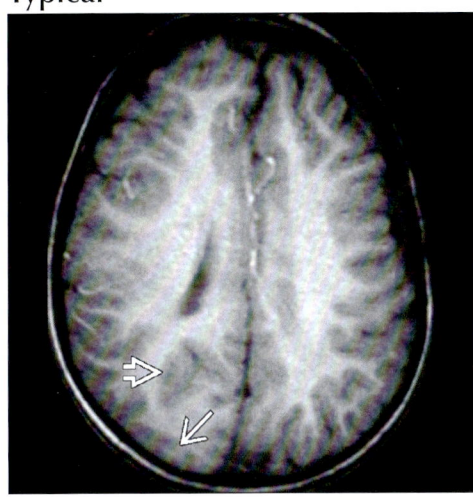

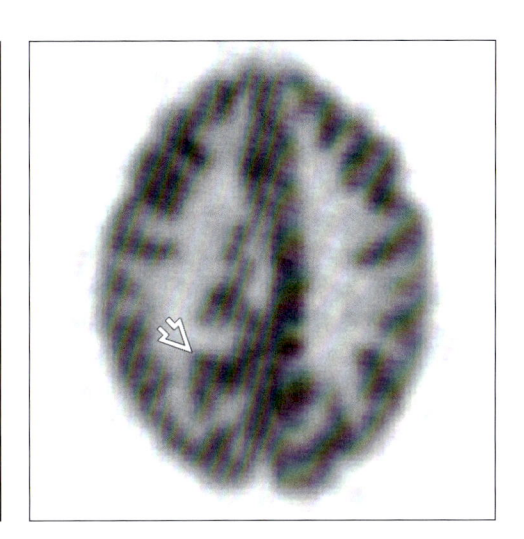

(Left) Axial T1WI MR in a seizure patient shows heterotopic gray matter in right parietal/occipital region ⇨. Note thinning of overlying cortex ➔. (See next 3 images). (Right) Same patient as previous image. Interictal FDG PET demonstrates iso-cortical metabolism in region of right posterior parietal/occipital heterotopic gray matter ⇨. (See next image).

Typical

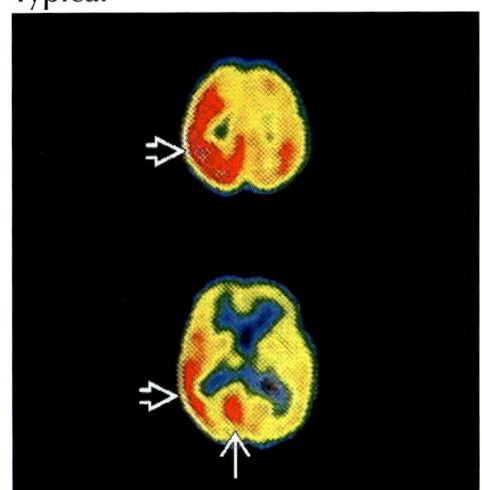

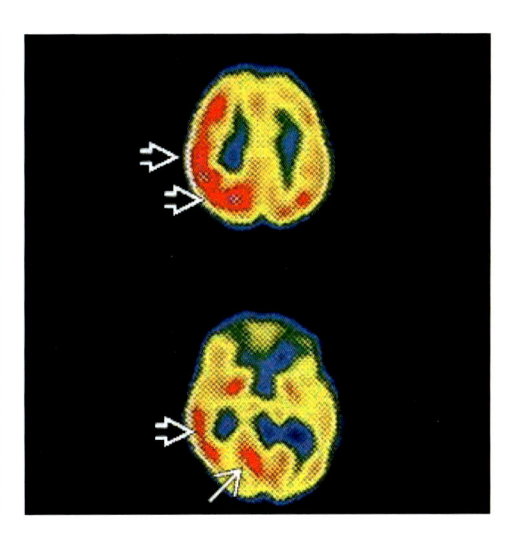

(Left) Ictal Tc-99m HMPAO axial SPECT (same patient as previous image) shows increased uptake in HGM ⇨. Spread to ipsilateral cortex ➔ is minimized by rapid injection (< 1 min) after seizure onset. (Right) Ictal Tc-99m axial HMPAO SPECT (same patient as previous image) shows increased uptake in HGM ⇨. Spread to ipsilateral cortex ➔ is minimized by rapid injection (< 1 min) after seizure onset.

Typical

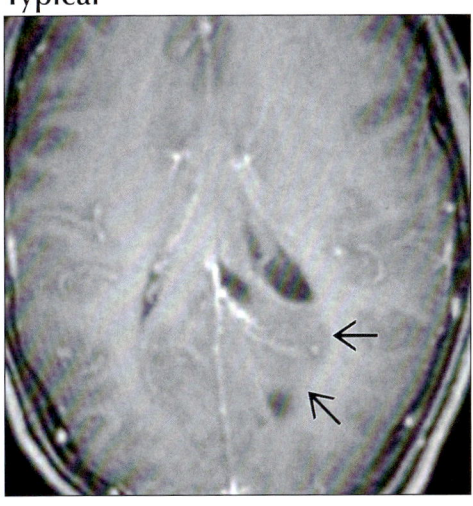

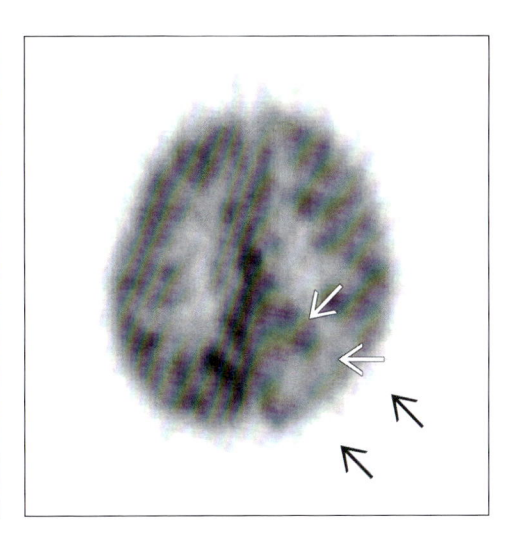

(Left) Axial T1WI MR shows heterotopic gray matter in left paramedian parietal/occipital region ➔. See companion FDG PET of same patient in next image. (Right) Axial FDG PET (same patient as previous image) demonstrates iso-cortical metabolism in region of HGM ⇨. Note hypometabolism in overlying cortex ➔, more common with large regions of HGM.

HETEROTOPIC GRAY MATTER

Typical

(Left) Coronal T1WI MR in patient with intractable seizures shows complex paramedian parietal regions of asymmetry and HGM (including site shown by ➡). See next three images. (Right) Same seizure patient as at left. Coronal interictal FDG PET shows iso-cortical metabolism in region of heterotopic gray matter ➡.

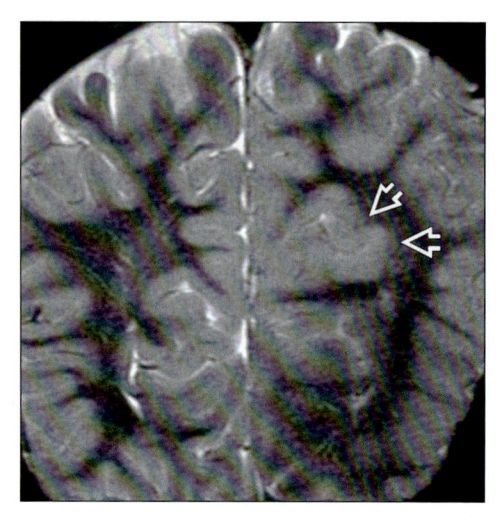

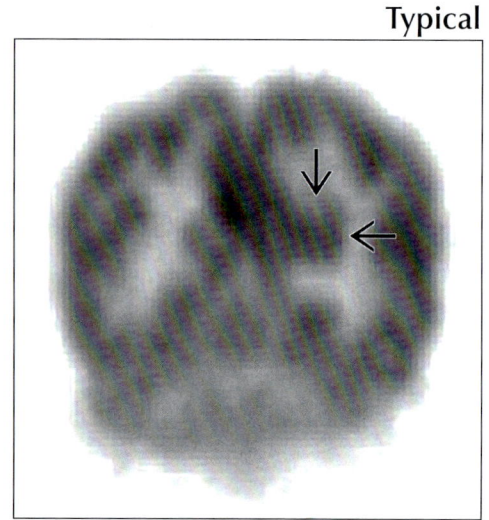

Typical

(Left) Ictal Tc-99m HMPAO axial SPECT (same patient as previous image) shows increased uptake in HGM ➡. There is also spread to ipsilateral cortex ➡ despite timely injection after seizure onset. (Right) Ictal Tc-99m HMPAO axial SPECT (same patient as previous image) shows increased uptake in HGM ➡. There is also spread to ipsilateral cortex ➡ despite timely injection after seizure onset.

Other

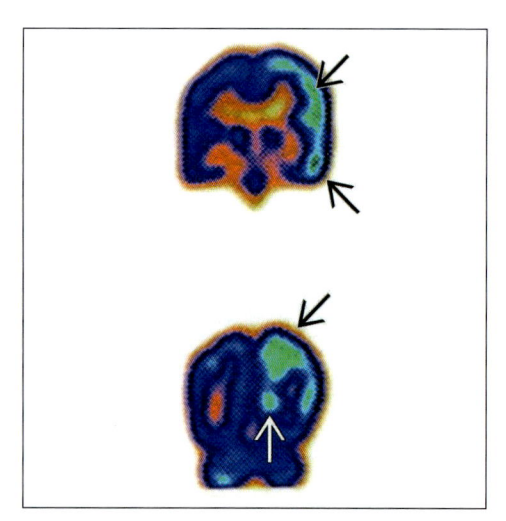

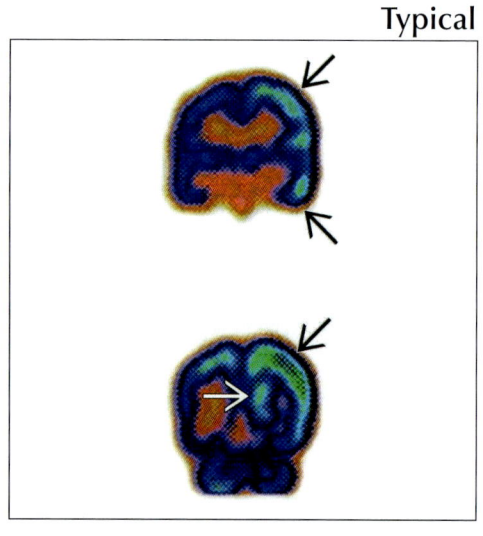

(Left) Tumor mimicking HGM. T1 C+ MR demonstrates enhancement in region of tumor recurrence ➡ 6 months after XRT for glioma. See FDG PET at right. (Right) Tumor mimicking HGM (same patient as previous image). Axial FDG PET shows mild uptake in region of tumor ➡ recurrence 6 months after XRT for glioma. Tumor can mimic HGM on PET; HGM does not enhance on MR.

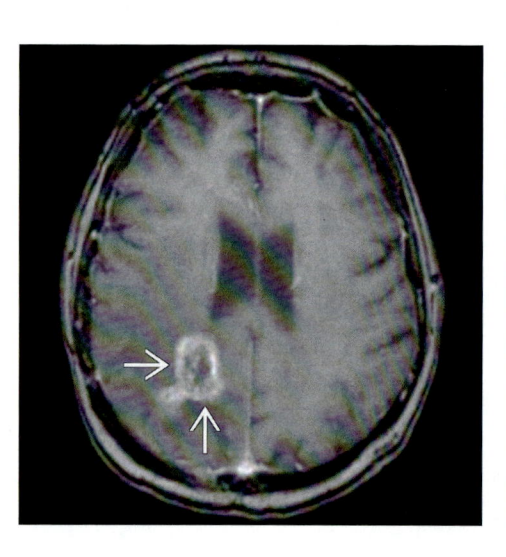

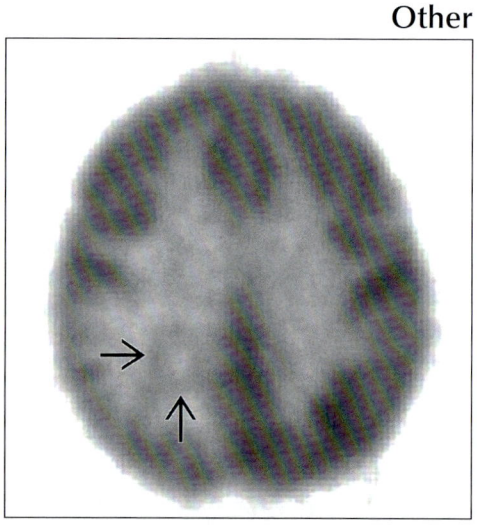

HETEROTOPIC GRAY MATTER

Typical

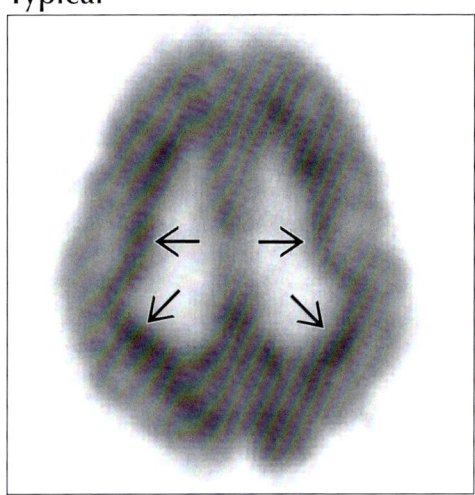

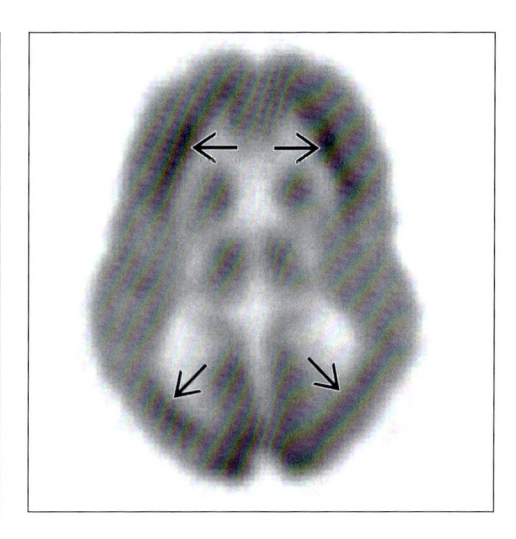

(Left) Band heterotopia: Axial FDG PET. There is a band of continuous hypermetabolism ➔ along the inner margin of gray matter. Note lack of normal gyri/sulci. Same patient as next 5 images. **(Right)** Band heterotopia: Axial FDG PET. There is a band of continuous hypermetabolism along the inner margin of gray matter ➔. Normal gyral/sulcal pattern is lacking.

Typical

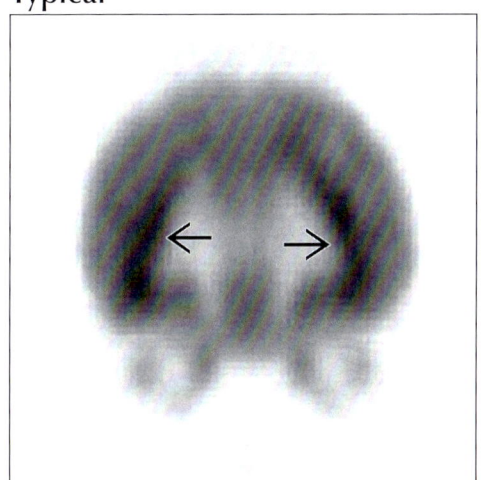

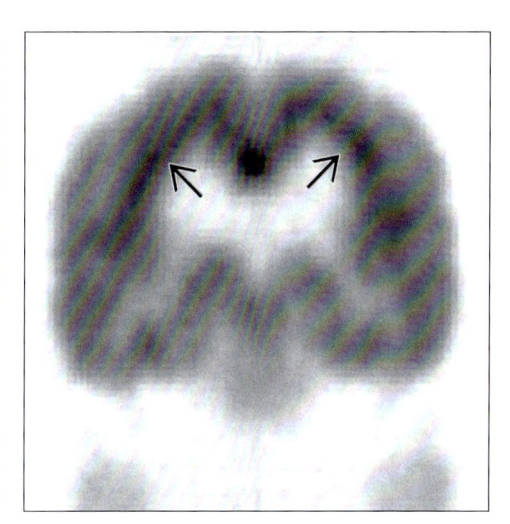

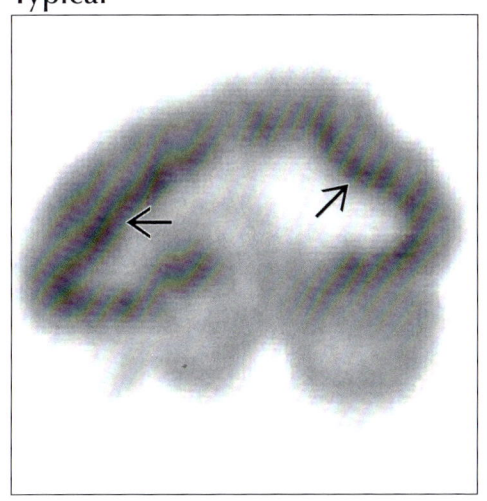

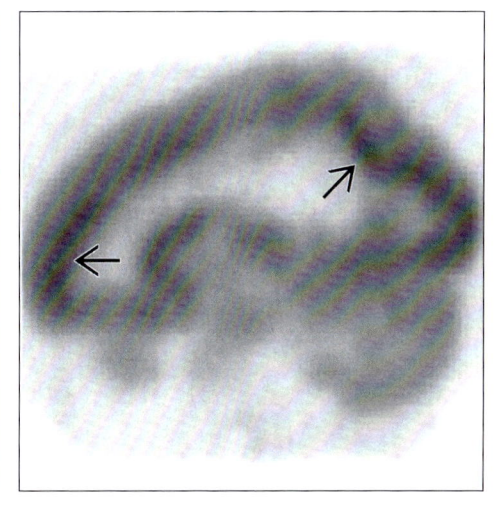

(Left) Band heterotopia: Coronal FDG PET. There is a band of hypermetabolism along the inner margin of gray matter ➔. Normal gyral/sulcal pattern is lacking. **(Right)** Band heterotopia: Coronal FDG PET. There is a band of hypermetabolism along the inner margin of gray matter ➔. Normal gyral/sulcal pattern is lacking.

Typical

(Left) Band heterotopia: Sagittal FDG PET. There is a band of hypermetabolism along the inner margin of the gray matter ➔. The normal gyral/sulcal pattern is lacking. **(Right)** Band heterotopia: Sagittal FDG PET. There is a band of hypermetabolism along the inner margin of the gray matter ➔. The normal gyral/sulcal pattern is lacking.

BRAIN INFECTION & INFLAMMATION

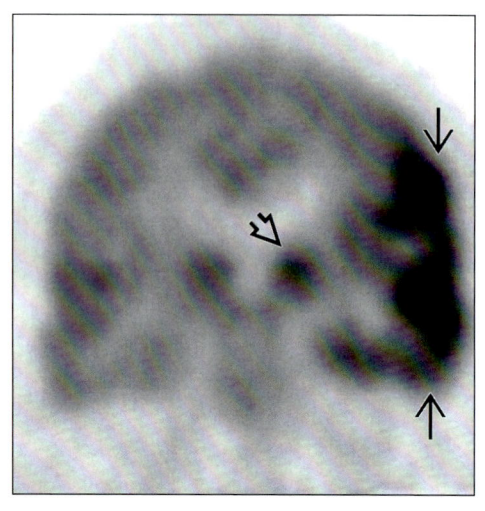

Coronal F-18 FDG PET shows hypermetabolic activity in left temporal lobe ➡ and basal ganglia ⇨, typical for acute herpes simplex encephalitis (HSE).

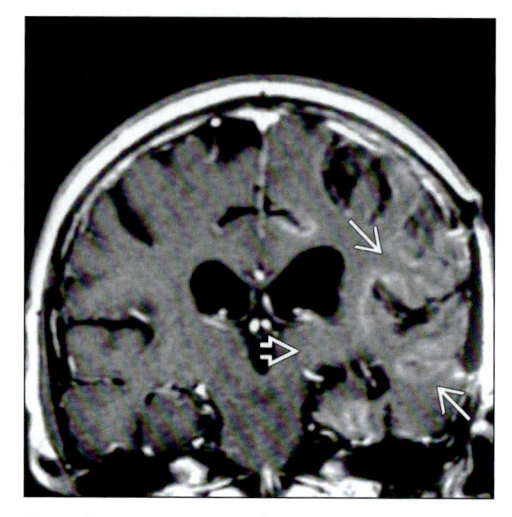

Coronal T1 C+ MR of patient at left shows enhancement of left temporal lobe ➡ and basal ganglia ⇨, corresponding to hypermetabolism on PET in patient with HSE.

TERMINOLOGY

Abbreviations and Synonyms
- Herpes simplex encephalitis (HSE)
- Rasmussen encephalitis (RE)
- Creutzfeldt-Jakob disease (CJD), transmissible spongiform encephalopathy (TSE)
- Progressive multifocal leukoencephalopathy (PML)
- Opportunistic infection (OI)

Definitions
- HSE: Parenchymal infection caused by herpes simplex virus type 1 (HSV-1)
- Cerebral abscess: Focal pyogenic infection (bacterial, fungal, parasitic)
- Cerebritis: Brain inflammation due to infectious/noninfectious causes
- Encephalitis: Inflammation caused by various pathogens (most common = viral)
- RE: Chronic, unilateral brain inflammation, etiology unclear
- PML: Subacute demyelinating OI

IMAGING FINDINGS

General Features
- Best diagnostic clue
  - HSE: Abnormal MR signal and enhancement of medial temporal and inferior frontal lobes; cingulate gyrus and contralateral temporal lobe highly suggestive
  - Cerebral abscess: Depending on acuity, MR or CT enhancing ring, central low density, peripheral edema
  - Cerebritis: Acute = enhancement CT, MR; chronic = atrophy, hyperintensity on T2 MR
    - Acute: Enhancement on CT, MR
    - Chronic: Hyperintense T2 MR, atrophy
  - RE: Unilateral cerebral atrophy
  - OI: Variable appearance, most hyperintense on T2
- Location
  - HSE: Limbic system most typically (temporal lobes, insula, subfrontal, cingulate gyri)
    - Cerebral convexities, asymmetrical, basal ganglia often spared, atypical in children
    - Usually bilateral; can be asymmetrical
    - Children atypical: Primarily cerebral hemispheres

DDx: Brain Infection and Inflammation

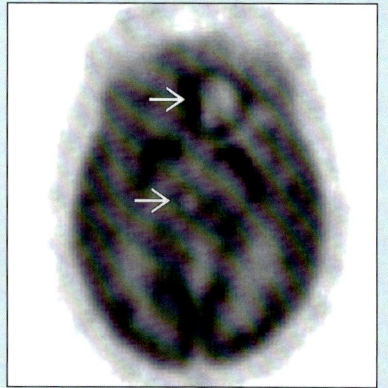

Primary CNS Lymphoma

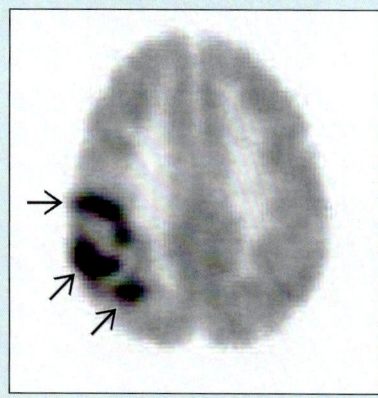

High Grade Glioma

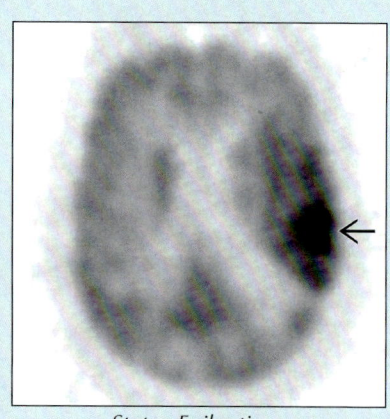

Status Epilepticus

BRAIN INFECTION & INFLAMMATION

Key Facts

Imaging Findings
- Hypermetabolic on F-18 FDG PET: Acute cerebritis (any cause), acute HSE, acute OI, abscess (centrally hypometabolic in subacute stage), limbic encephalitis
- Isometabolic on F-18 FDG PET: Subacute encephalitis
- Hypometabolic on FDG PET: Toxoplasmosis, PML, CJD (patchy hypometabolism), RE, chronic/burned out infection/inflammation
- F-18 FDG PET: Limited ability to distinguish ring-enhancing lesions; however, toxoplasmosis = hypometabolic
- Tc-99m ECD or HMPAO SPECT: Hypometabolic for most conditions
- In-111 leukocytes: Inferior to F-18 FDG PET, relatively insensitive for nonpyogenic/chronic bacterial infections
- Tc-99m glucoheptonate blood brain barrier (BBB) scan: Focal breakdown in BBB ⇒ increased activity

Top Differential Diagnoses
- Limbic Encephalitis
- Neoplasm
- Ischemia
- Status Epilepticus

Diagnostic Checklist
- Immediate empiric antibiotics if infection suspected
- Stroke or tumor may mimic, history often helpful
- Consider limbic encephalitis if all clinical tests negative, subacute onset of symptoms
- F-18 FDG PET: Useful for equivocal or problem cases
- MR most sensitive (FLAIR and DWI) for diagnosis

  - Cerebral abscess: Primarily gray-white junction, supratentorial, also atypical locations
  - Atypical infectious encephalitis: Any location
  - RE: Entire hemisphere, worse pre-central and inferior frontal
- Morphology
  - RE: Focal first, then hemispheric
  - Abscess: Ring enhancement = capsular stage

Nuclear Medicine Findings
- PET
  - Hypermetabolic on F-18 FDG PET: Acute cerebritis (any cause), acute HSE, acute OI, abscess (centrally hypometabolic in subacute stage), limbic encephalitis
  - Isometabolic on F-18 FDG PET: Subacute encephalitis
  - Hypometabolic on FDG PET: Toxoplasmosis, PML, CJD (patchy hypometabolism), RE, chronic/burned out infection/inflammation
  - F-18 FDG PET: Limited ability to distinguish ring-enhancing lesions; however, toxoplasmosis = hypometabolic
- SPECT
  - Tc-99m ECD or HMPAO SPECT: Hypometabolic for most conditions
  - In-111 leukocytes: Inferior to F-18 FDG PET, relatively insensitive for nonpyogenic/chronic bacterial infections
- Tc-99m glucoheptonate blood brain barrier (BBB) scan: Focal breakdown in BBB ⇒ increased activity

CT Findings
- CECT: Enhancement, mass effect, hemorrhage

MR Findings
- T1WI
  - Decreased signal in gray and white matter, loss of gray-white junction, mass effect
  - Subacute hemorrhage ⇒ increased signal in edematous brain
  - Chronic: Atrophy and encephalomalacia
- T2WI
  - Increased signal
  - Subacute hemorrhage ⇒ increased signal in edematous brain
- FLAIR: Hyperintense
- DWI: May be hyperintense (restricted diffusion)
- T1 C+: Parenchymal, meningeal enhancement (may not be seen in early HSE)

Imaging Recommendations
- Best imaging tool
  - MR > CT; however, false negatives in first few days of OI, HSE
  - F-18 FDG PET for problem-solving in unclear cases after MR/CT
- Protocol advice
  - F-18 FDG PET
    - 10 mCi F-18 FDG IV
    - After injection, patient should rest in darkened room
    - Whole-brain image at 45-60 min
    - Fuse PET images to correlative MR: Increases sensitivity/specificity of PET findings

DIFFERENTIAL DIAGNOSIS

Limbic Encephalitis
- Rare paraneoplastic syndrome associated with primary tumor, often lung
- Imaging may be indistinguishable from HSE on MR and F-18 FDG PET
- Subacute symptom onset (weeks to months) vs. acute in HSE

Neoplasm
- Low grade gliomas often hypometabolic on F-18 FDG PET
- High grade gliomas hypermetabolic on F-18 FDG PET
- Metastases iso- or hypermetabolic to normal brain
- Primary CNS lymphoma hypermetabolic, ring-like on F-18 FDG PET

BRAIN INFECTION & INFLAMMATION

Ischemia
- Typical vascular distribution (MCA, ACA, PCA)
- Acute onset
- F-18 FDG PET and Tc-99m ECD/HMPAO SPECT: Decreased uptake centrally; may have increased peripheral uptake = "luxury perfusion" equivalent

Status Epilepticus
- Seizure focus
  - Ictal scan: Increased activity on F-18 FDG PET or Tc-99m ECD/HMPAO SPECT
  - Interictal scan: Decreased activity on F-18 FDG PET or Tc-99m ECD/HMPAO SPECT
- Active seizures may disrupt BBB, cause signal abnormalities and enhancement
- Temporal lobe epilepsy hyperperfusion may mimic herpes encephalitis

PATHOLOGY

General Features
- Etiology
  - HSE: HSV-1 infection, reactivation (adults), primary (infants and children)
  - Immunocompromised: OI, HSE
  - Underlying malignancy: Limbic encephalitis
  - CJD
    - Inherited mutations in prion protein
    - Acquired from infected prion-containing material

Gross Pathologic & Surgical Features
- Encephalitis, cerebritis, acute pyogenic: Unencapsulated vascular congestion, hemorrhage, necrosis, edema
- Subacute abscess: Peripheral capsule, necrotic core

CLINICAL ISSUES

Presentation
- Most common signs/symptoms
  - Fever
  - Headache
  - Seizure
  - Altered mental status, focal or diffuse neurologic deficit (< 30%)
  - May progress to coma and death
  - CJD: Rapidly progressive dementia

Demographics
- Gender: M = F

Natural History & Prognosis
- Mortality: 50-70% (viral); 0-30% (abscess)
- Rapid diagnosis, early treatment can decrease mortality, may improve outcome (HSE, OI)
- In general, survival complicated by memory difficulties, hearing loss, medically intractable epilepsy, personality changes
- CJD: Unrelenting dementia, death
- RE: Hemiplegia, cognitive impairment in most cases

Treatment
- Infectious: Antivirals/antibiotics, anti-seizure medications
- Abscess: Surgical drainage, antibiotics, anti-seizure medications
- Aseptic: Corticosteroids, anti-seizure medications, antiviral agents, alpha-interferon, immunoglobulin

DIAGNOSTIC CHECKLIST

Consider
- Immediate empiric antibiotics if infection suspected
- Stroke or tumor may mimic, history often helpful
- Consider limbic encephalitis if all clinical tests negative, subacute onset of symptoms

Image Interpretation Pearls
- F-18 FDG PET: Useful for equivocal or problem cases
  - Ring-enhancing lesions on MR: Toxoplasmosis vs. lymphoma
  - Determine acuity of infection/inflammation
- MR most sensitive (FLAIR and DWI) for diagnosis

SELECTED REFERENCES

1. Floeth FW et al: 18F-FET PET Differentiation of Ring-Enhancing Brain Lesions. J Nucl Med. 47(5):776-782, 2006
2. Fauser S et al: FDG-PET and MRI in potassium channel antibody-associated non-paraneoplastic limbic encephalitis: correlation with clinical course and neuropsychology. Acta Neurol Scand. 111(5):338-43, 2005
3. Küker W et al: Diffusion-weighted MRI in herpes simplex encephalitis. Neuroradiology. 46:122-5, 2004
4. Lee BY et al: FDG-PET findings in patients with suspected encephalitis. Clin Nucl Med. 29(10):620-5, 2004
5. Scheid R et al: Serial 18F-fluoro-2-deoxy-D-glucose positron emission tomography and magnetic resonance imaging of paraneoplastic limbic encephalitis. Arch Neurol. 61(11):1785-9, 2004
6. Chiapparini L et al: Diagnostic imaging in 13 cases of Rasmussen's encephalitis: can early MRI suggest the diagnosis? Neuroradiology. 45(3):171-83, 2003
7. Engler H et al: Multitracer study with positron emission tomography in Creutzfeldt-Jakob disease. Eur J Nucl Med Mol Imaging. 30(1):85-95, 2003
8. Fiorella DJ et al: (18)F-fluorodeoxyglucose positron emission tomography and MR imaging findings in Rasmussen encephalitis. AJNR Am J Neuroradiol. 22(7):1291-9, 2001
9. Kassubek J et al: Limbic encephalitis investigated by 18FDG-PET and 3D MRI. J Neuroimaging. 11(1):55-9, 2001
10. Leonard JR et al: MR imaging of herpes simplex type 1 encephalitis in infants and young children: a separate pattern of findings. AJR Am J Roentgenol. 174(6):1651-5, 2000
11. Weiner SM et al: Alterations of cerebral glucose metabolism indicate progress to severe morphological brain lesions in neuropsychiatric systemic lupus erythematosus. Lupus. 9(5):386-9, 2000
12. Hoffman JM et al: FDG-PET in differentiating lymphoma from nonmalignant central nervous system lesions in patients with AIDS. J Nucl Med. 34(4):567-75, 1993
13. Hanson MW et al: FDG-PET in the selection of brain lesions for biopsy. J Comput Assist Tomogr. 15(5):796-801, 1991

BRAIN INFECTION & INFLAMMATION

IMAGE GALLERY

Variant

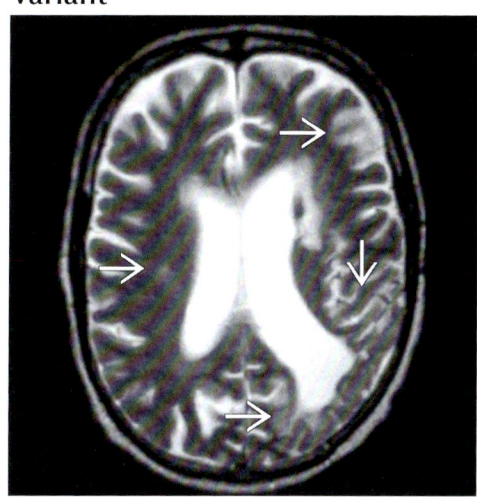

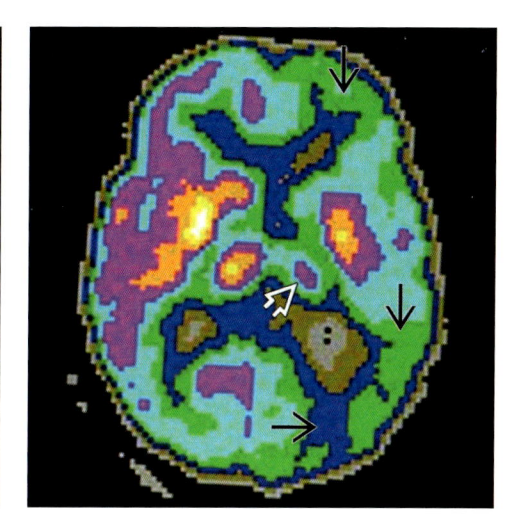

(Left) Axial T2 MR shows nonspecific, subtle areas of increased signal ➡ in patient with early CJD. With disease progression, findings become more obvious. *(Right)* Axial F-18 FDG PET in patient with CJD. Large areas of marked hypometabolism in cortex ➡, basal ganglia ➡. PET findings are often much more striking than MR/CT.

Typical

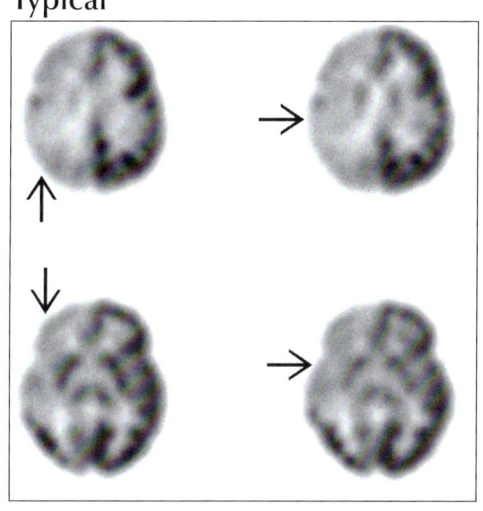

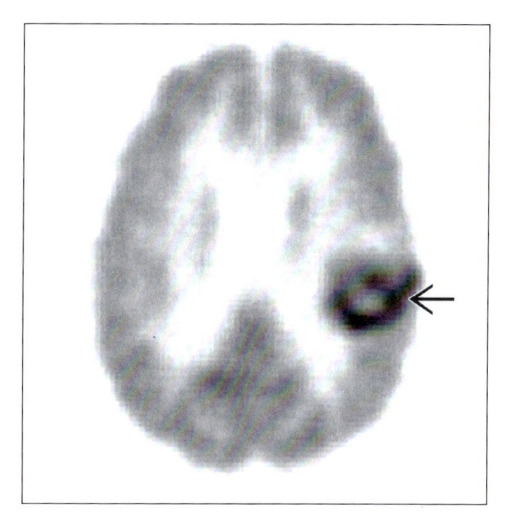

(Left) Axial F-18 FDG PET in patient with Rasmussen encephalitis (RE) shows diffuse right hemispheric hypometabolism ➡. Late in disease, diffuse hemicerebral atrophy occurs. *(Right)* Axial FDG PET shows ring of hypermetabolism in left parietal lobe ➡, typical appearance for cerebral abscess. Central necrosis/hypometabolism occurs in subacute (capsular) stage.

Typical

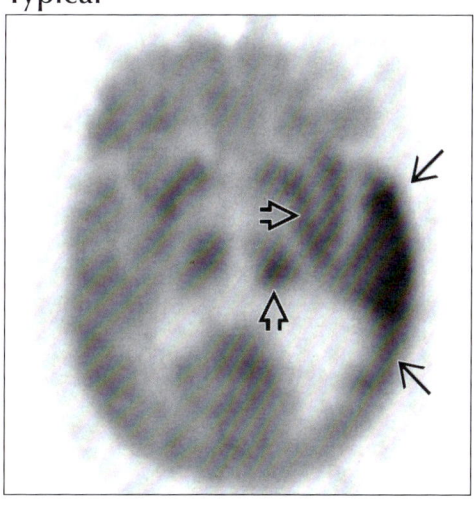

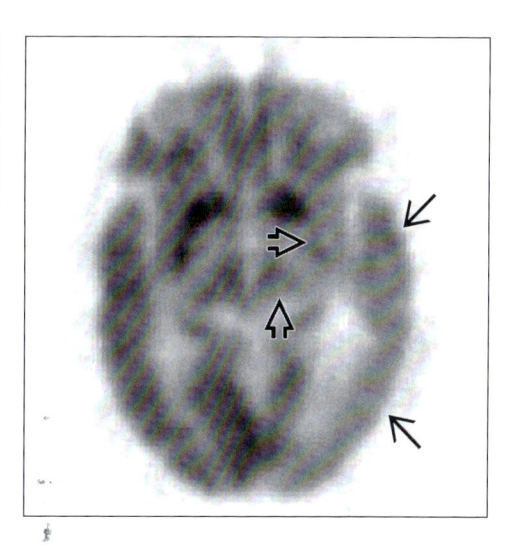

(Left) Axial F-18 FDG PET in early cerebritis shows hypermetabolism in left temporal/parietal lobes ➡ and basal ganglia ➡ in patient with HSE. *(Right)* Six months later, axial F-18 FDG PET in patient at left shows hypometabolism in left temporal/parietal lobes ➡ and basal ganglia ➡, typical of late findings after HSE episode.

PSYCHIATRY, DRUG ADDICTION & FORENSICS

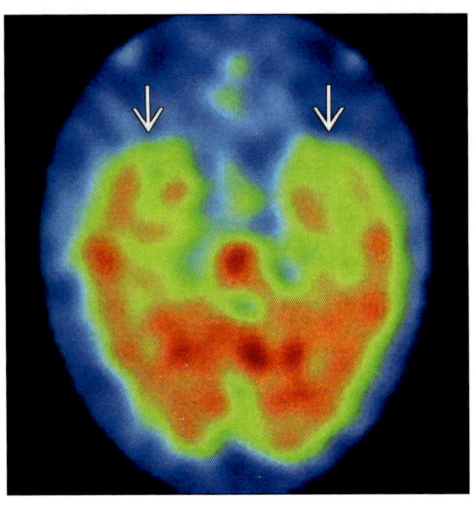

Axial brain SPECT shows decreased activity over the temporal tips ➔ in a symptomatic adult post head trauma with negative anatomic studies. This is a typical finding.

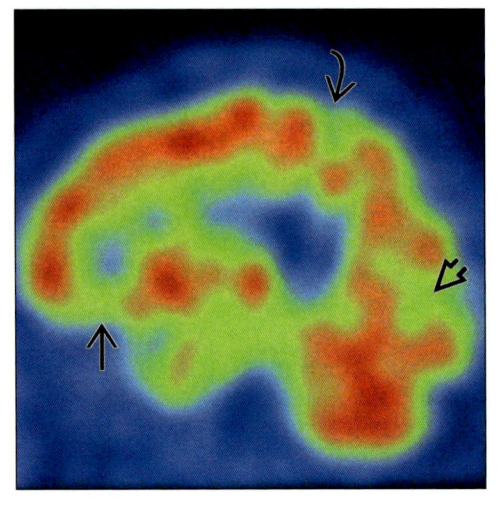

Sagittal brain SPECT (in the same patient as left) shows decreased activity over the floor of the frontal lobe ➔, a typical finding. Other abnormalities are occipital ➔ and parietal ➔.

TERMINOLOGY

Definitions
- Brain imaging attempting to show functional rather than anatomic abnormalities

IMAGING FINDINGS

General Features
- Best diagnostic clue
  - Depends on the specific diagnosis
  - Resting versus stress studies can be valuable especially with ADD

Nuclear Medicine Findings
- Head injury: Patients with symptoms and negative anatomic studies often have abnormal SPECT scans
  - Location of abnormality dependent on mechanism of injury
    - Typical post-trauma distribution in tips of temporal lobes and floor of frontal lobes
    - Location of abnormality will vary with mechanism of injury
  - Nuclear imaging is more sensitive than CT or MR, and may correlate better with clinical findings
- Obsessive-compulsive disorder (OCD): Increased activity in anterior cingulate is most commonly described
  - Also variably described are increased orbitofrontal cortex, increased basal ganglia, increased medial frontal, decreased frontal, decreased right caudate, decreased right thalamus
- Schizophrenia: Decreased activity in frontal lobes, referred to as hypofrontality, is most commonly described
  - Variably described are decreased basal ganglia, decreased temporal lobes, decreased left temporal lobe
  - Some studies show increased activity in visual or auditory cortex if tracer is injected during visual or auditory hallucinations
  - Some findings are likely related to effect of drugs used for treatment or recreation
  - SPECT patterns in mental illness may relate more closely with specific symptoms such as hallucinations than with specific psychiatric diagnoses

DDx: Marijuana Acute Exposure Effect

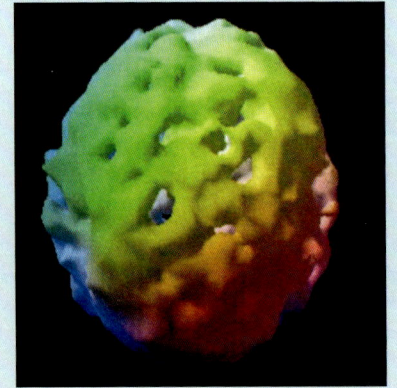

Top Surface Map

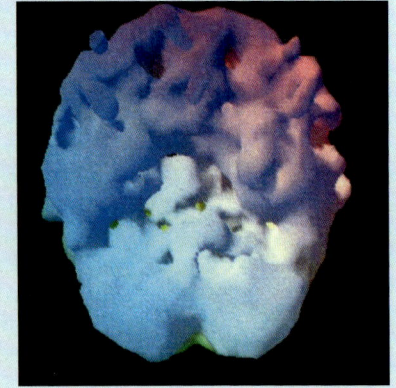

Base Surface Map

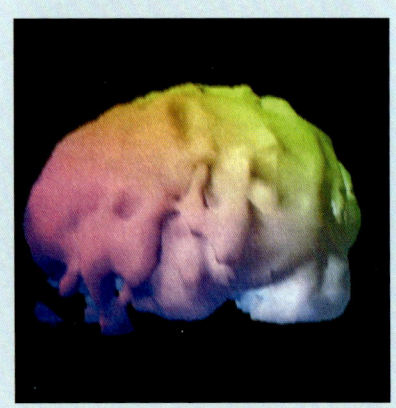

Lat Surface Map

PSYCHIATRY, DRUG ADDICTION & FORENSICS

Key Facts

Imaging Findings
- Head injury: Patients with symptoms and negative anatomic studies often have abnormal SPECT scans
- Obsessive-compulsive disorder (OCD): Increased activity in anterior cingulate is most commonly described
- Schizophrenia: Decreased activity in frontal lobes, referred to as hypofrontality, is most commonly described
- Depression: Decreased activity in frontal lobes is most commonly reported finding
- Panic disorder and anxiety: Frontal hypoactivity has been described as well as basal ganglia hyperactivity
- Substance abuse: Diffuse cortical decreased activity seen with substances such as alcohol, marijuana, barbiturates, pain killers, narcotics, and nicotine
- Criminal and antisocial behavior: Decreased prefrontal, frontal, and temporal activity are most commonly described
- Violence: Increased cingulate activity, decreased prefrontal activity, temporal lobe increases and decreases often on the left, increased caudate and/or thalamic activity have been described
- Attention deficit disorder (ADD): Normal or decreased activity frontal and/or temporal lobes at baseline the most commonly described finding
- Toxic exposure and multiple chemical sensitivity: Variety of findings have been described in this controversial area including patchy cortical increases or decreases, and overall decreased cortical activity

---

- SPECT findings that cross clinical classification boundaries are often associated with common symptoms
- Depression: Decreased activity in frontal lobes is most commonly reported finding
  - Variably described are decreased frontal poles, temporal lobes, anterior cingulate, left caudate
  - Severe depression may show generalized decreased cortical activity
  - Hypoactive areas often improve secondary to an attention task
    - Task can be a standard mental performance task such as the Conner Performance Task
    - Mental tasks such as math problems can be easily designed for individual patients if desired
    - Task is administered from 10 minutes pre to 10 minutes post tracer injection
    - Typical ADD response to stress, worsening in frontal and temporal lobes, is the opposite of depression
  - Patients depressed on a vascular basis from excessive antihypertensive medication will show same decreased frontal pattern
    - Scan will normalize upon adjustment of medication and improvement of symptoms
- Panic disorder and anxiety: Frontal hypoactivity has been described as well as basal ganglia hyperactivity
- Substance abuse: Diffuse cortical decreased activity seen with substances such as alcohol, marijuana, barbiturates, pain killers, narcotics, and nicotine
  - Focal decreased activity seen most commonly with cocaine and crack
    - Focal hypoactivity also seen with inhaled glue, paint, and solvents
    - Abnormalities reverse if due to vascular spasm or persist if due to infarction
  - Pre-existing mental problems that predispose toward substance abuse may themselves cause perfusion abnormalities
    - Some pre-existing abnormalities may improve with non prescribed drugs and illegal substances
  - Decreased frontal lobe activity in depression often improved by stimulants
  - Increased temporal lobe activity in violent patients may normalize with depressants
- Criminal and antisocial behavior: Decreased prefrontal, frontal, and temporal activity are most commonly described
- Violence: Increased cingulate activity, decreased prefrontal activity, temporal lobe increases and decreases often on the left, increased caudate and/or thalamic activity have been described
- Attention deficit disorder (ADD): Normal or decreased activity frontal and/or temporal lobes at baseline the most commonly described finding
  - Hypoactive or normal frontal and/or temporal lobes at rest often worsen secondary to an attention task
  - Attention task details described above under depression
- Toxic exposure and multiple chemical sensitivity: Variety of findings have been described in this controversial area including patchy cortical increases or decreases, and overall decreased cortical activity

Imaging Recommendations
- Best imaging tool
  - ECD SPECT, Ceretec SPECT, and FDG PET
    - Normal distribution and abnormal findings vary with the modality
    - Best to adopt a single modality and SPECT agent and develop familiarity with it
  - SPECT: Numerous reports of findings, although definitive research has not yet confirmed diagnostic/therapeutic value
  - FDG PET: Less clinical experience in use for psychiatry, drug abuse or forensics than SPECT
  - MRI/fMRI/CT: No consistent findings
- Protocol advice
  - PET: 10 mCi FDG (fasting), image at 60 min
  - SPECT: 20-30 mCi, image at 60-90 min
  - Normal distribution on SPECT and PET varies with environment
    - Infants and children have different normal appearance from adults

PSYCHIATRY, DRUG ADDICTION & FORENSICS

- SPECT normal distribution slightly different for HMPAO vs ECD
- ECD normal distribution varies slightly over time
- HMPAO: Amount of blood pool activity varies with time to imaging; consistent timing important
- Eyes should be consistently closed or open especially with SPECT, preferably open
- Movement, visual and auditory stimuli will affect the normal distribution
- Standard environment with SPECT should be maintained for 10 minutes after injection
- SPECT imaging should be performed on multiple head cameras
- Medications affecting brain function should be discontinued if possible unless effect is being assessed
- SPECT collimation, filtering and image processing should be consistent
- Image display parameters should be kept consistent, preferably using computer monitors over printed images
  - Studies can be viewed in grayscale or color
  - Beware of step color scales
- Interpretation criteria should be consistent whether subjective, semiquantitative, or quantitative
  - Beware of normal databases as screening of participants often does not consider psychiatric conditions, drugs, differences in equipment, acquisition, processing
  - Subjective assessment is an acceptable protocol if consistently applied
  - Reference should be made to a normal structure, often cerebellum, assuming no known cerebellar abnormality or cerebellar diaschisis
  - If cerebellum is abnormal, reference structures can be pons or homotopic contralateral regions
- Additional nuclear medicine imaging options: Receptor imaging technologies not yet in practical use
- Correlative imaging features: Functional imaging abnormalities may or may not have anatomic correlates

DIAGNOSTIC CHECKLIST

Image Interpretation Pearls
- PET and SPECT normal distribution differ
  - Basal ganglia, thalamus and cerebellum hotter relative to cerebral cortex on SPECT than on PET
  - After early childhood, anterior to posterior gradient on PET but not SPECT
    - PET frontal > occipital uptake to age 30 or 40, then frontal < occipital
- Forensic and ethical issues
  - Functional brain imaging in forensic situations such as criminal cases and personal injury is controversial
  - Diagnostic patterns for many psychiatric diagnoses are not generally agreed upon and have not been confirmed
    - Scan findings often relate more to specific symptoms and less to disease classifications
  - Delineating brain scan abnormalities is not same as determining cause or prognosis
  - Brain scan abnormalities are often unequivocal, but etiology or chronology may not be as clear cut
  - Care should be taken attempting to extrapolate appearance of brain at time of imaging to its state at prior time when an antisocial action occurred
- Tracer can be injected during mental tasks, or under the effects of prescription drugs, recreational drugs, or alcohol

SELECTED REFERENCES

1. Oner O et al: Regional cerebral blood flow in children with ADHD: changes with age. Brain Dev. 27(4):279-85, 2005
2. Smith DJ et al: The use of single photon emission computed tomography in depressive disorders. Nucl Med Commun. 26(3):197-203, 2005
3. Benabarre A et al: Clinical value of 99mTc-HMPAO SPECT in depressed bipolar I patients. Psychiatry Res. 132(3):285-9, 2004
4. Carey PD et al: Single photon emission computed tomography (SPECT) of anxiety disorders before and after treatment with citalopram. BMC Psychiatry. 4:30, 2004
5. Graff-Guerrero A et al: Correlation between cerebral blood flow and items of the Hamilton Rating Scale for Depression in antidepressant-naive patients. J Affect Disord. 80(1):55-63, 2004
6. Hendler T et al: Brain reactivity to specific symptom provocation indicates prospective therapeutic outcome in OCD. Psychiatry Res. 124(2):87-103, 2003
7. Parsey RV et al: Applications of positron emission tomography in psychiatry. Semin Nucl Med. 33(2):129-35, 2003
8. Volkow ND et al: Positron emission tomography and single-photon emission computed tomography in substance abuse research. Semin Nucl Med. 33(2):114-28, 2003
9. Kaya GC et al: Technetium-99m HMPAO brain SPECT in children with attention deficit hyperactivity disorder. Ann Nucl Med. 16(8):527-31, 2002
10. Soderstrom H et al: Reduced frontotemporal perfusion in psychopathic personality. Psychiatry Res. 114(2):81-94, 2002
11. Brower MC et al: Neuropsychiatry of frontal lobe dysfunction in violent and criminal behaviour: a critical review. J Neurol Neurosurg Psychiatry. 71(6):720-6, 2001
12. Camargo EE: Brain SPECT in neurology and psychiatry. J Nucl Med. 42(4):611-23, 2001
13. Videbech P et al: The Danish PET/depression project: PET findings in patients with major depression. Psychol Med. 31(7):1147-58, 2001
14. Soderstrom H et al: Reduced regional cerebral blood flow in non-psychotic violent offenders. Psychiatry Res. 98(1):29-41, 2000
15. Amen DG et al: High resolution brain SPECT imaging of marijuana smokers with AD/HD. J Psychoactive Drugs. 30(2):209-14, 1998
16. Amen DG et al: Visualizing the firestorms in the brain: an inside look at the clinical and physiological connections between drugs and violence using brain SPECT imaging. J Psychoactive Drugs. 29(4):307-19, 1997
17. Amen DG et al: Brain SPECT findings and aggressiveness. Ann Clin Psychiatry. 8(3):129-37, 1996

PSYCHIATRY, DRUG ADDICTION & FORENSICS

IMAGE GALLERY

Typical

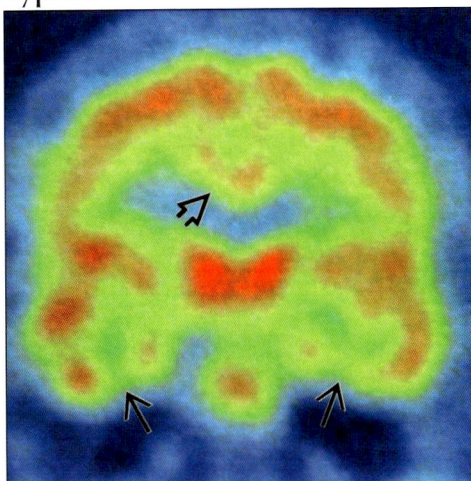

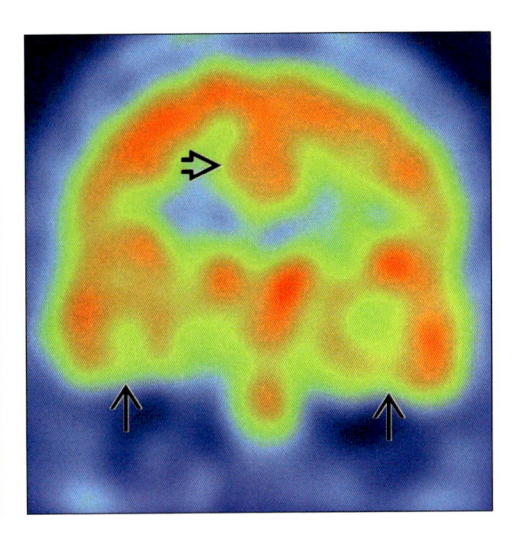

(Left) Coronal brain SPECT shows relative decreased activity over the anterior cingulate gyrus ⇨ in a depressed adult. Bilateral temporal lobe defects → are also present. *(Right)* Coronal brain SPECT shows a normal amount of labeling of the anterior cingulate gyrus ⇨. Bilateral temporal lobe defects are incidentally noted → in this schizophrenic adult.

Typical

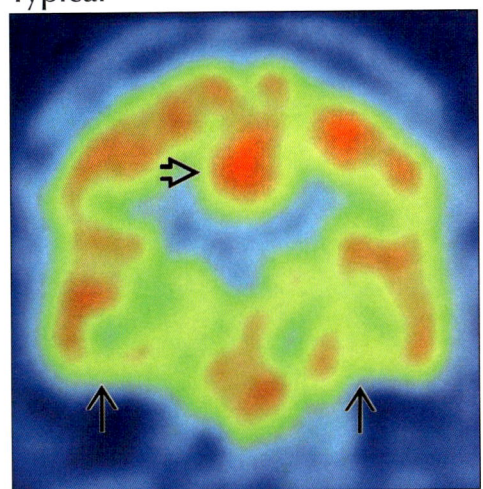

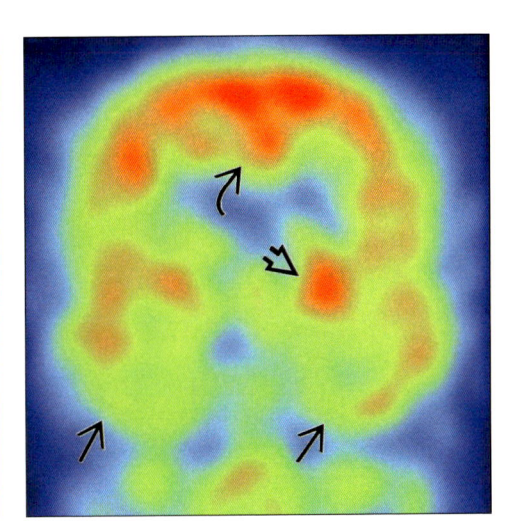

(Left) Coronal brain SPECT shows abnormally increased activity in the anterior cingulate gyrus ⇨ in this adult with obsessive compulsive disorder. Bilateral temporal defects → are also seen. *(Right)* Coronal brain SPECT shows a hot left caudate nucleus ⇨ in this adult with OCD. Also seen are bilateral temporal lobe defects →. Anterior cingulate labeling ⇨ is borderline.

Typical

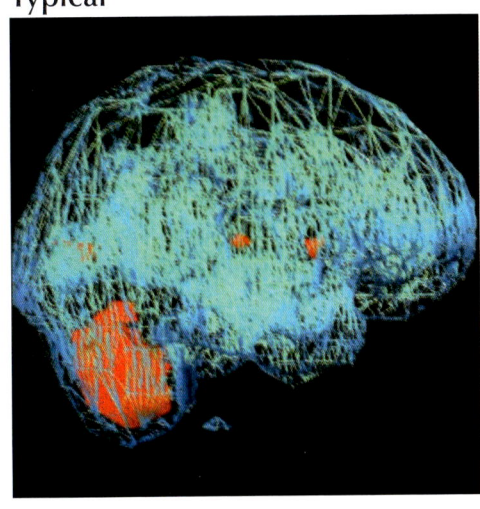

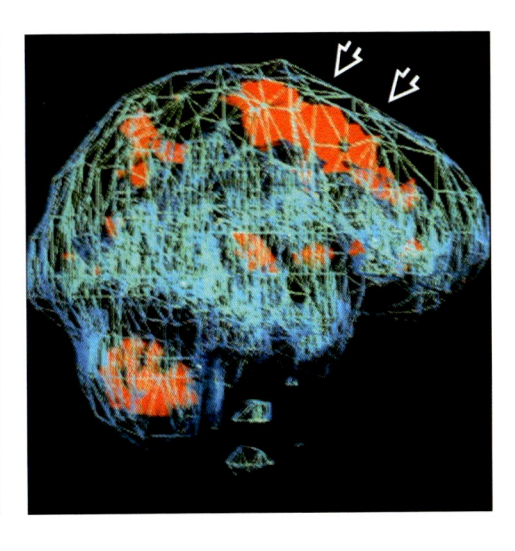

(Left) Right lateral brain SPECT shows no hot foci in adult with obsessive compulsive disorder on a study injected at rest. *(Right)* Right lateral brain SPECT (in the same patient as left) shows increased activity along the cingulate gyrus ⇨ on another study with tracer injection during performance of a mental attention task.

PSYCHIATRY, DRUG ADDICTION & FORENSICS

Typical

(Left) Coronal brain SPECT shows bilateral frontal decreased activity ➔ in this depressed adult. See next image. *(Right)* Sagittal brain SPECT (in the same patient as left) shows frontal lobe decreased activity between the arrows ➔. This nonspecific finding can also be seen in other disorders.

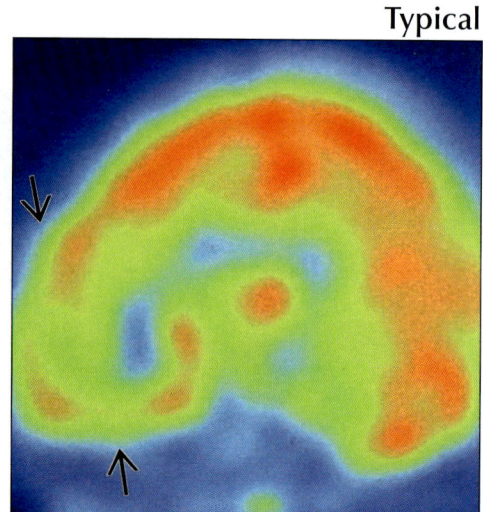

Typical

(Left) Coronal brain SPECT shows bilateral decreased temporal activity ➔ as well as a hot right caudate nucleus ➔ in an adult with a history of criminal violence. *(Right)* Axial brain SPECT shows much less than average cerebellar activity ➔. The cerebellum should not be used as an internal standard in this patient.

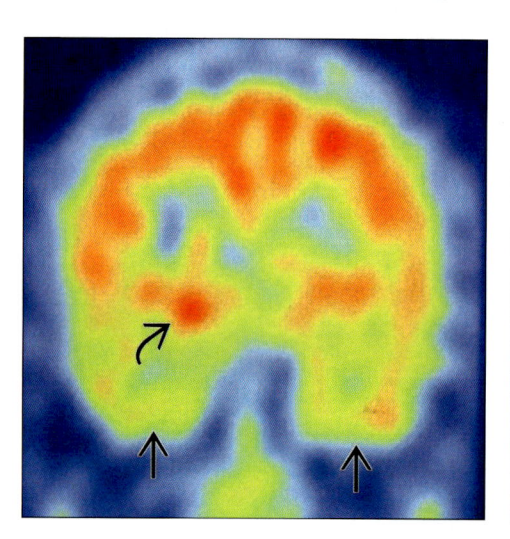

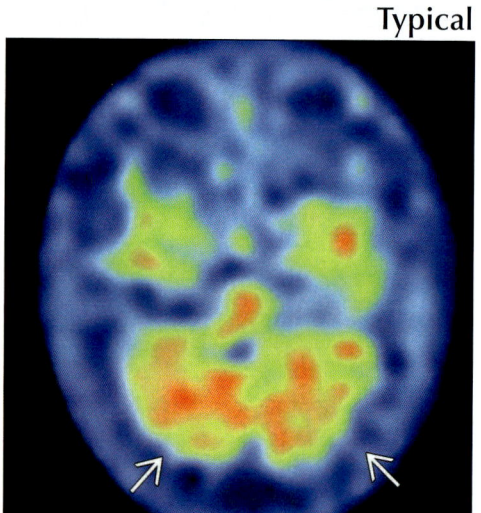

Typical

(Left) Brain SPECT on base surface map of a rest injected study shows decreased bilateral frontal and temporal activity ➔ in a depressed adult. *(Right)* Brain SPECT on base surface map (of same patient as left) injected during performance of an attention task shows significant improvement typical of depression.

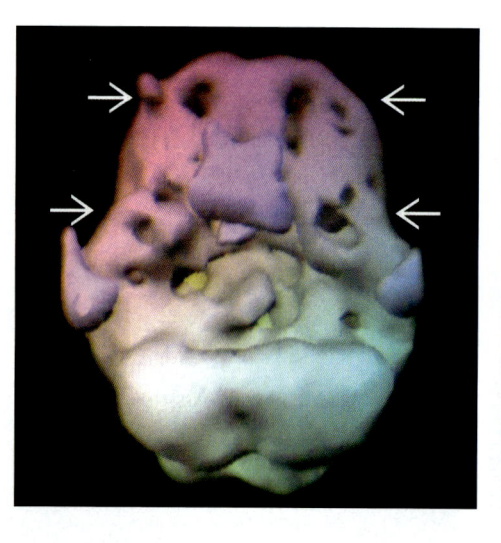

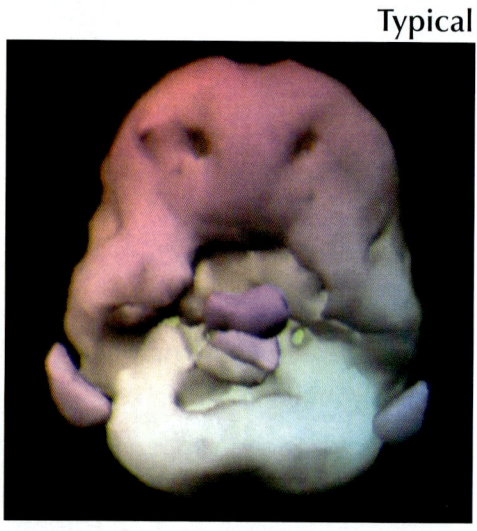

PSYCHIATRY, DRUG ADDICTION & FORENSICS

Typical

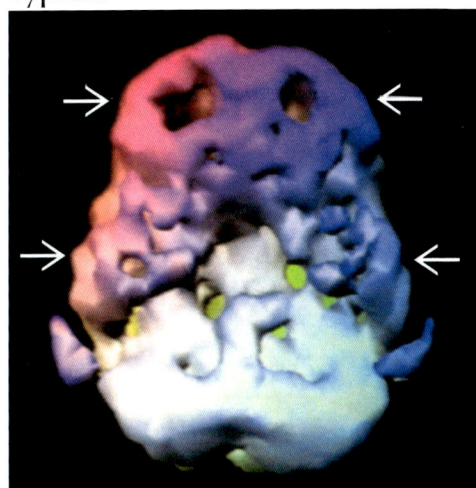

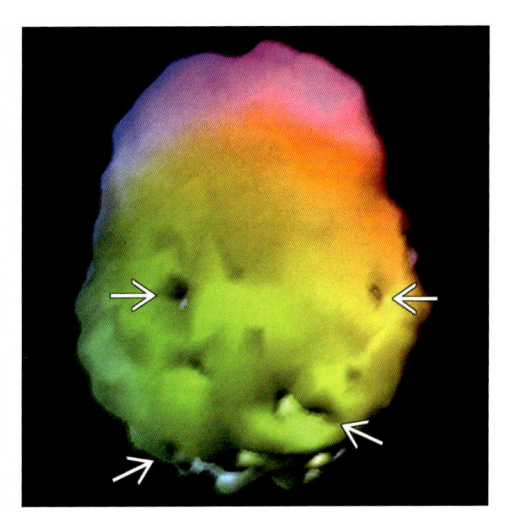

(Left) Brain SPECT on base surface map of a murderer shows significant defects in both frontal and temporal lobes ➡. **(Right)** Brain SPECT on this vertex surface map (same patient at left) shows additional bilateral parietal and occipital defects ➡.

Typical

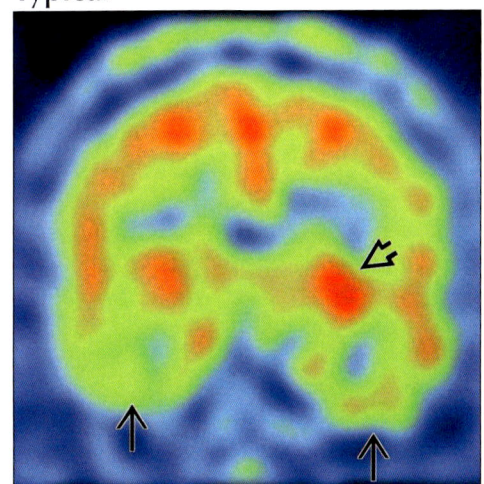

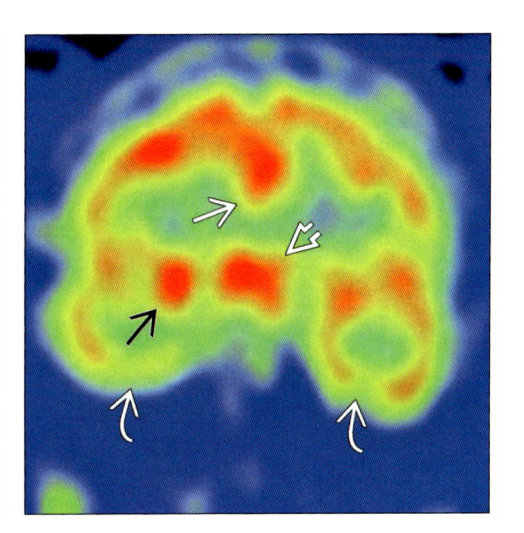

(Left) Coronal brain SPECT shows a left temporal hot spot ➡ coupled with bilateral temporal defects ➡ in an adult with a history of violent behavior. **(Right)** Coronal brain SPECT shows increased thalamic ➡, cingulate ➡, and caudate ➡ activity as well as bilateral temporal decreased activity ➡ in an adult with a history of violence.

Typical

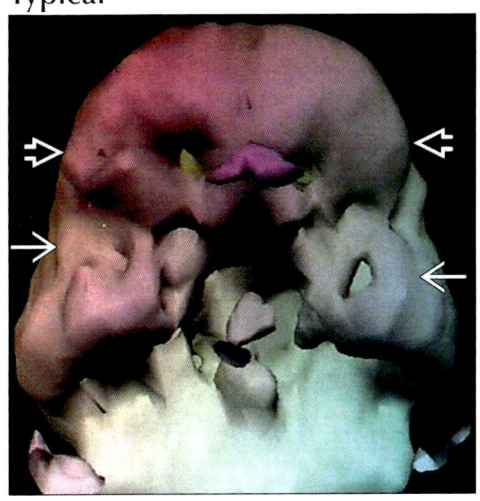

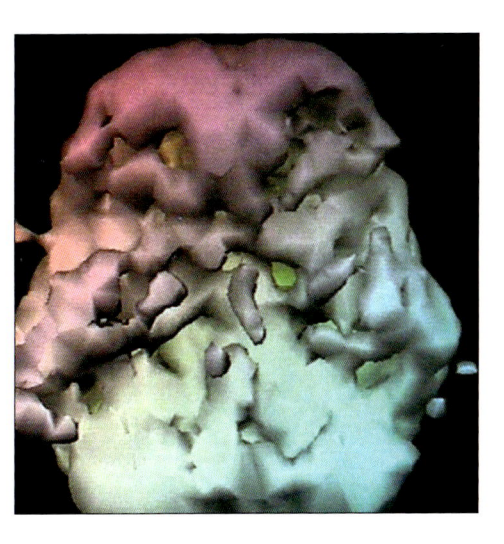

(Left) Brain SPECT on base surface map shows a child with ADD injected in a resting state. Defects in both temporal lobes ➡ and smaller defects ➡ in both frontal lobes are seen. **(Right)** Brain SPECT on base surface map (same patient at left) shows severe worsening of the temporal and frontal defects when injected with tracer while performing an attention task.

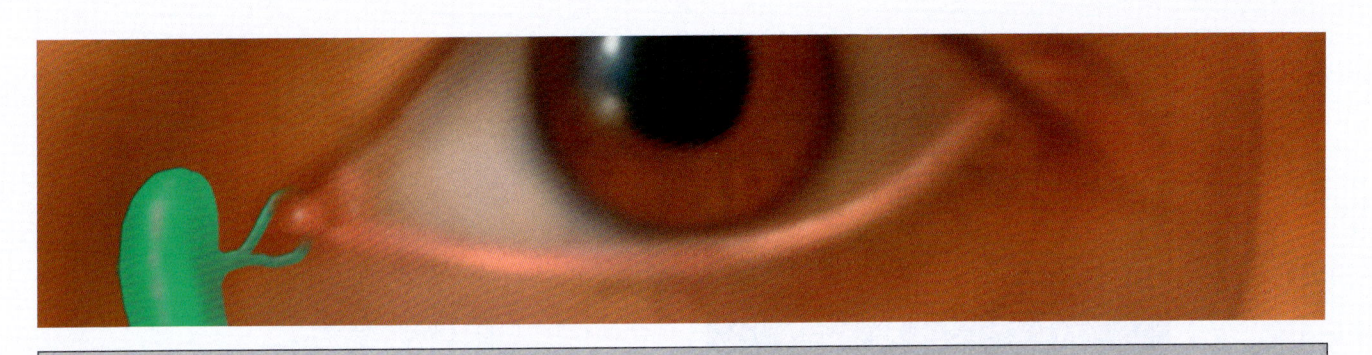

SECTION 6: Head and Neck

Squamous Cell Carcinoma of the Head and Neck

SCCHN, Staging 6-2
SCCHN, Primary Unknown 6-6
SCCHN, Therapeutic Assessment/Restaging 6-8

Miscellaneous Primary Head and Neck Tumors

Parotid and Salivary Tumors 6-12
Neuroendocrine Tumors, Head & Neck 6-14

Miscellaneous

Lacrimal Complex Dysfunction 6-18

SCCHN, STAGING

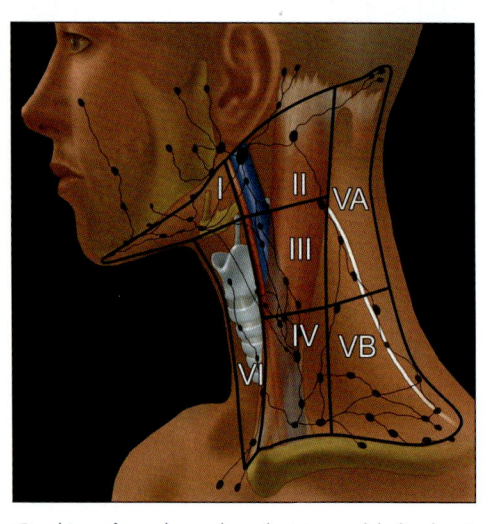

Graphic of neck nodes depicts nodal levels. I: Submental-submandibular; II: High jugular; III: Mid-jugular; IV: Low jugular; VA and VB: High and low spinal accessory; VI: Anterior cervical.

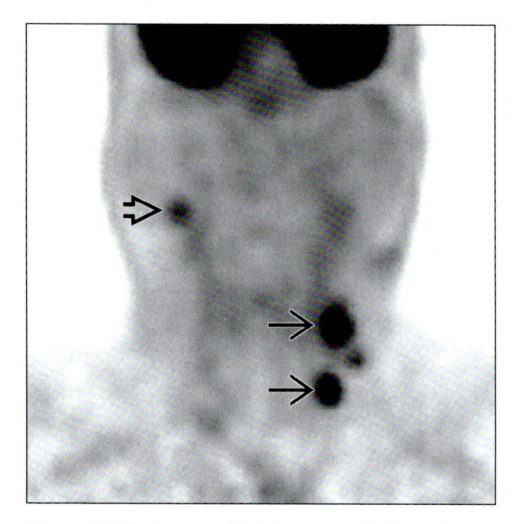

Coronal PET shows multiple hypermetabolic malignant level III, IV nodes in the left neck ➔. A single contralateral level II node in the right neck ➔ led to bilateral neck dissections.

TERMINOLOGY

Abbreviations and Synonyms
- Squamous cell carcinoma of the head and neck (SCCHN), lymph node staging, squamous cell carcinoma (SCCa) nodes

Definitions
- Assessment of primary, regional and distant malignancy from tumors of squamous cell origin in the head and neck

IMAGING FINDINGS

General Features
- Best diagnostic clue
  ○ Intensely FDG-avid nodes in the neck on PET or PET/CT
  ○ Enlarged or necrotic lymph nodes in the neck +/- enhancement on CT
- Location
  ○ Primary squamous cell lesion may involve any mucosal surface; commonly involving the base of tongue, tonsils or adenoids
  ○ Lymph node metastases involve neck nodes in expected drainage pattern based on primary tumor
- Size
  ○ Early primary SCCHN may be undetectable (unknown primary SCCHN)
  ○ Lymph node metastases may range in size from normal (< 1 cm) to several centimeters
  ○ Different CT size criteria for abnormal; ≥ 1 cm for most nodes; ≥ 1.5 cm for level I-II nodes; ≥ 8 mm for retropharyngeal nodes; FDG PET can detect smaller positive nodes
- Morphology
  ○ When large enough, some degree of mass effect, abnormal enhancement or necrosis
  ○ Fatty hilum usually denotes benign lesion on CT (may be positive on PET)
  ○ Indistinct borders usually denote extranodal spread

Nuclear Medicine Findings
- PET
  ○ Squamous cell carcinoma almost always FDG avid

DDx: Asymmetrical FDG Activity in a Patient Newly Diagnosed with SCCHN

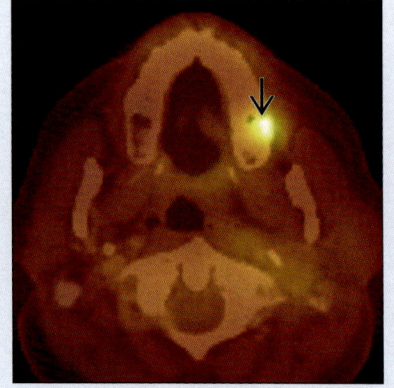

Dental Abscess

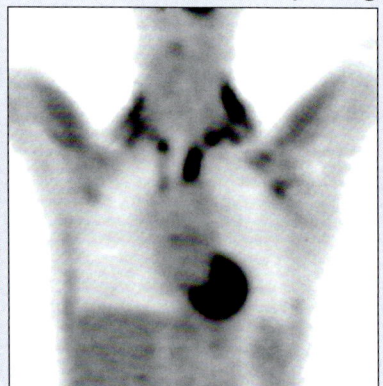

Muscle/Brown Fat

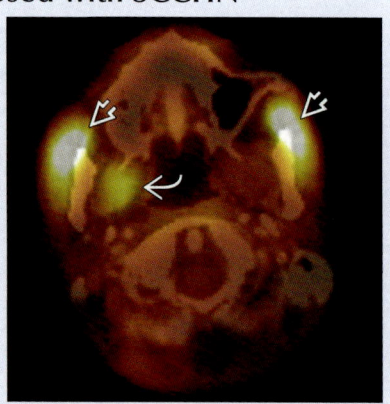

Muscle Activity

SCCHN, STAGING

Key Facts

Terminology
- Assessment of primary, regional and distant malignancy from tumors of squamous cell origin in the head and neck

Imaging Findings
- Intensely FDG-avid nodes in the neck on PET or PET/CT
- Enlarged or necrotic lymph nodes in the neck +/- enhancement on CT
- Lymph node metastases involve neck nodes in expected drainage pattern based on primary tumor
- When large enough, some degree of mass effect, abnormal enhancement or necrosis
- Look for primary lesion along the mucosal surfaces and evidence for nodal or distant spread
- Combined PET/CT may offer additional localization information and improve interpreting physician confidence level
- Extended field FDG PET staging may detect disease outside of the head and neck in up to 21%

Clinical Issues
- Nodal metastases best prognostic factor for SCCHN
- Radical, modified radical, or selective neck dissection

Diagnostic Checklist
- Consider PET or PET/CT for patients at substantial risk of metastatic disease, both nodal and hematogenous
- Know physiologic FDG uptake patterns in the neck to avoid misinterpretation

---

  - Look for primary lesion along the mucosal surfaces and evidence for nodal or distant spread

CT Findings
- CECT: Early enhancement, rim-enhancement, central necrosis or indistinct borders

Imaging Recommendations
- Best imaging tool
  - CECT with PET
  - Combined PET/CT may offer additional localization information and improve interpreting physician confidence level
    - Overall sensitivity and specificity of FDG PET and PET/CT > 90%; PET/CT sensitivity 96% and specificity 98%
    - PET/CT more helpful for radiation therapy planning; can lead to changes in gross tumor volume
    - Extended field FDG PET staging may detect disease outside of the head and neck in up to 21%
- Protocol advice
  - High resolution PET/CT from top of head to carina using IV CT contrast (should duplicate standard head and neck CT protocol)
  - Scan with arms down on PET/CT to avoid beam hardening artifact; use neck immobilization device
  - Scan in mask for radiation planning PET/CT
    - Display images with PET intensity kept low-moderate (avoid "blooming")
  - Pretreatment with benzodiazepines in patients with excessive muscular FDG uptake on FDG PET
  - Warm patients before and after injection of FDG to reduce brown fat FDG activity

DIFFERENTIAL DIAGNOSIS

Asymmetrical Muscle Activity
- Correlate PET with CT; pretreatment with benzodiazepines may reduce muscle uptake

Abscess or Supportive Nodes
- Usually has central necrosis; identicle in appearance to necrotic lymph node
- FDG PET not helpful for differentiation; biopsy required

Brown Fat
- Measure the Hounsfield units (HU) using CT; diagnostic if HU measure -50 to -150

Metastatic Disease from Thyroid or Melanoma
- May look identicle to squamous cell carcinoma

Lymphoma
- Difficult to differentiate from SCCHN based on imaging; associated mucosal lesion favors SCCHN

Reactive Nodes
- Tend to be normal morphology to minimally enlarged, symmetrical and low level FDG uptake
- May be associated with diffuse tonsillar uptake if recent upper respiratory or viral infection
- Careful history for recent upper respiratory infection is advisable

PATHOLOGY

General Features
- General path comments
  - American Joint Committee on Cancer (AJCC) and American Academy of Otolaryngology-Head and Neck Surgery (AAO-HNS) nodal level classification scheme
    - Level IA: Submental nodes between anterior digastrics; level IB: Submandibular, lateral to IA anterior to the posterior margin of submandibular gland (SMG)

SCCHN, STAGING

- Level IIA: Upper internal jugular nodes; IIA: Anterior, lateral or posterior and touching the jugular vein; level IIB: Posterior not touching jugular
- Level III: Mid internal jugular nodes, extend from inferior hyoid to cricoid arch
- Level IV: Low internal jugular nodes, extend from cricoid arch to the level of the clavicle
- Level V: Spinal accessory group, nodes in the posterior triangle; level VA: Above cricoid; level VB: Below inferior cricoid border
- Level VI: Upper visceral nodes; between the carotid arteries from bottom of the hyoid to the top of the manubrium
- Level VII: Superior mediastinal nodes; between the carotid arteries from below the top of the manubrium above the inominate vein
- Supraclavicular nodes: At or caudal to the level of the clavicle and lateral to the carotid artery
- Retropharyngeal nodes: Within 2 cm of the skull base medial to the carotid arteries
- Parotid: Nodes within the parotid gland
- Etiology: Smoking, chewing tobacco, alcohol abuse
- Associated abnormalities: Risk factor also predispose to esophageal and lung cancer

CLINICAL ISSUES

Presentation
- Most common signs/symptoms: May present with pain associated with primary mass or neck mass

Demographics
- Age: Generally > 40-45
- Gender: M > F

Natural History & Prognosis
- Nodal metastases best prognostic factor for SCCHN
  - Unilateral nodal involvement 50% reduction in prognosis; bilateral nodal involvement 75% reduction in prognosis
  - Carotid artery involvement or encasement dismal prognosis 100% mortality

Treatment
- Radical, modified radical, or selective neck dissection
  - Radical neck dissection: Excision of levels I-V lymph nodes, sternocleidomastoid muscle (SCM), intenal jugular vein (IJV) and cranial nerve XI
  - Modified radical neck dissection: Excision of levels I-V lymph nodes +/- cranial nerve XI
  - Selective neck dissection: Excision of selective nodal groups
- Radiation therapy +/- chemotherapy

DIAGNOSTIC CHECKLIST

Consider
- Consider PET/CT in patients with primary tumors that are prone to bilateral metastases; often less conspicuous on conventional imaging
  - Primary tumors of the nasopharynx, tongue base, and supraglottis
- Consider PET or PET/CT for patients at substantial risk of metastatic disease, both nodal and hematogenous
  - Patients with T3 or T4 lesions of the oral cavity, oropharynx, or larynx

Image Interpretation Pearls
- Know physiologic FDG uptake patterns in the neck to avoid misinterpretation

SELECTED REFERENCES

1. Dammann F et al: Rational diagnosis of squamous cell carcinoma of the head and neck region: comparative evaluation of CT, MRI, and 18FDG PET. AJR Am J Roentgenol. 184(4):1326-31, 2005
2. Dobert N et al: The prognostic value of FDG PET in head and neck cancer. Correlation with histopathology. Q J Nucl Med Mol Imaging. 49(3):253-7, 2005
3. Yen TC et al: Staging of untreated squamous cell carcinoma of buccal mucosa with 18F-FDG PET: comparison with head and neck CT/MRI and histopathology. J Nucl Med. 46(5):775-81, 2005
4. Zanation AM et al: Use, accuracy, and implications for patient management of [18F]-2-fluorodeoxyglucose-positron emission/computerized tomography for head and neck tumors. Laryngoscope. 115(7):1186-90, 2005
5. Daisne JF et al: Tumor volume in pharyngolaryngeal squamous cell carcinoma: comparison at CT, MR imaging, and FDG PET and validation with surgical specimen. Radiology. 233(1):93-100, 2004
6. Schoder H et al: Positron emission imaging of head and neck cancer, including thyroid carcinoma. Semin Nucl Med. 34(3):180-97, 2004
7. Goerres GW et al: Impact of whole body positron emission tomography on initial staging and therapy in patients with squamous cell carcinoma of the oral cavity. Oral Oncol. 39(6):547-51, 2003
8. Schmid DT et al: Impact of positron emission tomography on the initial staging and therapy in locoregional advanced squamous cell carcinoma of the head and neck. Laryngoscope. 113(5):888-91, 2003
9. Schwartz DL et al: Staging of head and neck squamous cell cancer with extended-field FDG-PET. Arch Otolaryngol Head Neck Surg. 129(11):1173-8, 2003
10. Sigg MB et al: Staging of head and neck tumors: [18F]fluorodeoxyglucose positron emission tomography compared with physical examination and conventional imaging modalities. J Oral Maxillofac Surg. 61(9):1022-9, 2003
11. Brink I et al: Lymph node staging in extracranial head and neck cancer with FDG PET--appropriate uptake period and size-dependence of the results. Nuklearmedizin. 41(2):108-13, 2002
12. Hannah A et al: Evaluation of 18 F-fluorodeoxyglucose positron emission tomography and computed tomography with histopathologic correlation in the initial staging of head and neck cancer. Ann Surg. 236(2):208-17, 2002
13. Stoeckli SJ et al: Is there a role for positron emission tomography with 18F-fluorodeoxyglucose in the initial staging of nodal negative oral and oropharyngeal squamous cell carcinoma. Head Neck. 24(4):345-9, 2002
14. Kresnik E et al: Evaluation of head and neck cancer with 18F-FDG PET: a comparison with conventional methods. Eur J Nucl Med. 28(7):816-21, 2001

SCCHN, STAGING

IMAGE GALLERY

Variant

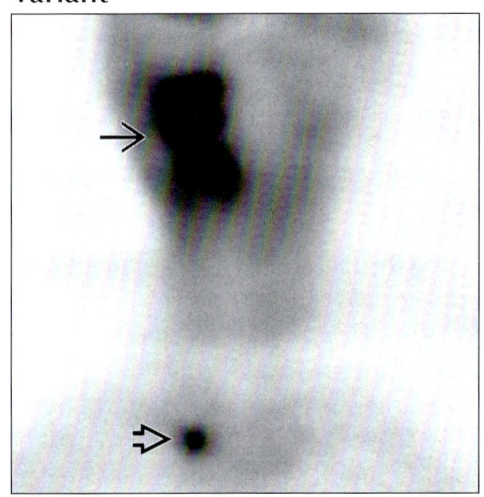

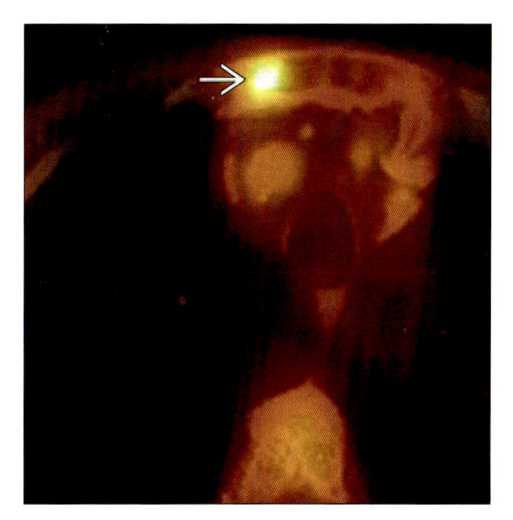

(Left) Coronal PET shows large hypermetabolic oral cavity mass ➔. A single lesion outside of the neck is also identified, although poorly localized ➔. *(Right)* Axial fused PET CT easily localizes the abnormality in the previous figure to a single hypermetabolic focus in the sternum ➔ compatible with metastatic disease.

Typical

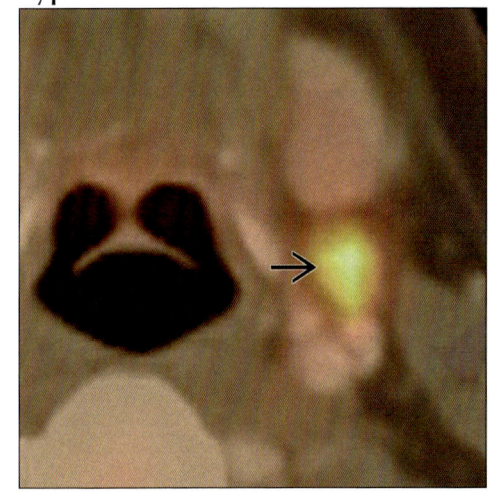

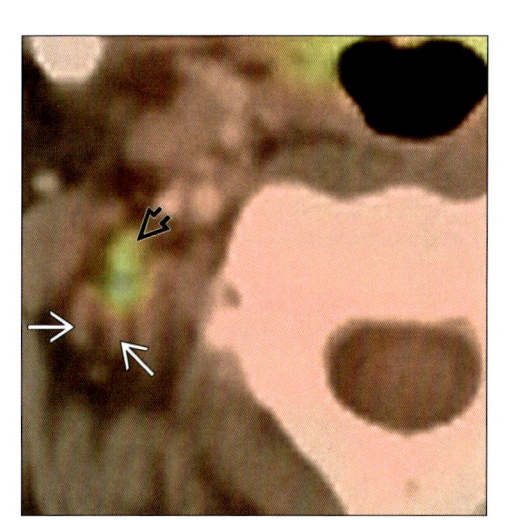

(Left) Axial fused PET CT shows a single hypermetabolic level II lymph node ➔ in the left neck correlating to a mildly enlarged lymph node in this patient who was diagnosed with a left-sided SCCHN. *(Right)* Axial fused PET CT in same patient as previous image shows several normal-sized level II lymph nodes in the contralateral neck ➔. However, only one of the lymph nodes shows FDG activity ➔.

Typical

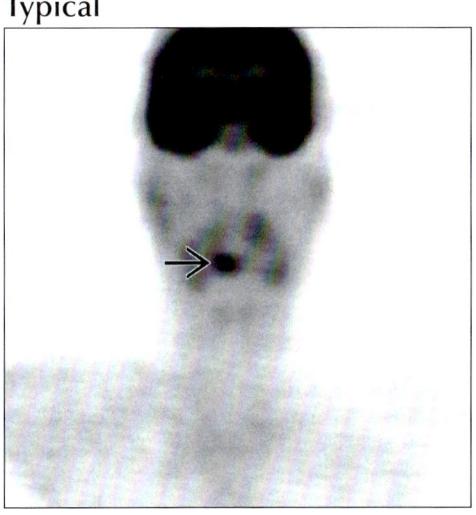

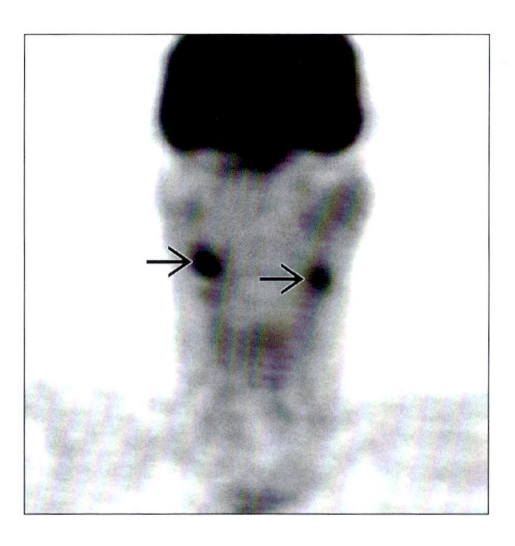

(Left) Coronal PET shows focal intense FDG uptake ➔ poorly localized in this patient with newly diagnosed laryngeal carcinoma. *(Right)* Coronal PET in the same patient as previous image shows bilateral level II lymph nodes ➔ leading to bilateral radical neck dissections in this patient.

SCCHN, PRIMARY UNKNOWN

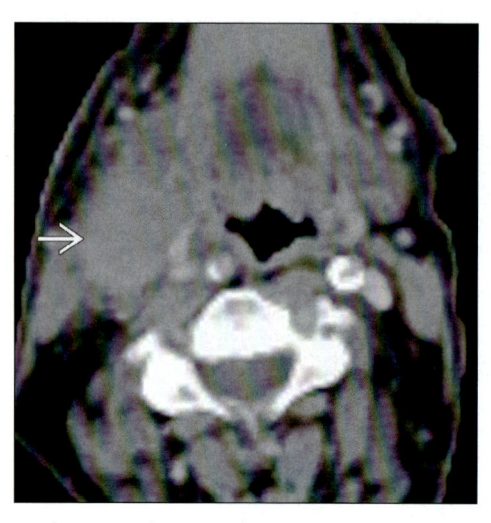

Axial CECT shows a large mass in the right parapharyngeal space ➔. No mucosal lesion is identified on the CT portion of this PET/CT exam. Same patient as next image.

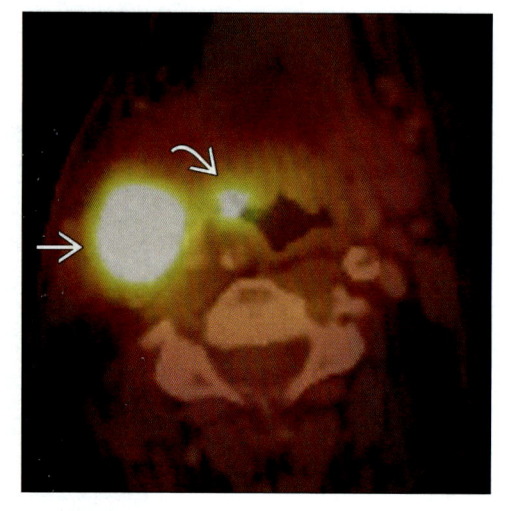

Axial fused PET CT shows the large right parapharyngeal mass ➔ seen on CT. Additional lesion also present along the right mucosal surface ➔. Directed biopsy was positive.

TERMINOLOGY

Abbreviations and Synonyms
- Unknown mucosal primary

Definitions
- Metastatic squamous cell carcinoma of the neck without an identifiable mucosal primary lesion
- Some definitions include undetectable mucosal lesions by clinical exam while others include negative anatomical imaging

IMAGING FINDINGS

General Features
- Best diagnostic clue
  - PET shows asymmetrical focal fluorodeoxyglucose (FDG) uptake, with or without an identifiable abnormality on CT
    - Fused PET/CT images often helpful for determining whether potential FDG abnormalities are mucosal lesions
    - Helpful for directing clinicians to areas for directed biopsies
- Location: Mucosal surfaces of the oropharynx, nasopharynx and hypopharynx
- Size: A few millimeters to several centimeters
- Morphology
  - CT findings: Usually enough to show typical abnormalities on anatomical imaging
    - May show subtle necrosis, enhancement or mass effect

Nuclear Medicine Findings
- FDG PET typically shows focal asymmetrical FDG uptake in the mucosal primary

Imaging Recommendations
- Best imaging tool
  - Combined PET/CT
    - Sensitivity for PET and PET/CT 26-43% in cases where primary has eluded diagnosis
    - Sensitivity for PET/CT similar, but better for accurate localization of lesion and directed biopsy recommendations
- Protocol advice
  - Contrast-enhanced CT with PET/CT

DDx: Muscular Uptake of FDG Uptake in the Head and Neck

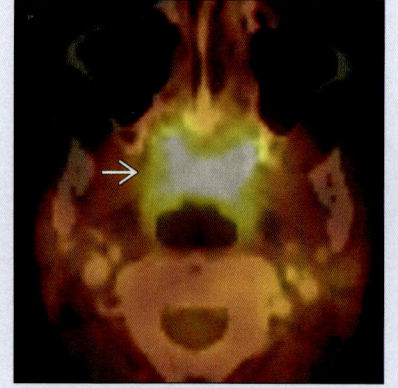

Palate FDG Uptake

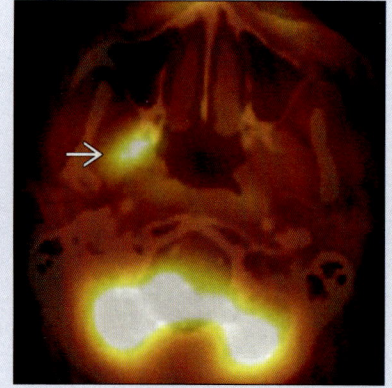

Medial Pterygoid

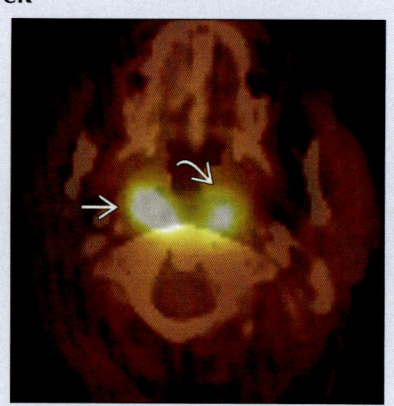

Symmetrical NHL

SCCHN, PRIMARY UNKNOWN

Terminology
- Unknown mucosal primary

Imaging Findings
- PET shows asymmetrical focal fluorodeoxyglucose (FDG) uptake, with or without an identifiable abnormality on CT
- Location: Mucosal surfaces of the oropharynx, nasopharynx and hypopharynx

Key Facts
- FDG PET typically shows focal asymmetrical FDG uptake in the mucosal primary
- Sensitivity for PET and PET/CT 26-43% in cases where primary has eluded diagnosis

Clinical Issues
- Surgical resection for the primary lesion and metastatic neck lesions +/- radiation therapy

- Scan with arms down to avoid beam hardening artifact on CT
- High resolution PET/CT from top of head to carina

DIFFERENTIAL DIAGNOSIS

Physiologic Activity
- Benign tonsil FDG uptake typically will be symmetrical but can be intense
- Muscle activity may be asymmetrical

Symmetrical Mucosal Involvement with Other Malignancy
- CT may show asymmetrical mass effect

Non-Hodgkin Lymphoma (NHL)
- May mimic tonsilar inflammatory disease

CLINICAL ISSUES

Presentation
- Other signs/symptoms: One or more neck masses, with or without pain

Natural History & Prognosis
- PET and PET/CT can help direct biopsy
- If all imaging is negative, patients are usually followed with serial imaging evaluation

Treatment
- Surgical resection for the primary lesion and metastatic neck lesions +/- radiation therapy
- Whole neck irradiation if mucosal primary is not identified

DIAGNOSTIC CHECKLIST

Consider
- PET or PET/CT evaluation after negative exam prior to random biopsies
- MRI may provide additional information

Image Interpretation Pearls
- Look for asymmetrical FDG activity

SELECTED REFERENCES
1. Freudenberg LS et al: Dual modality of 18F-fluorodeoxyglucose-positron emission tomography/computed tomography in patients with cervical carcinoma of unknown primary. Med Princ Pract. 14(3):155-60, 2005
2. Miller FR et al: Positron emission tomography in the management of unknown primary head and neck carcinoma. Arch Otolaryngol Head Neck Surg. 131(7):626-9, 2005
3. AAssar OS et al: Metastatic head and neck cancer: role and usefulness of FDG PET in locating occult primary tumors. Radiology. 210(1):177-81, 1999

IMAGE GALLERY

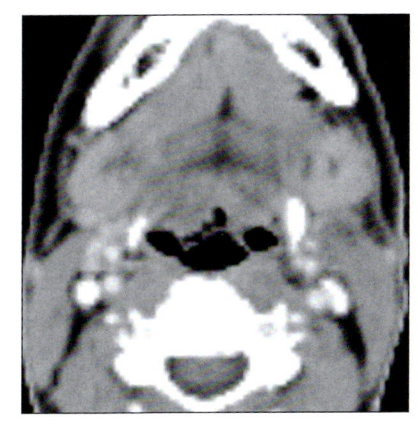

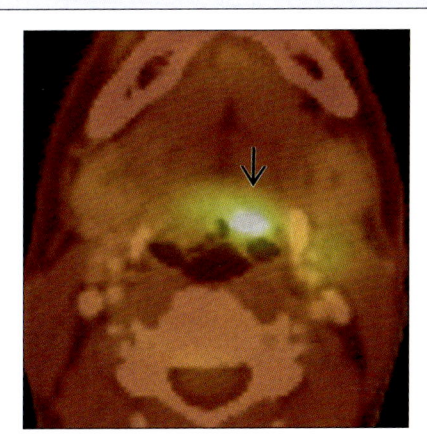

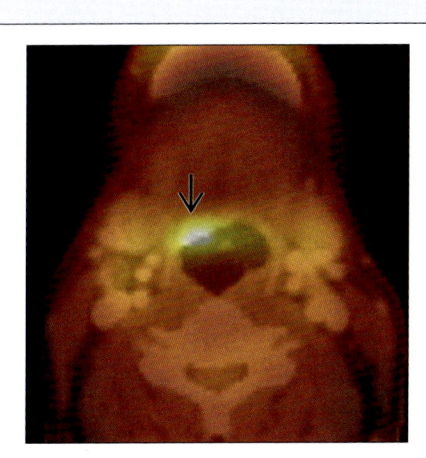

(Left) Axial CECT shows no abnormalities. The mucosal surfaces show no evidence of tumor. Same patient as next image. *(Center)* Axial fused PET/CT shows a focal asymmetrical area of FDG uptake in the left base of tongue ➔ not seen on the CT portion of the exam, confirmed to be the primary mucosal lesion. *(Right)* Axial fused PET/CT shows focal area of intense FDG uptake in the right base of tongue ➔ confirmed to be the primary mucosal lesion not identified on the CT portion of the exam.

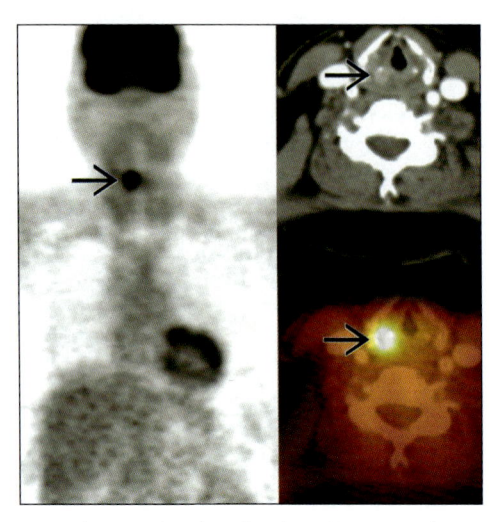

SCCHN, THERAPEUTIC ASSESSMENT/RESTAGING

Coronal PET and axial CT/fused PET/CT images show a focal intensely FDG avid laryngeal tumor ➔ prior to radiation therapy.

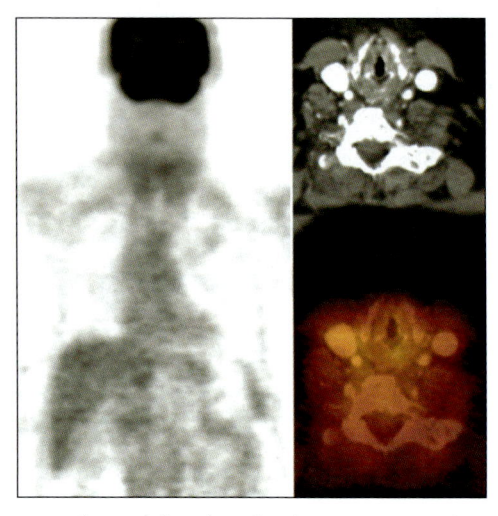

Coronal PET and axial CT/fused PET/CT images show no residual FDG activity approximately 8 weeks following radiation therapy.

TERMINOLOGY

Abbreviations and Synonyms
- Squamous cell carcinoma of the head and neck (SCCHN)

Definitions
- Restaging of SCCHN following chemotherapy, radiation or other therapies

IMAGING FINDINGS

General Features
- Best diagnostic clue: Intense FDG activity in or around treated primary tumor with corresponding CT evidence of residual tumor
- Location
  - Assessment of primary and metastatic lesions following therapy
  - Also assess for new lesions
- Size
  - Variable
    - Following surgery, no detectable tumor should be present; variable amounts of post-surgical change
    - Following chemoradiation, metabolic response may precede reductions in tumor volume

Nuclear Medicine Findings
- PET
  - PET/CT is more accurate than PET and CT separately, PET is more accurate than CT alone
    - FDG PET sensitivity and specificity for residual disease 90% and 83%
    - PET/CT sensitivity, specificity and accuracy 98%, 92% and 94%
    - PET/CT decreases equivocal lesions by ~ 50%; provides improved biopsy localization information
    - 74% better localization with PET/CT compared to PET in regions previously treated; 58% for untreated regions
  - Post surgery: Usually wait 4-6 weeks after to reevaluate with PET and PET/CT to avoid false positive studies due to inflammation

DDx: Inflammation/Infection Mimicking SCCHN

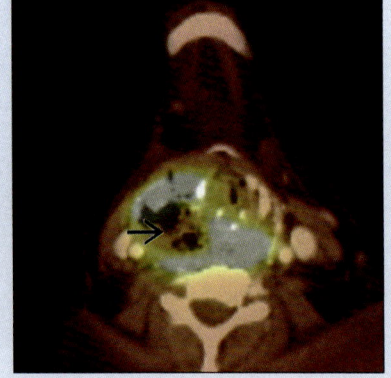

Neck Abscess 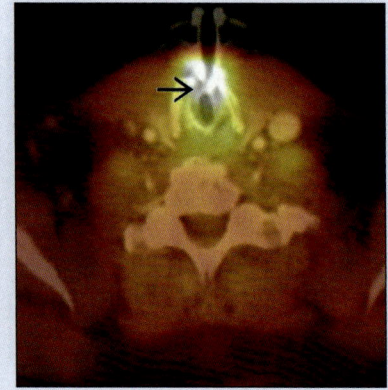   *Peristomal Inflammation* 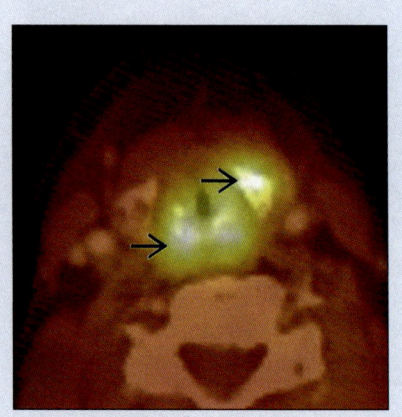   *XRT Inflammation*

SCCHN, THERAPEUTIC ASSESSMENT/RESTAGING

Key Facts

Terminology
- Restaging of SCCHN following chemotherapy, radiation or other therapies

Imaging Findings
- Best diagnostic clue: Intense FDG activity in or around treated primary tumor with corresponding CT evidence of residual tumor
- Following chemoradiation, metabolic response may precede reductions in tumor volume
- Accuracy of CT ranges from 50-70%
- CT may show enhancement, necrosis or mass effect with residual/recurrent tumor
- PET/CT is more accurate than PET and CT separately, PET is more accurate than CT alone
- Pitfalls and limitations
  - Several structures in the neck with variable physiologic FDG activity

Top Differential Diagnoses
- Residual/Recurrent Malignancy
- Abscess Formation
- Radiation-Induced Inflammation
- Asymmetrical Muscle/Brown Fat

Diagnostic Checklist
- General scanning guidelines
- Wait at least 3-5 weeks following surgery
- When in doubt determining post-therapy FDG uptake vs. tumor, perform short term follow-up
- Also consider dual-time point PET exam

  - Reevaluation following surgery may be particularly helpful in cases where surgical margins are positive
  o Post radiation
    - Positive PET 1 month after XRT has a positive predictive value of ~ 100%
    - Negative PET 1 month after XRT has a negative predictive value much lower (14%) early; fewer false negatives with longer follow up period
  o Post chemotherapy (approximately 1 month after completion): Sensitivity and specificity of FDG PET 90% and 83%
    - Little data evaluating early response to chemotherapy
  o Pitfalls and limitations
    - Several structures in the neck with variable physiologic FDG activity
    - Common muscles with asymmetrical FDG activity: Medial and lateral pterygoids, sternocleidomastoid, strap muscles and mylohyoid
    - Glands: Salivary glands (submandibular and parotid); asymmetrical if unilateral resection; can also have intense FDG activity following some chemo regimens
    - Lymphoid tissue: Lingual tonsils, palatine tonsils and adenoids (Waldeyer ring)
    - Brown fat: Can be symmetrical or asymmetrical; can be focal anywhere in the neck
    - FDG PET may not detect small areas of residual/recurrent disease leading to early false negative exams after therapy
    - Cartilage necrosis may be FDG avid indefinitely
    - Cricoarytenoids typically FDG avid and often asymmetric

CT Findings
- CECT
  o Post therapy neck difficult to interpret
    - Accuracy of CT ranges from 50-70%
    - Loss of fat planes and extensive post surgical changes reduce the specificity of CT
    - Distortion of normal anatomy can be due to bony-cartilaginous necrosis, edema and desmoplastic changes
    - CT may show enhancement, necrosis or mass effect with residual/recurrent tumor
    - Best method of detection using CECT is serial exams

Imaging Recommendations
- Best imaging tool: Combined PET/CT
- Protocol advice
  o Scan with arms down, CECT, and neck immobilization device
  o Consider dual-time point imaging to help differentiate between inflammatory and neoplastic FDG activity

DIFFERENTIAL DIAGNOSIS

Residual/Recurrent Malignancy
- Often indistinguishable from abscess/inflammation
- Short-term serial evaluation very helpful

Abscess Formation
- Often indistinguishable from tumor; correlate clinically
- Usually requires biopsy for differentiation

Radiation-Induced Inflammation
- FDG uptake from inflammation usually present for 4-8 weeks following therapy
- Osteoradionecrosis can cause false positive early before frank necrosis when PET becomes negative
- Dual-time point PET imaging at 1 hour and 3 hour post FDG injection may be helpful in differentiating tumor vs. inflammation
  o FDG uptake from 1-3 h: Tumor may increase; inflammation may plateau or decrease

Asymmetrical Muscle/Brown Fat
- Measure Hounsfield units (HU); if -50 to -150 compatible with brown fat
- Can be focal and asymmetrical

SCCHN, THERAPEUTIC ASSESSMENT/RESTAGING

- Warm patient before FDG injection to reduce brown fat uptake of FDG

CLINICAL ISSUES

Presentation
- Most common signs/symptoms: Symptoms of residual/recurrent tumor overlap with post-treatment complications; most common pain
- Other signs/symptoms: Mass on clinical exam

Demographics
- Age: > 50
- Gender: M > F

Natural History & Prognosis
- FDG has prognostic implications for SCCHN
  - SUV > 9 poorer prognosis for initial staging 22% 3 year survival vs. 73% for SUV ≤ 9
  - Reevaluation with FDG PET in the early phase of treatment (in one study) was associated with tumor response, survival and local control

Treatment
- Biopsy areas that appear suspicious on PET or PET/CT vs. short-term interval follow-up PET or PET/CT

DIAGNOSTIC CHECKLIST

Consider
- General scanning guidelines
  - Wait at least 3-5 weeks following surgery
  - Wait 6-12 weeks following radiation therapy; less false positives and false negatives with later follow-up periods
  - Wait 1 month after chemo

Image Interpretation Pearls
- When in doubt determining post-therapy FDG uptake vs. tumor, perform short term follow-up
  - Post treatment inflammation almost always resolves on short-term follow up exam
- Also consider dual-time point PET exam

SELECTED REFERENCES

1. Branstetter BF 4th et al: Head and neck malignancy: is PET/CT more accurate than PET or CT alone? Radiology. 235(2):580-6, 2005
2. Kapoor V et al: Role of 18FFDG PET/CT in the treatment of head and neck cancers: posttherapy evaluation and pitfalls. AJR Am J Roentgenol. 184(2):589-97, 2005
3. Nam SY et al: Early evaluation of the response to radiotherapy of patients with squamous cell carcinoma of the head and neck using 18FDG-PET. Oral Oncol. 41(4):390-5, 2005
4. Ryan WR et al: Positron-emission tomography for surveillance of head and neck cancer. Laryngoscope. 115(4):645-50, 2005
5. Yao M et al: Can post-RT FDG PET accurately predict the pathologic status in neck dissection after radiation for locally advanced head and neck cancer? In regard to Rogers et al. (Int J Radiat Oncol Biol Phys 2004;58:694-697). Int J Radiat Oncol Biol Phys. 61(1):306-7; author reply 307, 2005
6. Yen RF et al: Whole-body 18F-FDG PET in recurrent or metastatic nasopharyngeal carcinoma. J Nucl Med. 46(5):770-4, 2005
7. Allal AS et al: Prediction of outcome in head-and-neck cancer patients using the standardized uptake value of 2-[18F]fluoro-2-deoxy-D-glucose. Int J Radiat Oncol Biol Phys. 59(5):1295-300, 2004
8. Conessa C et al: FDG-PET scan in local follow-up of irradiated head and neck squamous cell carcinomas. Ann Otol Rhinol Laryngol. 113(8):628-35, 2004
9. Kubota K et al: FDG-PET delayed imaging for the detection of head and neck cancer recurrence after radio-chemotherapy: comparison with MRI/CT. Eur J Nucl Med Mol Imaging. 31(4):590-5, 2004
10. Liu SH et al: False positive fluorine-18 fluorodeoxy-D-glucose positron emission tomography finding caused by osteoradionecrosis in a nasopharyngeal carcinoma patient. Br J Radiol. 77(915):257-60, 2004
11. McCollum AD et al: Positron emission tomography with 18F-fluorodeoxyglucose to predict pathologic response after induction chemotherapy and definitive chemoradiotherapy in head and neck cancer. Head Neck. 26(10):890-6, 2004
12. Rogers JW et al: Can post-RT neck dissection be omitted for patients with head-and-neck cancer who have a negative PET scan after definitive radiation therapy? Int J Radiat Oncol Biol Phys. 58(3):694-7, 2004
13. Schmidt M et al: 18F-FDG PET for detecting recurrent head and neck cancer, local lymph node involvement and distant metastases. Comparison of qualitative visual and semiquantitative analysis. Nuklearmedizin. 43(3):91-101;quiz 102-4, 2004
14. Schoder H et al: Head and neck cancer: clinical usefulness and accuracy of PET/CT image fusion. Radiology. 231(1):65-72, 2004
15. Schwartz DL et al: FDG-PET prediction of head and neck squamous cell cancer outcomes. Arch Otolaryngol Head Neck Surg. 130(12):1361-7, 2004
16. Swisher SG et al: 2-Fluoro-2-deoxy-D-glucose positron emission tomography imaging is predictive of pathologic response and survival after preoperative chemoradiation in patients with esophageal carcinoma. Cancer. 101(8):1776-85, 2004
17. Yao M et al: The role of post-radiation therapy FDG PET in prediction of necessity for post-radiation therapy neck dissection in locally advanced head-and-neck squamous cell carcinoma. Int J Radiat Oncol Biol Phys. 59(4):1001-10, 2004
18. Yao M et al: Value of FDG PET in assessment of treatment response and surveillance in head-and-neck cancer patients after intensity modulated radiation treatment: a preliminary report. Int J Radiat Oncol Biol Phys. 60(5):1410-8, 2004
19. Fukui MB et al: PET/CT imaging in recurrent head and neck cancer. Semin Ultrasound CT MR. 24(3):157-63, 2003
20. Kunkel M et al: Detection of recurrent oral squamous cell carcinoma by [18F]-2-fluorodeoxyglucose-positron emission tomography: implications for prognosis and patient management. Cancer. 98(10):2257-65, 2003
21. Yen RF et al: 18-fluoro-2-deoxyglucose positron emission tomography in detecting residual/recurrent nasopharyngeal carcinomas and comparison with magnetic resonance imaging. Cancer. 98(2):283-7, 2003
22. Minn H et al: Prediction of survival with fluorine-18-fluoro-deoxyglucose and PET in head and neck cancer. J Nucl Med. 38(12):1907-11, 1997

SCCHN, THERAPEUTIC ASSESSMENT/RESTAGING

IMAGE GALLERY

Typical

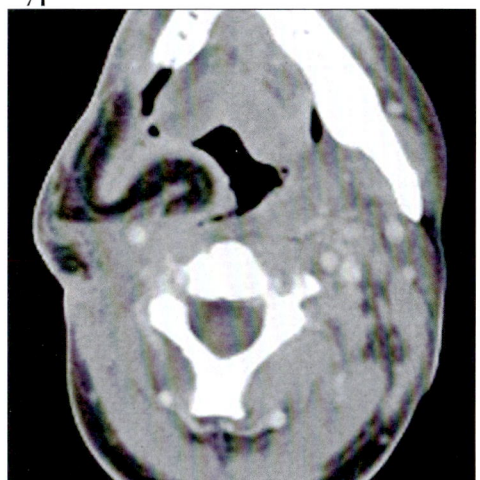

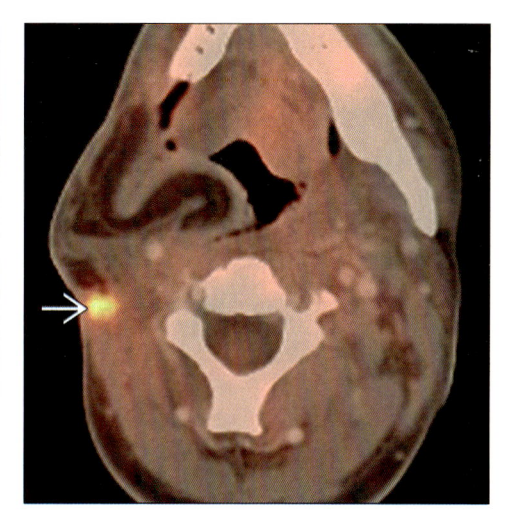

(Left) Axial CECT shows no evidence of residual/recurrent tumor. Note extensive post-operative changes, loss of fat planes, and difficulty assessing the area surrounding the flap. (Right) Axial fused PET/CT shows a focal hypermetabolic area in the posterolateral portion of the flap ➡ consistent with residual/recurrent tumor.

Typical

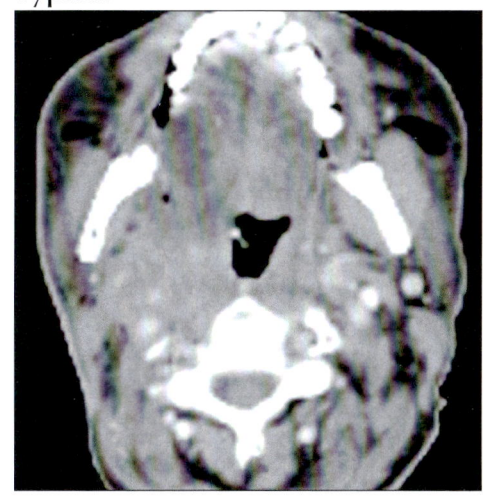

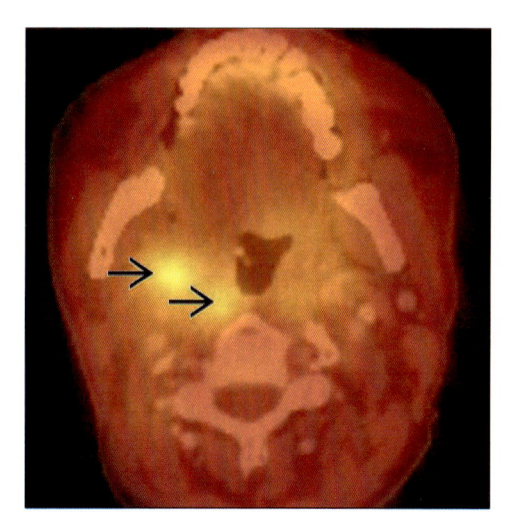

(Left) Axial CECT shows extensive post-operative changes with no definite evidence for residual/recurrent tumor approximately 3 months following resection. (Right) Axial fused PET/CT shows two foci of moderate FDG activity in the right parapharyngeal area ➡ without an identifiable CT abnormality compatible with residual/recurrent tumor.

Typical

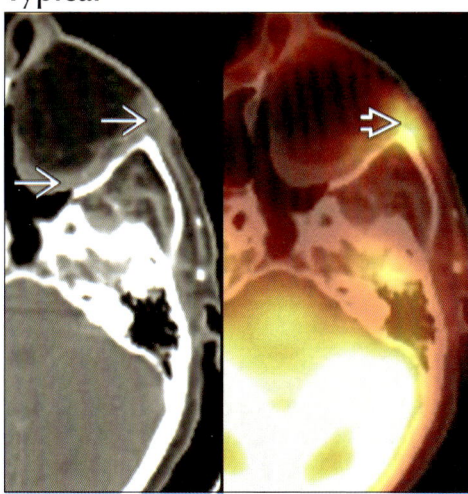

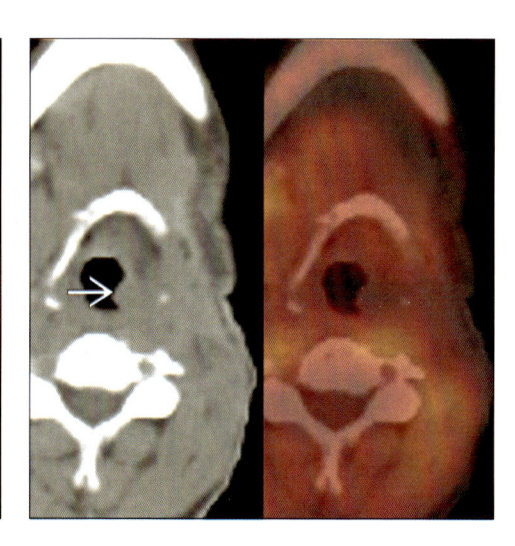

(Left) Axial CT shows thickening along the posterolateral flap borders ➡ 6 weeks after surgery. PET/CT shows the residual/recurrent tumor only along the lateral flap border ➡. (Right) Axial CT shows an area adjacent to the trachea ➡ worrisome for tumor on an MR in this patient with a known recurrence. PET/CT shows no FDG uptake saving patient a tracheostomy.

PAROTID AND SALIVARY TUMORS

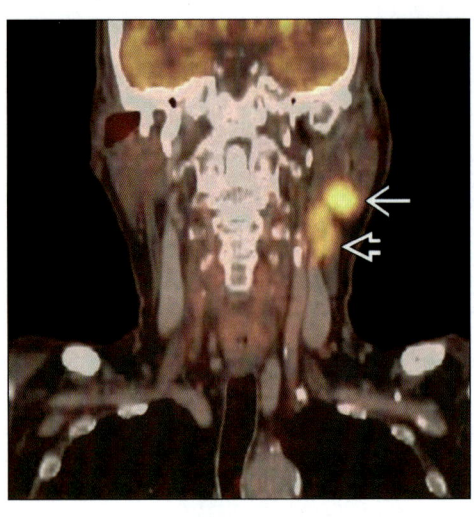

Coronal fused FDG PET/CT demonstrates hypermetabolic left parotid mass ➡ and adjacent lymph nodes ⇨. Biopsy revealed malignant mixed salivary tumor.

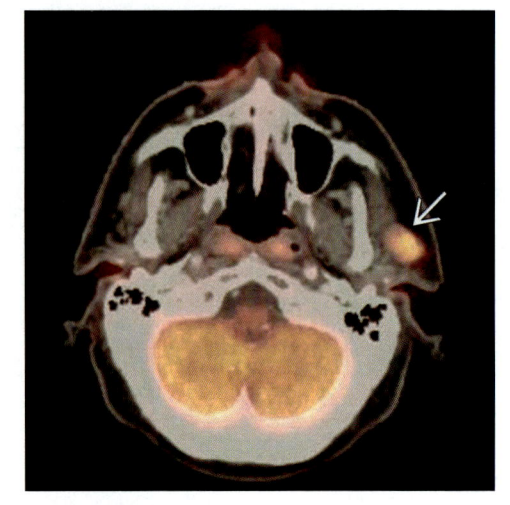

Axial fused FDG PET/CT demonstrates hypermetabolic mass in superior portion of left parotid gland ➡ confirmed at biopsy to be a Warthin tumor (often as metabolically active as cancers).

TERMINOLOGY

Abbreviations and Synonyms
- Benign mixed tumors (BMT) or pleomorphic adenoma; Warthin tumor; parotid carcinoma (mucoepidermoid and adenoid cystic), primary lymphoma

Definitions
- Tumors of the parotid and submandibular glands (salivary glands)

IMAGING FINDINGS

General Features
- Best diagnostic clue: Negative Tc-99m pertechnetate and positive FDG PET
- Location: Tumors within the parotid space
- Size: Variable from few millimeters to several centimeters

Nuclear Medicine Findings
- PET: General: Sensitivity and specificity 75% and 67%; 30% false positive rate for malignancy (mostly due to Warthin tumor)
- Ga-67 Scintigraphy: Sensitivity and specificity for differentiation of benign from malignant parotid masses 58% and 72%

CT Findings
- CECT: Variable, fairly low sensitivity and specificity

Imaging Recommendations
- Best imaging tool: Nuclear medicine: Combination FDG PET or PET/CT and salivary gland scintigraphy with Tc-99m pertechnetate

DIFFERENTIAL DIAGNOSIS

Benign Mixed Tumor or Pleomorphic Adenoma
- Can be positive or negative on FDG PET; tends to be less FDG avid than primary parotid malignancies and Warthin tumor

DDx: FDG Uptake in the Parotid

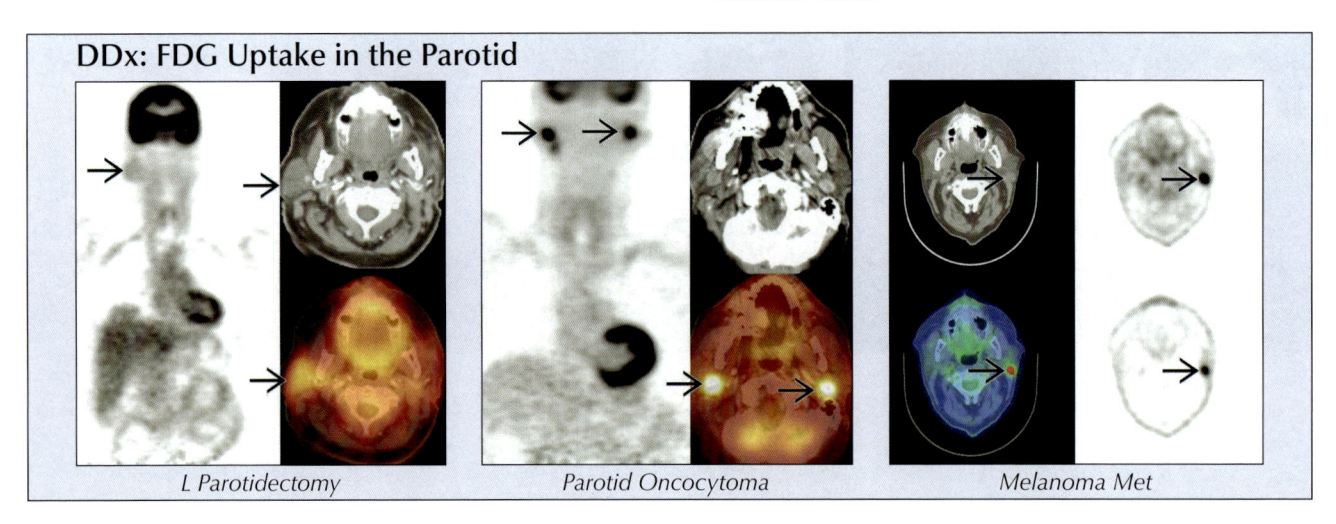

L Parotidectomy   *Parotid Oncocytoma*   *Melanoma Met*

PAROTID AND SALIVARY TUMORS

Key Facts

Terminology
- Benign mixed tumors (BMT) or pleomorphic adenoma; Warthin tumor; parotid carcinoma (mucoepidermoid and adenoid cystic), primary lymphoma

Imaging Findings
- Best diagnostic clue: Negative Tc-99m pertechnetate and positive FDG PET
- Location: Tumors within the parotid space

- PET: General: Sensitivity and specificity 75% and 67%; 30% false positive rate for malignancy (mostly due to Warthin tumor)
- Ga-67 Scintigraphy: Sensitivity and specificity for differentiation of benign from malignant parotid masses 58% and 72%
- Best imaging tool: Nuclear medicine: Combination FDG PET or PET/CT and salivary gland scintigraphy with Tc-99m pertechnetate

Warthin Tumor
- Tend to be positive on both FDG PET and Tc-99m pertechnetate

Primary Parotid Carcinoma (Adenoid Cystic or Mucoepidermoid)
- Almost always FDG avid

Non-Hodgkin Lymphoma
- Higher grade tumors more FDG avid

Parotid Metastases
- FDG avidity will depend on the primary lesion

CLINICAL ISSUES

Presentation
- Most common signs/symptoms: Cheek mass +/- pain
- Other signs/symptoms: Occasional VII nerve paralysis

Demographics
- Age: BMT > 35
- Gender: BMT M:F = 1:2

Treatment
- Options, risks, complications: Presurgical evaluation depends on clinical exam as well as radiologic work-up
- Depends on cell type
- Resection or preservation of facial nerve
- Extended radiation or superficial parotidectomy
- Additional radical neck dissection

DIAGNOSTIC CHECKLIST

Consider
- Scintigraphy first; if negative consider FDG PET or PET/CT
- FNA may be most cost effective approach; sensitivity 64-92% and specificity 75-100%
  - May increase risk of recurrence secondary to "spillage"

Image Interpretation Pearls
- Primary parotid carcinoma almost always positive on FDG PET; Warthin tumor commonly positive on FDG PET; BMT occasionally positive on FDG PET

SELECTED REFERENCES
1. Uchida Y et al: Diagnostic value of FDG PET and salivary gland scintigraphy for parotid tumors. Clin Nucl Med. 30(3):170-6, 2005
2. Horiuchi M et al: Four cases of Warthin's tumor of the parotid gland detected with FDG PET. Ann Nucl Med. 12(1):47-50, 1998
3. Matsuda M et al: Positron emission tomographic imaging of pleomorphic adenoma in the parotid gland. Acta Otolaryngol Suppl. 538:214-20, 1998
4. Okamura T et al: Fluorine-18 fluorodeoxyglucose positron emission tomography imaging of parotid mass lesions. Acta Otolaryngol Suppl. 538:209-13, 1998
5. Keyes JW Jr et al: Salivary gland tumors: pretherapy evaluation with PET. Radiology. 192(1):99-102, 1994

IMAGE GALLERY

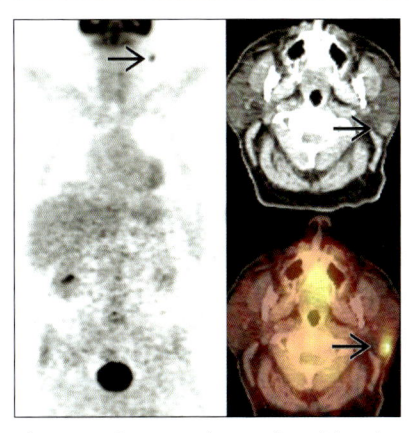

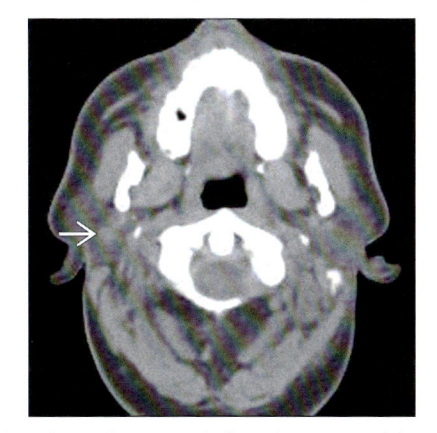

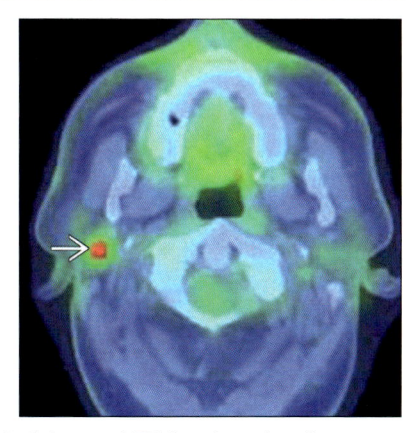

(Left) Coronal PET, axial CT and axial fused PET/CT show a hypermetabolic enhancing nodule in the left parotid ➔ found incidentally in a patient with colon cancer. Path showed Warthin tumor. (Center) Axial NECT shows a soft tissue attenuation nodule in the right parotid ➔. (Right) Axial fused PET/CT shows intense FDG activity corresponding to the right parotid mass ➔ in the previous figure. Pathology was benign.

NEUROENDOCRINE TUMORS, HEAD & NECK

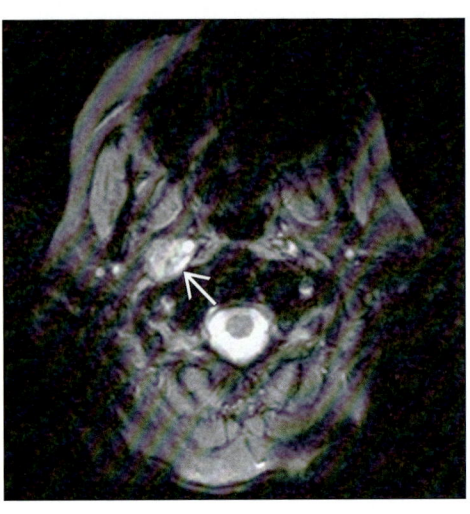

Axial GRE MRI shows carotid space mass ➡, found incidentally. Patient had elevated serum gastrin levels. See In-111 octreotide scan at right.

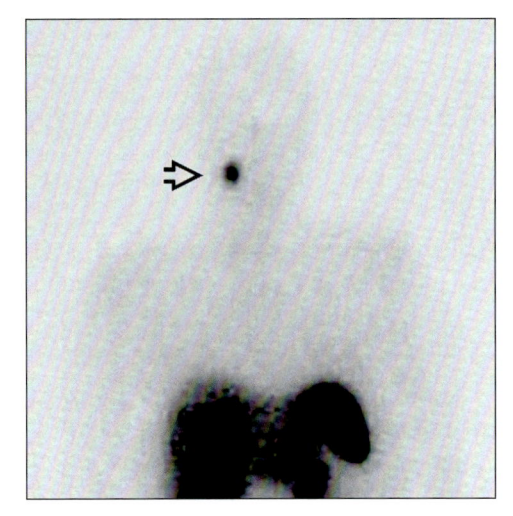

Same patient as left image. Anterior planar view of In-111 octreotide (pentatreotide) scan. Increased uptake at site of carotid space mass ➢ confirms presence of neuroendocrine tumor.

TERMINOLOGY

Abbreviations and Synonyms
- Neuroendocrine tumors (NET), small cell undifferentiated carcinoma, Merkel cell carcinoma (MCC)

Definitions
- Heterogeneous group of tumors of neuroendocrine origin
- Merkel cells first described by Frederick Merkel in 1875
  - Believed to be slow-acting mechanoreceptors in the basal layer of the epidermis
  - Provide information about touch and hair movement

IMAGING FINDINGS

General Features
- Best diagnostic clue: Aggressive cutaneous mass (MCC) or mass involving the structures listed below (NET)
- Location
  - Sun exposed skin (head and neck 50%) with most common location being periorbital area (MCC); about 40% occur along the extremities
  - MCC is thought to arise from hair follicles or dermal Merkel cells, although no definite evidence
  - Salivary glands, larynx, sinonasal cavity, upper esophagus and oral cavity for non-MCC NET tumors
  - Staging for MCC
    - IA disease confined to skin < 2 cm in diameter
    - IB disease confined to skin > 2 cm in diameter
    - Involvement in regional lymph nodes
    - Metastatic disease
- Size: Range in size from a few millimeters to several centimeters, average less than 2 cm
- Morphology: MCC: Firm violaceous or reddish nodular papule or plaque +/- ulceration

Nuclear Medicine Findings
- FDG PET usually shows intense uptake within primary and metastatic lesions for MCC
  - Several case studies and small series showing most MCC to be intensely FDG avid; occasional false negative
- For non-MCC NET, FDG may show variability

DDx: Cutaneous Mass

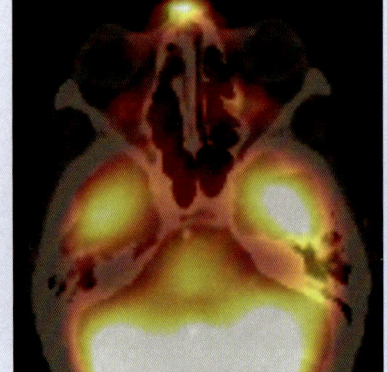

Nasal Melanoma

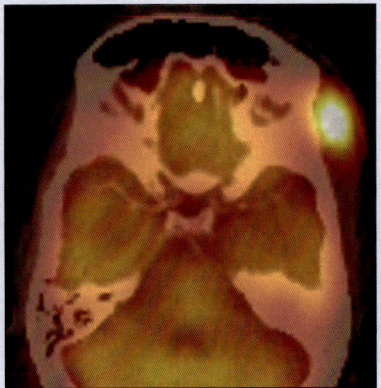

Squamous Cell Cancer

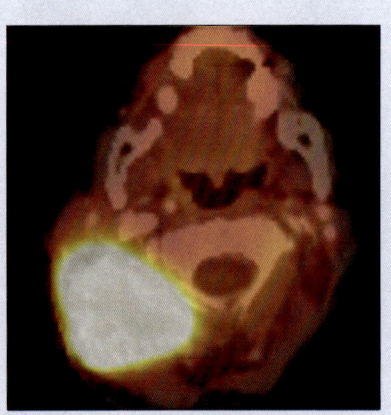

Lymphoma

NEUROENDOCRINE TUMORS, HEAD & NECK

Key Facts

Terminology
- Neuroendocrine tumors (NET), small cell undifferentiated carcinoma, Merkel cell carcinoma (MCC)

Imaging Findings
- Best diagnostic clue: Aggressive cutaneous mass (MCC) or mass involving the structures listed below (NET)
- Morphology: MCC: Firm violaceous or reddish nodular papule or plaque +/- ulceration
- FDG PET usually shows intense uptake within primary and metastatic lesions for MCC
- Some head and neck NET may show very little FDG activity
- FDG PET may influence management in up to 25% of patients

Top Differential Diagnoses
- Metastatic Disease from Small Cell Carcinoma of the Lung
- Melanoma
- Cutaneous Lymphoma
- Squamous Cell Carcinoma

Clinical Issues
- Usually painless reddish ulcerated plaque on the skin near the orbits with MCC
- Can be mistaken for basal cell carcinoma, amelanotic melanoma, squamous cell carcinoma and cutaneous lymphoma

Diagnostic Checklist
- Contrast-enhanced CT or FDG PET/CT, particularly in MCC

  - Some head and neck NET may show very little FDG activity
    - Metastatic lesions may show photopenia compared to background normal activity
  - F-DOPA PET also shows some variability in the uptake

Imaging Recommendations
- Best imaging tool
  - CT scan with contrast or PET/CT with contrast
  - FDG PET likely helpful in MCC; other head and neck NET may have less FDG activity
  - FDG PET overall sensitivity for all NET approximately 76%
  - FDG PET may influence management in up to 25% of patients
- Protocol advice: IV contrast for CT; arms down for PET or PET/CT
- Additional nuclear medicine imaging options
  - Octreotide not well evaluated for NET tumors of the head and neck, but several studies suggesting its utility in NET outside the head and neck
- Correlative imaging features
  - CT findings
    - Primary lesion may show necrosis, enhancement or mass effect for both MCC and non-MCC NET
    - Lymphadenopathy range 1.2-11 cm; mean 4.2 cm

DIFFERENTIAL DIAGNOSIS

Metastatic Disease from Small Cell Carcinoma of the Lung
- Non-MCC NET may be indistinguishable by imaging; look for primary lung lesions

Melanoma
- Primary MCC usually more red in color
- Immunohistochemically positive for S100 protein and thyroid transcription factor-1

Cutaneous Lymphoma
- B or T-cell origin, may be localized or involve other organs and sites

Squamous Cell Carcinoma
- Usually mucosal surface involved

PATHOLOGY

General Features
- Genetics
  - Chromosomal rearrangements on chromosomes 1, 3 and 5 for MCC
  - Loss of more than one tumor suppressor gene
- Etiology
  - Idiopathic or iatrogenic immunosuppression has been implicated
  - Sunlight (UVB index correlated to the incidence of MCC)
  - Exposure to arsenic and methoxsalen and UV treatment for psoriasis also implicated
  - Also documented in patients with congenital ectodermal dysplasia, Cowden disease and Hodgkin
- Epidemiology: MCC annual incidence 0.42 per 100,000 for Caucasian populations; about 1/20th this figure for African-American populations
- Associated abnormalities: Possible association between squamous cell and basal cell carcinoma

Gross Pathologic & Surgical Features
- Reddish papule or plaque that often demonstrates dermal invasion
- Can present with multiple satellite lesions from spread through the dermal lymphatics

Microscopic Features
- Sheets, ribbons or nests of small round blue cells
- Neurosecretory granules can be demonstrated in most lesions
- Immunohistochemistry helpful for differentiation from lymphoma, Ewing sarcoma, melanoma and basal cell carcinoma

NEUROENDOCRINE TUMORS, HEAD & NECK

- Positive for cytokeratin 20, neurofilaments, chromogranin, CAM 5.2 and synaptophysin
- Negative for S100 and leukocyte common antigen
- KIT receptor tyrosine kinase (CD117) expressed in 95% of MCCs

CLINICAL ISSUES

Presentation
- Most common signs/symptoms
  - Usually painless reddish ulcerated plaque on the skin near the orbits with MCC
  - Also have shiny surface, often with telangiectasia
  - Can be mistaken for basal cell carcinoma, amelanotic melanoma, squamous cell carcinoma and cutaneous lymphoma
- Other signs/symptoms: Pain may be secondary symptom

Demographics
- Age: Most common between the ages of 69 and 82; only 5% of cases occur before age 50
- Gender: M:F = 1.5:1
- Ethnicity: MCC rarely in non-Caucasian patients

Natural History & Prognosis
- 30-60% mortality rate in patients with MCC in most studies
  - 5 year outcomes for MCC are as follows: Local control 94%, locoregional control 80% and survival 37%
- 5 year survival for small cell arising from the major salivary glands is 46%

Treatment
- Wide local excision and lymph node dissection
  - Adjuvant chemotherapy and/or radiotherapy may be beneficial

DIAGNOSTIC CHECKLIST

Consider
- Contrast-enhanced CT or FDG PET/CT, particularly in MCC

SELECTED REFERENCES

1. Acebo E et al: Merkel cell carcinoma: a clinicopathological study of 11 cases. J Eur Acad Dermatol Venereol. 19(5):546-51, 2005
2. Allen PJ et al: Merkel cell carcinoma: prognosis and treatment of patients from a single institution. J Clin Oncol. 23(10):2300-9, 2005
3. Chang DT et al: Merkel cell carcinoma of the skin with leptomeningeal metastases. Am J Otolaryngol. 26(3):210-3, 2005
4. Deganello A et al: Infrahyoid myocutaneous flap reconstruction after wide local excision of a Merkel cell carcinoma. Acta Otorhinolaryngol Ital. 25(1):50-3; discussion 53-4, 2005
5. Deichmann M et al: The chemoresistance gene ABCG2 (MXR/BCRP1/ABCP1) is not expressed in melanomas but in single neuroendocrine carcinomas of the skin. J Cutan Pathol. 32(7):467-73, 2005
6. Fernandez-Figueras MT et al: Prognostic significance of p27Kip1, p45Skp2 and Ki67 expression profiles in Merkel cell carcinoma, extracutaneous small cell carcinoma, and cutaneous squamous cell carcinoma. Histopathology. 46(6):614-21, 2005
7. Leong SP: Selective sentinel lymphadenectomy for malignant melanoma, Merkel cell carcinoma, and squamous cell carcinoma. Cancer Treat Res. 127:39-76, 2005
8. Llombart B et al: Clinicopathological and immunohistochemical analysis of 20 cases of Merkel cell carcinoma in search of prognostic markers. Histopathology. 46(6):622-34, 2005
9. McAfee WJ et al: Merkel cell carcinoma. Cancer. 104(8):1761-4, 2005
10. McNiff JM et al: CD56 staining in Merkel cell carcinoma and natural killer-cell lymphoma: magic bullet, diagnostic pitfall, or both? J Cutan Pathol. 32(8):541-5, 2005
11. Pagella F et al: Merkel cell carcinoma of the auricle. Am J Otolaryngol. 26(5):324-6, 2005
12. Poulsen M: Merkel cell carcinoma of skin: diagnosis and management strategies. Drugs Aging. 22(3):219-29, 2005
13. Poulsen MG et al: Does chemotherapy improve survival in high-risk stage I and II merkel cell carcinoma of the skin? Int J Radiat Oncol Biol Phys. 2005
14. Schmalbach CE et al: Reliability of sentinel lymph node biopsy for regional staging of head and neck Merkel cell carcinoma. Arch Otolaryngol Head Neck Surg. 131(7):610-4, 2005
15. Sidhu GS et al: Merkel cells, normal and neoplastic: an update. Ultrastruct Pathol. 29(3-4):287-94, 2005
16. Talbot JN et al: 6-[F-18]Fluoro-L- -DOPA Positron Emission Tomography in the Imaging of Merkel Cell Carcinoma: Preliminary Report of Three Cases with 2-Deoxy-2-[F-18]Fluoro-D: -Glucose Positron Emission Tomography or Pentetreotide-(111In) SPECT Data. Mol Imaging Biol. 2005
17. Veness MJ et al: Merkel cell carcinoma: improved outcome with adjuvant radiotherapy. ANZ J Surg. 75(5):275-81, 2005
18. Veness MJ: Merkel cell carcinoma: improved outcome with the addition of adjuvant therapy. J Clin Oncol. 23(28):7235-6; author reply 7237-8, 2005
19. Wilson LD et al: Merkel cell carcinoma: improved outcome with the addition of adjuvant therapy. J Clin Oncol. 23(28):7236-7; author reply 7237-8, 2005
20. Yao M et al: Merkel cell carcinoma: two case reports focusing on the role of fluorodeoxyglucose positron emission tomography imaging in staging and surveillance. Am J Clin Oncol. 28(2):205-10, 2005
21. Bickle K et al: Merkel cell carcinoma: a clinical, histopathologic, and immunohistochemical review. Semin Cutan Med Surg. 23(1):46-53, 2004
22. Lehrer MS et al: Merkel cell carcinoma. Curr Treat Options Oncol. 5(3):195-9, 2004
23. Mendenhall WM et al: Merkel cell carcinoma. Laryngoscope. 114(5):906-10, 2004
24. Poulsen M: Merkel-cell carcinoma of the skin. Lancet Oncol. 5(10):593-9, 2004
25. Suarez C et al: Merkel cell carcinoma of the head and neck. Oral Oncol. 40(8):773-9, 2004
26. Ikawa F et al: Brain metastasis of Merkel cell carcinoma. Case report and review of the literature. Neurosurg Rev. 22(1):54-7, 1999
27. Longo F et al: Neuroendocrine (Merkel cell) carcinoma of the oral mucosa: report of a case with immunohistochemical study and review of the literature. J Oral Pathol Med. 28(2):88-91, 1999
28. Skidmore RA Jr et al: Nonmelanoma skin cancer. Med Clin North Am. 82(6):1309-23, vi, 1998

NEUROENDOCRINE TUMORS, HEAD & NECK

IMAGE GALLERY

Variant

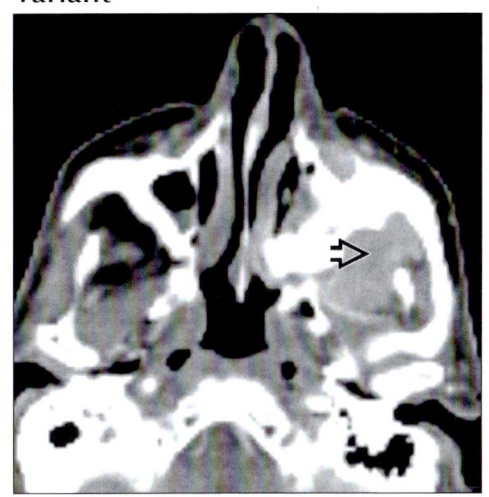

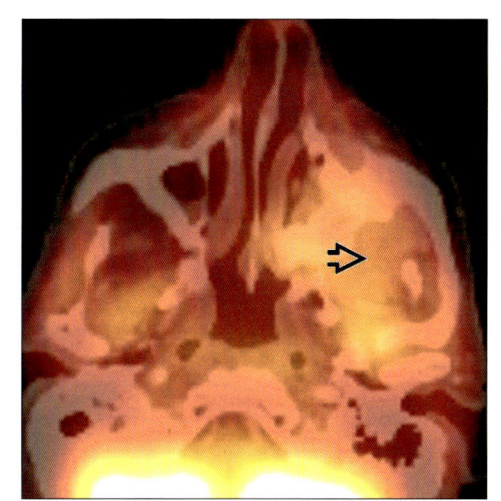

(Left) Axial CECT shows a large partially enhancing mass ⇨ due to a neuroendocrine tumor. *(Right)* Axial fused PET/CT shows little FDG activity in the area of the enhancing mass ⇨. Many neuroendocrine tumors, such as this, are poorly FDG avid.

Variant

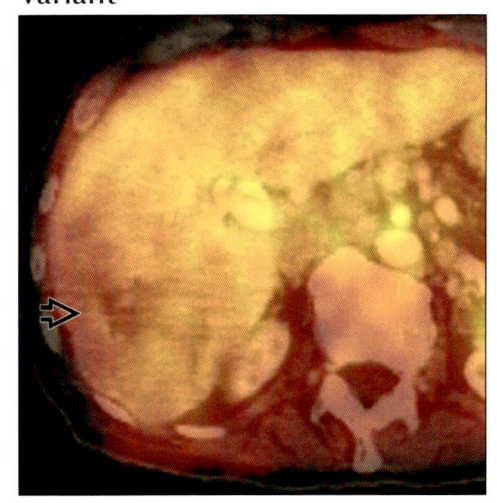

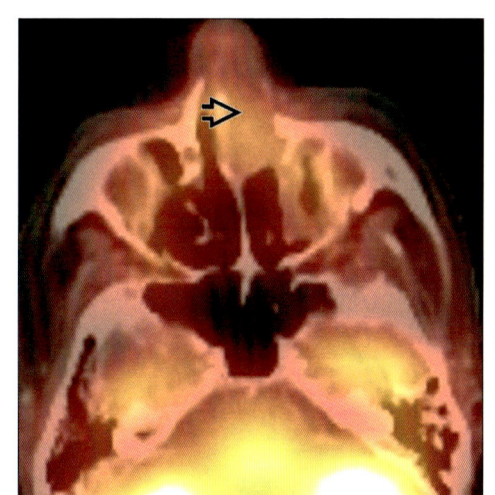

(Left) Axial fused PET/CT shows a low attenuation mass ⇨ in the liver with FDG activity that is below background liver (photopenic), typical of many metastatic neuroendocrine tumors. *(Right)* Axial fused PET/CT shows non-FDG avid mass in the left nasal cavity ⇨. Biopsy showed neuroendocrine tumor.

Typical

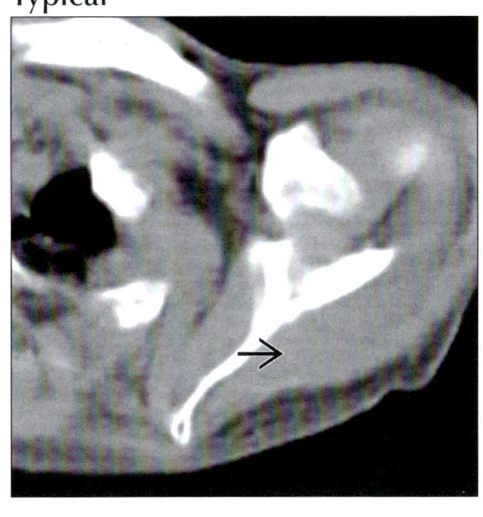

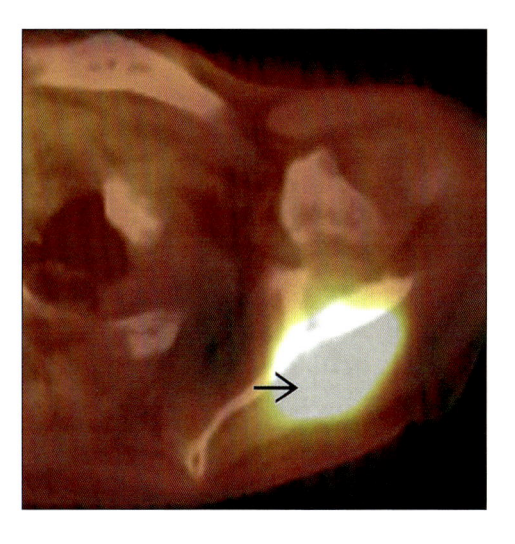

(Left) Axial CECT shows no definite evidence for a lesion → in the suprascapularis muscle. *(Right)* Axial fused PET/CT shows intense FDG activity in suprascapularis muscle, invading bone →. Biopsy showed metastatic neuroendocrine tumor from a primary head and neck neuroendocrine tumor.

LACRIMAL COMPLEX DYSFUNCTION

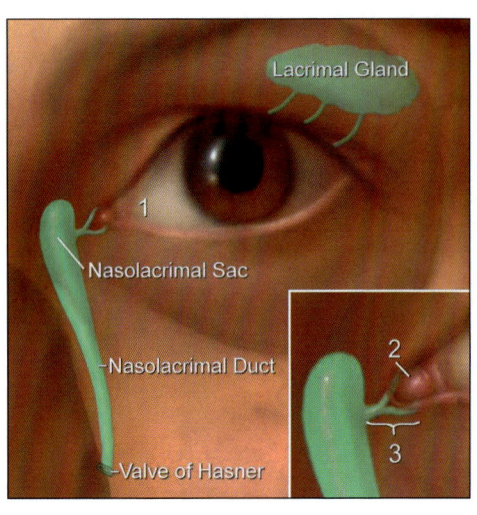

Graphic of left lacrimal complex. 1) Inner canthus; 2) ampulla; 3) superior, inferior, and common canaliculi.

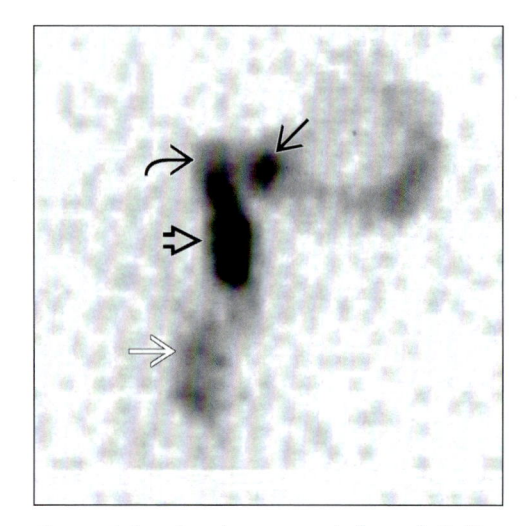

Dacryoscintigraphy shows normal flow of Tc-99m pertechnetate through left lacrimal complex: Inner canthus and canaliculi ➡, nasolacrimal sac ➚, nasolacrimal duct ⮞, nostril ➡.

TERMINOLOGY

Definitions
- Partial or complete functional obstruction at canaliculi, nasolacrimal sac, nasolacrimal duct

IMAGING FINDINGS

General Features
- Best diagnostic clue: Images are visually evaluated; there is no quantitative data to distinguish normal vs. abnormal

Imaging Recommendations
- Best imaging tool: Dacryoscintigraphy
- Protocol advice
  ○ Dacryoscintigraphy
    ▪ Evaluate lacrimal complex dysfunction after mechanical etiology ruled out
    ▪ Absence of radiotracer activity distal to functional obstruction
    ▪ Tc-99m pertechnetate: 0.1 mCi/mL normal saline: 1-2 drops per eye
    ▪ Examine less symptomatic eye first
    ▪ Capture radioactive tears with tissue paper to decrease contamination of skin over lacrimal complex
    ▪ Pinhole collimator over eye and nose for 15 minutes
  ○ Normal
    ▪ Symmetrical passage of activity from inner canthus to lacrimal sac, lacrimal duct and nasopharynx
  ○ Abnormal
    ▪ Completely obstructed: Failure to pass beyond a specific structure signifies obstruction at that site
    ▪ Partial obstruction may result in delayed or diminished transit (compare to normal eye)
- Correlative imaging
  ○ CT/MR: Evaluate anatomy and/or mechanical etiology for obstruction
  ○ Contrast dacryocystography: Radio-opaque dye injected into lacrimal complex

DDx: Lacrimal Complex Dysfunction

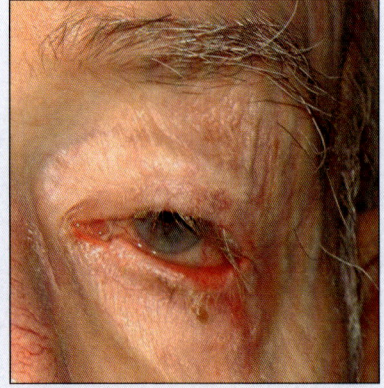

Ectropion (Courtesy P. Yeatts, MD)

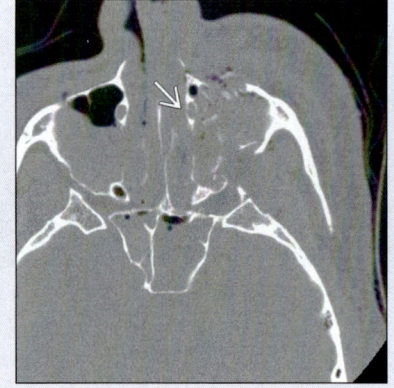

Nasolacrimal Fracture

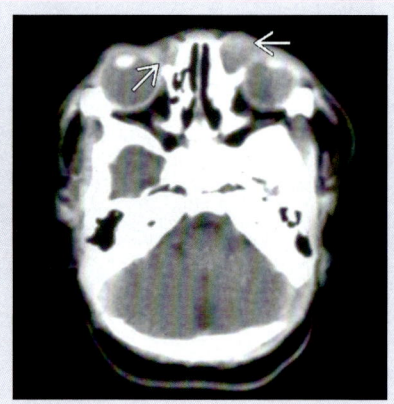

Lacrimal Mucoceles

LACRIMAL COMPLEX DYSFUNCTION

Key Facts

Terminology
- Partial or complete functional obstruction at canaliculi, nasolacrimal sac, nasolacrimal duct

Imaging Findings
- Dacryoscintigraphy
- Evaluate lacrimal complex dysfunction after mechanical etiology ruled out
- Absence of radiotracer activity distal to functional obstruction

- Tc-99m pertechnetate: 0.1 mCi/mL normal saline: 1-2 drops per eye
- Capture radioactive tears with tissue paper to decrease contamination of skin over lacrimal complex

Pathology
- Nasolacrimal duct stenosis
- Aberrant or blocked punctum lacrimale
- Lacrimal excretion pump dysfunction

DIFFERENTIAL DIAGNOSIS

Anatomic Abnormality
- Ectropion, entropion, trichiasis, trauma, congenital

Mass Effect
- Neoplasm, congenital, lacrimal stones

Overproduction of Tears
- Corneal irritation, drug-induced, psychogenic

PATHOLOGY

General Features
- Etiology
  - Congenital: Usually resolves by 1 year of age
  - Acquired: Age-related change, infection (dacryocystitis), inflammatory disease (e.g. granulomatous), neoplasm, surgical complication, trauma

Gross Pathologic & Surgical Features
- Nasolacrimal duct stenosis
- Aberrant or blocked punctum lacrimale
- Lacrimal excretion pump dysfunction

Microscopic Features
- Fibrosis, scarring

CLINICAL ISSUES

Presentation
- Most common signs/symptoms: Epiphora: Overflow of tears from eye

Treatment
- Probe through lower canaliculus into lacrimal complex
- Balloon dacryoplasty to dilate incomplete obstruction
- Dacryocystorhinostomy: Creation of epithelialized tract between lacrimal sac and nose
- Treat underlying cause

SELECTED REFERENCES

1. Chung YA et al: The clinical value of dacryoscintigraphy in the selection of surgical approach for patients with functional lacrimal duct obstruction. Ann Nucl Med. 19(6):479-83, 2005
2. Goldberg D: Nasolacrimal duct obstruction. Ophthalmology. 112(6):1173-4; author reply 1174, 2005
3. Marr JE et al: Management of childhood epiphora. Br J Ophthalmol. 89(9):1123-6, 2005
4. Wormald PJ et al: Investigation and endoscopic treatment for functional and anatomical obstruction of the nasolacrimal duct system. Clin Otolaryngol Allied Sci. 29(4):352-6, 2004
5. Zilelioglu G et al: Quantitative lacrimal scintigraphy after dacryocystorhinostomy. Ophthalmic Surg Lasers Imaging. 35(1):37-40, 2004
6. Soparkar CN et al: Evaluation of the lacrimal sac. Ophthalmology. 110(12):2434-5; author reply 2435-6, 2003

IMAGE GALLERY

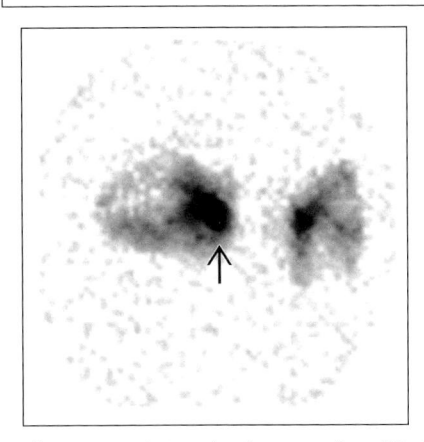

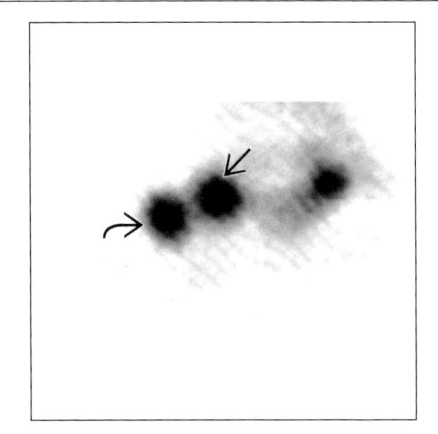

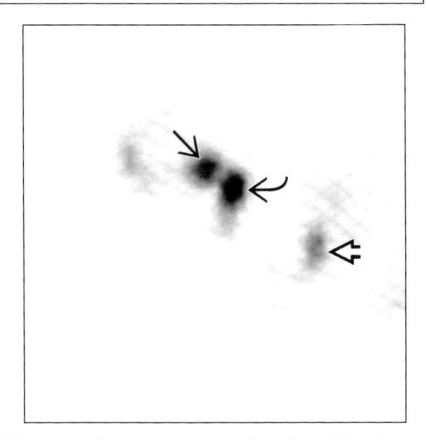

(Left) Dacryoscintigraphy shows pooling of Tc-99m pertechnetate at right inner canthus ➔, signifying canalicular system dysfunction. *(Center)* Radiotracer activity at left inner canthus ➔ and lacrimal sac ➔. No activity distal to lacrimal sac signifies site of dysfunction. *(Right)* Radiotracer activity in right inner canthus ➔ and nasolacrimal sac and duct ➔. No activity in right nostril signifies distal nasolacrimal duct dysfunction. Unobstructed left lacrimal complex with activity evident in left nostril ➔.

Verträge

8.6.   18.4.
2. 10.
2. 11.
24.12
27. 13.
28. 12.

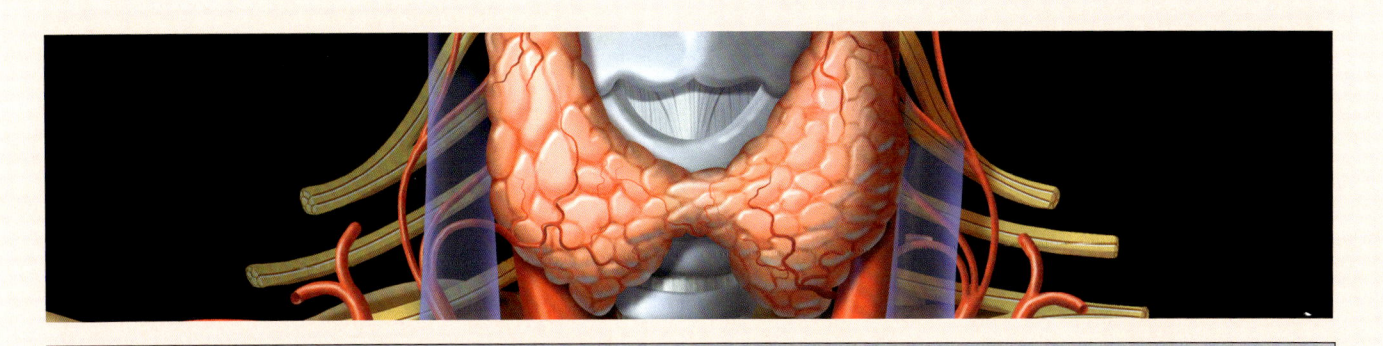

SECTION 7: Thyroid/Parathyroid

Introduction and Overview

Thyroid Overview	7-2

Parathyroid

Parathyroid Adenoma, Typical	7-6
Parathyroid Adenoma, Ectopic	7-10

Hyperthyroidism

Graves Disease	7-12
Hashimoto Thyroiditis	7-16
Multinodular Goiter	7-20
Thyroid Adenoma, Hyperfunctioning	7-24
Subacute Thyroiditis	7-28
I-131 Hyperthyroid Therapy	7-32

Thyroid, Benign Miscellaneous

Ectopic Thyroid	7-36
Congenital Hypothyroidism	7-40
Benign Thyroid Conditions, PET	7-44

Thyroid Cancer

Well-Differentiated Thyroid Cancer	7-48
I-131 Thyroid Cancer Therapy	7-54
Well-Differentiated Thyroid Cancer, PET	7-58
Medullary Thyroid Cancer	7-62

THYROID OVERVIEW

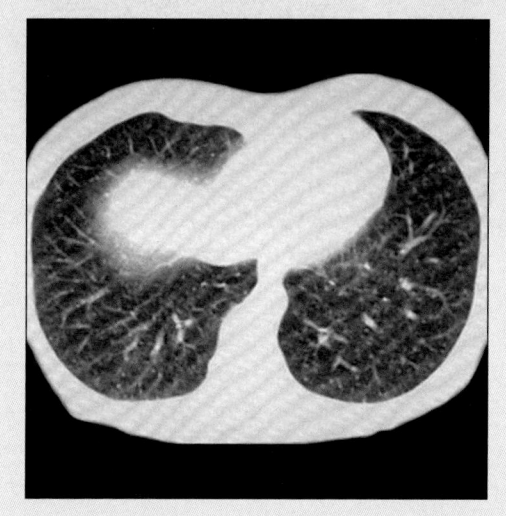

Axial NECT shows innumerable miliary nodules throughout both lungs in patient with metastatic papillary thyroid cancer.

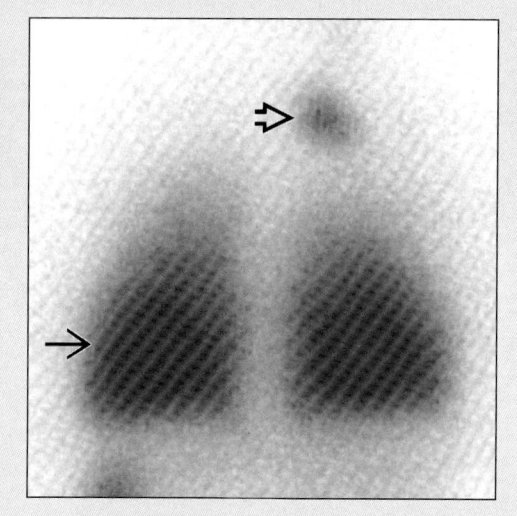

Posterior I-131 scan (same patient as previous image) shows metastatic papillary thyroid cancer with uptake throughout both lungs ➔ and in lower right neck ▷.

TERMINOLOGY

Definitions
- Radioactive iodine uptake (RAIU) by thyroid or thyroid remnant

RADIOPHARMACEUTICALS

Tc-99m Pertechnetate
- Purpose: Used for thyroid scan only
  - Inadequate for accurate RAIU: Trapped but not organified
- Radiopharmaceutical characteristics
  - Energy: 140 KeV (88%), gamma
  - T½: 6.03 h
- Dose (IV)
  - Adults: 74-370 MBq (2-10 mCi)
  - Children: 1-5 MBq/kg (0.015-.07 mCi/kg)
- Dosimetric data
  - Adult
    - Target organ (upper large intestine): 0.062 mGy/MBq (0.23 rad/mCi)
    - Effective dose: 0.013 mSv/MBq (0.048 rem/mCi)
  - Child (5 year old)
    - Target organ: 0.21 mGy/MBq (0.78 rad/mCi)
    - Effective dose: 0.04 mSv/MBq (0.15 rem/mCi)

Na I-123
- Purpose: RAIU; thyroid scan; whole body scan (for thyroid cancer)
- Dose (oral)
  - Thyroid scan
    - Adults: 3.7-22.2 MBq (100-600 µCi)
    - Children: 0.1-0.3 MBq/kg (.003-0.01 mCi/kg)
  - Whole body scan (for thyroid cancer): Image at 24 h
    - Adults and children: 37-74 MBq (1-2 mCi)
  - RAIU
    - Adults: 3.7-7.4 MBq (100-200 µCi)
    - Children: 3.7-7.4 MBq (100-200 µCi)
- Radiopharmaceutical characteristics
  - Energy: 159 KeV (83%), gamma
  - T½: 13 h
- Dosimetric data
  - Adult hyperthyroid
    - Target organ (thyroid): 1.9 mGy/MBq (7.0 rad/mCi)
    - Effective dose: 0.075 mSv/MBq (0.28 rem/mCi)
  - Child (5 year old) hyperthyroid
    - Target organ (thyroid): 9.8 mGy/MBq (36 rad/mCi)
    - Effective dose: 0.45 mSv/MBq (1.3 rem/mCi)
  - Adult athyroidal
    - Target organ (bladder wall): 0.09 mGy/MBq (0.33 rad/mCi)
    - Effective dose: 0.013 mSv/MBq (0.048 rem/mCi)
- Imaging time after administration
  - Thyroid scan: 4, 6 or 24 h (all acceptable)
  - Whole body scan: 24 h
  - RAIU: 24 h (optional 2, 4 h)

Na I-131
- Purpose: RAIU for hyperthyroidism, RAIU by thyroid remnant for thyroid cancer, whole body scan, hyperthyroid and thyroid cancer treatment
- Dose (oral)
  - RAIU
    - Adult: 0.15-0.37 MBq (4-10 µCi)
    - Children: 0.15-0.37 MBq (4-10 µCi)
  - Whole body scan (for thyroid cancer pretherapy, surveillance)
    - Adults and children: 74-370 MBq (2-10 mCi)
  - Hyperthyroid treatment (typical ranges)
    - Graves disease: 370-555 MBq (8-15 mCi)
    - Toxic adenoma, multinodular goiter: 740-1110 MBq (20-33 mCi)
  - Thyroid cancer treatment (depends on clinical scenario)
    - Ablation of thyroid bed remnant: 2.75-5.5 GBq (75-150 mCi)
    - Treatment of presumed metastatic disease to neck, mediastinum: 5.55-7.4 GBq (150-200 mCi)

THYROID OVERVIEW

Key Facts

Radiopharmaceuticals
- Tc-99m pertechnetate: Used for thyroid scan only
- Na I-123: Used for RAIU and thyroid scan for hyperthyroidism; RAIU and whole body scan for thyroid cancer
- Na I-131: Used for RAIU for hyperthyroidism, RAIU by thyroid remnant for thyroid cancer, whole body scan, hyperthyroid and thyroid cancer treatment

NRC Regulatory Guide 8.39: Release of Patients Administered Radioactive Materials
- Activity at or below which patients can be released post I-131 therapy: 33 mCi
- Measured dose rate at 1 meter below which patients can be released post I-131 therapy: 7 mrem/hr at 1 meter
- Activity above which patients must receive written radiation safety precautions: 7 mCi; 2 mrem/hr at 1 meter
- Activity at which written instructions or a record if I-131 administered to a breastfeeding woman: 0.0004 mCi (instructions); 0.002 mrem/hr (record)
  - Complete cessation of breastfeeding recommended x 2 months prior to treatment
- Activity above which early release calculations/procedures must be observed: 33 mCi

Required for Early Release for > 33 mCi I-131
- Maximum bystander dose ≤ 5 mSv (500 mrem), dose rate at 1 meter ≤ 48.5 mrem/h for dose < 221 mCi
- Able to understand and follow radiation safety precautions

- Treatment of distant metastases: > 7.4 GBq (200 mCi) often given, may require dosimetry to keep 48 h whole body retention < 4.44 GBq (120 mCi); lung retention < 2.96 GBq (80 mCi)
- Radiopharmaceutical characteristics
  - Beta decay < 0.61 MeV; average 0.192 MeV; travels 0.8 mm in tissue
  - Gamma emission: 364 KeV (82%); 285 KeV (6%)
  - $T\frac{1}{2}$ = 8.06 days
- Dosimetric data
  - Adult hyperthyroid
    - Target organ (thyroid): 210 mGy/MBq (780 rad/mCi)
    - Effective dose: 6.6 mSv/MBq (24.0 rem/mCi)
  - Child (5 year old) hyperthyroid
    - Target organ (thyroid): 1,100 mGy/MBq (4,100 rad/mCi)
    - Effective dose: 34 mSv/MBq (130.0 rem/mCi)
  - Adult athyroidal
    - Target organ (bladder wall): 0.61 mGy/MBq (2.3 rad/mCi)
    - Effective dose: .072 mSv/MBq (0.27 rem/mCi)

TYPES OF STUDIES

Thyroid Scan
- Indications
  - Most common: Confirm toxic autonomous thyroid nodule with normal-range uptake measurement
  - Palpable nodule, multinodular goiter: To exclude malignancy, usually examined with ultrasound first; thyroid scan not first test of choice

Whole Body Scan
- Indications
  - Thyroid cancer
    - Whole body survey for thyroid cancer metastases

Thyroid Uptake Measurement
- Indications
  - Hyperthyroidism
    - Helpful in diagnosis and I-131 therapy dose determinations
  - Thyroid cancer
    - Estimate of residual thyroid tissue post-thyroidectomy
    - Helpful with dosimetry

I-131 Therapy
- Hyperthyroidism: Graves disease, toxic adenoma, toxic multinodular goiter
- Thyroid cancer: Post-thyroidectomy remnant ablation, residual/metastatic disease
- Low-iodine diet: Used at least 2 weeks prior to I-131 therapy for thyroid cancer
  - Avoid the following
    - Iodized salt, dairy products, seafood, seaweed, sea kelp, canned fruit or vegetables, chocolate, commercially made bread, white flour, FDC red dye #3, multivitamins with iodine

NUCLEAR REGULATORY COMMISSION (NRC)

Federal Regulatory Agency
- Regulates nuclear material and reactor by-product material
- 10CFR Part 20: Code of Federal Regulations sets radiation protection standards including dose limits, safety procedures, and waste disposal
- 10CFR Part 35: Medical use of by-product material regulations and training standards for authorized users (AU) and radiation safety officers (RSO)
  - Authorized user
    - Licensed physician, dentist or podiatrist named on site radiation license, responsible for by-product material use
    - Others may work with by-product material under direct AU supervision
  - Radiation safety officer
    - Provides institutional oversight to ensure compliance with NRC regulations

THYROID OVERVIEW

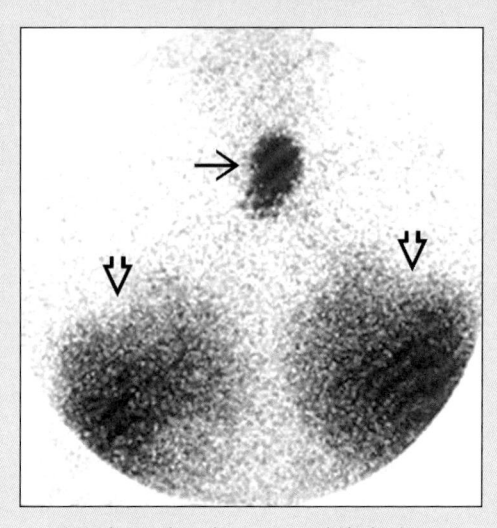

Anterior planar chest from I-131 whole body scan in thyroid cancer patient shows residual uptake in thyroid bed →. Note intense uptake in lactating breasts ▷ as patient ceased breastfeeding only 2 weeks prior.

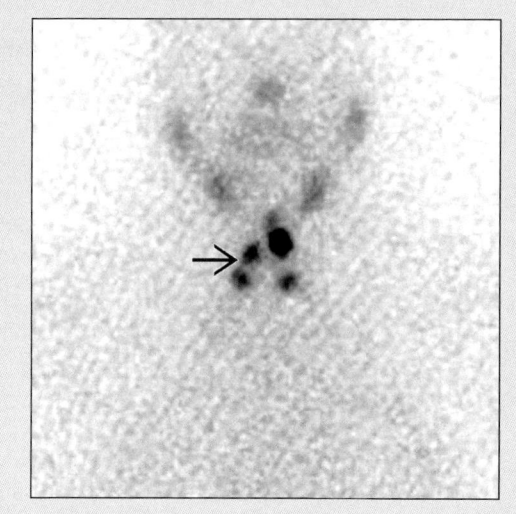

Anterior planar I-123 scan following thyroidectomy for thyroid cancer shows multiple foci of uptake in thyroid bed bilaterally →, likely residual thyroid tissue.

NRC Regulatory Guide 8.39: Release of Patients Administered Radioactive Materials
- Activity at or below which patients can be released post I-131 therapy: 33 mCi
- Measured dose rate at 1 meter below which patients can be released post I-131 therapy: 7 mrem/hr at 1 meter
- Activity above which patients must receive written radiation safety precautions: 7 mCi; 2 mrem/hr at 1 meter
- Activity at which written instructions or record if I-131 administered to breastfeeding woman: 0.0004 mCi (instructions); 0.002 mrem/hr (record)
  - Complete cessation of breastfeeding recommended 2 months prior to treatment
- Activity above which early release calculations/procedures must be observed: 33 mCi

NRC Regulatory Guide 8.39: Records of Release of Patients Administered Radioactive Materials
- None required: < 33 mCi I-131; < 7 mrem/hr
- Record of release based on measured dose rate, bystander dose; delayed release of patient based on radioactive decay calculation
- Record: Patient identifier, radiopharmaceutical administered, route and administered activity, date of administration, measured dose rate/release calculations as required

NRC Agreement State Program
- NRC relinquishes to states portions of its regulatory authority to license and regulate radioisotope use and administration
- "Agreement state"
  - Agreement signed by state governor and NRC that transfers NRC authority to state in accordance with act 274b of the Atomic Energy Act of 1954

Written Directive
- Required by NRC
- Include patient name, dosage, route of administration, dated and signed by AU for dose > 30 µCi (1.1 MBq)

Outpatient vs. Inpatient Therapy
- Outpatient treatment indicated for patients receiving < 33 mCi (1.22 GBq) I-131
- Approved for higher dose I-131, if certain criteria met
  - Release calculations: Maximum bystander dose ≤ 5 mSv (500 mrem), dose rate at 1 meter ≤ 48.5 mrem/h for dose < 221 mCi
  - Able to understand/observe radiation safety precautions
- Radiation safety precautions: Typical (for administered activity > 33 mCi, dose, patient specific calculations of exact precautions is required)
  - Not required for doses < 7 mCi
  - First 2-3 days: Reduce radiation dose to others by containing bodily waste
    - Be conscious of I-131 excretion in tears, mucous, saliva, sweat, menstrual blood, urine, feces
    - Have sole use of toilet, if possible; flush twice with lid down after use
    - Dispose of tissues, sanitary/incontinence products in separate receptacle, place in outside garbage
    - Wash hands often; take shower each day
    - Do not share bed or bath linens
    - Do not share eating utensils, plates, glasses; use disposable ware
    - No open-mouth kissing, sexual activity
  - First 2-3 days: Maintain distance from other people
    - Maintain 6-foot distance from infants/children, women who may be pregnant, adults
    - No public transportation, public events (movies, concerts, places of worship, etc.), work venues
    - Short duration car trips (< 4 h) with adults OK
    - Otherwise, do not be closer than 6 feet to any one person for > 5 minutes total per day
  - First 7 days: Sleep alone, maintain 6-foot distance from infants/children, women who may be pregnant
    - Continue to limit time on public transportation, public events, work venues as not always apparent who may be pregnant

THYROID OVERVIEW

IMAGE GALLERY

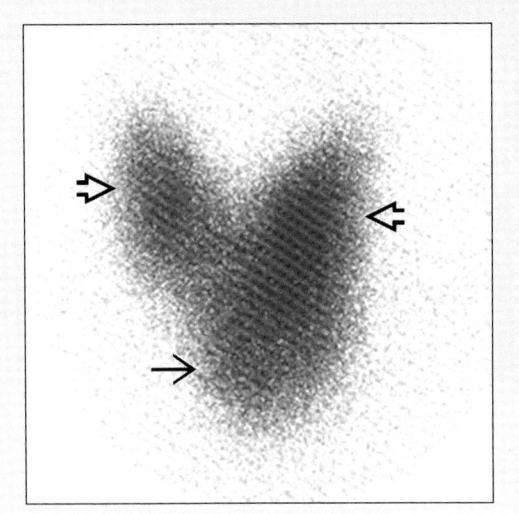

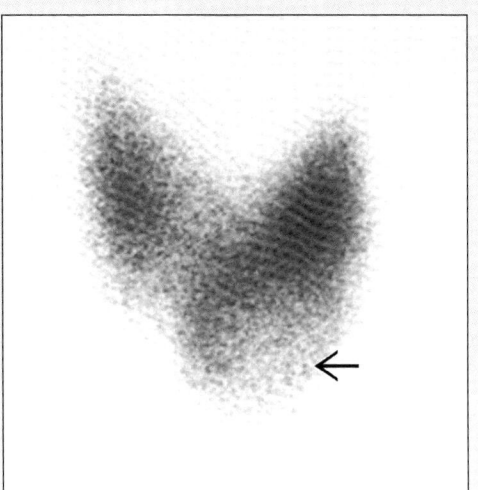

(Left) Anterior Tc-99m pertechnetate scan in patient with left lower lobe nodule shows similar uptake in nodule ⇒ and normal thyroid ⇒. (Right) I-123 scan (same patient as previous image) shows cold nodule ⇒. This "discordant" nodule may be an adenoma or thyroid cancer. This was biopsy-proven papillary thyroid cancer.

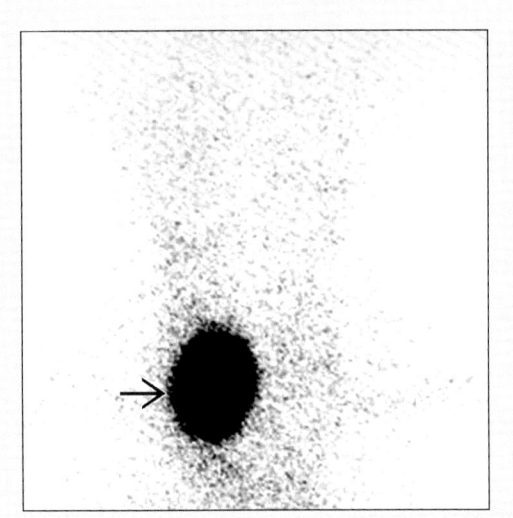

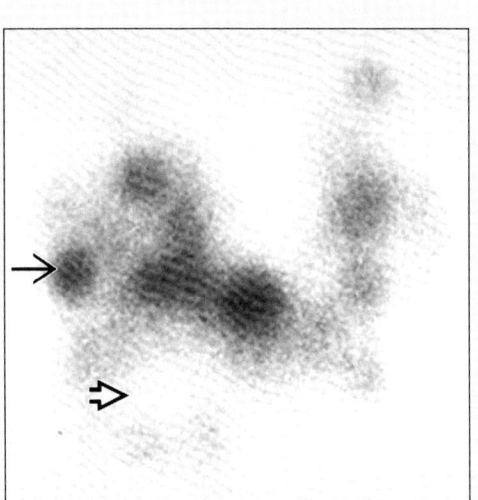

(Left) Anterior planar I-123 scan shows intense uptake in right thyroid nodule ⇒ with suppression of normal thyroid, due to hyperfunctioning thyroid adenoma (toxic nodule). (Right) Anterior I-123 thyroid scan shows enlarged thyroid with multiple hot ⇒ and cold ⇒ nodules, a typical appearance of multinodular goiter.

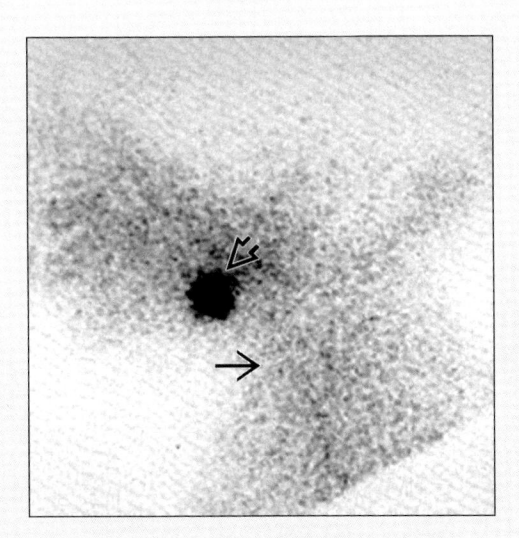

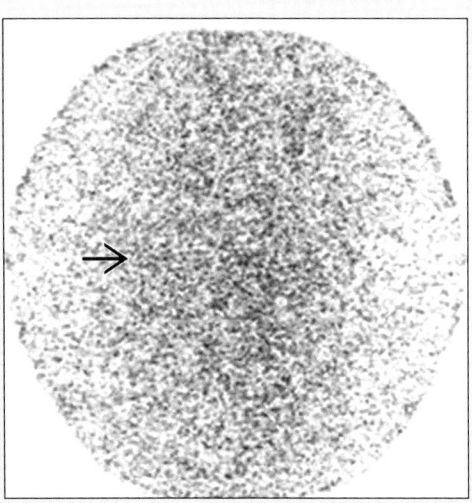

(Left) Lateral Tc-99m pertechnetate scan of neck in hypothyroid infant shows absence of normal thyroid tissue ⇒ and focus of activity at tongue base ⇒ in a sublingual thyroid. (Right) Anterior I-123 scan of neck in patient with neck tenderness and hyperthyroidism following an upper respiratory illness. No thyroid uptake evident ⇒ and RAIU was < 1%, characteristic findings of subacute thyroiditis.

PARATHYROID ADENOMA, TYPICAL

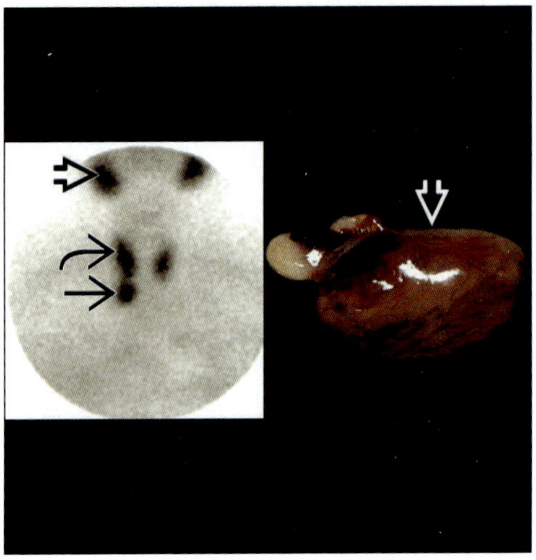

Tc-99m MIBI shows parathyroid adenoma ⇒ inferior to inferior pole of right thyroid lobe ⇒. Activity also evident in salivary glands ⇒. Gross specimen: 1.5 cm brown-tan parathyroid adenoma ⇒.

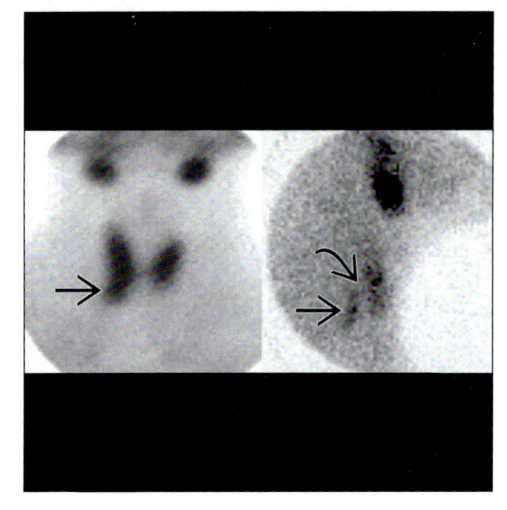

Anterior and lateral Tc-99m MIBI shows low-lying right superior parathyroid adenoma ⇒ separated from posterior thyroid by photopenic space ⇒ due to thyrothymic ligament.

TERMINOLOGY

Definitions
- Primary hyperparathyroidism: Hypercalcemia due to increased production of parathyroid hormone (PTH) by parathyroid gland(s)
  - Parathyroid adenoma: 75-85% of primary hyperparathyroidism cases
  - Parathyroid hyperplasia: 10-15%
  - Parathyroid carcinoma: 0.5-5%

IMAGING FINDINGS

General Features
- Best diagnostic clue: Focus of increased activity not conforming to thyroid on parathyroid scintigraphy
- Location
  - Perithyroidal (90-95%)
    - Posterior or inferior to thyroid (most common)
    - Subcapsular (3-8%): Under fibrous capsule surrounding thyroid
    - Intrathyroidal (2%): Within thyroid parenchyma
  - Ectopic (5-10%)
    - Parathyroid glands also found in carotid sheath, mediastinum, great vessels, cardiac border due to embryological dysgenesis
- Size: 0.5-5 g
- Morphology
  - Well-circumscribed nodule
  - May undergo cystic degeneration
- Number
  - Single, double, supernumerary

Nuclear Medicine Findings
- Dual-phase Tc-99m sestamibi parathyroid scintigraphy
  - Early images
    - 10-20 minutes post injection
    - Thyroid and parathyroid adenoma evident
  - Delayed images
    - 90 minutes post-injection
    - 60% of adenomas retain radiotracer longer than thyroid
  - SPECT
    - When planar images inadequate for localization
    - SPECT after early images, prior to delayed images
    - Define spatial orientation of adenoma compared to thyroid before tracer washout

DDx: Mimics of Parathyroid Adenoma on Parathyroid Scintigraphy

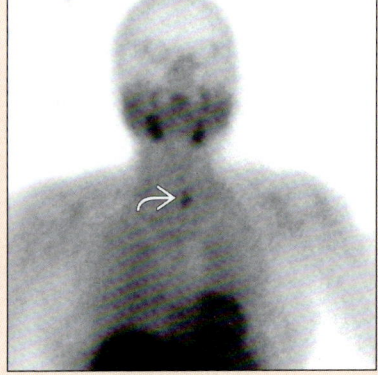

Thyroid Cancer

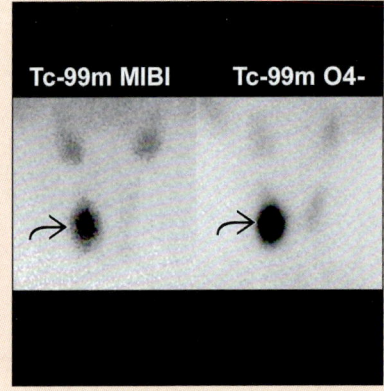

Thyroid Adenoma

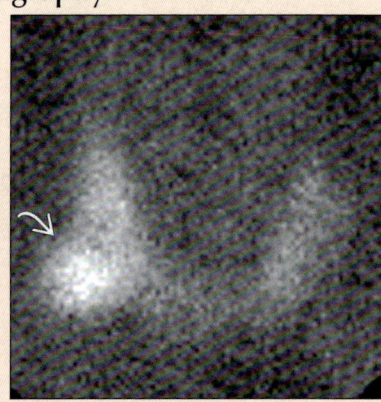

Parathyroid Cancer

PARATHYROID ADENOMA, TYPICAL

Key Facts

Terminology
- Primary hyperparathyroidism: Hypercalcemia due to increased production of parathyroid hormone (PTH) by parathyroid gland(s)
- Parathyroid adenoma: 75-85% of primary hyperparathyroidism cases
- Parathyroid hyperplasia: 10-15%
- Parathyroid carcinoma: 0.5-5%

Imaging Findings
- Best diagnostic clue: Focus of increased activity not conforming to thyroid on parathyroid scintigraphy
- Perithyroidal (90-95%)
- Posterior or inferior to thyroid (most common)
- Subcapsular (3-8%): Under fibrous capsule surrounding thyroid
- Intrathyroidal (2%): Within thyroid parenchyma
- Ectopic (5-10%)
- Parathyroid glands also found in carotid sheath, mediastinum, great vessels, cardiac border due to embryological dysgenesis
- Single, double, supernumerary

Top Differential Diagnoses
- Benign Thyroid Pathology
- Parathyroid Carcinoma
- Other Malignancy
- Infection/Inflammation

Clinical Issues
- Minimally invasive parathyroidectomy
- Unilateral cervical exploration
- Bilateral cervical exploration

- Better to localize activity posterior to thyroid, in tracheoesophageal groove, or ectopic site

Imaging Recommendations
- Best imaging tool: Dual-phase Tc-99m sestamibi parathyroid scintigraphy
- Protocol advice
  - Anterior planar image with parallel hole collimator over neck and chest
    - Screen for ectopic adenomas from base of skull to inferior heart border
  - Anterior planar image over thyroid with converging collimator
    - Best image to lateralize adenoma
  - Lateral planar image with pinhole collimator
    - Gives anteroposterior location of adenoma relative to thyroid
  - Anterior oblique planar
    - Useful when anterior images inadequate for lateralization
  - SPECT
    - Increases contrast in adenoma
    - May show smaller adenoma
    - Confirm tracheoesophageal groove location
    - Identify ectopic parathyroid adenomas
- Dual-tracer parathyroid scintigraphy
  - Radiopharmaceutical taken up by thyroid and parathyroid adenoma: Image first
    - Tc-99m sestamibi or Tl-201
  - Radiopharmaceutical taken up by thyroid only: Inject and image second at typically higher doses
    - Iodine-123 or Tc-99m pertechnetate
  - Digital or visual subtraction leads to identification of parathyroid adenoma
- Correlative imaging features: Parathyroid adenoma
  - Ultrasound
    - Homogeneous, hypoechoic, hypervascular mass
    - Cystic regions may occur
    - Surrounded by thin echogenic rim (fat) if intrathyroidal
  - MR
    - T1 low intensity
    - T2 similar or higher intensity than fat
  - CECT
    - Homogeneous, enhancing mass

DIFFERENTIAL DIAGNOSIS

Benign Thyroid Pathology
- Thyroid adenoma
- Multinodular goiter
- Ectopic thyroid

Parathyroid Carcinoma
- Scintigraphic appearance identical to parathyroid adenoma, unless lymphadenopathy evident on images
- Regional lymph node metastases at presentation as high as 17%
- Heterogeneous, often calcified nodules

Other Malignancy
- Thyroid
- Lung
- Lymphoma
- Head and neck

Infection/Inflammation
- Benign lymphadenopathy
- Abscess

PATHOLOGY

General Features
- Genetics
  - 95% of cases sporadic
  - 5%: Multiple endocrine neoplasia syndromes (MEN-1, MEN-2a), familial hypocalciuric hypercalcemia
- Etiology: Increased parathyroid hormone production causes mobilization of calcium from bones and renal conservation of calcium
- Epidemiology
  - Incidence in US: 25 cases per 100,000
  - Prevalence: 1 in 500 to 1 in 1,000

PARATHYROID ADENOMA, TYPICAL

- Associated abnormalities
  - Osteitis fibrosa cystica: Resorption of bone, especially distal phalanges; increased alkaline phosphatase
  - Brown tumors: Fibrous lytic lesions of bone
  - Metastatic calcification of organs
  - Nephrolithiasis
  - Peptic ulcer disease (usually with MEN-1)
  - Weakness
  - Gout and pseudogout
  - Anemia
  - Mental confusion
  - Arrhythmia

Gross Pathologic & Surgical Features
- Well-circumscribed, soft, tan nodule
- May show cystic degeneration
- 0.5-5 g

Microscopic Features
- Fibrous capsule
- Predominately chief cells
- Nests of oxyphil cells
- Rarely oxyphil cells predominate

CLINICAL ISSUES

Presentation
- Most common signs/symptoms
  - Hypercalcemia on routine blood chemistry
  - Mental confusion, sleep disorders
  - Bone pain: Compression fractures
  - Renal colic: Nephrolithiasis

Demographics
- Age: Peak incidence > 50 years
- Gender: M:F = 1:3

Treatment
- Minimally invasive parathyroidectomy
  - Very small incision (0.5 inch)
  - Distinction between superior or inferior origin important so dissection does not extend over recurrent laryngeal nerve and fascial planes
  - First localize parathyroid adenoma in right or left neck
  - Then localize parathyroid adenoma in anteroposterior plane as compared to thyroid
    - Posteriorly displaced adenomas: Superior in origin
    - Inferiorly displaced adenomas: Inferior in origin
    - Closely apposed to thyroid: Mid- to superior pole of thyroid lobe = superior in origin; inferior pole of thyroid lobe = inferior in origin
- Unilateral cervical exploration
  - Incision from midline neck laterally (1-2 inches)
  - Important to localize parathyroid adenoma in right or left neck
- Bilateral cervical exploration
  - Historically popular treatment
  - Still used in cases of hyperparathyroidism with
    - Concurrent multinodular goiter, thyroid adenomas
    - Recurrent hyperparathyroidism
    - Negative parathyroid scan (adenoma with no uptake, hyperplasia)

DIAGNOSTIC CHECKLIST

Image Interpretation Pearls
- False negatives
  - Radiotracer may wash out of adenoma before delayed images; however, early planar images may be adequate for localization
  - SPECT images obtained after washout from parathyroid adenoma
  - Photopenic nodule posterior to or inferior to thyroid suggests cystic degeneration or necrosis
  - Limited field of view: Image from carotid sheath to inferior cardiac border
  - Avoid satisfaction of search: Multiple adenomas may be present
- False positives
  - Thyroid adenomas
  - Multinodular goiter
  - Asymmetric activity in salivary glands can resemble ectopic parathyroid adenoma in carotid sheath
  - Single or multiple foci in lateral neck suggest lymphadenopathy and malignant etiology (parathyroid carcinoma, thyroid cancer)

SELECTED REFERENCES

1. Baliski CR et al: Selective unilateral parathyroid exploration: an effective treatment for primary hyperparathyroidism. Am J Surg. 189(5):596-600; discussion 600, 2005
2. Cohen MS et al: Outpatient minimally invasive parathyroidectomy using local/regional anesthesia: a safe and effective operative approach for selected patients. Surgery. 138(4):681-7; discussion 687-9, 2005
3. Gilat H et al: Minimally invasive procedure for resection of a parathyroid adenoma: the role of preoperative high-resolution ultrasonography. J Clin Ultrasound. 33(6):283-7, 2005
4. Kleinpeter KP et al: Is parathyroid carcinoma indeed a lethal disease? Ann Surg Oncol. 12(3):260-6, 2005
5. Kraas J et al: The scintigraphic appearance of subcapsular parathyroid adenomas. Clin Nucl Med. 30(4):213-7, 2005
6. Mehta NY et al: Relationship of technetium Tc 99m sestamibi scans to histopathological features of hyperfunctioning parathyroid tissue. Arch Otolaryngol Head Neck Surg. 131(6):493-8, 2005
7. Palestro CJ et al: Radionuclide imaging of the parathyroid glands. Semin Nucl Med. 35(4):266-76, 2005
8. Shi H et al: Parathyroid and bone scintigraphy in hyperparathyroidism. Clin Nucl Med. 30(11):769-70, 2005
9. Clark P et al: Providing optimal preoperative localization for recurrent parathyroid carcinoma: a combined parathyroid scintigraphy and computed tomography approach. Clin Nucl Med. 29(11):681-4, 2004
10. Smith JR et al: Radionuclide imaging of the parathyroid glands: patterns, pearls, and pitfalls. Radiographics. 24(4):1101-15, 2004
11. Clark PB et al: Enhanced scintigraphic protocol required for optimal preoperative localization before targeted minimally invasive parathyroidectomy. Clin Nucl Med. 28(12):955-60, 2003

PARATHYROID ADENOMA, TYPICAL

IMAGE GALLERY

Typical

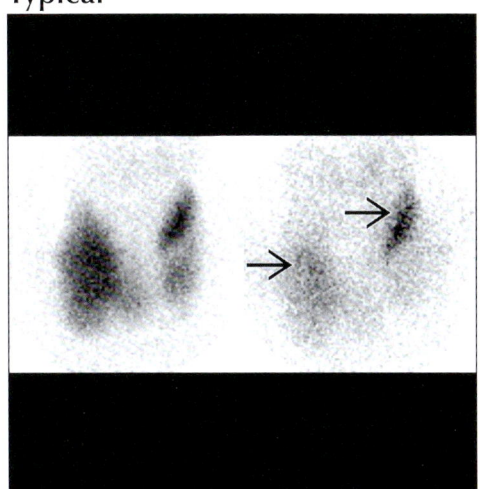

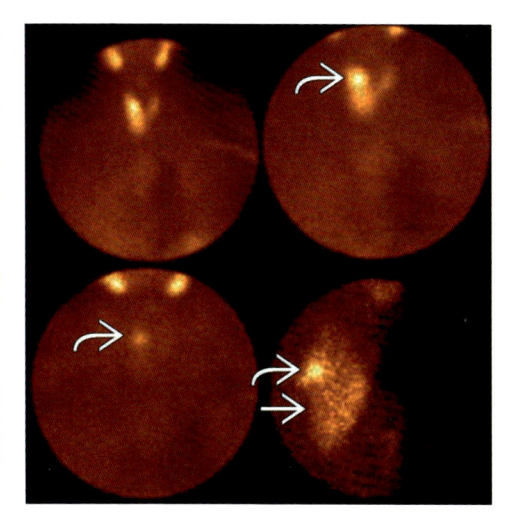

(Left) Tc 99m sestamibi parathyroid scan 15 min (lt) and 90 min (rt) shows delayed washout of MIBI from bilateral foci ➡, consistent with either parathyroid or thyroid adenomas. Tc-99m 04- or I-123 is indicated. *(Right)* Tc-99m MIBI 15 min (upper lt & rt), 90 min (lower lt), & 15 min rt lat pinhole (lower rt) shows delayed washout from right superior parathyroid adenoma ➡ close to posterior aspect of thyroid ➡.

Variant

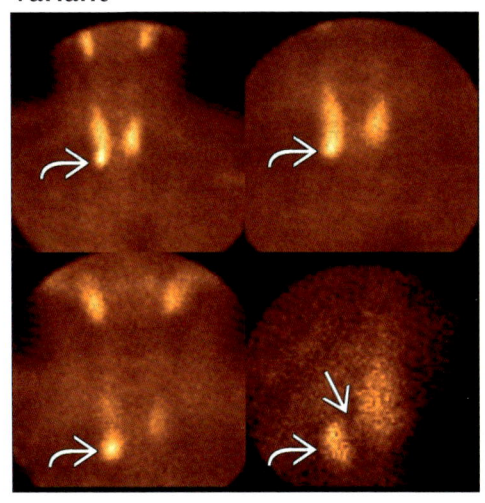

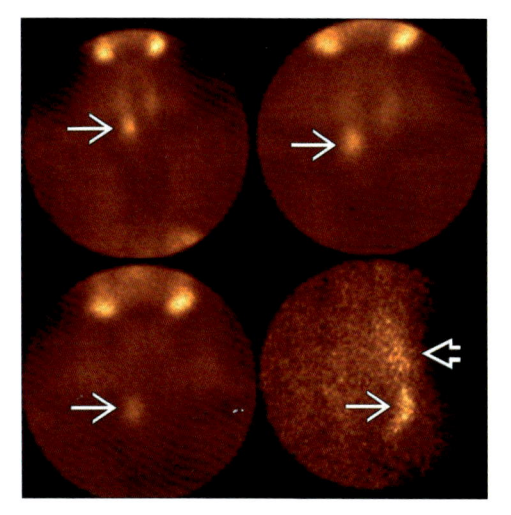

(Left) Tc-99m MIBI 15 min (upper lt & rt), 90 min (lower lt), & 15 min rt lat pinhole (lower rt) shows low-lying right superior parathyroid adenoma ➡, separated from thyroid by photopenic gap ➡. *(Right)* Tc-99m MIBI 15 min (upper lt & rt), 90 min (lower lt), & 15 min rt lat pinhole (lower rt) shows right inferior parathyroid adenoma ➡, in same vertical plane as thyroid gland ➡.

Typical

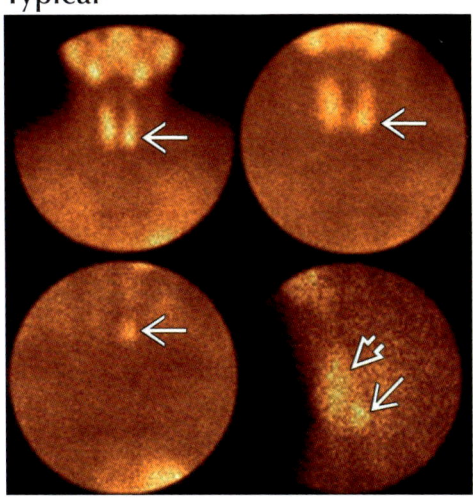

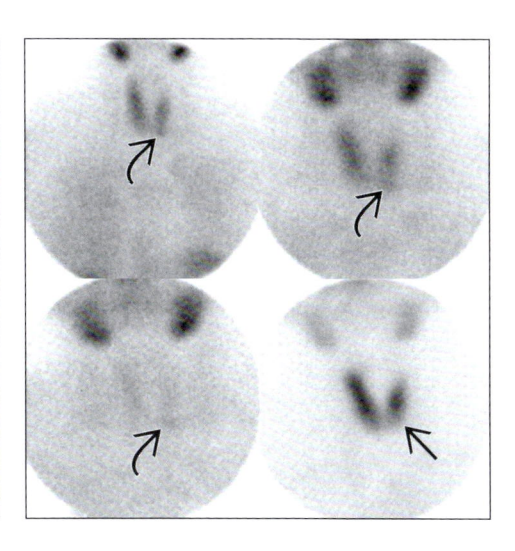

(Left) Tc-99m MIBI 15 min (upper lt & rt), 90 min (lower lt), & 15 min lt lat pinhole (lower rt) shows typical location of left inferior parathyroid adenoma ➡, close to posterior aspect of thyroid ➡. *(Right)* Right lateral parathyroid scan Subtle lt inferior subcapsular parathyroid adenoma: 15 min Tc-99m O4- thyroid scan (lower rt) shows subtle cool region ➡ which shows MIBI uptake ➡.

PARATHYROID ADENOMA, ECTOPIC

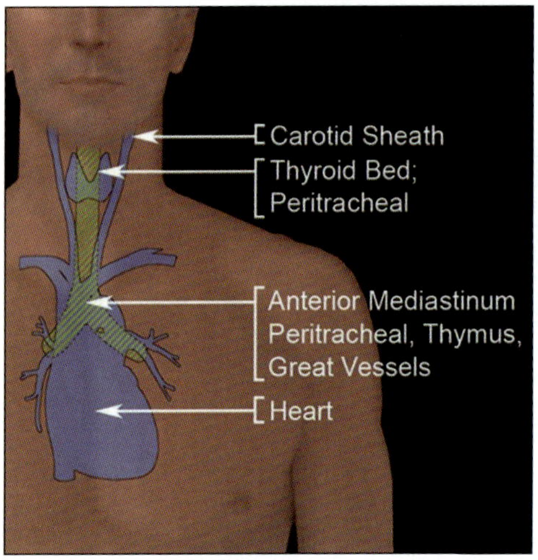

Anterior graphic shows possible locations of ectopic parathyroid adenomas. Up to 10% of solitary parathyroid adenomas are ectopic.

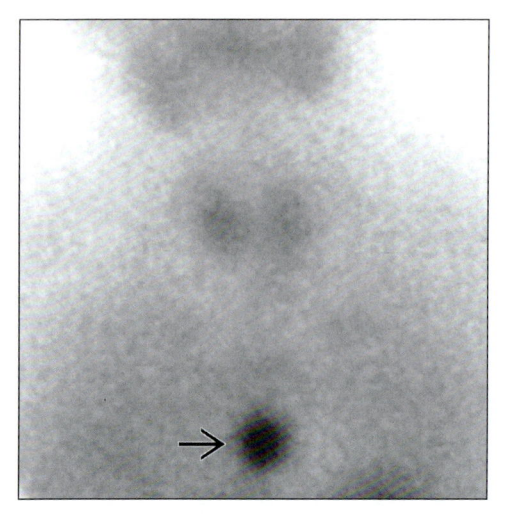

Anterior parathyroid scan shows focal increased activity ➡ overlying the mediastinum. At surgery, an intrathymic parathyroid adenoma was resected.

TERMINOLOGY

Definitions
- Parathyroid adenoma arising from aberrantly located parathyroid gland

IMAGING FINDINGS

General Features
- Best diagnostic clue: Focal increased activity in neck or thorax on parathyroid scintigraphy
- Location
  - Carotid sheath, thoracic inlet, mediastinum, great vessels, cardiac border
    - Up to 10% of solitary parathyroid adenomas ectopic
- Number
  - Single, double, supernumerary

Imaging Recommendations
- Best imaging tool: Tc-99m sestamibi parathyroid scintigraphy
- Protocol advice
  - Survey neck and thorax with parallel hole collimator
    - Include carotid sheath ⇒ inferior cardiac border
  - SPECT
    - Increases contrast
    - 3D localization of ectopic adenoma
- Tc-99m sodium pertechnetate scintigraphy
  - Distinguish ectopic parathyroid from salivary glands and/or ectopic thyroid
  - Compare to parathyroid scintigraphy
- Correlative imaging features: Parathyroid adenoma
  - F-18 FDG PET: Focal increased activity
  - CECT: Homogeneous, enhancing mass
  - T1WI MR: Hypointense; T2WI MR: Similar or higher intensity than fat

DIFFERENTIAL DIAGNOSIS

Benign Thyroid Pathology
- Ectopic thyroid
- Multinodular goiter

Malignancy
- Head and neck
- Thyroid

DDx: Mimics of Ectopic Parathyroid Adenoma on Parathyroid Scintigraphy

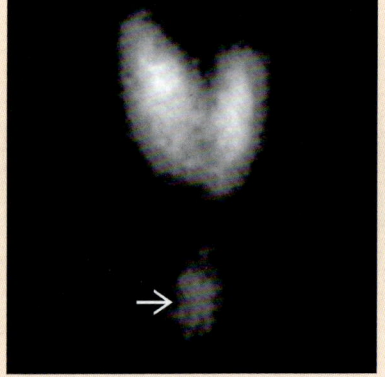

Substernal Thyroid 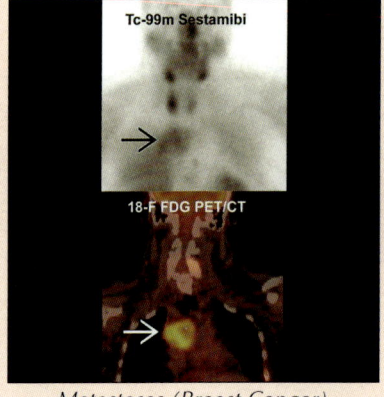 | *Metastases (Breast Cancer)* 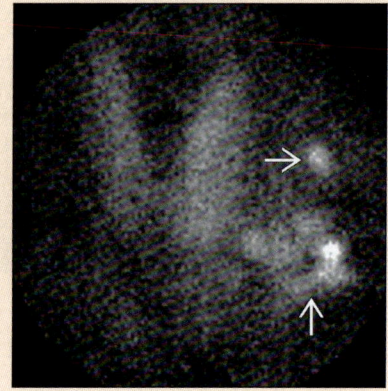 | *Lymphoma*

PARATHYROID ADENOMA, ECTOPIC

Key Facts

Terminology
- Parathyroid adenoma arising from aberrantly located parathyroid gland

Imaging Findings
- Best diagnostic clue: Focal increased activity in neck or thorax on parathyroid scintigraphy
- Carotid sheath, thoracic inlet, mediastinum, great vessels, cardiac border
- Up to 10% of solitary parathyroid adenomas ectopic

- Best imaging tool: Tc-99m sestamibi parathyroid scintigraphy

Top Differential Diagnoses
- Benign Thyroid Pathology
- Malignancy
- Infection/Inflammation

Clinical Issues
- Directed surgical resection most common treatment

- Parathyroid
- Lung
- Lymphoma
- Thymoma

Infection/Inflammation
- Benign lymphadenopathy
- Abscess

PATHOLOGY

General Features
- Embryology
  - Superior parathyroid glands arise from fourth branchial complex with thyroid
    - Early developmental arrest leaves ectopic parathyroids around carotid sheath
  - Inferior parathyroid glands arise from third branchial complex and descend with thymus
    - Leads to ectopic parathyroids in anterior mediastinum and thorax

CLINICAL ISSUES

Treatment
- Directed surgical resection most common treatment
- Ablation: Radiofrequency or alcohol

DIAGNOSTIC CHECKLIST

Image Interpretation Pearls
- False negatives
  - SPECT obtained after tracer washout from adenoma
  - Photopenic nodule: Cystic degeneration or necrosis of adenoma
  - Limited field of view: Image from carotid sheath to inferior cardiac border
  - Avoid satisfaction of search: Multiple adenomas may be present
- False positives
  - Asymmetric activity in salivary glands can resemble ectopic parathyroid adenoma in carotid sheath
  - Single or multiple foci in lateral neck suggest lymphadenopathy and malignancy

SELECTED REFERENCES

1. Palestro CJ et al: Radionuclide imaging of the parathyroid glands. Semin Nucl Med. 35(4):266-76, 2005
2. Clark P et al: Providing optimal preoperative localization for recurrent parathyroid carcinoma: a combined parathyroid scintigraphy and computed tomography approach. Clin Nucl Med. 29(11):681-4, 2004
3. Smith JR et al: Radionuclide imaging of the parathyroid glands: patterns, pearls, and pitfalls. Radiographics. 24(4):1101-15, 2004
4. Clark PB et al: Enhanced scintigraphic protocol required for optimal preoperative localization before targeted minimally invasive parathyroidectomy. Clin Nucl Med. 28(12):955-60, 2003

IMAGE GALLERY

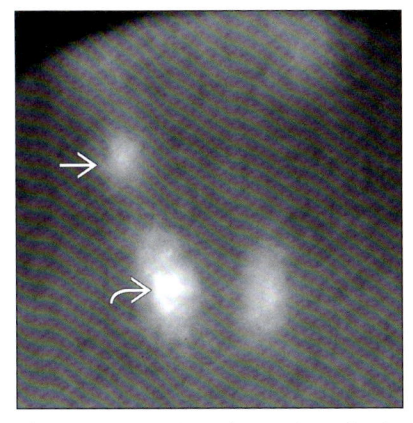

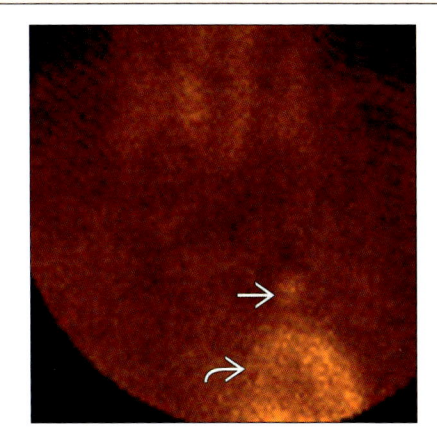

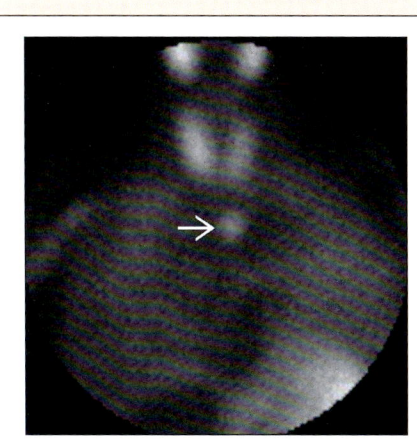

(Left) Anterior parathyroid scan shows focal increased activity ➡ inferior to right mandible, superior to right thyroid lobe ➡. Location in carotid sheath confirmed at surgery. *(Center)* Anterior parathyroid scan shows focal increased activity ➡ over left hemithorax, superior to heart ➡. This pericardial parathyroid adenoma was located superior to mid left ventricle. *(Right)* Anterior parathyroid scan shows focal increased activity inferior to the thyroid ➡. This adenoma was posterior to the sternum at surgery.

GRAVES DISEASE

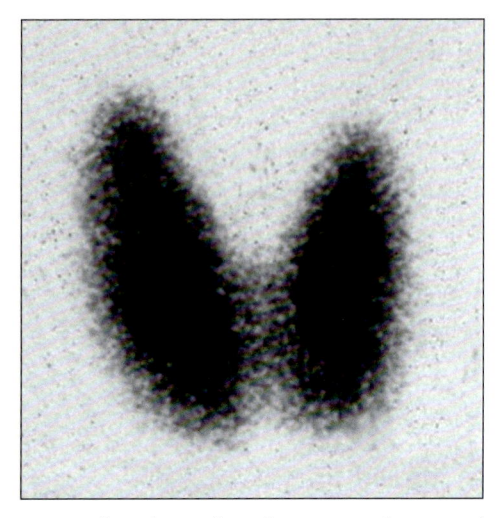

Anterior thyroid scan shows homogeneously increased thyroid uptake with smooth contours classic for Graves disease.

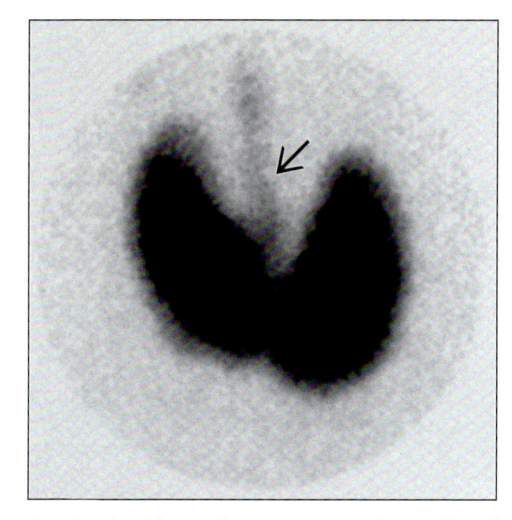

Anterior thyroid scan shows intense uptake in enlarged thyroid with prominent pyramidal lobe ➔, a frequent finding in Graves disease.

TERMINOLOGY

Abbreviations and Synonyms
- Diffuse toxic goiter

Definitions
- Autoimmune thyrotoxicosis induced by thyroid stimulating antibodies (TSAs)
- Thyroid functions autonomously, independent of pituitary thyrotropin stimulating hormone (TSH)

IMAGING FINDINGS

General Features
- Best diagnostic clue: Homogeneously enlarged thyroid with markedly increased radiotracer uptake
- Morphology: Diffuse, symmetric enlargement of both thyroid lobes

Nuclear Medicine Findings
- Tc-99m pertechnetate or iodine-123 scan shows homogeneously increased uptake with high target-to-background levels
- Superimposed nodules occur in 5-10%
  - Iodine deficiency or radiation exposure: ↑ Nodules
  - If nodules: Consider Marine-Lenhart syndrome
- Radioactive iodine uptake measurement: Diagnosis and therapy planning
  - ↑ Radioactive iodine uptake almost always present (> 35-40%); usually higher than other hyperthyroidism causes
  - If uptake exceeds 50-80%, Graves diagnosis confirmed

Ultrasonographic Findings
- Grayscale Ultrasound
  - Enlarged thyroid with thickened isthmus
  - Typically homogeneous without focal nodularity
- Color Doppler: Vascularity increased over normal tissue

Imaging Recommendations
- Best imaging tool
  - Thyroid scan
    - Tc-99m pertechnetate: 3-5 mCi (111-185 MBq) IV; image at 20 minutes
    - Iodine-123: 100-400 µCi (3.7-14.8 MBq) po; image at 4 hrs

DDx: Thyrotoxicosis

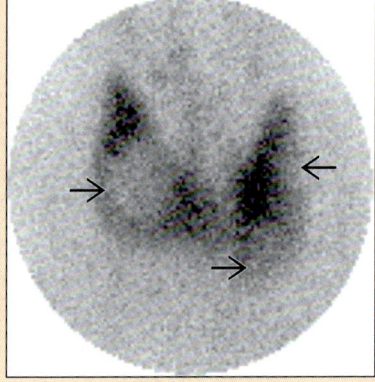

| Multinodular Goiter | Subacute Thyroiditis | Toxic Adenoma |

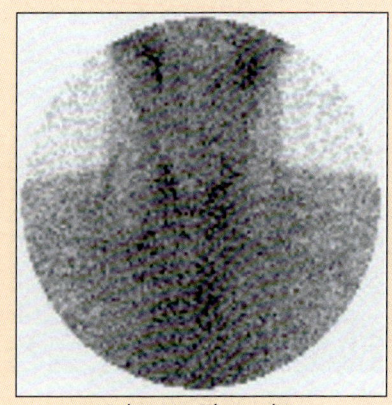

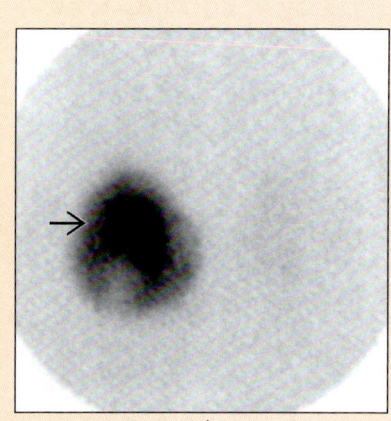

GRAVES DISEASE

Key Facts

Terminology
- Diffuse toxic goiter
- Autoimmune thyrotoxicosis induced by thyroid stimulating antibodies (TSAs)

Imaging Findings
- Tc-99m pertechnetate or iodine-123 scan shows homogeneously increased uptake with high target-to-background levels
- Superimposed nodules occur in 5-10%
- ↑ Radioactive iodine uptake almost always present (> 35-40%); usually higher than other hyperthyroidism causes
- If uptake exceeds 50-80%, Graves diagnosis confirmed

Top Differential Diagnoses
- Subacute Thyroiditis
- Multinodular Goiter, Toxic Adenoma
- Hashimoto disease with "Hashitoxicosis"
- Medication/Contrast Effects
- Non-Thyroid Endogenous Sources

Pathology
- Most common cause of hyperthyroidism
- ↓ TSH most sensitive
- Elevated T4, T3 despite ↓ TSH typical
- Anti-thyroid antibodies: Anti-TSH receptor in serum

Clinical Issues
- Most common: 3rd-5th decade
- Gender: M < F (1:7-8)

- Protocol advice
  - Correlate thyroid imaging with physical exam
  - Review history of medications, diet, family history
  - Stop antithyroid medications 5-7 days before scan
  - Delay scan 6-8 weeks after IV iodinated contrast (interferes with thyroid uptake)
  - Perform I-123 or I-131 uptake measurement at 4/24 hours
    - Aids in diagnosis and therapeutic dose determination
    - I-123 allows simultaneous uptake calculation with scan
    - Can use 5-10 µCi (0.2-0.4 MBq) I-131 for uptake if planning Tc-99m scan
    - 24 hour uptake usually reserved for cases very high 4 hour uptake
    - High turnover in high uptakes; not all trapped iodine organified, so lower 24 hour measurement more indicative of true uptake
    - Patients with high iodine turnover may require higher-dose radioactive iodine therapy

DIFFERENTIAL DIAGNOSIS

Subacute Thyroiditis
- Self-limiting postviral autoimmune thyrotoxicosis
  - Autoimmune thyroid stimulation ⇒ hormone release, suppressing TSH
  - Clinical diagnosis difficult in prolonged cases or when prior upper respiratory illness not apparent
- Very low or absent radioactive iodine uptake
- Medical symptom management; not treated with radioactive iodine

Multinodular Goiter, Toxic Adenoma
- Autonomous nodule(s) may be difficult to palpate
- Normal to elevated radioactive iodine uptake; nodularity on scan
- Generally requires higher levels of I-131 for therapy

Hyperthyroid Autoimmune Thyroiditis
- Hashimoto disease with "Hashitoxicosis"
  - Chronic thyroiditis characterized by anti-thyroid antibodies: Anti-thyroperoxidase, anti-thyroglobulin, and anti-mitochondrial antibodies
  - 3-5% develop transient thyrotoxicosis
- Silent thyroiditis, postpartum thyroiditis
  - Painless, self-limited autoimmune thyrotoxicosis characterized by lymphocytic infiltration
- Not treated with radioactive iodine

Medication/Contrast Effects
- Thyroiditis factitia: Exogenous thyroid hormone
  - Low radioiodine uptake due to thyroid suppression by exogenous hormone ingestion; no autonomous thyroid function
- Amiodarone-induced thyroiditis: Effects may last weeks to months
- Jod-Basedow phenomenon: Iodine-induced thyrotoxicosis in endemic (iodine-deficient)/nonendemic goiter, other diseases, normal thyroid

Non-Thyroid Endogenous Sources
- Pheochromocytoma
- Trophoblastic tumors
- Metastatic thyroid cancer

PATHOLOGY

General Features
- Genetics
  - Frequent familial history of autoimmune thyroiditis: Graves, Hashimoto, or postpartum thyroiditis
  - Genetic susceptibility: Several human leukocyte antigen (HLA) haplotypes and gene for CTLA4 which helps code for T-cell down regulation
- Etiology: Susceptibility increased by combined genetic and environmental factors; history of triggering event such as surgery may be elicited
- Epidemiology
  - Most common cause of hyperthyroidism
    - 70-80% of thyrotoxicosis

GRAVES DISEASE

- In US 30:100,000 persons per year
- Associated abnormalities
  - Thyroid function laboratory findings
    - ↓ TSH most sensitive
    - Elevated T4, T3 despite ↓ TSH typical
  - Anti-thyroid antibodies: Anti-TSH receptor in serum
    - Anti-thyrotropin receptor antibodies ↑ thyroid hormone production
    - Antibodies to thyroglobulin, thyroid peroxidase, and sodium-iodide symporter frequently detected

Gross Pathologic & Surgical Features
- Enlarged, soft, vascular
  - Thyroid weighs 50-150 g (normal 15-20 g)

Microscopic Features
- Stromal follicular hyperplasia, vascular congestion, retention of lobular architecture; lymphocytic invasion occurs early

CLINICAL ISSUES

Presentation
- Most common signs/symptoms
  - Anxiety, weight loss, heat intolerance, tremor, palpitations
  - Graves ophthalmopathy
    - Exophthalmos, diplopia: Seen in 25-30% patients
    - Treat with high-dose glucocorticoids
    - Orbital CT or MR may be needed in cases of ophthalmopathy
    - Effects of I-131 therapy controversial; rare cases of ↑ ophthalmopathy with radioiodine therapy reported, may be coincidental
- Other signs/symptoms
  - Dermopathy and acropachy
  - Menstrual irregularities, infertility
  - Elderly: Diagnosis may be difficult, presenting with cardiac symptoms, weight loss

Demographics
- Age
  - Most common: 3rd-5th decade
    - Can occur any age, even in children
- Gender: M < F (1:7-8)

Natural History & Prognosis
- Presents with moderate/severe hyperthyroidism
  - Cardiac complications: Heart failure, arrhythmia (atrial fibrillation)
  - Thyrotoxic crisis/storm: Rare but potentially life-threatening acute thyroid hormone discharge
    - Most often in untreated patients under stress (surgery, concomitant illness)
    - Can be caused by radioactive iodine therapy, especially in debilitated
  - Osteoporosis

Treatment
- Antithyroid medication: Propylthiouracil (PTU) or Methimazole (Tapazole)
  - Often used temporarily (side effects or relapse in over 50% of patients)
  - Rare agranulocytosis (0.2-0.5%), hepatic dysfunction
- Radioactive iodine (I-131)
  - Empiric standard dose or calculated dose: Typically 5-15 mCi I-131 po
  - Calculated dose based on uptake measurement and thyroid size
    - 100-180 µCi/g thyroid tissue divided by 4/24-hr uptake
    - Higher doses for large goiter, low uptake value, or repeat therapy
  - Immediate post-therapy side effects rare but include
    - Radiation thyroiditis: Locally inflamed thyroid (treat with acetaminophen, corticosteroids)
    - Thyroid storm: Treat with beta-blockers
  - Effectiveness of therapy slow (weeks-months)
  - 10% require retreatment after 6-12 months
  - Hypothyroidism is goal of therapy (difficult to achieve euthyroidism, may under treat hyperthyroidism if attempted)
    - Life-long thyroid hormone replacement required
- Thyroidectomy
  - Hemithyroidectomy: Patients often suffer recurrence
  - As with radioactive iodine therapy, total thyroidectomy requires life-long thyroid hormone replacement
  - Risks: Laryngeal nerve trauma, bleeding, infection, scar, death
  - Often reserved for patients with large, compressive goiters
  - Used in patients with contraindications to other therapy
    - Medical: Hepatic disease, medically refractive hyperthyroidism
    - Radioactive iodine: Unable to follow radiation safety precautions, patient bias against radiation treatment

DIAGNOSTIC CHECKLIST

Consider
- For treatment and diagnosis, often do not need a thyroid scan
  - High radioactive iodine uptake measurement (> 50-80%) at 4/24 hours = Graves disease

SELECTED REFERENCES

1. Ando T et al: Thyrotropin receptor antibodies: new insights into their actions and clinical relevance. Best Pract Res Clin Endocrinol Metab. 19(1):33-52, 2005
2. Baldini M et al: Relationship between the sonographic appearance of the thyroid and the clinical course and autoimmune activity of Graves' disease. J Clin Ultrasound. 33(8):381-5, 2005
3. Cooper DS: Antithyroid drugs. N Engl J Med. 3;352(9):905-17, 2005
4. Vemulakonda US et al: Therapy dose calculation in Graves' disease using early I-123 uptake measurements. Clin Nucl Med. 21(2):102-5, 1996

GRAVES DISEASE

IMAGE GALLERY

Typical

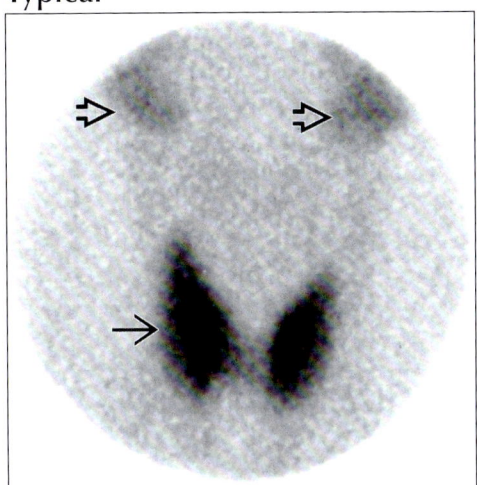

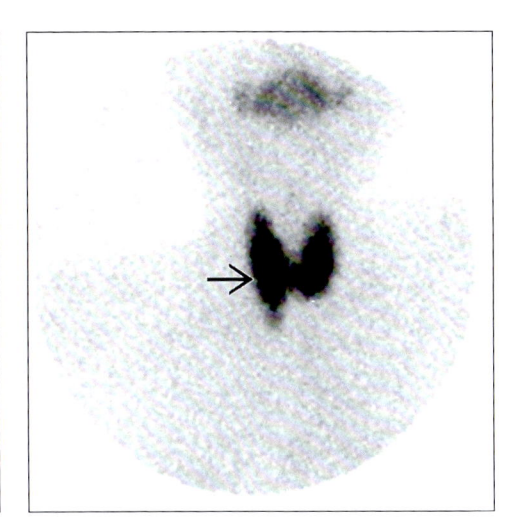

(Left) Anterior thyroid scan shows mild thyroid enlargement ➔ but normal background and salivary ⇨ activity. In the hyperthyroid patient with increased radioactive iodine uptake, this signifies early Graves disease. *(Right)* Anterior thyroid scan shows enlarged thyroid ➔ with high target-to-background activity and no salivary activity, classic Graves disease findings.

Variant

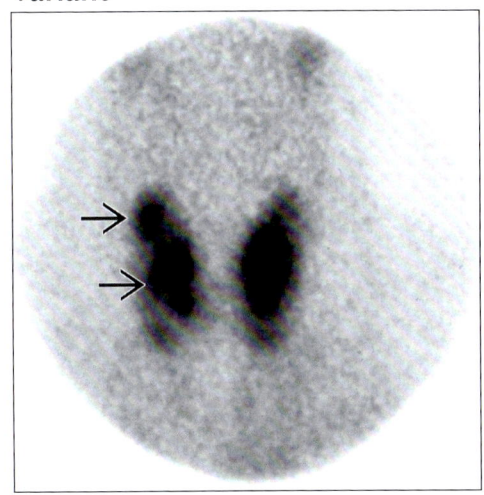

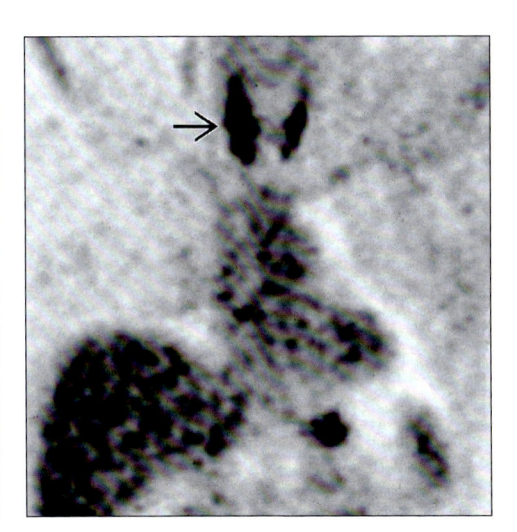

(Left) Anterior thyroid scan in Graves disease patient shows enlarged, nodular thyroid ➔. Clinical examination and antibody levels help differentiate Graves with superimposed nodules from multinodular goiter. *(Right)* Coronal PET shows homogeneously increased thyroid activity ➔ suggesting diffuse thyroid disease, such as Graves disease.

Other

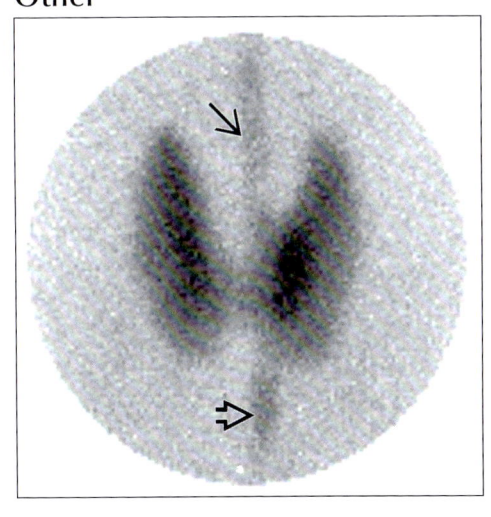

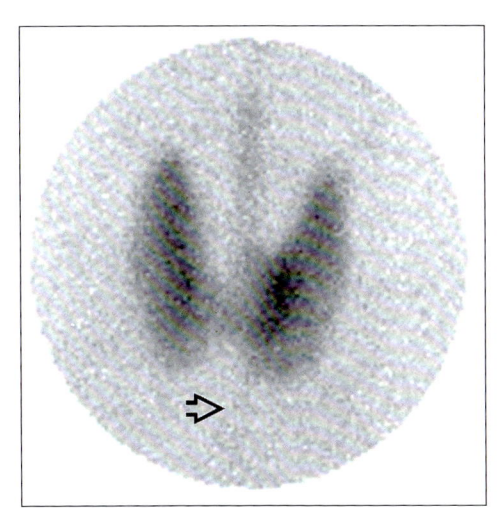

(Left) Anterior thyroid scan in patient with Graves disease. Note large pyramidal lobe ➔ and radiotracer extending from thyroid inferiorly ⇨. Same patient as next image. *(Right)* Anterior thyroid scan in same patient as previous image shows inferior activity no longer present ⇨. The patient swallowed a glass of water and was re-imaged to distinguish thyroid from retained tracer in esophagus.

HASHIMOTO THYROIDITIS

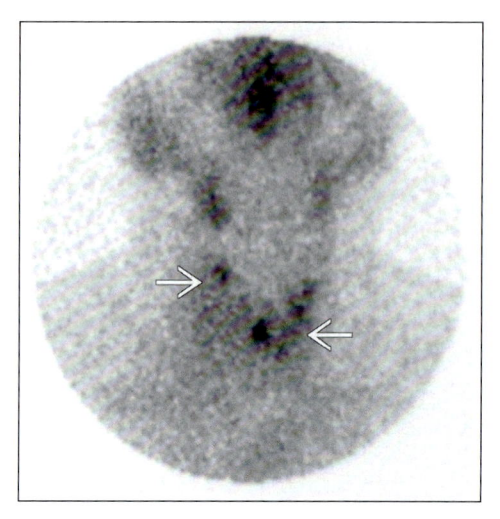

Anterior thyroid scan shows diffuse activity (low target-to-background) in Hashimoto thyroiditis patient with superimposed goiter ➡.

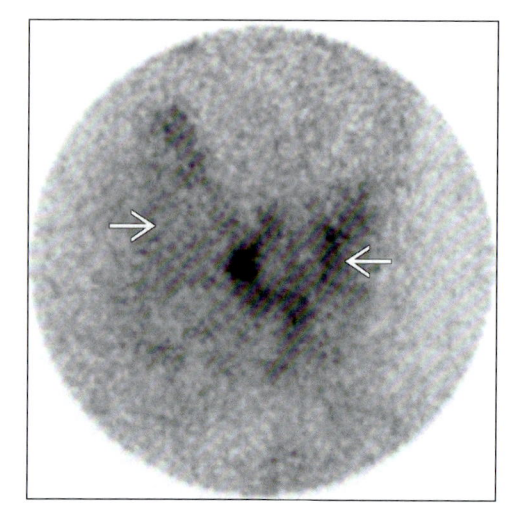

Anterior pinhole thyroid scan shows heterogeneous uptake ➡ typical in patients with Hashimoto thyroiditis.

TERMINOLOGY

Abbreviations and Synonyms
- Chronic thyroiditis, chronic lymphocytic thyroiditis

Definitions
- Part of spectrum of autoimmune thyroid diseases
- Cellular and humoral-mediated thyroid destruction

IMAGING FINDINGS

General Features
- Best diagnostic clue: Diffusely enlarged thyroid in hypothyroid patient
- Size
  - Variable
  - Most common: Moderate goiter

Nuclear Medicine Findings
- Tc-99m pertechnetate or I-123 scan: Pattern highly variable
  - Early: Normal or mildly increased activity (similar to Graves disease)
  - Progression: Patchy/heterogeneous activity (mimics multinodular goiter)
  - End-stage: May show little uptake
  - Nodules: Concurrent adenoma (hot) or cancer (cold) can occur
- I-123 or I-131 uptake: Variable, depending on stage
  - Most common: Low-normal or decreased uptake, due to tissue destruction in later stages
  - Transient thyrotoxicosis, "Hashitoxicosis" with increased uptake occurs in 3-5%

CT Findings
- CECT: Symmetrically enlarged, decreased density, no calcification or necrosis

MR Findings
- Nonspecific: Heterogeneous signal frequent, relationship to clinical stage unclear

Ultrasonographic Findings
- Grayscale Ultrasound
  - Enlarged thyroid with diffusely decreased/heterogeneous echogenicity or heterogeneous echogenicity
  - Increased flow on color Doppler often present

DDx: Goiter

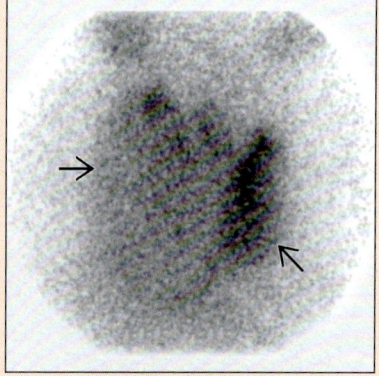

Diffuse Nontoxic Goiter

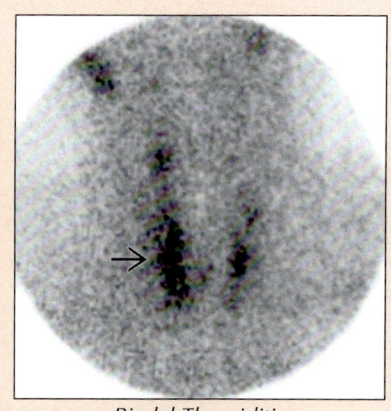

Riedel Thyroiditis

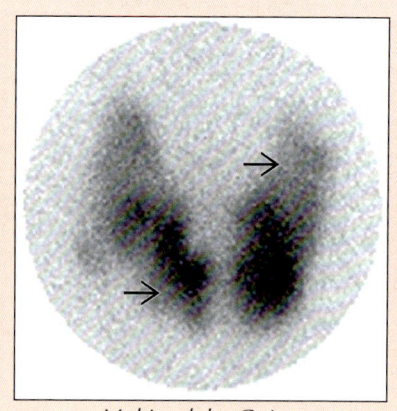

Multinodular Goiter

HASHIMOTO THYROIDITIS

Key Facts

Terminology
- Chronic thyroiditis, chronic lymphocytic thyroiditis
- Part of spectrum of autoimmune thyroid diseases
- Cellular and humoral-mediated thyroid destruction

Imaging Findings
- Tc-99m pertechnetate or I-123 scan: Pattern highly variable
- I-123 or I-131 uptake: Variable, depending on stage

Top Differential Diagnoses
- Diffuse Nontoxic or Endemic Goiter
- Riedel Struma: Fibrous Invasive Thyroiditis
- Multinodular Goiter
- Invasive/Infiltrative Disease
- Recovering Subacute Thyroiditis
- Medication Effects

Pathology
- US: Most common cause of hypothyroidism
- Worldwide: 2nd leading cause of hypothyroidism (iodine deficiency = 1st)

Clinical Issues
- Hypothyroidism
- Goiter
- Other signs/symptoms: Hyperthyroidism or Hashitoxicosis (rare)

Diagnostic Checklist
- Radioactive iodine uptake: Increased, normal or decreased
- Hashimoto thyroiditis on scan: May mimic Graves, multinodular goiter, nontoxic goiter, or other autoimmune thyroiditis

---

  o Late: Ill-defined nodularity

Imaging Recommendations
- Best imaging tool
  o Nuclear medicine: Thyroid scan and radioactive iodine uptake
  o Most common: Ultrasound (can often exclude malignancy)
- Protocol advice
  o Stop thyroid replacement before scan
    - 4-6 weeks for levothyroxine (T4 or Synthroid)
    - 2-3 weeks for triiodothyronine (T3 or Cytomel)
  o IV iodinated contrast: Delay uptake and scan for 6-8 weeks
  o History: Medication, family history
  o Thyroid scan
    - I-123: Image 4 hrs after 100-400 µCi po
    - Tc-99m pertechnetate: 3-5 mCi IV after 4/24 hr radioactive iodine uptake performed; image at 20 minutes
    - High resolution planar and pinhole collimators
    - Correlate physical exam with images
  o Radioactive iodine uptake
    - Measure at 4/24 hrs
    - 100-400 µCi I-123 (can scan and perform uptake with same dose)
    - 5-10 µCi I-131 po (scan with Tc-99m pertechnetate after 4/24 hr uptake)

DIFFERENTIAL DIAGNOSIS

Diffuse Nontoxic or Endemic Goiter
- Endemic: Found in regions with iodine deficiency (e.g., mountains); associated with goitrogen exposure
- Sporadic: Enzymatic defect, iodine deficiency, goitrogen exposure

Riedel Struma: Fibrous Invasive Thyroiditis
- Hypercellular infiltrate causing thick fibrotic bands, hypothyroidism in 30-40%
- Histology can usually distinguish from Hashimoto
- May involve orbit, mediastinum, biliary tract

Multinodular Goiter
- Diffusely nodular, enlarged thyroid
- Normal or increased radioactive iodine uptake

Invasive/Infiltrative Disease
- Invasive thyroid carcinoma: Poorly marginated or invasive lesion
  o Adenopathy often present on CT
- Lymphoma
- Amyloid, hemochromatosis, progressive systemic sclerosis (scleroderma)

Recovering Subacute Thyroiditis
- Self-limited post-viral autoimmune thyrotoxicosis
- Scan may show patchy uptake after acute phase

Medication Effects
- Lithium-induced hypothyroidism
  o Inhibits uptake of iodine, release of thyroid hormone
  o Autoimmune thyroiditis (20-40%) and goiter (50%) with long term therapy
- Amiodarone
  o Effects may last weeks to months
  o Hyperthyroidism: Due to high levels of iodine in drug
  o Hypothyroidism: Thyroiditis and inhibited conversion of T4 to T3 (associated with ↑ interleukin-6)
- Alpha interferon
  o Induces thyroid autoimmunity in 10-20% with anti-thyroid antibodies

PATHOLOGY

General Features
- Genetics
  o Family history common
    - 1° relatives: Anti-thyroid antibodies more common than general population
  o Associated immune-modifying genes: CTLA-4 and several human leukocyte antigen (HLA) haplotypes

HASHIMOTO THYROIDITIS

- Etiology
  - Genetic and environmental factors
  - Autoimmune process mediated by cellular and humoral mechanisms
    - Early stage: Lymphoid infiltration
    - Elevated anti-thyroid antigen antibodies in 85-90%
    - Most common antibodies: Anti-thyroperoxidase, anti-thyroglobulin
    - Also anti-TSH receptor blocking and anti-mitochondrial antibodies
    - Possible overlap with Graves disease
  - Similar to other autoimmune thyroid diseases such as post-partum and silent thyroiditis
- Epidemiology
  - US: Most common cause of hypothyroidism
  - Worldwide: 2nd leading cause of hypothyroidism (iodine deficiency = 1st)
- Associated abnormalities
  - Other autoimmune disease
    - Lupus, Sjögren syndrome, progressive systemic sclerosis (scleroderma), rheumatoid arthritis, type 1 diabetes mellitus, Addison disease, pernicious anemia, chronic active hepatitis
  - Lymphoma
    - Up to 70-80% increased risk of developing non-Hodgkin lymphoma

Gross Pathologic & Surgical Features
- Thyroid usually enlarged; firm or rock-hard

Microscopic Features
- Diffuse lymphocytic and plasma cell infiltration
- Atrophic follicles without colloid
- Fibrosis, septations common
- Antibodies to thyroid antigens
  - Antithyroid peroxidase (anti-TPO), antithyroglobulin
  - TSH-receptor blocking antibodies and thyroid-stimulating antibodies (less common)

CLINICAL ISSUES

Presentation
- Most common signs/symptoms
  - Hypothyroidism
    - Fatigue
    - Constipation
    - Dry skin/hair
    - Cold intolerance
    - Constipation
  - Goiter
    - Hoarse voice
    - Neck pressure
- Other signs/symptoms: Hyperthyroidism or Hashitoxicosis (rare)

Demographics
- Age
  - Peak incidence: 4th-6th decades
    - Peak 10-15 years later in men
- Gender: M:F = 1:10

Natural History & Prognosis
- Hyperthyroid, euthyroid, or hypothyroid depending stage
- Hyperthyroidism or Hashitoxicosis in early stage
  - T4 and T3 leak into circulation when cell membranes damaged
  - Rare
- Hypothyroidism
  - Develops insidiously
  - May be subclinical
    - Elevated TSH, normal thyroid hormone levels
- Prognosis
  - Good if diagnosed early
    - If on thyroid replacement, patient can lead normal life
  - Myxedema coma
    - Rare complication affecting untreated hypothyroid patient
    - Severe stress or illness precipitates
    - High mortality rate
    - Poor prognosis despite steroid therapy

Treatment
- Life-long thyroid hormone replacement

DIAGNOSTIC CHECKLIST

Consider
- Thyroid scan often not needed
  - Diagnosis made with clinical/lab findings
- Check anti-thyroid antibody levels

Image Interpretation Pearls
- Radioactive iodine uptake: Increased, normal or decreased
- Hashimoto thyroiditis on scan: May mimic Graves, multinodular goiter, nontoxic goiter, or other autoimmune thyroiditis

SELECTED REFERENCES

1. Ban Y et al: Genetic susceptibility in thyroid autoimmunity. Pediatr Endocrinol Rev. 3(1):20-32, 2005
2. Sahlmann CO et al: Quantitative thyroid scintigraphy for the differentiation of Graves' disease and hyperthyroid autoimmune thyroiditis. Nuklearmedizin. 43(4):124-8, 2004
3. Smith JR et al: Radionuclide imaging of the thyroid gland: patterns, pearls, and pitfalls. Clin Nucl Med. 29(3):181-93, 2004
4. Intenzo CM et al: Scintigraphic features of autoimmune thyroiditis. Radiographics. 21(4):957-64, 2001
5. Tollin SR et al: The utility of thyroid nuclear imaging and other studies in the detection and treatment of underlying thyroid abnormalities in patients with endogenous subclinical thyrotoxicosis. Clin Nucl Med. 25(5):341-7, 2000
6. Intenzo CM et al: Clinical, laboratory, and scintigraphic manifestations of subacute and chronic thyroiditis. Clin Nucl Med. 18(4):302-6, 1993
7. Ramtoola S et al: The thyroid scan in Hashimoto's thyroiditis: the great mimic. Nucl Med Commun. 9(9):639-45, 1988

HASHIMOTO THYROIDITIS

IMAGE GALLERY

Typical

Typical

Typical

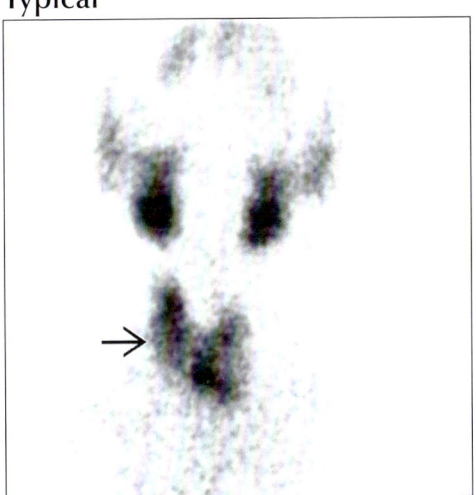

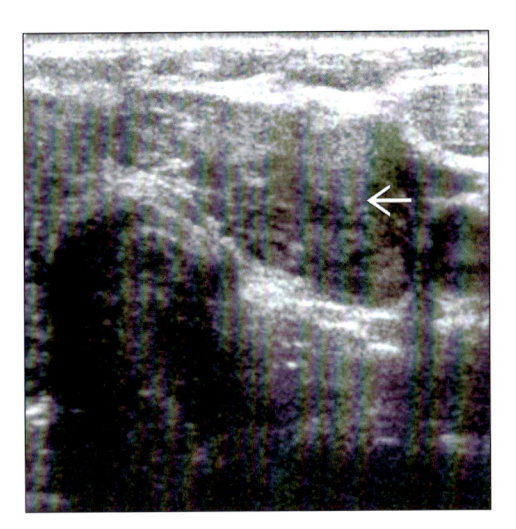

(Left) Anterior thyroid scan shows slightly enlarged, irregular thyroid ➡ with low-normal uptake in early Hashimoto thyroiditis. No nodules were present at ultrasound. (Right) Transaxial thyroid ultrasound shows diffuse coarse echogenicity of thyroid ➡ in patient with Hashimoto thyroiditis.

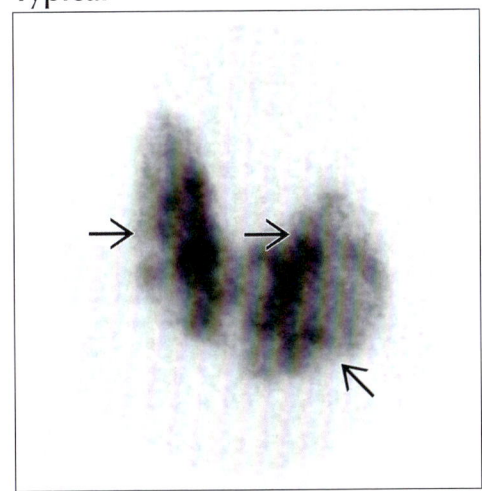

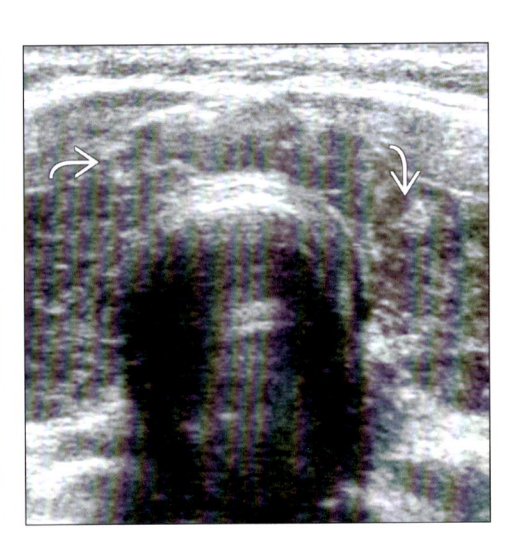

(Left) Pinhole anterior thyroid scan shows irregular uptake ➡ in patient with Hashimoto thyroiditis mimicking multinodular goiter. (Right) Transaxial ultrasound shows enlarged thyroid with diffuse heterogeneous echotexture ➡.

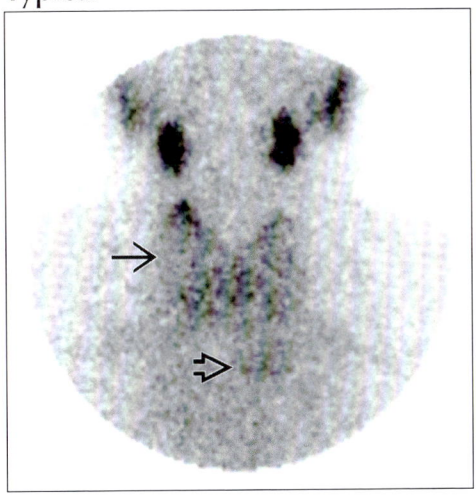

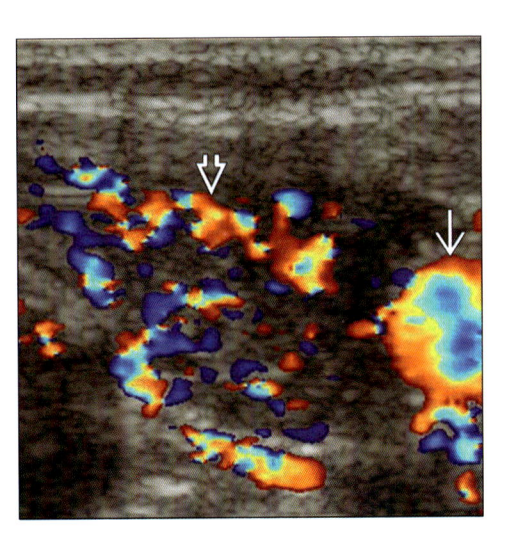

(Left) Anterior thyroid scan shows Hashimoto thyroiditis ➡ with substernal goiter ▷. (Right) Color Doppler ultrasound shows increased thyroid vascularity ➡ of Hashimoto thyroiditis adjacent to the carotid artery ➡.

MULTINODULAR GOITER

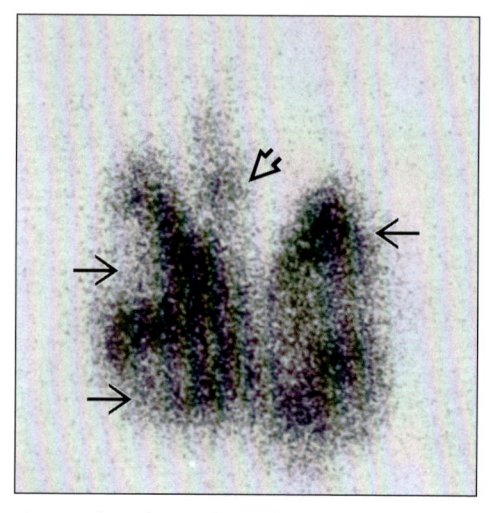

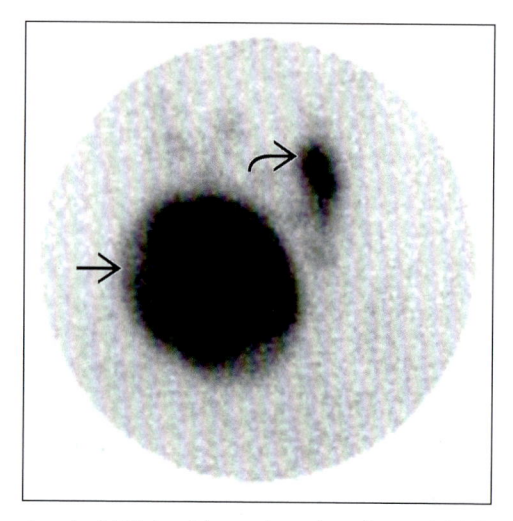

Anterior thyroid scan shows thyroid enlargement and bilateral nodules ⇨ in a patient with multinodular goiter. Note pyramidal lobe also evident ⇨.

Anterior I-123 thyroid scan shows large hot nodule ⇨ and small nodule ⇨ which suppresses adjacent thyroid, making small cold nodules more difficult to see.

TERMINOLOGY

Abbreviations and Synonyms
- Multinodular goiter (MNG)
- Euthyroid: Adenomatous goiter, nontoxic nodular goiter, colloid nodular goiter
- Hyperthyroid: Toxic nodular goiter, Plummer disease (one or more nodules)

Definitions
- Adenomatous thyroid hyperplasia ⇒ nodules in enlarged thyroid
  - Many nodules become autonomous
  - Some nodules become toxic ⇒ toxic nodular goiter

IMAGING FINDINGS

General Features
- Best diagnostic clue: Diffusely enlarged thyroid with multiple nodules
- Location: Thyroid enlargement extends substernally in > 1/3 cases (common cause anterior mediastinal mass)
- Size: Moderate > very large

Nuclear Medicine Findings
- Radioiodine uptakes often normal to slightly ↑: Higher therapeutic I-131 doses required
- Heterogeneous radiotracer uptake with irregular, nodular thyroid contour
  - Discrete nodules may be hot (increased activity), cold (photopenic), warm, or isointense/not visualized
  - Most nodules cold
- Hot nodules: Autonomous toxic adenomas suppress normal thyroid
- Warm nodules: Increased uptake, no thyroid suppression
- Dominant cold nodules: Require follow-up (biopsy if not cystic on ultrasound)

CT Findings
- NECT
  - Circumscribed regions of low attenuation from colloid or degenerating cysts
  - High attenuation with hemorrhage, calcification
- CECT: Inhomogeneously enhancing, enlarged thyroid with multiple cystic and solid masses

DDx: Thyrotoxicosis and Goiter

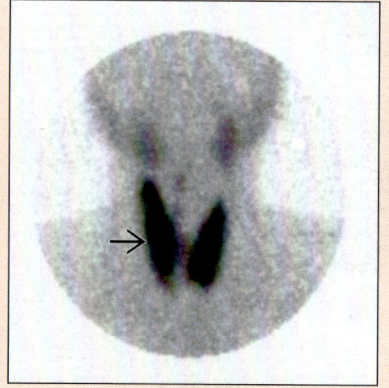

Graves Disease

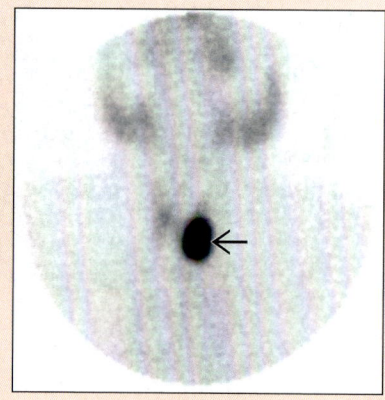

Toxic Adenoma

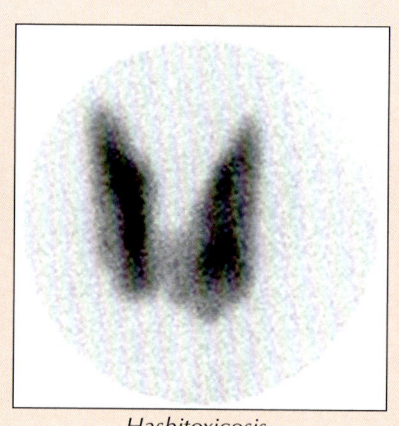

Hashitoxicosis

MULTINODULAR GOITER

Key Facts

Terminology
- Adenomatous thyroid hyperplasia ⇒ nodules in enlarged thyroid
- Many nodules become autonomous
- Some nodules become toxic ⇒ toxic nodular goiter

Imaging Findings
- Heterogeneous radiotracer uptake with irregular, nodular thyroid contour
- Discrete nodules may be hot (increased activity), cold (photopenic), warm, or isointense/not visualized
- Most nodules cold

Top Differential Diagnoses
- Graves Disease
- Hashitoxicosis
- Toxic or Autonomous Nodule
- Post-Viral Subacute Thyroiditis
- Cancer
- Reidel Thyroiditis

Clinical Issues
- Rx dose: Typically 20-25 mCi (740-925 MBq) I-131
- Requires weeks to months to become fully effective
- Multiple doses may be required
- Subtotal or total thyroidectomy recommended for very large, compressive goiter

Diagnostic Checklist
- Elderly: MNG + subclinical hyperthyroidism common
- Radioactive iodine treatment for symptomatic (cardiac) relief

Ultrasonographic Findings
- Grayscale Ultrasound
  - Hypoechoic solid nodules, anechoic cysts, hyperechoic fibrotic or post hemorrhagic regions
  - Focal hyperechoic calcifications showing distal shadowing

Imaging Recommendations
- Best imaging tool
  - Depends on clinical question
  - Thyroid uptake and scan
    - Hyperthyroid patient: Diagnosis and I-131 therapy planning
    - Substernal mass: Confirms thyroid goiter
    - Large/dominant nodule: Characterizes function (thus cancer risk)
  - Ultrasound
    - Dominant nodule +/- enlarging: Direct fine needle aspiration (FNA), identify adenopathy
  - CECT: Assess substernal goiter or airway compression
- Protocol advice
  - Thyroid uptake
    - 100-400 µCi (3.7-14.8 MBq) I-123 orally for uptake and scan, or 5-10 µCi (185-370 kBq) I-131 uptake with Tc-99m pertechnetate scan
    - Measure uptake 4/24 hrs post radioiodine administration po
    - Helpful for diagnosis in difficult cases and for therapy planning
  - Thyroid scan with Tc-99m pertechnetate
    - 3-5 mCi (111-185 MBq) IV, delay imaging 20 minutes
    - Must be done after thyroid uptake (Tc-99m emissions interfere)
  - Thyroid scan with I-123
    - 100-400 µCi (3.7-14.8 MBq) I-123 po
    - Convenience of scan and uptake in one dose often worth added expense of I-123 (cyclotron-produced)
    - Identifies discordant nodules (5%) falsely hot on Tc-99m pertechnetate but actually cold (lack of organification)
  - Image anteriorly with parallel and pinhole collimators
- Additional nuclear medicine imaging options
  - Tc-99m sestamibi: Thyroid adenomas may show increased uptake and delayed clearance mimicking parathyroid adenoma
  - FDG PET
    - Benign adenomas, thyroid cancer may show abnormal, focal ↑ uptake requiring biopsy follow-up
    - Metastatic well-differentiated thyroid cancer: Usually I-131 avid (PET often falsely negative)

DIFFERENTIAL DIAGNOSIS

Graves Disease
- Diffuse toxic goiter: Uptake > 50-80% (usually much higher than other thyroid diseases)
- Graves requires less I-131 for treatment compared with MNG (10-15 mCi vs. 20-25 mCi I-131)

Hashitoxicosis
- Autoimmune chronic thyroiditis; + anti-thyroid antibodies
- Hashimoto typically a hypofunctional goiter; often similar appearance to MNG
- 3-5% patients experience early transient thyrotoxicosis

Toxic or Autonomous Nodule
- Plummer disease: Single or multiple toxic nodules
- Toxic nodule suppresses surrounding thyroid
- Resistance to I-131 therapy requires higher/multiple doses (20-25 mCi I-131)

Post-Viral Subacute Thyroiditis
- Self-limiting autoimmune thyroiditis which may cause thyrotoxicosis
- Very low or absent radiotracer uptake (uptake needed to prevent inappropriate I-131 therapy)

MULTINODULAR GOITER

Cancer
- Primary thyroid cancer, metastasis, thyroid lymphoma: Discrete cold nodule, ill-defined mass

Riedel Thyroiditis
- Benign invasive fibrosis causing diffuse thyroid enlargement; leads to hypothyroidism

PATHOLOGY

General Features
- Genetics
  - Sporadic (rarely germ-line) mutations in thyroid stimulating hormone (TSH) receptor
  - Often family history of recurrent thyroiditis, goiter
- Etiology
  - Genetic and environmental factors
  - Iodine deficiency alone insufficient to cause MNG (may accelerate development)
  - Radiation exposure: ↑ Thyroid nodule development and thyroid cancer risk
- Epidemiology
  - US: Second most common cause of hyperthyroidism (Graves #1)
  - Toxic nodules: Most common cause of hyperthyroidism endemic regions
  - Worldwide incidence: 1-4%
  - Nodular development 5-15x more common in women with palpable nodules (5-6% population > 40 years of age)

Gross Pathologic & Surgical Features
- Enlarged, firm thyroid with variable size nodules, cysts

Microscopic Features
- Normal sized follicles with macro- and microfollicles
- Degenerating follicles cause infarction, hemorrhage and calcification

CLINICAL ISSUES

Presentation
- Most common signs/symptoms
  - Large neck mass with palpable nodules
    - Thyrotoxicosis may be insidious
    - Weight loss
    - Anxiety
    - Palpitations
    - Menstrual irregularity
- Other signs/symptoms
  - Elderly: Cardiac symptoms may be only sign
    - Atrial fibrillation, congestive heart failure
    - Subclinical hyperthyroidism (normal T4/T3 but suppressed TSH): Frequent cardiac symptoms ⇒ treatment
  - Patients often present years after disease process begins

Demographics
- Age
  - MNG peaks 5th-7th decades
  - Hyperthyroidism + MNG peaks 6th-7th decades
- Gender: M:F = 1:3-4

Natural History & Prognosis
- Gradual nodular growth, goiter formation
- Prognosis good if diagnosed and properly treated
- Nontoxic nodular goiter
  - Colloid nodules and cysts: Usually cold, benign
  - Warm nodular adenomas: Develop slowly, some become autonomous
  - No initial suppression of normal thyroid by autonomous adenomas
  - High incidence of subclinical hyperthyroidism, suppressed TSH
- Multinodular goiter
  - 10% of autonomous nodules may become toxic
  - Toxic nodules: ↑ Uptake in palpable nodules with surrounding thyroid suppression
  - Insidious development of clinical hyperthyroidism may occur over years
- Thyroid cancer risk 5% in MNG, lower than solitary cold nodule
  - Cancer risk solitary cold nodule overall 15-20%, ranging from 5% up to surgical reports of 40%
  - Cancer risk in hot nodule < 1%

Treatment
- No therapy for small nonpalpable nodules in asymptomatic patient
- Medical therapy for thyrotoxicosis
  - Thyroid blockers
    - Propylthiouracil (PTU)
    - Methimazole
  - Beta-blockers
    - Cardioprotective
    - Symptomatic relief
- Radioactive iodine ablation
  - Rx dose: Typically 20-25 mCi (740-925 MBq) I-131
  - Requires weeks to months to become fully effective
  - Multiple doses may be required
  - Subtotal or total thyroidectomy recommended for very large, compressive goiter

DIAGNOSTIC CHECKLIST

Consider
- Elderly: MNG + subclinical hyperthyroidism common
  - Radioactive iodine treatment for symptomatic (cardiac) relief
- Radioactive iodine Rx of MNG with 20-25 mCi (740-925 MBq) I-131
  - May require multiple doses

SELECTED REFERENCES

1. Smith JR et al: Radionuclide imaging of the thyroid gland: patterns, pearls, and pitfalls. Clin Nucl Med. 29:181-94, 2004
2. Intenzo CM et al: Scintigraphic manifestations of thyrotoxicosis. Radiographics. 23(4):857-69, 2003
3. Marqusee E et al: Usefulness of ultrasonography in the management of nodular thyroid disease. Ann Intern Med. 133(9):696-700, 2000

MULTINODULAR GOITER

IMAGE GALLERY

Typical

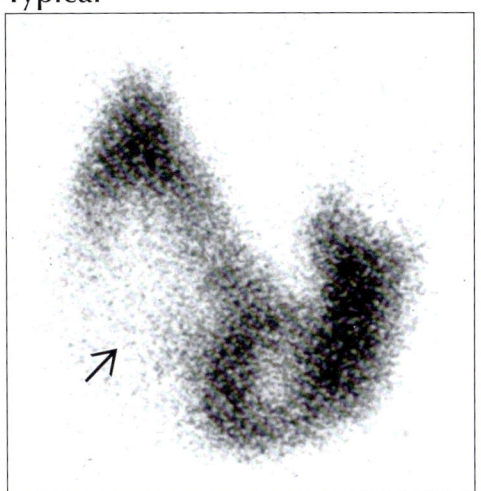

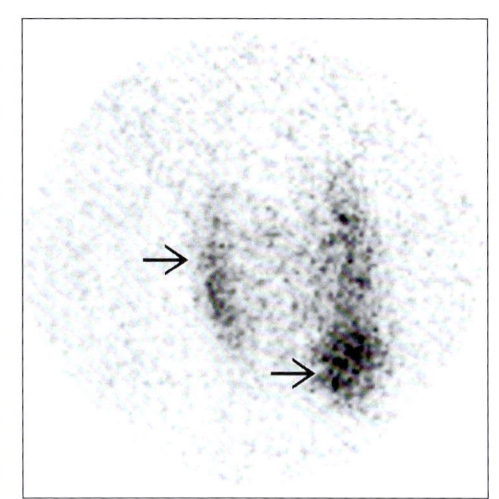

(Left) Anterior I-123 thyroid scan showing multinodular goiter with dominant cold nodule ➔ which was papillary thyroid cancer on biopsy. *(Right)* Anterior I-123 thyroid scan shows patchy heterogeneous uptake ➔ in a patient with MNG. This pattern often seen in older patients or end-stage MNG.

Variant

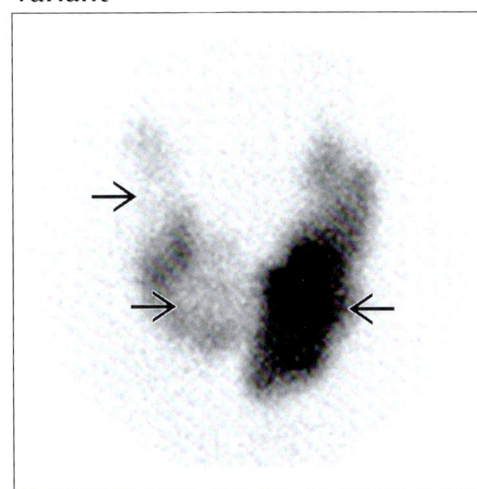

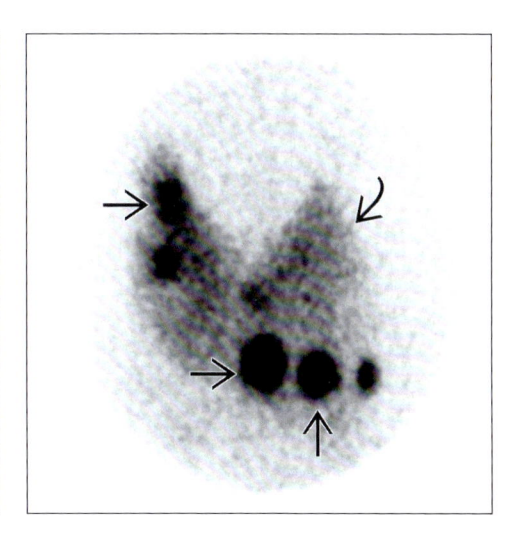

(Left) Anterior I-333 thyroid scan shows asymmetrically increased uptake with nodularity ➔ in patient with MNG. *(Right)* Anterior I-123 thyroid scan shows MNG with predominantly hot nodules ➔ that do not cause suppression of normal thyroid ➔.

Typical

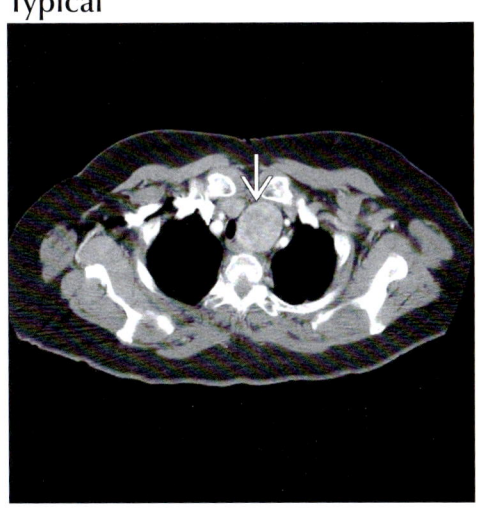

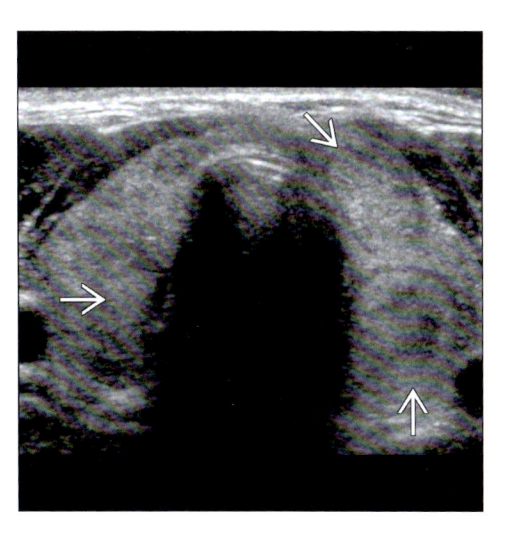

(Left) Axial CECT shows heterogeneously enhancing substernal goiter ➔ in patient with MNG. *(Right)* Transaxial ultrasound shows multiple discrete nodules ➔ in patient with MNG.

THYROID ADENOMA, HYPERFUNCTIONING

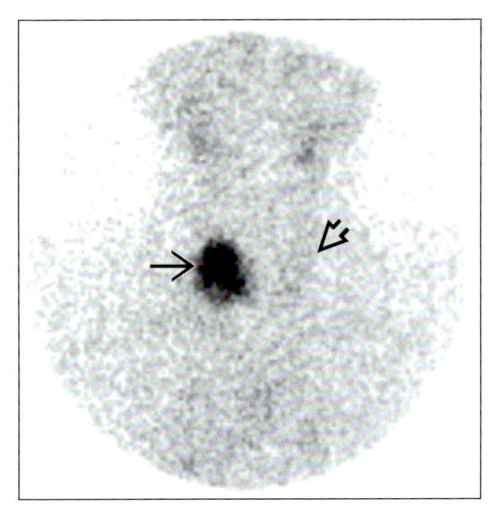

Anterior thyroid scan shows large hot nodule ➡ in right thyroid lobe. Note little uptake in normal thyroid tissue ➡ as thyroid hormone released by toxic nodule suppresses TSH, inhibiting radiotracer uptake.

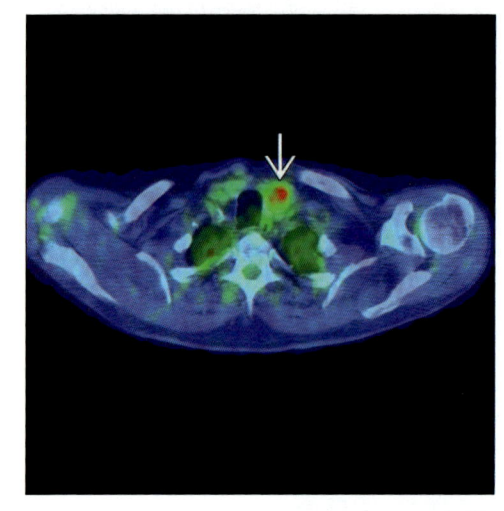

Axial fused PET/CT shows FDG avid thyroid nodule ➡. The differential for such nodules includes thyroid cancer, MNG, and benign adenoma (as in this case).

TERMINOLOGY

Abbreviations and Synonyms
- Plummer disease: Solitary toxic nodule or toxic multinodular goiter (MNG)

Definitions
- Follicular adenomas: Neoplasms arising from epithelial cells; usually well-encapsulated, benign, autonomous
  - Thyrotoxicosis results from hyperfunctioning nodule releasing thyroid hormone
  - 15-40% of thyroid nodules
  - Most nodules are not adenomas but are hyperplasia: Non-neoplastic adenomatous hyperplasia; usually poorly encapsulated, focal adenomatous/colloidal

IMAGING FINDINGS

General Features
- Best diagnostic clue
  - Large solitary nodule with ↑ activity (hot)
  - Little or no uptake in remaining thyroid
- Size: Usually > 2-3 cm

Nuclear Medicine Findings
- I-123 or Tc-99m pertechnetate scan: Single, usually large hot nodule; minimal or no activity in remaining thyroid
  - Overall cancer risk in hot nodule < 4% (< 1% in hyperthyroid patient with toxic hot nodule)
- If remaining thyroid unsuppressed, nodule better described as warm (not hot)
  - Patients usually euthyroid = nontoxic nodule
  - Caution: Hot or warm nodules on Tc-99m pertechnetate scan that do not suppress remaining thyroid may be discordantly cold on I-123
    - Discordant nodules: Same risk of cancer as other cold nodules (~ 15-20%)
- Palpable nodules not evident on scan = indeterminate
  - Have cancer risk similar to cold nodule
- Multinodular goiter (MNG)
  - Multiple nodules, > 1 hot nodule

CT Findings
- NECT
  - Well-circumscribed hypodense nodule
  - Often incidental finding
- CECT

DDx: Thyrotoxicosis with Nodules

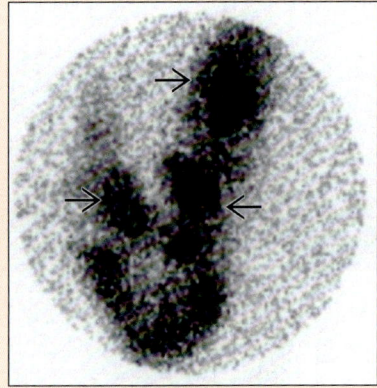

Toxic Multinodular Goiter 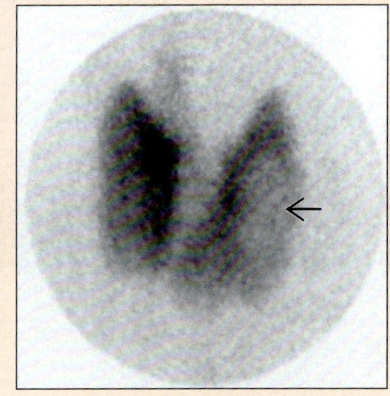 | Graves + Cystic Nodule 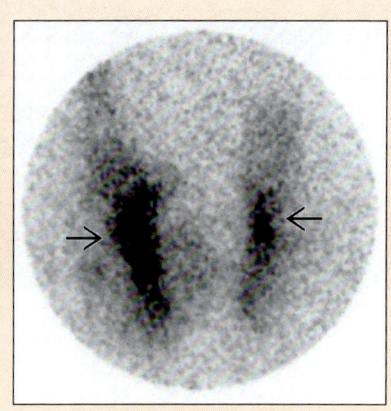 | Hashimoto Thyroiditis

THYROID ADENOMA, HYPERFUNCTIONING

Key Facts

Terminology
- Plummer disease: Solitary toxic nodule or toxic multinodular goiter (MNG)
- Follicular adenomas: Neoplasms arising from epithelial cells; usually well-encapsulated, benign, autonomous
- Thyrotoxicosis results from hyperfunctioning nodule releasing thyroid hormone

Imaging Findings
- I-123 or Tc-99m pertechnetate scan: Single, usually large hot nodule; minimal or no activity in remaining thyroid
- Overall cancer risk in hot nodule < 4% (< 1% in hyperthyroid patient with toxic hot nodule)

Top Differential Diagnoses
- Toxic Multinodular Goiter
- Graves Disease
- Hashimoto Thyroiditis
- Unilobar Thyroid Agenesis
- Thyroid Cancer
- Subacute Thyroiditis

Clinical Issues
- Medical therapy: Thyroid-blocking propylthiouracil (PTU) or methimazole
- Often used to achieve protective euthyroid state before radioiodine ablation, thyroidectomy
- Radioiodine ablation: 25-30 mCi (925-1110 MBq) I-131 usually effective
- Surgical treatment: Lobectomy or nodule excision

- Hypodense enhancing nodule
- May appear similar to MNG
- Enhancement varies with size (large nodules can degenerate)

MR Findings
- T1WI
  - Iso- to hypointense
  - Hemorrhage may cause hyperintensity
  - Often incidental finding
- T2WI: Classically hyperintense

Other Modality Findings
- FDG PET: Focal accumulation in benign and malignant nodules
  - Risk of malignancy ≤ 50%; biopsy under ultrasound
  - FDG avid benign adenomas: Most often nontoxic, part of MNG

Ultrasonographic Findings
- Grayscale Ultrasound
  - Small nodules: Isoechoic or hypoechoic
  - Larger nodules: Heterogeneous
  - Well circumscribed, hypoechoic ring (halo sign) typical
  - Hemorrhage may ⇒ calcifications
  - Microcalcifications raise suspicion for malignancy
- Color Doppler: ↑ Blood flow (greater at periphery)

Imaging Recommendations
- Best imaging tool: Tc-99m pertechnetate or I-123 thyroid scan
- Protocol advice
  - Hold thyroid-blocking medications 5-7 days
  - Delay scan 6-8 weeks after IV iodinated contrast (e.g., CECT)
  - Thyroid scan dose
    - Tc-99m pertechnetate: 3-5 mCi (111-185 MBq) IV; imaging at 20 minutes
    - I-123: 200-400 µCi (7.4-14.8 MBq) po; images at 4-6 or 24 hrs
  - Extend patient's neck
  - Image with anterior pinhole collimator
    - Anterior, RAO, LAO
    - Mark palpable nodule(s) and obtain additional image
- Additional nuclear medicine imaging options
  - Thyroid uptake measurement with 5-10 µCi (185-370 KBq) I-131 po
    - Measure at 4-6 hrs with probe (24 hr uptake not usually needed)
    - May be only mildly increased, high-normal
    - Less helpful in I-131 therapy planning than with Graves, MNG: Dose often empirically chosen
    - Successful therapy: High and often multiple I-131 doses, usually ≥ 25 mCi (925 MBq)

DIFFERENTIAL DIAGNOSIS

Toxic Multinodular Goiter
- Thyrotoxicosis + nodules (adenomatous hyperplasia and adenomas)
- May present with one dominant or palpable lesion
- Smaller nodules often clinically inapparent

Graves Disease
- May present with palpable mass from goiter, superimposed nodule, cyst

Hashimoto Thyroiditis
- Usually low, normal thyroid function tests
- 5% develop Hashitoxicosis
- May be nodular in later stages

Unilobar Thyroid Agenesis
- Presents as unilateral mass in euthyroid patient

Thyroid Cancer
- Palpable nodule, mass in euthyroid patient
- Usually cold on thyroid scan
- Thyroid cancer + hyperthyroidism rare

Subacute Thyroiditis
- Post-viral autoimmune thyrotoxicosis
- No nodules

THYROID ADENOMA, HYPERFUNCTIONING

PATHOLOGY

General Features
- Etiology
  - Acquired mutations in TSH receptor ⇒ ↑ thyroid activation
  - ↑ Toxicity of thyroid nodules in iodine-deficient regions
- Epidemiology
  - Palpable nodules: 5-7% females and 1-2% males (most asymptomatic)
    - Toxic nodular goiter: 58% of cases; leading cause of hyperthyroidism in endemic regions
    - Solitary toxic nodule: 10% of cases
  - In US, Graves disease is most common cause of hyperthyroidism with toxic nodular goiter (15-30%)

Gross Pathologic & Surgical Features
- Well-encapsulated, firm nodule

Microscopic Features
- Variably sized thyroid follicles (macro and microfollicles)
- Hemorrhage
- Fibrosis
- Calcification
- Cystic degeneration

CLINICAL ISSUES

Presentation
- Most common signs/symptoms
  - Weight loss
  - Palpitations
  - Tachycardia
  - Heat intolerance
  - Amenorrhea
  - Unilateral palpable thyroid nodule
  - Minimal thyroid tissue palpable on contralateral side
- Other signs/symptoms
  - Elderly may present with only cardiac disease
    - Atrial fibrillation
    - Congestive heart failure

Demographics
- Age
  - Middle-age
  - Toxicity usually 4th-6th decades
- Gender: M < F = 1:3

Natural History & Prognosis
- Initially, follicular adenomas small, asymptomatic, slow-growing
- Larger nodules begin to function autonomously
  - Independent of TSH stimulation
  - No longer suppressed by T3 suppression test
- Some autonomous nodules function at very high level ⇒ thyrotoxicosis
  - Usually euthyroid until nodule 2.5-3.0 cm
  - Increased endogenous T4/T3 ↓ TSH release by pituitary feedback mechanisms
  - Decreased TSH ⇒ normal thyroid tissue suppression
- Prognosis good with treatment
- Rare risk of malignancy in toxic nodules (< 1%)

Treatment
- Medical therapy: Thyroid-blocking propylthiouracil (PTU) or methimazole
  - Often used to achieve protective euthyroid state before radioiodine ablation, thyroidectomy
  - Usually only successful in short term (thyrotoxicosis almost always recurs)
- Radioiodine ablation: 25-30 mCi (925-1110 MBq) I-131 usually effective
  - More radio-resistant than Graves
    - Higher I-131 doses used
    - May require multiple treatments
  - Risk of thyroid crisis/storm after treatment
    - Beta blocker or thyroid-blocking medications protective
  - Postablative hypothyroidism
    - Occurs less frequently than with Graves treatment
    - Suppressed thyroid relatively protected
    - < 10% of patients hypothyroid by 5 years
- Surgical treatment: Lobectomy or nodule excision
  - Common therapy for large toxic nodules
  - More successful treatment of solitary toxic nodules than MNG, Graves
  - Recurrent thyrotoxicosis, hypothyroidism after surgery very rare

DIAGNOSTIC CHECKLIST

Consider
- Toxic nodule usually refers to one hyperfunctioning nodule
- Multiple nodules = MNG
- Higher I-131 doses required, as toxic nodule relatively radioresistant
  - ≥ 25 mCi (925 MBq) I-131
- Only ~ 1 in 10 patients become hypothyroid as suppressed thyroid tissue protected from I-131 uptake
- Surgical treatment common for large toxic nodules

SELECTED REFERENCES
1. Erdogan MF et al: Effect of radioiodine therapy on thyroid nodule size and function in patients with toxic adenomas. Nucl Med Commun. 25(11):1083-7, 2004
2. Erdogan MF et al: Effect of radioiodine therapy on thyroid nodule size and function in patients with toxic adenomas. Nucl Med Commun. 25(11):1083-7, 2004
3. Pacini F et al: Management of thyroid nodules: a clinicopathological, evidence-based approach. Eur J Nucl Med Mol Imaging. 31(10):1443-9, 2004
4. Pacini F et al: Management of thyroid nodules: a clinicopathological, evidence-based approach. Eur J Nucl Med Mol Imaging. 31(10):1443-9, 2004
5. Burch HB et al: Diagnosis and management of the autonomously functioning thyroid nodule: the Walter Reed Army Medical Center experience, 1975-1996. Thyroid. 8(10):871-80, 1998

THYROID ADENOMA, HYPERFUNCTIONING

IMAGE GALLERY

Other

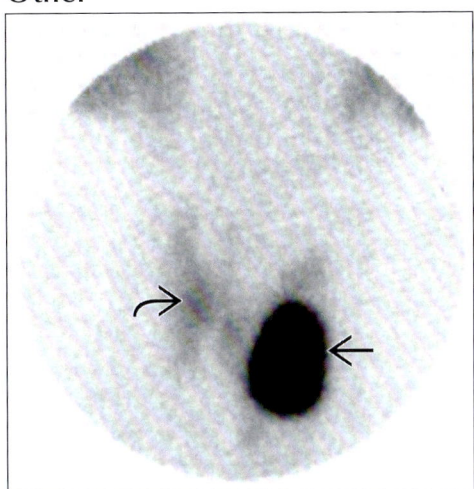

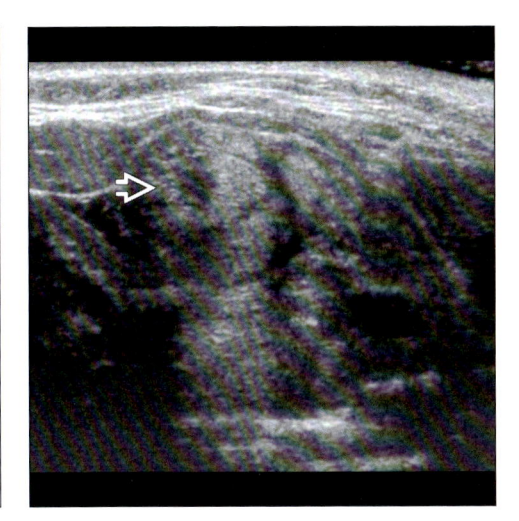

(Left) Anterior thyroid scan shows large toxic nodule ➡ in left thyroid lobe with moderate suppression of remaining thyroid ➡ in hyperthyroid patient. *(Right)* Transverse ultrasound shows heterogeneous, well-circumscribed nodule ➡, consistent with toxic adenoma in a hyperthyroid patient.

Typical

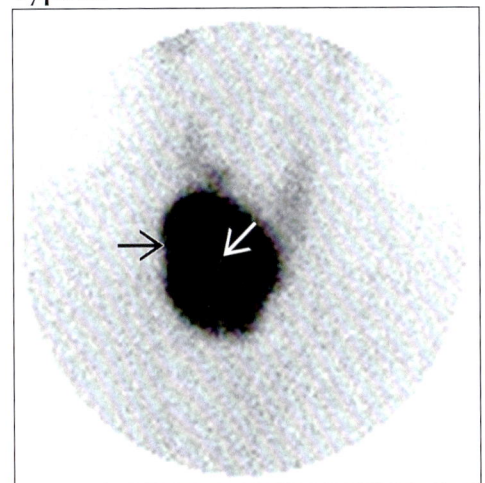

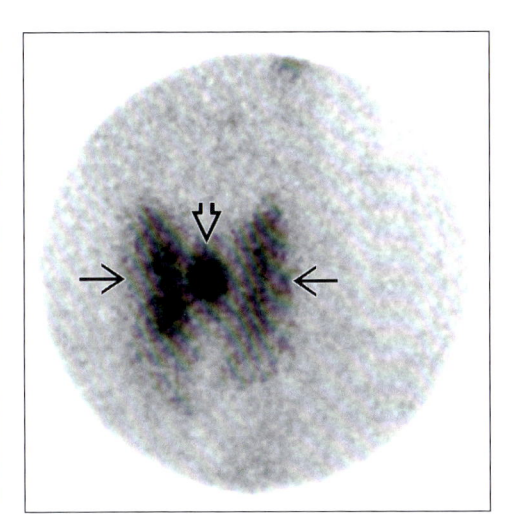

(Left) Anterior thyroid scan shows large autonomous adenoma ➡ with central degeneration ➡, more common in larger nodules. *(Right)* Anterior thyroid scan shows focal hot nodule ➡ that does not suppress surrounding thyroid ➡. While this nodule may be autonomous, it is not toxic.

Variant

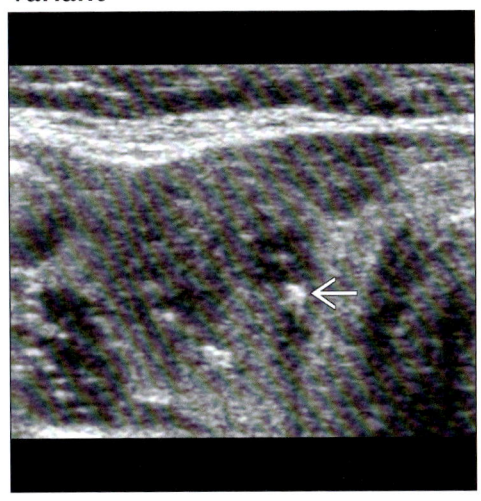

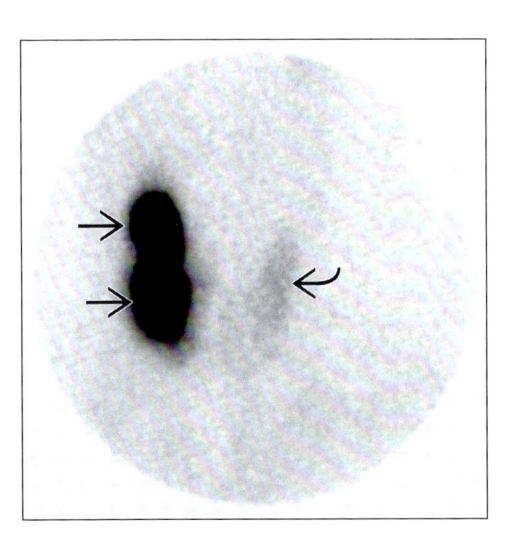

(Left) Transaxial ultrasound shows thyroid nodule with microcalcifications ➡, raising concern for thyroid malignancy instead of autonomous nodule. *(Right)* Anterior thyroid scan shows two hot nodules ➡ in right thyroid that suppress uptake in left thyroid lobe ➡. While they are toxic, when > 1 nodule present, MNG is more appropriate term.

SUBACUTE THYROIDITIS

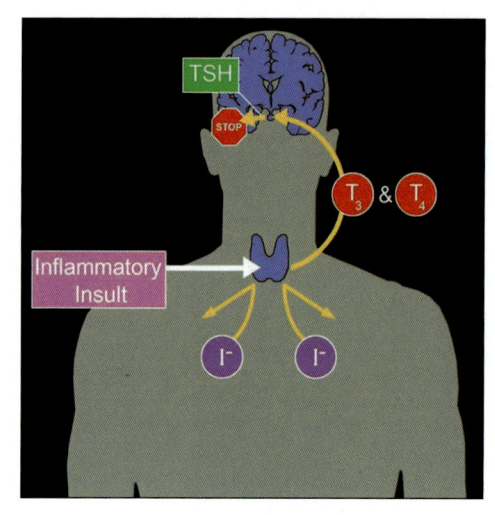

Diagrammatic graphic of subacute thyroiditis effects.

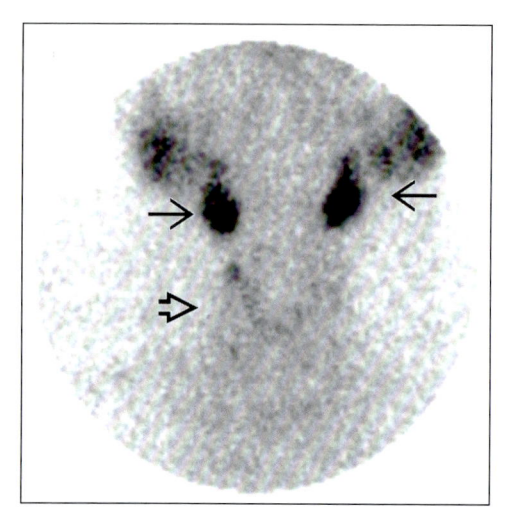

Anterior thyroid scan shows nearly absent thyroid activity ⇨ with normal salivary activity → in patient with subacute thyroiditis.

TERMINOLOGY

Abbreviations and Synonyms
- Subacute thyroiditis (SAT)
- Subacute granulomatous thyroiditis (SGT): de Quervain thyroiditis, painful thyroiditis
- Subacute lymphocytic thyroiditis (SLT): Painless/silent thyroiditis, postpartum lymphocytic thyroiditis
- Radioactive iodine (RAI)

Definitions
- Inflammatory thyroid disorder with 3-phase clinical course
  - Transient hyperthyroidism from preformed thyroid hormone release
  - Hypothyroidism
  - Spontaneous return to euthyroidism
- Two main subgroups
  - SGT
    - Associated with viral infection
    - de Quervain or painful thyroiditis
  - SLT
    - Appears to be autoimmune-mediated
    - Painless, silent thyroiditis
  - Postpartum thyroiditis: Similar to SLT, typically 1-6 months postpartum

IMAGING FINDINGS

General Features
- Best diagnostic clue: Very low thyroid RAI uptake + clinical hyperthyroidism

Nuclear Medicine Findings
- In acute phase SAT, thyroid RAI uptake very low (often < 1% at 24 hours)
  - Uptake key to differentiating SAT from other causes of hyperthyroidism (e.g., Graves)
  - Uptake improves with recovery phase, eventually normalizes
  - RAI therapy contraindicated (self-limited disease)
- Thyroid scan shows very low, absent thyroid activity in early SAT
  - Most common: Thyroid diffusely involved
  - Can occur in one lobe
  - Can show patchy activity in less severe, recovery phase of SAT

DDx: Thyrotoxicosis

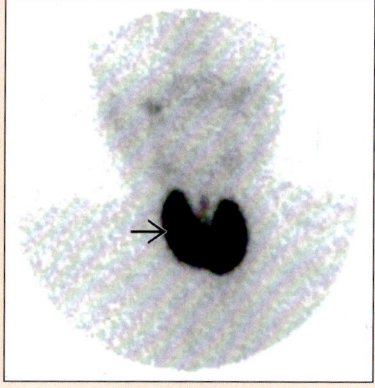

Graves Disease

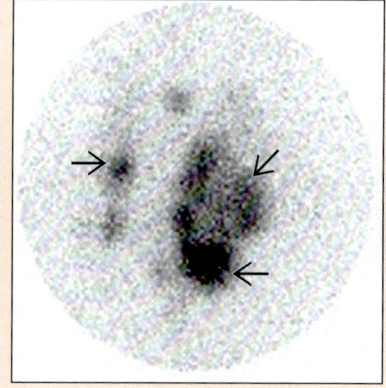

Multinodular Goiter

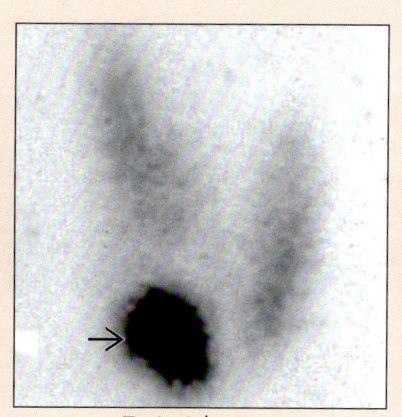

Toxic Adenoma

SUBACUTE THYROIDITIS

Key Facts

Terminology
- Subacute thyroiditis (SAT)
- Inflammatory thyroid disorder with 3-phase clinical course

Imaging Findings
- Best diagnostic clue: Very low thyroid RAI uptake + clinical hyperthyroidism
- In acute phase SAT, thyroid RAI uptake very low (often < 1% at 24 hours)
- Uptake key to differentiating SAT from other causes of hyperthyroidism (e.g., Graves)
- Uptake improves with recovery phase, eventually normalizes
- RAI therapy contraindicated (self-limited disease)
- Thyroid scan shows very low, absent thyroid activity in early SAT

Top Differential Diagnoses
- Graves Disease
- Toxic Multinodular Goiter & Toxic Adenoma
- Hashimoto Disease
- Infiltrative Thyroid Diseases
- Acute Thyroiditis
- Iatrogenic Factors

Diagnostic Checklist
- Major cause of hyperthyroidism with very low uptake
- Important to distinguish from other causes of hyperthyroidism because RAI therapy contraindicated
- Most often, low thyroid uptake enough to diagnose SAT
- Uptake may be normal in recovery phase of SAT
- Thyroid scan necessary only in diagnostic dilemmas

CT Findings
- NECT
  - Normal: Thyroid hyperdense due to concentration of iodine
  - SAT: Thyroid slightly less dense than normal, may be unrecognized if clinical history unknown
- CECT: Moderate thyroid enhancement in early SAT

MR Findings
- T1WI: Slightly increased signal in early SAT
- T2WI: Markedly increased T2 signal with early SAT

Ultrasonographic Findings
- Grayscale Ultrasound
  - Acute phase: Hypoechoic, nonechoic regions 2° inflammation, tissue damage
  - Recovery phase: Isoechoic with slight increased vascularity; resolution of hypoechoic regions
- Color Doppler
  - Slight increase in overall flow
  - Absent vascularity in nonechoic regions

Imaging Recommendations
- Best imaging tool
  - Thyroid uptake
  - Scan often not necessary
- Protocol advice
  - Exclude iatrogenic causes for false positive (low uptake) study
    - Delay study 6-8 weeks following IV iodinated contrast (e.g., CECT)
    - Stop thyroid-blocking medications (propylthiouracil or methimazole) 5-7 days
    - Stop thyroid replacement, if any: 4-6 weeks for thyroxine (T4), 2-3 weeks for triiodothyronine (T3) effects to clear
  - Thyroid uptake measurement 4, 24 hours after radioiodine
    - 100-400 μCi (3.7-14.8 MBq) I-123 po for uptake; scan also possible at 4 hours, if needed
    - 5-10 μCi (0.19-0.37 MBq) I-131 po for uptake
  - Thyroid scan
    - Very low uptake measurements (1-5%) virtually diagnostic of SAT; scan only if diagnosis unclear
    - Uptake dose of I-123 can also be used for scan
    - Tc-99m pertechnetate: 3-5 mCi (111-185 MBq), image at 20 min (after I-123 uptake measurement)
- Additional nuclear medicine imaging options
  - Tc-99m sestamibi, Tc-99m tetrofosmin and Thallium-201: Diffusely increased thyroid uptake with delayed washout in acute SAT

DIFFERENTIAL DIAGNOSIS

Graves Disease
- Hyperthyroidism + high uptake measurement (> 50-80%)

Toxic Multinodular Goiter & Toxic Adenoma
- Hyperthyroidism + normal to elevated thyroid uptake

Hashimoto Disease
- Hyperthyroidism or Hashitoxicosis may develop < 5% of cases
- Thyroid uptake may be low with hypothyroidism, elevated with hyperthyroidism

Infiltrative Thyroid Diseases
- Lymphoma, leukemia, amyloid, tuberculosis, metastatic adenocarcinoma may present with enlarged thyroid, hyperthyroidism

Acute Thyroiditis
- Suppurative thyroid disease: Patients have fever, ↑ white blood count
- More common in immunocompromised patients

Iatrogenic Factors
- Amiodarone may ⇒ hyperthyroidism, hypothyroidism lasting weeks to months (iodine effect, follicular cell injury)
- Iodinated contrast: Low RAI uptake after IV contrast; may ⇒ hyperthyroidism (Jod-Basedow iodine effect)
- Thyroiditis factitia: Exogenous thyroid hormone ingestion may ⇒ hyperthyroidism, low RAI uptake

SUBACUTE THYROIDITIS

- Thyroid trauma (biopsy, surgery, seatbelt injury, vigorous palpation) ⇒ transient thyroid hormone release
- Interferon and radiation therapy can induce thyroiditis

PATHOLOGY

General Features
- Etiology
  - Inflammatory process with cellular infiltration of thyroid
    - Causes follicular cell destruction, thyroid hormone release
  - SGT associated with viral upper respiratory illness
    - Many viruses implicated: Mumps, coxsackievirus, adenovirus, measles, influenza
  - SLT: Part of spectrum of autoimmune thyroid disorders
    - Often considered a variant of Hashimoto disease
- Epidemiology: 20-25% hyperthyroidism, 10% hypothyroidism caused by SAT

Microscopic Features
- Inflammatory cell infiltrates, predominantly lymphocytes
- Disrupted follicular cells around colloid
- SGT also contains numerous multinucleated giant cells

CLINICAL ISSUES

Presentation
- Most common signs/symptoms
  - SGT: Enlarged painful thyroid gland and markedly elevated erythrocyte sedimentation rate
  - SLT: Nontender, mild thyromegaly
- Other signs/symptoms
  - Hyperthyroidism
    - Nervousness
    - Heat intolerance
    - Weight loss
    - Palpitations
    - Sinus tachycardia
    - Atrial fibrillation
  - Hypothyroidism
    - Often mild, asymptomatic

Demographics
- Age: May occur at any age
- Gender: M < F (1:2 in SLT; 1:5 in SGT)

Natural History & Prognosis
- Hyperthyroidism usually lasts < 2-3 months
- Hypothyroidism follows, typically lasting 2-4 months
  - Increased circulating thyroid hormone prevents iodine uptake and new hormone synthesis by suppressing TSH
  - Depletion of preformed hormone in colloid may also occur
- 90-95% euthyroid within 6 months (hypothyroidism occasionally permanent)
- Relapsing clinical course not infrequent in SAT

Treatment
- RAI therapy contraindicated
  - With SAT, hyperthyroidism self-limited
  - Important to distinguish from Graves disease, which is treated with RAI
- Thyroid blocking thioamides (propylthiouracil and methimazole) not indicated
  - Symptoms caused by excess hormone release not increased synthesis
- Symptomatic treatment for neck pain
  - Often only treatment needed
  - Non-steroidal pain medication occasionally sufficient
    - Acetaminophen
    - Ibuprofen
  - Prednisone 40-60 mg po QD often needed for 4-6 weeks
  - Aspirin contraindicated
    - May ↑ symptoms by displacing thyroid hormone from thyroid binding globulin
- Thyrotoxicosis may require beta blockers
  - Control arrhythmia, tachycardia
  - Propranolol until symptoms abate
    - 10-40 mg po q4-8 hours
- Iodine decreases peripheral conversion of T4 to T3 (more active)
  - Saturated solution of potassium iodide (SSKI)
    - 2 drops in water po TID
    - Administer dose of oral iodinated contrast agent (iopanoic acid or ipodate)
  - May improve thyrotoxicosis symptoms if beta blockers not tolerated
- Thyroid hormone replacement
  - If transient or permanent hypothyroidism
  - Thyroxine

DIAGNOSTIC CHECKLIST

Consider
- Major cause of hyperthyroidism with very low uptake
- Important to distinguish from other causes of hyperthyroidism because RAI therapy contraindicated
- Most often, low thyroid uptake enough to diagnose SAT
- Uptake may be normal in recovery phase of SAT
- Thyroid scan necessary only in diagnostic dilemmas

Image Interpretation Pearls
- In cases of no radiopharmaceutical uptake by thyroid, double-check to exclude causes of iatrogenic false positive scan
- Although usually affects both thyroid lobes, SAT can be confined to one lobe

SELECTED REFERENCES
1. Cooper DS: Hyperthyroidism. Lancet. 362(9382):459-68, 2003
2. Intenzo CM et al: Clinical, laboratory, and scintigraphic manifestations of subacute and chronic thyroiditis. Clin Nucl Med. 18(4):302-6, 1993

SUBACUTE THYROIDITIS

IMAGE GALLERY

Typical

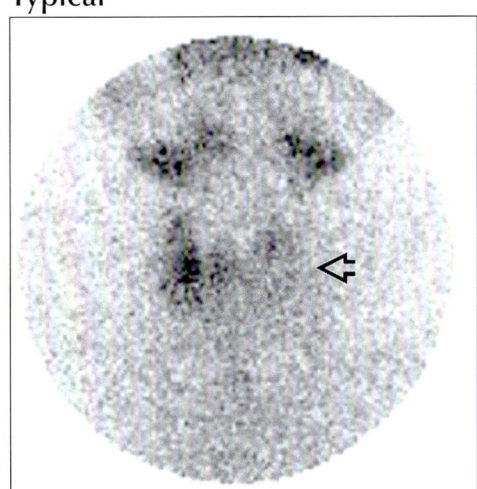

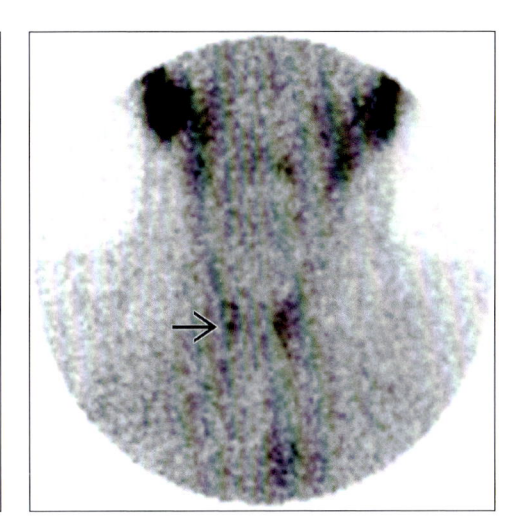

(Left) Anterior thyroid scan shows subacute thyroiditis confined to left thyroid lobe ⇨. This could be mistaken for cold nodule if clinical history, low radioactive iodine uptake not known. *(Right)* Anterior thyroid scan with Tc-99m pertechnetate. Thyroid uptake → in this patient with subacute thyroiditis is very low.

Typical

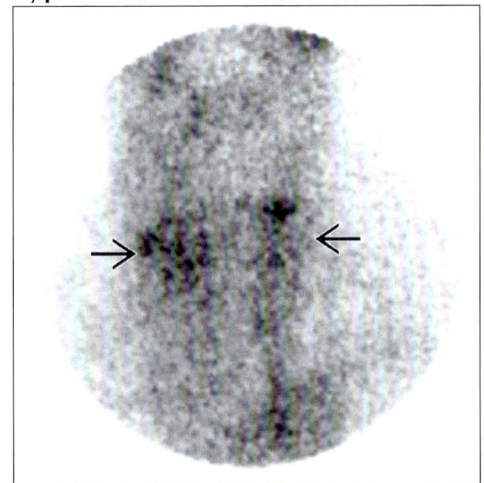

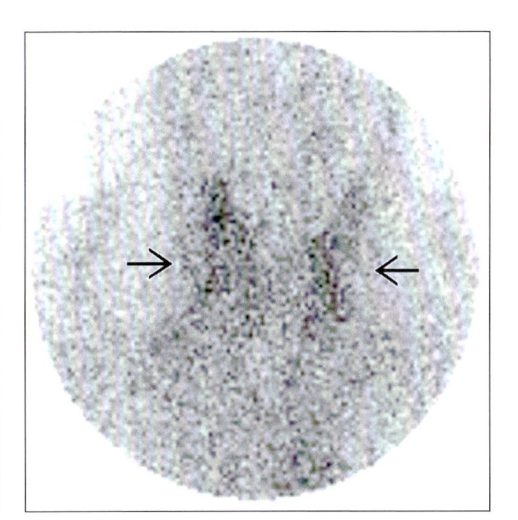

(Left) Anterior thyroid scan shows patchy uptake in thyroid → during early recovery from subacute thyroiditis. *(Right)* Anterior thyroid scan shows diffuse, low-level thyroid uptake →, which may be seen in mild or recovery phase of subacute thyroiditis.

Other

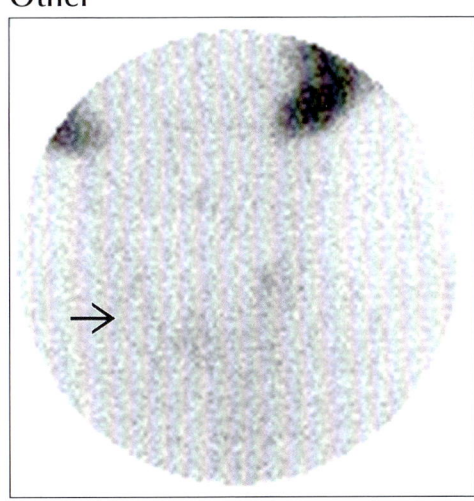

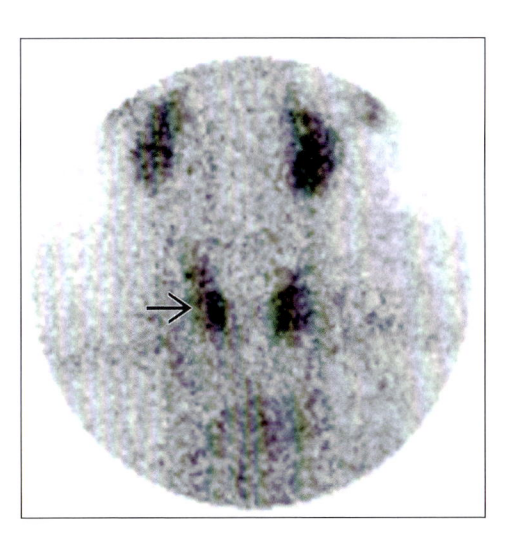

(Left) Anterior thyroid scan shows little thyroid uptake → due to recent IV administration of CT contrast. The effects of iodinated contrast can mimic appearance of subacute thyroiditis. *(Right)* Anterior thyroid scan in patient with amiodarone-induced thyrotoxicosis shows low-normal thyroid uptake →. The appearance of amiodarone-induced thyroid disease varies and may be difficult to distinguish from subacute thyroiditis.

I-131 HYPERTHYROID THERAPY

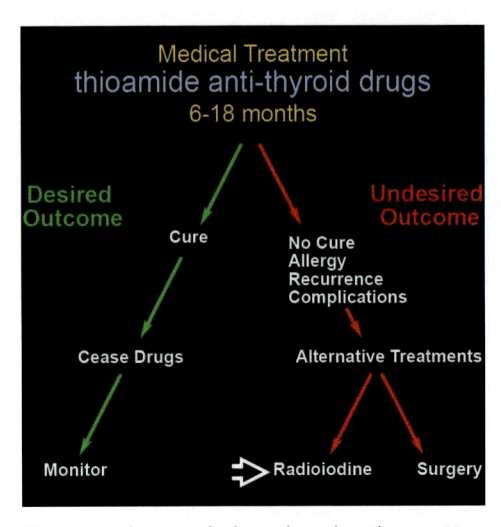

Decision-making tree for hyperthyroidism therapy. Note I-131 therapy ⇨ usually performed after trial of anti-thyroid drugs.

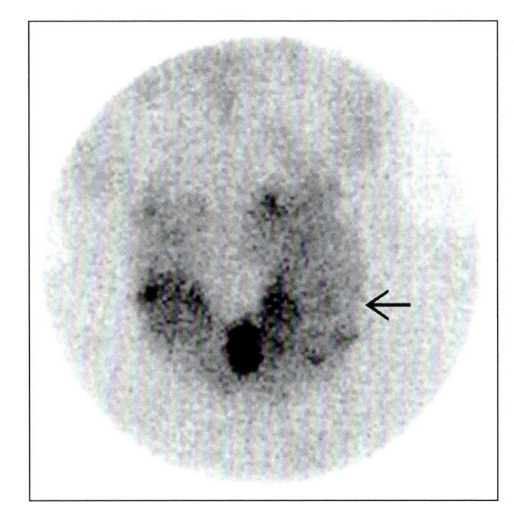

Anterior thyroid scan shows toxic multinodular goiter ⇨. Large nodular goiters are more difficult to treat with I-131. Even high doses may not reduce compressive symptoms.

TERMINOLOGY

Synonyms
- Radioiodine (RAI) therapy
- Thyroid ablation

Definitions
- Hyperthyroidism: ↑ Circulating thyroid hormone (thyrotoxicosis) from diseases that increase hormone production/release
- I-131 therapy: Targeted thyroid follicular cell destruction for hyperthyroidism caused by Graves disease, autonomous nodules, nodular goiters

PRE-PROCEDURE

Indications
- Graves disease (diffuse toxic goiter)
  - Responds well to RAI, favored therapy in US
  - Diffusely increased activity with radioiodine uptake (RAIU) usually very high (> 50-80%)
- Multinodular goiter (MNG)
  - May be asymptomatic requiring no therapy or cause hyperthyroidism (toxic nodular goiter)
  - Thyroid scan: Multiple hot and/or cold nodules, RAIU varies from normal to moderately elevated
  - Subclinical hyperthyroidism (↓ TSH, normal T4) may require treatment where risk of side effects high (e.g., elderly)
- Toxic adenoma (TA)
  - Autonomously hyperfunctioning adenomatous tumor
  - Scan shows one hot nodule suppressing remaining thyroid, RAIU normal to ↑

Contraindications
- Pregnancy
  - I-131 crosses placenta with fetal thyroid concentration beginning 10-12th gestational week
  - I-131 administration can ⇒ fetal death, hypothyroidism
- Breastfeeding
  - Breastfeeding patients must be counseled to terminate breastfeeding and wait 2 months before RAI to avoid radiation dose to breasts
  - Breastfeeding cannot be resumed post RAI therapy
  - Breastfeeding future offspring OK
- Low RAIU thyrotoxicosis etiologies are not treated with I-131
  - Subacute thyroiditis: Self-limited post-inflammatory process may be difficult to diagnose clinically but is differentiated by ↓↓ RAIU
  - Drug-induced thyrotoxicosis
    - Thyroiditis factitia: Prescribed or surreptitiously ingested thyroid hormone ⇒ clinical hyperthyroidism but ↓↓ RAIU
    - Amiodarone: May cause hyperthyroidism (up to 10%) lasting months
    - Iodine-induced hyperthyroidism: Usually due to IV contrast in patients with MNG, endemic goiter
- Hashitoxicosis: Rare hyperthyroidism in early Hashimoto disease
  - Diagnosis usually made clinically; ↑ thyroid antibodies

Getting Started
- Things to Check
  - Diagnosis clearly established by physical exam, lab findings, overall clinical picture
    - Suppressed TSH < 0.1 mU/L most sensitive test, ↑ thyroid hormone (T4 and T3) varies
    - RAIU (I-123 or I-131) to confirm diagnosis or aid I-131 therapy planning
    - RAIU normal values vary by lab: 4-6 hr ~ 5-15%, and 24 hr ~ 10-30%

I-131 HYPERTHYROID THERAPY

Key Facts

Terminology
- Radioiodine (RAI) therapy
- I-131 therapy: Targeted thyroid follicular cell destruction for hyperthyroidism caused by Graves disease, autonomous nodules, nodular goiters

Procedure
- Dose determination: Depends on diagnosis, desired outcome, gland size, RAIU
- Carefully confirm patient identity, verify dose on-site in dose calibrator
- Administer therapy in isolated dosing area
- Send outpatient directly home
- Therapy report includes therapy justification, pregnancy test, informed consent, administered dose, any complications, and patient follow-up

Post-procedure
- Response to I-131 occurs slowly as stores of hormone are depleted with some response by 2-4 weeks, maximal effect by 3-4 months
- Monitor condition: Side effects more common in large glands with high RAIU
- Plan continuous surveillance for hypothyroidism

Problems & Complications
- Fetal I-131 exposure resulting in fetal demise or neonatal hypothyroidism
- Thyroid storm frequently fatal medical emergency from surgery, illness or I-131 therapy in poorly controlled hyperthyroid patients
- Nausea and vomiting
- Radiation thyroiditis

- Consider low iodine diet 10 days - 2 weeks; not commonly required
- Females of child-bearing age questioned about possible pregnancy
  - Document negative βHCG serum pregnancy test (< 24 hrs old)
  - Exceptions only with extreme care (e.g., documented hysterectomy)
- Patient understanding and cooperation
  - Legally able to participate in informed consent process
  - Able to understand and follow radiation safety instructions
  - Uses toilet independently, no incontinence
  - Incontinence/dialysis require special decisions concerning storage and disposal of contaminated material and exposure to personnel
- Outpatient therapy
  - Patient must not pose a risk to family members or caregivers
  - NRC mandates no bystander receive an exposure > 5 mSv (0.5 rem) in any year
  - Release patients: Dose rate at 1 m ≤ 0.07 mSv/hr (7 mrem/hr) or activity ≤ 1.2 GBq (33 mCi)
  - State regulations may be more stringent
- Written directive required
  - Written order includes patient name, dosage, and route of administration, dated and signed by AU for doses > 30 µCi (1.1 MBq)
- Medications
  - Do not use medications that decrease I-131 uptake
    - Iodinated contrast: 2-4 weeks after CT, up to 8 weeks others
    - Iodine-containing supplements (kelp), cough medications: 1-2 weeks
    - Thyroid hormone replacement: 4-6 weeks T4; 2-3 weeks T3
  - Antithyroid thioamide drugs: Propylthiouracil (PTU) 3-5 days; methimazole 5-7 days

Patient Consent
- Written informed consent required prior to I-131 therapy
- Both verbal and written radiation safety instructions must be given
- List I-131 side effects
- List physician emergency phone number
- Provide written document verifying radioactive therapy in case of detection by monitoring devices at secure institutions during travel/work

PROCEDURE

Procedure Steps
- Dose determination: Depends on diagnosis, desired outcome, gland size, RAIU
  - Calculated doses to deliver 80-200 µCi (2.96-7.4 MBq) per gram thyroid may be used but have no proven benefit
    - (Desired dose x gland weight) divided by RAIU fraction (% uptake/100)
    - Use higher doses for larger glands, low uptake, and Graves with rapid I-131 turnover (high RAIU at 4 hrs diminishing by 24 hrs)
  - Graves disease
    - Generally responds well to I-131
    - Empiric 5-12 mCi (185-444 MBq) doses, euthyroid state possible
    - Attempts to achieve euthyroid state may be futile as hypothyroidism typical eventually from autoimmune gland destruction
    - High doses of 15 mCi (555 MBq) result in more rapid hypothyroidism, fewer retreatments, more predictable replacement hormone timing
  - Toxic adenomas, nodular goiters
    - Require higher doses than Graves, typically by more than 50%
    - Empiric doses of 20-29 mCi (740-1073 MBq) or more are routine
    - Calculated doses use upper end of range, 200 µCi (7.4 MBq)/gram
    - Reports of recombinant TSH (rhTSH) increasing I-131 effectiveness

I-131 HYPERTHYROID THERAPY

- Carefully confirm patient identity, verify dose on-site in dose calibrator
- Prevent volatilized RAI exposure from liquid I-131
  - Use capsule dose of I-131
  - If liquid dose, open in ventilated fume hood, rapidly contain spills
- Administer therapy in isolated dosing area
- Observe for emesis 15-30 min
- Send outpatient directly home
- Check 24 hr thyroid uptake of technologists/physicians preparing or administering liquid I-131

Findings and Reporting

- Therapy report includes therapy justification, pregnancy test, informed consent, administered dose, any complications, and patient follow-up
- Medical events exposing patients to unintended radiation must be reported to the NRC, patient and referring physician for specific cases
  - Doses exceed 5 rem (0.05 Sv) effective dose equivalent or 50 rem (0.5 Sv) to an organ/skin **and** given incorrectly (wrong patient, route, agent)
  - Dose involving > 5 rem (0.05 Sv) effective dose equivalent or 50 rem (0.5 Sv) to any organ/skin **and** differs by > 20% from prescribed
  - "Misadministration" terminology no longer used

Alternative Procedures/Therapies

- Medical therapy alternative: PTU or methimazole
  - Often first line therapy or to reduce thyroid storm risk before surgery/I-131
  - Graves: Often responds initially but permanent remission low (10-34%)
  - Nodular goiter: Remission rare & up to 95% relapse in 2 years
  - Adverse effects frequent although serious complications rare
    - Allergy (rash, pruritics, fever) 1-5%, fatal agranulocytosis (0.2-0.5%), hepatitis, vasculitis, polyarthritis
- Surgical resection
  - Mortality nearly zero, other complications (hemorrhage, recurrent laryngeal nerve damage, hypocalcemia) rare, 1-4%
  - Graves and MNG: Subtotal/total thyroidectomy less effective than I-131 but used occasionally for cosmetic reasons or compressive symptoms
  - TA: Nodule resection usually curative with little risk recurrence or hypothyroidism

POST-PROCEDURE

Expected Outcome

- Response to I-131 occurs slowly as stores of hormone are depleted with some response by 2-4 weeks, maximal effect by 3-4 months
- Approximately 10% of patients require I-131 retreatment
  - 2nd dose usually higher (20-30%) and can be repeated at 3-6 months

Things To Do

- Monitor condition: Side effects more common in large glands with high RAIU
  - β-blocker (propranolol): Often used for transient ↑ hormone release without altering I-131 effects
  - Non-steroidal agents (acetaminophen) for minor neck tenderness
  - Steroids (dexamethasone): For first signs worsening neck pain or possible thyroid storm
  - May restart PTU/methimazole 2-3 days after I-131 therapy as relief is slow
- Plan continuous surveillance for hypothyroidism

PROBLEMS & COMPLICATIONS

Complications

- Most feared complication(s)
  - Fetal I-131 exposure resulting in fetal demise or neonatal hypothyroidism
  - Thyroid storm frequently fatal medical emergency from surgery, illness or I-131 therapy in poorly controlled hyperthyroid patients
    - Presents with fever, irritability, vomiting, diarrhea, and hypotension
    - Treated aggressively with fluids, β-blockers, and steroids
- Other complications
  - Nausea and vomiting
  - Radiation thyroiditis
    - Painful neck and/or transient increase hyperthyroid symptoms from hormone release and autoimmune factors
  - Hypothyroidism most frequent complication, may occur after several months or many years
    - Hypothyroidism requires life-long thyroid hormone replacement
    - Incidence in 1st year correlates with I-131 dose but occurs in majority of patients after 10-25 yrs regardless of dose
  - Worsening Graves exophthalmos rare, treated with steroids
  - Cancer
    - No increased risk of secondary cancers, including thyroid cancer or leukemia, at doses used for hyperthyroidism
    - Occasional thyroid cancer case reports suggest an association with the underlying thyroid disease/nodules rather than I-131 exposure
  - Reproduction
    - No ↓ fertility or ↑ risk of genetic diseases noted in children

SELECTED REFERENCES

1. Franklyn JA: The management of hyperthyroidism. N Engl J Med. 330(24):1731-8, 1994

I-131 HYPERTHYROID THERAPY

IMAGE GALLERY

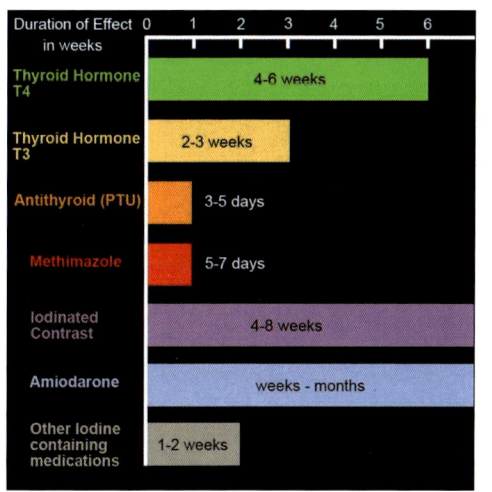

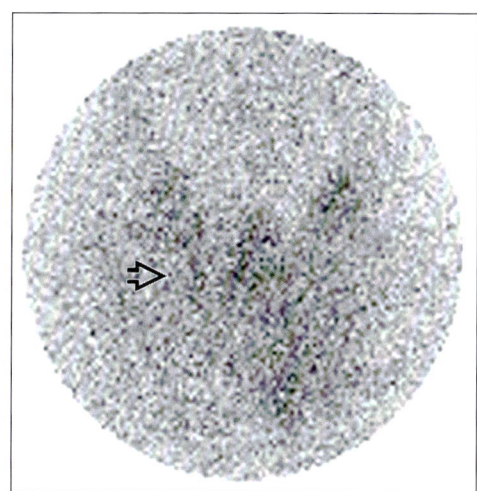

(Left) Graphic shows common iatrogenic causes of low I-131 thyroid uptake and duration of effect on I-131 uptake resulting from TSH suppression or elevated iodine stores. **(Right)** Anterior thyroid scan shows low thyroid uptake ⇨ from subacute thyroiditis. This patient did not receive I-131 therapy as Graves was excluded.

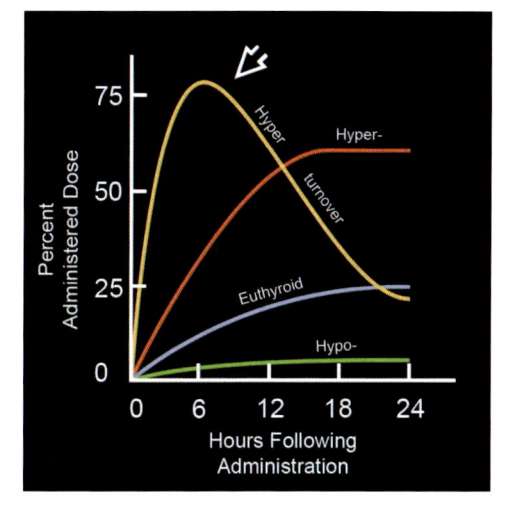

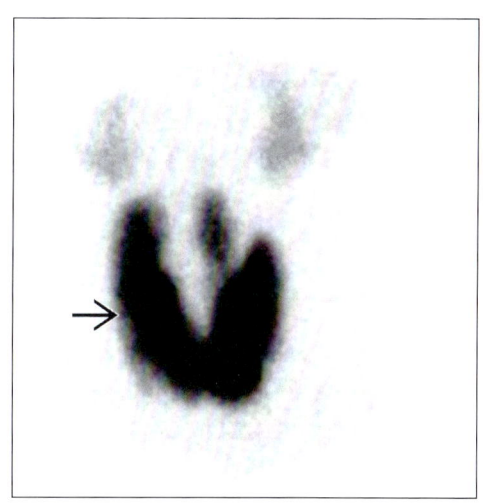

(Left) Graphic shows I-131 retention in different thyroid states. 24 hr uptakes are more accurate in Graves disease patients with a very high 4 hr uptake ⇨ as rapid washout may follow. **(Right)** Anterior thyroid scan shows marked enlargement and intense thyroid uptake → in patient with Graves disease. After I-131 therapy, these patients are at risk for thyroid storm.

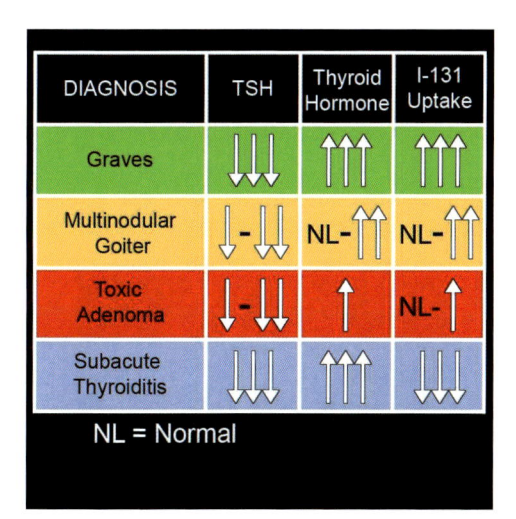

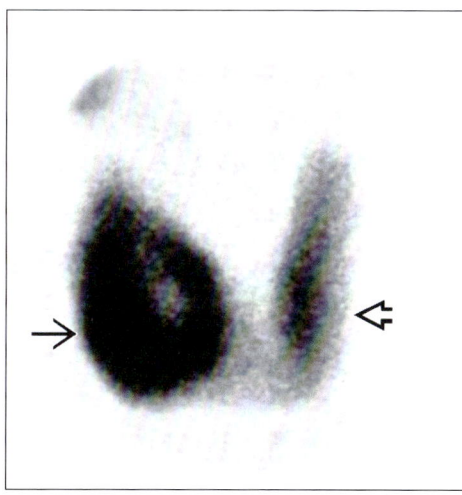

(Left) Graphic shows relationship of clinical parameters in hyperthyroidism. Note I-131 thyroid uptake differentiates subacute thyroiditis (not treated with RAI) from causes of hyperthyroidism that are treated with I-131. **(Right)** Anterior thyroid scan shows a toxic adenoma → causing suppression of remaining thyroid ⇨. Such large adenomas are most frequently treated with surgery.

ECTOPIC THYROID

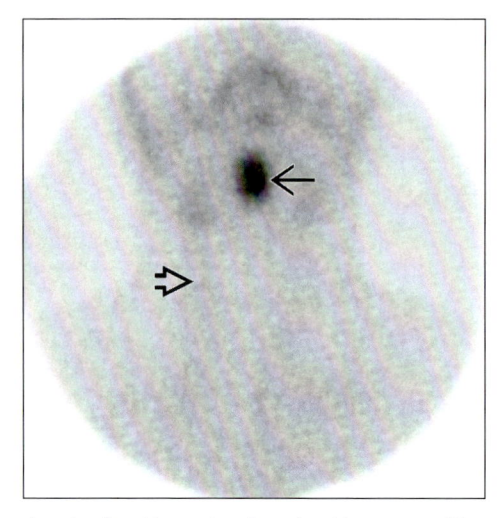

Anterior thyroid scan in a hypothyroid teenager with a lingual thyroid ➔ confirms the diagnosis. No thyroid tissue in thyroid bed ⇨.

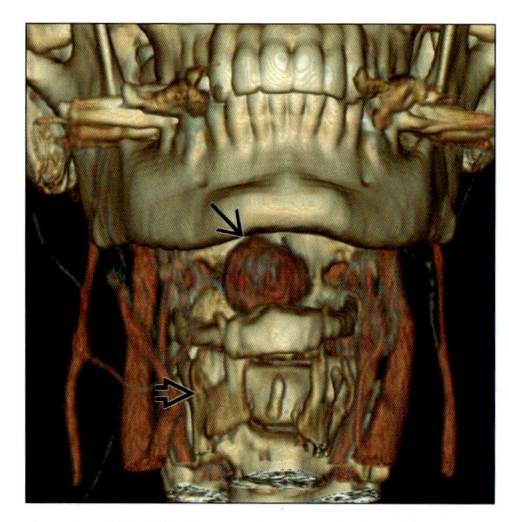

Anterior 3D MR shows absence of thyroid tissue in thyroid bed ⇨ and a well-circumscribed ectopic thyroid ➔.

TERMINOLOGY

Abbreviations and Synonyms
- Ectopic thyroid
  - Lingual thyroid
  - Sublingual thyroid
- Thyroid dysgenesis

Definitions
- Aberrantly located thyroid associated with hypothyroidism and/or mass

IMAGING FINDINGS

General Features
- Best diagnostic clue
  - Radiotracer uptake in lingual mass
  - No activity in expected thyroid location
- Location
  - Usually one focus of ectopic thyroid; may be multiple
  - Most ectopic thyroid found midline in thyroglossal duct tract
    - 90% in foramen cecum region in base of tongue
  - Atypical locations for ectopic thyroid
    - Sublingual thyroid (above hyoid, below base of tongue): Majority of remaining ectopic cases
    - Intratracheal, intralaryngeal: May cause airway compression
    - Intrapericardial
    - Intraesophageal
    - Struma ovarii
- Size: 1-3 cm

Nuclear Medicine Findings
- I-123 or Tc-99m pertechnetate thyroid scan
  - Diagnose and localize ectopic thyroid
  - Focus of activity in ectopic location (e.g., base of tongue)
  - No activity in thyroid bed
  - Ectopic thyroid = only thyroid tissue in > 70% cases
- Tc-99m sestamibi parathyroid scan
  - Tc-99m sestamibi taken up by thyroid as well as parathyroid adenoma, heart, cancers, etc.
  - May show abnormal activity in unsuspected ectopic thyroid

DDx: Masses in Floor of Mouth

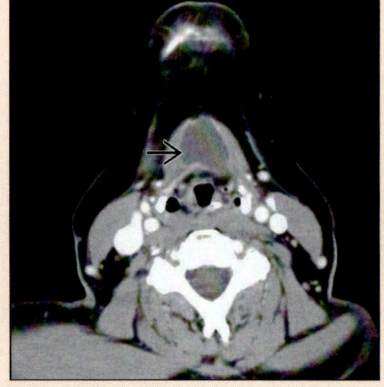

Thyroglossal Duct Cyst

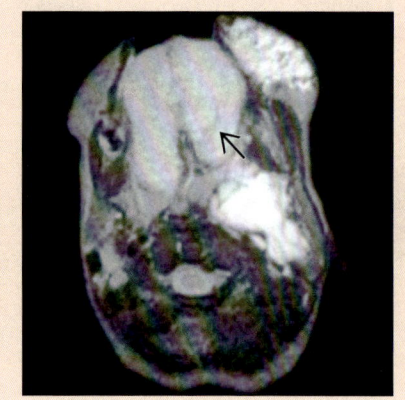

Lymphangioma

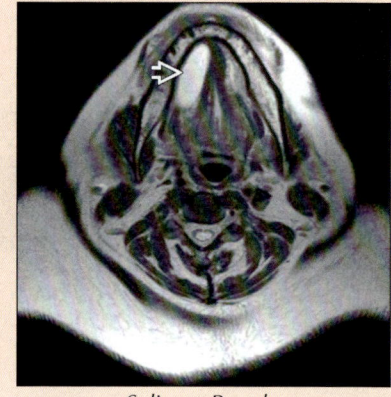

Salivary Ranula

ECTOPIC THYROID

Key Facts

Terminology
- Aberrantly located thyroid associated with hypothyroidism and/or mass

Imaging Findings
- Radiotracer uptake in lingual mass
- No activity in expected thyroid location
- Usually one focus of ectopic thyroid; may be multiple
- Most ectopic thyroid found midline in thyroglossal duct tract
- Tc-99m pertechnetate or I-123 thyroid scan
- Use marker views to confirm activity location; landmarks often unclear in infants

Top Differential Diagnoses
- Congenital Head or Neck Masses
- Thyroglossal duct cyst
- Venous vascular malformations
- Dermoid or epidermoid of tongue
- Lymphangioma
- Branchial cleft cysts
- Salivary ranula
- Primary Congenital Hypothyroidism
- Central Hypothyroidism

Clinical Issues
- Laboratory screen shows abnormally ↑ TSH
- Signs/symptoms of hypothyroidism in newborns nonspecific
- Classic hypothyroid symptoms occur later in untreated patients
- Untreated hypothyroidism ⇒ retarded growth, mental development
- Thyroid hormone replacement required

CT Findings
- NECT
  - Well-circumscribed midline mass
  - High density
- CECT
  - Well-circumscribed midline mass
  - Homogeneous dense enhancement

MR Findings
- T1WI: Hyperintense midline mass (relative to tongue)
- T2WI: Hyperintense midline mass
- T1 C+: Homogeneous enhancement of midline mass

Imaging Recommendations
- Best imaging tool
  - Tc-99m pertechnetate or I-123 thyroid scan
    - Confirms presence of ectopic thyroid
  - CECT for oropharyngeal mass assessment
    - Identifies pathology, related abnormalities (e.g., tracheal compression)
- Protocol advice
  - Stop thyroid hormone replacement prior to thyroid scan
    - 6-8 weeks for levothyroxine (T4)
    - 2-3 weeks for triiodothyronine (T3)
  - Delay scan 4-6 weeks if IV contrast recently administered (e.g., prior CECT)
  - Tc-99m pertechnetate thyroid scan
    - Adults: 3-5 mCi (111-185 MBq) IV
    - Children: 30 µCi/kg (1.1 MBq/kg) IV
    - Image at 15-20 minutes
    - Tc-99m pertechnetate preferred in infants, small children due to compliance issues with oral I-123
  - I-123 thyroid scan
    - Adults: 100-400 µCi (3.7-14.8 MBq) po
    - Children: 30-120 µCi (1.1-4.6 MBq) po
    - Image at 4-6 hours
    - 4, 24 hour uptake can also be obtained if desired
  - Images
    - Anterior parallel hole collimator image for newborns
    - Anterior pinhole collimator for magnification helpful in older patients
    - Lateral images useful to localize ectopic thyroid in anteroposterior plane
    - Consider sedation, papoose board restraint for children to reduce motion artifact
  - Use marker views to confirm activity location; landmarks often unclear in infants

DIFFERENTIAL DIAGNOSIS

Congenital Head or Neck Masses
- Thyroglossal duct cyst
  - Paramedian location
  - Most near hyoid (20-25% suprahyoid)
- Venous vascular malformations
  - Multilobulated with phleboliths
  - Variable enhancement
- Dermoid or epidermoid of tongue
  - Dermoid: Fat density NECT with high T1 signal MR
  - Epidermoid: Fluid density CT with high T2 signal MR
- Lymphangioma
  - Uniloculated or multiloculated non-enhancing cystic mass with high T2 signal
  - Usually posterior cervical but affects all neck spaces
  - May be very large
- Branchial cleft cysts
  - Usually excluded by lateral location
- Salivary ranula
  - Lentiform retention cyst from traumatic/inflammatory insult to minor salivary gland
  - Typically older patient

Primary Congenital Hypothyroidism
- Congenital enzymatic defects (partial or complete) affect various steps in iodine transport and organification

Central Hypothyroidism
- Pituitary disorders = rare cause of hypothyroidism

ECTOPIC THYROID

- ○ Insufficient or defective thyrotropin stimulating hormone (TSH)
- Hypothalamic deficiency of thyrotropin releasing hormone (TRH)
  - ○ Destruction by mass, infection, infiltrative processes (sarcoid)
  - ○ Rare, but may be seen in adults

PATHOLOGY

General Features
- Etiology
  - ○ Fetal thyroid descent arrested between 3rd-7th gestational week
  - ○ Development likely relates to hypoplastic gland
    - Abnormal thyroid tissue shows frequent migration failure in studies
    - Underlying abnormal thyroid may help explain hypofunctional status
  - ○ Hereditary or environmental factors may play role
- Epidemiology
  - ○ 1:100,000 incidence
  - ○ Causes 75% of pediatric non-goiter-related hypothyroidism
- Associated abnormalities: Rare reports of thyroid cancer arising from ectopic thyroid

Gross Pathologic & Surgical Features
- Mobile paramedian mass at base of tongue, sublingual, other atypical ectopic locations

Microscopic Features
- Normally sized follicles interdigitate with musculoskeletal fibers

CLINICAL ISSUES

Presentation
- Most common signs/symptoms
  - ○ Laboratory screen shows abnormally ↑ TSH
  - ○ Signs/symptoms of hypothyroidism in newborns nonspecific
    - Bradycardia
    - Respiratory distress
    - Hypothermia
    - Hyperbilirubinemia
    - Poor feeding
  - ○ Classic hypothyroid symptoms occur later in untreated patients
    - Delayed growth
    - Delayed bone maturation (delayed bone age may be detected in newborns)
    - Dry skin/hair
    - Puffy facies
    - Constipation
- Other signs/symptoms
  - ○ Compressive mass effect (especially if ectopic thyroid enlarging due to suboptimal thyroid hormone suppression)
    - Stridor
    - Dysphagia

Demographics
- Age: Newborn or child

Natural History & Prognosis
- Up to 57% of cases detected in first year of life
- Ectopic tissue may maintain euthyroid state at first; duration variable
- Ectopic thyroid enlarges to compensate for decreasing level of endogenous thyroid hormone
- Hypothyroidism ensues
- Untreated hypothyroidism ⇒ retarded growth, mental development
- Prognosis good with early detection
  - ○ Normal intellectual development in 80% of patients if treatment initiated by 3 months of age
- Prognosis poor if therapy delayed for 1 year
  - ○ Normal intellectual development in 10% of patients

Treatment
- Thyroid hormone replacement required
  - ○ Maintain euthyroidism
  - ○ Suppress enlargement
- Surgical excision if enlarging ectopic thyroid obstructive
  - ○ Transoral approach requires splitting tongue
  - ○ May use median or lateral pharyngeal approach
  - ○ Autotransplantation of ectopic thyroid into large trunk muscles, extremities
    - Some have been successfully performed
    - Some argue against given slight risk of cancer, persistent need for hormonal replacement
- Successful I-131 ablation reported; minimal experience

DIAGNOSTIC CHECKLIST

Consider
- If no thyroid uptake in newborn, check for exogenous thyroid hormone administration before diagnosing agenesis

Image Interpretation Pearls
- Use markers to delineate landmarks on thyroid scan for optimal localization
- CECT useful for anatomic correlation
- Pooling of saliva on Tc-99m pertechnetate scan may interfere with interpretation: Administer water/formula and re-image

SELECTED REFERENCES

1. Kobayashi H et al: Utility of computed tomography in identifying an ectopic thyroid in infants and pre-school children. Endocr J. 52(2):189-92, 2005
2. Eugster EA et al: Definitive diagnosis in children with congenital hypothyroidism. J Pediatr. 144(5):643-7, 2004
3. Buyukgebiz A: Congenital hypothyroidism clinical aspects and late consequences. Pediatr Endocrinol Rev. 1 Suppl 2:185-90; discussion 190, 2003
4. Takashima S et al: MR imaging of the lingual thyroid. Comparison to other submucosal lesions. Acta Radiol. 42(4):376-82, 2001
5. Guarisco JL: Congenital head and neck masses in infants and children. Part II. Ear Nose Throat J. 70(2):75-82, 1991

ECTOPIC THYROID

IMAGE GALLERY

Typical

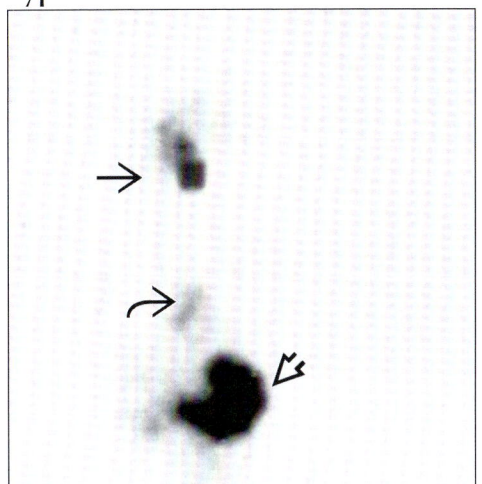

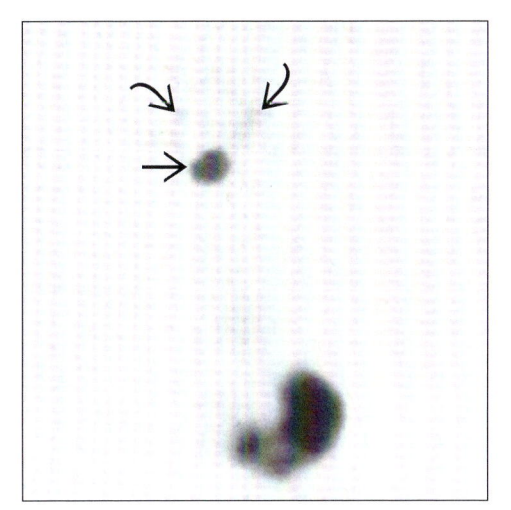

(Left) Anterior thyroid scan in newborn with hypothyroidism shows activity ➔ in neck region which is difficult to localize. Normal radiotracer activity in stomach ▷ and distal esophagus ➘. (Right) After repositioning of same patient as previous image, activity is now better localized to floor of mouth ➔ just below salivary gland ➘ landmarks.

Typical

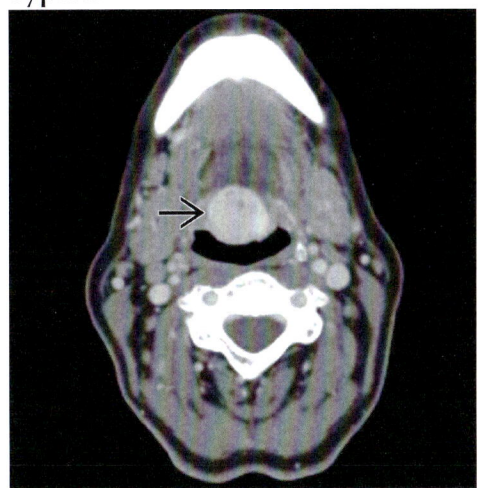

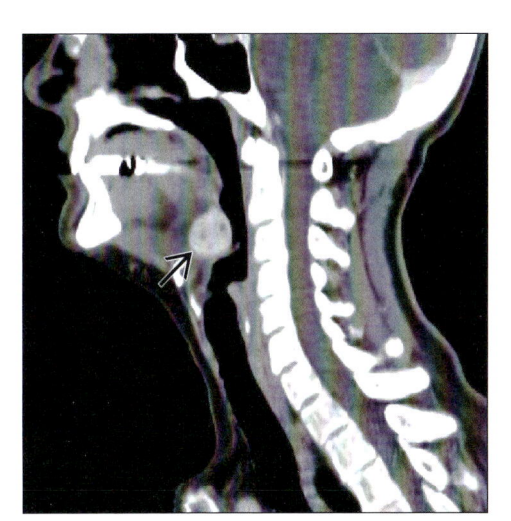

(Left) Axial CECT demonstrates a homogeneous enhancement in an ectopic lingual thyroid ➔. (Right) Lateral CECT in same patient as previous image shows enhancement of ectopic thyroid in tongue base ➔.

Variant

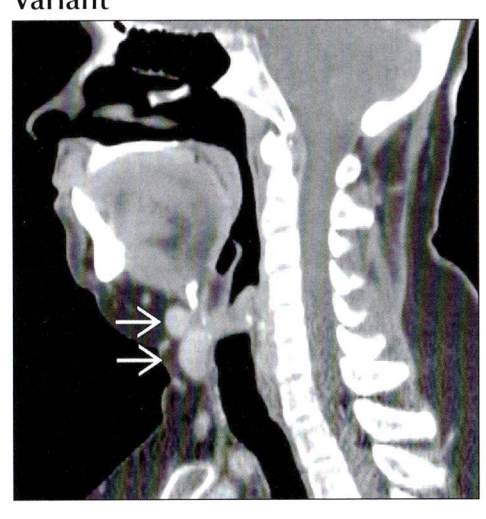

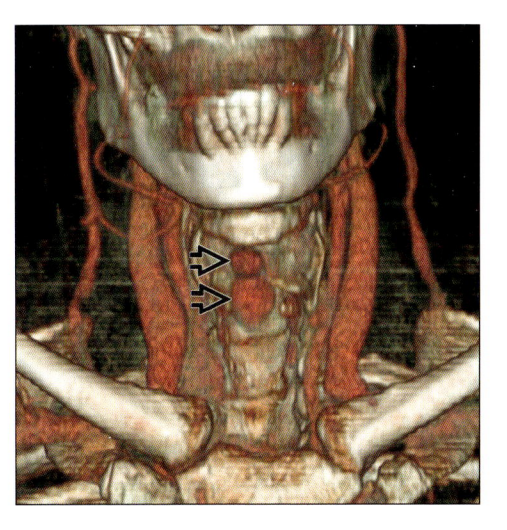

(Left) Lateral CECT shows two adjacent foci of thyroid tissue ➔ in the thyroglossal duct tract in patient with sublingual ectopic thyroid. (Right) Anterior 3D MR of same patient as previous image shows two well-circumscribed midline masses ▷ without normal thyroid tissue configuration.

CONGENITAL HYPOTHYROIDISM

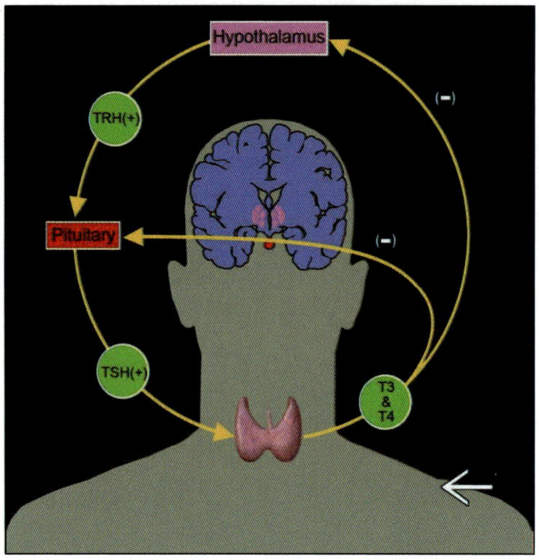

Graphic shows hypothalamic-pituitary-thyroid axis. Note that T3 and T4 inhibit hypothalamic and pituitary stimulation of thyroid.

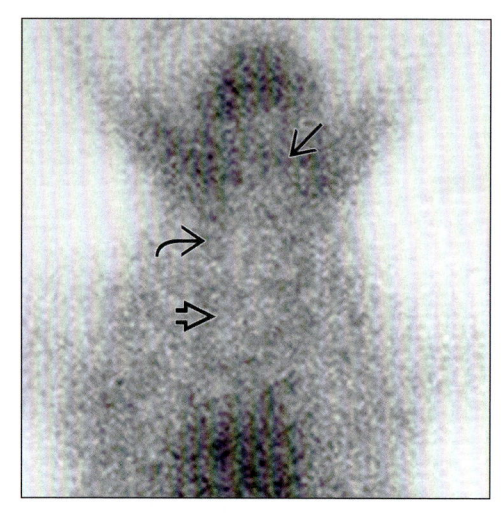

Anterior thyroid scan shows no uptake of radiotracer in oropharynx, neck or mediastinum in patient with congenital absence of thyroid.

TERMINOLOGY

Abbreviations and Synonyms
- Congenital hypothyroidism (CH), cretinism

Definitions
- Inadequate thyroid hormone production
  - Abnormal thyroid formation, ectopic thyroid
  - Inborn error of metabolism
  - Iodine deficiency

IMAGING FINDINGS

General Features
- Best diagnostic clue
  - ↑ TSH (> 20-30 mU/L) on 2nd-3rd day of life
  - Appearance on thyroid scan

Nuclear Medicine Findings
- I-123 or Tc-99m pertechnetate thyroid scan
  - Diagnose and localize ectopic thyroid
    - Ectopic: Focal uptake in abnormal location, most often midline at base of tongue
  - Thyroid agenesis: No uptake in thyroid bed; rarely from central hypothyroidism causing ↓ TSH
  - Inborn error of thyroid hormone metabolism: Bilobed thyroid gland in expected location
- Perchlorate washout: Rarely done
  - Identifies discrepancies between iodide trapping and organification occurring in congenital enzymatic deficiencies
  - After dose of I-123, I-131: Uptake measured at 1-2 hrs and hourly following 1 g potassium perchlorate
  - Washout > 10% suggests organification defect
  - Abnormal values also with chronic thyroiditis, propylthiouracil use

Radiographic Findings
- Bone age useful in CH evaluation
- Lateral knee radiograph: Absence of distal femoral epiphysis at 36 weeks gestational age indicates prenatal hypothyroidism; poor prognostic sign

CT Findings
- NECT: Ectopic thyroid: Well-circumscribed, high density mass, usually midline and at tongue base
- CECT: Homogeneous dense enhancement of ectopic thyroid tissue

DDx: Low Thyroid Uptake in Children

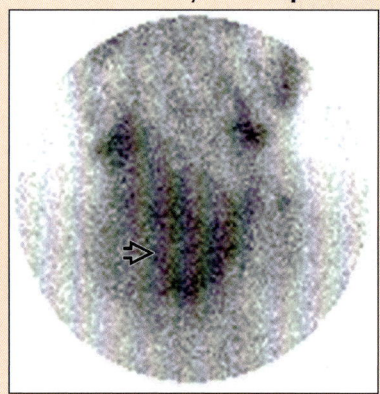

| Diffuse Nontoxic Goiter | Subacute Thyroiditis | Recent IV Contrast |

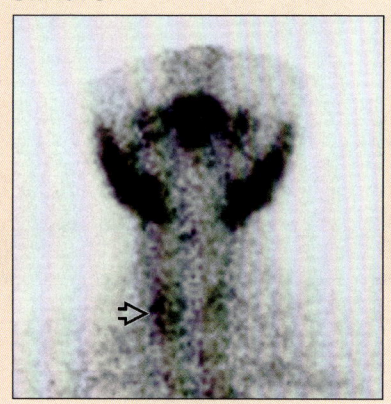

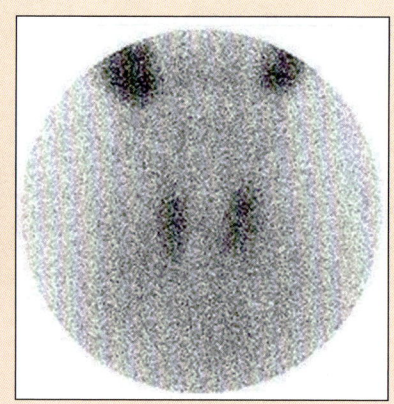

CONGENITAL HYPOTHYROIDISM

Key Facts

Imaging Findings
- I-123 or Tc-99m pertechnetate thyroid scan
- Ectopic: Focal uptake in abnormal location, most often midline at base of tongue
- Thyroid agenesis: No uptake in thyroid bed; rarely from central hypothyroidism causing ↓ TSH
- Inborn error of thyroid hormone metabolism: Bilobed thyroid gland in expected location
- Ideally, stop thyroid hormone replacement prior to thyroid scan or uptake
- If infant started on thyroid hormone for a few days, scan may be diagnostic on hormone

Top Differential Diagnoses
- Thyroid Dysgenesis
- Dyshormonogenesis

- Central Hypothyroidism: Pituitary or Hypothalamic Dysfunction
- Iodine Deficiency
- Maternal Factors
- Autoimmune Thyroiditis (Hashimoto)

Clinical Issues
- Most CH neonates: Full or post term, asymptomatic
- Untreated CH: Clinically evident hypothyroidism within weeks
- Severe growth and mental retardation if hypothyroidism uncorrected
- Even with early therapy, developmental delays common
- Primary hypothyroidism occurring after age 2 usually results in less severe retardation and symptoms
- Treat with immediate thyroid hormone replacement

Ultrasonographic Findings
- Grayscale Ultrasound
  - Absence of normal thyroid in neck
  - May not detect ectopic thyroid tissue

Imaging Recommendations
- Best imaging tool
  - Tc-99m pertechnetate or I-123 thyroid scan
    - Detect and localize ectopic thyroid
    - Visualize enlarged thyroid tissue in thyroid bed (organification defect)
    - Diagnose thyroid agenesis
- Protocol advice
  - Ideally, stop thyroid hormone replacement prior to thyroid scan or uptake
    - 4-6 weeks for levothyroxine (T4, Synthroid)
    - 2-3 weeks for triiodothyronine (T3, Cytomel)
    - If infant started on thyroid hormone for a few days, scan may be diagnostic on hormone
  - Delay scan 4-8 weeks after iodinated contrast administration
  - Tc-99m pertechnetate thyroid scan
    - Infant: 200-300 µCi (7.4-11.1 MBq) IV
    - Adults and adolescents: 3-5 mCi (111-185 MBq) IV
    - Image at 15-20 minutes
  - I-123 thyroid scan
    - Dose: Child 30-120 µCi (1.1-4.4 MBq), adults 100-400 µCi (3.7-14.8 MBq) orally
    - Image 4-6 hours, uptake can also be obtained at 4, 24 hrs
  - Images
    - Newborns: Parallel hole collimator, anterior
    - Children, adolescents, adults: Survey neck and mediastinum for ectopic thyroid with parallel hole collimator, anterior; pinhole collimator for magnification, ↑ sensitivity
    - Oblique or lateral images may help localize ectopic tissue in anteroposterior plane
    - Consider sedation for children or papoose restraint for infants to reduce motion artifact
  - Use marker views to identify thyroid bed or confirm activity location

DIFFERENTIAL DIAGNOSIS

Thyroid Dysgenesis
- Cause of 70-75% CH
- Abnormal thyroid gland development includes gland formation and descent
- Ectopic thyroid (25-50% of CH)
  - 90% found base of tongue in region of foramen cecum
  - Sometimes multiple, can occur anywhere in thyroglossal duct tract
  - May present with enlarging lingual mass requiring thyroid hormone suppression
  - Thyroid hormone production low despite presence of functioning tissue
    - Clinically, ↓ T4, ↑ TSH; some thyroglobulin detectable
    - Hormone production insufficient to sustain normal development
    - Occasionally sufficient hormone production to delay presentation until adolescence
- Agenesis or hypoplasia (20-50% of CH)
  - Thyroid scan typically demonstrates absent thyroid tissue uptake
  - Severe hypothyroidism: ↓ T4, ↑ TSH with undetectable thyroglobulin

Dyshormonogenesis
- Cause of 4-15% CH
- Defects may occur in biosynthesis, secretion, or utilization of thyroid hormone
- Enzymatic abnormalities
  - Peroxidase: Organification and coupling defects may be seen
  - Thyroglobulin: Defective synthesis or proteolysis causing ↓ release into circulation
  - Dehalogenase: Defective iodide reuse/recirculation results in depleted stores
- Deficient iodide trapping due to sodium-iodide symporter defects
- TSH resistance: Abnormal TSH receptor (TSH-R) on follicular cell membrane

CONGENITAL HYPOTHYROIDISM

- Peripheral thyroid hormone resistance: T3 receptor defect in peripheral cell nucleus

Central Hypothyroidism: Pituitary or Hypothalamic Dysfunction
- Cause of 10-15% CH
- Secondary hypothyroidism from decreased pituitary TSH
- Isolated or panhypopituitarism may be less severe symptoms than primary hypothyroidism
- Tertiary hypothyroidism from low hypothalamic TRH rare in children

Iodine Deficiency
- Iodine deficiency should be suspected in endemic regions or with a family history of goiter
- May or may not initially demonstrate goiter

Maternal Factors
- Autoimmune thyroiditis: TSH-R blocking antibodies may be present (e.g. Hashimoto disease)
  - Maternal IgG antibodies may cross placenta and block fetal thyroid
  - Antibody half life brief (1 week), usually resolves by 2-3 weeks
- Hyperthyroidism medication: Antithyroid thioamides, propylthiouracil (PTU), methimazole, act on fetus
- I-131 therapy for hyperthyroidism or cancer
  - I-131 crosses placenta, concentrates in fetal thyroid beginning 10-12 weeks gestational age ⇒ fetal demise, hypothyroidism

Autoimmune Thyroiditis (Hashimoto)
- Usually presents at adolescence but may occur anytime, including childhood
- Hypothyroid symptoms usually develop insidiously

PATHOLOGY

General Features
- Genetics
  - Thyroid gland dysgenesis (sporadic and familial) sometimes associated with abnormal genes (e.g., PAX8)
  - Multiple defects found in abnormal hormone synthesis and response
- Etiology: Most cases sporadic with inherited diseases rare and etiology most often unknown
- Epidemiology
  - Incidence: Worldwide 1:3,000-1:4,000 live births
  - Racial differences in CH largely of unclear etiology
    - 1/3 less frequent in blacks than whites
    - Increased prevalence in Hispanics (3:1)
  - Iodine deficiency: Location in endemic regions or socioeconomic factors
- Associated abnormalities
  - Congenital defects, cardiac atrial or ventricular septal defects, congenital deafness
  - Pendred syndrome
    - Sensorineural deafness and partial thyroid organification defect

CLINICAL ISSUES

Presentation
- Most common signs/symptoms: CH infants most commonly symptom free at presentation
- Other signs/symptoms
  - Prolonged jaundice
  - Large fontanelles
  - Umbilical hernia
  - Birth weight abnormality
    - Low (< 2,000 g)
    - High (> 4,500 g)
  - Hypothyroidism
    - Hypotonia
    - Myxedema
    - Macroglossia
    - Large fontanelle
  - ↓ Feeding/activity, anemia, hoarse cry

Demographics
- Age: CH is present at birth, most diagnosed < 2-3 weeks of age
- Gender: M:F = 1:2 (Hispanics 1:3)

Natural History & Prognosis
- Most CH neonates: Full or post term, asymptomatic
- Untreated CH: Clinically evident hypothyroidism within weeks
  - Severe growth and mental retardation if hypothyroidism uncorrected
- Even with early therapy, developmental delays common
  - Thyroid hormone exerts influence on early fetal brain development
  - Infants presenting with signs of hypothyroidism have lower IQs (10-20 points)
- Primary hypothyroidism occurring after age 2 usually results in less severe retardation and symptoms

Treatment
- Treat with immediate thyroid hormone replacement
  - Frequently monitor levothyroxine (T4) levels

SELECTED REFERENCES
1. Lafranchi S: Thyroid hormone in hypopituitarism, Graves' disease, congenital hypothyroidism, and maternal thyroid disease during pregnancy. Growth Horm IGF Res. 16 Suppl:20-4, 2006
2. Eugster EA et al: Definitive diagnosis in children with congenital hypothyroidism. J Pediatr. 144(5):643-7, 2004
3. Schoen EJ et al: The key role of newborn thyroid scintigraphy with isotopic iodide (123I) in defining and managing congenital hypothyroidism. Pediatrics. 114(6):e683-8, 2004
4. el-Desouki M et al: Thyroid scintigraphy and perchlorate discharge test in the diagnosis of congenital hypothyroidism. Eur J Nucl Med. 22(9):1005-8, 1995
5. Guarisco JL: Congenital head and neck masses in infants and children. Part II. Ear Nose Throat J. 70(2):75-82, 1991

CONGENITAL HYPOTHYROIDISM

IMAGE GALLERY

Typical

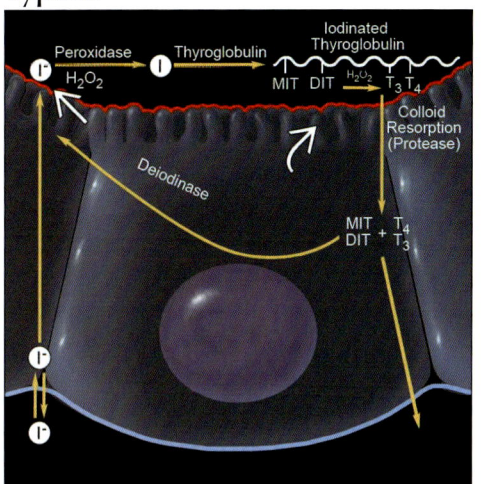

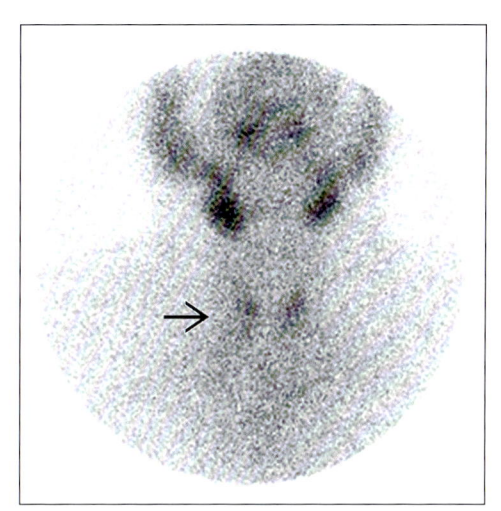

(Left) Graphic shows thyroid hormone production by thyroid follicles. Note iodide is trapped ➡ by the thyroid and organified ➡, playing an essential role in thyroid hormone production. (Right) Anterior thyroid scan shows bilobed thyroid gland in thyroid bed ➡ with very low uptake in a 13 year old with worsening hypothyroidism, likely due to an organification defect.

Typical

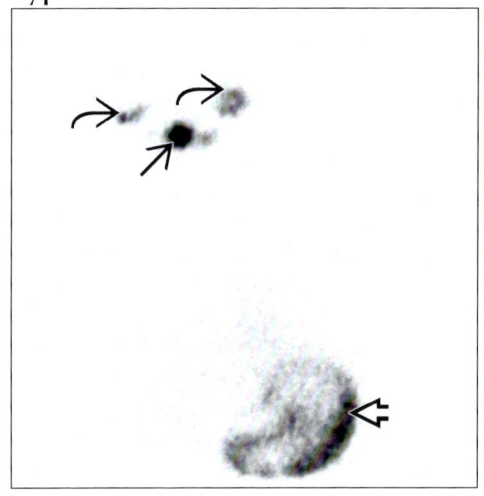

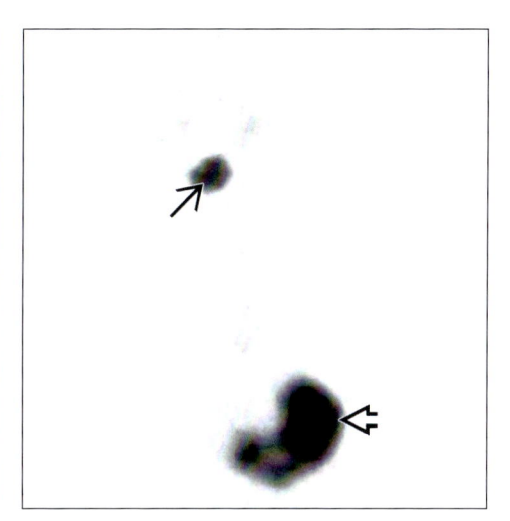

(Left) Anterior thyroid scan of 2 week old infant shows lingual thyroid ➡, normal uptake in stomach ⇨ and salivary glands ➡. (Right) Anterior image at 45 minutes in same patient at previous image shows continued radiotracer accumulation in stomach ⇨ and ectopic thyroid ➡ with washout of most salivary activity.

Typical

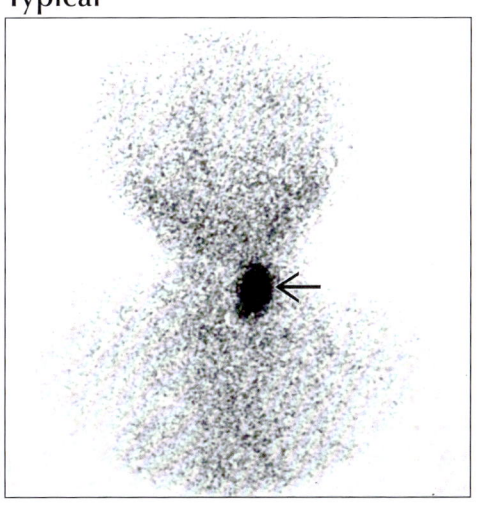

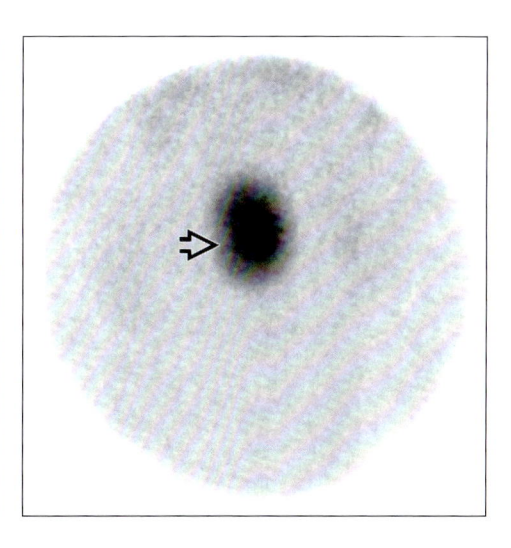

(Left) Anterior I-123 thyroid scan shows unilateral uptake ➡ in patient with hemiagenesis of thyroid. Differential considerations could include hemithyroidectomy or large toxic adenoma. (Right) Anterior thyroid scan shows sublingual ectopic thyroid ⇨ in floor of mouth with a characteristic rounded configuration in 10 year old patient with hypothyroidism.

BENIGN THYROID CONDITIONS, PET

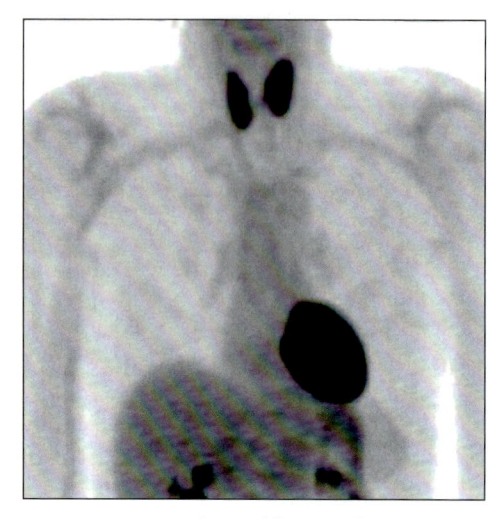

Anterior PET MIP shows diffuse uptake in enlarged thyroid gland, most consistent with Hashimoto thyroiditis. May be subclinical.

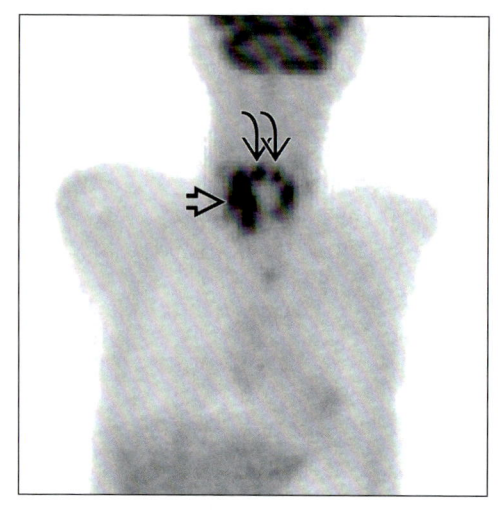

Anterior PET MIP shows lumpy-bumpy configuration with hot and cold regions consistent with multinodular goiter ⇨. Vocal cord activity is also visible ➔.

TERMINOLOGY

Definitions
- Non-malignant causes of thyroid uptake on FDG PET scans

IMAGING FINDINGS

General Features
- Best diagnostic clue: Moderate to marked increased activity relative to adjacent soft tissues
- Location
  - Thyroid gland
  - May be substernal
- Morphology
  - Diffuse increased uptake
  - Cold (hypometabolic) nodule
  - Hot (hypermetabolic) nodule
  - Multiple nodules
  - Mild diffuse ↑ uptake in skeletal muscle

Nuclear Medicine Findings
- PET
  - Normal
    - Normal: No significant uptake above background
  - Diffuse uptake is usually Hashimoto thyroiditis: May be subclinical
  - Multinodular goiter (MNG)
    - MNG: Bilateral hot or cold nodules
    - MNG: Enlarged "lumpy bumpy" thyroid configuration
  - Adenoma
    - Adenoma often hypermetabolic nodule; may also be low or moderate uptake; less uptake in small nodules due to volume averaging
    - FNA: Distinguish adenoma from well differentiated thyroid cancer, although thyroid cancer usually more hypermetabolic
  - Graves disease
    - Graves disease: Usually normal to mildly increased diffuse thyroid uptake
    - Graves disease: May show marked skeletal muscle uptake of FDG (psoas & abdominal muscles)
  - Hashimoto thyroiditis
    - Hashimoto thyroiditis: Usually more hypermetabolic than Graves disease on FDG PET

DDx: Thyroid Cancer

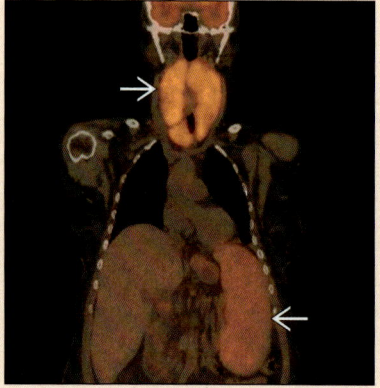

Lymphoma

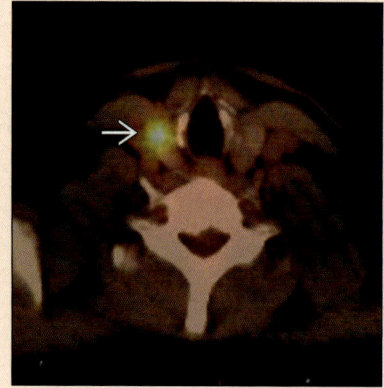

Well-Differentiated Thyroid Cancer

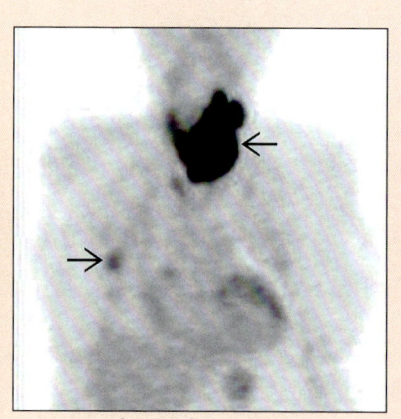

Anaplastic Thyroid Cancer

BENIGN THYROID CONDITIONS, PET

Key Facts

Imaging Findings
- Normal: No significant uptake above background
- MNG: Bilateral hot or cold nodules
- MNG: Enlarged "lumpy bumpy" thyroid configuration
- Adenoma often hypermetabolic nodule; may also be low or moderate uptake; less uptake in small nodules due to volume averaging
- FNA: Distinguish adenoma from well differentiated thyroid cancer, although thyroid cancer usually more hypermetabolic
- Graves disease: Usually normal to mildly increased diffuse thyroid uptake
- Graves disease: May show marked skeletal muscle uptake of FDG (psoas & abdominal muscles)
- Hashimoto thyroiditis: Usually more hypermetabolic than Graves disease on FDG PET
- Subacute thyroiditis: Diffuse FDG uptake, often markedly hypermetabolic

Top Differential Diagnoses
- Adjacent Metastatic or Reactive Lymph Node
- Metastases to Thyroid
- Well-Differentiated Thyroid Cancer
- Lymphoma
- Anaplastic Thyroid Cancer
- Subacute Thyroiditis
- Infection (Acute Thyroiditis)
- Normal Extrathyroidal Tissues
- Parathyroid Adenoma
- Tracheostomy Site

- Uptake (in both Hashimoto and Graves thyroiditis) is proportional to anti-thyroid antibody levels
- Hypermetabolism of the thyroid in hyperthyroid, euthyroid and hypothyroid phases of Hashimoto thyroiditis
  - Associated with other autoimmune & paraneoplastic disorders
- Subacute thyroiditis: Diffuse FDG uptake, often markedly hypermetabolic

Imaging Recommendations
- Best imaging tool: Hypermetabolic nodules need fine needle aspiration
- Protocol advice: PET/CT is useful for differentiation between a thyroid nodule and extrathyroidal malignant or reactive disease lymph nodes
- Additional nuclear medicine imaging options
  - Iodine or Tc-99m pertechnetate scans may be inadequate for characterization, especially of smaller nodules

DIFFERENTIAL DIAGNOSIS

Adjacent Metastatic or Reactive Lymph Node
- Anatomic information from PET/CT is useful for differentiation

Metastases to Thyroid
- While rare, can happen, especially from lung and breast primaries

Well-Differentiated Thyroid Cancer
- Cannot be differentiated from adenoma; must undergo FNA to distinguish
- Thyroid cancer is typically more hypermetabolic than adenomas, but there is great overlap

Lymphoma
- Hypermetabolic, diffuse or focal; often with additional sites of malignancy elsewhere
- Has been known to coexist with Hashimoto thyroiditis (particularly MALT lymphoma)
- Difficult to distinguish between thyroiditis and lymphoma by pathology

Anaplastic Thyroid Cancer
- Marked uptake, usually diffuse; extremely rapid growth

Subacute Thyroiditis
- Often follows upper respiratory infection
- Tender thyroid gland
- Markedly hypermetabolic
- Thyroid usually normal size or only minimally enlarged
- Diagnostic confirmation by radioiodine uptake: Usually very low

Infection (Acute Thyroiditis)
- Clinical symptoms suggest infection
- Can undergo rapid growth (may be indistinguishable from anaplastic thyroid cancer)
- Fever and elevated leukocyte count are expected

Normal Extrathyroidal Tissues
- Vocalis muscle: May involve one side only if unilateral vocal cord paralysis
- Cricoarytenoid muscle and cartilage: Often quite intense and asymmetrical
  - Particularly hypermetabolic due to cartilage necrosis following radiotherapy

Parathyroid Adenoma
- FDG PET is often positive in parathyroid adenoma and hyperplasia
- Greatest challenge is when parathyroid adenoma is subcapsular
- Additional imaging
  - Sestamibi scan may be positive in parathyroid adenoma, thyroid adenoma and thyroid cancer
  - Ultrasound recommended to differentiate (intracapsular parathyroid adenoma is surrounded by a thin hyperechoic rim)

BENIGN THYROID CONDITIONS, PET

- C-11 methionine may be superior to FDG PET in identifying parathyroid adenomas

Tracheostomy Site
- Midline hypermetabolic focus

PATHOLOGY

General Features
- Epidemiology
  - Incidence of increased thyroid uptake on PET scan reported to be 2-3%
    - Approximately equally split between nodular and diffuse pattern
  - Frequency of nodules increases throughout life
  - Single nodules are four times more common in females
- Associated abnormalities
  - Autoimmune disorders
    - Sjögren syndrome (uptake also in salivary tissue)
    - Rheumatoid arthritis
    - Polymyositis, dermatomyositis
    - Lupus
  - Paraneoplastic disorders
    - Thyroiditis and generalized or focal polymyositis/dermatomyositis
  - Diffuse muscle uptake in hyperthyroidism (especially Graves disease)

CLINICAL ISSUES

Presentation
- Most common signs/symptoms: Increased thyroid uptake on PET scan often incidental in asymptomatic patient

DIAGNOSTIC CHECKLIST

Image Interpretation Pearls
- Hypermetabolic solitary nodule
  - Fine needle aspiration recommended (even for small nodules) to distinguish adenoma from well-differentiated thyroid cancer
  - No other imaging studies can distinguish adenoma from carcinoma
  - Consider parathyroid adenoma for posterior nodules
- Diffuse increased FDG uptake
  - Diffuse uptake in asymptomatic, euthyroid patient is probably subclinical thyroiditis
    - Beyond thyroid function tests, no further work-up is necessary
  - Hyperthyroidism from Hashimoto disease is usually markedly hypermetabolic
    - Both in hyperthyroid (Hashitoxicosis), euthyroid and hypothyroid phases
  - Graves disease is variable in FDG uptake but usually increased over normal
    - Often associated with diffuse skeletal muscle uptake
  - Subacute thyroiditis is markedly hypermetabolic
- Lumpy-bumpy thyroid with multiple nodules
  - Probably multinodular goiter
  - Consider thyroid cancer if enlarging
- Thyroid uptake may be associated with other systemic disorders
  - Paraneoplastic thyroiditis: Often associated with focal or regional myositis
  - Autoimmune disease, such as Sjögren syndrome, Lupus, Rheumatoid arthritis, Polymyositis, Dermatomyositis

SELECTED REFERENCES

1. Biro E et al: Association of systemic and thyroid autoimmune diseases. Clin Rheumatol. [Epub ahead of print] Oct 25, 2005
2. Kim TY et al: 18F-fluorodeoxyglucose uptake in thyroid from positron emission tomogram (PET) for evaluation in cancer patients: high prevalence of malignancy in thyroid PET incidentaloma. Laryngoscope. 115(6):1074-8, 2005
3. Yi JG et al: Focal uptake of fluorodeoxyglucose by the thyroid in patients undergoing initial disease staging with combined PET/CT for non-small cell lung cancer. Radiology. 236(1):271-5, 2005
4. Chen YK et al: Elevated 18F-FDG uptake in skeletal muscles and thymus: a clue for the diagnosis of Graves' disease. Nucl Med Commun. 25(2):115-21, 2004
5. Kresnik E et al: Fluorine-18-fluorodeoxyglucose positron emission tomography in the preoperative assessment of thyroid nodules in an endemic goiter area. Surgery. 133(3):294-9, 2003
6. Cohen MS et al: Risk of malignancy in thyroid incidentalomas identified by fluorodeoxyglucose-positron emission tomography. Surgery. 130(6):941-6, 2001
7. Ramos CD et al: Incidental focal thyroid uptake on FDG positron emission tomographic scans may represent a second primary tumor. Clin Nucl Med. 26(3):193-7, 2001
8. Lawson MA et al: Three Cases of Primary Hyperparathyroidism (PHP) with Prior Failed Surgery Where Culprit Lesions Were Identified by 11C-Methionine Positron Emission Tomography (PET) and Accurately Localized with PET-MRI Coregistration. Clin Positron Imaging. 3(1):31-36, 2000
9. Boerner AR et al: Glucose metabolism of the thyroid in Graves' disease measured by F-18-fluoro-deoxyglucose positron emission tomography. Thyroid. 8(9):765-72, 1998
10. Borner AR et al: F-18-FDG PET of the thyroid gland in Graves' disease] Nuklearmedizin. 37(7):227-33, 1998
11. Cook GJ et al: [11C]Methionine positron emission tomography for patients with persistent or recurrent hyperparathyroidism after surgery. Eur J Endocrinol. 139(2):195-7, 1998
12. Yasuda S et al: Chronic thyroiditis: diffuse uptake of FDG at PET. Radiology. 207(3):775-8, 1998
13. Neumann DR et al: Regional body FDG-PET in postoperative recurrent hyperparathyroidism. J Comput Assist Tomogr. 21(1):25-8, 1997
14. Neumann DR et al: Comparison of FDG-PET and sestamibi-SPECT in primary hyperparathyroidism. J Nucl Med. 37(11):1809-15, 1996
15. Fujitake J et al: Localized polymyositis associated with chronic thyroiditis. J Rheumatol. 1994 Jun;21(6):1147-9. Localized polymyositis associated with chronic thyroiditis. J Rheumatol. 21(6):1147-9, 1994
16. Mazzaferri EL: Management of a solitary thyroid nodule. N Engl J Med. 328(8):553-9, 1993

BENIGN THYROID CONDITIONS, PET

IMAGE GALLERY

Typical

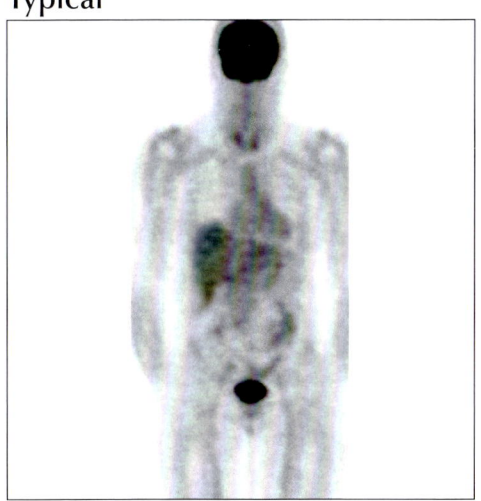

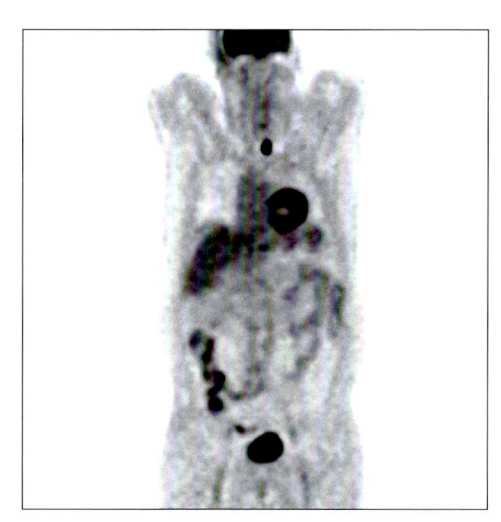

(**Left**) Coronal PET MIP shows mild diffuse uptake within the thyroid gland in a patient with an indeterminate pulmonary nodule. Associated skeletal muscle uptake is present. Consider Graves disease. (**Right**) Coronal PET shows an FDG avid nodule in the left thyroid lobe. As high as 50% of these are cancer. Most of the remainder are adenomas, often hyperfunctioning. FNA is needed.

Other

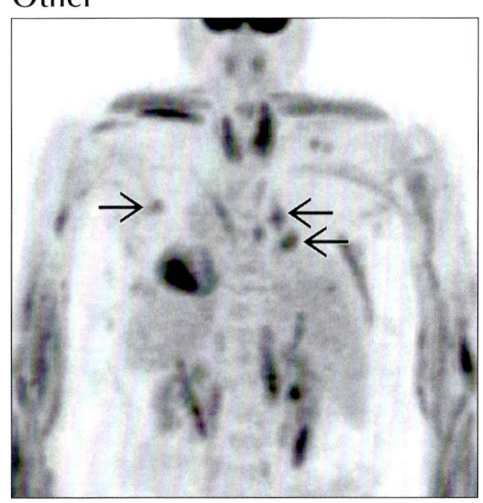

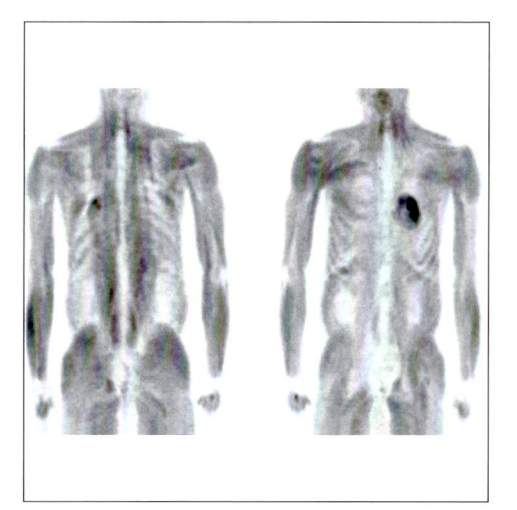

(**Left**) Posterior PET MIP in a patient with lung cancer ⇒ demonstrates diffuse thyroid uptake associated with focal uptake in skeletal muscles, an association seen with polymyositis or paraneoplastic syndrome. (**Right**) Anterior and posterior PET MIP images demonstrate diffuse skeletal muscle uptake, which can be seen with Graves disease. Thyroid uptake is variable but usually greater than normal.

Variant

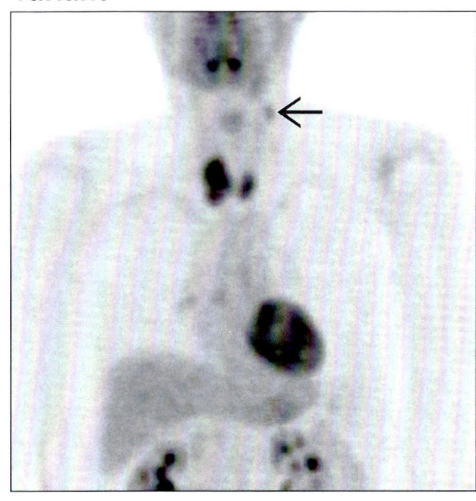

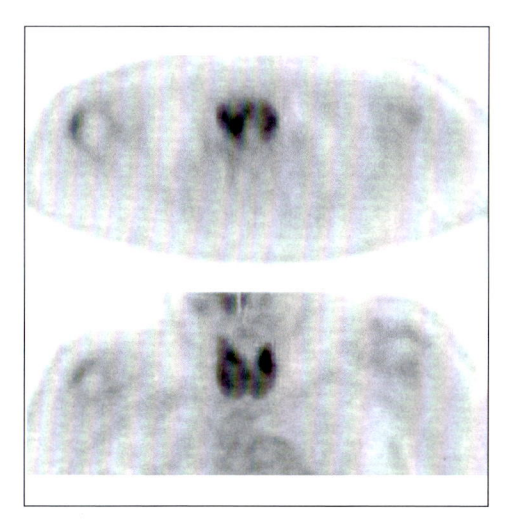

(**Left**) Anterior PET MIP shows asymmetrical uptake in both thyroid lobes, typical for multinodular goiter but was bilateral well-differentiated thyroid cancer in this case. Note met to left neck node ⇒. (**Right**) Transaxial and coronal PET shows typical appearance for multinodular goiter, with lumpy-bumpy thyroid and both hot and cold nodules.

WELL-DIFFERENTIATED THYROID CANCER

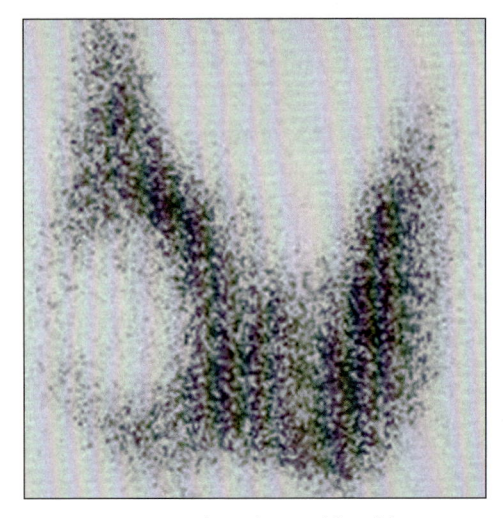

Anterior I-123 scan shows large cold nodule (10-20% chance of thyroid cancer).

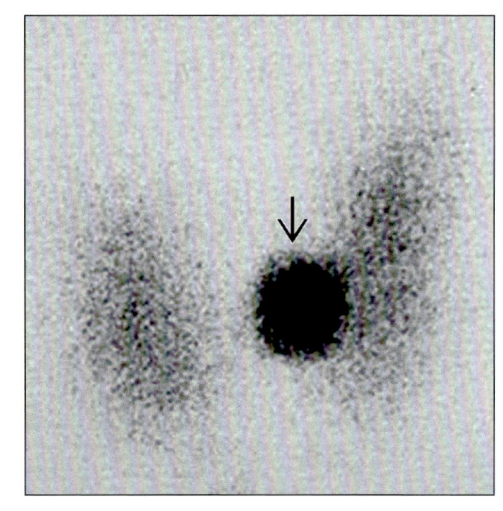

Anterior I-123 scan of thyroid with marker ➡ shows cold nodule in isthmus. Radioiodine scans for thyroid nodules require palpation and marking of nodule.

TERMINOLOGY

Abbreviations and Synonyms
- Well-differentiated thyroid cancer (WDTC)

Definitions
- Thyroid cancer of papillary, follicular, or mixed origin
- Not medullary or anaplastic cell types
- Radioiodine scan: I-123 or I-131 thyroid or whole body scintigraphy
- Stimulated scan: I-123 or I-131 whole body scan with elevated TSH due to thyroid hormone withdrawal or Thyrogen administration

IMAGING FINDINGS

General Features
- Best diagnostic clue
  - Palpable thyroid nodule without hyperthyroidism
  - Primary
    - Primary: Cold nodule on radioiodine scan
    - Primary: Solid or mixed characteristics on ultrasound
  - Residual thyroid after surgery
    - Focal uptake in thyroid bed, thyroglossal duct
  - Extrathyroidal spread of tumor
    - Focal non-physiologic uptake of radioiodine, lung mets may be diffuse
- Location
  - Residual local disease
    - Uptake in thyroid bed after surgery usually normal thyroid tissue
  - Local recurrence: Thyroid bed, cervical nodes
  - Extrathyroidal spread
    - Follicular WDTC: Hematogenous spread to lungs, bones
    - Papillary WDTC: Lymphatic spread to cervical/mediastinal nodes, lung
- Size
  - Metastatic cervical nodes may not be enlarged
  - Lung metastases: Microscopic, miliary or nodules
  - Bone mets can be very large
- Morphology
  - Lymph nodes
    - Metastatic rounded +/- calcification; fatty hilum: Benign
  - Thyroid bed recurrence: Variable morphology

DDx: False Positive Uptake on Radioiodine Scan

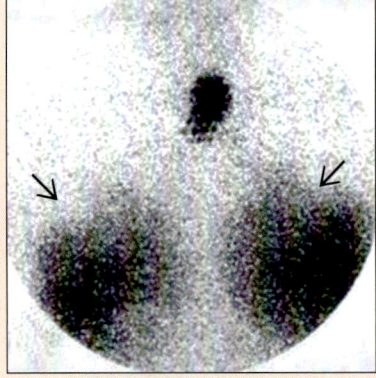

Lactating Breasts

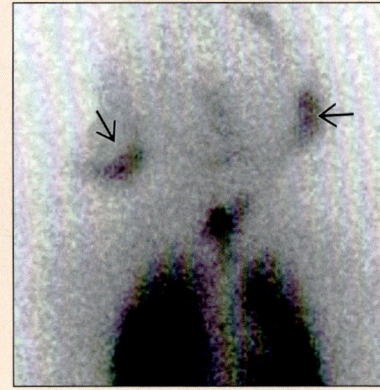

Perspiration (Hair)

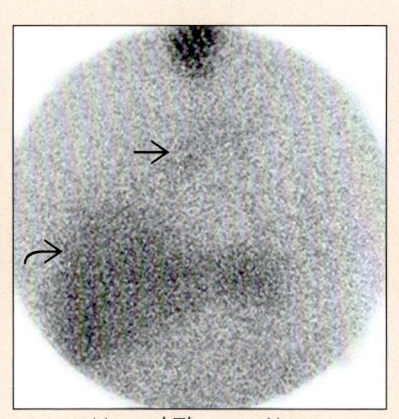

Normal Thymus, Liver

WELL-DIFFERENTIATED THYROID CANCER

Key Facts

Imaging Findings
- Primary: Cold nodule on radioiodine scan
- Primary: Solid or mixed characteristics on ultrasound
- Uptake in thyroid bed after surgery usually normal thyroid tissue
- Follicular WDTC: Hematogenous spread to lungs, bones
- Papillary WDTC: Lymphatic spread to cervical/mediastinal nodes, lung
- Cold nodule on I-123 scan: May be hot/warm on Tc-99m O4-
- Normal: Salivary glands, saliva, nasopharynx
- Cervical nodes: Focal radioiodine uptake
- Lung mets: Diffuse or focal (may be inapparent by CT)
- Bone mets may be inapparent by conventional bone scan
- Diffuse liver uptake rarely metastatic: Metabolized radiolabeled thyroid hormone
- Non-iodine avid WDTC
- FDG PET (stimulated scan more sensitive)
- Low iodine diet 2 weeks prior to scan
- Withhold thyroxine 4-6 weeks
- May give Cytomel for 1 month, then withdraw 2-3 weeks prior to scan
- I-131 2-3 mCi day 1, whole body scan day 3-4
- I-123, 800-1000 µCi day 1, whole body scan day 2
- Oblique neck images or Tc-99m O4- scan if salivary gland vs. lymph node
- Non-iodine avid tumor: Tc-99m Sestamibi or FDG PET: Best if TSH elevated
- Thyroglobulin > 2.0 ng/mL indicates thyroid tissue

- o Bone mets classically lytic
- o Lung mets microscopic, miliary, larger nodules

Nuclear Medicine Findings
- Primary
  - o Cold nodule on I-123 scan: May be hot/warm on Tc-99m O4-
  - o May appear extrathyroidal if connected by stalk
- Extrathyroidal neck
  - o Normal: Salivary glands, saliva, nasopharynx
  - o Cervical nodes: Focal radioiodine uptake
- Extracervical metastases
  - o Focal uptake not due to normal physiologic structure
  - o Lung mets: Diffuse or focal (may be inapparent by CT)
  - o Bone mets may be inapparent by conventional bone scan
  - o Diffuse liver uptake rarely metastatic: Metabolized radiolabeled thyroid hormone

Imaging Recommendations
- Best imaging tool
  - o Primary tumor (pre-operative)
    - I-123 scan or ultrasound
  - o Residual cervical disease (post-operative)
    - Stimulated radioiodine scan
  - o Cervical recurrence
    - High-resolution ultrasound
    - Stimulated radioiodine scan
  - o Distant metastases
    - Stimulated radioiodine scan
  - o Non-iodine avid WDTC
    - FDG PET (stimulated scan more sensitive)
- Protocol advice
  - o Low iodine diet 2 weeks prior to scan
  - o Withdrawal scan
    - Withhold thyroxine 4-6 weeks
    - May give Cytomel for 1 month, then withdraw 2-3 weeks prior to scan
    - TSH > 30 mU/L initial evaluation, > 40 mU/L surveillance scans
    - I-131 2-3 mCi day 1, whole body scan day 3-4
    - I-123, 800-1000 µCi day 1, whole body scan day 2
  - o Thyrogen (recombinant human TSH) stimulated scan
    - May be slightly less sensitive than withdrawal scan but doubtful clinical impact
    - FDA approval for scanning; therapy currently off-label for use of Thyrogen
    - Typical protocol: Thyrogen 0.9 mg day 1 and day 2, radioiodine day 3, scan day 4-6
    - For I-131 treatment when TSH low from hypopituitarism or surgically unresectable thyroid
  - o Oblique neck images or Tc-99m O4- scan if salivary gland vs. lymph node
  - o Non-iodine avid tumor: Tc-99m Sestamibi or FDG PET: Best if TSH elevated
  - o 1 week post-therapy scan more sensitive than pre-therapy scan
    - Better assessment of disease burden for surveillance
  - o Tc-99m pertechnetate not recommended (may show uptake in solid tumors)
- Correlative tests
  - o Serum thyroglobulin (Tg)
    - Complementary to radioiodine scan, best if TSH high
    - Thyroglobulin > 2.0 ng/mL indicates thyroid tissue
    - Anti-Tg antibodies interfere with assay

DIFFERENTIAL DIAGNOSIS

Normal Physiologic Uptake
- Salivary glands, alimentary and urinary tract

Contamination
- Urine, perspiration, nasal secretions, saliva
- Suspected iodine contamination, check urine level (want < 200 µg/L)

Infection/Inflammation, Other Tumors
- Infection or other tumors may be radioiodine avid

WELL-DIFFERENTIATED THYROID CANCER

Thymus
- Due to iodine trapping within cystic Hassall bodies

PATHOLOGY

General Features
- Genetics
  - Most cases occur in isolation
  - Can occur familially or with Gardner syndrome
- Etiology: Head and neck irradiation as child, nuclear "fallout", question Hashimoto thyroiditis
- Epidemiology
  - Of all thyroid cancers: 80% papillary, 10% follicular
  - 20 year latency for papillary
  - Estimated 25,690 new cases of thyroid cancer in the United States for 2005
  - Estimated 1,490 deaths from thyroid cancer in the United States for 2005

Gross Pathologic & Surgical Features
- Papillary: Whitish invasive neoplasm, ill-defined margins
  - Fine needle biopsy often diagnostic
- Follicular: Brown encapsulated neoplasm
  - Fibrosis, hemorrhage, cystic change common

Microscopic Features
- Papillary
  - Fine needle aspiration biopsy usually diagnostic
  - Neoplastic epithelial papillae, complex arborization, nuclei empty ground-glass appearance, nuclear grooves, pseudoinclusions, psammoma bodies
- Follicular
  - Tumor and vascular invasion, may require special stains
  - Neoplastic follicular cells, solid, trabecular, follicular growth
  - Immunohistochemical staining for thyroglobulin, cytokeratins

CLINICAL ISSUES

Presentation
- Most common signs/symptoms: Painless neck mass most common
- Other signs/symptoms: Hoarseness, dysphagia, airway obstruction

Demographics
- Age: Papillary 34-40 years; follicular 40-70 years
- Gender: M < F = 1:3

Natural History & Prognosis
- 10 year survival
  - 93% papillary
    - Prognosis good, most dependent on tumor size (< 2.5 cm)
  - 85% follicular
    - More aggressive, older age group
  - 75% Hürthle cell
    - Follicular variant, less iodine avid but I-131 may still be effective
- Worse prognosis
  - Age < 20 years, > 45 years
  - Tumor size > 2.5 cm
  - Extracapsular extension, microvascular invasion
  - Distant mets
  - Delay in treatment > 12 months

Treatment
- Surgery
  - Total thyroidectomy: Usually for cancers > 1 cm
  - Hemithyroidectomy: Difficult to monitor serum thyroglobulin or radioiodine scans
- I-131 ablation and therapy
- TSH suppression
  - Slightly supraphysiologic doses of levothyroxine to suppress TSH (~ .01 mU/L)
- External beam radiation
  - More effective for bone metastases than I-131

SELECTED REFERENCES

1. Besic N et al: Aggressiveness of Therapy and Prognosis of Patients with Hurthle Cell Papillary Thyroid Carcinoma. Thyroid. 16(1):67-72, 2006
2. Jemal A et al: Cancer statistics, 2005. CA Cancer J Clin. 55(1):10-30, 2005
3. Hilditch TE et al: Self-stunning in thyroid ablation: evidence from comparative studies of diagnostic 131I and 123I. Eur J Nucl Med Mol Imaging. 29(6):783-8, 2002
4. Mazzaferri EL et al: Management of papillary and follicular (differentiated) thyroid cancer: new paradigms using recombinant human thyrotropin. Endocr Relat Cancer. 9(4):227-47, 2002
5. Mandel SJ et al: Superiority of iodine-123 compared with iodine-131 scanning for thyroid remnants in patients with differentiated thyroid cancer. Clin Nucl Med. 26(1):6-9, 2001
6. Mitchell G et al: False positive 131I whole body scans in thyroid cancer. Br J Radiol. 73(870):627-35, 2000
7. Seabold JE et al: Comparison of 99mTc-methoxyisobutyl isonitrile and 201Tl scintigraphy for detection of residual thyroid cancer after 131I ablative therapy. J Nucl Med. 40(9):1434-40, 1999
8. Hundahl SA et al: A National Cancer Data Base report on 53,856 cases of thyroid carcinoma treated in the U.S., 1985-1995. Cancer. 83(12):2638-48, 1998
9. Alam MS et al: Value of combined technetium-99m hydroxy methylene diphosphonate and thallium-201 imaging in detecting bone metastases from thyroid carcinoma. Thyroid. 7(5):705-12, 1997
10. Chung JK et al: Clinical significance of hepatic visualization on iodine-131 whole-body scan in patients with thyroid carcinoma. J Nucl Med. 38(8):1191-5, 1997
11. Ladenson PW et al: Comparison of administration of recombinant human thyrotropin with withdrawal of thyroid hormone for radioactive iodine scanning in patients with thyroid carcinoma. N Engl J Med. 337(13):888-96, 1997
12. Vermiglio F et al: Iodine concentration by the thymus in thyroid carcinoma. J Nucl Med. 37(11):1830-1, 1996
13. Willis LL et al: Mediastinal uptake of I-131 in a hiatal hernia mimicking recurrence of papillary thyroid carcinoma. Clin Nucl Med. 18(11):961-3, 1993

WELL-DIFFERENTIATED THYROID CANCER

IMAGE GALLERY

Typical

Typical

Typical

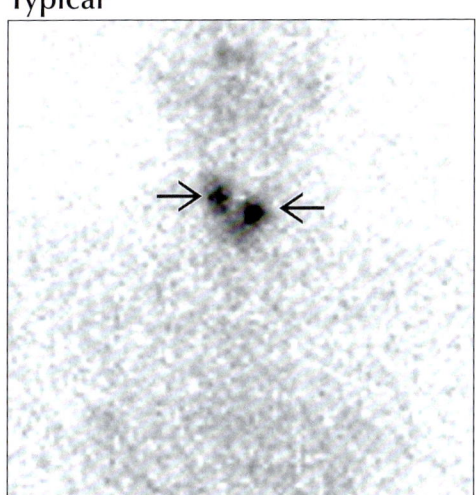

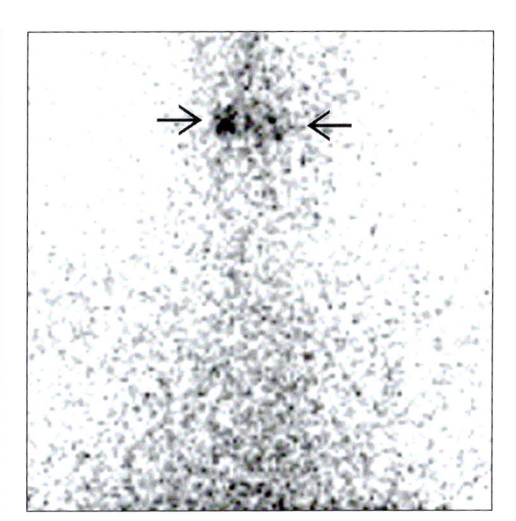

(Left) Anterior I-131 whole body scan following thyroidectomy shows uptake in the thyroid bed, likely related to residual normal thyroid tissue ➔. Patient treated with 100 mCi I-131. See next image. (Right) I-131 whole body scan in same patient as previous image 1 year later shows resolution of activity in the thyroid bed. Note asymmetrical uptake in submandibular glands ➔, common following I-131 treatment.

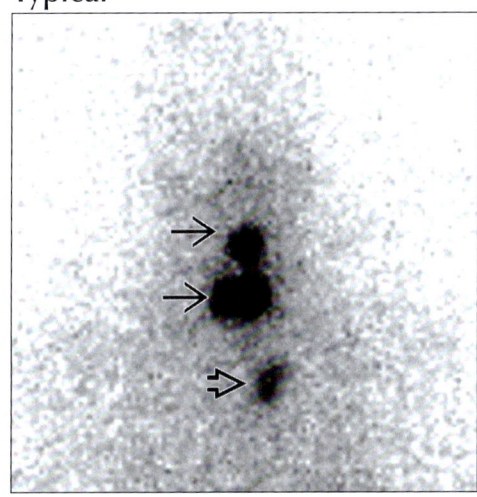

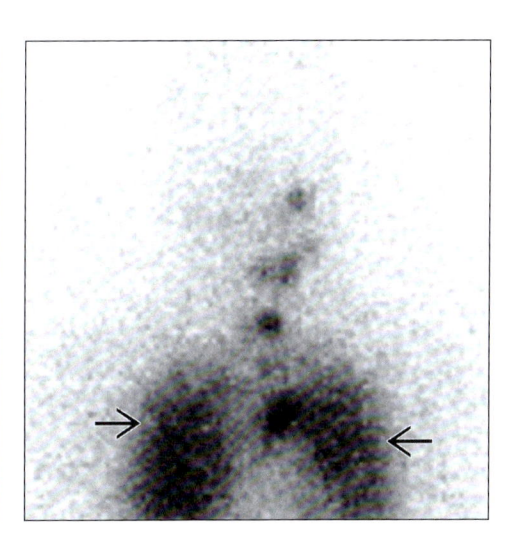

(Left) Anterior whole body I-131 scan shows several sites in anterior neck ➔, and one in upper mediastinum ⇨, but nothing in the lungs. Patient was treated with 150 mCi I-131. See next image. (Right) Anterior whole body scan 1 week after treatment in the same patient as previous image shows diffuse uptake in the lungs consistent with metastatic pulmonary disease ➔. Post-therapy scan is more sensitive than pretherapy scan.

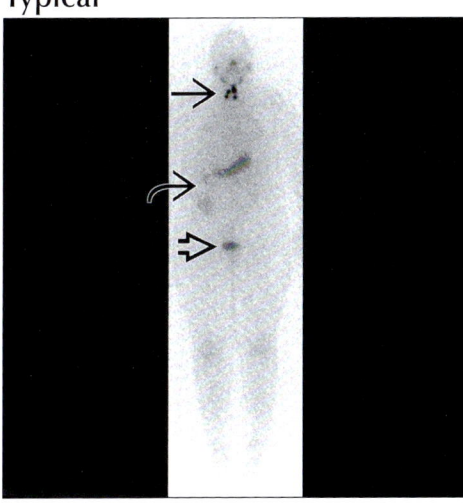

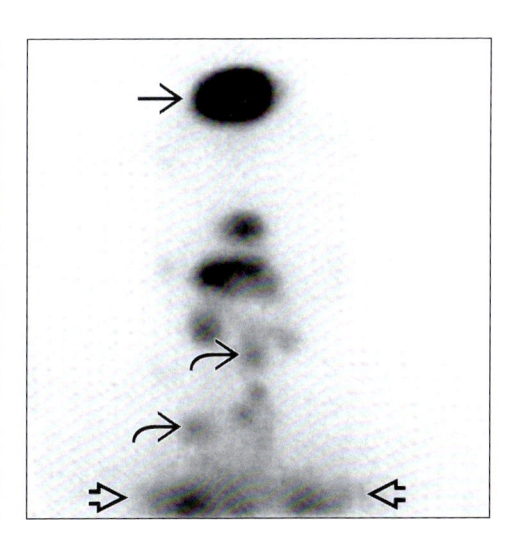

(Left) Anterior whole body radioiodine scan shows residual activity in thyroid bed (normal thyroid vs. thyroid cancer) ➔, physiologic uptake in stomach and intestine ➔, bladder ⇨. (Right) Anterior radioiodine scan of head and neck shows metastatic disease to skull ➔, neck ➔, and top of lungs ⇨. The skull metastasis was large and lytic.

WELL-DIFFERENTIATED THYROID CANCER

Variant

(Left) Anterior I-131 scan of the head and neck following thyroidectomy for WDTC shows marked uptake in the chest. See next image.
(Right) Axial NECT of the same patient as previous image shows large substernal goiter ➡.

Variant

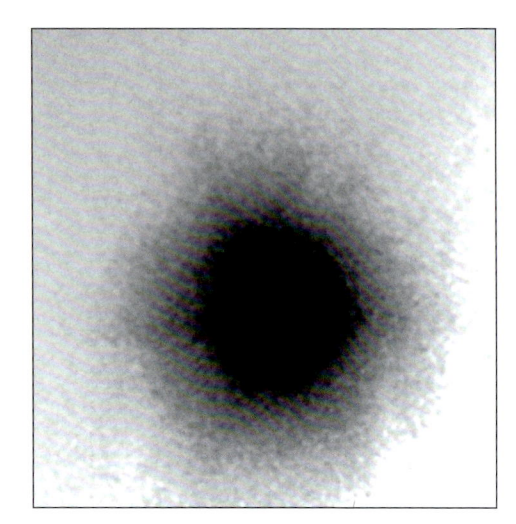

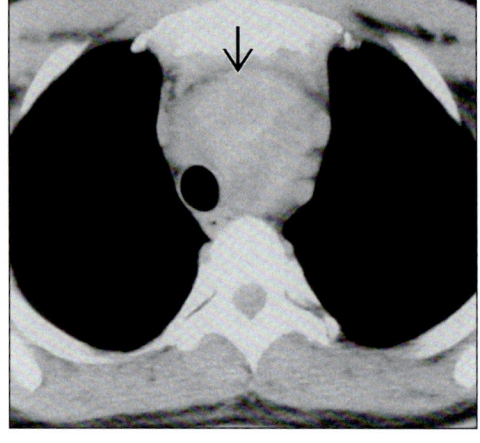

(Left) I-131 scan in a patient with elevated Tg following thyroidectomy and prior I-131 treatment. No abnormal sites were identified. Note normal uptake in nose ➡ and mouth ➡. See next image.
(Right) Anterior Tc-99m sestamibi scan same patient as previous image demonstrates focus of abnormal activity in lower left neck ➡, undetected by radioiodine scan. At surgery, this was recurrent WDTC.

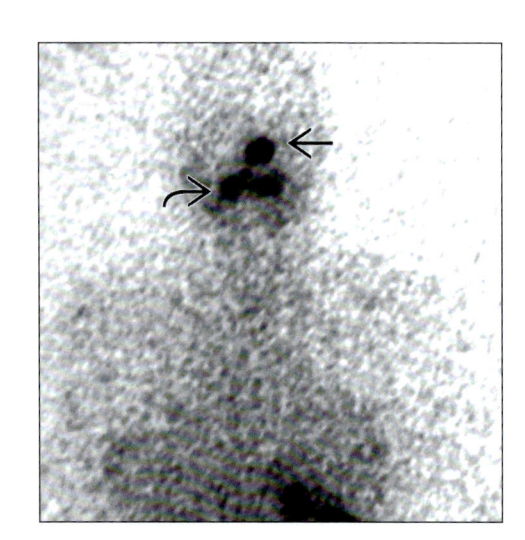

Variant

(Left) Tc-99m pertechnetate scan of thyroid in patient with new deviation of trachea on CXR. Scan shows normal uptake in prominent inferior pole of left lobe ➡. See next image. **(Right)** Scan repeated with I-123 (same patient as previous image), which now shows cold nodule in inferior pole of left thyroid lobe ➡. At surgery, this was WDTC. This is classical "discordant nodule".

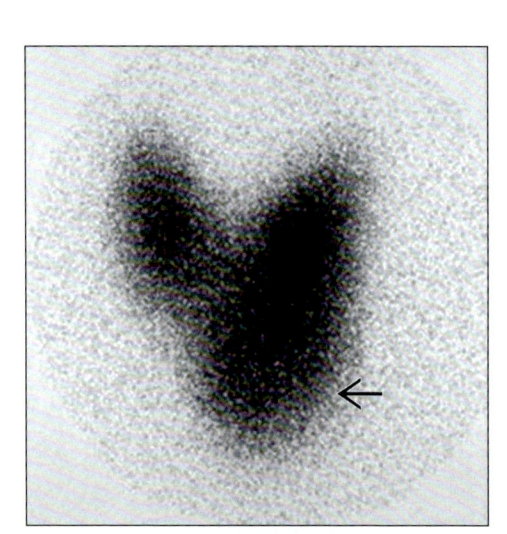

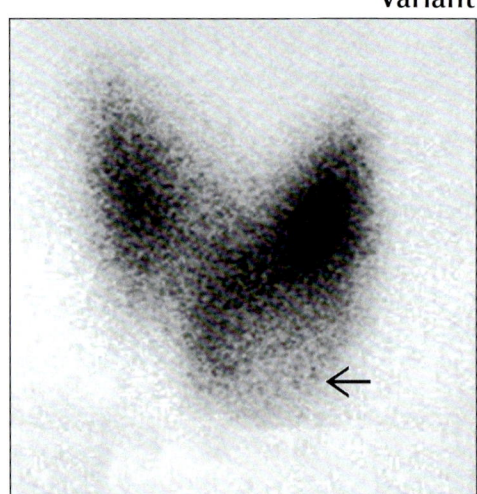

WELL-DIFFERENTIATED THYROID CANCER

Variant

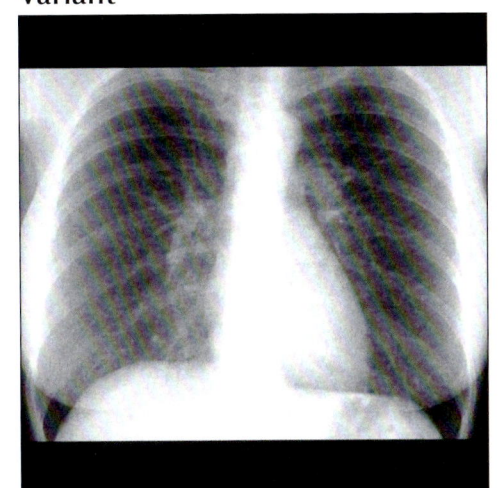

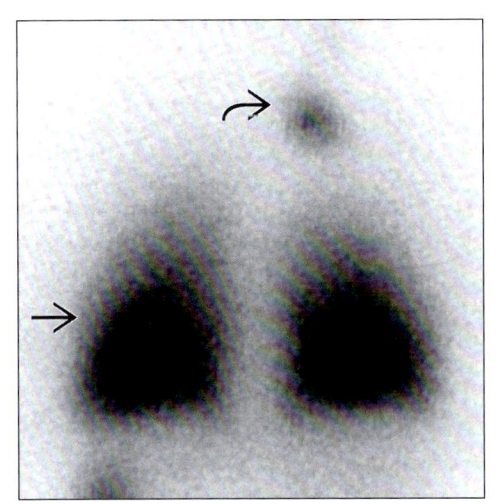

(Left) PA normal CXR in 20 year old patient with history of papillary thyroid cancer, previously treated with 150 mCi I-131. Tg was markedly elevated. Same patient as next 2 images. (Right) Posterior radioiodine scan of lower neck, and chest shows intense uptake in lungs ➔, as well as lower right neck ➔, consistent with recurrent and metastatic WDTC. See next image.

Variant

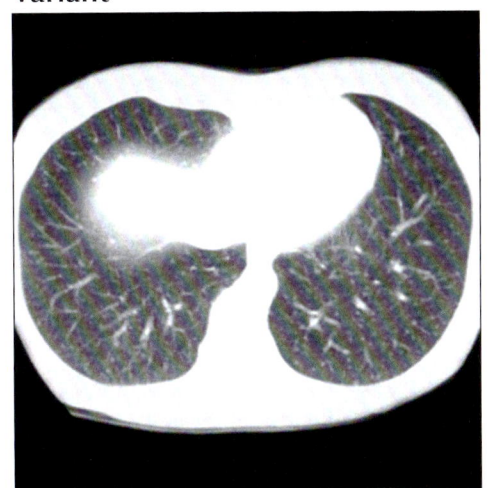

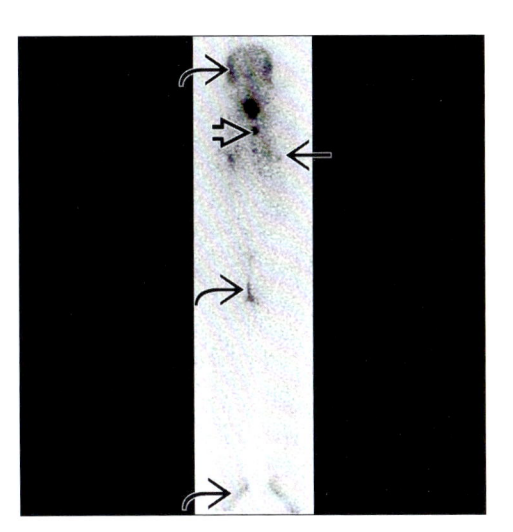

(Left) Axial NECT in same patient as previous 2 images demonstrates many miliary nodules in the lung bases, consistent with metastatic WDTC. (Right) Posterior whole body radioiodine scan shows metastatic disease in the lungs ➔ and mediastinum ➔, and lower neck. Also shown are contamination due to perspiration ➔ in the scalp, gluteal cleft and feet.

Variant

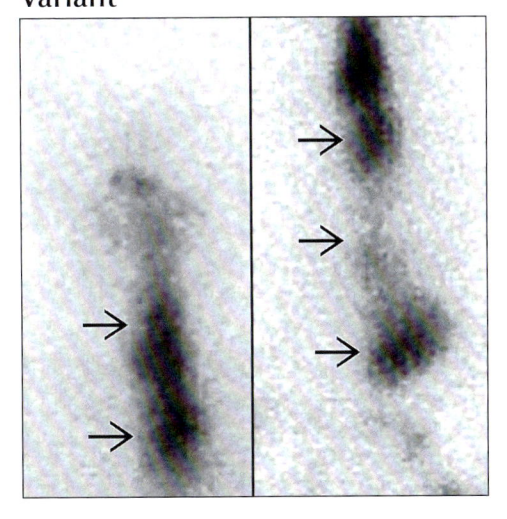

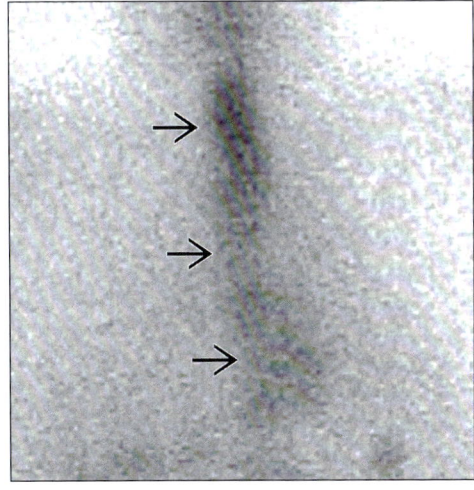

(Left) Anterior radioiodine scan of the neck and chest demonstrates intense uptake in thoracic stomach ➔, a normal variant, in patient with a gastroesophageal pull-through for previous esophageal cancer. See next image. (Right) Repeat upright imaging following administration of water in the same patient as previous image. Note washout of the activity in the thoracic stomach ➔. Radioiodine is actively secreted by gastric mucosa.

I-131 THYROID CANCER THERAPY

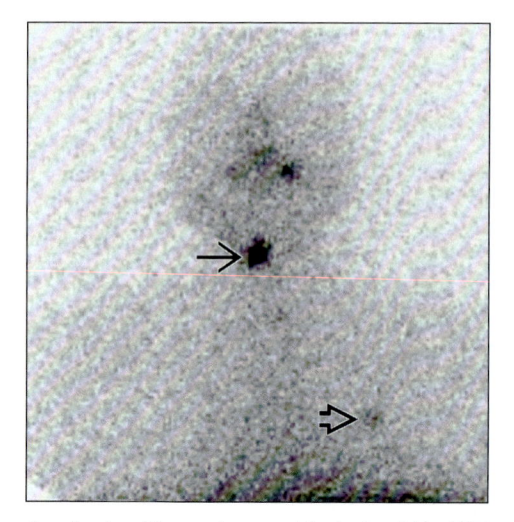

Anterior thyroid scan shows activity in thyroid bed ➡ and in a metastatic ⇨ lung nodule. This patient was treated with 200 mCi I-131.

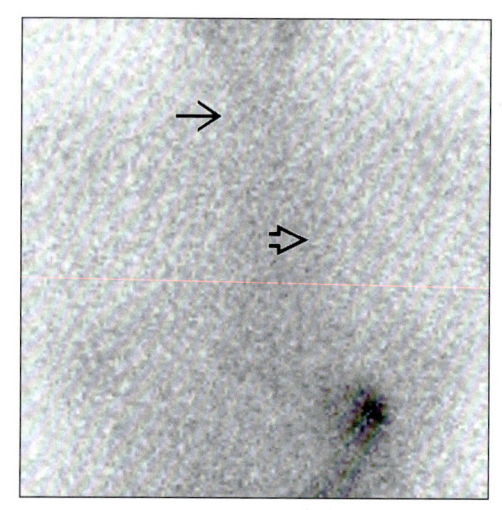

Anterior thyroid scan in same patient as previous image one year later shows normal scan, with resolution of thyroid bed ➡ and lung ⇨ activity.

TERMINOLOGY

Abbreviations
- Serum thyrotropin (TSH)
- Radioactive iodine (RAI)

Definitions
- Papillary, follicular, Hürthle cell, mixed thyroid cancer, anaplastic
  - < 45 years old
    - Stage I: Any tumor size, nodes +/-, no metastases
    - Stage II: Any tumor size, nodes +/-, + metastases
  - > 45 years old
    - Stage I: Tumor < 2 cm (limited to thyroid), - nodes, no metastases
    - Stage II: Tumor 2-4 cm (limited to thyroid), - nodes, no metastases
    - Stage III: Tumor size > 4 cm with no or minimal extrathyroidal extension or + level VI nodes, no metastases
    - Stage IV A: Extrathyroidal extension of differentiated tumor, surgically resectable anaplastic tumor; + level VI, cervical, superior mediastinal nodes; no metastases
    - Stage IV B: Unresectable tumor, +/- nodes, no metastases
    - Stage IV C: + Metastases
- Anaplastic, medullary
  - Not amenable to RAI therapy
- RAI treatment with I-131
  - High-energy beta emissions travel 0.8 mm, ablate thyroid tissue
  - Non-thyroid tissues minimally affected
  - Whole-body scan (WBS) scan can be done using gamma emissions

PRE-PROCEDURE

Indications
- Post-thyroidectomy remnant ablation
  - RAI ablation recommended for
    - Select stage I patients (multifocal disease, nodal metastases, extrathyroidal, vascular invasion, or more aggressive histology)
    - All patients < 45 yrs old with stage II
    - Most patients > 45 yrs old with stage II
    - Stage III/IV disease
  - If lobectomy only, RAI ablation not recommended
  - Dose: Usually 100-150 mCi, depending on surgical pathological findings
- Recurrent or residual disease
  - Detected on physical exam, WBS, ultrasound, CT, MR
  - Regional lymphadenopathy
  - Distant metastases (lungs, bones)
  - Elevated serum thyroglobulin with unknown anatomic site
  - Higher dose RAI: 150-200 mCi
    - RAI alone or as adjunct to surgery

Contraindications
- Pregnancy
- Breastfeeding within 2 months of treatment

Getting Started
- Things to Check
  - Pre-therapy WBS
    - Low to moderate risk patients: WBS may not be needed, controversial
    - High risk patients: Evaluate for distant metastases, locoregional disease
    - Recurrence: WBS to detect sites of disease, confirm disease is RAI-avid
  - RAI thyroid uptake measurement

I-131 THYROID CANCER THERAPY

Key Facts

Terminology
- Radioactive iodine (RAI)

Pre-procedure
- Patient follows low-iodine diet for 1-2 weeks
- Thyroid hormone withdrawal or recombinant human TSH (rhTSH) stimulation
- TSH > 30 mU/L if thyroid hormone withdrawal
- Negative pregnancy test
- Recent iodine load
- Inpatient versus outpatient therapy

Procedure
- I-131 capsule given po in nuclear medicine clinic
- If patient unable to swallow capsule, liquid I-131 administered via straw or feeding tube
- Inpatients often treated in hospital room
- Review radiation safety precautions
- Confirm that patient able to follow radiation safety guidelines
- Explain risks, benefits and indications of RAI with patient
- Obtain written informed consent
- Confirm patient name, date of birth
- Administer I-131 po
- Document administered dose
- Radiation safety release calculations/dose meter reading

Post-procedure
- Better prognosis: Age < 45 yrs
- Better prognosis: Small tumor, papillary/follicular
- Better prognosis: Females
- Better prognosis: Immediate treatment

- ≥ 5% uptake in remnant ⇒ lower therapy dose
- Patient follows low-iodine diet for 1-2 weeks
- Thyroid hormone withdrawal or recombinant human TSH (rhTSH) stimulation
- Laboratory tests
  - TSH > 30 mU/L if thyroid hormone withdrawal
  - Negative pregnancy test
  - Complete blood count if previously treated with high doses of I-131
- Recent iodine load
  - Contrast for angiogram, CT; high dietary iodine (e.g., sea kelp supplements)
  - Urine iodine level, should be < 200 microgram/L for RAI treatment
- Inpatient versus outpatient therapy
  - Nuclear Regulatory Commission guidelines: Can be treated as outpatient if total effective dose equivalent to any other individual does not exceed 5.0 mSv
  - Most treated as outpatients
  - Inpatient treatment for very high doses, contraindications to early release (e.g., unable to follow radiation safety precautions)
- Medications
  - Thyroid hormone withdrawal pre-WBS, therapy
    - Off levothyroxine for 4-6 weeks (half life of T4 is 2 weeks)
    - Alternatively give triiodothyronine (shorter T½) for 2-4 weeks, then triiodothyronine withdrawal for 2 weeks
  - Or stimulate thyroid tissue with rhTSH
    - Currently FDA approved for scan, not therapy
    - Used prior to RAI therapy in patients with contraindication to withdrawal (e.g., psychiatric illness, elderly)
    - Avoids hypothyroid symptoms as patient stays on thyroid hormone
    - Decreased RAI dose to blood due to faster body clearance
- Low iodine diet
  - < 50 micrograms/day
  - Start 1-2 weeks prior to treatment
- Dose of RAI (in general)
  - Low risk: 100 mCi
  - Higher risk, recurrent/residual disease: 125-200 mCi
  - Occasionally treat with > 200-300 mCi (recurrent, aggressive disease)
- Isolation for inpatients: Room prepped by radiation safety office, nuclear medicine technologist
- Treatment of appropriate patients as outpatients: Must follow radiation safety precautions

PROCEDURE

Patient Position/Location
- Best procedure approach
  - I-131 capsule given po in nuclear medicine clinic
  - If patient unable to swallow capsule, liquid I-131 administered via straw or feeding tube
    - Stringent radiation safety precautions required to avoid contaminating personnel with liquid
  - Inpatients often treated in hospital room

Procedure Steps
- Patient NPO 3-4 hrs prior to treatment
- Outpatient
  - Consultation
    - Review radiation safety precautions
    - Confirm that patient able to follow radiation safety guidelines
    - Explain risks, benefits and indications of RAI with patient
  - Obtain written informed consent
  - Confirm patient name, date of birth
  - Administer I-131 po
- Inpatient
  - Vitals and physical examination by nurses, physicians prior to treatment
  - Consultation as above
  - Obtain written informed consent
  - Confirm patient name, date of birth
  - Administer I-131 po
  - Measure dose rate 1 meter away from patient
  - Calculate dose rate needed for discharge

I-131 THYROID CANCER THERAPY

- Post-procedure instructions for patient
  o Resume low-iodine diet 2 hrs following I-131 ingestion
    ▪ Normal diet may be resumed 48 hrs post RAI
  o Encourage fluid intake
    ▪ Frequent urination ⇒ lower radiation dose to genitourinary tract
  o Begin using sour candy, gum 24-48 hrs post treatment
    ▪ Reduces stasis of I-131 in salivary glands
    ▪ Reported increased salivary damage if given earlier than 24 hours
  o Resume thyroid hormone 48-72 hrs post RAI therapy; continue thyroid hormone if rhTSH used

Findings and Reporting
- Document administered dose
- Radiation safety release calculations/dose meter reading

Alternative Procedures/Therapies
- Radiologic
  o Thyroid radiofrequency ablation, embolization
    ▪ Few case reports for nonsurgical thyroidectomy patients
- Surgical
  o Thyroidectomy = primary treatment for thyroid cancer
  o Recurrent disease in neck may be treated with surgery + RAI
- Other
  o External beam radiation
    ▪ Considered for gross tumor therapy when surgery, RAI not effective (non-iodine-avid disease, anaplastic)
    ▪ Palliation of bone metastases causing pain, pathologic fracture, neurologic compromise
  o Chemotherapy: Little data to support use

POST-PROCEDURE

Expected Outcome
- Prognosis
  o Better prognosis: Age < 45 yrs
  o Better prognosis: Small tumor, papillary/follicular
  o Better prognosis: Females
  o Better prognosis: Immediate treatment
- Locoregional disease
  o Single dose of I-131: ~ 65% effective in eradicating disease
- Distant metastatic disease
  o Single dose of I-131
    ▪ 33% effective for lung metastases
    ▪ 7% effective for bone metastases

Things To Do
- Post-therapy WBS
  o 7-10 days following RAI therapy
  o Detects additional sites of disease ≤ 26% of patients

Things To Avoid
- Pregnancy
  o In males and females, avoid pregnancy for 6 months

PROBLEMS & COMPLICATIONS

Problems
- Nausea
  o Common; prescribe antiemetic
- Diarrhea
  o Rare
- Salivary gland complications
  o Xerostomia: Sour candy, gum use (> 24 hrs post RAI) may prevent
  o Radiation parotitis: Worse in older patients, not common
- Change in sense of taste
  o Usually returns to normal in 1-6 months
- Sore throat
  o Due to local radiation dose from thyroid bed
  o Throat lozenges for symptomatic relief
- Radiation thyroiditis
  o Mild neck pain
  o More common when significant residual thyroid
  o Treat with nonsteroidal anti-inflammatory medication or corticosteroids

Complications
- Most feared complication(s)
  o Radiation lung fibrosis
    ▪ If diffuse pulmonary metastases, consider dosimetry
  o Bone marrow suppression
    ▪ Consider dosimetry for very large doses, especially in children or renal insufficiency
- Other complications
  o Infertility
    ▪ Possible very small risk of permanent infertility with multiple high doses in males
  o Anaplastic transformation of differentiated tumors
    ▪ Few reported cases
  o Secondary malignancies
    ▪ Very low risk; dose-related

SELECTED REFERENCES

1. Cooper DS et al: Management Guidelines for Patients with Thyroid Nodules and Differentiated Thyroid Cancer. Thyroid. [Epub ahead of print] No abstract available, 2006
2. Pacini F et al: Radioiodine ablation of thyroid remnants after preparation with recombinant human thyrotropin in differentiated thyroid carcinoma: results of an international, randomized, controlled study. J Clin Endocrinol Metab. 91(3):926-32, 2006
3. Nakada K et al: Does lemon candy decrease salivary gland damage after radioiodine therapy for thyroid cancer? J Nucl Med. 46(2):261-6, 2005
4. Robbins RJ et al: The evolving role of (131)I for the treatment of differentiated thyroid carcinoma. J Nucl Med. 46 Suppl 1:28S-37S, 2005
5. Rubino C et al: Second primary malignancies in thyroid cancer patients. Br J Cancer. 89(9):1638-44, 2003
6. Mazzaferri EL et al: Management of papillary and follicular (differentiated) thyroid cancer: new paradigms using recombinant human thyrotropin. Endocr Relat Cancer. 9(4):227-47, 2002
7. Parthasarathy KL et al: Treatment of thyroid carcinoma: emphasis on high-dose 131I outpatient therapy. J Nucl Med Technol. 30(4):165-71; quiz 172-3, 2002

I-131 THYROID CANCER THERAPY

IMAGE GALLERY

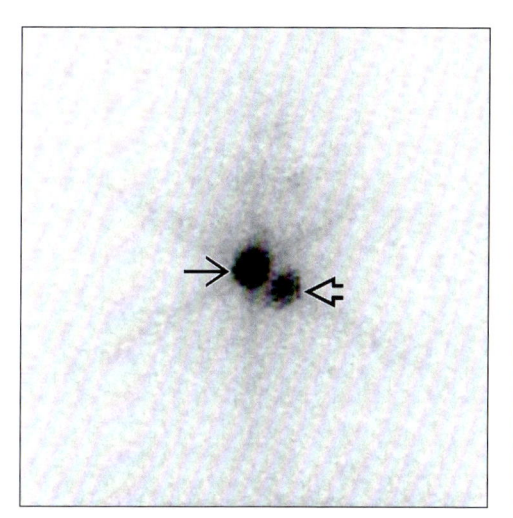

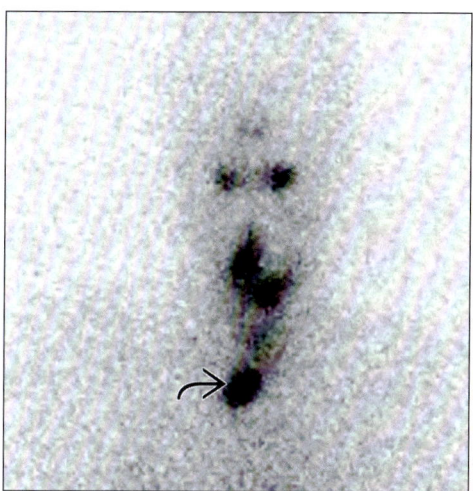

(Left) Anterior thyroid scan shows thyroid bed activity ➔ and lymphadenopathy ⇨. This patient received 150 mCi I-131. *(Right)* Anterior thyroid scan (of same patient as previous image) post-therapy, shows a third focus of activity ➔ which may represent additional metastatic thyroid cancer or normal substernal thyroid tissues.

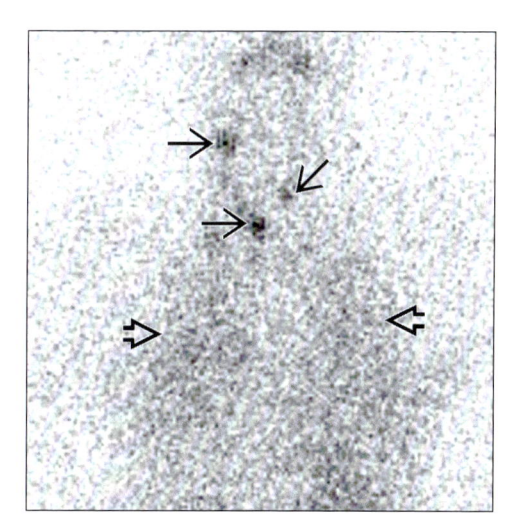

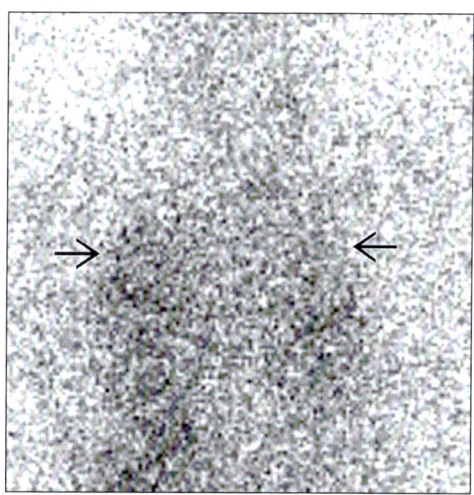

(Left) Anterior thyroid scan shows three foci of disease in the neck ➔ and diffuse lung activity ⇨ in patient with metastatic follicular thyroid carcinoma. Body dosimetry was performed to ensure no more than 80 mCi would be delivered to the lungs. *(Right)* Posterior thyroid scan of same patient as previous image shows extensive lung metastases ➔.

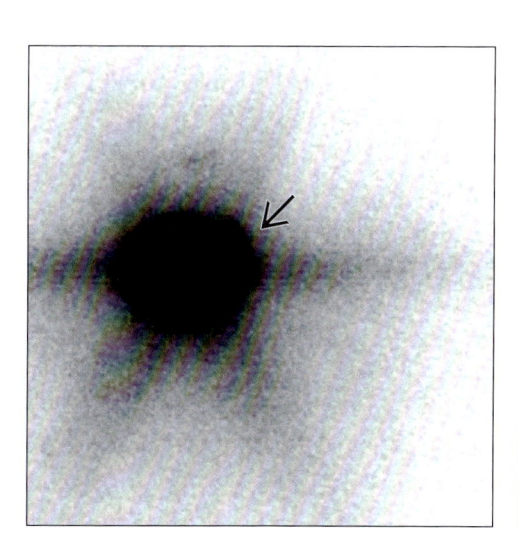

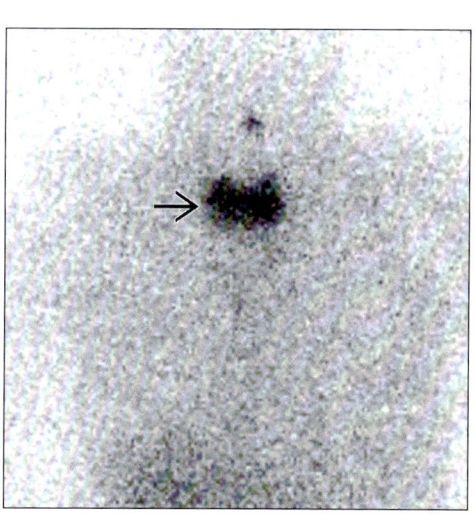

(Left) Anterior thyroid scan 7 days post RAI therapy with 40 mCi I-131 shows large amount of uptake in thyroid ➔. This patient was not a surgical candidate; RAI was given in lieu of surgery. *(Right)* Anterior thyroid scan of same patient as previous image 7 months later shows residual thyroid activity ➔ in neck. The patient was given a second dose of I-131 (100 mCi). This is an uncommon treatment approach, as several RAI administrations are often needed.

WELL-DIFFERENTIATED THYROID CANCER, PET

Coronal fused PET/CT shows focal uptake in superior left thyroid bed ➔ consistent with recurrent thyroid cancer. Patient had prior thyroidectomy and I-131 therapy. I-131 scan was negative.

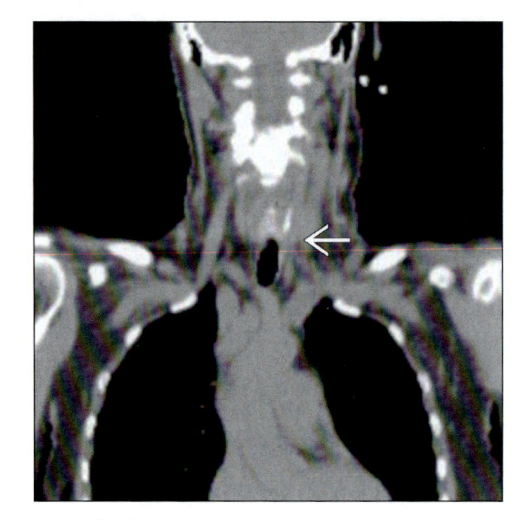

Coronal NECT in same patient as previous image with recurrent thyroid cancer in left thyroid bed. Site of recurrence inapparent by CT ➔. Iodinated contrast contraindicated if I-131 therapy contemplated.

TERMINOLOGY

Abbreviations and Synonyms
- Well-differentiated thyroid cancer (WDTC)

Definitions
- Thyroid carcinoma of papillary and/or follicular cell origin

IMAGING FINDINGS

General Features
- Best diagnostic clue
  - Focal asymmetrically increased uptake on FDG PET due to normal structure or inflammatory condition
  - Not due to normal structure or inflammatory condition
- Location
  - Primary well-differentiated thyroid cancer
    - Focal area of uptake in the thyroid gland (usually found incidentally when FDG PET performed for another reason)
    - Focal uptake in thyroid nodule ~ 50% chance of malignancy
  - Recurrence
    - Typically in the thyroid bed
  - Metastatic disease
    - Cervical and mediastinal lymph nodes
    - Distant metastases to bone, lungs and mediastinum
- Size
  - Metastatic cervical nodes often are not enlarged
  - Lung metastases may be inapparent by CT (diffuse microscopic)
- Morphology
  - Metastatic nodes may not be abnormal in morphology by CT or ultrasound
  - Typical conformation of thymus can help differentiate from anterior mediastinal nodal metastases

Nuclear Medicine Findings
- FDG PET Scan

DDx: Thyroid Cancer

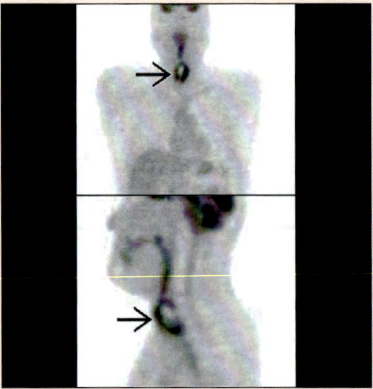

Tracheostomy Site

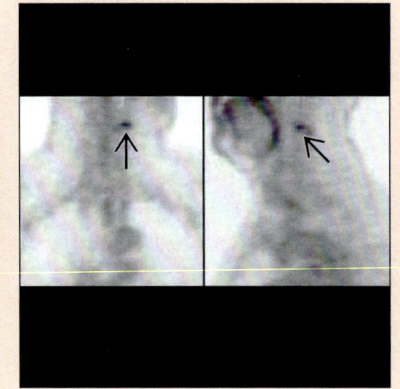

Degenerative Facet

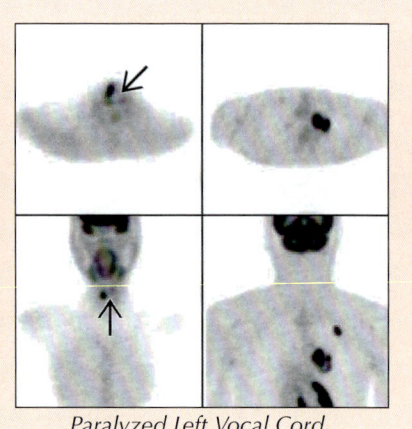

Paralyzed Left Vocal Cord

WELL-DIFFERENTIATED THYROID CANCER, PET

Key Facts

Imaging Findings
- PET scan indicated & approved for reimbursement by CMS in patients with thyroidectomy, radioactive I-131 therapy, elevated serum thyroglobulin, but negative I-131 whole body scan
- Best FDG PET yield: Patients with stimulated thyroglobulin > 10 mU/L
- FDG uptake by WDTC is often only moderate (mean SUV ~ 2.5 at 60 min)
- Elevated thyrotropin (TSH) nearly doubles SUV in sites of WDTC over suppressed state
- High resolution neck ultrasound: Preferred method for surveillance following I-131 therapy by most endocrinologists
- FNA of any suspicious lymph nodes can be accomplished at the time of ultrasound
- FDG PET should optimally be performed with elevated TSH
- Optimized dosage schedule for rhTSH is not yet established, but Medicare pays for two injections; we recommend 0.9 gm IM on day 1 and day 2, and FDG PET on day 3-5 (all acceptable)

Clinical Issues
- If pre-Rx I-131 scan negative, consider giving therapeutic I-131 if Tg ↑: Often effective if post-Rx I-131 scan proves positive
- Non-iodine avid recurrence: FDG PET may help identify areas ammenable to surgical removal

Diagnostic Checklist
- Focal uptake in thyroid may represent thyroid cancer (~ 50%)

- o PET scan indicated & approved for reimbursement by CMS in patients with thyroidectomy, radioactive I-131 therapy, elevated serum thyroglobulin, but negative I-131 whole body scan
  - In these situations, approximately 50% of patients will have site of identifiable tumor by FDG PET
- o Best FDG PET yield: Patients with stimulated thyroglobulin > 10 mU/L
- o FDG uptake by WDTC is often only moderate (mean SUV ~ 2.5 at 60 min)
- o Elevated thyrotropin (TSH) nearly doubles SUV in sites of WDTC over suppressed state
- o Combined PET/CT is useful for differentiating lymph node metastases, muscle uptake, and hypermetabolic brown fat
- FDG PET can follow a negative I-131 or I-123 whole body scan in patients with elevated thyroglobulin (Tg)
  - o I-131 or I-123 whole body scan should be performed prior to injection of FDG, if both scans performed on same day
- Additional nuclear medicine imaging options
  - o High resolution neck ultrasound: Preferred method for surveillance following I-131 therapy by most endocrinologists
    - FNA of any suspicious lymph nodes can be accomplished at the time of ultrasound
    - Typically done when TSH (thyrogen or hypothyroid) stimulated Tg is > 10 mU/L (some use 2 mU/L cut off)
    - Operator dependent and time consuming but excellent results in experienced hands
    - FDG PET can be reserved for cases where site of tumor is inapparent, or where high-resolution ultrasound is difficult
  - o I-123 or I-131 whole body scan
    - May be completely normal with extensive metastatic disease, indicating tumor has become less well differentiated and/or non non-iodine avid
  - o Tc-99m MIBI (sestamibi)
    - Useful in identifying sites of non-iodine avid well-differentiated thyroid cancer
    - Most practitioners feel that sestamibi is inferior to FDG PET

Imaging Recommendations
- Best imaging tool
  - o I-123 or I-131 whole body scan when tumor is iodine avid
  - o FDG PET scan for non iodine avid tumor
- Protocol advice
  - o FDG PET should optimally be performed with elevated TSH
    - TSH increases thyrocyte metabolism, glucose transport, hexokinase I levels, and overall glycolysis
    - TSH elevation can be accomplished by either thyroid hormone withdrawal (hypothyroid state) or administration of recombinant human TSH (rhTSH, "thyrogen")
    - Optimized dosage schedule for rhTSH is not yet established, but Medicare pays for two injections; we recommend 0.9 gm IM on day 1 and day 2, and FDG PET on day 3-5 (all acceptable)

DIFFERENTIAL DIAGNOSIS

Benign Thyroid Conditions
- Increased FDG uptake in incidentally-identified thyroid nodule
  - o 50% chance of malignancy
  - o Others are benign nodules, usually follicular adenomas

Other Cancers of Head and Neck
- Squamous cell carcinoma of the head and neck
- Neuroendocrine tumors
- Metastases
- Anaplastic thyroid cancer
- Lymphoma of thyroid gland
- Medullary thyroid cancer

Normal/Benign Extrathyroidal Structures
- Asymmetrical muscle uptake

WELL-DIFFERENTIATED THYROID CANCER, PET

- ○ Valium prior to injection may reduce
- ○ Gentle support of head during uptake interval
- Vocal cords
  - ○ Avoid talking during uptake interval
- Cricoarytenoids
  - ○ Often asymmetrical
- Tonsillar and adenoid tissue
  - ○ Careful history regarding upper respiratory infection, allergies
- Reactive lymph nodes
  - ○ Often in presence of enhanced tonsillar FDG uptake
- Salivary glands
  - ○ FDG uptake often asymmetrical if patient treated previously with I-131
  - ○ Accessory sites of salivary tissue may be difficult to distinguish from lymph nodes
    - ▪ Pertechnetate scan may be helpful in defining (cannot do on same day after FDG injection)
- Degenerative arthritis of cervical spine
  - ○ Facet joints may be quite focal in FDG uptake
- Tracheostomy sites

CLINICAL ISSUES

Presentation
- Most common signs/symptoms: Palpable neck mass
- Other signs/symptoms
  - ○ Hoarseness
  - ○ Dysphagia
  - ○ Bone pain (bone mets)
  - ○ Cough (lung or mediastinal mets)
  - ○ Elevated Tg levels after definitive treatment of WDTC
    - ▪ TSH-stimulated thyroglobulin levels more sensitive

Demographics
- Age: Thyroid cancer occurs over a wide range of ages, including pediatric patients
- Gender: Females predominate for all histologies

Natural History & Prognosis
- Best prognosis females 20-40 years
- Intensely FDG avid tumor is a poor prognostic indicator
- 96% of patients with WDTC are curable with current treatment strategies
  - ○ Most favorable prognosis in papillary or papillary-follicular cell types
- Size of primary nodule is more important than presence of lymph node involvement in prognosis of papillary thyroid cancer
  - ○ < 2.5 cm primary: Excellent prognosis
    - ▪ Necessity for definitive surgery and radioiodine therapy has not been well established
    - ▪ Ablation of thyroid remnant with ~ 30 mCi I-131 is often desirable to enable long term thyroglobulin assessment
  - ○ Extracervical disease is rarely curable

Treatment
- If pre-Rx I-131 scan negative, consider giving therapeutic I-131 if Tg ↑: Often effective if post-Rx I-131 scan proves positive
- Non-iodine avid recurrence: FDG PET may help identify areas ammenable to surgical removal
- Surgery or external beam radiation are other options

DIAGNOSTIC CHECKLIST

Image Interpretation Pearls
- Focal uptake in thyroid may represent thyroid cancer (~ 50%)
- Residual or recurrent thyroid cancer is often only moderate in FDG uptake (SUV 2.0-3.0): Can be improved with TSH stimulation

SELECTED REFERENCES

1. David A et al: Clinical value of different responses of serum thyroglobulin to recombinant human thyrotropin in the follow-up of patients with differentiated thyroid carcinoma. Thyroid. 15(2):158-64, 2005
2. Hooft L et al: [18F]fluorodeoxyglucose uptake in recurrent thyroid cancer is related to hexokinase i expression in the primary tumor. J Clin Endocrinol Metab. 90(1):328-34, 2005
3. Kim TY et al: 18F-fluorodeoxyglucose uptake in thyroid from positron emission tomogram (PET) for evaluation in cancer patients: high prevalence of malignancy in thyroid PET incidentaloma. Laryngoscope. 115(6):1074-8, 2005
4. Macapinlac HA: FDG-PET in head and neck, and thyroid cancer. Chang Gung Med J. 28(5):284-95, 2005
5. Robbins RJ et al: Real-time Prognosis for Metastatic Thyroid Carcinoma Based on FDG-PET Scanning. J Clin Endocrinol Metab. 2005
6. Yi JG et al: Focal uptake of fluorodeoxyglucose by the thyroid in patients undergoing initial disease staging with combined PET/CT for non-small cell lung cancer. Radiology. 236(1):271-5, 2005
7. Chin BB et al: Recombinant human thyrotropin stimulation of fluoro-D-glucose positron emission tomography uptake in well-differentiated thyroid carcinoma. J Clin Endocrinol Metab. 89(1):91-5, 2004
8. Menzel C et al: The influence of thyroglobulin on functional imaging in differentiated thyroid cancer. Nucl Med Commun. 25(3):239-43, 2004
9. Scanga DR et al: Value of FDG PET imaging in the management of patients with thyroid, neuroendocrine, and neural crest tumors. Clin Nucl Med. 29(2):86-90, 2004
10. Zhuang H et al: Investigation of thyroid, head, and neck cancers with PET. Radiol Clin North Am. 42(6):1101-11, viii, 2004
11. Boer A et al: FDG PET imaging in hereditary thyroid cancer. Eur J Surg Oncol. 29(10):922-8, 2003
12. Szakall S Jr et al: 18F-FDG PET detection of lymph node metastases in medullary thyroid carcinoma. J Nucl Med. 43(1):66-71, 2002
13. Van Tol KM et al: Better yield of (18)fluorodeoxyglucose-positron emission tomography in patients with metastatic differentiated thyroid carcinoma during thyrotropin stimulation. Thyroid. 12(5):381-7, 2002
14. Helal BO et al: Clinical impact of (18)F-FDG PET in thyroid carcinoma patients with elevated thyroglobulin levels and negative (131)I scanning results after therapy. J Nucl Med. 42(10):1464-9, 2001

WELL-DIFFERENTIATED THYROID CANCER, PET

IMAGE GALLERY

Typical

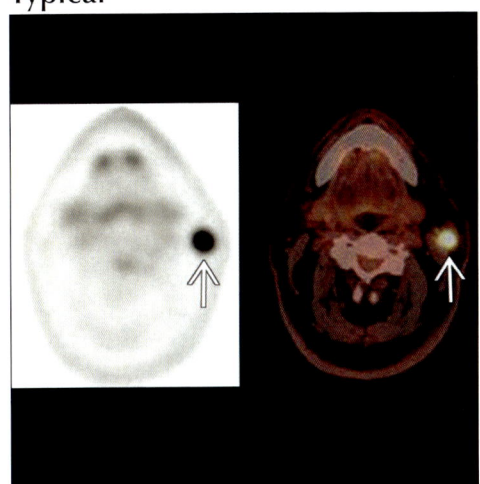

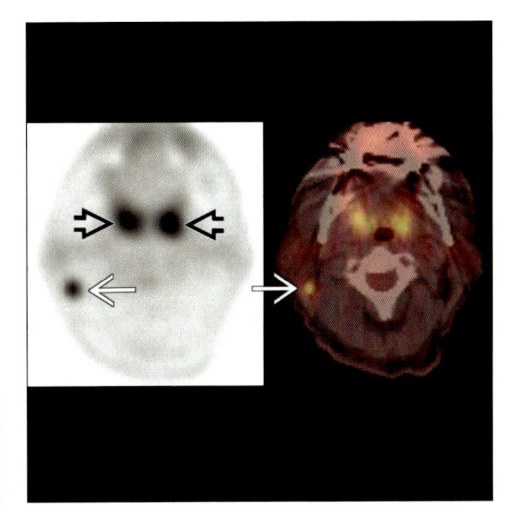

(Left) Axial PET and fused PET/CT images demonstrate intense focus of activity in subcutaneous node in left neck ➡. Focus was non-iodine avid metastatic papillary follicular thyroid cancer. *(Right)* Axial PET and fused PET/CT images demonstrate FDG avid 1 cm high right level II node ➡ proved metastatic WDTC. I-131 scan negative. Note marked uptake in normal adenoid tissue ➡.

Variant

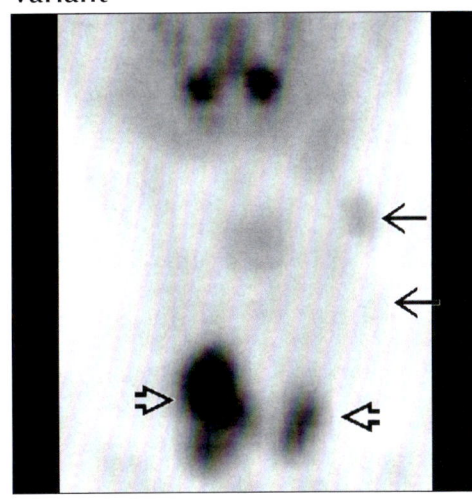

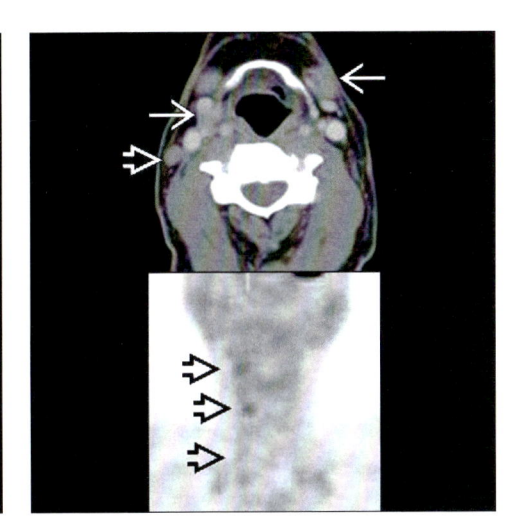

(Left) Anterior MIP PET image of neck with bilateral lobular FDG-avid WDTC ➡ (initially presumed to be multinodular goiter) and faint uptake in metastatic left neck nodes ➡. *(Right)* Axial CT and coronal FDG PET without TSH stimulation demonstrate only mild-moderate FDG uptake in sites of nodal metastatic WDTC ➡, ➡. Other CT sites ➡ were post-therapy inflammation.

Other

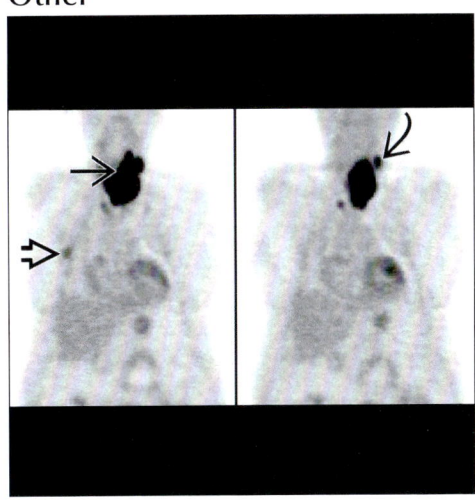

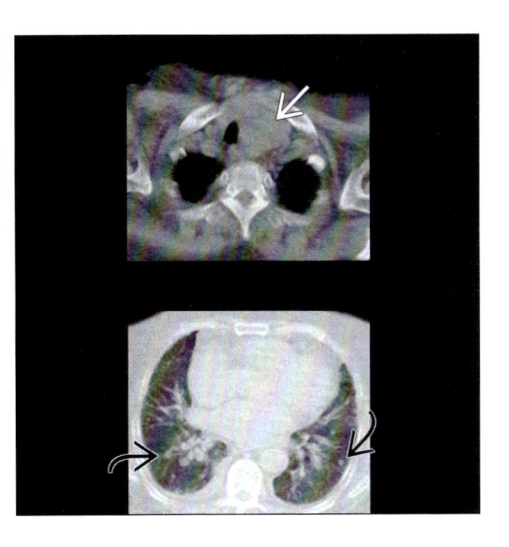

(Left) Axial and coronal PET with FDG uptake in anaplastic thyroid cancer ➡ with cervical nodal ➡ and lung ➡ metastases. Tumor grew over 2 month interval. *(Right)* Axial soft tissue and lung windows from CT of patient at left demonstrates markedly enlarged thyroid mass ➡ and multiple lung metastases ➡. Diagnosis was anaplastic thyroid cancer.

MEDULLARY THYROID CANCER

Coronal FDG PET shows hypermetabolic foci in upper lumbar vertebra ➔, left sacroiliac region ➔ and left lung ➔ in a patient with metastatic medullary thyroid cancer. Same patient as next image.

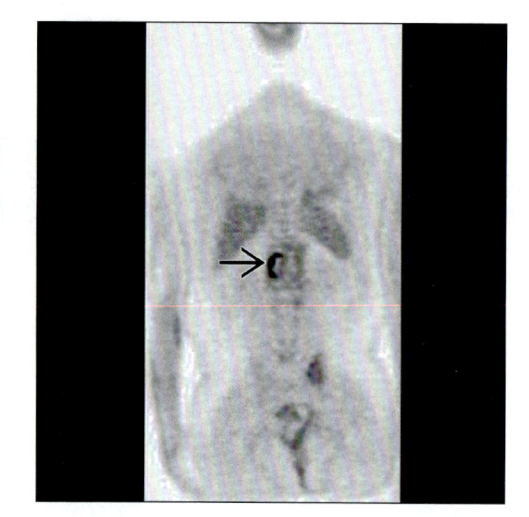

Coronal FDG PET, same patient as previous after radiation therapy shows hypermetabolic rim ➔ in upper lumbar vertebra, probably residual sacroiliac tumor. Other sites may be post treatment inflammation.

TERMINOLOGY

Abbreviations and Synonyms
- Abbreviation: Medullary thyroid carcinoma (MTC)

Definitions
- Rare neuroendocrine malignancy arising from thyroid parafollicular "C-cells"

IMAGING FINDINGS

General Features
- Best diagnostic clue: Solid lesions in thyroid gland with nodal metastases; ± calcifications
- Location
  - Within thyroid gland, no lobar predisposition
  - Frequently multifocal
    - 2/3 of sporadic cases, almost all familial cases
  - Nodal metastases: Level VI and superior mediastinum
    - Retropharyngeal nodes, levels III and IV (mid and low internal jugular chain)
- Size: 2-25 mm
- Morphology
  - Solid, usually well-circumscribed mass in thyroid gland
  - More infiltrative type seen with familial forms

Nuclear Medicine Findings
- Nuclear medicine methods: For detection of recurrent disease when cross-section imaging negative
  - FDG PET: Sensitivity 70-100%, specificity 79-90%
    - Also positive in well-differentiated and anaplastic thyroid cancer, thyroiditis, other malignancies
  - In-111 octreotide (pentetreotide, Octreoscan): Sensitivity 25-41%, specificity 92%
    - Also positive in many neuroendocrine tumors
  - Sestamibi or Myoview: Sensitivity 25-40%, specificity 100%
    - Also positive in thyroid and parathyroid adenomas, various malignancies
  - Tc-99m pentavalent (V) DMSA: Sensitivity 33-40%, specificity 78%
  - In same series as nuclear techniques: Sensitivity/specificity MR (82/67%), CT (50/20%)
  - I-131/I-123 Methyiodobenzylguanidine (MIBG): Limited reports, can be positive in MTC

DDx: Mimics of Medullary Thyroid Cancer

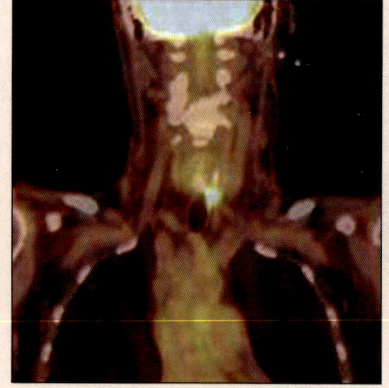

Thyroid Cancer

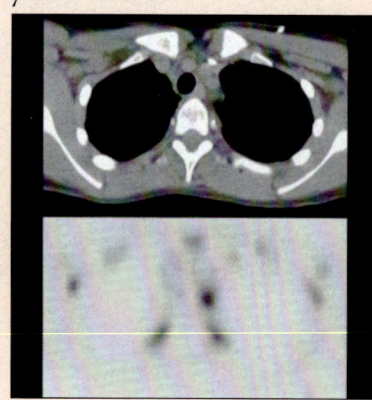

Hypermetabolic Brown Fat

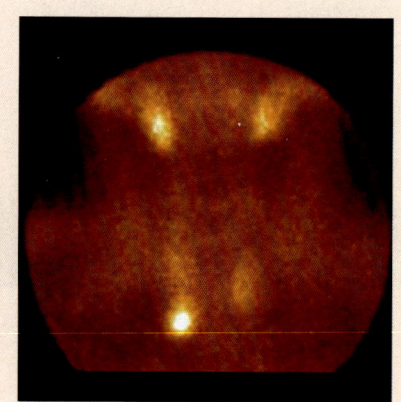

Parathyroid Adenoma (Sestamibi)

MEDULLARY THYROID CANCER

Key Facts

Terminology
- Abbreviation: Medullary thyroid carcinoma (MTC)
- Rare neuroendocrine malignancy arising from thyroid parafollicular "C-cells"

Imaging Findings
- FDG PET: Sensitivity 70-100%, specificity 79-90%
- Not iodine avid: Scanning and treatment with radioiodine not effective

Top Differential Diagnoses
- Multinodular Goiter (MNG)
- Follicular Adenoma
- Thyroid Non-Hodgkin Lymphoma (NHL)
- Well-Differentiated Thyroid Carcinoma
- Parathyroid Adenoma

Pathology
- Sporadic (~ 85%) or hereditary, familial forms (15%)
- Type 2 multiple endocrine neoplasia (MEN) syndromes
- Familial medullary thyroid carcinoma (FMTC)

Clinical Issues
- Clinical Profile: Middle-age patient with lower neck mass or patient with family history of MEN has tumor found on screening exam
- Familial type almost always multifocal and bilateral
- 2/3 of sporadic cases are bilateral
- Up to 75% have lymphadenopathy at presentation
- Mainstay of MTC treatment is complete resection of local and regional disease

---

- Most helpful for suspected recurrence
  - Elevated tumor markers but no gross disease on cross-sectional imaging
- Not iodine avid: Scanning and treatment with radioiodine not effective

CT Findings
- CECT
  - No contraindication to iodinated contrast as with epithelial thyroid tumors
  - Solid low density well-circumscribed mass in thyroid; may be multifocal (familial types)
  - Fine, punctate calcifications in tumor and nodal metastases

MR Findings
- Irregular margins and extraglandular extension; often well-defined

Ultrasonographic Findings
- Grayscale Ultrasound
  - Hypoechoic, irregular intrathyroidal mass with microcalcifications
  - Lymph nodes frequently detected
- Color Doppler: Hypervascularity with irregular arrangement of vessels

Imaging Recommendations
- Best imaging tool
  - High resolution ultrasound (US) is most frequent initial tool for evaluation of thyroid nodule
    - FNA can be performed at same time
  - MR or FDG PET/CT for cases where cross-sectional imaging negative (similar performance)
  - CECT may have better performance in mediastinum than MR
- Protocol advice
  - Consider PET/CT protocol with high resolution technique, iodinated contrast
  - CECT, must extend to carina in order to evaluate mediastinal nodes

DIFFERENTIAL DIAGNOSIS

Multinodular Goiter (MNG)
- Diffusely enlarged gland with multiple nodules, course calcifications

Follicular Adenoma
- Solitary mass without evidence of invasion, no adenopathy

Thyroid Non-Hodgkin Lymphoma (NHL)
- Diffuse enlargement of gland with infiltrative mass
- Rarely see calcifications in mass or in nodes

Well-Differentiated Thyroid Carcinoma
- Similar imaging features to MTC on CT, US, MR, nuclear methods (except radioiodine)

Parathyroid Adenoma
- Similar features on Tc-99m sestamibi, Myoview; usually extrathyroidal

PATHOLOGY

General Features
- General path comments
  - Arises from parafollicular "C-cells" of thyroid that secrete calcitonin
    - "C-cells" derived from ultimobranchial bodies
- Genetics
  - Sporadic (~ 85%) or hereditary, familial forms (15%)
  - Associated with mutations of RET proto-oncogene on chromosome 10q11.2
    - Found in familial (100%) and sporadic (40-60%) cases
    - Screening for RET mutations is performed for family members of patients with MTC
- Etiology
  - No identified exogenous cause and not related to other thyroid conditions
  - Type 2 multiple endocrine neoplasia (MEN) syndromes

MEDULLARY THYROID CANCER

- Autosomal dominant
- MEN 2A: Multifocal MTC, pheochromocytoma, parathyroid hyperplasia, hyperparathyroidism
- MEN 2B: Multifocal MTC, pheochromocytoma, mucosal neuromas of lips, tongue, GI tract, conjunctiva; younger patients, more aggressive tumors
  - Familial medullary thyroid carcinoma (FMTC)
    - Autosomal dominant condition where only neoplasm is MTC
    - Later onset, more indolent course than MEN syndromes
- Epidemiology
  - 5-10% all thyroid gland malignancies
  - ≤ 14% thyroid cancer deaths
  - 10% pediatric thyroid malignancies (MEN 2)

Gross Pathologic & Surgical Features
- Solid, firm, well-circumscribed but non-encapsulated
  - Tan/pink cut section, calcifications may be evident
- Necrosis and hemorrhage only with larger lesions

Microscopic Features
- Proliferation of large atypical round to polygonal cells with granular cytoplasm
- Cells separated by vascular stroma, hyalinized collagen and amyloid
- Stains strongly for calcitonin (80%)
- Also stains for carcinoembryonic antigen (CEA), chromogranin A and neuron-specific enolase

CLINICAL ISSUES

Presentation
- Most common signs/symptoms
  - Painless thyroid nodule
  - Other signs/symptoms
    - Less commonly dysphagia, hoarseness, pain
    - Uncommonly presents with paraneoplastic syndromes: Cushing or carcinoid syndromes
    - Rarely presents with diarrhea from elevated calcitonin, though often an associated symptom
  - Elevated serum calcitonin
    - Used as screening tool, for estimation of extent of disease and as baseline for post-operative monitoring
- Clinical Profile: Middle-age patient with lower neck mass or patient with family history of MEN has tumor found on screening exam

Demographics
- Age
  - Sporadic form: Mean age = 50 years
  - Familial form: Mean age = 30 years
  - Can occur in children, especially with MEN 2B
- Gender: M < F in Caucasians and in children

Natural History & Prognosis
- Familial type almost always multifocal and bilateral
- 2/3 of sporadic cases are bilateral
- Up to 75% have lymphadenopathy at presentation
- Indicators of better prognosis
  - Female gender, younger age at surgery
  - FMTC and MEN 2A syndromes
  - Tumor < 10 cm, no nodes, early stage disease
  - Normal preoperative CEA levels, complete surgical resection
- Overall 5 year survival = 72%; 10 year = 56%

Treatment
- Prophylactic thyroidectomy performed if familial RET mutation detected
  - FMTC and MEN 2A perform thyroidectomy at age 5-6
  - MEN 2B perform thyroidectomy during infancy
- Mainstay of MTC treatment is complete resection of local and regional disease
  - Total thyroidectomy with level VI nodal dissection ± superior mediastinal nodes
  - Node levels II-V resected if positive nodes in lateral neck
- Adjuvant radiation therapy
  - XRT used if extensive soft tissue invasion or extracapsular nodal spread

DIAGNOSTIC CHECKLIST

Consider
- Consider familial syndromes with multifocal tumors or young patient

Image Interpretation Pearls
- Imaging appearance may exactly mimic differentiated thyroid carcinoma
- PET/CT and MR best performance for detection of recurrence: PET and CECT allows detection of distant mets

SELECTED REFERENCES

1. Khan N et al: Review of fluorine-18-2-fluoro-2-deoxy-D-glucose positron emission tomography (FDG-PET) in the follow-up of medullary and anaplastic thyroid carcinomas. Cancer Control. 12(4):254-60, 2005
2. Li S et al: The radionuclide molecular imaging and therapy of neuroendocrine tumors. Curr Cancer Drug Targets. 5(2):139-48, 2005
3. Bustillo A et al: Octreotide scintigraphy in the head and neck. Laryngoscope. 114(3):434-40, 2004
4. de Groot JW et al: Impact of 18F-fluoro-2-deoxy-D-glucose positron emission tomography (FDG-PET) in patients with biochemical evidence of recurrent or residual medullary thyroid cancer. Ann Surg Oncol. 11(8):786-94, 2004
5. Massoll N et al: Diagnosis and management of medullary thyroid carcinoma. Clin Lab Med. 24(1):49-83, 2004
6. Schoder H et al: Positron emission imaging of head and neck cancer, including thyroid carcinoma. Semin Nucl Med. 34(3):180-97, 2004
7. Clayman GL et al: Medullary thyroid cancer. Otolaryngol Clin North Am. 36(1):91-105, 2003
8. Solbiati L et al: Ultrasound of thyroid, parathyroid glands and neck lymph nodes. Eur Radiol. 11(12):2411-24, 2001
9. Dorr U et al: The contribution of somatostatin receptor scintigraphy to the diagnosis of recurrent medullary carcinoma of the thyroid. Semin Oncol. 21(5 Suppl 13):42-5, 1994

MEDULLARY THYROID CANCER

IMAGE GALLERY

Typical

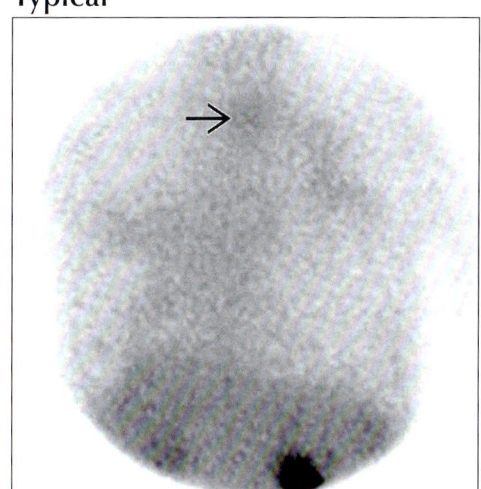

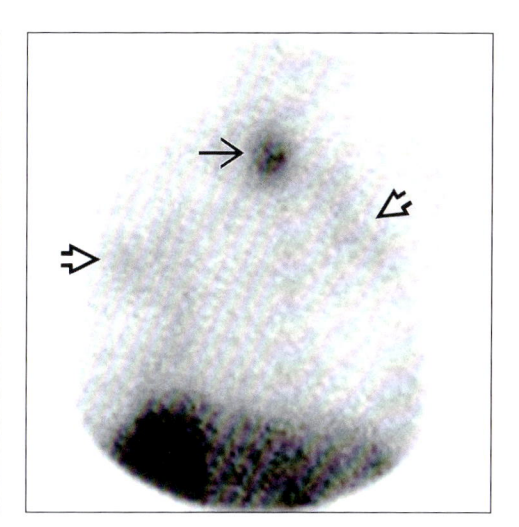

(Left) Anterior planar chest, In-111 octreoscan at 4 h post tracer injection. Vague uptake in lower neck ➡ at site of MTC. Vague uptake in chest is known inflammatory disease. Same patient as next image. *(Right)* Anterior planar chest, In-111 octreoscan at 24 h post tracer injection. Significant uptake in lower neck ➡ at site of MTC. Mild uptake in chest ⇨ is known inflammatory disease.

Variant

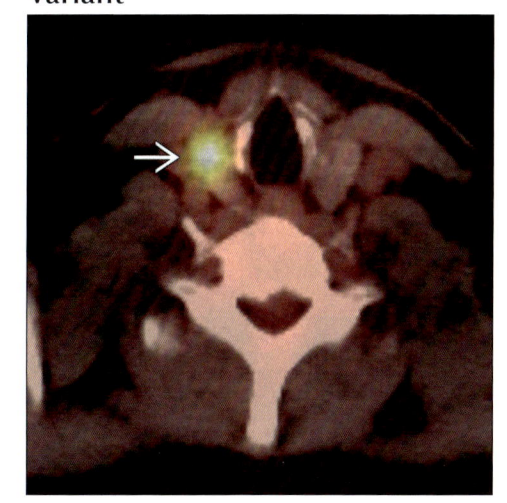

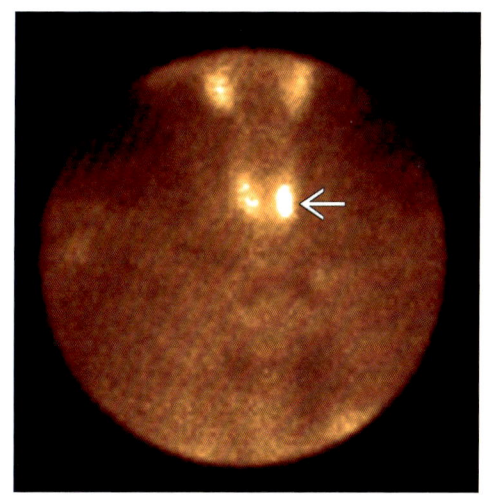

(Left) Fused transaxial FDG PET/CT shows focal hypermetabolic mass ➡ in right thyroid lobe in patient with medullary thyroid cancer. *(Right)* Anterior planar chest Tc-99m sestamibi scan performed for parathyroid adenoma localization shows focal uptake ➡ in lower right thyroid lobe. Medullary thyroid cancer at biopsy.

Typical

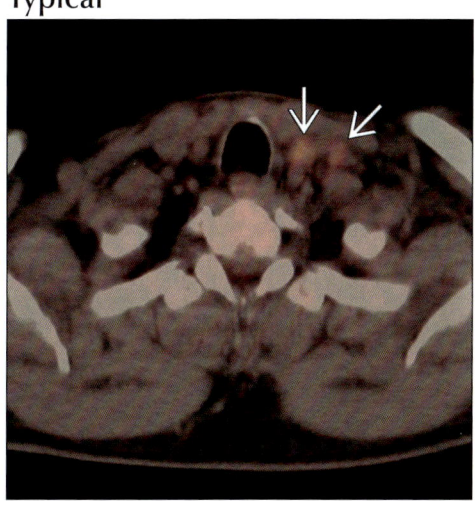

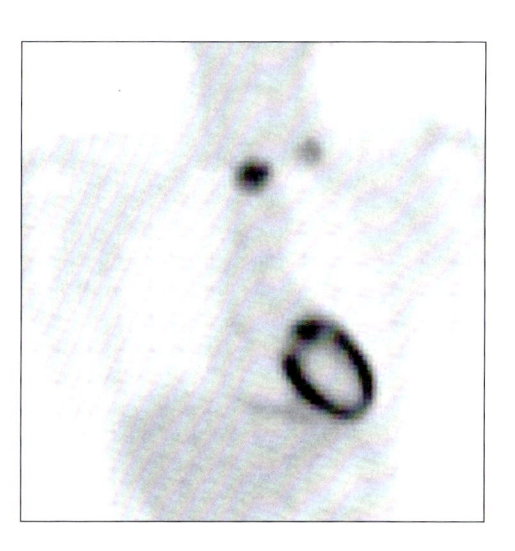

(Left) Transaxial fused FDG PET/CT shows hypermetabolic left level IV metastatic nodes ➡ in patient with elevated calcitonin 1 year post thyroidectomy for MTC. *(Right)* Coronal FDG PET in patient with breast cancer shows unsuspected uptake in thyroid bed and left lower neck, proven at biopsy to be MTC. No breast cancer mets were identified.

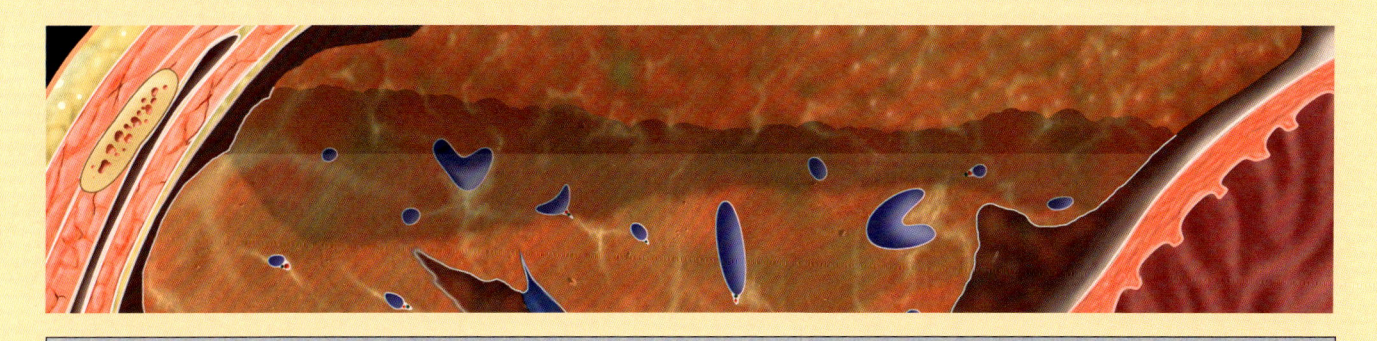

SECTION 8: Gastrointestinal

Introduction and Overview
GI Anatomy & Imaging Issues	8-2

Biliary
Acute Calculous Cholecystitis	8-4
Acute Acalculous Cholecystitis	8-10
Chronic Cholecystitis	8-16
Biliary Leak	8-20
Common Bile Duct Obstruction	8-22
Choledochal Cyst	8-24
Biliary Bypass Obstruction	8-28
Biliary Atresia	8-30
Cholangiocarcinoma	8-34
Gallbladder Cancer	8-38

Hepatic
Focal Nodular Hyperplasia	8-42
Hepatic Cirrhosis	8-46
Hypersplenism	8-52
Hepatic Metastases	8-56
Hepatoblastoma	8-60
Hepatocellular Carcinoma	8-64
Cavernous Hemangiomas	8-70

Adrenal
Adrenal Malignancy	8-74
Pheochromocytoma	8-80
Neuroblastoma	8-84

Spleen
Asplenia/Polysplenia Syndromes	8-90
Accessory & Ectopic Splenic Tissue	8-94

Oropharynx & Esophagus
Esophageal Cancer	8-98
Esophageal Dysmotility	8-102

Stomach
Gastritis	8-106
Gastric Emptying Disorders	8-108
Gastric Carcinoma	8-112

Intestine
Intestinal Cancer, Primary and Staging	8-116
Intestinal Cancer, Therapy Eval./Restaging	8-120
Meckel Diverticulum	8-122
GI Bleeding Localization	8-126
Inflammatory Bowel Disease	8-130

Pancreas
Pancreatitis	8-134
Pancreatic Adenocarcinoma	8-136
Islet Cell Tumors	8-140

Miscellaneous
Intraabdominal Infection	8-144
Carcinoid Tumor	8-150
GI Stromal Tumors	8-154
Peritoneal Systemic Shunt Evaluation	8-158
Diaphragmatic Patency Determination	8-162
Intraarterial Hepatic Pump Evaluation	8-164

GI ANATOMY & IMAGING ISSUES

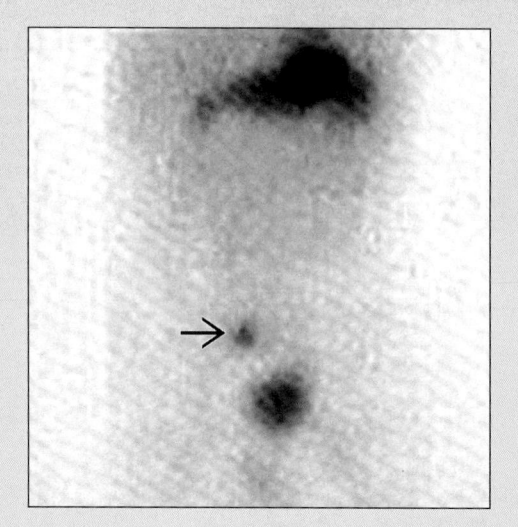

Anterior planar Tc-99m pertechnetate scan in a child with recurrent lower GI bleed demonstrates focal increased uptake ➔ in the right lower quadrant, consistent with Meckel diverticulum.

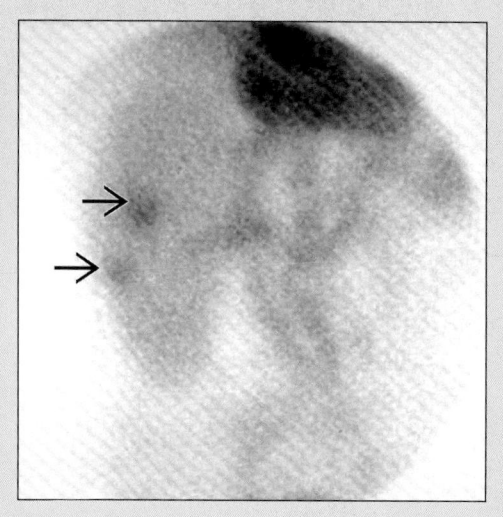

Anterior planar Tc-99m RBC scan 90 minutes post injection demonstrates increased uptake at two sites in the liver ➔, consistent with cavernous hemangiomas.

TERMINOLOGY

Definitions
- Disease affecting the esophagus, stomach, small and large bowel, pancreas, liver, spleen, adrenal glands, mesentery, and peritoneum

PATHOLOGY-BASED IMAGING ISSUES

Key Concepts or Questions
- Wide variety of diagnostic imaging options may be applied to same diseases: Nuclear medicine, plain radiography, fluoroscopic contrast, CT, MR, ultrasound (US), angiography
- Clear definition of clinical question is critical in choosing appropriate imaging approach
- Nuclear medicine imaging must be applied in the context of other correlative imaging studies
  - To choose the best test for a given patient and clinical question
  - To ensure the most cost-effective approach when confronted with "competing" modalities
  - To result in greatest accuracy by consolidating information from complementary imaging studies

Imaging Approaches
- Disorders of esophageal motility
  - Radionuclide esophagram
- Disorders of gastric emptying
  - Quantitative determination of emptying of radioactive meal
    - Dual-labeling methods of both solid and liquid may help differentiate gastroparesis from partial gastric outlet obstruction
- Hepatobiliary disease
  - Acute cholecystitis: Hepatobiliary scan
    - Morphine augmentation for non-visualization of gallbladder at 45 min: Must see small bowel before administration
    - Acalculous cholecystitis: Gallbladder may fill in ~ 15%
  - Chronic cholecystitis/gallbladder dysfunction: Hepatobiliary scan with gallbladder ejection fraction (GBEF)
    - Broad range of normal (10-90%), but most patients with gallbladder dysfunction have GBEF < 35%
  - Biliary atresia: Hepatobiliary scan with 24 h delayed imaging
- Hepatocellular disease
  - Tc-99m sulfur colloid (liver-spleen) scan can display patterns suggestive of specific disease in some cases: Most patterns nonspecific
  - Tagged red blood cell (RBC) scan for cavernous hemangiomas
  - Liver-spleen or hepatobiliary scan for focal nodular hyperplasia
- Splenic imaging
  - Hypersplenism
    - Infiltrative diseases may show decreased Tc-99m sulfur colloid uptake in spleen
    - Cr-51 labeled RBCs: Permits determination of increased red cell destruction, splenic sequestration
    - FDG PET: Focal uptake more specific for tumor than diffuse
  - Splenosis, splenule, accessory spleen, asplenia & polysplenia syndromes
    - Heat-damaged RBC scan highly sensitive and specific
- GI oncology
  - Carcinoma
    - FDG PET: Sensitive and specific for staging, restaging although reimbursement issues limit utilization
    - False negative FDG PET: Highly mucinous adenocarcinomas, hepatocellular carcinoma (HCC), very small lesions (especially in liver)
    - False positive FDG PET: Inflammation, normal physiologic uptake
  - Carcinoid

GI ANATOMY & IMAGING ISSUES

Key Facts

Wide Variety of Nuclear Medicine Imaging Options May Be Applied to Same Diseases
- Clear definition of clinical question critical in choosing the appropriate imaging approach
- Nuclear medicine imaging must be applied in the context of other correlative imaging studies
- Ensures the most cost-effective approach when confronted with anatomic imaging modalities
- Greatest accuracy achieved by consolidating information from complementary imaging studies

GI Nuclear Medicine Provides Unique Info in Several Clinical Scenarios
- GI bleeding scan to direct angiography/intervention
- Hepatobiliary scan with CCK to diagnose chronic cholecystitis (↓ gallbladder EF)
- Optimal staging of GI malignancy (e.g., FDG PET)
- Localize/diagnose Meckel diverticulum

- More aggressive disease usually quite FDG-avid: But not typically a reimbursed indication for PET
- Variable uptake with In-111 Octreoscan: May be predictive of responsiveness to Sandostatin treatment
  - Islet cell tumors (e.g., gastrinoma, insulinoma, glucagonoma)
    - In-111 Octreoscan: Preferably combined with SPECT; SPECT fusion to CT or MR highly recommended
  - Pheochromocytoma
    - Sensitivity greater with MIBG than Octreoscan, although image quality better with latter
  - HCC
    - HCC often poorly FDG-avid, or similar to normal liver: Reduction in SUV may nonetheless signify therapeutic response
    - Ga-67 citrate scintigraphy may be useful in problem cases
  - Adrenal metastases
    - FDG activity > liver = most likely malignant
    - NP-59, I-131 or I-123 MIBG for secreting adrenal tumors in problematic cases
  - GI lymphoma, GIST tumors: FDG PET excellent for staging and evaluating response to treatment
- Gastrointestinal bleeding
  - Localization of acute bleeding
    - Tagged RBC scan vastly preferred over Tc-99m sulfur colloid
    - Visualized activity must be observed for sufficient interval to allow identification of site of origin
    - Best used to direct angiography/embolization to specific vascular territory
- Meckel diverticulum
  - Tc-99m pertechnetate scan identifies diverticula containing gastric mucosa
  - Pretreatment with cimetidine critical to prevent gastric excretion of tracer
  - Oblique imaging with bladder empty important to identify diverticula near bladder
- Infection
  - In-111 WBC preferred over Tc-99m HMPAO WBC or Ga-67 for most abdominal infection imaging
- Inflammatory bowel disease
  - Tc-99m HMPAO WBC scan with early imaging (1-4 h) typically preferred for active disease

IMAGE GUIDED THERAPIES

Intrahepatic Radioembolization
- Y-90 microspheres
  - Pre-therapy embolization scan with Tc-99m MAA to prevent embolization of extrahepatic structures
    - Quantify intratumoral vascular shunt to lungs
    - Identify extrahepatic organs supplied by accessory vessels arising from hepatic arterial supply

RELATED REFERENCES

1. Maurer AH et al: Update on gastrointestinal scintigraphy. Semin Nucl Med. 36(2):110-8, 2006

IMAGE GALLERY

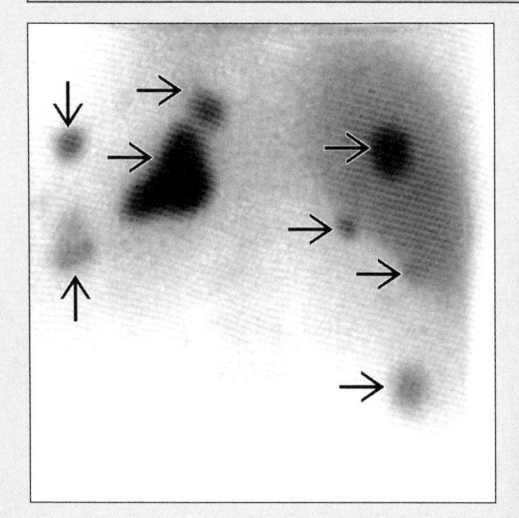

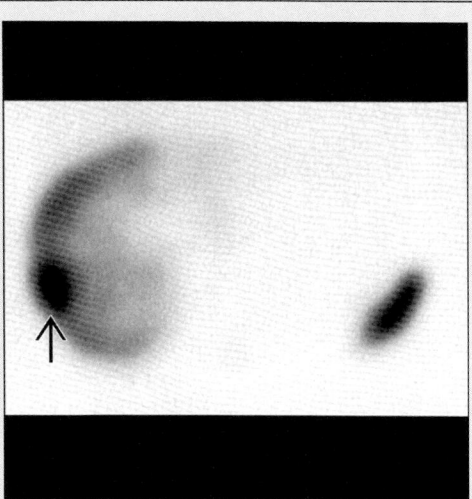

(Left) Posterior planar heat-damaged RBC scan in patient with prior history of splenectomy due to splenic trauma, demonstrates multiple foci of increased uptake ➔, consistent with splenosis. *(Right)* Transaxial Tc-99m sulfur colloid SPECT scan of abdomen (in patient with lateral right hepatic lobe mass on CT) shows focal increased uptake in mass ➔, consistent with focal nodular hyperplasia.

ACUTE CALCULOUS CHOLECYSTITIS

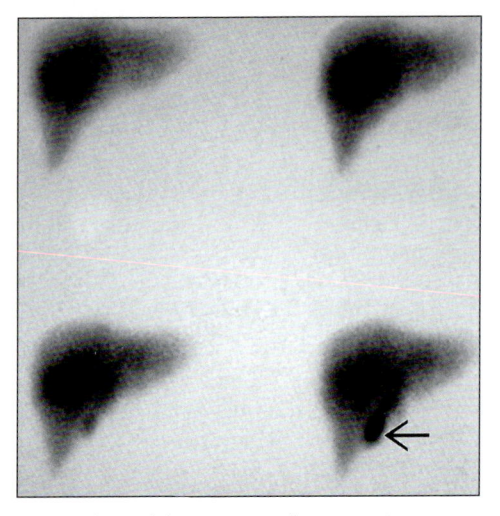

Normal hepatobiliary scintigraphy 5-20 minutes post injection. Gallbladder visualizes ➡. See next image.

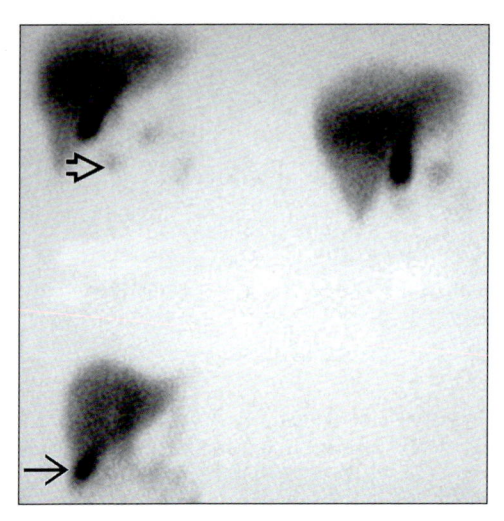

Normal hepatobiliary scintigraphy 30-35 minutes post injection. Gallbladder ➡ and duodenum ⇨ visualize.

TERMINOLOGY

Abbreviations and Synonyms
- Acute calculous cholecystitis (ACC)

Definitions
- Cholecystitis in the presence of, and assumed induced by, cholelithiasis

IMAGING FINDINGS

General Features
- Best diagnostic clue
  - Ultrasound: Cholelithiasis, gallbladder wall thickening and pericholecystic fluid
  - Tc-99m diisopropyliminodiacetic acid derivative (IDA) scan: Absence of gallbladder visualization sensitive for ACC, specificity lower
  - Gallbladder visualization with IDA scan virtually excludes ACC
  - If gallbladder visualizes on IDA scan: Stimulated cholecystokinin (CCK) (Cholecystokinin, Sincalide, Kinevac) study should be performed with gallbladder ejection fraction to exclude gallbladder dysfunction
- Location: Right upper quadrant, gallbladder fossa

Nuclear Medicine Findings
- Non visualization of the gallbladder on IDA scan
  - Morphine cholescintigraphy (MC) may be useful, see protocol advice

Imaging Recommendations
- Best imaging tool
  - Ultrasound
    - US: First line of imaging, no radiation, less expensive but inherent limitations
    - US: Operator dependent, nonspecific
    - US limited in obese patients
  - IDA scan inconclusive or negative ultrasound cases
    - Scintigraphic evaluation more sensitive than ultrasound
  - MRCP: Alternative to IDA scan when common bile duct (CBD) obstruction suspected
- Protocol advice

DDx: Duodenal Bulb Mimicking Gallbladder in Patient with Hepatic Metastases

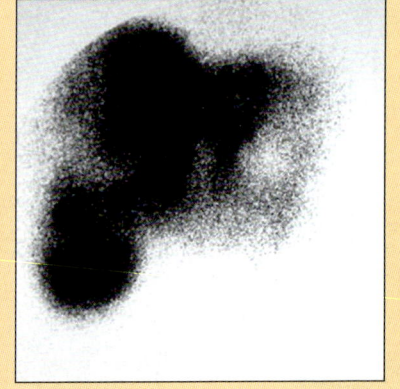

5 Minutes Post Injection 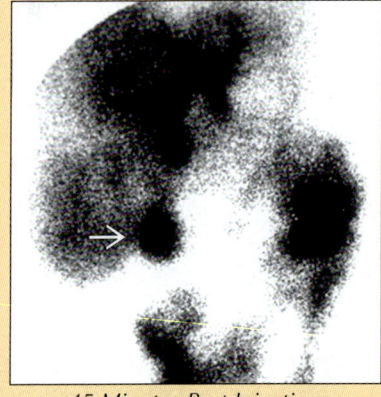   *45 Minutes Post Injection* 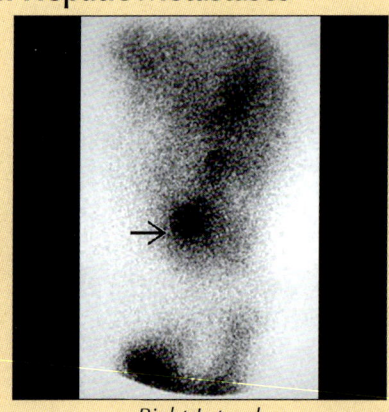   *Right Lateral*

ACUTE CALCULOUS CHOLECYSTITIS

Key Facts

Imaging Findings
- Ultrasound: Cholelithiasis, gallbladder wall thickening and pericholecystic fluid
- Tc-99m diisopropyliminodiacetic acid derivative (IDA) scan: Absence of gallbladder visualization sensitive for ACC, specificity lower
- Gallbladder visualization with IDA scan virtually excludes ACC
- If gallbladder visualizes on IDA scan: Stimulated cholecystokinin (CCK) (Cholecystokinin, Sincalide, Kinevac) study should be performed with gallbladder ejection fraction to exclude gallbladder dysfunction
- Non visualization of the gallbladder on IDA scan
- Visualization of gut, but not gallbladder at 45 min: Administer morphine sulfate (MSO4, 0.04 milligrams/kg IV over 1-3 minutes)

- Patients NPO > 24 hours should be given CCK prior to IDA scan
- In-111 or Tc-99m labeled white blood cell (WBC) scan confirms infection in equivocal cases

Top Differential Diagnoses
- Chronic Calculous Cholecystitis
- Complete Common Bile Duct (CBD) Obstruction
- Non-Fasting Normal
- Prolonged Fasting

Diagnostic Checklist
- Beware of duodenal bulb accumulation simulating gallbladder visualization
- Right lateral imaging should be performed
- Oral administration of water helps resolve difficult cases

- ○ Visualization of gut, but not gallbladder at 45 min: Administer morphine sulfate (MSO4, 0.04 milligrams/kg IV over 1-3 minutes)
    - Image x 45 min after MSO4: If no gallbladder activity, study may be stopped
    - If hepatic dysfunction or MSO4 contraindication, delayed imaging for up to 4-24 h
    - Must see small bowel before MSO4 is administered
- ○ Current IDA derivatives effective for bilirubin levels up to 20-30 mg/dl
- ○ The patient should be NPO except water for 4-6 hours prior to study
- ○ Patients NPO > 24 hours should be given CCK prior to IDA scan
    - To empty potentially full, atonic gallbladder
    - CCK: 0.02 micrograms/kg IV over 3-10 minutes at least 30 minutes prior to IDA scan
    - Some recommend 30 minute infusion to avoid gallbladder spasm and pain
- Additional nuclear medicine imaging options
    - ○ In-111 or Tc-99m labeled white blood cell (WBC) scan confirms infection in equivocal cases
        - 2-4 h (Tc-99m WBC), 24 hour (Tc-99m, In-111) images
        - In-111 WBC scan allows imaging after recent IDA scan despite residual Tc-99m
- Correlative imaging features (ultrasound, CT, MR)
    - ○ Cholelithiasis
    - ○ Gallbladder wall thickening, (greater than 3.5 mm)
    - ○ Gallbladder hydrops (transverse diameter > 5 cm, often pear-shaped
    - ○ Pericholecystic fluid
    - ○ CBD dilatation if associated CBD obstruction

DIFFERENTIAL DIAGNOSIS

Chronic Calculous Cholecystitis
- Gall bladder may not visualize secondary to chronic dysfunction and dyskinesia
    - ○ Both successfully treated with surgical intervention; distinction may be academic

Complete Common Bile Duct (CBD) Obstruction
- Ultrasound evaluation for intra and extrahepatic biliary dilation
- MRCP or ERCP in challenging cases
- With CBD obstruction, gallbladder may or may not visualize

Non-Fasting Normal
- Postprandial gallbladder contraction prevents tracer accumulation and visualization

Postcholecystectomy
- Both patients and referring services may be unclear as to prior surgical status

Prolonged Fasting
- May result in atonic, distended, or sludge-filled gallbladder
- Pretreat with CCK to empty gallbladder

Severe Hepatocellular Disease
- Delayed imaging (to 24 h) may be necessary

Rare Causes of Nonvisualization of the Gallbladder
- Extrinsic/intrinsic compression of gallbladder
    - ○ Abscess, gallbladder carcinoma, gallbladder torsion, choledochocele
- Hepatic dysfunction
    - ○ Hyperalimentation, AIDS cholangitis, hepatitis, alcoholism, cirrhosis, sepsis
- Congenital biliary abnormalities
    - ○ Gallbladder agenesis, intrahepatic gallbladder
- Inflammatory syndromes
    - ○ Kawasaki, Dengue shock, Dubin Johnson, Rotor syndromes

Other Causes of Right Upper Quadrant Pain
- Ascending cholangitis
- Acute pancreatitis
- Hepatic abscess
- Peptic ulcer disease

ACUTE CALCULOUS CHOLECYSTITIS

- Acute myocardial infarction
- Retrocecal appendicitis
- Pyelonephritis
- Pericarditis

PATHOLOGY

General Features
- Genetics
  - Increased risk of cholecystitis in patients with gallstones
    - Patients with first degree relatives with histories of gallstones
    - Native Americans (e.g., Pima Indians) and Scandinavians
- Etiology
  - Cystic duct obstruction secondary to gallstone impaction
    - Vascular congestion and edema of gallbladder wall, then cellular infiltration by polymorphonuclear leukocytes
    - 10-35% of cholelithiasis patients progress to complications requiring cholecystectomy
    - Many spontaneously resolve in first week with resultant chronic post inflammatory changes
    - Asymptomatic cholelithiasis does not require prophylactic intervention
  - Risk factors for cholelithiasis
    - Obesity, rapid or cyclic weight loss, diabetes mellitus, pregnancy, hemolytic diseases, increasing age, total parenteral nutrition (TPN), post menopausal estrogens and ceftriaxone
- Epidemiology
  - Cholecystitis is one of the most common surgeries in United States
    - Approximately 10% of US adult population has cholelithiasis; increases with age

Microscopic Features
- Inflammation and lymphocytic infiltration

CLINICAL ISSUES

Presentation
- Most common signs/symptoms
  - Right upper quadrant pain, epigastric pain radiating to the right epichondrium
    - Pain elicited by eating a fatty meal
    - Murphy sign: Pain elicited by palpating the subcostal region causing suspension of inspiration
- Other signs/symptoms
  - Gamma-glutamyl transpeptidase (GGT) elevation is associated with cholecystitis
    - GGT of 90 units/l has 1 in 3 chance of choledocholithiasis
    - One in 30 chance of bile duct obstruction when GGT less than 90 units/l

Demographics
- Age: Most common in the 4th and 5th decades
- Gender
  - 4:1 = M:F ratio during reproductive years
  - Male-to-female ratio increases as patient age increases

Natural History & Prognosis
- Untreated disease progresses and can result in severe complications including
  - Choledocholithiasis, gallbladder rupture, abscesses, peritonitis, gallstone ileus, biliary peritonitis, acute gallstone pancreatitis, sepsis, multi-organ dysfunction, multi-organ failure

Treatment
- Since the 1990's, early laparoscopic cholecystectomy has become treatment of choice for patients with ACC
  - Percutaneous and endoscopic cholecystostomy achieve similar mortality, avoiding risky anesthesia
  - Antibiotic and supportive therapy useful in isolated cases due to infectious etiologies, particularly in the elderly or otherwise frail
  - Oral dissolution therapy has very limited efficacy
    - Recurrent cholelithiasis: 25% within 5 years

DIAGNOSTIC CHECKLIST

Consider
- Complete common duct obstruction
- Acute pancreatitis
- High grade hepatocellular disfunction

Image Interpretation Pearls
- Beware of duodenal bulb accumulation simulating gallbladder visualization
  - Right lateral imaging should be performed
    - Shows a down-turning "hockey stick" configuration of gallbladder in anterior/inferior aspect of liver (major fissure of liver)
  - Oral administration of water helps resolve difficult cases
    - Clearing tracer pooling in the duodenal bulb
    - Water does not result in contraction of gallbladder

SELECTED REFERENCES

1. Schirmer BD et al: Cholelithiasis and cholecystitis. J Long Term Eff Med Implants. 15(3):329-38, 2005
2. Soderlund C et al: Bile duct injuries at laparoscopic cholecystectomy: a single-institution prospective study. Acute cholecystitis indicates an increased risk. World J Surg. 29(8):987-93, 2005
3. Tan YM et al: Dengue Shock syndrome presenting as acute cholecystitis. Dig Dis Sci. 50(5):874-5, 2005
4. Vetrhus M et al: Quality of life and pain in patients with acute cholecystitis. Results of a randomized clinical trial. Scand J Surg. 94(1):34-9, 2005
5. Papi C et al: Timing of cholecystectomy for acute calculous cholecystitis: a meta-analysis. Am J Gastroenterol. 99(1):147-55, 2004
6. Ziessman HA: Acute cholecystitis, biliary obstruction, and biliary leakage. Semin Nucl Med. 33(4):279-96, 2003
7. Bellows CF et al: Am Fam Physician. 2005 Aug 15;72(4):637-42. Review. PMID: 16127953 [PubMed - indexed for MEDLINE] 2: Hanbidge AE, Buckler PM, O'Malley ME, Wilson SR.

ACUTE CALCULOUS CHOLECYSTITIS

IMAGE GALLERY

Other

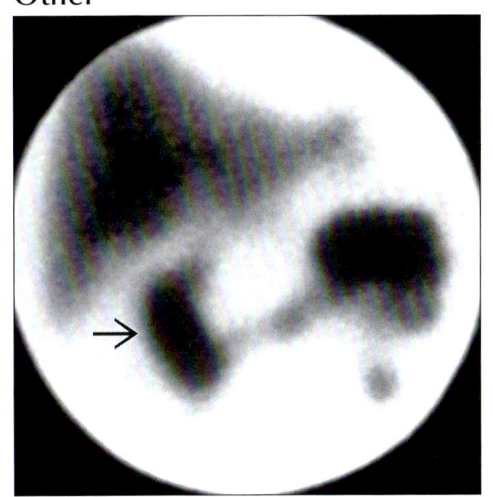

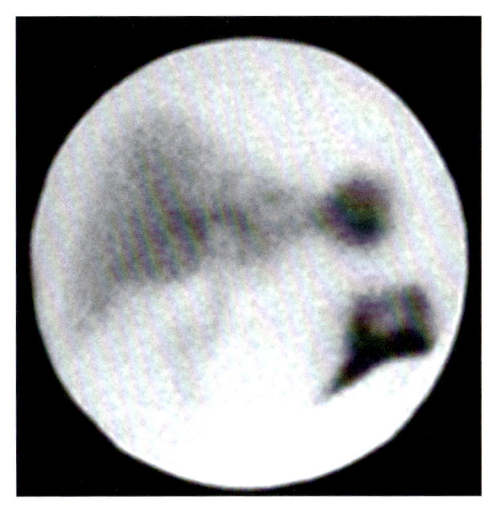

(Left) Anterior hepatobiliary scintigraphy 45 minutes post injection. Duodenum ➡, but no gallbladder visualizes. See next image post morphine. *(Right)* Hepatobiliary scan at 80 minutes post injection in same patient as previous image. Morphine sulfate (IV) was given at 45 minutes post injection. Non-visualization of gallbladder confirms acute cholecystitis.

Typical

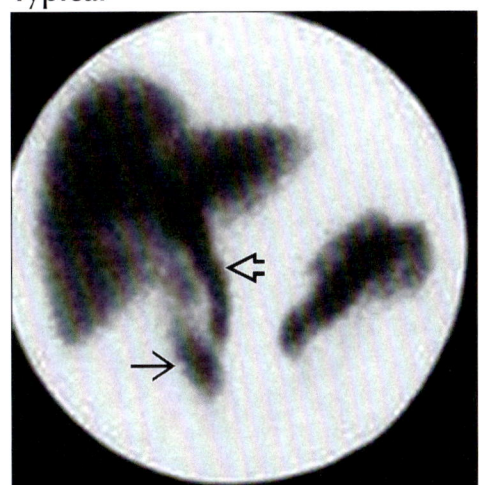

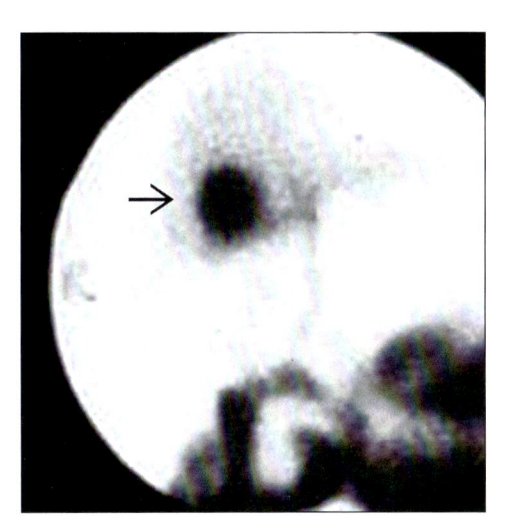

(Left) Anterior hepatobiliary scintigraphy 45 minutes post injection. Duodenum ➡, and common bile duct ▷, but no gallbladder visualizes. See next image post morphine. *(Right)* Hepatobiliary scan at 60 minutes post injection in same patient as previous image. Morphine sulfate (IV) was given at 45 minutes post injection. Gallbladder visualizes ➡, confirming patency of cystic duct.

Other

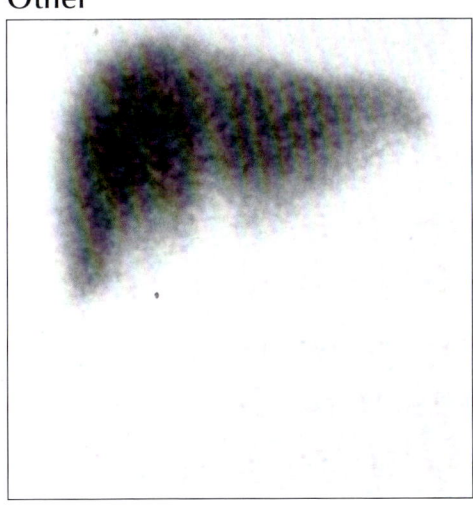

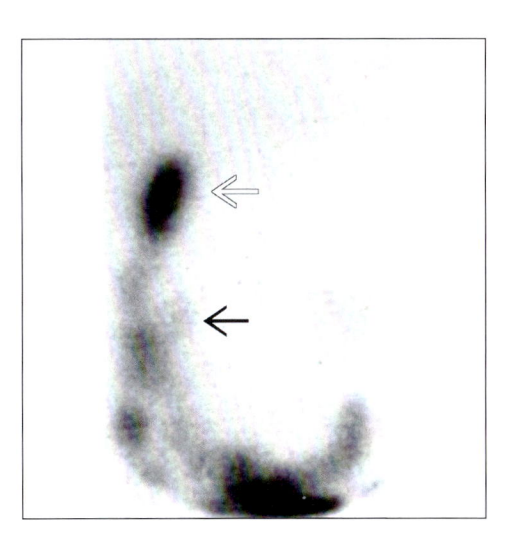

(Left) Anterior hepatobiliary scan 4 hours post injection in young woman with gallstones and acute right upper quadrant pain. No extrahepatic excretion, consistent with common bile duct obstruction. See next image. *(Right)* Anterior image at 24 h in same patient as previous image. Resolution of pain. CBD stone passed. Gallbladder ➡ and gut visualizes ➡. Gallbladder visualization is variable in CBD obstruction.

ACUTE CALCULOUS CHOLECYSTITIS

(**Left**) Anterior hepatobiliary scan 35-60 minutes post injection of tracer. "Nubbin sign" ➡ is thought to be due to pooling of tracer in portion of cystic duct distal to site of obstructing stone. (**Right**) Anterior hepatobiliary scan during first 40 minutes post injection. CBD ➡ and duodenum ➡ visualize, but no gallbladder. Same patient as in next 4 images.

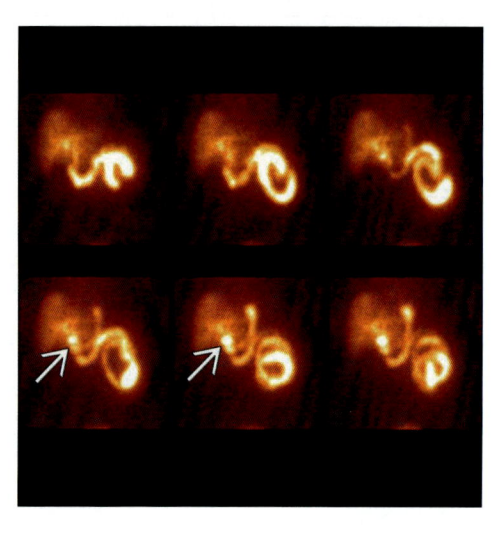

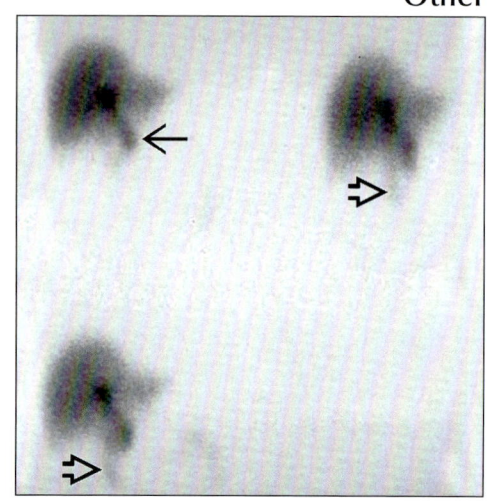

(**Left**) Anterior IDA scan in same patient as previous image, after morphine sulfate given IV. A structure visualizes that is not in the typical location of the gallbladder ➡. See next image. (**Right**) Anterior IDA scan in same patient as previous, 120 min post injection (morphine given at 60 min). Marked uptake at structure not typical in location for gallbladder ➡. See next for right lateral.

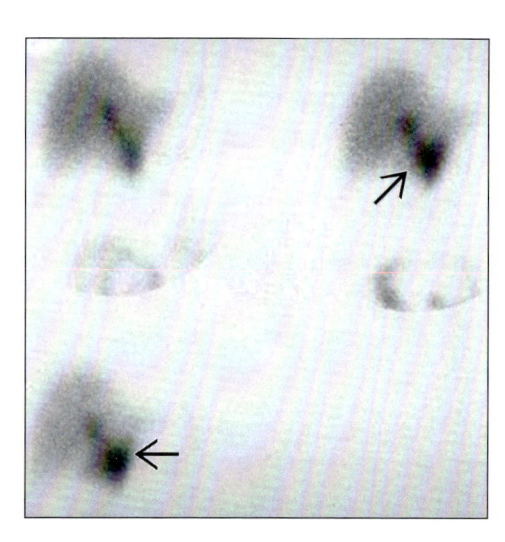

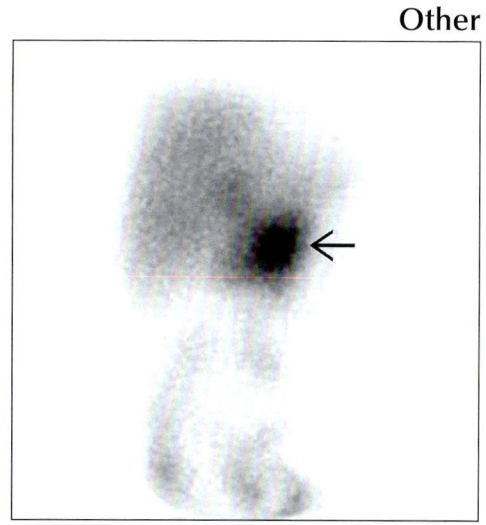

(**Left**) Right lateral IDA scan in same patient as previous, 120 minutes post injection (morphine given at 60 minutes). Right lateral confirms visualization of gallbladder ➡. See next image. (**Right**) Repositioned anterior image same patient as previous image confirms gallbladder in typical location ➡. Patient was positioned obliquely for initial imaging. Patient positioning is critical!

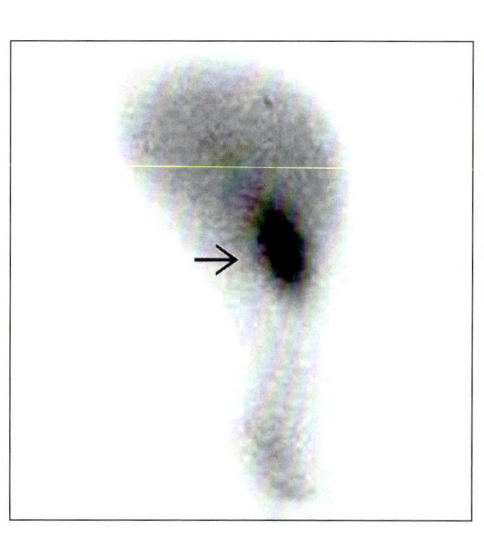

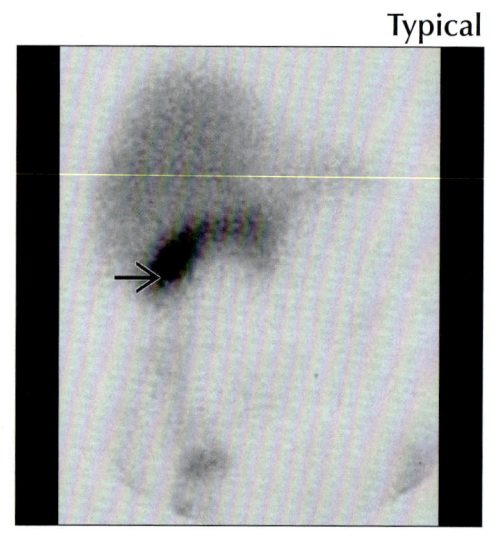

ACUTE CALCULOUS CHOLECYSTITIS

Typical

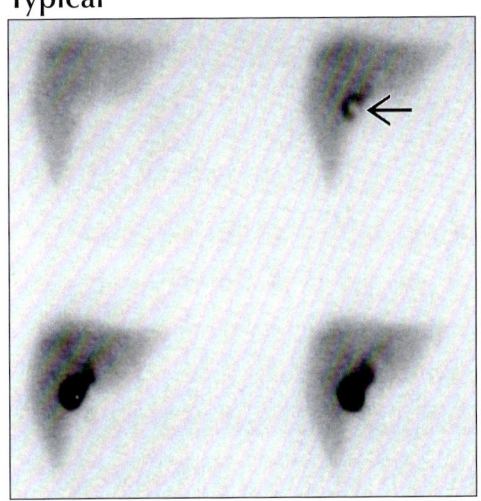

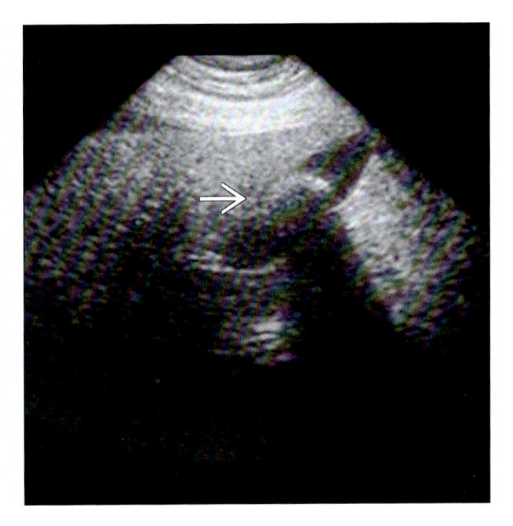

(Left) Anterior hepatobiliary scan 0-20 minutes post injection demonstrates filling defect in gallbladder ➔. See next image. (Right) Ultrasound of right upper quadrant in same patient as left. Filling defect in gallbladder is confirmed to be large gallstone ➔.

Other

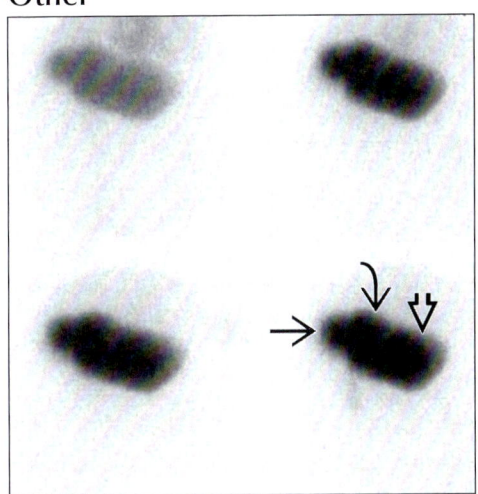

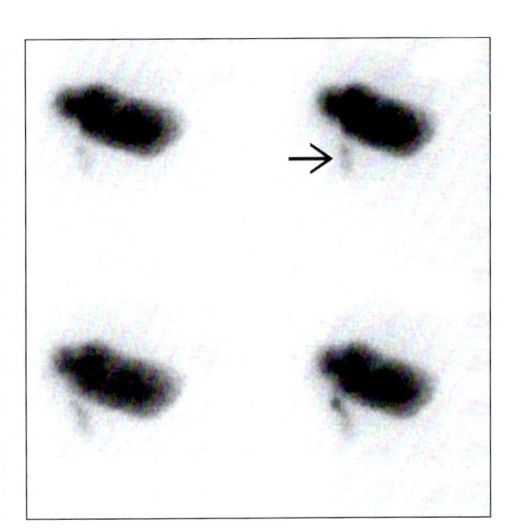

(Left) Anterior hepatobiliary scan at 0-20 minutes in patient with agenesis of right lobe of the liver. Caudate lobe ➔, medial ➔, and lateral ➔ segments of left lobe are identifiable. See next image. (Right) Anterior hepatobiliary scan at 25-40 minutes in same patient as previous image. Common bile duct, but not gallbladder, visualizes ➔. See next image.

Other

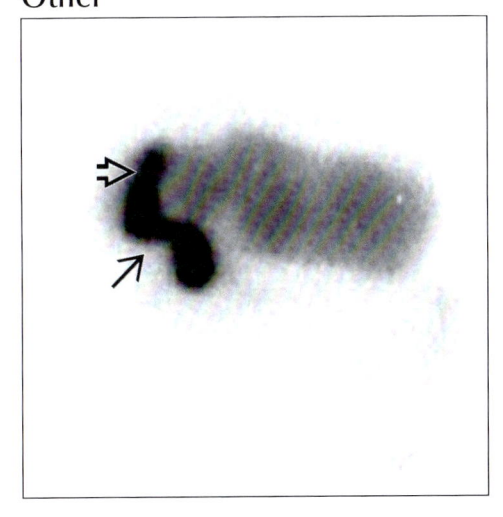

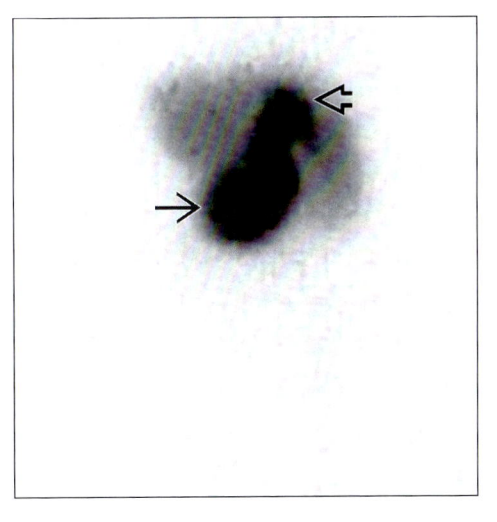

(Left) Anterior hepatobiliary scan at 60 minute post injection (15 minutes after morphine sulfate IV) in same patient as previous image demonstrates filling of gallbladder ➔ and cystic duct ➔. See next image. (Right) Right lateral IDA scan in same patient as previous image confirms filling of gallbladder ➔ and cystic duct ➔. Gallbladder is not positioned anteriorly, as in normals, resulting in lateral configuration seen on anterior imaging, left.

ACUTE ACALCULOUS CHOLECYSTITIS

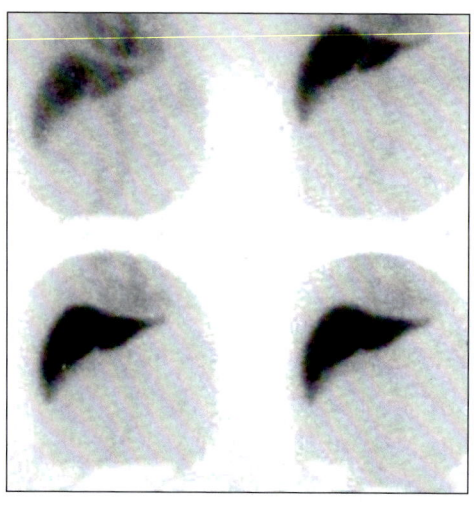

Heart transplant with gangrenous gallbladder due to acalculous cholecystitis. Anterior images obtained at 5-20 minutes demonstrate absence of extrahepatic activity.

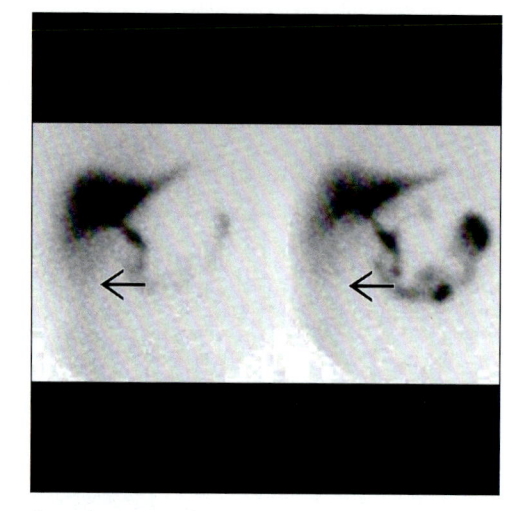

Same heart transplant patient as left. Anterior images obtained at 45-55 minutes demonstrate faint activity in right pericolic gutter ➡, bile leak from perforated gangrenous gallbladder.

TERMINOLOGY

Abbreviations and Synonyms
- Acute acalculous cholecystitis (AAC)
- Acute acalculous biliary disease
- Cystic duct syndrome

Definitions
- Acute cholecystitis in the absence of cholelithiasis

IMAGING FINDINGS

General Features
- Best diagnostic clue
  - Hepatobiliary scintigraphy (IDA scan): Non visualization of gallbladder with "rim sign" of inflammation around gallbladder fossa
  - Ultrasound: Thickening [edema (+/-) air] in gallbladder wall, no stones
  - CT: Thickening of gallbladder wall, pericholecystic stranding, no stones

Nuclear Medicine Findings
- Hepatobiliary Scintigraphy
  - Angiographic sequence
    - Hyperemic "blush" on vascular phase of IDA scan in gallbladder fossa due to inflammation
  - Serial imaging
    - Non visualization of gallbladder in 85%
    - Gallbladder may visualize in 15% of patients with AAC but usually small gallbladder, delayed visualization or only after morphine sulfate
    - "Rim sign" of inflammation and decreased clearance of tracer from liver around gallbladder fossa
    - Bile leak in cases of associated gallbladder perforation
  - Non-diagnostic
    - Visualization of gallbladder
    - Failure to visualize any extrahepatic structures (sepsis, acute hepatitis, drug or hyperalimentation-induced intrahepatic cholestasis, common duct obstruction)
- Labeled Leukocyte Scintigraphy: Increased uptake of labeled cells in gallbladder wall/gallbladder fossa

DDx: Gallbladder Mass Mimicking Thickening due to AAC

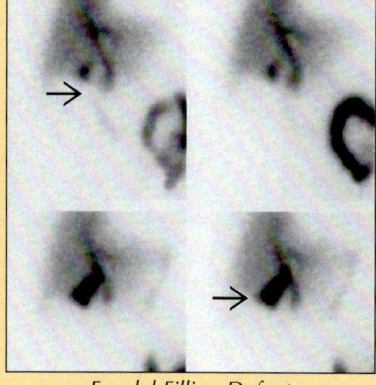

Fundal Filling Defect 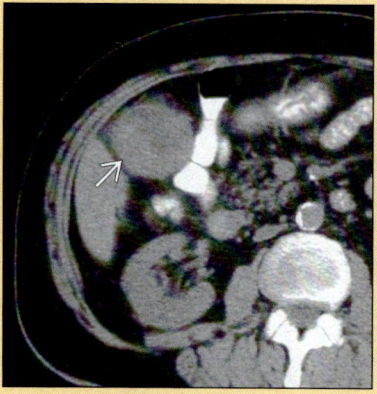   *Gallbladder Mass* 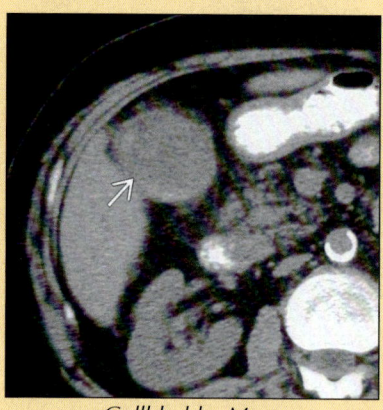   *Gallbladder Mass*

ACUTE ACALCULOUS CHOLECYSTITIS

Key Facts

Imaging Findings
- Hyperemic "blush" on vascular phase of IDA scan in gallbladder fossa due to inflammation
- Non visualization of gallbladder in 85%
- Gallbladder may visualize in 15% of patients with AAC but usually small gallbladder, delayed visualization or only after morphine sulfate
- "Rim sign" of inflammation and decreased clearance of tracer from liver around gallbladder fossa
- Bile leak in cases of associated gallbladder perforation
- Labeled Leukocyte Scintigraphy: Increased uptake of labeled cells in gallbladder wall/gallbladder fossa
- CT and US: Gallbladder wall thickness of > 5 cm, pericholecystic fluid, air in gallbladder wall, sludge

Clinical Issues
- Fever, right upper quadrant pain, and vomiting

- Presenting symptoms and laboratory values are frequently nonspecific; presentation may be insidious
- High index of suspicion with bacterial sepsis, severe trauma including surgical trauma and burns, multiple transfusions, diabetes mellitus and severe debilitation
- Delays in diagnosis are common and associated with high morbidity/mortality

Diagnostic Checklist
- In very ill, septic or immunocompromised patients
- Labeled leukocyte scan in cases where other modalities non-diagnostic, equivocal, or discordant
- 15% of patients with AAC with demonstrate visualization of the gallbladder on IDA scan

---

- Correlative imaging features
  - CT and US: Gallbladder wall thickness of > 5 cm, pericholecystic fluid, air in gallbladder wall, sludge

Imaging Recommendations
- Best imaging tool
  - Ultrasonography (US)
    - Usually first line imaging modality employed
    - Sensitivity 50%, specificity 94%, accuracy 75%
  - Hepatobiliary scintigraphy
    - Used in equivocal US cases but probably superior to US
    - Regarded as positive if the gallbladder cannot be visualized
    - Sensitivity 67%, specificity 100%, accuracy 86%
  - Tc-99m HMPAO or In-111 oxine labeled white blood cell (WBC) scintigraphy
    - When discordant or equivocal results by other modalities
- Protocol advice
  - Hepatobiliary scintigraphy
    - NPO x 6 hr prior to scan
    - No narcotics x 4 hr prior to scan
    - Pretreatment with CCK (.02 ug/kg over 10 minutes) if NPO for > 24 hr or sludge in gallbladder, wait 30 minutes to inject tracer
    - Tc-99m iminodiacetic acid (IDA) derivative (such as mebrofenin) 5 mCi IV
    - Immediate anterior angiographic phase x 1 min (4 seconds/frame)
    - Serial anterior dynamic imaging x 45 minutes (5 minutes/frame)
    - Morphine (morphine sulfate) administered IV (0.02 mg/kg over 1 minute) at 45 minutes if gut, but no gallbladder, visualized
    - Additional dynamic imaging (5 min/frame) x 45 more minutes
    - Right lateral view to confirm anterior location of gallbladder
    - Water by mouth to washout suspected duodenal bulb activity (can mimic gallbladder)
    - Delayed imaging (up to 24 hr) if slow hepatic transit due to hepatocellular disease or severe intrahepatic cholestasis
  - Labeled WBC scintigraphy: Either Tc-99m or In-111 labeled WBCs are acceptable
    - Tc-99m HMPAO labeled WBCs: Angiographic phase, then 2 hr, 4 hr, 24 hr imaging (later images compromised by normal gut activity)
    - In-111 oxine labeled WBCs: 24 hr imaging (may allow additional evaluation of abdomen)

DIFFERENTIAL DIAGNOSIS

Acute Calculous Cholecystitis (ACC)
- Stones seen by alternative imaging: US is best
- AAC is more likely the result of severe systemic disease while ACC represents local gallbladder disease

Medications, Drug Use
- Delayed transit of IDA through biliary system
- Cannot be differentiated by imaging alone: Requires clinical correlation

Other Intraabdominal Disorders
- Hepatitis, pancreatitis
  - Delayed transit of IDA through biliary system
  - Plain films, CT or MR may be revealing imaging studies; correlative laboratory values are highly contributory

PATHOLOGY

General Features
- Etiology
  - Primary mechanisms are seeding of gallbladder wall with bacteria, ischemia/reperfusion, or effects of eicosanoid proinflammatory mediators
  - Edema of gallbladder wall and cystic duct follows, with secondary obstruction of cystic duct in 85% of patients
  - Intrinsic or extrinsic cystic duct obstruction

ACUTE ACALCULOUS CHOLECYSTITIS

- Intrinsic obstruction secondary to inspissated gallbladder bile/sludge or obstructive inflammatory material
- Extrinsic obstruction secondary to lymphadenopathy, mass, fibrosis or abscess
  - Opiate treatments can reduce gallbladder motility and contribute to the development of AAC
- Epidemiology
  - Immunocompromised state, CHF, burns, trauma, ischemic bowel, septic, hypovolemic, diabetic, elderly
  - Vasculopathic/vasculitic, post-operative, malnourishment (especially parenteral nutrition), bile stasis, opioid therapy, positive-pressure ventilation, total parenteral nutrition
  - Approximately 2 per 1,000 admissions to the SICU, incidence appears to be increasing, perhaps because of increased suspicion prompting evaluation
  - Not limited to surgical or injured patients and can be seen in children
- Associated abnormalities: Sepsis, multi-organ dysfunction, perforation of gallbladder

Gross Pathologic & Surgical Features
- Gallbladder may be edematous, hemorrhagic, necrotic, gangrenous (may extend into cystic duct)

Microscopic Features
- Bile infiltration of gallbladder wall, lymphatic dilation, leukocyte margination of blood vessels
- Inflammation and lymphocytic infiltration
- Fibrosis and edema
- Intense vascular injury in the muscularis and serosa
- May include frank necrosis and gangrene

CLINICAL ISSUES

Presentation
- Most common signs/symptoms
  - Fever, right upper quadrant pain, and vomiting
  - Presenting symptoms and laboratory values are frequently nonspecific; presentation may be insidious
  - High index of suspicion with bacterial sepsis, severe trauma including surgical trauma and burns, multiple transfusions, diabetes mellitus and severe debilitation
- Other signs/symptoms
  - Leukocytosis, hyperamylasemia, abnormal aminotransferases
    - Leukocyte count and liver function tests may be normal
    - Right upper quadrant tenderness may not necessarily be present

Natural History & Prognosis
- Delays in diagnosis are common and associated with high morbidity/mortality
- Minimal clinical manifestations may rapidly progress to gangrene with perforation
- Mortality and morbidity are high
  - Mortality variably listed as 30-45%
- High incidence of gangrene, gallbladder perforation, and abscess
  - Bile peritonitis, subacute pericholecystic abscess, chronic perforation, cholecystenteric fistula

Treatment
- Antibiotic and supportive therapy is critical due to infectious etiology of most cases
- Prompt surgical treatment: Cholecystectomy, cholecystotomy
  - Delays in treatment are associated with high morbidity/mortality
- Cholecystostomy is an alternative, although percutaneous and endoscopic cholecystostomy produce similar mortality
  - Avoids high risk of general anesthesia for laparotomy or laparoscopy and should be considered as a definitive treatment in critically ill patients

DIAGNOSTIC CHECKLIST

Consider
- In very ill, septic or immunocompromised patients
- Labeled leukocyte scan in cases where other modalities non-diagnostic, equivocal, or discordant

Image Interpretation Pearls
- Inflammatory change of the gallbladder wall without obvious source of obstruction (by US, CT, MRCP)
- 15% of patients with AAC with demonstrate visualization of the gallbladder on IDA scan

SELECTED REFERENCES

1. Laurila J et al: Histopathology of acute acalculous cholecystitis in critically ill patients. Histopathology. 47(5):485-92, 2005
2. Owen CC et al: Acute Acalculous Cholecystitis. Curr Treat Options Gastroenterol. 8(2):99-104, 2005
3. Hoffmann JC et al: Gallbladder involvement of Henoch-Schonlein purpura mimicking acute acalculous cholecystitis. Digestion. 70(1):45-8, 2004
4. Laurila J et al: Acute acalculous cholecystitis in critically ill patients. Acta Anaesthesiol Scand. 48(8):986-91, 2004
5. Pozo MJ et al: Chemical mediators of gallbladder dysmotility. Curr Med Chem. 11(13):1801-12, 2004
6. Dabus Gde C et al: Percutaneous cholecystostomy: a nonsurgical therapeutic option for acute cholecystitis in high-risk and critically ill patients. Sao Paulo Med J. 121(6):260-2, 2003
7. Owen CC et al: Gallbladder polyps, cholesterolosis, adenomyomatosis, and acute acalculous cholecystitis. Semin Gastrointest Dis. 14(4):178-88, 2003
8. Wang NC et al: Acute acalculous cholecystitis and pancreatitis in a patient with concomitant leptospirosis and scrub typhus. J Microbiol Immunol Infect. 36(4):285-7, 2003
9. Mariat G et al: Contribution of ultrasonography and cholescintigraphy to the diagnosis of acute acalculous cholecystitis in intensive care unit patients. Intensive Care Med. 26(11):1658-63, 2000
10. Kalliafas S et al: Acute acalculous cholecystitis: incidence, risk factors, diagnosis, and outcome. Am Surg. 64(5):471-5, 1998

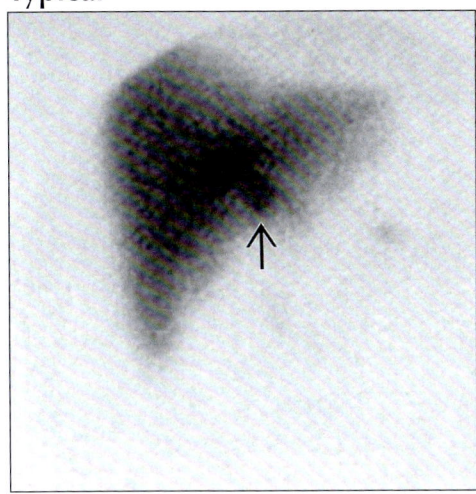

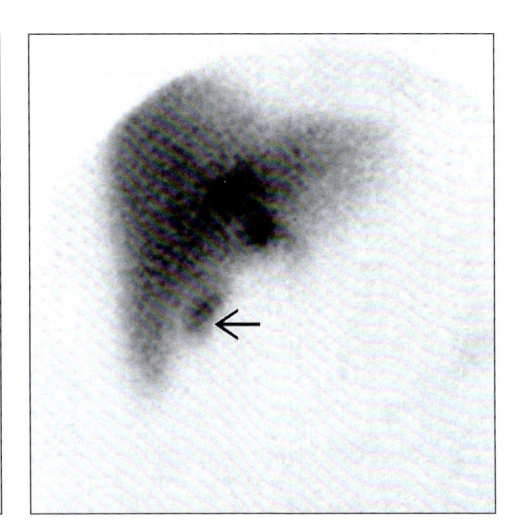

ACUTE ACALCULOUS CHOLECYSTITIS

IMAGE GALLERY

Typical

(Left) Heart transplant patient with acalculous cholecystitis. Anterior image from hepatobiliary scan at 20 min shows faint duodenal activity ➡. Same as next three images. *(Right)* Heart transplant patient with acalculous cholecystitis. Anterior image from hepatobiliary scan at 50 min shows presumed gallbladder activity ➡. (See next image).

Typical

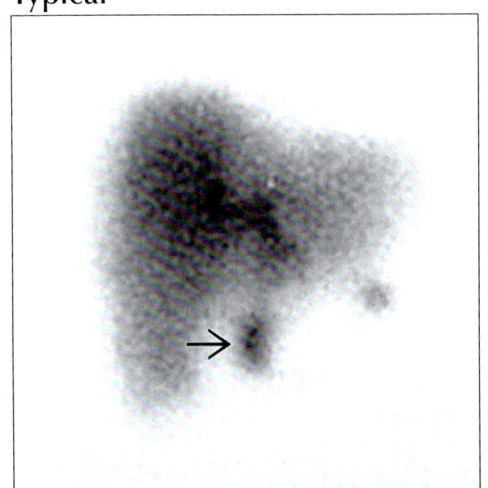

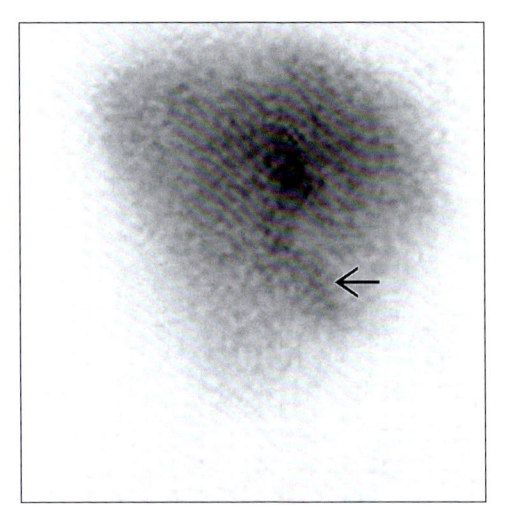

(Left) Same patient as previous image. RAO image from hepatobiliary scan at 50 min demonstrates possible gallbladder activity ➡. (See next image). *(Right)* Same patient as left. Right lateral image from hepatobiliary scan at 50 min confirms gallbladder activity ➡.

Typical

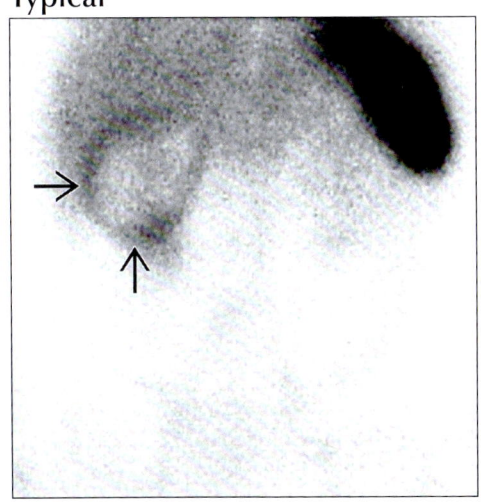

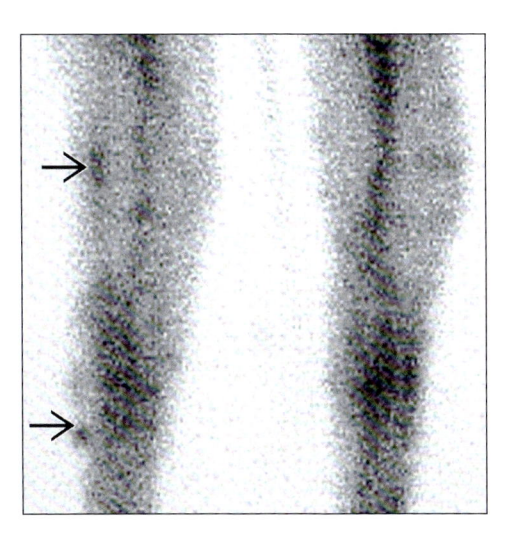

(Left) Bone marrow transplant patient without gallstones. Anterior Tc-99m HMPAO leukocyte scan at 2 hours post injection shows uptake in gallbladder wall ➡ consistent with AAC. *(Right)* Same patient as left. Increased uptake in firm subcutaneous septic emboli nodules on lower extremities ➡.

ACUTE ACALCULOUS CHOLECYSTITIS

(Left) In-111 leukocyte scan of anterior abdomen shows Intense activity in gallbladder wall ➡ due to AAC (Courtesy F. Datz, MD). *(Right)* Anterior images from a hepatobiliary scan at 52-60 minutes post injection in a diabetic patient with acalculous cholecystitis demonstrates lack of gallbladder activity and a positive "rim sign" ➡.

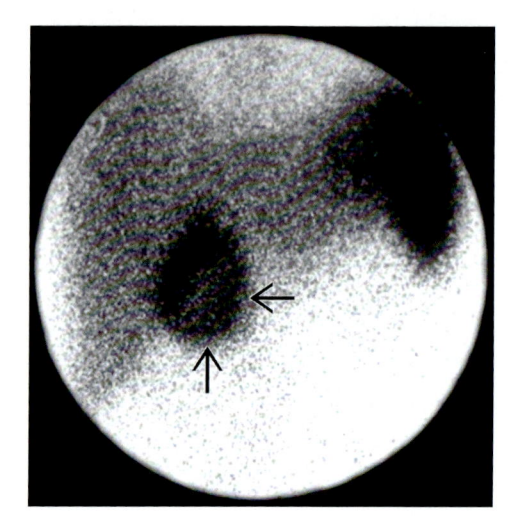

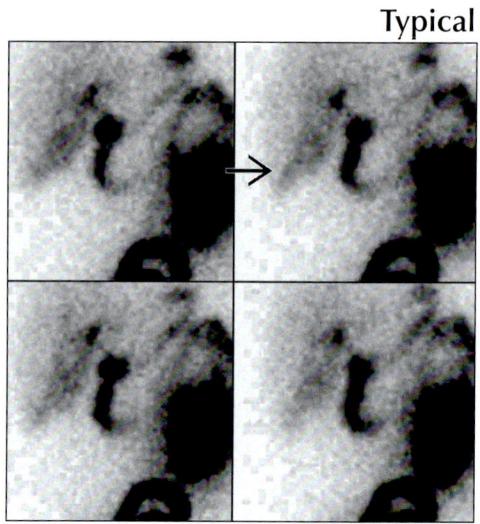

(Left) Septic diabetic patient with AAC. Hepatobiliary scan over 5-20 minutes shows duodenal bulb activity ➡ mimicking gallbladder. *(Right)* Same septic diabetic patient as left. Following oral water, activity in duodenal bulb decreases ➡.

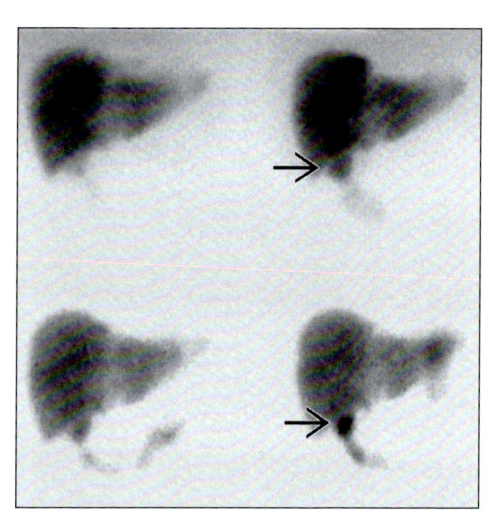

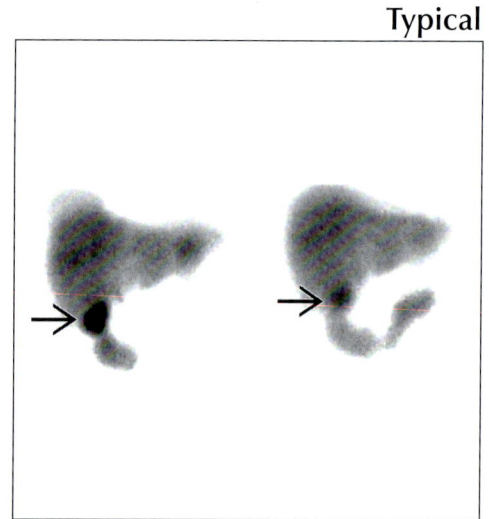

(Left) AIDS patient with acute acalculous cholecystitis. Hepatobiliary scan at 40-50 minutes demonstrates activity in duodenal bulb, mimicking gallbladder ➡. *(Right)* Same patient as left. Oral water washes out duodenal bulb activity ➡.

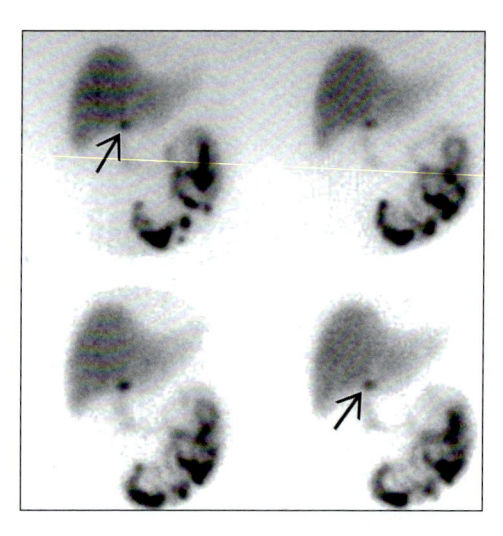

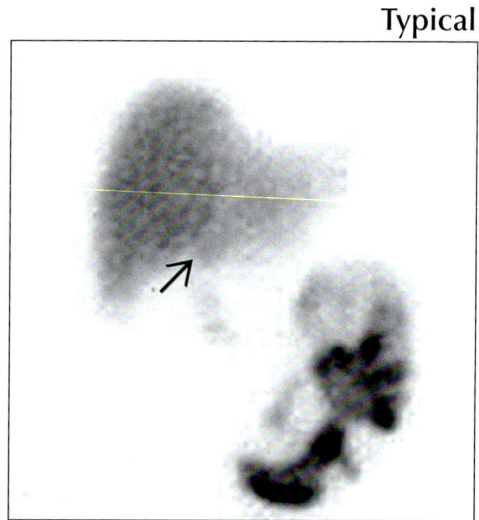

ACUTE ACALCULOUS CHOLECYSTITIS

Other

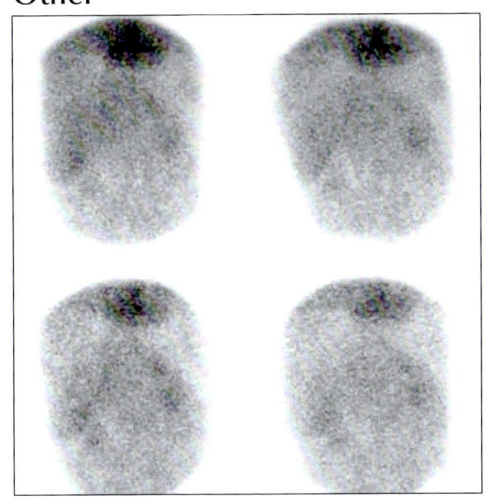

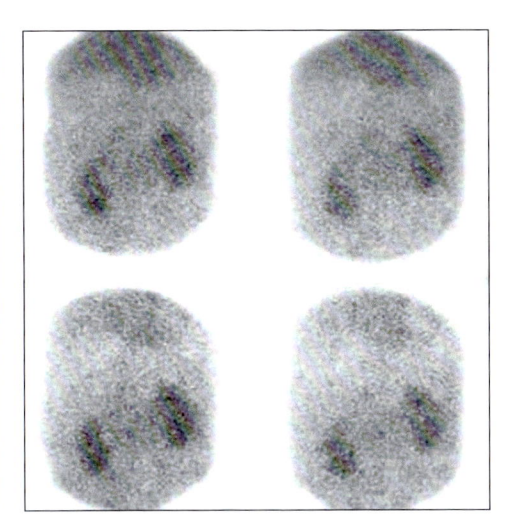

(Left) Patient with severe chemical (alcohol) hepatitis mimicking AAC. Hepatobiliary scan 5-10 minutes post injection demonstrates faint activity in liver, likely blood pool, which subsequently fades. Same as next 4 images. *(Right)* Hepatobiliary scan with additional images at 60-70 minutes shows progressive clearing of blood pool activity, marked kidney activity (vicarious renal excretion), in patient with severe chemical (alcohol) hepatitis.

Other

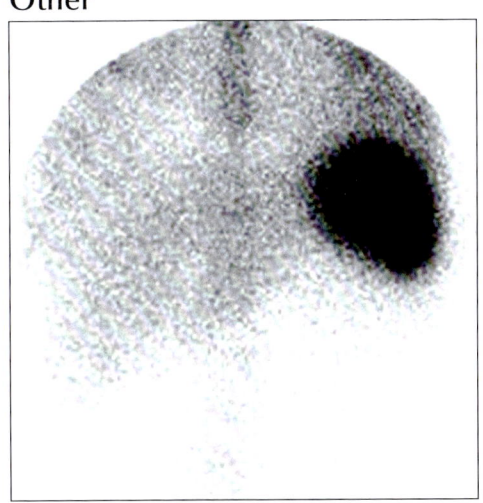

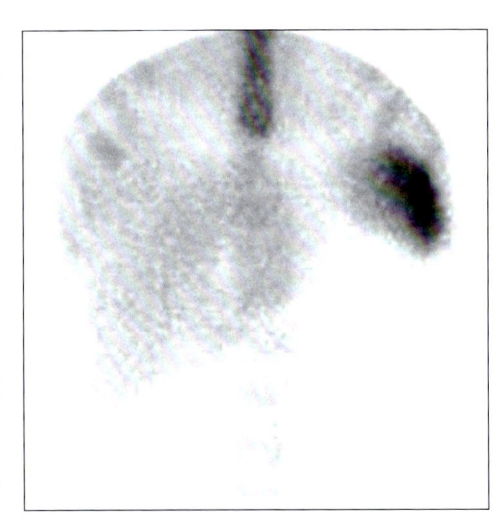

(Left) Patient with severe chemical hepatitis mimicking AAC. In-111 leukocyte scan in same patient shows overall reduced liver activity. No focal uptake in gallbladder fossa to suggest cholecystitis. *(Right)* Patient with severe chemical hepatitis mimicking AAC (same patient as previous 3 images). Tc-99m sulfur colloid liver spleen scan confirms severely compromised hepatic function by colloid shift to spleen, bone marrow.

Other

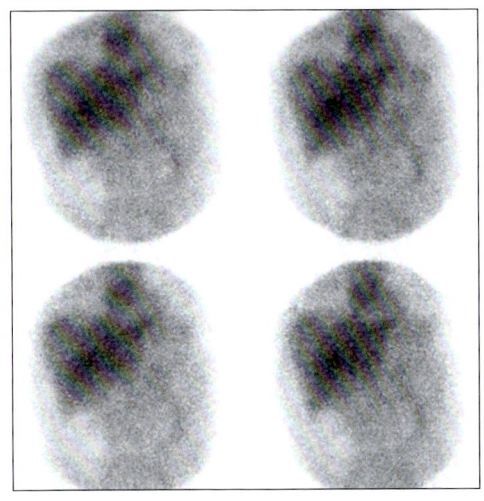

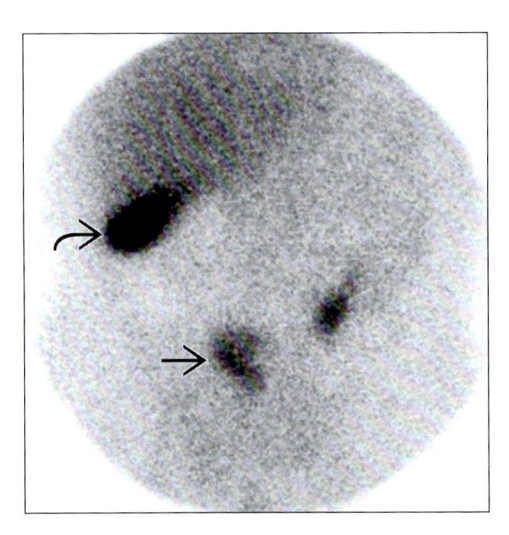

(Left) Severe cirrhosis mimicking AAC. Hepatobiliary scan at 50-55 minutes shows high background and blood pool, no extrahepatic excretion. *(Right)* Severe cirrhosis mimicking AAC (same patient as previous image). Anterior 24 hr scan shows excretion into gut ➡ and gallbladder ➡. Visualization delayed secondary to poor hepatic function, (severe cirrhosis) not cholecystitis.

CHRONIC CHOLECYSTITIS

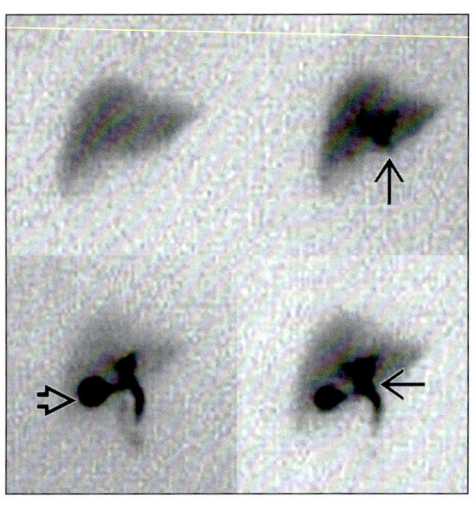

Anterior hepatobiliary scintigraphy shows sequential visualization of normal biliary tree ⇒ and GB ⇒.

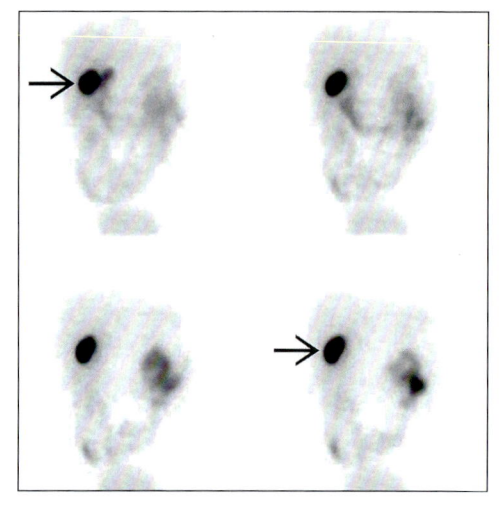

Anterior hepatobiliary scintigraphy shows no GB contraction on sequential imaging ⇒. GBEF was < 10%.

TERMINOLOGY

Abbreviations and Synonyms
- Chronic cholecystitis (CC)
- Chronic acalculous cholecystitis (CAC)
- Chronic calculous cholecystitis (CCC)
- Gallbladder (GB)
- Gallbladder ejection fraction (GBEF)

Definitions
- Gallbladder dysfunction: Biliary colic, spasm, dyskinesia
- Chronic cholecystitis: Chronic GB inflammation producing right upper quadrant (RUQ) pain
- Cholescintigraphy: Hepatobiliary scan, IDA scan

IMAGING FINDINGS

General Features
- Best diagnostic clue
  - Normal IDA scan: Gut visualizes by 60 minutes, gallbladder prior to gut
  - Findings of CC gallbladder dysfunction are nonspecific: Visualization of GB after gut, delayed visualization of GB > 1h, visualization of GB only after morphine sulfate (MSO4)
  - ↓ GB ejection fraction (GBEF) on cholecystokinin (CCK)-stimulated cholescintigraphy
    - CCK: Hormone secreted by upper small intestine mucosa that induces GB contraction, sphincter of Oddi relaxation, ↑ intestinal motility
    - Although normal GBEF(2 SD) is very broad: 10-90%; most patients with GB dysfunction have an EF < 35%
    - GBEF ≤ 60% may be associated with CC; can be treated with cholecystectomy if symptoms ≥ 1 yr

Imaging Recommendations
- Best imaging tool
  - Cholescintigraphy with Tc-99m labeled iminodiacetic acid (IDA) derivatives utilizing CCK (Sincalide)
    - Recommended if equivocal ultrasound findings, persistent clinical suspicion, chronic RUQ pain of unknown etiology

DDx: Right Upper Quadrant Pain

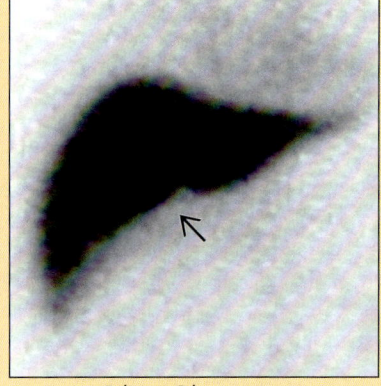

Biliary Obstruction 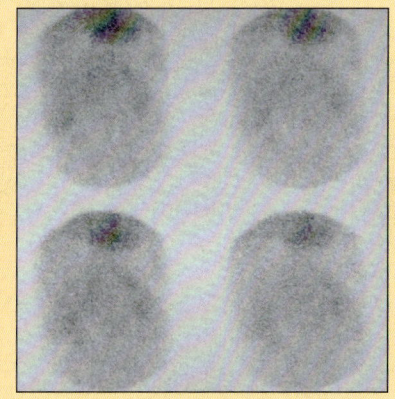 | *Hepatitis* 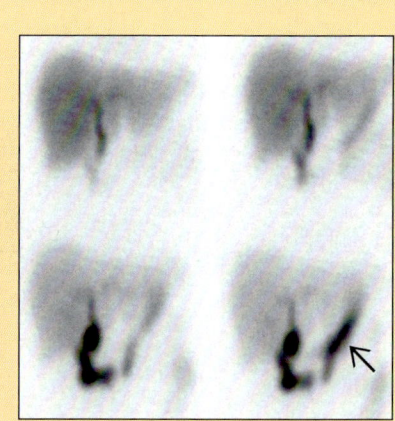 | *Biliary Gastric Reflux*

CHRONIC CHOLECYSTITIS

Key Facts

Terminology
- Chronic cholecystitis: Chronic GB inflammation producing right upper quadrant (RUQ) pain
- Cholescintigraphy: Hepatobiliary scan, IDA scan

Imaging Findings
- Normal IDA scan: Gut visualizes by 60 minutes, gallbladder prior to gut
- Findings of CC gallbladder dysfunction are nonspecific: Visualization of GB after gut, delayed visualization of GB > 1h, visualization of GB only after morphine sulfate (MSO4)
- ↓ GB ejection fraction (GBEF) on cholecystokinin (CCK)-stimulated cholescintigraphy
- Although normal GBEF(2 SD) is very broad: 10-90%; most patients with GB dysfunction have an EF < 35%
- GBEF determination

Top Differential Diagnoses
- Acute Cholecystitis
- Biliary or Pancreatic Sphincter Dysfunction
- Biliary Duodenogastric Reflux
- Hepatitis

Clinical Issues
- Open or laparoscopic cholecystectomy: Current treatments of choice

Diagnostic Checklist
- Opioid intake immediately before study must be excluded before attributing ↓ GBEF to chronic cholecystitis
- Patients with normal GBEF may progress to ↓ GBEF over period of years

---

  - ↓ GBEF (< 35%) may be associated with many drugs and comorbid factors: Morphine, calcium channel blockers, oral contraceptives, octreotide, erythromycin
  - CCK can replicate symptoms in CC and irritable bowel syndrome
  - Symptom replication with CCK does not equal CC
 - Ultrasonography: First-line imaging in cases of suspected cholecystitis
- Protocol advice
 - Dose: 5-8 mCi (185-296 MBq) of Tc-99m IDA (e.g., HIDA, DISIDA)
 - Patient NPO 4-6 hrs prior
  - Allows relaxation of GB (contracted GB may not take up radiotracer)
  - If patient NPO > 24 hrs, administer 0.01-0.02 µg/kg CCK IV 30 minutes prior to cholescintigraphy to empty GB
  - Duration of CCK effect is 20 min
  - May inject IDA 30 min after CCK infusion complete
 - Opiate agonists: Withhold 6 hrs prior to IDA scan
  - Can cause sphincter of Oddi spasm
  - Opiate antagonists (Narcan, Naloxone) can be used for reversal if necessary
 - If no GB activity x 45 min, can administer MSO4 (0.04 mg/kg) to fill GB
  - If MSO4 contraindicated, delayed imaging x 4 h (24 h if hepatocellular disease)
 - GBEF determination
  - At 45 min (or after visualization of GB if GB visualization is delayed): Administer 0.02-0.04 µg/kg CCK IV
  - Infuse slowly (over ~ 3 minutes) to prevent cystic duct spasm
  - Some advocate infusion over 30 minutes
  - Rapid CCK injection may produces pain/cramping

DIFFERENTIAL DIAGNOSIS

Acute Cholecystitis
- Nonvisualization of GB on cholescintigraphy

Biliary or Pancreatic Sphincter Dysfunction
- Sphincter of Oddi dysfunction, biliary dyskinesia or obstruction, post-cholecystectomy syndrome
- Milwaukee diagnostic criteria
 - Episodic epigastric or right upper quadrant pain lasting 45 min or longer
 - Elevated hepatic enzymes (1.5 x transaminases)
 - Dilated biliary duct (> 12 mm)
- Hypertonic sphincter of Oddi manometry variable, may be transiently normal at time of manometry

Biliary Duodenogastric Reflux
- Evaluate tracer transit for retrograde filling of proximal duodenum and gastric lumen
- Associated with pyloroplasty/resection, biliary/gastric surgery, or primary pyloric failure
- Biliary reflux gastritis
 - Gastric erosions, hyperemia, metaplasia, neoplasia and frank carcinomatous degeneration

Hepatitis
- Poor hepatic extraction and biliary excretion 2° to hepatocellular dysfunction
 - Persistent blood pool activity of IDA

Occult Biliary Lithiasis, Microlithiasis
- Diagnosis of exclusion

Chronic or Autoimmune Pancreatitis
- Laboratory values, patient history and CT may be helpful
- Biopsy can be inconclusive or misleading

Peptic Ulcer Disease
- Clinical history and Helicobacter pylori evaluations helpful

CHRONIC CHOLECYSTITIS

Bowel Disease
- Irritable bowel syndrome, sprue, celiac disease, gluten intolerance, gluten-sensitive enteropathy, nontropical sprue
- Patient history, serology, histology and clinical response contributory
- Absence of human leukocyte antigen (HLA) class II molecules DQ2 or DQ8 has very high negative predictive value

Appendicitis
- Elongated vermiform appendix or ectopic cecum can ⇒ right upper quadrant pain

Bowel Ischemia
- Laboratory values, conventional or CT angiogram helpful

Abscess
- Hepatic, renal, perirenal, pararenal, intraperitoneal

Local Mass Effect
- Periductal pancreatic adenocarcinoma
- CT, MR useful if ultrasound inconclusive
- Tumor or lymphadenopathy about ampulla of Vater, pancreatic head, or biliary ductal system

Intraperitoneal Adhesions
- Check surgical history

PATHOLOGY

General Features
- Etiology
  - Chronic GB inflammation due to cholelithiasis
  - Chronic GB inflammation without cholelithiasis
    - Microlithiasis may be present in some cases
  - GB dysfunction
  - Cholesterolosis
  - Cystic duct stenosis
  - Etiology of ↓ GBEF uncertain
- Epidemiology: Typically middle-aged, obese, females
- Associated abnormalities
  - Diabetes mellitus
  - Sickle cell disease
  - Irritable bowel syndrome
  - Pancreatic insufficiency
  - Sprue
  - Achalasia

Microscopic Features
- Chronic inflammatory and fibrotic changes of GB wall including lymphocytic infiltration

CLINICAL ISSUES

Presentation
- Most common signs/symptoms: Chronic intermittent RUQ pain

Demographics
- Age: Fourth and fifth decades
- Gender: Female more common

Natural History & Prognosis
- Chronic abdominal pain presents diagnostic dilemma for clinicians
- Extensive testing and evaluation common without diagnosis

Treatment
- Open or laparoscopic cholecystectomy: Current treatments of choice
- Surgeons reluctant to undertake operative intervention
- Often good surgical result in patients with intractable chronic RUQ pain with ↓ GBEF

DIAGNOSTIC CHECKLIST

Consider
- Opioid intake immediately before study must be excluded before attributing ↓ GBEF to chronic cholecystitis
- Patients with normal GBEF may progress to ↓ GBEF over period of years

Image Interpretation Pearls
- GB nonvisualization may be 2° to viscous biliary fluid in a chronically dysfunctional GB: False positive for acute cholecystitis

SELECTED REFERENCES

1. Hsu PI et al: A Prospective Randomized Trial of Esomeprazole- versus Pantoprazole-Based Triple Therapy for Helicobacter pylori Eradication. Am J Gastroenterol. 100(11):2387-92, 2005
2. Levine MS et al: Diseases of the esophagus: diagnosis with esophagography. Radiology. 237(2):414-27, 2005
3. Meize-Grochowski R: Celiac disease: a multisystem autoimmune disorder. Gastroenterol Nurs. 28(5):394-402, 2005
4. Kim CW et al: [A case of chronic acalculous cholecystitis diagnosed by delayed contrast emptying in gallbladder] Korean J Gastroenterol. 43(5):320-3, 2004
5. Krishnamurthy GT et al: Constancy and variability of gallbladder ejection fraction: impact on diagnosis and therapy. J Nucl Med. 45(11):1872-7, 2004
6. Jagannath SB et al: A long-term cohort study of outcome after cholecystectomy for chronic acalculous cholecystitis. Am J Surg. 185(2):91-5, 2003
7. Majeski J: Gallbladder ejection fraction: an accurate evaluation of symptomatic acalculous gallbladder disease. Int Surg. 88(2):95-9, 2003
8. Merg AR et al: Mechanisms of impaired gallbladder contractile response in chronic acalculous cholecystitis. J Gastrointest Surg. 6(3):432-7, 2002
9. Chen PF et al: The clinical diagnosis of chronic acalculous cholecystitis. Surgery. 130(4):578-81; discussion 581-3, 2001
10. Ziessman HA: Cholecystokinin cholescintigraphy: clinical indications and proper methodology. Radiol Clin North Am. 39(5):997-1006, ix, 2001

CHRONIC CHOLECYSTITIS

IMAGE GALLERY

Typical

Typical

Typical

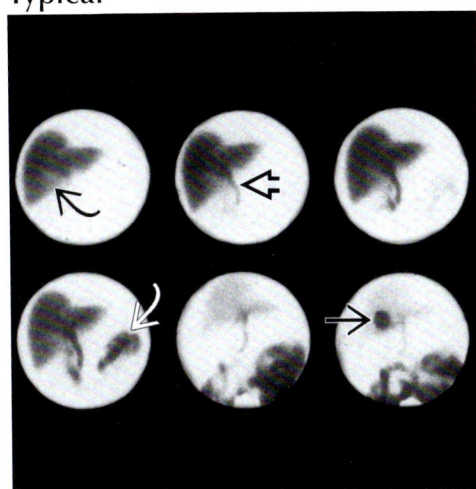

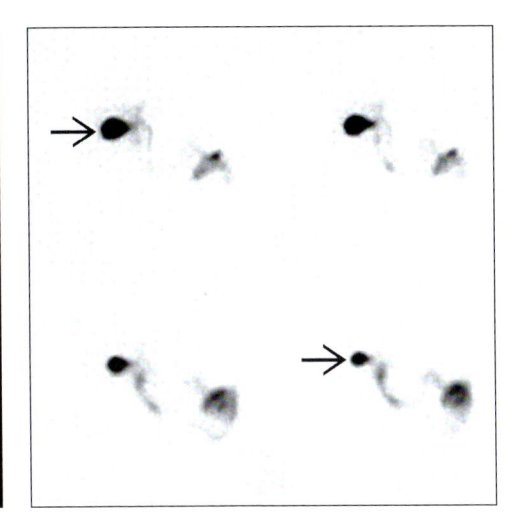

(Left) Anterior hepatobiliary scintigraphy shows normal hepatic ➔, biliary ➔, and small bowel ➔ visualization. No GB activity until 90 minutes ➔ suggests chronic cholecystitis. (Right) In same patient as previous image, administration of CCK resulted in normal gallbladder contraction (GBEF of 80%) ➔. Findings do not support chronic cholecystitis or gallbladder dysfunction.

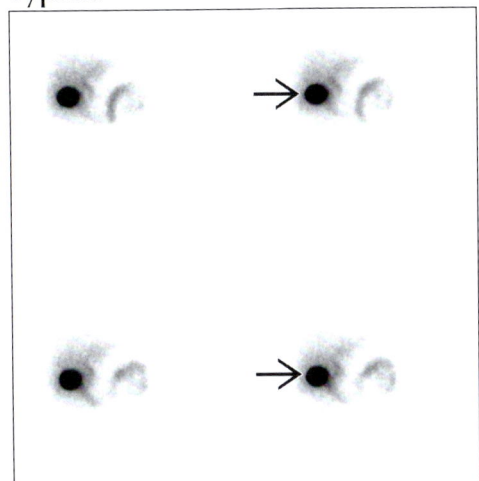

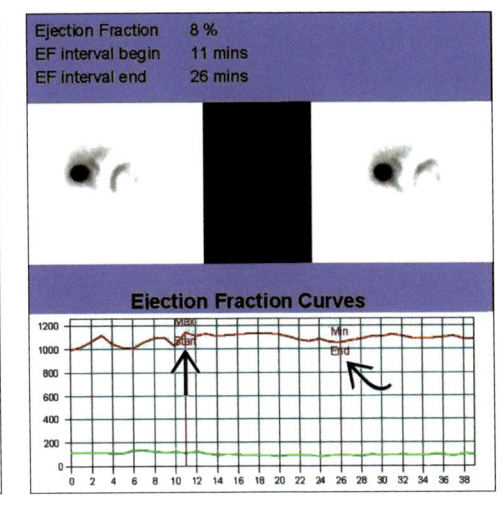

(Left) Anterior hepatobiliary scintigraphy shows no GB contraction on sequential imaging ➔. (Right) Anterior GB time-activity-curve in same patient as previous image. Note little change in maximum ➔ to minimum ➔ counts, signifying decreased GBEF.

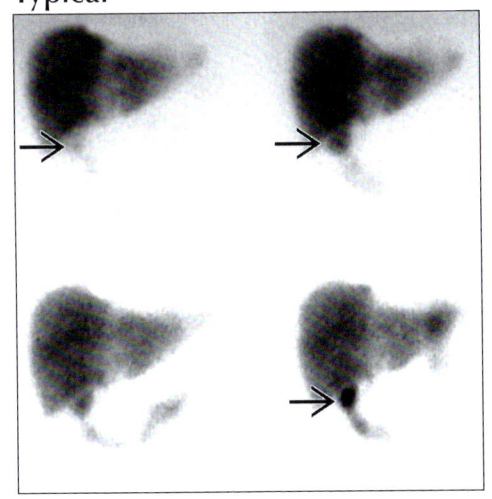

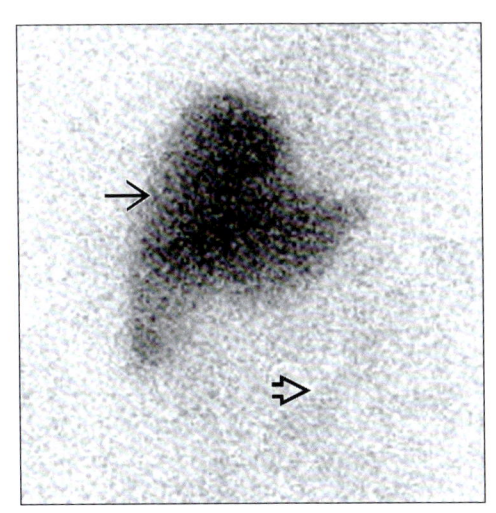

(Left) Anterior hepatobiliary scintigraphy shows sequential images with tracer accumulation in region of GB fossa ➔. Activity in duodenal bulb can mimic GB activity, as in this case. (Right) Anterior hepatobiliary scintigraphy shows normal hepatic uptake ➔ and low background counts ➔ indicating severe cholestasis. This patient had high grade biliary obstruction.

BILIARY LEAK

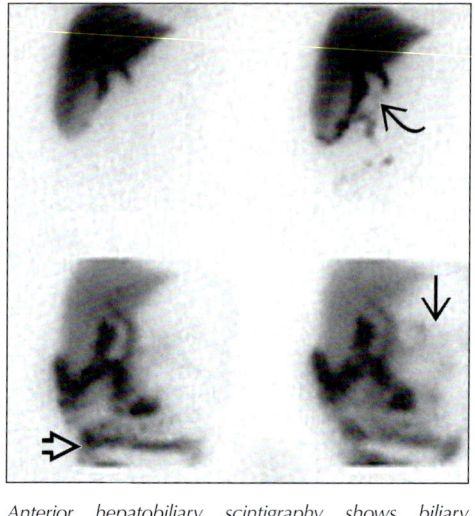

Anterior hepatobiliary scintigraphy shows biliary extravasation from hepatic hilum ⇨ into Morrison pouch ➡ and peritoneal cavity ⇨.

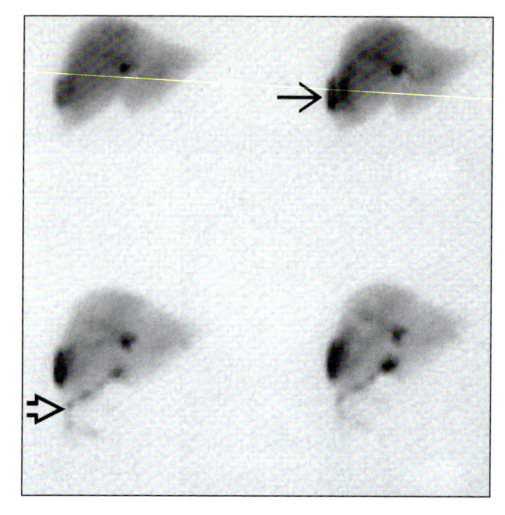

Anterior hepatobiliary scintigraphy shows tracer subjacent to lateral hepatic capsule ➡ in a biloma with free-flowing tracer inferior to right hepatic lobe ⇨.

TERMINOLOGY

Definitions
- Bile extrinsic to biliary tree and bowel, usually within peritoneal cavity or biloma (focal bile collection)

IMAGING FINDINGS

General Features
- Location
  - Usually within peritoneal cavity; can be retroperitoneal
  - Near cystic stump following cholecystectomy
  - Near biliary enteric anastomosis after orthotopic liver transplant
    - 5-10% cases: Bile leakage following drain removal post liver transplant
  - In vicinity of hepatic violations secondary to penetrating trauma, liver surgery
- Morphology: Usually free-flowing unless biloma (contained fluid collection)

Nuclear Medicine Findings
- Extravasation of Tc-99m IDA outside biliary system
  - Often starts in gallbladder fossa, porta hepatis
    - Tracer frequently tracks inferior to right hepatic lobe ⇒ right paracolic gutter/Morrison pouch, over liver dome or freely into peritoneum

Imaging Recommendations
- Best imaging tool
  - Tc-99m IDA hepatobiliary cholescintigraphy
    - Fluid collections identified by US, CT or otherwise are thus characterized
- Protocol advice
  - 5 mCi 185 MBq Tc-99m IDA derivative (e.g., HIDA, DISIDA)
  - Sequential one minute acquisitions to 60 minutes
  - Static images at 2-4 hr, 24 hr
- Additional nuclear medicine imaging options
  - Oblique, lateral: Localize abnormalities in anteroposterior plane
  - Right lateral decubitus: Facilitates tracer pooling away from central bile duct and enteric system

DDx: Extraductal Fluid

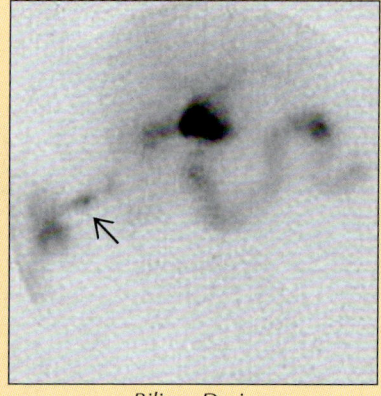

Biliary Drain

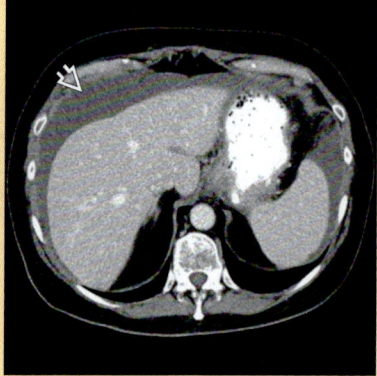

Ascites

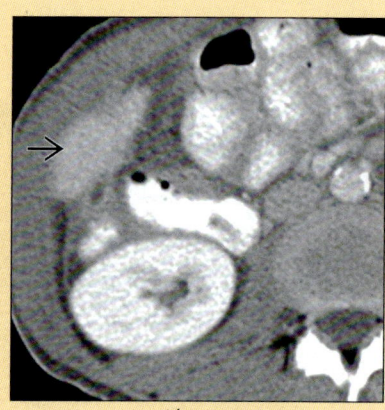

Abscess

BILIARY LEAK

Key Facts

Terminology
- Bile extrinsic to biliary tree and bowel, usually within peritoneal cavity or biloma (focal bile collection)

Top Differential Diagnoses
- Ascites
- Abscess
- Pancreatitis

Pathology
- Most often post procedural: Cholecystectomy or liver transplant
- Also in iatrogenic, blunt, penetrating trauma to right upper quadrant/epigastrium

Clinical Issues
- Most common signs/symptoms: Fluid collection, pain, fever: Bile peritonitis

DIFFERENTIAL DIAGNOSIS

Ascites
- Chronic liver disease, cirrhosis; no tracer accumulation

Abscess
- Enhancing wall on CECT, may contain gas in up to 50% of cases; no tracer accumulation

Pancreatitis
- Associated pancreatic abnormalities/laboratory values

Midgut malrotation
- May mimic IDA extravasation in subhepatic region

PATHOLOGY

General Features
- Etiology
  - Most often post procedural: Cholecystectomy or liver transplant
    - Biliary anatomy can be highly variable; anomalous ducts may be unrecognized, particularly at laparoscopic cholecystectomy
  - Also in iatrogenic, blunt, penetrating trauma to right upper quadrant/epigastrium
    - Blunt liver injury: Leaks associated with hepatic abbreviated injury score of ≥ 4
  - Gangrenous gallbladder: Perforation
- Associated abnormalities
  - Variant biliary anatomy
    - Subvesical bile duct of Luschka and cystohepatic duct: Incomplete resorption of embryonic biliary duct plexus

CLINICAL ISSUES

Presentation
- Most common signs/symptoms: Fluid collection, pain, fever: Bile peritonitis

Treatment
- Small, slow leaks: Conservative therapy
- Larger leaks
  - Surgical revision
  - Endoscopic stent
  - Percutaneous transhepatic biliary drainage

DIAGNOSTIC CHECKLIST

Image Interpretation Pearls
- Delayed images (≤ 24 hr) can help in equivocal cases

SELECTED REFERENCES
1. Pacholczyk M et al: Biliary complications following liver transplantation: single-center experience. Transplant Proc. 38(1):247-9, 2006
2. Wahl WL et al: Diagnosis and management of bile leaks after blunt liver injury. Surgery. 138(4):742-7; discussion 747-8, 2005

IMAGE GALLERY

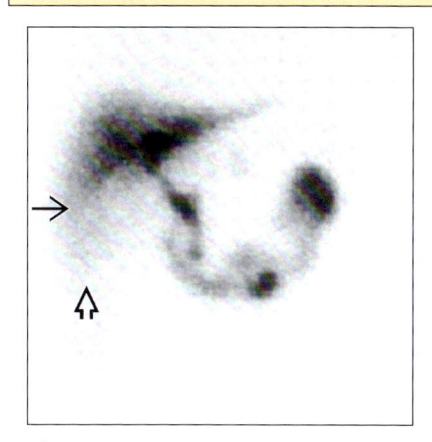

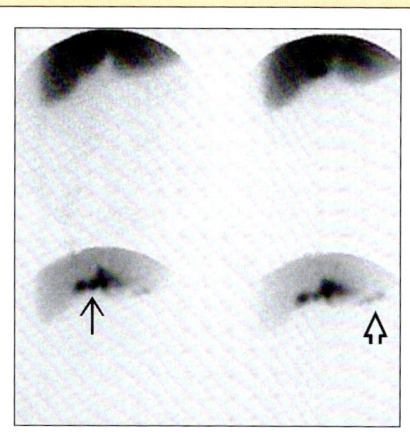

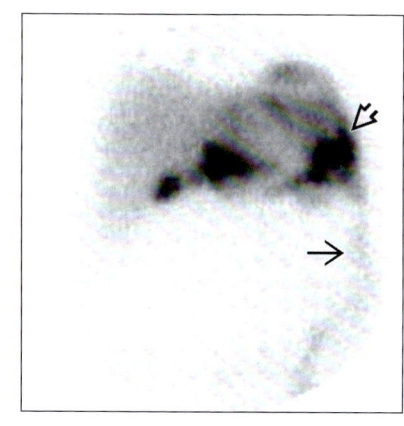

(Left) Anterior hepatobiliary scintigraphy shows smearing of inferior margin of right hepatic lobe ➔ extending inferiorly along paracolic gutter ⇨ in patient with ruptured gangrenous cholecystitis. (Center) Anterior hepatobiliary scintigraphy shows tracer in hepatic hilum ➔ with tracking toward left hepatic lobe ⇨ indicating biliary leak. (Right) Anterior hepatobiliary scintigraphy at 2 hr shows tracer collecting around left hepatic lobe ⇨ with free drainage into left paracolic gutter ➔.

COMMON BILE DUCT OBSTRUCTION

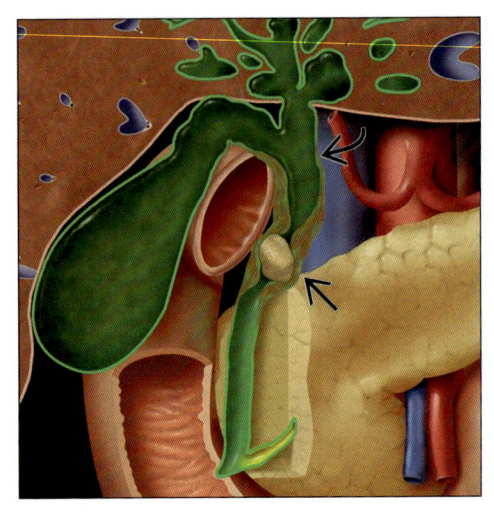

Coronal graphic shows common duct stone ➡ with mural inflammation near pancreatic head resulting in mild diffuse upstream biliary dilation ➡.

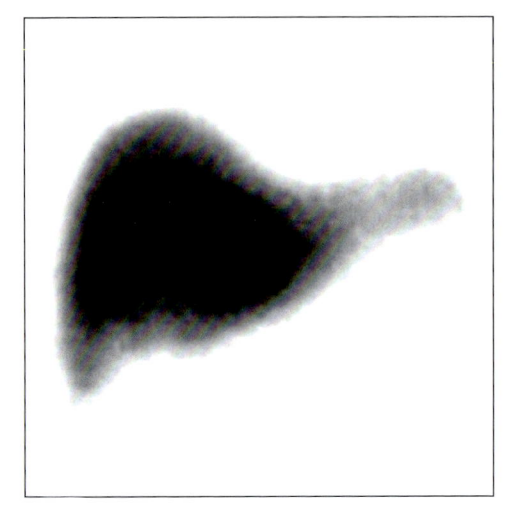

Anterior hepatobiliary scan at 2 h shows no activity in GB, CBD, duodenum due to high grade obstruction from choledocholithiasis. Low blood pool activity makes hepatocellular disease unlikely.

TERMINOLOGY

Definitions
- Common bile duct (CBD) obstruction: Luminal stenosis, intraluminal blockage, extraluminal compression

IMAGING FINDINGS

General Features
- Best diagnostic clue
  - IDA scan: Absence of visualization of small bowel
  - MRCP: Visualization of obstructing stone or mass with proximal CBD dilation

Nuclear Medicine Findings
- Hepatobiliary Scintigraphy
  - Cholescintigraphy shows obstruction before biliary dilation evident by conventional imaging
    - Positive for obstruction: Absence of visualization of duodenum, small bowel
  - Normal study precludes obstruction
  - IDA scan cannot be used to diagnose partial obstruction, only complete obstruction
  - False positives: Prolonged fasting, gallbladder dysfunction (pooling in gallbladder)
  - Visualization of gallbladder is variable in presence of isolated common bile duct visualization

CT Findings
- Proximal ductal dilatation
- Secondary signs: Pancreatitis, gallstones, pancreatic ductal stones

MR Findings
- MRCP: May be normal early, more sensitive than US

Other Modality Findings
- ERCP or percutaneous cholangiography: 90% sensitivity, invasive, potential for intervention

Ultrasonographic Findings
- US: Frequently first evaluation; shadowing lithiasis absent ~ 25-80%
  - Biliary dilation nonspecific, often delayed finding

DDx: No Biliary to Bowel Transit

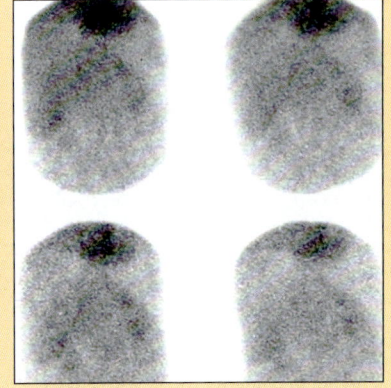

Alcoholic Hepatitis 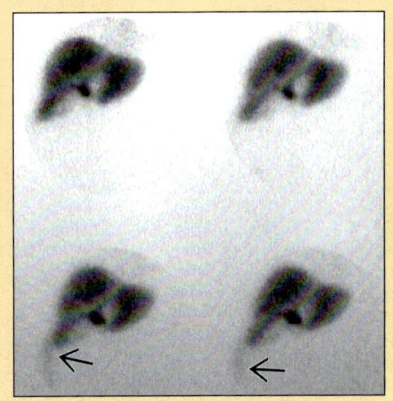 | *Biliary Leak* 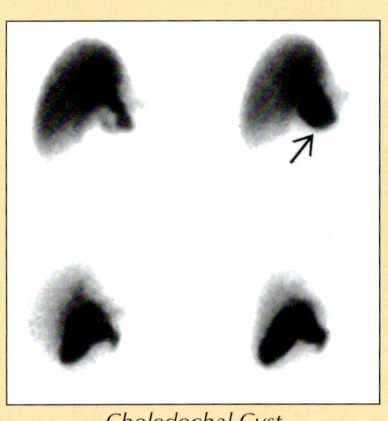 | *Choledochal Cyst*

COMMON BILE DUCT OBSTRUCTION

Key Facts

Terminology
- Common bile duct (CBD) obstruction: Luminal stenosis, intraluminal blockage, extraluminal compression

Imaging Findings
- Cholescintigraphy shows obstruction before biliary dilation evident by conventional imaging
- Normal study precludes obstruction

Pathology
- Etiology: Choledocholithiasis (most common), pancreatic duct stones, benign stricture, neoplasm, parasites, sludge/debris

Diagnostic Checklist
- High grade obstruction: Persistent hepatogram, no biliary excretion, > 2 hour transit to small bowel
- Partial CBD obstruction: Cannot be reliably diagnose by IDA scan

Imaging Recommendations
- Best imaging tool: MRCP, IDA scan
- Protocol advice
  - 5-8 mCi (185-296 MBq) of Tc-99m IDA preparation: Image 1-4 h, as necessary
  - Visualization of GB but not small bowel: Give oral fatty challenge or cautious IV CCK
- Correlative imaging features (MRCP, CT, US): Biliary stricture/truncation or upstream dilation; intraductal calculus, thrombus or mass; extraductal mass/compression inducing obstruction

DIFFERENTIAL DIAGNOSIS

Opioid Medication
- Contracts sphincter of Oddi; stop x 4-6 hrs

Chronic Dilation
- Previous obstruction, chronic cholelithiasis, surgery

Hepatocellular Disease/Cholestasis
- ↓ Extrahepatic excretion of IDA, ↑ blood pool

PATHOLOGY

General Features
- Etiology: Choledocholithiasis (most common), pancreatic duct stones, benign stricture, neoplasm, parasites, sludge/debris

CLINICAL ISSUES

Presentation
- Most common signs/symptoms: RUQ pain, fever, ↑ liver function tests
- Other signs/symptoms
  - Early: ↑ Serum alkaline phosphatase
  - Late: Hyperbilirubinemia, jaundice, biliary cirrhosis

DIAGNOSTIC CHECKLIST

Image Interpretation Pearls
- Non-visualization of small bowel + high blood pool: Severe hepatocellular disease
- High grade obstruction: Persistent hepatogram, no biliary excretion, > 2 hour transit to small bowel
- Partial CBD obstruction: Cannot be reliably diagnose by IDA scan
  - Biliary-bowel transit normal in ≤ 50% of cases of partial CBD obstruction

SELECTED REFERENCES
1. Schirmer BD et al: Cholelithiasis and cholecystitis. J Long Term Eff Med Implants. 15(3):329-38, 2005
2. Rubens DJ: Hepatobiliary imaging and its pitfalls. Radiol Clin North Am. 42(2):257-78, 2004
3. Ziessman HA: Acute cholecystitis, biliary obstruction, and biliary leakage. Semin Nucl Med. 33(4):279-96, 2003

IMAGE GALLERY

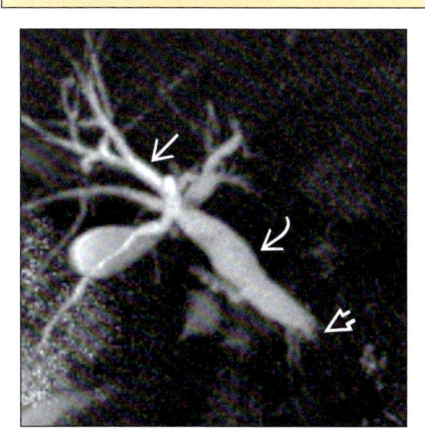

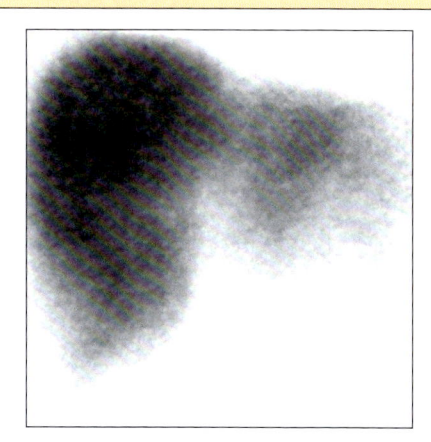

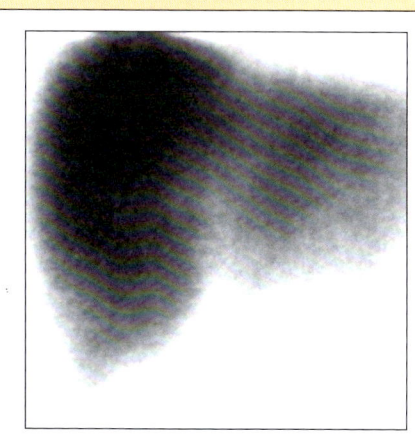

(Left) Coronal oblique MRCP shows normal intrahepatic ducts ➡, dilated extrahepatic duct ➡, ductal truncation ➡ at pancreas, denoting biliary dilatation due to obstruction at level of pancreas. *(Center)* Anterior hepatobiliary scan at 20 min in patient with jaundice post cholecystectomy shows good hepatic tracer extraction and clearing of blood pool. See next image. *(Right)* Anterior hepatobiliary scan at 90 min in same patient at left shows increased tracer in liver with no biliary excretion, indicating high grade obstruction due to CBD stone.

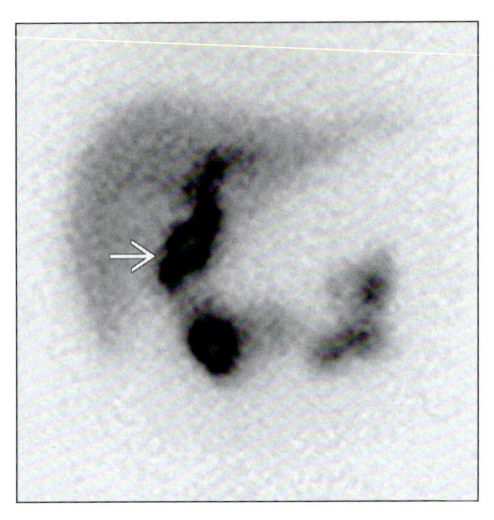

CHOLEDOCHAL CYST

Anterior Tc-99m hepatobiliary scan shows tracer accumulation in ectatic fusiform extrahepatic CBD ➔ with subsequent decompression into small bowel: Type I choledochal cyst.

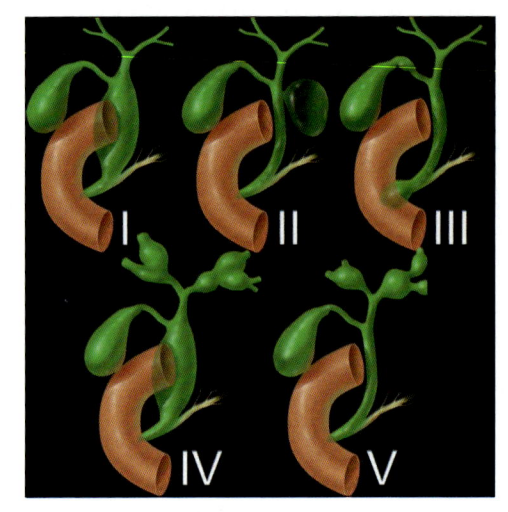

Graphic demonstrates choledochal cyst classification scheme: I-fusiform extrahepatic CBD; II- saccular; III-choledochocele; IV-multifocal; V-multiple intrahepatic (Caroli disease).

TERMINOLOGY

Abbreviations and Synonyms
- Choledochal cyst, choledochocele, choledochal diverticulum, Caroli disease
  - Family of abnormalities involving various configurations of biliary tree dilation
  - Common bile duct (CBD)

Definitions
- Fusiform, cystic, or saccular dilation of intrahepatic and extrahepatic biliary tree
  - Not a true cyst by strict definition

IMAGING FINDINGS

General Features
- Best diagnostic clue
  - Accumulation and retention of tracer within cystic structure on Tc-99m hepatobiliary scintigraphy
  - Accumulation and retention of contrast or fluid signal within cystic structure on ERCP or MRCP, respectively
  - Accessory cystic structure on cross sectional or ultrasound (US) imaging
- Location: Biliary tree, usually extrahepatic common bile duct
- Size: 2-20 cm, may be larger
- Morphology
  - Typically fusiform, less commonly saccular
  - Visser classification: Descriptive with corresponding characteristic profiles
    - Choledochal cyst, choledochal diverticulum, choledochocele, Caroli disease
  - Todani types I-V
    - Type I: Cystic dilatation of part or all of extrahepatic biliary tree (80-90% of cases)
    - Type II: Diverticulum (extrahepatic, supraduodenal)
    - Type III: Choledochocele (cystic dilatation of intramural duodenal segment of CBD)
    - Type IV: Multiple intra and extrahepatic cysts
    - Type V: Caroli disease (isolated dilatation of segments of intrahepatic bile ducts) also known as communicating cavernous biliary ectasia

DDx: Enlarged Bile Ducts

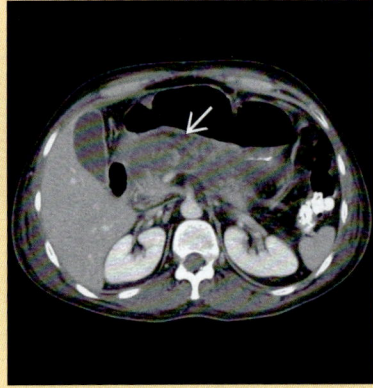

Pancreatitis 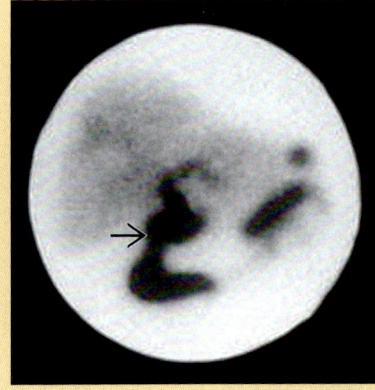 *Duodenal Pooling* 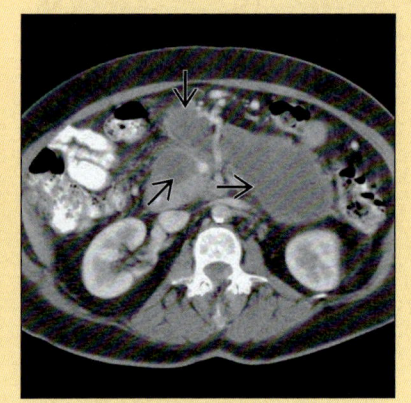 *Pancreatic Pseudocysts*

CHOLEDOCHAL CYST

Key Facts

Terminology
- Fusiform, cystic, or saccular dilation of intrahepatic and extrahepatic biliary tree
- Not a true cyst by strict definition

Imaging Findings
- Accumulation and retention of tracer within cystic structure on Tc-99m hepatobiliary scintigraphy
- Initially photopenic region usually overlying porta hepatis on IDA scan
- Delayed tracer accumulation with prolonged stasis in affected segment of biliary tree
- May necessitate imaging up to 24 hours to demonstrate filling of cyst
- Infants may benefit from premedication to enhance hepatic tracer excretion

Clinical Issues
- Cholangitis, jaundice and pancreatitis common
- Other signs/symptoms: RUQ or mid epigastric mass
- Usually identified during childhood
- Gender: F:M ~ 4:1
- Complications largely 2° to compression of adjacent structures

Diagnostic Checklist
- Use IDA scan to evaluate unknown childhood jaundice or cystic structures in RUQ
- Evaluates for biliary continuity in ambiguous cases
- Nonvisualization of gallbladder may occur as large choledochal cysts may compress

Nuclear Medicine Findings
- Tc-99m hepatobiliary scintigraphy (IDA scan)
  - Initially photopenic region usually overlying porta hepatis on IDA scan
  - Delayed tracer accumulation with prolonged stasis in affected segment of biliary tree
  - May require delayed imaging to 24 h to demonstrate

Imaging Recommendations
- Best imaging tool
  - MRCP with contrast enhanced sequences
    - Non-enhancing fluid signal in biliary tree dilation: T1 hypointense; T2 hyperintense
    - Absence of ductal stone, extrinsic compression
  - CECT: Fluid density biliary tree dilation in absence of ductal stone, extrinsic compression
  - ERCP: Contrast opacification of dilated duct
- Protocol advice
  - Standard Tc-99m HIDA scintigraphy protocol
    - Dose: 5-8 mCi (185-296 MBq) of Tc-99m IDA
    - May necessitate imaging up to 24 hours to demonstrate filling of cyst
- Infants may benefit from premedication to enhance hepatic tracer excretion
  - Phenobarbital 2.5mg/kg BID for 5 to 7 days
  - Ursodeoxycholic acid (UDCA) 10 mg/kg po q/12 hr for 2-3 days

DIFFERENTIAL DIAGNOSIS

Biliary Obstruction
- Cholelithiasis
- Bile duct tumor, ampullary tumor
- Pancreatic pseudocyst
- Pancreatic neoplasm
- Recurrent pyogenic cholangitis
  - May be associated with profound cholelithiasis conforming to configuration of dilated duct
  - Most common in Asians, associated with parasites and gram-bacterial infection

Pancreatic Pseudocyst
- History of pancreatitis
- Frequently associated with pancreas +/-normal biliary tree
- No IDA accumulation

Post-Operative Change
- Common bile duct frequently enlarged post cholecystectomy but should not exceed 10-12 mm

Hepatic Cyst
- No extrahepatic biliary dilation or central dot sign of portal vasculature on CECT or US
- No HIDA accumulation

Mesenteric or Omental Cyst
- No HIDA accumulation
- Thin wall and septations (best seen on US)

Biloma
- Biliary leak with loculation

PATHOLOGY

General Features
- Genetics
  - Not yet characterized
    - Exception: Caroli disease; autosomal recessive, associated with unbalanced translocation between chromosomes 3 and 8 and other abnormalities
- Etiology
  - Congenital, rarely familial
    - Related to partial/total arrest of remodeling of embryonic ductal plate
    - Genetic and non-genetic causes remain unidentified
    - Often associated with pancreaticobiliary maljunction
  - Choledochocele
    - Wall of CBD herniates into duodenum: Intraduodenal choledochal cyst

CHOLEDOCHAL CYST

- Possibly 2° to inflammatory scarring, stenosis following stone passage or congenital narrowing
- Epidemiology: Usually identified in infancy or childhood as a result of biliary obstruction
- Associated abnormalities
  - Associated with anomalous junction of pancreatic duct and biliary tree in > 90% of cases, often common junction in sphincter of Oddi
  - Increased incidence of cholangiocarcinoma, estimated risk 20 times of average population
  - Increased risk for pancreatitis

CLINICAL ISSUES

Presentation
- Most common signs/symptoms
  - Cholangitis, jaundice and pancreatitis common
    - Chronic right upper quadrant (RUQ) or epigastric pain
    - Intermittent fever
    - Pruritus
    - Vomiting
    - Labs: ↑ Bilirubin, alkaline phosphatase, {gamma}-glutamyl transferase, transaminases, serum amylase
- Other signs/symptoms: RUQ or mid epigastric mass

Demographics
- Age
  - Usually identified during childhood
    - 25% during first year
    - Most prior to age 10
- Gender: F:M ~ 4:1
- Ethnicity: Most common in patients of Asian descent

Natural History & Prognosis
- Cholestasis of lithogenic bile salts
  - ⇒ Jaundice, pain, cholelithiasis, and cholangitis
  - Abscess, perforation, peritonitis may develop
- Complications largely 2° to compression of adjacent structures
  - Cholestasis, cholelithiasis, cholangitis
  - Pancreatitis, 30-70% of patients
  - Biliary rupture/leak, peritonitis
  - Biliary cirrhosis and portal hypertension
  - Duodenal obstruction
- Malignant transformation
  - Usually cholangiocarcinoma
  - Most common in choledochal cysts types I and IV

Treatment
- Sphincterotomy
  - May be successful in more distal type III choledochal cysts (choledochocele)
- Complete surgical biliary excision in cases not amenable to sphincterotomy
  - Includes cholecystectomy with hepaticojejunostomy or Roux-en-Y hepaticojejunostomy
  - Roux-en-Y hepaticojejunostomy currently preferred because of ↓ post-op bilious gastritis 2° to duodenogastric bile reflux
  - Incomplete resection vulnerable to malignant transformation
- Percutaneous drainage
  - Temporizing measure in patients with acute complications
- Internal drainage procedures with incomplete or no cystectomy associated with ↑ risk of malignant transformation
  - Now supplanted by excision and revision as above

DIAGNOSTIC CHECKLIST

Image Interpretation Pearls
- Use IDA scan to evaluate unknown childhood jaundice or cystic structures in RUQ
  - Especially in the newborn and children
  - Evaluates for biliary continuity in ambiguous cases
    - Also useful to establish integrity of biliary enteric anastomosis post-operatively
  - Nonvisualization of gallbladder may occur as large choledochal cysts may compress
    - May result in false positive for acute cholecystitis
    - Compare with other imaging modalities
- Complete and accurate evaluation requires combinations of US, CT, MRI/MRCP, ERCP
- US
  - Dilated segment or segments of biliary tree
  - Especially RUQ cystic structure in fetal abdomen
  - As early as 25 weeks gestation
- MRCP: Fluid signal ectasia of biliary tree in absence of causative mass or lesion
- CECT
  - Dilated segment or segments of biliary tree separate from gallbladder
  - Caroli disease demonstrates dilated intrahepatic bile ducts
    - Central dot sign: Enhancing portovascular structures surrounded by ectatic biliary radicals
- UGI
  - Choledochocele, incidental finding of well-defined, smooth filling defect on medial wall of descending duodenum
  - Choledochal cyst, diverticulum or Caroli disease likely occult on UGI

SELECTED REFERENCES

1. Clifton MS et al: Prenatal diagnosis of familial type I choledochal cyst. Pediatrics. 117(3):e596-600, 2006
2. Lee HC et al: Biliary cysts in children--long-term follow-up in Taiwan. J Formos Med Assoc. 105(2):118-24, 2006
3. Stipsanelli E et al: Spontaneous rupture of a type IV(A) choledochal cyst in a young adult during radiological imaging. World J Gastroenterol. 12(6):982-986, 2006
4. Desmet VJ: [Cystic diseases of the liver. From embryology to malformations] Gastroenterol Clin Biol. 29(8-9):858-60, 2005
5. Shimotakahara A et al: Roux-en-Y hepaticojejunostomy or hepaticoduodenostomy for biliary reconstruction during the surgical treatment of choledochal cyst: which is better? Pediatr Surg Int. 21(1):5-7, 2005
6. Poddar U et al: Ursodeoxycholic acid-augmented hepatobiliary scintigraphy in the evaluation of neonatal jaundice. J Nucl Med. 45(9):1488-92, 2004
7. Visser BC et al: Congenital choledochal cysts in adults. Arch Surg. 139(8):855-60; discussion 860-2, 2004

CHOLEDOCHAL CYST

IMAGE GALLERY

Typical

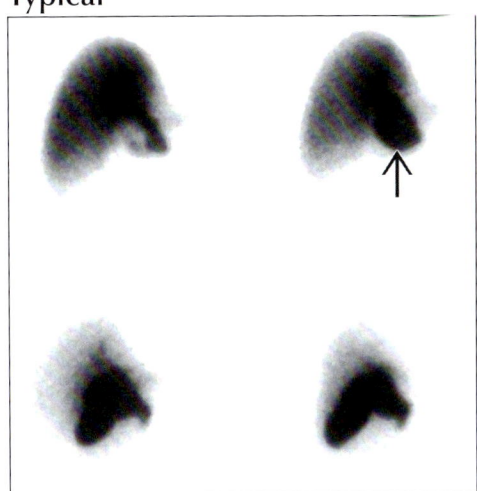

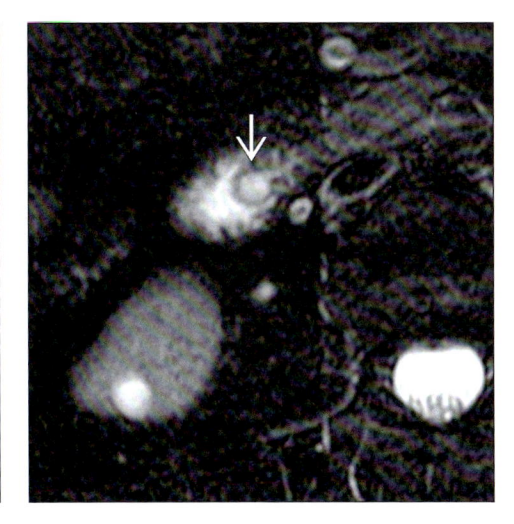

(Left) Hepatobiliary scintigraphy shows progressive tracer accumulation within cystic structure ➡ involving the extrahepatic bile duct in patient with type I choledochal cyst. *(Right)* Axial FSE T2MR shows choledochocele intruding into duodenal lumen ➡. Patient had no upstream biliary stasis.

Typical

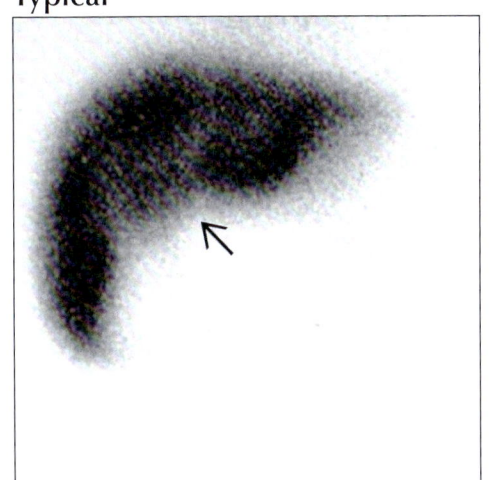

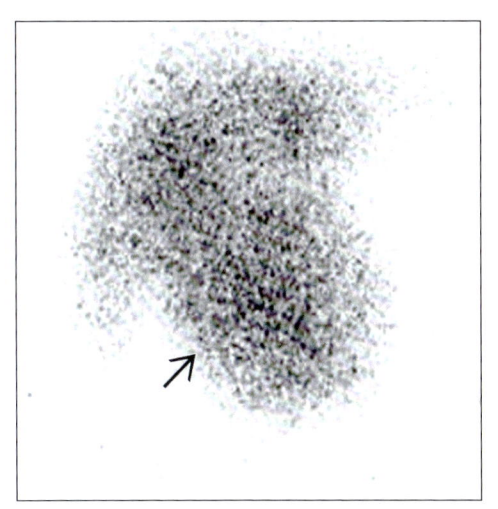

(Left) Anterior planar hepatobiliary scintigraphy at 1 h shows prompt hepatic extraction of tracer without biliary excretion ➡. See next image. *(Right)* 24 h delayed anterior planar hepatobiliary scintigraphy (same patient as previous image) shows filling of a cystic, dilated structure ➡ confirming biliary continuity and indicating choledochal cyst.

Other

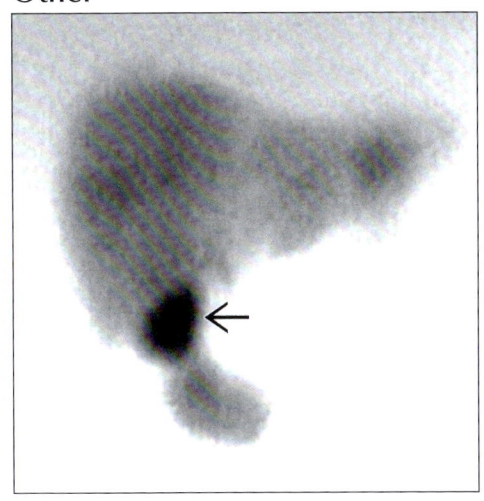

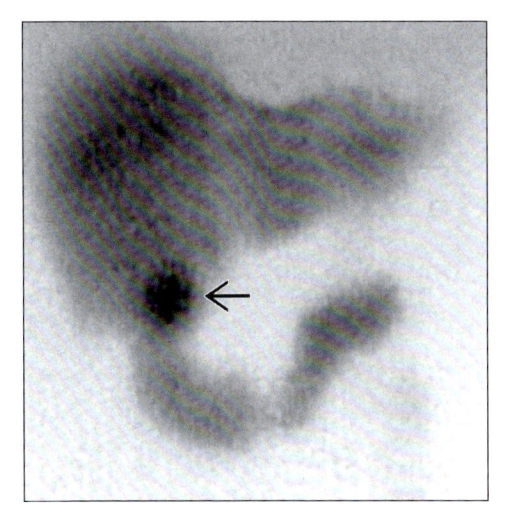

(Left) Anterior hepatobiliary scintigraphy shows tracer accumulation ➡ near level of ampulla of Vater. See next image. *(Right)* Anterior hepatobiliary scintigraphy in same patient at left after ingesting water shows interval clearance of activity ➡, indicating that it represented duodenal pooling, not choledochal cyst.

BILIARY BYPASS OBSTRUCTION

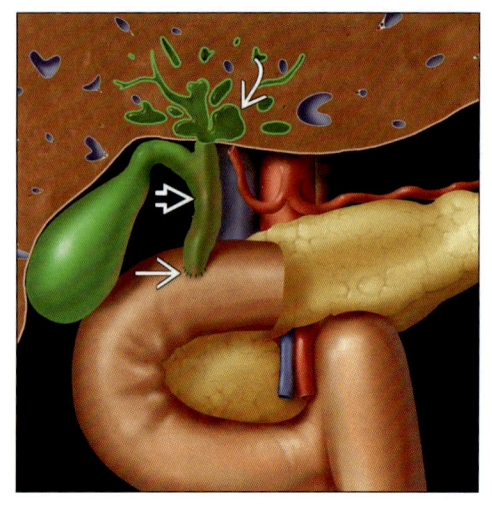

Coronal graphic shows post-surgical stenosis at choledochoduodenostomy ➡ with diffuse upstream dilation of intrahepatic biliary tree ➡ and extrahepatic bile duct ➡.

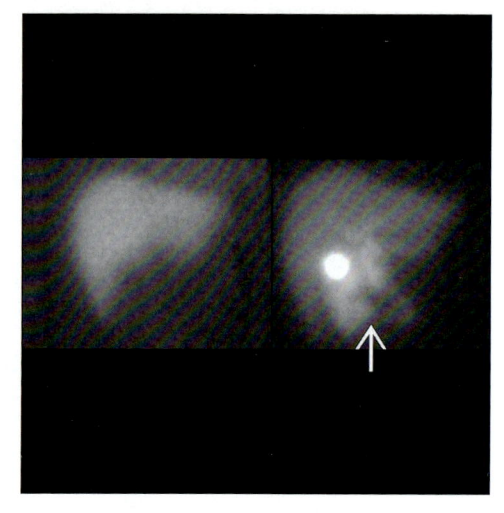

IDA scan at 10 and 90 minutes shows delayed transit through the small bowel in presence of partial obstruction ➡ following Roux-en-Y choledochojejunostomy.

TERMINOLOGY

Definitions
- Partial or complete obstruction of resected, reanastomosed biliary tree or its segments

IMAGING FINDINGS

General Features
- Best diagnostic clue
  - Biliary stasis or decreased ductal clearance
  - Dilation of biliary tree alone insufficient
    - Many non-obstructed patients display persistent biliary dilation following bypass (> 20%)

Nuclear Medicine Findings
- Persistent tracer in biliary system
- Delayed clearance of tracer through biliary system (partial obstruction)

Imaging Recommendations
- Best imaging tool
  - Hepatobiliary scintigraphy shows absent, ↓ bile flow noninvasively
  - Hepatobiliary scintigraphy most accurate imaging
- Protocol advice
  - 5-8 mCi (185-296 MBq) of Tc-99m IDA (or derivative) IV
  - Maneuver patient to facilitate drainage if activity transit appears inappropriate
  - CCK augments biliary excretion and washout, improves specificity
  - Region of interest time-activity curve calculated over CBD or segment of biliary tree in question
    - Biliary tree should drain sequentially despite increasing accumulation in small bowel
    - Exclude positional pooling in small bowel with postural maneuvers
  - Must exclude failed or improper imaging
- Correlative imaging features
  - US, CECT, MRCP and ERCP: Useful in initial evaluation of new-onset biliary dilation
    - Post-operative or chronic dilation cannot be reliably distinguished from obstruction
    - Bowel contents and postoperative changes may obfuscate areas of concern

DDx: Nonobstructive Hepatic Pathology

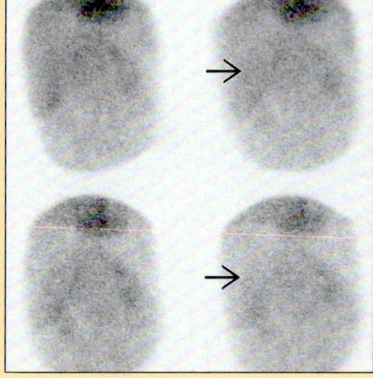

Chemical Hepatitis

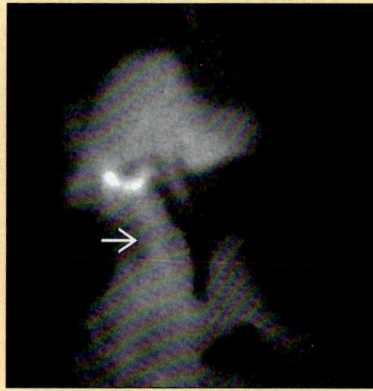

Bile Leak

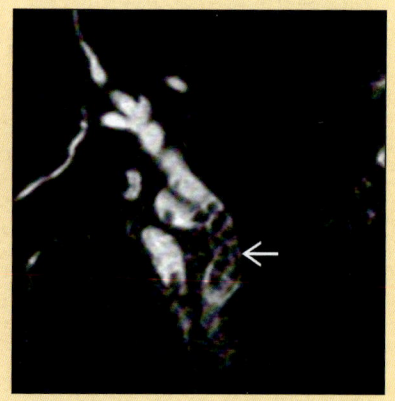

Nonobstructive Choledocholithiasis

BILIARY BYPASS OBSTRUCTION

Key Facts

Terminology
- Partial or complete obstruction of resected, reanastomosed biliary tree or its segments

Imaging Findings
- Dilation of biliary tree alone insufficient
- Many non-obstructed patients display persistent biliary dilation following bypass (> 20%)
- Hepatobiliary scintigraphy shows absent, ↓ bile flow noninvasively

Clinical Issues
- Most common signs/symptoms: RUQ pain, fever, jaundice

Diagnostic Checklist
- Transit to small bowel by 1 hour ≈ patency
- Retention/increasing tracer at 1 hour ≈ obstruction
- No excretion ≈ total obstruction vs. severe hepatic dysfunction

DIFFERENTIAL DIAGNOSIS

Post-Operative Dilation
- Capacious bile ducts after cholecystectomy, resolution of previous obstruction, choledochal cyst

Bile Leak
- Post-operative tracer extravasation on hepatobiliary scintigraphy

Poor Hepatic Washout
- 2° to severe cellular dysfunction (e.g., hepatitis)

PATHOLOGY

General Features
- Etiology
  - Benign or malignant disease requiring biliary bypass
    - Stenosis of biliary enteric anastomosis
    - Hepatic allograft or post-Whipple evaluations
    - Retained stone, sludge or debris
    - Stent occlusion, collapse, migration

Gross Pathologic & Surgical Features
- Post-surgical anatomy can vary
  - Choledocho-jejunostomy vs. -duodenostomy, intrahepatic choledochojejunostomy
    - Upstream dilation may not be present, therefore conventional imaging of limited accuracy
    - Partial stenosis, obstruction most likely at anastomosis

CLINICAL ISSUES

Presentation
- Most common signs/symptoms: RUQ pain, fever, jaundice

Treatment
- Endoscopic biliary stenting
- Percutaneous transhepatic biliary drainage, stenting
- Surgical revision of bypass

DIAGNOSTIC CHECKLIST

Image Interpretation Pearls
- Transit to small bowel by 1 hour ≈ patency
  - Retention/increasing tracer at 1 hour ≈ obstruction
  - No excretion ≈ total obstruction vs. severe hepatic dysfunction

SELECTED REFERENCES

1. Zeissman HA et al: Nuclear Medicine: The Requisites. 3rd ed. C.V. Mosby, Boston. 185-7, 2006
2. Chahal P et al: Cholangiocarcinoma. Curr Treat Options Gastroenterol. 8(6):493-502, 2005
3. Hammarstrom LE: Role of palliative endoscopic drainage in patients with malignant biliary obstruction. Dig Surg. 22(5):295-304; discussion 305, 2005
4. Lucas MH et al: Positional biliary stasis: scintigraphic findings following biliary-enteric bypass surgery. J Nucl Med. 36(1):104-6, 1995

IMAGE GALLERY

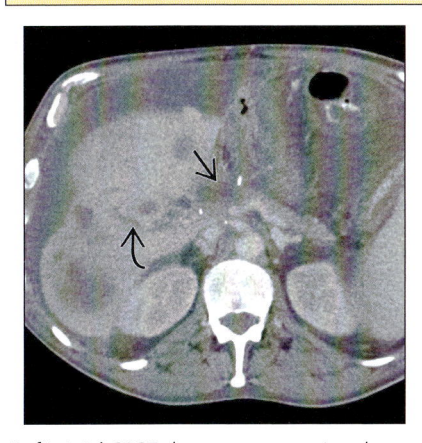

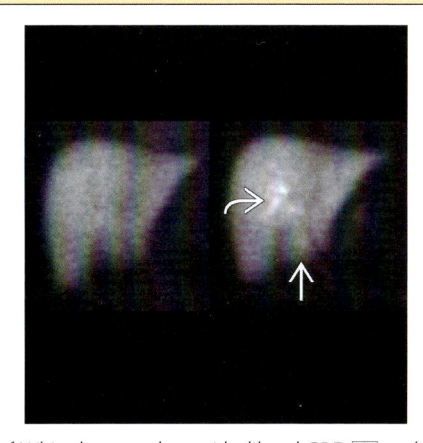

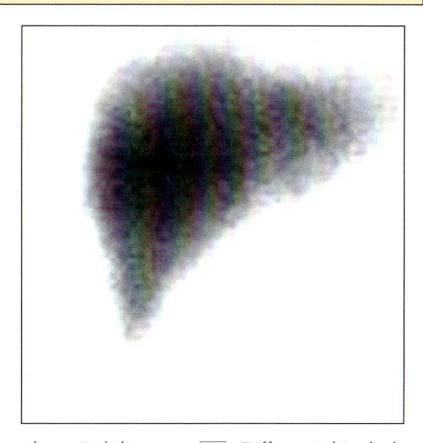

(Left) Axial CECT shows post-operative change of Whipple procedure with dilated CBD ➔ and intrahepatic biliary tree ➔. Differential includes post-operative dilation vs. obstruction, best evaluated with hepatobiliary scan. (Center) Hepatobiliary scan at 5 and 60 min shows pooling in subhepatic region ➔, dilated intrahepatic ducts ➔, no antegrade transit in patient with obstructed Kasai anastomosis. (Right) Hepatobiliary scan at 60 min shows no extrahepatic biliary excretion in patient with completely obstructed choledochojejunostomy and acute pancreatitis.

BILIARY ATRESIA

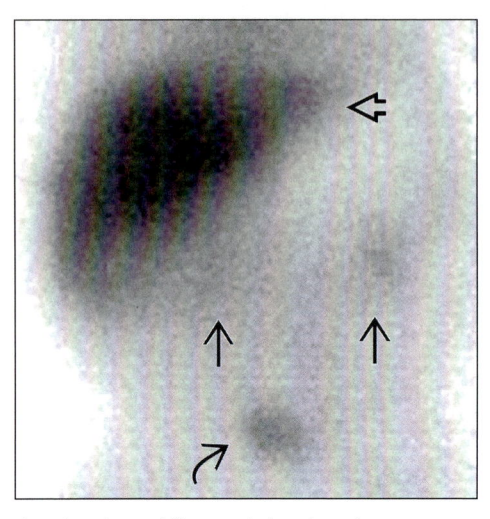

Anterior hepatobiliary scintigraphy shows prompt hepatic tracer extraction ⇦ on early image. Normal kidneys ➔ and bladder ➔ are also seen. No bowel is visualized. See next image.

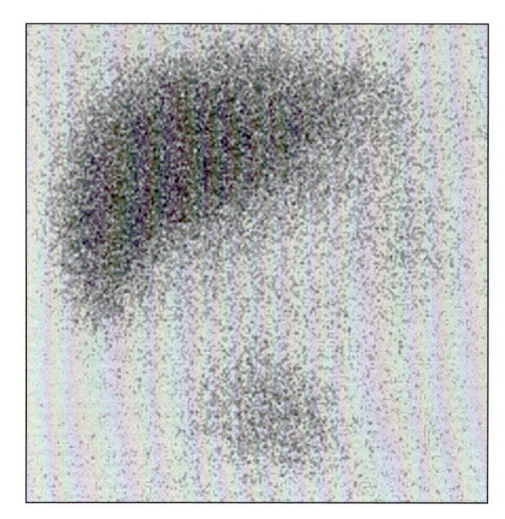

Anterior hepatobiliary scintigraphy at 24 hours shows persistent hepatic activity and faint bladder visualization but no bowel. This is a typical appearance in this patient with BA.

TERMINOLOGY

Abbreviations and Synonyms
- Biliary atresia (BA), Tc-99m iminodiacetic acid derivative (IDA)

Definitions
- Idiopathic inflammatory process of the bile ducts resulting in cholestasis, progressive fibrosis of the biliary tract, and eventually biliary cirrhosis

IMAGING FINDINGS

General Features
- Best diagnostic clue: Cholestasis with non visualization of biliary tree or bowel on early or delayed IDA images

Nuclear Medicine Findings
- Hepatobiliary Scintigraphy
  o Normal
    ▪ Rapid disappearance of IDA from blood pool with prompt and uniform uptake within liver with maximum activity typically reached by 5 minutes
    ▪ In normal neonates, gallbladder, hepatic and common bile ducts are often not seen
    ▪ Bowel activity is normally seen by 40 minutes
  o Neonatal hepatitis
    ▪ Poor uptake by liver, high blood pool, +/- visualization of extrahepatic structures
  o Biliary atresia
    ▪ Non visualization of the bowel with persistent hepatic activity on delayed imaging
    ▪ In neonates, with good concentration of tracer by liver, and low blood pool > 30 minutes distinguishes from neonatal hepatitis
    ▪ Biliary atresia after 3 months of age may show reduced hepatic extraction and delayed clearance from blood pool from liver failure

Imaging Recommendations
- Best imaging tool
  o Hepatobiliary scintigraphy with Tc-99m IDA (typically mebrofenin)

DDx: Total Parenteral Nutrition Induced Cholestasis: Mimics Biliary Atresia

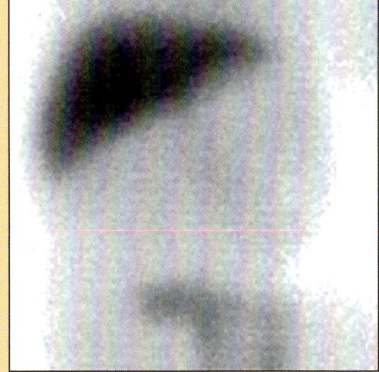

TPN Early Image

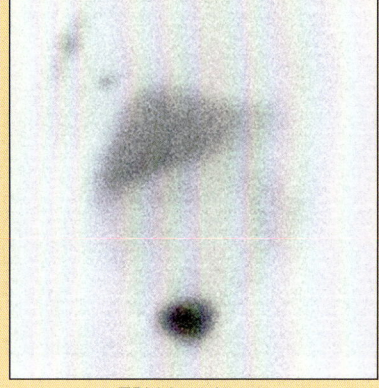

TPN Late Image

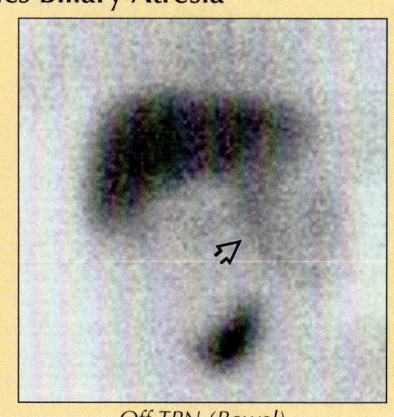

Off TPN (Bowel)

BILIARY ATRESIA

Key Facts

Terminology
- Idiopathic inflammatory process of the bile ducts resulting in cholestasis, progressive fibrosis of the biliary tract, and eventually biliary cirrhosis

Imaging Findings
- Best diagnostic clue: Cholestasis with non visualization of biliary tree or bowel on early or delayed IDA images
- Sensitivity and negative predictive value for excluding biliary atresia is virtually 100% when intestinal or extrahepatic biliary activity is seen
- Premedication with phenobarbital is essential
- Continuous gamma camera acquisition for the first hour is recommended to allow for subsequent viewing of continuous data in cine format

Pathology
- Epidemiology: Reported incidence ranges from 1 in 8,000 live births to 1 in 18,000 live births

Clinical Issues
- Persistent jaundice beyond 3 weeks of age in full term infants and 4 weeks of age in pre-term infants
- Prompt diagnosis is crucial for surgical success
- Untreated infants die of liver failure within 1-2 years

Diagnostic Checklist
- Following abnormal studies consider confirming the blood level and repeating the scan following additional phenobarbital as needed to attain adequate levels

---

- Sensitivity and negative predictive value for excluding biliary atresia is virtually 100% when intestinal or extrahepatic biliary activity is seen
- False positives due to hyperalimentation, neonatal hepatitis
- Protocol advice
  o Premedication with phenobarbital is essential
    - 2.5 mg/kg bid x 5 days
    - Phenobarbital stimulates the hepatic transport system for organic anions and induces microsomal enzymes
  o Alternative premedication is ursodeoxycholic acid (20 mg/kg in two divided doses for 2-3 days) to optimize bile flow
  o Tc-99m IDA: 2-3 mCi injected intravenously
  o Continuous gamma camera acquisition for the first hour is recommended to allow for subsequent viewing of continuous data in cine format
    - Static images at any desired time interval can be generated from this data set
    - Faint mobile bowel activity is often more easily or only visualized on cine loops compared with static images
  o Additional anterior static images 4-24 hours post-injection, or until bowel visualized
- Correlative imaging features
  o Ultrasound
    - A fibrotic triangular cord cranial to the portal vein bifurcation plus a small measured gallbladder length is suggestive of biliary atresia
    - Useful in demonstrating other causes of neonatal cholestasis
  o Magnetic resonance cholangiopancreatography (MRCP) and CT are not standard of practice

DIFFERENTIAL DIAGNOSIS

Neonatal Hepatitis
- Accounts for approximately 1/3 of cases of neonatal cholestasis
- Suspect in patients < 2 month old
- Hepatic uptake of IDA is typically delayed
- Bowel activity may not be seen on initial scan with the likelihood of appearance increasing on subsequent scans

Inspissated Bile Syndrome/Cystic Fibrosis
- Nuclear scan findings can be identical to biliary atresia

Cholestasis Secondary to Total Parenteral Nutrition (TPN)
- Typically in premature infants with scan findings that mimic biliary atresia but improve with cessation of TPN

Choledochal Cyst
- Usually a photopenic defect inferiorly in early images which slowly accumulates tracer over time

Alagille Syndrome
- Paucity or absence of intralobular bile ducts
- Slow washout peripherally with normal washout centrally and visualization of bowel

Alpha-1 Antitrypsin Deficiency
- Most common inherited cause of neonatal cholestasis with a clinical presentation similar to biliary atresia

Caroli Disease
- Dilation of the intrahepatic ducts that appear as photopenic areas within the liver which later accumulate activity

Choledocholithiasis
- While the condition is rare in this age group, mechanical obstruction can always mimic other causes of cholestasis

PATHOLOGY

General Features
- Genetics: No known genetic predilection

BILIARY ATRESIA

- Etiology: Congenital biliary atresia is of unknown etiology but suspected to originate from prenatal biliary duct inflammation
- Epidemiology: Reported incidence ranges from 1 in 8,000 live births to 1 in 18,000 live births
- Associated abnormalities
  - Alagille syndrome (syndromic biliary atresia)
    - Autosomal dominant disorder characterized by chronic cholestasis, characteristic facies, skeletal anomalies, cardiac anomalies, ocular anomalies, renal abnormalities, developmental delay, growth retardation, pancreatic insufficiency
  - Polysplenia syndrome
    - Including situs inversus, poly- or asplenia, cardiovascular malformations and anomalies of the portal vein and hepatic artery

Gross Pathologic & Surgical Features

- Diagnosis confirmed at surgery by presence of a fibrotic biliary remnant and definition of absent proximal and distal bile duct patency by cholecystocholangiography
- Cirrhosis may be present if diagnosis is delayed

Microscopic Features

- Inflammation and fibrosing stricture of the hepatic or common bile ducts, periductal inflammation of intrahepatic bile ducts, and progressive destruction of the intrahepatic biliary tree
- Anatomically classified into three types
  - 1: Atresia involving the common bile duct and a patent proximal system
  - 2: Atresia involving the hepatic duct but with patent proximal ducts
  - 3: Atresia involving the right and left hepatic ducts at the porta hepatis (most common)

CLINICAL ISSUES

Presentation

- Most common signs/symptoms
  - Persistent jaundice beyond 3 weeks of age in full term infants and 4 weeks of age in pre-term infants
  - Cholestasis with conjugated hyperbilirubinemia
- Other signs/symptoms
  - Acholic stools
  - Late developments include failure to thrive after initial normal weight gain, pruritus, and coagulopathy

Demographics

- Age: Neonates
- Gender: M:F = 1:1.4

Natural History & Prognosis

- Prompt diagnosis is crucial for surgical success
  - Untreated infants die of liver failure within 1-2 years
- 4 year survival rate is 40% for neonates undergoing Kasai portoenterostomy
- Jaundice free patients following Kasai have a 10 year survival of nearly 90%
- 70-80% will eventually require liver transplantation
  - Despite successful surgery (Kasai), progressive inflammation and fibrosis of biliary ducts develops to varying degrees in all patients, leading to biliary cirrhosis in the majority of patients

Treatment

- Kasai portoenterostomy
  - Removal of atretic tissue with a Roux-en-Y anastomosis made between the jejunum and the hilum of the liver
  - Success dependent on age at surgery, anatomical findings, luminal size of the bile ducts, and the experience of the surgeon
    - If performed prior to 60 days of age 91% of infants maintain bile flow
    - If performed after 3 months of age 17% maintain bile flow
- Liver transplantation
  - Patients who remain jaundiced following Kasai usually either die or require transplantation by 8 years of age

DIAGNOSTIC CHECKLIST

Image Interpretation Pearls

- Early liver blood pool activity can mimic active tracer uptake
- The standard phenobarbital protocol will not always produce the desired blood level of > 15 ug/ml
  - Following abnormal studies consider confirming the blood level and repeating the scan following additional phenobarbital as needed to attain adequate levels

SELECTED REFERENCES

1. Davenport M: Biliary atresia. Semin Pediatr Surg. 14(1):42-8, 2005
2. Lykavieris P et al: Outcome in adulthood of biliary atresia: a study of 63 patients who survived for over 20 years with their native liver. Hepatology. 41(2):366-71, 2005
3. Mack CL et al: Unraveling the pathogenesis and etiology of biliary atresia. Pediatr Res. 57(5 Pt 2):87R-94R, 2005
4. Davenport M et al: The outcome of the older (> or =100 days) infant with biliary atresia. J Pediatr Surg. 39(4):575-81, 2004
5. Venigalla S et al: Neonatal cholestasis. Semin Perinatol. 28(5):348-55, 2004
6. Charearnrad P et al: The effect of phenobarbital on the accuracy of technetium-99m diisopropyl iminodiacetic acid hepatobiliary scintigraphy in differentiating biliary atresia from neonatal hepatitis syndrome. J Med Assoc Thai. 86 Suppl 2:S189-94, 2003
7. Kobayashi H et al: Biliary atresia. Semin Neonatol. 8(5):383-91, 2003
8. Benya EC: Pancreas and biliary system: imaging of developmental anomalies and diseases unique to children. Radiol Clin North Am. 40(6):1355-62, 2002
9. Spivak W et al: Diagnostic utility of hepatobiliary scintigraphy with 99mTc-DISIDA in neonatal cholestasis. J Pediatr. 110(6):855-61, 1987
10. Gerhold JP et al: Diagnosis of biliary atresia with radionuclide hepatobiliary imaging. Radiology. 146(2):499-504, 1983

BILIARY ATRESIA

IMAGE GALLERY

Typical

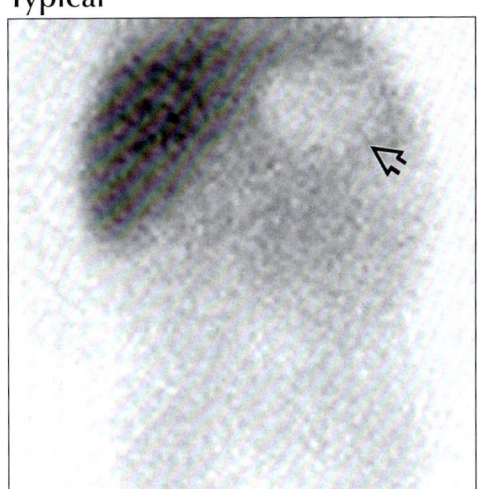

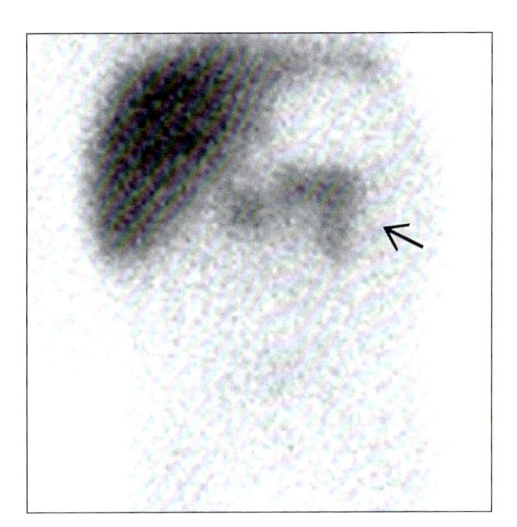

(Left) Anterior hepatobiliary scintigraphy shows normal hepatic extraction by 15 minutes post-injection. Gas in the stomach ⊳ is commonly seen. See next image. *(Right)* Anterior hepatobiliary scintigraphy at one hour in same patient shows tracer clearly present in bowel ➔. This normal hepatic transit of tracer excludes biliary atresia.

Other

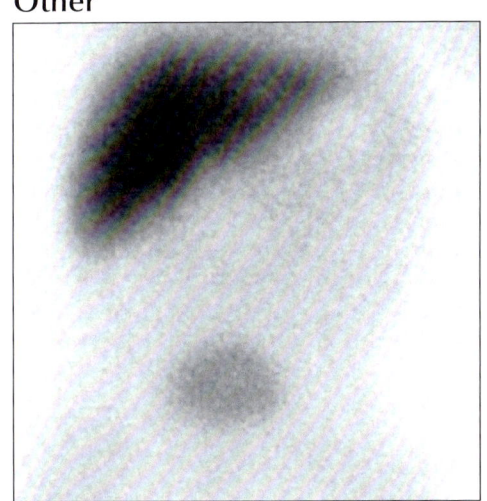

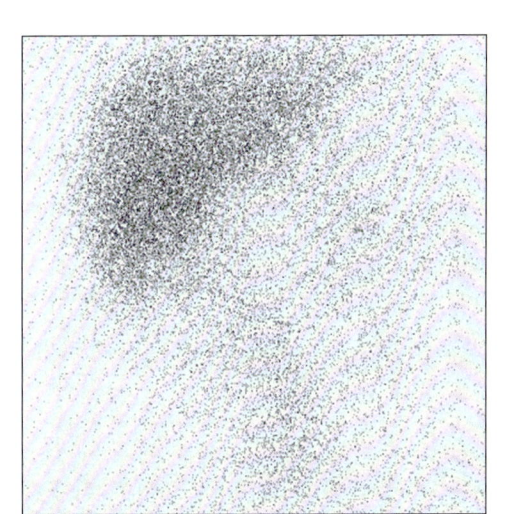

(Left) Anterior hepatobiliary scintigraphy shows retention of hepatic activity, urinary excretion, and no bowel at one hour. See next image. *(Right)* Anterior hepatobiliary scintigraphy 24 hour image in same patient shows persistent hepatic activity, very faint urinary tract activity and no bowel. Pathology showed Alagille syndrome.

Typical

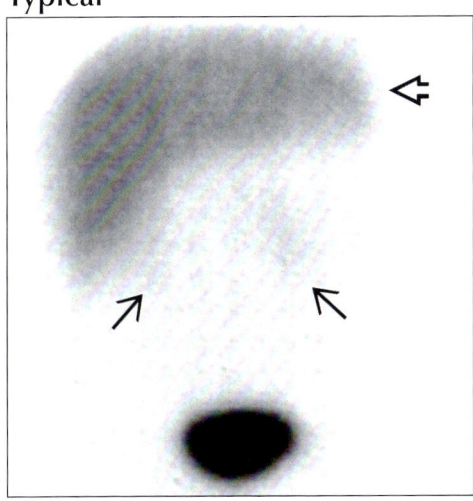

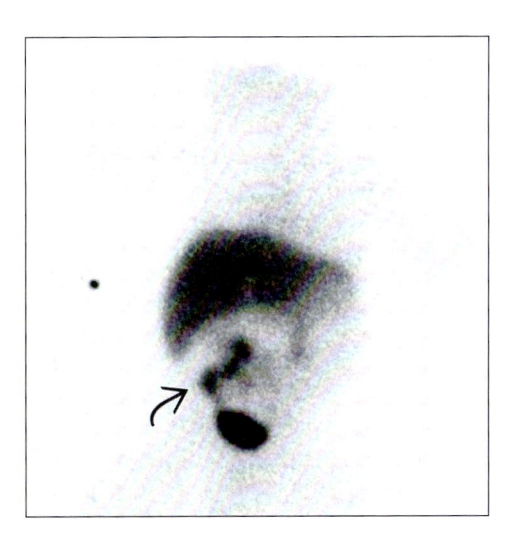

(Left) Anterior hepatobiliary scintigraphy shows at 24 hours retention of tracer in liver ⊳ with no visualization of bowel. Faint renal activity ➔. See next image. *(Right)* Anterior hepatobiliary scintigraphy in same patient shows bowel activity ➔ on early imaging following Kasai portoenterostomy. (Courtesy S. O'Hara, MD).

CHOLANGIOCARCINOMA

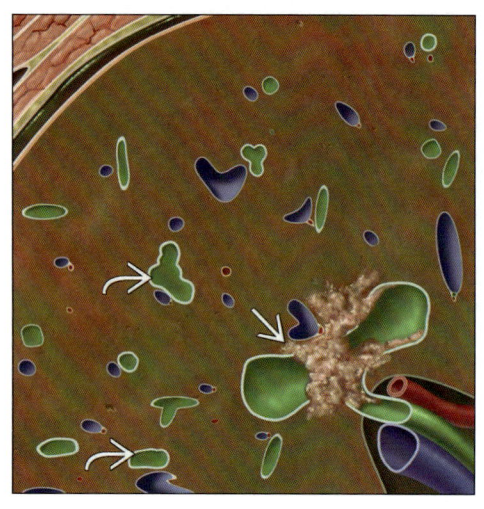

Graphic shows central hilar Klatskin cholangiocarcinoma at confluence of common bile duct ➡ with peripheral intrahepatic ductal dilatation ➡.

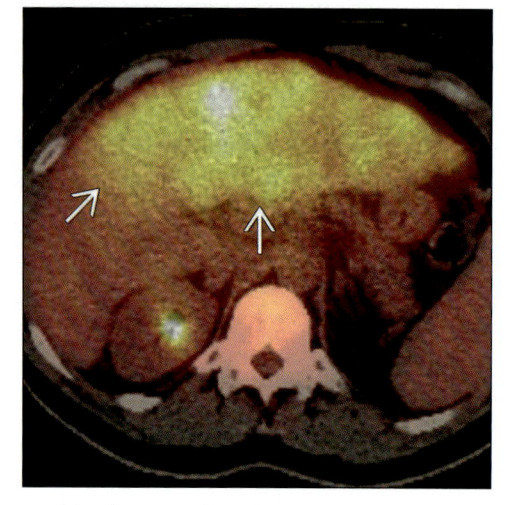

Axial fused PET/CT shows hypermetabolic activity in a large peripheral cholangiocarcinoma ➡ in left and right hepatic lobes.

TERMINOLOGY

Abbreviations and Synonyms
- Cholangiocarcinoma (CC), Klatskin tumor, malignant bile duct tumor

Definitions
- Malignancy that arises from ductular epithelium of intrahepatic biliary tree, extrahepatic bile ducts
  - Note: Gallbladder cancer 9x more common than CC

IMAGING FINDINGS

General Features
- Best diagnostic clue
  - PET: Hypermetabolic activity corresponding to primary tumor in liver, extrahepatic metastatic disease
  - Ultrasound (US), CT, MR: For hilar lesions (Klatskin tumor), bile duct obstruction with small central mass
- Location
  - Extrahepatic tumors (87-92% of CC): Proximal, middle, distal ductal tumors
  - Extrahepatic tumor at bifurcation of proximal common hepatic duct = Klatskin tumor
  - Intrahepatic tumors (8-13% of CC) arise from small ducts
  - Nodular or papillary type most common in distal duct and periampullary region
  - Intrahepatic tumors have tendency for perineural spread; spread to liver, peritoneum, lung extremely rare
  - Extrahepatic tumors spread to celiac nodes in ~ 16% of cases
- Size
  - 5-20 cm at presentation
  - More central lesions (Klatskin) smaller at diagnosis
- Morphology: Variable

Nuclear Medicine Findings
- PET
  - Peripheral CC: Intensely hypermetabolic activity, may be ring-shaped
  - Hilar CC: Low activity with focal nodular or linear branching pattern

DDx: Variable and Non-FDG Avid Hepatic Lesions

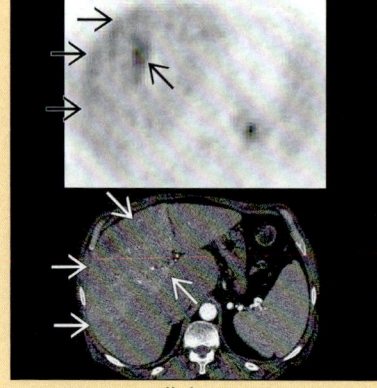

Hepatocellular Carcinoma

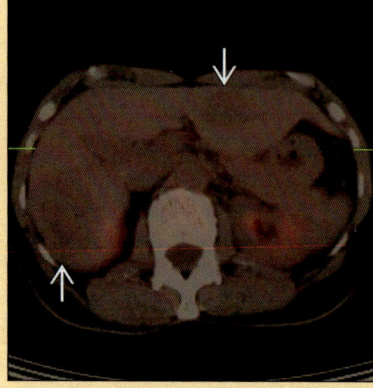

Cavernous Hemangiomas

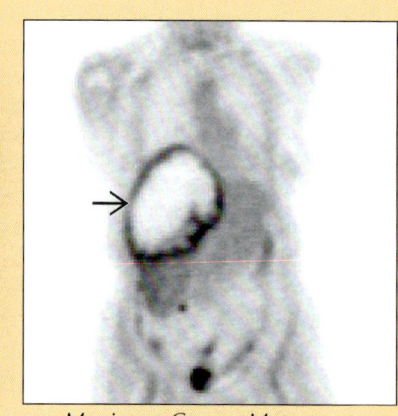

Mucinous Cancer Metastases

CHOLANGIOCARCINOMA

Key Facts

Terminology
- Cholangiocarcinoma (CC), Klatskin tumor, malignant bile duct tumor
- Malignancy that arises from ductular epithelium of intrahepatic biliary tree, extrahepatic bile ducts

Imaging Findings
- Peripheral CC: Intensely hypermetabolic activity, may be ring-shaped
- Hilar CC: Low activity with focal nodular or linear branching pattern
- PET sensitivity 61-90% for primary CC; 85% for nodular, 18% for infiltrating
- PET sensitivity for distant mets 65-70%, but for regional or hepatoduodenal mets only 13%

Top Differential Diagnoses
- Hepatocellular Carcinoma (HCC)
- Primary Sclerosing Cholangitis (PSC)
- Focal Nodular Hyperplasia (FNH)
- Cavernous Hemangioma
- Pancreatic Carcinoma

Diagnostic Checklist
- Ability of PET to detect distant metastases alters surgical management (reportedly up to 30% of cases)
- In general, FDG activity in primary tumor variable: Larger more peripheral lesions detected more often
- False positive on PET due to inflammation, e.g., intrahepatic stone, biliary stent
- False negative on PET with mucinous adenocarcinomas

- Lower FDG uptake may be related to tumor size or arrangement of fibrous stroma and mucin pool in tumor
  - PET sensitivity 61-90% for primary CC; 85% for nodular, 18% for infiltrating
  - PET sensitivity for distant mets 65-70%, but for regional or hepatoduodenal mets only 13%
  - False negatives with mucinous adenocarcinomas
  - False positive due to foci of inflammation, e.g., intrahepatic stone
  - Not reliable for early diagnosis of CC in patients with primary sclerosing cholangitis (PSC)
- Hepatobiliary Scintigraphy: Focal photopenic lesion
- Tc-99m Sulfur Colloid: Focal photopenic lesion
- Ga-67 Scintigraphy: Variable Ga-67 uptake

CT Findings
- NECT
  - Hilar masses often not visible on NECT
  - Mass predominately hypoattenuating with irregular margins
  - Larger peripheral lesions may show isodense lesion with central low attenuation, scarring
- CECT
  - On dynamic CT or MR, peripheral CC seen as intrahepatic mass showing early peripheral rim-enhancement
  - Delayed enhancement with increasing attenuation seen in up to 74% of lesions, usually ↑ CT sensitivity/specificity
  - Sensitivity reported as low as 50%, particularly for smaller hilar lesions
  - Solitary small well-demarcated tumors difficult to differentiate from primary hepatocellular carcinoma (HCC)

Imaging Recommendations
- Best imaging tool
  - PET for staging distant metastases; characterizing peripheral CC
  - CT: Similar to US for demonstrating ductal dilation, large mass lesions; staging regional/distant metastases
  - US first-line technique for evaluating primary tumor, may detect intrahepatic tumors in up to 87%
  - MRCP/ERCP: Sensitivity of 71-81% for malignancy in malignant stenoses

DIFFERENTIAL DIAGNOSIS

Hepatocellular Carcinoma (HCC)
- NECT typically shows an iso- or hypodense mass
- Shows early enhancement on CECT (vs. late enhancement in CC)
- Variable FDG uptake with ~ 50% having little/no FDG uptake due to ↑ glucose-6-phosphatase

Primary Sclerosing Cholangitis (PSC)
- Isolated dilation of intrahepatic bile ducts, known as skip dilations, strongly suggestive of PSC

Focal Nodular Hyperplasia (FNH)
- On NECT scans, FNH may appear as isoattenuating, slightly hypoattenuating mass
- After contrast administration, FNH becomes hyperattenuating relative to surrounding liver in arterial phase
- Larger lesions may have characteristic central scar

Cavernous Hemangioma
- On NECT, hemangiomas appear hypoattenuating relative to adjacent liver
- On arterial phase of CECT, small hemangiomas show intense, uniform enhancement, retain enhancement during portal venous phase
- On portal venous phase of CECT, characteristic peripheral nodular enhancement with continued centripetal filling in most larger lesions

Pancreatic Carcinoma
- Abrupt obstruction of pancreatic and/or distal common bile duct
- Look for dilated pancreatic duct distal to mass lesion

CHOLANGIOCARCINOMA

PATHOLOGY

General Features
- General path comments
  - Extent of duct involvement by perihilar tumors classified by Bismuth classification
  - > 95% are cancers of biliary tree and 90% of CC are adenocarcinomas
  - Hilar type
    - Develops from large bile ducts of hepatic hilum, symptomatic early due to central bile duct obstruction, jaundice
  - Peripheral type
    - Originates from interlobular bile ducts, tends to form mass, large size before becoming clinically apparent (no central biliary obstruction)
  - 60-70% of CC are Klatskin tumors
  - 20-30% arise in distal common bile duct
  - 5-10% are peripheral
  - Increased glucose transporter and hexokinase activity relative to surrounding tissue
- Etiology
  - Risk factors
    - PSC
    - Parasitic infection
    - Fibropolycystic liver disease
    - Intrahepatic biliary stones
    - Carcinogen exposure
    - Viral hepatitis
  - Known risk factors account for only a few cases of CC
  - Thorotrast (intravascular contrast agent used until 1950s) strongly associated; ↑ risk 300x many years after exposure
- Epidemiology
  - 2nd most common primary hepatic malignancy after HCC
  - Incidence of intrahepatic CC increasing worldwide, cause unclear
  - Incidence of extrahepatic CC declining
  - 10% prevalence of CC among PSC patients

CLINICAL ISSUES

Presentation
- Most common signs/symptoms
  - Obstructive jaundice (90%)
  - Abdominal pain (47%)
  - Palpable mass (18%)

Demographics
- Age: Peak incidence 7th decade
- Gender: Slight male predominance

Natural History & Prognosis
- Overall 5 year survival < 5%
- With aggressive surgical treatment, 5 year survival rate 22-32%, complication rates ≤ 36-59%, 60 day mortality 8-10%

Treatment
- Surgical resection = only curative treatment
- Intrahepatic and Klatskin tumors require liver resection
- Liver transplantation combined with chemoradiotherapy may improve survival
- Chemotherapy and radiotherapy generally ineffective for inoperable tumors
- Biliary drainage: Mainstay of palliation
- Photodynamic therapy: New palliative technique that may improve quality of life

DIAGNOSTIC CHECKLIST

Consider
- Ability of PET to detect distant metastases alters surgical management (reportedly up to 30% of cases)
- PET sensitivity for distant mets 65-70%,
- PET sensitivity for regional or hepatoduodenal mets ~ 13%

Image Interpretation Pearls
- In general, FDG activity in primary tumor variable: Larger more peripheral lesions detected more often
- In patients with biliary stents: 58% of cases have hypermetabolic activity along stent tract
- False positive on PET due to inflammation, e.g., intrahepatic stone, biliary stent
- False negative on PET with mucinous adenocarcinomas

SELECTED REFERENCES

1. Lee JD et al: Different glucose uptake and glycolytic mechanisms between hepatocellular carcinoma and intrahepatic mass-forming cholangiocarcinoma with increased (18)F-FDG uptake. J Nucl Med. 46(10):1753-9, 2005
2. Reinhardt MJ et al: Detection of Klatskin's tumor in extrahepatic bile duct strictures using delayed 18F-FDG PET/CT: preliminary results for 22 patient studies. J Nucl Med. 46(7):1158-63, 2005
3. Wakabayashi H et al: Significance of fluorodeoxyglucose PET imaging in the diagnosis of malignancies in patients with biliary stricture. Eur J Surg Oncol. 31(10):1175-9, 2005
4. Anderson CD et al: Fluorodeoxyglucose PET imaging in the evaluation of gallbladder carcinoma and cholangiocarcinoma. J Gastrointest Surg. 8(1):90-7, 2004
5. Kim YJ et al: Usefulness of 18F-FDG PET in intrahepatic cholangiocarcinoma. Eur J Nucl Med Mol Imaging. 30(11):1467-72, 2003
6. Fritscher-Ravens A et al: FDG PET in the diagnosis of hilar cholangiocarcinoma. Nucl Med Commun. 22(12):1277-85, 2001
7. Kluge R et al: Positron emission tomography with [(18)F]fluoro-2-deoxy-D-glucose for diagnosis and staging of bile duct cancer. Hepatology. 33(5):1029-35, 2001
8. Iwata Y et al: Clinical usefulness of positron emission tomography with fluorine-18-fluorodeoxyglucose in the diagnosis of liver tumors. Ann Nucl Med. 14(2):121-6, 2000
9. Keiding S et al: Dynamic 2-[18F]fluoro-2-deoxy-D-glucose positron emission tomography of liver tumours without blood sampling. Eur J Nucl Med. 27(4):407-12, 2000
10. Shiomi S et al: Combined hepatocellular carcinoma and cholangiocarcinoma with high F-18 fluorodeoxyglucose positron emission tomographic uptake. Clin Nucl Med. 24(5):370-1, 1999

CHOLANGIOCARCINOMA

IMAGE GALLERY

Typical

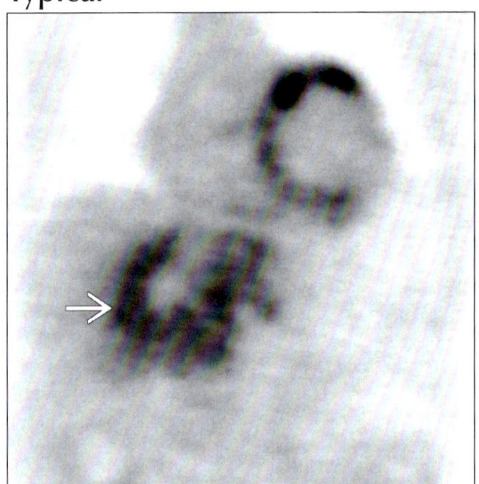

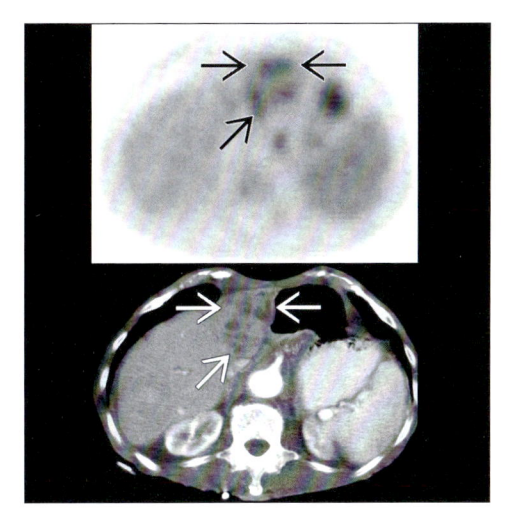

(Left) Coronal PET shows heterogeneous hypermetabolic activity in a large primarily left lobe hepatic lesion ➡ compatible with peripheral cholangiocarcinoma. *(Right)* Axial PET (top) and CECT (bottom) show dilated ➡, hypermetabolic ➡ left intrahepatic bile ducts in a patient with cholangiocarcinoma, consistent either with tumor extension or obstruction and infection.

Typical

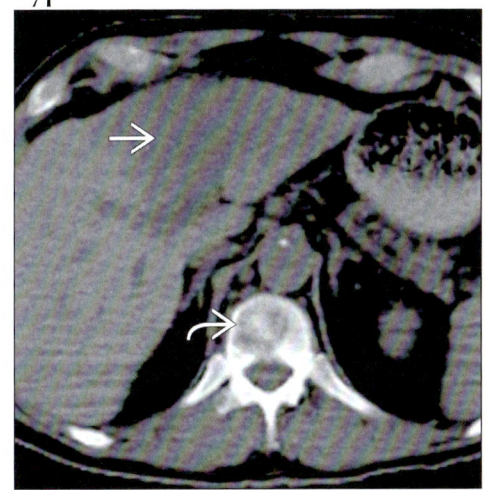

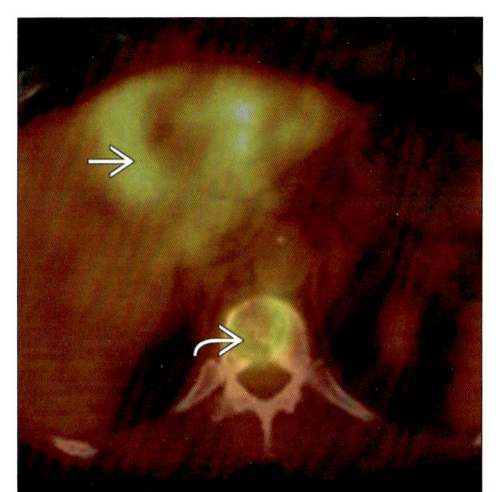

(Left) Axial NECT shows primary cholangiocarcinoma in left hepatic lobe ➡. Note lytic lesion in vertebral body ➡, representing metastatic disease. See next image. *(Right)* Axial fused PET/CT in same patient as previous image shows hypermetabolic activity in left hepatic lobe cholangiocarcinoma ➡ and vertebral body metastatic lesion ➡.

Other

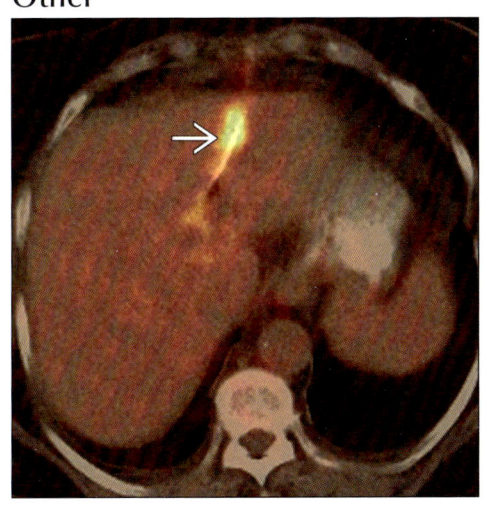

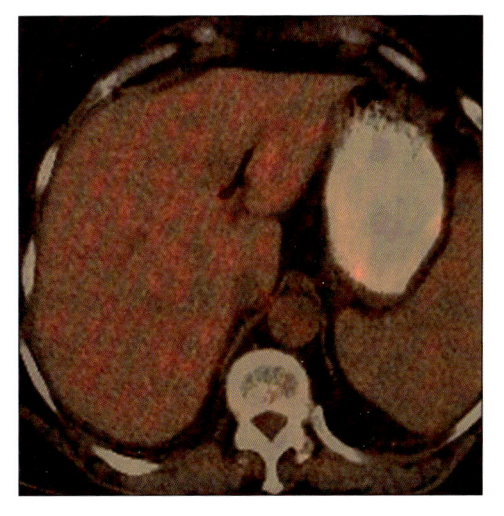

(Left) Axial fused PET/CT shows hypermetabolic surrounding a percutaneous catheter ➡, worrisome for tumor versus inflammation due to catheter placement. Same as next image. *(Right)* Axial fused PET/CT 5 weeks later in same patient as previous image shows complete resolution of hypermetabolic activity after catheter removal.

GALLBLADDER CANCER

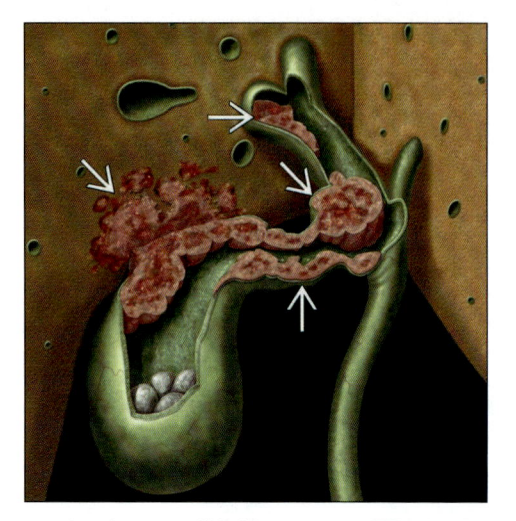

Graphic shows a gallbladder carcinoma ➡ infiltrating the liver along with bile duct in a patient with cholelithiasis.

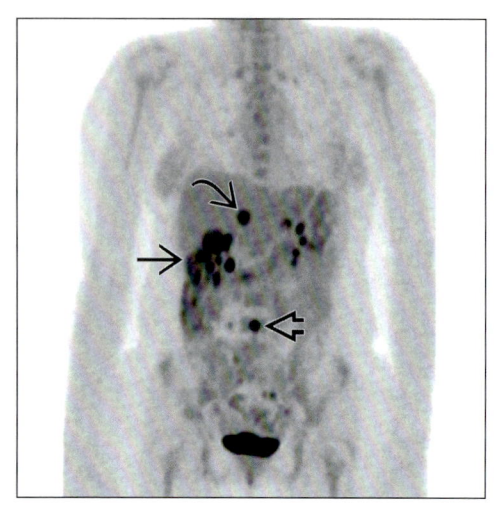

Coronal PET shows intense uptake in the gallbladder ➡ as well as in metastases in liver ➡ and a peritoneal lymph ➡ node from gallbladder carcinoma.

TERMINOLOGY

Definitions
- Epithelial malignancy arising from gallbladder (GB) mucosa

IMAGING FINDINGS

General Features
- Best diagnostic clue: GB mass with intense uptake often invading into liver
- Size
  - Rarely presents early as a generalized wall thickening or polypoid lesion
  - Usually presents as a large infiltrating mass due to delay in diagnosis

Nuclear Medicine Findings
- PET
  - Intense FDG uptake in the primary GB mass often directly extends into liver
  - Abnormal uptake along bile ducts with subserosal and regional lymph node invasion
  - PET often reveals disease in non-enlarged lymph nodes
  - Distant hematogenous metastasis and peritoneal seeding may occur
    - PET often identifies distant disease undetected on CT
    - Metastasis shows increased radiotracer uptake
  - Limited data on GB cancer, but data from other tumors suggests
    - PET identifies additional disease 15-35% of the time
    - Helps upstage patient or avoid unnecessary surgery in approximately 1/3
  - PET limitations in GB cancer diagnosis
    - False positives occur in any infectious and inflammatory processes
    - False negatives can occur in smaller lesions, especially less than 8-10 mm
    - Lower sensitivity for carcinomatosis; fusion to CT or PET CT improves this sensitivity
    - Highly mucinous tumors may be poorly FDG avid
  - PET appears most useful in identifying recurrent or metastatic disease

DDx: Gallbladder Carcinoma

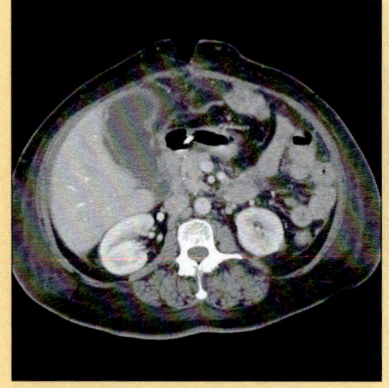

Chronic Cholecystitis 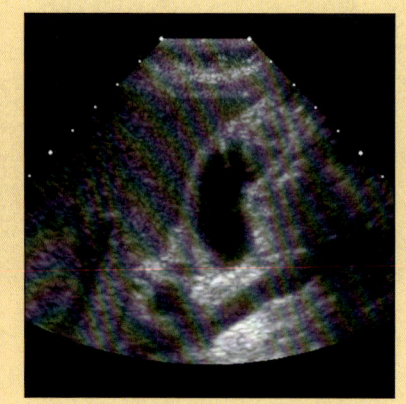 *Adenomyomatosis* 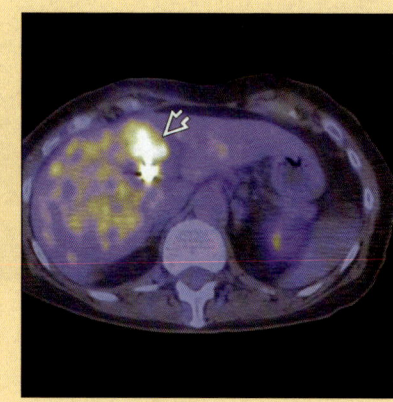 *Cholangiocarcinoma*

GALLBLADDER CANCER

Key Facts

Imaging Findings
- Usually presents as a large infiltrating mass due to delay in diagnosis
- Calcified gallstones in 65-75% of GB cancer patients
- Porcelain gallbladder frequently reported
- Intense FDG uptake in the primary GB mass often directly extends into liver
- Abnormal uptake along bile ducts with subserosal and regional lymph node invasion
- Distant hematogenous metastasis and peritoneal seeding may occur
- PET often identifies distant disease undetected on CT
- False positives occur in any infectious and inflammatory processes
- False negatives can occur in smaller lesions, especially less than 8-10 mm
- PET appears most useful in identifying recurrent or metastatic disease

Top Differential Diagnoses
- Chronic cholecystitis
- Cholangiocarcinoma
- Metastases
- Gallbladder Polyp
- Adenomyomatosis

Clinical Issues
- Very poor prognosis: 75% present at diagnosis with advanced disease and a 5 y survival rate of 4-12%
- Surgical resection is only curative therapy, but effectiveness limited as most patients present with advanced disease

CT Findings
- NECT
  - Calcified gallstones in 65-75% of GB cancer patients
    - < 1% of patents with gallstones develop GB cancer
  - Porcelain gallbladder frequently reported
    - Association may not be as strong as once believed
  - Thickened GB wall or mass
- CECT
  - Limited ability to differentiate early tumor from benign lesions
  - Because early diagnosis is rare, most patients present with obvious mass
    - Poorly enhancing GB mass often extends directly into liver
    - Hazy density around common bile duct from direct spread or periportal adenopathy
  - Advanced disease: Intraperitoneal metastasis and carcinomatosis
    - If whole body not scanned, may miss recurrent disease or late stage distant lung and bone metastasis
  - Tumor stage is often underestimated, including disease in non-enlarged regional and distant lymph nodes, small liver lesions and peritoneal seeding

MR Findings
- T1WI
  - Isointense or hypointense GB mass
  - Higher signal than liver background
- T2WI: Slightly increased signal to liver
- T1 C+
  - Rapidly enhancing GB mass often retains contrast
    - Must be differentiated from benign inflammatory polyps or thickening
  - Liver invasion may be more obvious with enhancement
- MRCP
  - Biliary dilation late, when common duct becomes obstructed
  - May provide some useful facts to help with staging

Ultrasonographic Findings
- Grayscale Ultrasound
  - Excellent screening tool often used as patients present with symptoms of biliary colic
  - Demonstrates infiltrative mass filling GB most commonly
  - Polypoid mass second most common finding
  - Differentiating malignancy from benign etiologies often not possible in early stages
  - Calcifications may obscure tumors
  - Not as useful for staging or detecting distant disease
  - Limited use in detecting recurrent disease

Imaging Recommendations
- Best imaging tool: CECT or PET CT
- Protocol advice
  - PET CT
    - To evaluate surgical candidates
    - To evaluate for recurrence or therapy response
    - Probably limited in early cancer detection
  - CECT suspicious GB lesions or known GB malignancy
  - F-18 FDG PET patient preparation
    - Fast at least 6 hours
    - Always check serum glucose: Delay scan if not normal or not < 200 in diabetics
    - No insulin within 2 hours of injection or muscle uptake will occur
    - Keep patients warm before injection and avoid strenuous exercise 24 hours prior to scan
  - Dose: 370-555 MB (10-15 mCi) F-18 FDG IV, allow 1 hour before scanning
  - Scan patient arms overhead for less artifact in liver and periportal region
  - Perform routine CT or transmission scan for attenuation correction followed by emission scan
  - Fusion to CT or PET CT preferred
  - Delay scan 4-6 weeks postoperatively to avoid false positives for recurrence
- Additional nuclear medicine imaging findings
  - Hepatobiliary (HIDA) scan shows no gallbladder filling

GALLBLADDER CANCER

DIFFERENTIAL DIAGNOSIS

Cholecystitis
- Chronic cholecystitis
  - Often confused with GB carcinoma clinically and on CECT or ultrasound
  - GB wall thickening, cholelithiasis, porcelain GB may also be seen in GB cancer
- Acute cholecystitis
  - Shows intense FDG uptake but is differentiated clinically
- Xanthomatous cholangitis
  - Benign inflammatory process
  - Confused with GB cancer by many imaging modalities
  - A few case reports of FDG uptake

Cholangiocarcinoma
- Pattern of spread may be similar to GB cancer but usually less localized

Metastases
- To gallbladder, periportal lymph nodes or liver

Gallbladder Polyp
- Benign polyps in 4-6% of the general population; most show no radiotracer uptake

Adenomyomatosis
- Look for Rokitansky-Aschoff sinuses; usually no radiotracer uptake PET

PATHOLOGY

General Features
- Associated abnormalities: Cholelithiasis, porcelain gallbladder

Microscopic Features
- Cellular classifications include: Adenocarcinoma (intestinal type, papillary, mucinous, clear cell), signet ring cell, adenosquamous, squamous cell, small cell, undifferentiated, carcinoma sarcoma, and carcinoma NOS
- F-18 FDG PET may show less uptake in mucinous tumors causing false negatives

Staging, Grading or Classification Criteria
- Stage I: Tumor limited to gallbladder
  - IA: T1 N0 M0 invades GB lamina propria
  - IB: T2 N0 M0 invades perimuscular connective tissue layer
- Stage II: Tumor invades serosa or has spread to regional lymph nodes
  - IIA: T3 N0 M0 tumor invades serosa/visceral peritoneum
  - IIB: T1-3 N1 M0
- Stage III: Involves main portal vein or hepatic artery, directly invades liver and/or adjacent organ: T4 N0-1 M0
- Stage IV: Tumor invades multiple organs, and/or distant metastases (any T, any N, M1)

CLINICAL ISSUES

Presentation
- Most common signs/symptoms: Biliary colic: RUQ pain, vomiting, weight loss, jaundice
- Other signs/symptoms: Elevated bilirubin and alkaline phosphatase when biliary obstruction present

Demographics
- Age: Peak incidence 6th and 7th decades
- Gender: M:F = 1:3 to 1:4

Natural History & Prognosis
- Very poor prognosis: 75% present at diagnosis with advanced disease and a 5 y survival rate of 4-12%
- Resected localized stage I disease 5 year survival approaches 100%

Treatment
- Surgical resection is only curative therapy, but effectiveness limited as most patients present with advanced disease
  - Cholecystectomy for lesions confined to gallbladder
    - GB cancer often found unexpectedly in postoperative specimens performed for supposed cholecystitis
  - Radical cholecystectomy with partial hepatectomy and regional lymph node dissection for more advanced disease
  - Only patients with disease beyond gastrohepatic ligament are not candidates for surgery (stage IVB)
- Radiation therapy and chemotherapy show very limited benefit
- Needle biopsy contraindicated as tumor seeding frequently occurs along needle tract

DIAGNOSTIC CHECKLIST

Image Interpretation Pearls
- Look for infiltration along biliary ducts, direct extension into liver, and portal node involvement
- Pitfall: Misregistered normal bowel activity onto liver or GB can be misleading without CT correlation for presence of mass lesions

SELECTED REFERENCES

1. Chander S et al: PET imaging of gallbladder carcinoma. Clin Nucl Med. 30(12):804-5, 2005
2. Wakabayashi H et al: Significance of fluorodeoxyglucose PET imaging in the diagnosis of malignancies in patients with biliary stricture. Eur J Surg Oncol. 31(10):1175-9, 2005
3. Anderson CD et al: Fluorodeoxyglucose PET imaging in the evaluation of gallbladder carcinoma and cholangiocarcinoma. J Gastrointest Surg. 8(1):90-7, 2004
4. Grand D et al: CT of the gallbladder: spectrum of disease. AJR Am J Roentgenol. 183(1):163-70, 2004
5. Rodriguez-Fernandez A et al: Positron-emission tomography with fluorine-18-fluoro-2-deoxy-D-glucose for gallbladder cancer diagnosis. Am J Surg. 188(2):171-5, 2004
6. Koh T et al: Differential diagnosis of gallbladder cancer using positron emission tomography with fluorine-18-labeled fluoro-deoxyglucose (FDG-PET). J Surg Oncol. 84(2):74-81, 2003

GALLBLADDER CANCER

IMAGE GALLERY

Typical

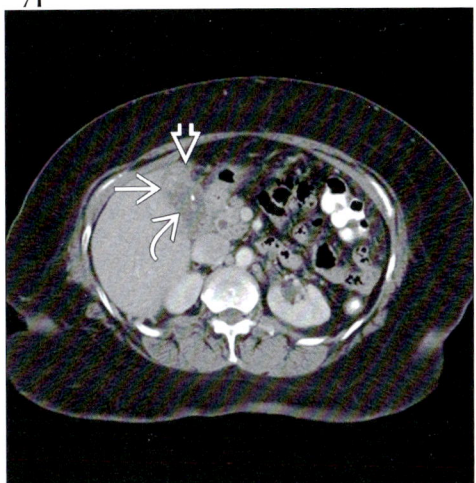

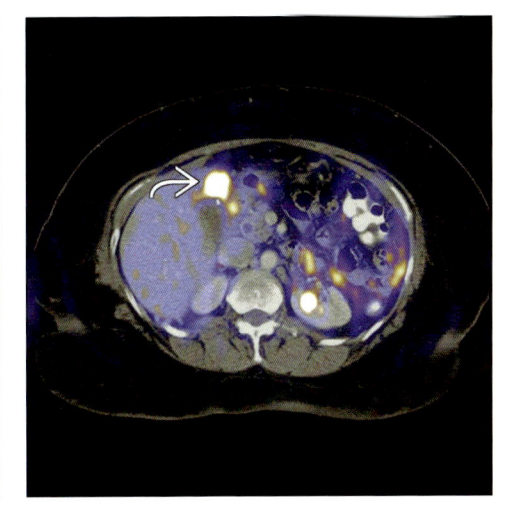

(Left) Axial CECT shows calcifications ⇨ and pericholecystic fluid ⇨ around a gallbladder mass proven to be polypoid gallbladder carcinoma ⇨.
(Right) Axial fused PET/CT at the same level as the previous CECT shows intense uptake in the mass ⇨, a polypoid gallbladder cancer.

Other

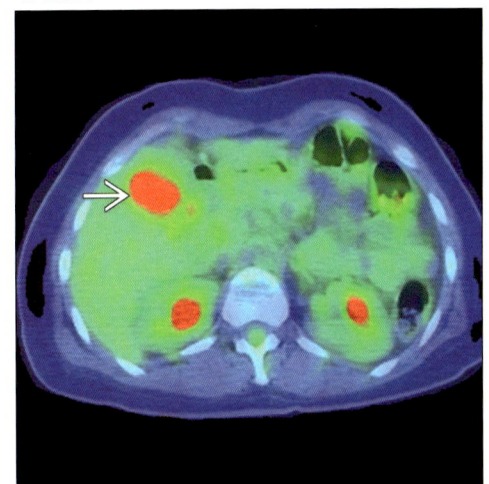

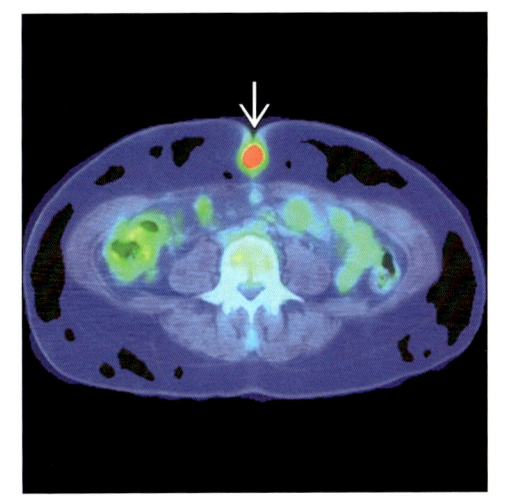

(Left) Axial fused PET/CT shows intense uptake in the infiltrating gallbladder carcinoma which fills the lumen of the gallbladder ⇨.
(Right) Axial fused PET/CT shows intense uptake beneath the umbilicus ⇨ probably caused by tumor seeding during laparoscopic biopsy of a gallbladder cancer.

Typical

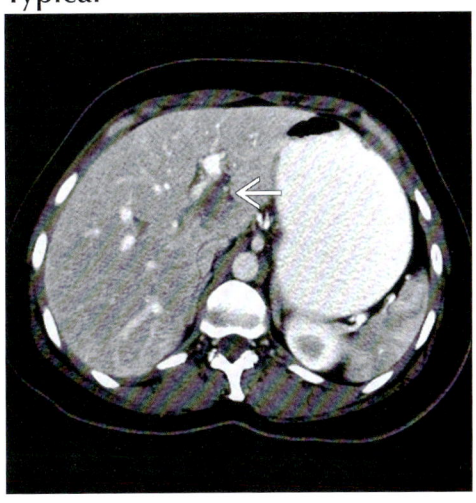

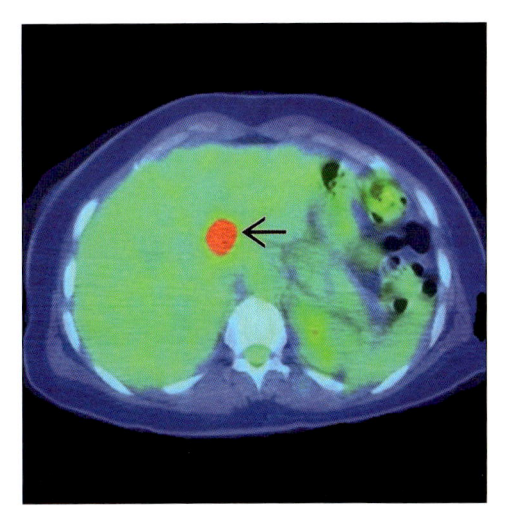

(Left) Axial CECT shows a hazy density and fullness around the biliary ducts ⇨ from spread of gallbladder cancer. See next image.
(Right) Axial fused PET/CT at the same level as the previous CECT shows intense uptake from the tumor ⇨.

FOCAL NODULAR HYPERPLASIA

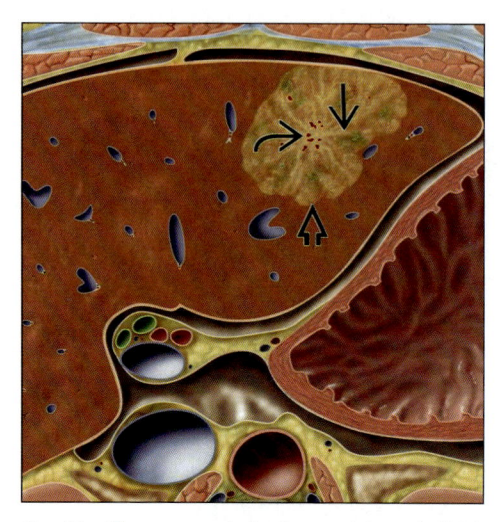

Graphic illustrates typical characteristics of FNH: Central vascularity ➔, radiating fibrous septae ➔, well-defined margins ➔ and absence of capsule.

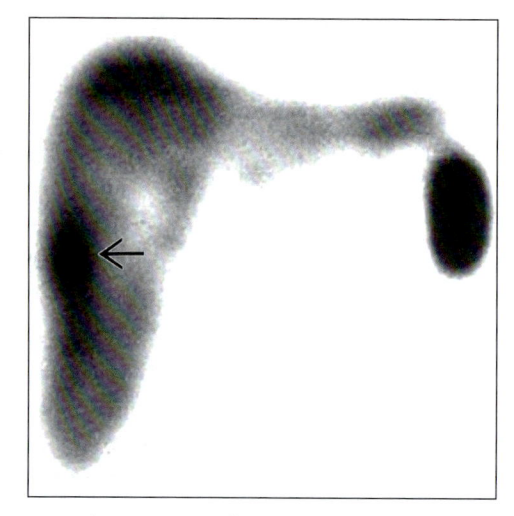

Coronal Tc-99m sulfur colloid SPECT shows subcapsular tracer accumulation in lateral portion of right hepatic lobe ➔.

TERMINOLOGY

Abbreviations and Synonyms
- Focal nodular hyperplasia (FNH)

Definitions
- Benign neoplastic or tumor-like hamartomatous malformation of the liver
  - Most common solid hepatic tumor

IMAGING FINDINGS

General Features
- Best diagnostic clue
  - Typical FNH: Fibrous central scar with radiating septae
    - Prominent arterial phase hyperattenuation with contrast forming a spoke-and-wheel pattern
    - Homogeneous: 90%; arterial hyperattenuation: 90%; central scar: 50%
    - Reports of central scar in fibrolamellar hepatocellular carcinoma (HCC), hepatic adenoma, intrahepatic cholangiocarcinoma
    - Occasionally pedunculated
- Location
  - Hepatic parenchyma
    - Right lobe > left (2:1)
- Size
  - Usually 2-5 cm
  - Occasionally > 10 cm
- Morphology
  - Well-defined proliferative mass of hepatocytes, biliary canaliculi, fibrous septae
    - 20% multiple
  - Telangiectatic FNH (atypical)
    - Inhomogeneous
    - Central scar absent
    - Uncharacteristically large

Nuclear Medicine Findings
- Problem solving modality if CECT, C+ MR nondiagnostic
- Tc-99m sulfur colloid (SC) scintigraphy
  - Traditional scintigraphic agent for FNH
  - DOSE: 4-6 mCi (148-220 MBq) Tc-99m SC
  - Presence of functioning Kupffer cells allows Tc-99m SC accumulation

DDx: Mimics of Focal Nodular Hyperplasia on Tc-99m Sulfur Colloid Scan

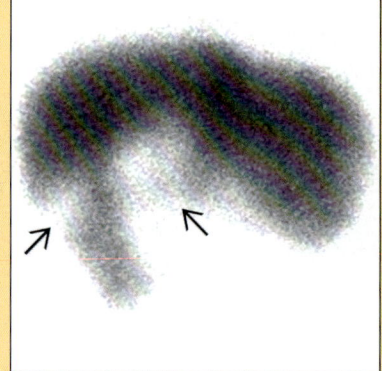

Metastases (Cold) 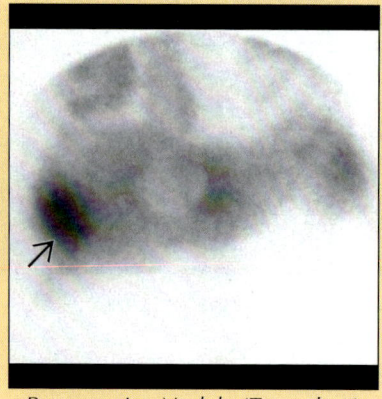 | *Regenerating Nodule (Transplant)* 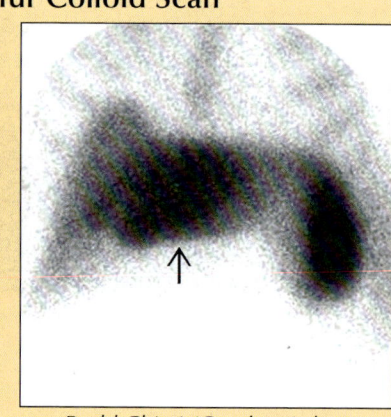 | *Budd-Chiari (Caudate Lobe)*

FOCAL NODULAR HYPERPLASIA

Key Facts

Imaging Findings
- Typical FNH: Fibrous central scar with radiating septae
- Right lobe > left (2:1)
- Usually 2-5 cm
- Tc-99m IDA scintigraphy
- Prompt tracer extraction 2° to ↑ vascularity
- Delayed clearance: Disorganized biliary canaliculi ⇒ poor tracer transit
- CECT, MR C+: Brightly enhancing on early arterial phase, delayed enhancement of central scar

Top Differential Diagnoses
- Hepatic Adenoma
- Hepatocellular Carcinoma (HCC) or Metastatic Disease
- Regenerative Nodules
- Hemangioma
- Superior Vena Cava Syndrome
- Budd Chiari Syndrome, Hepatic Venous Occlusive Disease

Diagnostic Checklist
- Practical limits of resolution are 1-2 cm for SPECT, 2-3 cm for planar scintigraphy
- Tc-99m HIDA: Early visualization with persistent tracer/delayed washout
- Functional hepatocytes extract tracer promptly; disorganized canaliculi prevent rapid excretion
- HCC: Initially cold to ≥ 1 hr, delayed fill-in can be seen (bile lakes)
- Tc-99m SC: Lesions with iso- or hyper-accumulation do not require biopsy

---

  - Approximately 2/3 of cases show iso or increased uptake relative to liver, 1/3 low uptake
- Tc-99m IDA scintigraphy
  - Typical findings (~ 90% FNH lesions)
    - Prompt tracer extraction 2° to ↑ vascularity
    - Delayed clearance: Disorganized biliary canaliculi ⇒ poor tracer transit
    - HCC can occasionally show delayed filling-in IDA

Imaging Recommendations
- Best imaging tool
  - CECT, MR C+: Brightly enhancing on early arterial phase, delayed enhancement of central scar
  - CECT
    - Early arterial homogeneous enhancement with hypoattenuating central scar
    - Central scar in 65% of FNH, easier to see in larger lesions
    - Delayed hyperattenuation of central scar: 80%
    - Well marginated, not encapsulated
  - MR
    - T1 and T2 hypointense
    - Central scar may be T2 hyperintense
    - Dynamic imaging is useful
    - Superparamagnetic iron oxide, sequestered by reticuloendothelial cells, contrast-enhancement increases specificity
  - US
    - Lesions often first detected incidentally at RUQ evaluation
    - Duplex Doppler should be applied
- Protocol advice
  - Standard Tc-99m HIDA scintigraphy protocol
    - Dose: 5-8 mCi (185-296 MBq) of Tc-99m IDA
    - Angiographic phase, dynamic, delayed anterior planar images
    - SPECT necessary in many, if not most cases
    - May be more accurate than Tc-99m sulfur colloid (SC)
- Additional nuclear medicine imaging options
  - PET not currently contributory
    - C11-acetate PET can be used to distinguish HCC from benign lesions but may show mild to moderate uptake in FNH

DIFFERENTIAL DIAGNOSIS

Hepatic Adenoma
- No central scar
- Associated with oral contraceptive use
- Frequently larger than FNH
  - Average 8-10 cm diameter
- Typically photopenic on Tc-99m HIDA (despite presence of hepatocytes)
- Photopenic on Tc-99m sulfur colloid
  - Kupffer cells, present in normal or ↓ quantities, but do not effectively accumulate Tc-99m SC
- More inclined to hemorrhage, therefore may present for potential resection

Hepatocellular Carcinoma (HCC) or Metastatic Disease
- Absent activity on HIDA and absent or ↓ accumulation of Tc-99m SC
- Larger the lesion, more likely HCC (not FNH)
- Fibrolamellar HCC in particular may have overlapping imaging features
  - Irregular or central scars, radiating septae
  - Associated with secondary signs of malignancy: Multiple lesions, adenopathy, local invasion, calcifications, metastases

Regenerative Nodules
- Cirrhotic patients
  - May include multiple regenerative nodules, macroregenerative nodules, or degenerative nodules

Hemangioma
- Peripheral nodular enhancement on CECT with characteristic progressive centripetal filling
- Delayed but persistent tracer accumulation on Tc-99m RBC scintigraphy

FOCAL NODULAR HYPERPLASIA

Superior Vena Cava Syndrome
- Tracer accumulation typically seen in left lobe 2° to collateralization

Budd Chiari Syndrome, Hepatic Venous Occlusive Disease
- Tc-99m SC accumulation usually most prominent in caudate 2° to direct drainage into inferior vena cava

PATHOLOGY

General Features
- Etiology
  - Hypothesized to be hyperplastic response to pre-existing abnormal vascularity
  - Associated with underlying vascular malformations
    - Hemangiomas, telangiectasias, arterial venous abnormalities
  - Not caused by oral contraceptives although hormonal stimulation may ⇒ growth
    - Hormonal and oral contraceptive cessation occasionally linked to ↓ size
- Epidemiology: Just less than 1% of normal population by large autopsy series
- Associated abnormalities
  - May be associated with benign intrahepatic vascular neoplasm in 20-25% of patients
  - Multiple lesions: ↑ Incidence of vascular malformations of other organs; meningiomas, astrocytomas

Gross Pathologic & Surgical Features
- Unencapsulated mass or nodule containing central scar, fibrovascular septations
- Arterial blood supply

Microscopic Features
- Normal hepatocytes, primitive bile ducts (variable), nodules of Kupffer cells invested by central stellate fibrous septae; associated with anomalous artery

CLINICAL ISSUES

Presentation
- Most common signs/symptoms: Usually asymptomatic, incidental finding
- Other signs/symptoms
  - Occasional hepatomegaly, abdominal mass
  - Complications unusual
    - Hemorrhage, infarction

Demographics
- Age
  - Usually 3rd or 4th decades
  - Rarely infantile or childhood
- Gender: M < F (1:4)

Natural History & Prognosis
- Usually benign course
- May cause pain secondary to mass effect
- Rarely hemorrhage (2-3%); hemoperitoneum
- No statistically significant increased risk of malignant transformation

Treatment
- Conservative management
- Suspension of hormonal stimulation (oral contraceptives)
- Surgical resection rare in clinically warranted cases

DIAGNOSTIC CHECKLIST

Consider
- Combining imaging modalities (CECT, US, MR, scintigraphy) often facilitates diagnosis
- FNA often nondiagnostic
  - Confident diagnostic imaging averts biopsy, resection and further unnecessary imaging

Image Interpretation Pearls
- Practical limits of resolution are 1-2 cm for SPECT, 2-3 cm for planar scintigraphy
- Tc-99m HIDA: Early visualization with persistent tracer/delayed washout
  - Functional hepatocytes extract tracer promptly; disorganized canaliculi prevent rapid excretion
  - HCC: Initially cold to ≥ 1 hr, delayed fill-in can be seen (bile lakes)
- Tc-99m SC: Lesions with iso- or hyper-accumulation do not require biopsy
  - 1/3: ↑ Tracer accumulation
  - 1/3: Isointense tracer accumulation
  - 1/3: Absent or ↓ tracer accumulation
    - Additional analysis required: HIDA, biopsy or other characterization

SELECTED REFERENCES

1. Zeissman HA et al: Nuclear Medicine-The Requisites in Radiology. 3rd Ed. 187-9, 2006
2. Huynh LT et al: The typical appearance of focal nodular hyperplasia in triple-phase CT scan, hepatobiliary scan, and Tc-99m sulfur colloid scan with SPECT. Clin Nucl Med. 30(11):736-9, 2005
3. Wanless I: The pathogenesis of focal nodular hyperplasia of the liver. Journal of Gastroenterology and Hepatology. 19, S342-3, 2004
4. Attal P et al: Telangiectatic focal nodular hyperplasia: US, CT, and MR imaging findings with histopathologic correlation in 13 cases. Radiology. 228(2):465-72, 2003
5. Brancatelli G et al: Focal nodular hyperplasia: CT findings with emphasis on multiphasic helical CT in 78 patients. Radiology. 219(1):61-8, 2001
6. Huang YE et al: A central scar in hepatic focal nodular hyperplasia detected on liver SPECT imaging. Clin Nucl Med. 26(4):367-9, 2001
7. Leconte I et al: Focal nodular hyperplasia: natural course observed with CT and MRI. J Comput Assist Tomogr. 24(1):61-6, 2000
8. Nguyen BN et al: Focal nodular hyperplasia of the liver: a comprehensive pathologic study of 305 lesions and recognition of new histologic forms. Am J Surg Pathol. 23(12):1441-54, 1999
9. Datz FL: Gamuts in Nuclear Medicine. 3rd ed. St. Louis, Mosby. 258, 1995

FOCAL NODULAR HYPERPLASIA

IMAGE GALLERY

Typical

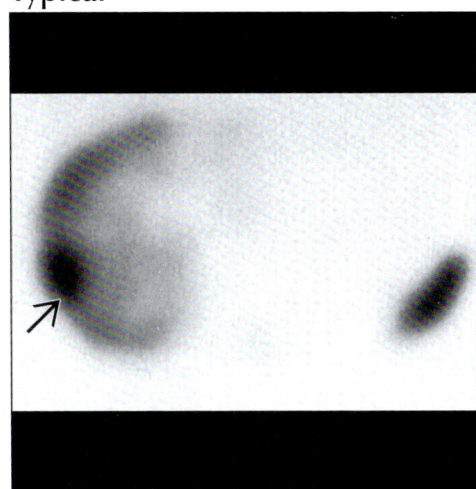

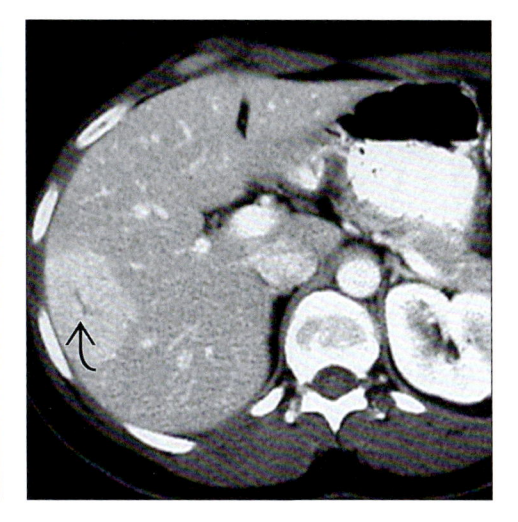

(Left) Axial Tc-99m sulfur colloid SPECT image of FNH shows focal subcapsular accumulation in periphery of right hepatic lobe ➡. Same as next image. *(Right)* Axial CECT of same patient as previous image shows FNH with early arterial phase enhancement and central hypoattenuating scar ➡.

Variant

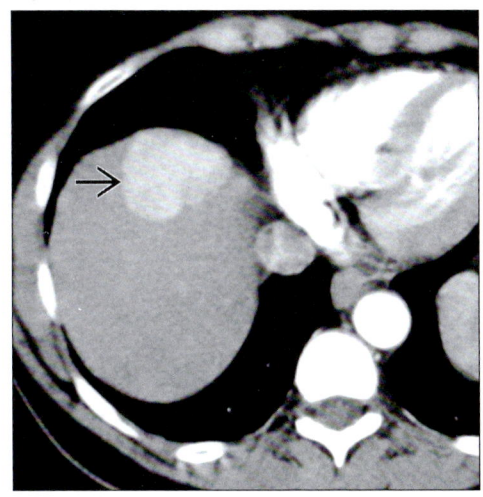

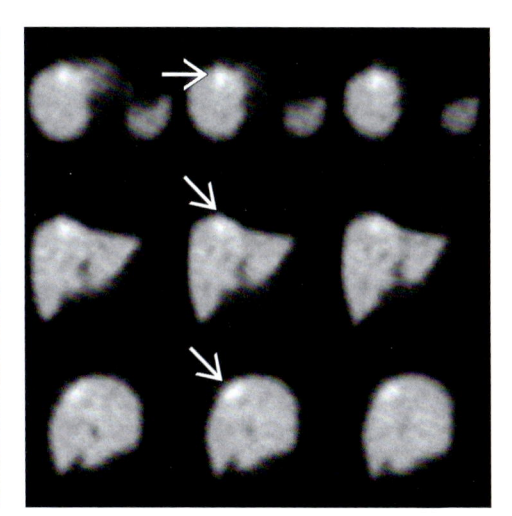

(Left) Axial CECT during arterial phase shows subcapsular enhancing hepatic mass without central scar ➡. Same as next image. *(Right)* Tc-99m sulfur colloid triplanar imaging of same patient as previous image shows tracer accumulation corresponding to CECT, indicating benign FNH ➡.

Typical

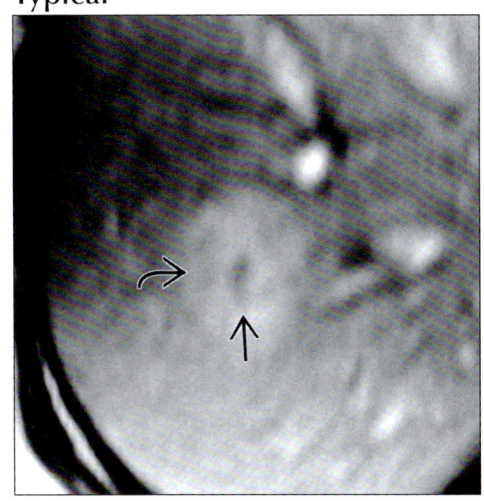

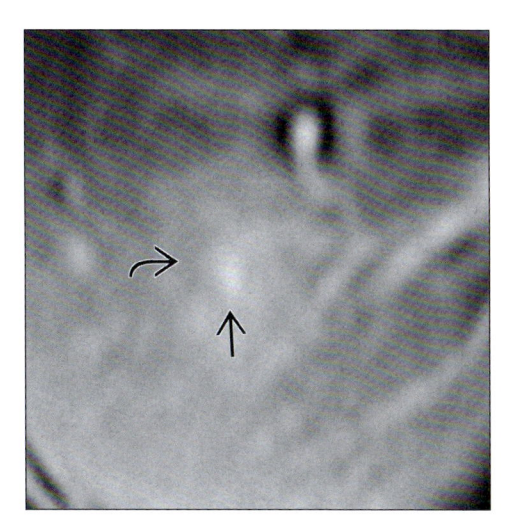

(Left) Axial T1 MR with contrast shows well circumscribed, unencapsulated lesion ➡ with central low signal ➡, suggesting FNH. *(Right)* Axial T2 MR of same patient as previous image shows mildly hyperintense, unencapsulated lesion ➡ with hyperintense central scar ➡, the typical appearance of FNH.

HEPATIC CIRRHOSIS

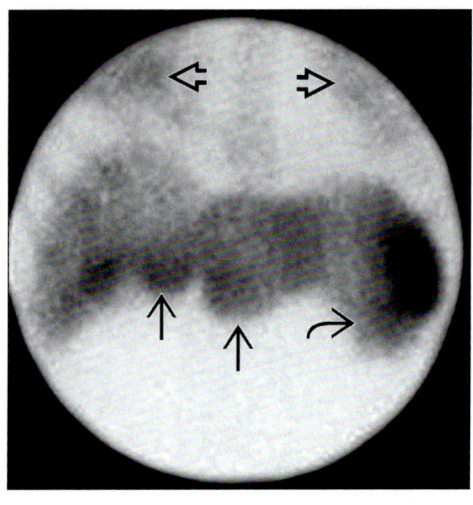

Typical signs of cirrhosis on sulfur colloid scan: ↓ Size Rt & medial Lt lobe liver, ↑ caudate, lateral Lt lobe liver ⇨ & spleen ⇨ ("Batman" sign), uptake in bone, lungs ⇨, photopenic defect from ascites.

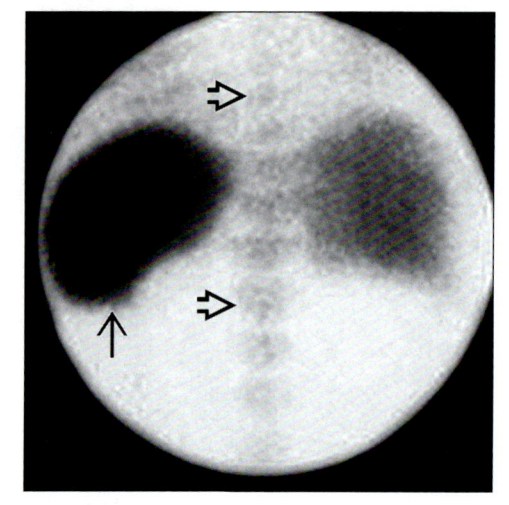

Posterior Tc-99m sulfur colloid scan shows increased uptake in spleen ⇨, relative to liver, and in bone marrow ⇨, signs of "colloid shift" typical of cirrhosis.

TERMINOLOGY

Definitions
- Chronic liver disease with diffuse parenchymal necrosis, fibrosis, regenerative nodules

IMAGING FINDINGS

General Features
- Best diagnostic clue: Nodular contour, wide fissures, hyperdense nodules (NECT) that disappear on CECT
- Location: Diffuse liver involving both lobes
- Size: Liver usually reduced in size
- Key concepts
  ○ Common end response of liver to a variety of insults and injuries
  ○ Classification of cirrhosis: Morphology, histopathology & etiology
    ▪ Micronodular (Laennec) cirrhosis: Alcoholism (60-70% cases in US)
    ▪ Macronodular (postnecrotic) cirrhosis: Viral hepatitis (10% in US; majority of cases worldwide)
    ▪ Mixed cirrhosis
  ○ 1 of 10 leading causes of death in Western world, 6th in US

Nuclear Medicine Findings
- Liver spleen scan: Tc-99m sulfur colloid (SC)
  ○ Liver spleen scan: Overall small liver, relative enlargement, increased uptake of left lobe, caudate & spleen ("Batman sign")
  ○ Spleen "hotter" than liver on posterior SC image: Sensitive but nonspecific
  ○ Uptake at normal intensities in red marrow: Colloid shift
  ○ Uptake of colloid in lungs: Unknown cause, possibly estrogen effect
  ○ Photopenic region between liver and lung or rib cage: Ascites
- VQ scan: Tc-99m MAA
  ○ Hepatopulmonary syndrome: Numerous arteriovenous connections result in effective R → L shunting on VQ scan
  ○ Uptake of Tc-99m MAA in brain, kidneys
- Hepatobiliary (HB) scan: Tc-99m Choletec
  ○ Normal HB scan: Visualization of gut by 1 h, gallbladder < 1 h

DDx: Mimics of Cirrhosis on Tc-99m Sulfur Colloid Scan

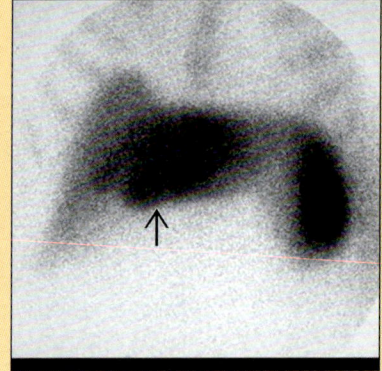

Budd-Chiari (Caudate Lobe) 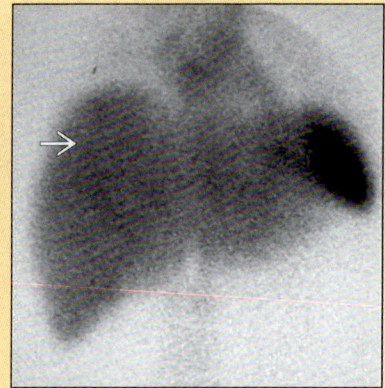   *Viral Hepatitis* 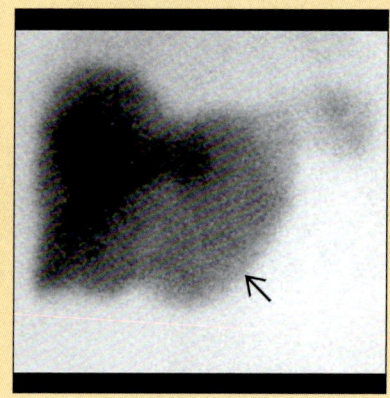   *Fatty Liver*

HEPATIC CIRRHOSIS

Key Facts

Terminology
- Chronic liver disease with diffuse parenchymal necrosis, fibrosis, regenerative nodules

Imaging Findings
- Liver spleen scan: Overall small liver, relative enlargement, increased uptake of left lobe, caudate & spleen ("Batman sign")
- Spleen "hotter" than liver on posterior SC image: Sensitive but nonspecific
- Uptake at normal intensities in red marrow: Colloid shift
- Uptake of colloid in lungs: Unknown cause, possibly estrogen effect
- Hepatopulmonary syndrome: Numerous arteriovenous connections result in effective R → L shunting on VQ scan
- Hepatobiliary scan in cirrhosis: Delayed time line for visualization of gut and gallbladder, often up to 24 h
- Tagged RBC Identification of active bleeding from coagulopathy and/or varices: Esophageal, gastric, rectal
- Spontaneous bacterial peritonitis: Increased labeled WBC uptake in ascites
- Occasional splenic uptake on bone scan in cirrhosis: Possibly due to microinfarcts of spleen or splenic siderosis

Top Differential Diagnoses
- Budd-Chiari Syndrome
- Treated Metastatic Disease
- Hepatic Sarcoidosis
- Hepatitis

- ○ Hepatobiliary scan in cirrhosis: Delayed time line for visualization of gut and gallbladder, often up to 24 h
- Tagged red cell scan: Tc-99m pertechnetate-labeled autologous red cells
  - ○ Tagged RBC Identification of active bleeding from coagulopathy and/or varices: Esophageal, gastric, rectal
- Gallium scan: Ga-67 citrate
  - ○ Increased uptake on Ga-67 in 80% of cases of hepatoma: Likely more often positive than with FDG PET
- WBC scan: In-111 oxine preferred over Tc-99m HMPAO for labeling
  - ○ Spontaneous bacterial peritonitis: Increased labeled WBC uptake in ascites
- Bone scan: Tc-99m diphosphonate (e.g., MDP)
  - ○ Occasional splenic uptake on bone scan in cirrhosis: Possibly due to microinfarcts of spleen or splenic siderosis
- Diaphragmatic patency evaluation: Tc-99m MAA
  - ○ Peritoneal → pleural flow with diaphragmatic rent

CT Findings
- Nodular liver contour, atrophy of right lobe & medial segment of left lobe
- Enlarged caudate lobe & lateral segment of left lobe
- Widened fissures between segments/lobes
- Regenerative nodules; fibrotic & fatty changes
- Varices, ascites, splenomegaly & peribiliary cysts
- Siderotic regenerative nodules: ↑ Attenuation on NECT; isoenhancement on CECT
- Dysplastic regenerative nodules
  - ○ NECT: Large nodules hyperdense (↑ iron + ↑ glycogen); small nodules isodense (undetected)
  - ○ CECT: Usually enhance as normal liver, sometimes hypervascular
- Fibrotic & fatty changes
  - ○ NECT: Fibrosis with diffuse lacework, thick bands, mottled areas of ↓ density; fatty changes with mottled areas of ↓ attenuation
  - ○ CECT: Fibrosis less evident due to isoenhancement; confluent fibrosis with delayed enhancement; fatty changes with low attenuation
- Cirrhosis-induced hepatocellular carcinoma (HCC)
  - ○ NECT: Hypodense or heterogeneous; ± fat
  - ○ CECT: Intense or heterogeneous enhancement arterial; iso- to hypodense venous/delayed, ± capsule enhancement

MR Findings
- Paramagnetic effect of iron within siderotic regenerative nodules: T1WI hypointense; T2WI increased conspicuity of ↓ signal
- Gamna-Gandy bodies (hemorrhagic siderotic splenic nodules): T1, T2WI, T2 GRE & FLASH images hypointense
- Dysplastic regenerative nodules: T1WI hyperintense; T2WI hypointense
- HCC nodule: T1WI isointense or hypointense; T1 C+ enhancement; T2WI hyperintense
- Fibrotic & fatty changes: T1WI: Fibrosis hypointense, fat hyperintense; T2WI: Fibrosis hyperintense, fat hypointense
- MR angiography: Varices, collateral channels (transhepatic, gastroesophageal, paraesophageal, paraumbilical, intrahepatic, splenorenal)

Ultrasonographic Findings
- Grayscale Ultrasound
  - ○ Increased liver echogenicity/loss of normal triphasic hepatic vein Doppler tracing/increased pulsatility of portal vein Doppler tracing and same as CT findings
  - ○ Nodular liver contour; increased liver echogenicity; enlarged caudate lobe & lateral segment of left lobe; atrophy of right lobe & medial segment of left lobe; regenerating nodules
  - ○ Portal hypertension (PHT): Portal vein (> 13 mm), splenic vein (> 11 mm); superior mesenteric vein (> 12 mm); coronary veins (> 7 mm)
  - ○ PHT: Increased pulsatility of portal vein Doppler tracing; dilated hepatic & splenic arteries with increased flow; portal cavernoma, ascites, splenomegaly & varices, siderotic nodules
- Color Doppler
  - ○ To determine portal vein patency, flow direction

HEPATIC CIRRHOSIS

- When portal venous flow pattern is hepatofugal: Patient not a candidate for splenorenal shunt
- To guide shunt procedures & to assess blood flow: Transjugular intrahepatic portosystemic shunt

Imaging Recommendations
- Best imaging tool: Helical NECT & CECT

DIFFERENTIAL DIAGNOSIS

Budd-Chiari Syndrome
- Liver-spleen scan similar pattern to cirrhosis

Treated Metastatic Disease
- Nodules may shrink and fibrose with treatment

Hepatic Sarcoidosis
- Hypointense nodules on T1 & T2WI MR

Hepatitis
- Diffusely ↓ hepatic, ↑ splenic uptake sulfur colloid

PATHOLOGY

General Features
- General path comments
  - Catalase oxidation of ethanol → membrane, protein damage → inflammatory cells → tissue destruction
  - Steatosis → hepatitis → cirrhosis
  - Regenerative (especially sideritic) nodules → dysplastic nodules → HCC
- Etiology
  - Alcohol (60-70%), chronic viral hepatitis B/C (10%); primary biliary cirrhosis (5%); hemochromatosis (5%); primary sclerosing cholangitis, drugs, cardiac causes; malnutrition, hereditary (Wilson)
  - Peds: Biliary atresia, hepatitis, α-1 antitrypsin deficiency
- Epidemiology
  - 3rd leading cause of death for men 34-54 years
  - Risk of HCC
    - US: Hepatitis C (cirrhosis) causes 30-50% of HCC
    - Japan: Hepatitis C (cirrhosis) 70% of HCC cases
    - 2.5 times higher in cirrhotic hepatitis B positive
    - Alcohol & primary biliary cirrhosis: 2-5 fold ↑ risk
  - Mortality due to complications: Ascites (50%); variceal bleeding (25%); renal failure (10%); bacterial peritonitis (5%); complications of ascites (10%)

Gross Pathologic & Surgical Features
- Alcoholic cirrhosis
  - Early stage: Large, yellow, fatty, micronodular liver
  - Late stage: Shrunken, brown-yellow, hard organ with macronodules
- Postnecrotic cirrhosis: Macronodular (> 3 mm to 1 cm); fibrous scars

Microscopic Features
- Portal-central, portal-portal fibrous bands; micro & macronodules; mononuclear cells; abnormal arteriovenous interconnections

CLINICAL ISSUES

Presentation
- Most common signs/symptoms
  - Alcoholic cirrhosis: May be clinically silent, 10-40% cases found at autopsy
  - Nodular liver, anorexia, malnutrition, weight loss
  - Signs of portal hypertension: Splenomegaly, varices, caput medusae
  - Fatigue, jaundice, ascites, encephalopathy
  - Gynecomastia & testicular atrophy in males, virilization in females
- Clinical Profile: Patient with history of alcoholism, nodular liver, jaundice, ascites & splenomegaly
- Lab data: Increase in liver function tests; anemia
  - Alcoholic cirrhosis: Severe increase in AST (SGOT)
  - Viral: Severe increase in ALT (SGPT)

Demographics
- Age: Middle & elderly age group
- Gender: M > F

Natural History & Prognosis
- Complications: Ascites, variceal hemorrhage, renal failure, coma, HCC due to hepatitis B, C & alcoholism
- Prognosis: 5 year survival < 50% in alcoholic cirrhosis; liver transplantation increases survival period

Treatment
- Alcoholic cirrhosis: Abstinence, decrease protein diet, multivitamins, prednisone, diuretics (for ascites)
- Management of complications & underlying cause
- Advanced stage: Liver transplantation

DIAGNOSTIC CHECKLIST

Consider
- Rule out other causes of "nodular dysmorphic liver"

Image Interpretation Pearls
- Nodular liver contour; lobar atrophy & hypertrophy
- Regenerative nodules, ascites, splenomegaly, varices

SELECTED REFERENCES

1. Shiramizu B et al: Correlation of single photon emission computed tomography parameters as a noninvasive alternative to liver biopsies in assessing liver involvement in the setting of HIV and hepatitis C virus coinfection: a multicenter trial of the Adult AIDS Clinical Trials Group. J Acquir Immune Defic Syndr. 33(3):329-35, 2003
2. Zuckerman E et al: Quantitative liver-spleen scan using single photon emission computerized tomography (SPECT) for assessment of hepatic function in cirrhotic patients. J Hepatol. 39(3):326-32, 2003
3. Dodd GD 3rd et al: Spectrum of imaging findings of the liver in end-stage cirrhosis: part I, gross morphology and diffuse abnormalities. AJR Am J Roentgenol. 173(4):1031-6, 1999
4. Friman L: Distribution of the extrahepatic uptake in liver diseases as recorded by scintigraphy. Acta Radiol Diagn (Stockh). 22(2):103-20, 1981

HEPATIC CIRRHOSIS

IMAGE GALLERY

Typical

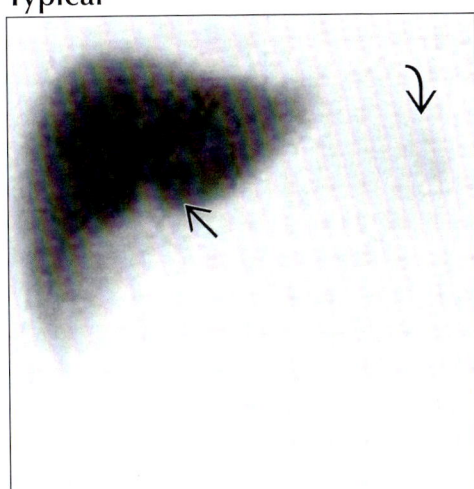

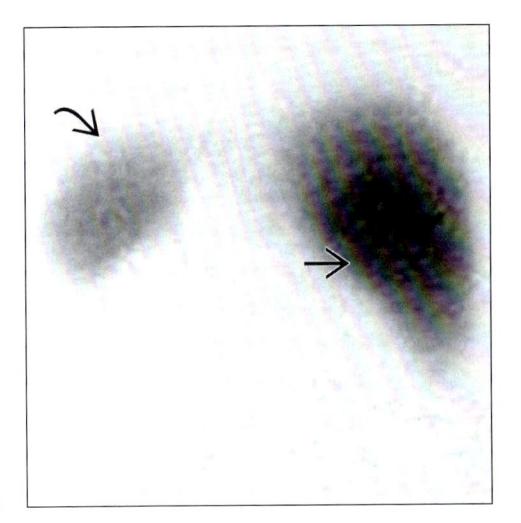

(Left) Anterior Tc-99m sulfur colloid scan demonstrates normal findings: Homogeneous liver activity ➡, spleen ➡ faintly seen on anterior view. See next image. *(Right)* Posterior Tc-99m sulfur colloid scan demonstrates normal findings: Homogeneous liver activity ➡, spleen ➡ less intense than liver (normal spleen:liver ratio is ≤ 1:1), lack of lung activity, lack of marrow activity at normal imaging intensities.

Other

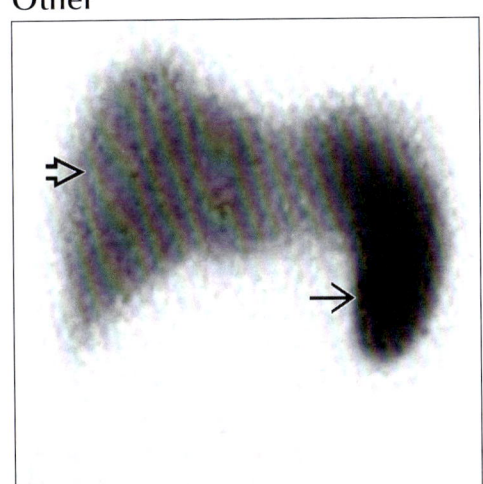

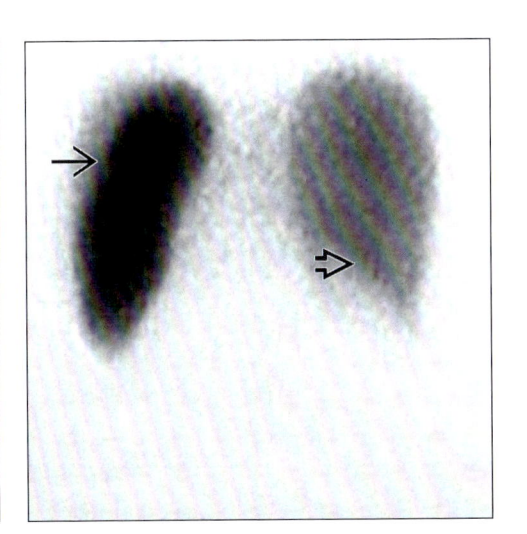

(Left) Anterior Tc-99m sulfur colloid scan of liver demonstrates splenomegaly ➡ and relatively normal appearing liver ➡. See next image. *(Right)* Posterior Tc-99m sulfur colloid scan demonstrates increased splenic ➡ to liver ➡ activity ratio (normal should be ≤ 1:1). Findings in this case due to Felty syndrome, not cirrhosis.

Typical

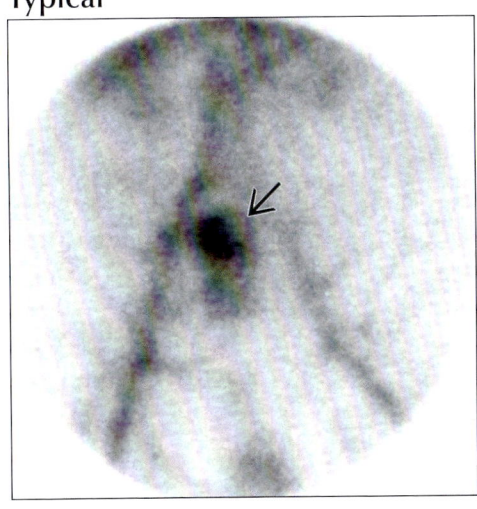

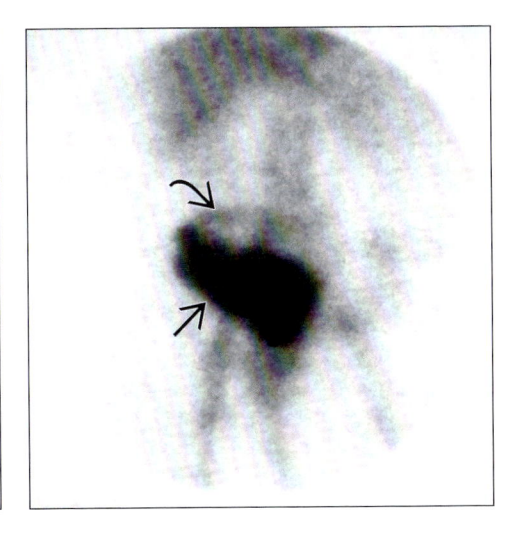

(Left) Tc-99m tagged RBC scan: Anterior abdomen & pelvis image at 10 minutes post injection in cirrhotic patient with rectal varices and lower GI bleed. Focus of uptake rapidly appeared just below aortic bifurcation ➡. See next image. *(Right)* Tc-99m tagged RBC scan: Anterior image of abdomen and pelvis 30 minutes post injection demonstrates intense uptake conforming to shape of rectum ➡ and distal sigmoid ➡, caused by active bleeding from rectal varix.

HEPATIC CIRRHOSIS

(Left) Tc-99m Choletec hepatobiliary scan in cirrhotic patient 50 minutes post injection shows blood pool activity ➡, unchanged from first image post injection. Delayed imaging indicated. See next 2 images. **(Right)** Tc-99m Choletec hepatobiliary scan in cirrhotic patient 4 h post injection shows visualization of gallbladder ➡, but not duodenum. Further delayed imaging recommended. See next image.

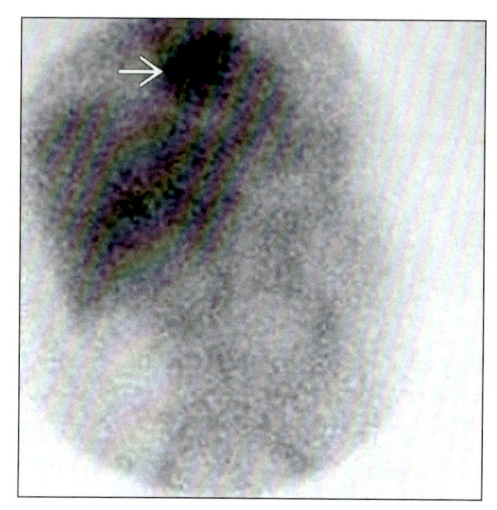

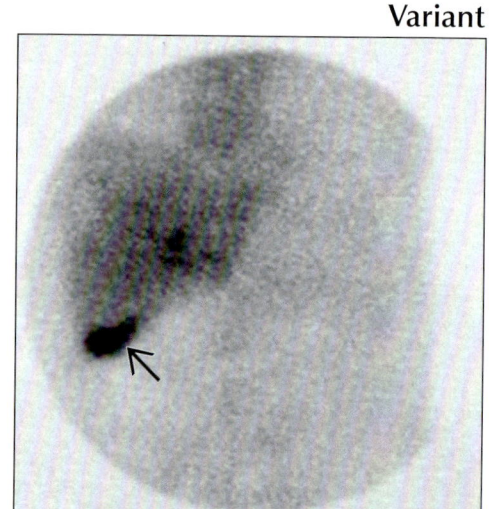

(Left) Tc-99m Choletec hepatobiliary scan in cirrhotic patient 18 h post injection shows both gallbladder ➡ and bowel ▹ activity. With cirrhosis, delayed imaging to 24 h is often indicated due to delayed transit. **(Right)** Anterior In-111 WBC scan of abdomen and pelvis in patient with ascites and fever shows diffuse increased uptake throughout abdomen ➡ consistent with spontaneous bacterial peritonitis.

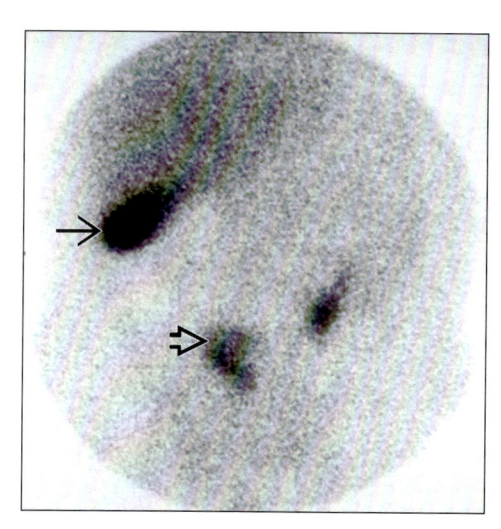

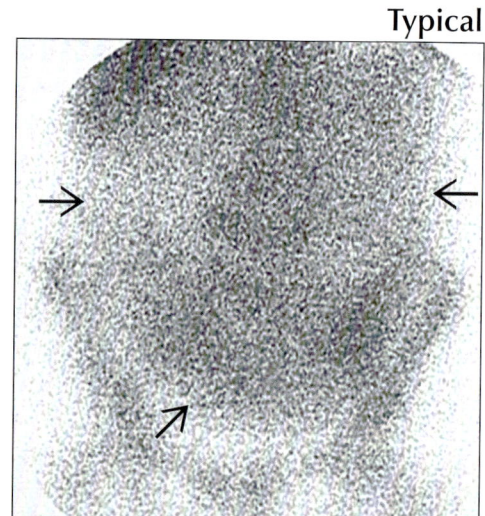

(Left) Graphic illustrates nodular surface of liver, fibrosis, relative enlargement of caudate lobe and lateral segment. **(Right)** Anterior Ga-67 scan in patient with chronic hepatitis B, cirrhosis and abdominal mass demonstrates heterogeneous increased uptake in hepatic mass ➡, proved hepatocellular carcinoma on biopsy.

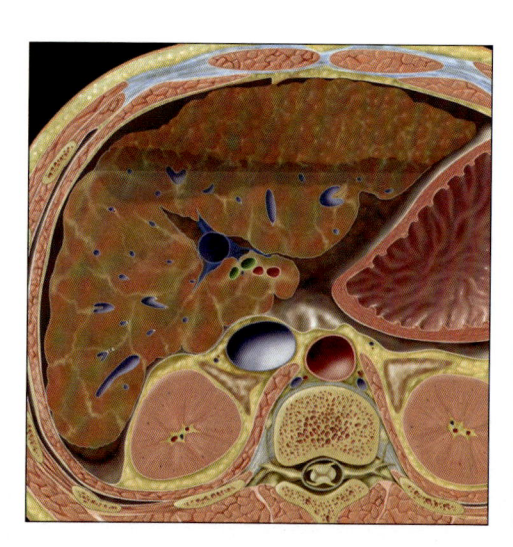

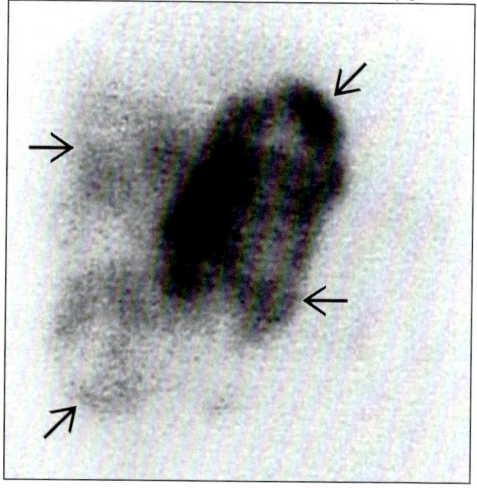

HEPATIC CIRRHOSIS

Typical

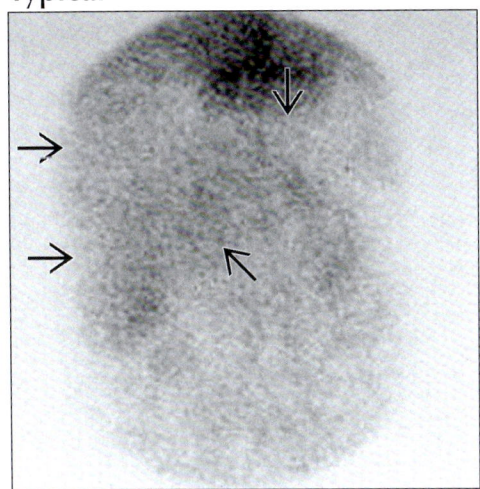

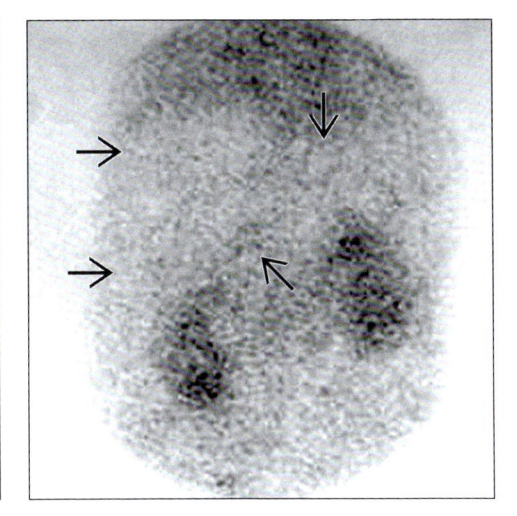

(Left) Tc-99m Choletec hepatobiliary scan in patient with cirrhosis and superimposed acute alcoholic hepatitis during first 5 min post injection shows faint blood pool activity in liver ➡ but no significant concentration of tracer. See next image. *(Right)* Tc-99m Choletec hepatobiliary scan in same patient as previous image 20 minutes post injection shows liver ➡ as photopenic defect, typical pattern for severe acute chemical hepatitis.

Typical

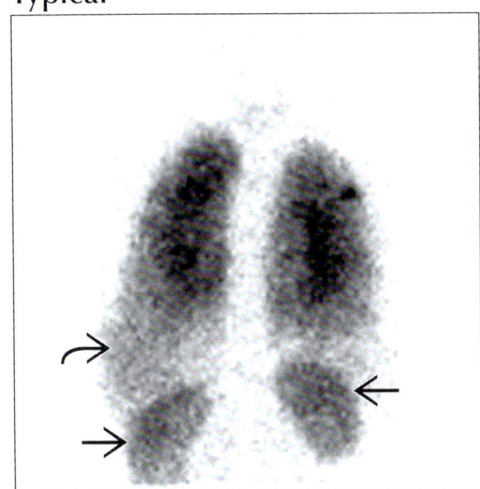

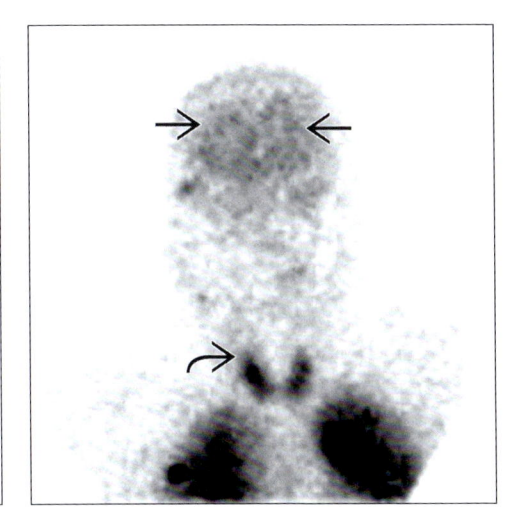

(Left) Tc-99m MAA perfusion lung scan: Posterior image shows uptake in spleen ➡ and kidneys ➡. See next image. *(Right)* Tc-99m MAA perfusion lung scan: Anterior image of head shows uptake in brain ➡. Patient had cirrhosis and hepatopulmonary syndrome (multiple small arteriovenous connections in lungs producing right → left shunt). Note free pertechnetate in thyroid ➡.

Typical

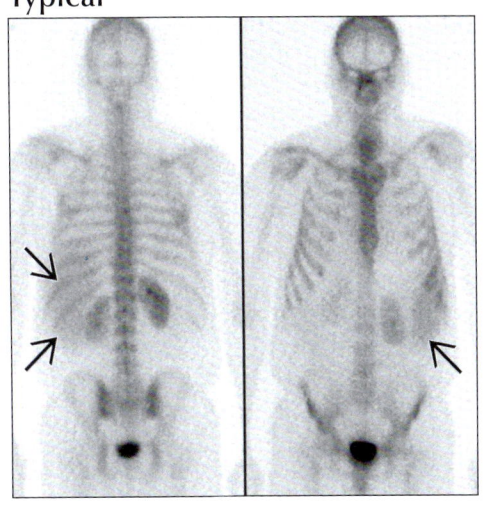

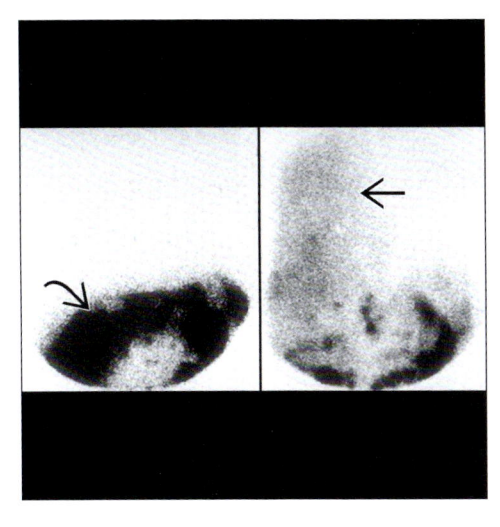

(Left) Tc-99m MDP bone scan: Posterior (left) and anterior (right) images in patient with cirrhosis show increased uptake in spleen ➡, likely due to secondary to splenic siderosis. *(Right)* Diaphragmatic patency scan with Tc-99m MAA injected intraperitoneally ➡ in cirrhotic patient with ascites and left pleural effusion. Posterior images immediately after injection (left). After left thoracentesis, activity is evident in left pleural space ➡, confirming diaphragmatic rent.

HYPERSPLENISM

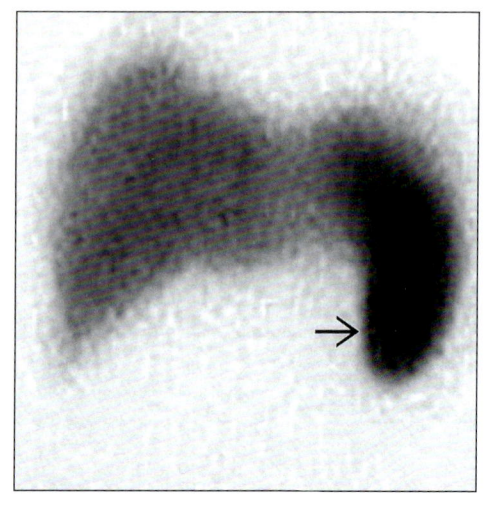

Anterior Tc-99m sulfur colloid scan of the upper abdomen shows splenomegaly ➔ with increased uptake, typical of liver disease or increased splenic function. Diagnosis was alcoholic liver disease.

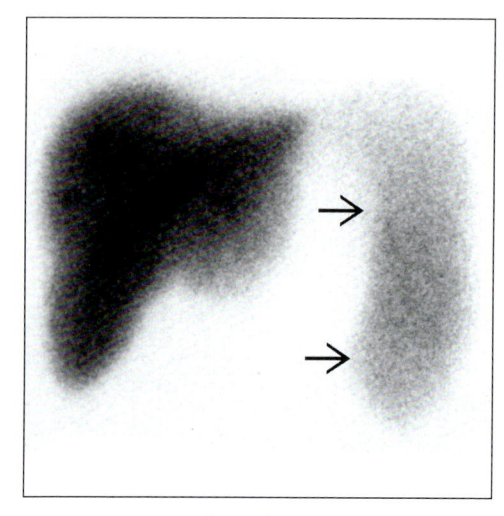

Anterior Tc-99m sulfur colloid scan of the upper abdomen shows splenomegaly ➔ with diffusely decreased splenic uptake, typical of infiltrative diseases. Diagnosis in this case was Gaucher disease.

TERMINOLOGY

Abbreviations and Synonyms
- Splenomegaly (SMG); hypersplenism (HS)

Definitions
- Splenomegaly: Enlarged spleen; volume > 500 cm³
- Hypersplenism (HS): Syndrome consisting of splenomegaly & pancytopenia in which bone marrow is either normal or hyperreactive

IMAGING FINDINGS

General Features
- Best diagnostic clue: Increased volume of spleen with convex medial border
- Size
  - Normal spleen in adult measures up to 13 cm; enlarged if it is 14 cm or longer
  - SMG: Anteroposterior (AP) diameter > two-thirds distance of AP diameter of abdominal cavity

Nuclear Medicine Findings
- Chromium-51 random RBC labeling: Definitive diagnosis of hypersplenism, splenic sequestration
  - Normal T1/2: 25-35 days
  - Normal spleen:precordium ratio < 2:1
  - Normal spleen:liver ratio < 1:1
  - Increased red cell destruction: T1/2 < 25 days
  - Active splenic sequestration: Spleen:liver ratio rises progressively to 2:1-4:1
  - Large spleen, no sequestration: Initial and stable spleen:precordium ratio > 2:1 (no progressive rise)
- Tc-99m sulfur colloid (SC) scan: Global assessment of splenic function
  - Normal posterior spleen:liver SC ratio ≤ 1:1
  - Enlarged spleen with increased SC uptake: Decreased hepatic function or increased splenic function
    - Cirrhosis/fibrosis, hepatitis, portal hypertension, chronic hemolytic anemias, Felty syndrome
  - Non-enlarged spleen with increased uptake: Acute viral hepatitis, iron deficiency, metastatic disease, reticuloendothelial stimulation (sepsis, infection), marrow stimulant drugs

DDx: Other Causes of Splenomegaly

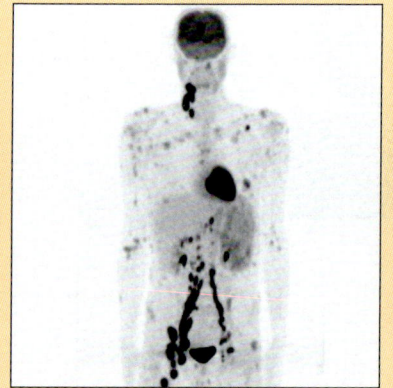

T-Cell Lymphoma

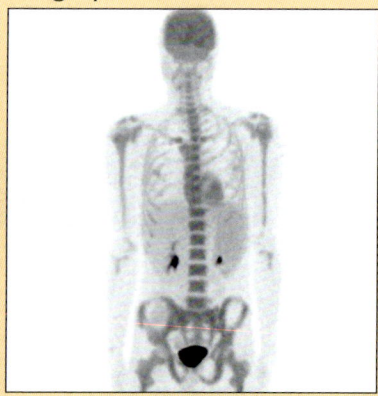

Marrow Stimulant Drugs

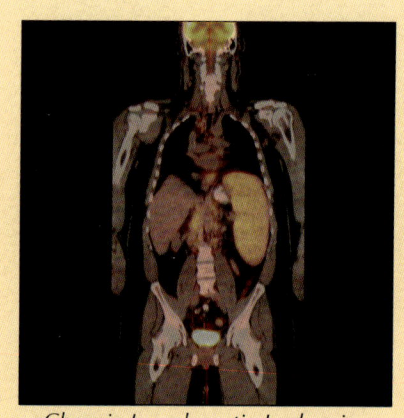

Chronic Lymphocytic Leukemia

HYPERSPLENISM

Key Facts

Terminology
- Splenomegaly: Enlarged spleen; volume > 500 cm³
- Hypersplenism (HS): Syndrome consisting of splenomegaly & pancytopenia in which bone marrow is either normal or hyperreactive

Imaging Findings
- Chromium-51 random RBC labeling: Definitive diagnosis of hypersplenism, splenic sequestration
- Normal T1/2: 25-35 days
- Increased red cell destruction: T1/2 < 25 days
- Active splenic sequestration: Spleen:liver ratio rises progressively to 2:1-4:1
- Large spleen, no sequestration: Initial and stable spleen:precordium ratio > 2:1 (no progressive rise)
- Tc-99m sulfur colloid (SC) scan: Global assessment of splenic function
- Normal posterior spleen:liver SC ratio ≤ 1:1
- Enlarged spleen with increased SC uptake: Decreased hepatic function or increased splenic function
- Enlarged spleen with decreased SC uptake: Infiltrative diseases of the spleen
- Sickle cell disease: Splenic uptake on bone scan with autoinfarction & splenic calcification; also with acute sickle crisis (increased kidney size and uptake also common)
- Uptake in spleen on bone scan: Can also be seen with leukemia, hemosiderosis, amyloidosis, splenic metastases, Wilson disease
- Diffuse splenic hypermetabolism on FDG PET: With most causes of SMG and HS; marrow stimulant drugs
- Focal splenic hypermetabolism on FDG PET: Malignant neoplasms, active granulomatous disease, abscess, acute infarction

---

- Enlarged spleen with decreased SC uptake: Infiltrative diseases of the spleen
  - Leukemia, diffuse lymphoma, myelofibrosis, glycogen storage disease, amyloidosis, metastatic disease, extensive granulomatous involvement
- Tc-99m bone scan: Increased uptake in spleen
  - Sickle cell disease: Splenic uptake on bone scan with autoinfarction & splenic calcification; also with acute sickle crisis (increased kidney size and uptake also common)
  - Uptake in spleen on bone scan: Can also be seen with leukemia, hemosiderosis, amyloidosis, splenic metastases, Wilson disease
- FDG PET: Normal spleen:liver ratio ≤ 1:1
  - Diffuse splenic hypermetabolism on FDG PET: With most causes of SMG and HS; marrow stimulant drugs
  - Focal splenic hypermetabolism on FDG PET: Malignant neoplasms, active granulomatous disease, abscess, acute infarction

CT Findings
- SMG: Medial margin of spleen is convex on CT
- Congestive SMG
  - Portal hypertension: SMG with varices, nodular shrunken liver, ascites
  - Splenic vein occlusion or thrombosis (often secondary to pancreatitis or pancreatic tumors)
  - Sickle-cell disease: Splenic sequestration; peripheral ↓ HU areas + areas ↑ attenuation, represent areas of infarct & hemorrhage
- Storage disorders
  - Gaucher disease: Spleen may have abnormal low attenuation; marked SMG, often extending into pelvis
  - Amyloidosis: Generalized or focal ↓ density on NECT & CECT
  - Primary hemochromatosis: Density of spleen is normal (unlike that of liver)
  - Hemosiderosis: Increased attenuation values in liver & spleen
- Space occupying lesions: Cysts, abscess, tumor
- Splenic infarction (veno-occlusion caused by sickling): SMG with focal infarcts; peripheral areas of low attenuation & hemorrhage associated with SMG
- Hemosiderosis: ↑ Attenuation of spleen (hemosiderin deposition); consequence of multiple blood transfusions (thalassemia, hemophilia)
- Splenic trauma: Splenic laceration or subcapsular hematoma; surrounding perisplenic hematoma (> 30 HU)
- Extramedullary hematopoiesis: Spleen may be diffusely enlarged; CECT: Focal masses of hematopoietic tissue that are isoattenuating relative to normal splenic tissue

MR Findings
- Portal hypertension: Multiple tiny (3-8 mm) foci of decreased signal; hemosiderin deposits; organized hemorrhage (Gamna-Gandy bodies or siderotic nodules)
- Sickle cell disease (splenic sequestration): Areas of abnormal signal intensity; hyperintense with dark rim on T1WI (subacute hemorrhage)
- Primary hemochromatosis: Normal signal & size of spleen
- Gaucher disease: Increased signal intensity on T1WI
- Extramedullary hematopoiesis: Focal hypointense nodules
- Hemosiderosis: ↓ Signal intensity of spleen on both T1 & T2WI
- Infarction: Peripheral, wedge-shaped areas of abnormal signal; low signal resulting from iron deposition

Ultrasonographic Findings
- Grayscale Ultrasound
  - SMG with normal echogenicity: Infection, congestion (portal HT), early sickle cell, H. spherocytosis, hemolysis, Felty syndrome, Wilson disease, polycythemia, myelofibrosis, leukemia
  - SMG with hyperechoic pattern: Leukemia, post-chemo & radiation therapy, malaria, TB, sarcoidosis, polycythemia, hereditary spherocytosis, portal vein thrombosis, hematoma, metastases

HYPERSPLENISM

- SMG with hypoechoic pattern: Lymphoma, multiple myeloma, chronic lymphocytic leukemia, congestion from portal HT, noncaseating granulomatous infection
- Sickle cell disease: Immediately after sequestration, peripheral hypoechoic areas seen
- Gaucher disease: Multiple, well-defined, discrete hypoechoic lesions; fibrosis or infarction

Imaging Recommendations
- Best imaging tool: Helical CT

DIFFERENTIAL DIAGNOSIS

Lymphoma & Metastases
- Lymphoma: Focal or diffuse hypermetabolism on FDG PET
- Metastases: Cold on Tc-99m SC, focally hypermetabolic on FDG PET

Primary Splenic Tumor
- Benign tumor: Hemangioma, hamartoma, lymphangioma
  - Typically cold on Tc-99m SC; low or isometabolic to spleen on FDG PET
- Malignant tumor: Angiosarcoma
  - Typically cold on Tc-99m SC; hypermetabolic on FDG PET (may be cold centrally)

Splenic Infection
- Cold on Tc-99m SC (small lesions inapparent), hypermetabolic on FDG PET

Granulomatous: Infectious and Non-Infectious
- Lesions of low attenuation on CT; hypermetabolic on FDG PET

PATHOLOGY

General Features
- Etiology
  - Congestive SMG: CHF, portal HT, cirrhosis, cystic fibrosis, splenic vein thrombosis, sickle cell (SC) sequestration
  - Neoplasm: Leukemia, lymphoma, metastases, primary neoplasm, Kaposi sarcoma
  - Storage disease: Gaucher, Niemann-Pick, gargoylism, amyloidosis, DM, hemochromatosis, histiocytosis
  - Infection: Hepatitis, malaria, mononucleosis, TB, typhoid, kala-azar, schistosomiasis, brucellosis
  - Hemolytic anemia: Hemoglobinopathy, hereditary spherocytosis, primary neutropenia, thrombocytopenic purpura
  - Extramedullary hematopoiesis: Osteopetrosis, myelofibrosis
  - Collagen disease: SLE, RA, Felty syndrome
  - Splenic trauma; sarcoidosis; hemodialysis

Microscopic Features
- Varies depending on underlying etiology

CLINICAL ISSUES

Presentation
- Most common signs/symptoms
  - Asymptomatic, splenomegaly, abdominal pain
  - Signs & symptoms related to underlying cause
- Lab data: Abnormal CBC (anemia, thrombocytopenia), LFT, antibody titers, cultures or bone marrow exam

Natural History & Prognosis
- Complications: Splenic rupture, shock & death
- HS: Usually develops as a result of SMG
- Splenic rupture, sequestration in SC disease: Poor prognosis

Treatment
- Treatment varies based on underlying condition
- Splenectomy in symptomatic & complicated cases

DIAGNOSTIC CHECKLIST

Consider
- SMG, usually a systemic cause rather than primary

Image Interpretation Pearls
- US can confirm presence of enlarged spleen or space occupying lesions
- CT & MR can further clarify abnormalities in size, shape & define parenchymal pathology
- Radioisotope scanning can diagnose HS & provide functional status of spleen

SELECTED REFERENCES

1. Ruiz-Hernandez G et al: [Splenic and bone marrow increased 18F-FDG uptake in a PET scan performed following treatment with G-CSF] Rev Esp Med Nucl. 23(2):124-6, 2004
2. Peck-Radosavljevic M: Hypersplenism. Eur J Gastroenterol Hepatol. 13(4):317-23, 2001
3. McCormick PA et al: Splenomegaly, hypersplenism and coagulation abnormalities in liver disease. Baillieres Best Pract Res Clin Gastroenterol. 14(6):1009-31, 2000
4. Carneskog J et al: The red cell mass, plasma erythropoietin and spleen size in apparent polycythaemia. Eur J Haematol. 62(1):43-8, 1999
5. Paterson A et al: A pattern-oriented approach to splenic imaging in infants and children. Radiographics. 19(6):1465-85, 1999
6. Israel O et al: Scintigraphic findings in Gaucher's disease. J Nucl Med. 27(10):1557-63, 1986
7. Shih WJ et al: Radiocolloid scintigraphy in Felty's syndrome. AJR Am J Roentgenol. 147(1):181-3, 1986
8. Bowdler AJ: Splenomegaly and hypersplenism. Clin Haematol. 12(2):467-88, 1983
9. Rao BK et al: Hepatic and splenic scintigraphy in idiopathic systemic amyloidosis. Eur J Nucl Med. 6(4):143-6, 1981
10. Mittelstaedt CA et al: Ultrasonic-pathologic classification of splenic abnormalities: gray-scale patterns. Radiology. 134(3):697-705, 1980
11. Davis G et al: Parameters of liver spleen scans as an indication of portal hypertension. Am J Gastroenterol. 65(1):31-6, 1976
12. Goy W et al: Splenic accumulation of 99mTc-diphosphonate in a patient with sickle cell disease: case report. J Nucl Med. 17(02):108-9, 1976

HYPERSPLENISM

IMAGE GALLERY

Typical

Typical

Typical

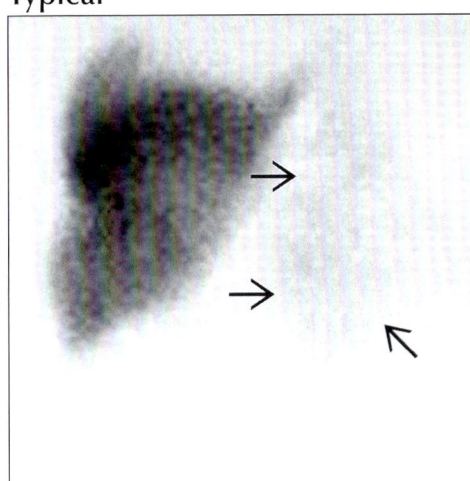

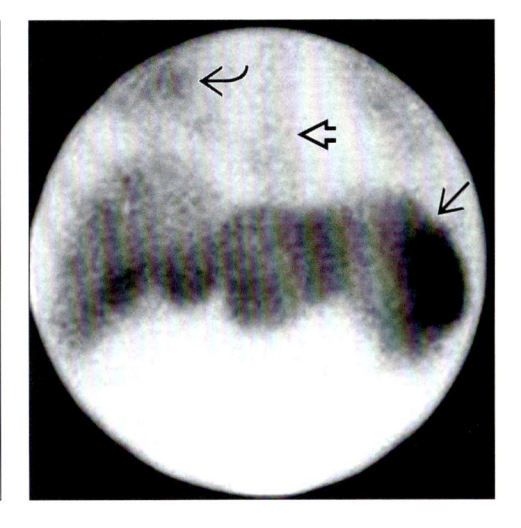

(Left) Anterior Tc-99m sulfur colloid scan of the upper abdomen shows splenomegaly with faint splenic uptake ➔, typical of infiltrative diseases. Diagnosis in this case was myelofibrosis. *(Right)* Anterior Tc-99m sulfur colloid scan of the upper abdomen shows splenomegaly ➔ with increased splenic uptake. Note small liver (larger left lobe), marrow uptake ➔, lung uptake ➔, & ascites, typical of cirrhosis.

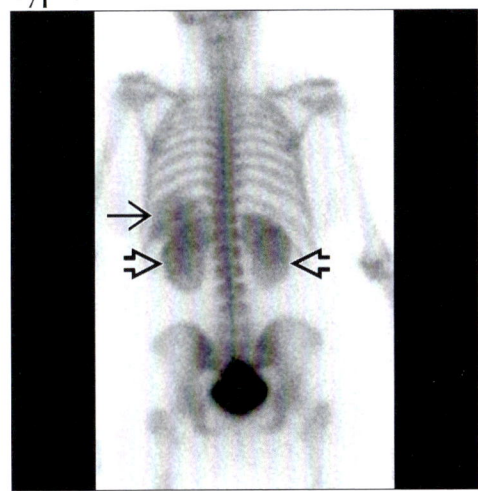

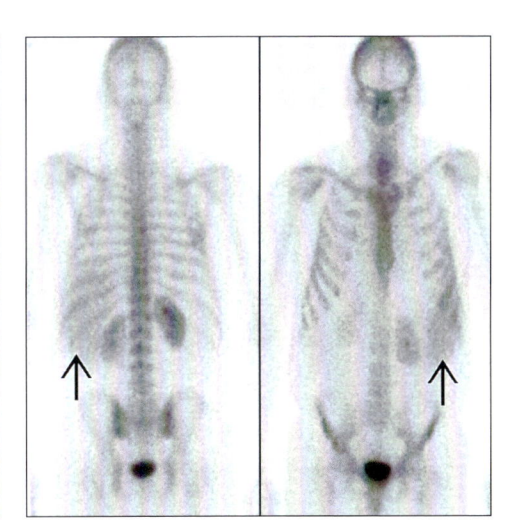

(Left) Posterior Tc-99m MDP bone scan demonstrates increased uptake in small spleen ➔ and in enlarged kidneys ➔, typical of sickle cell crisis. *(Right)* Posterior (left) and anterior (right) Tc-99m MDP bone scan demonstrates increased uptake in a large spleen ➔ in a patient with cirrhosis and splenic siderosis.

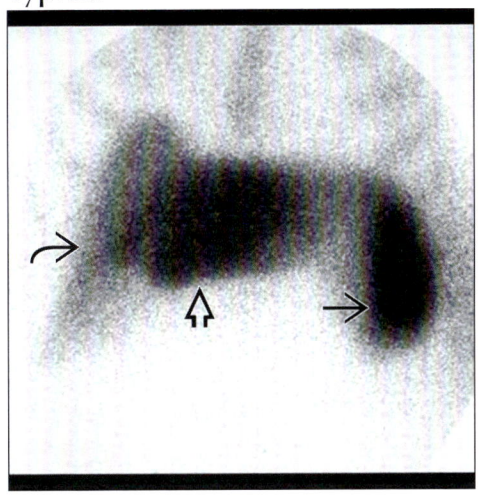

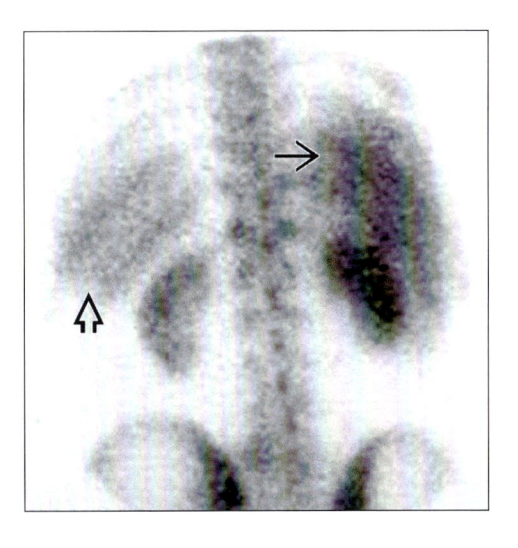

(Left) Anterior Tc-99m sulfur colloid scan of the upper abdomen shows splenomegaly ➔ with decreased uptake to right lobe of liver ➔ and hypertrophy of caudate lobe ➔ in a patient with Budd-Chiari syndrome. *(Right)* Posterior Tc-99m MDP bone scan image of abdomen shows uptake in both liver ➔ and spleen ➔, typical of metal or protein deposition diseases, such as Wilson disease, hemosiderosis, amyloidosis.

HEPATIC METASTASES

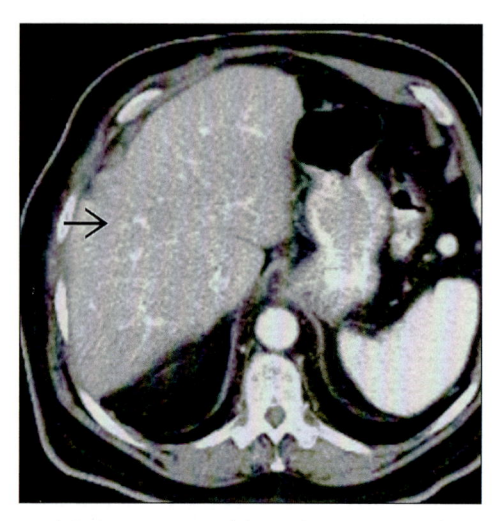

Axial CECT in patient with lung adenocarcinoma shows no metastases in liver ➔ despite good contrast enhancement technique.

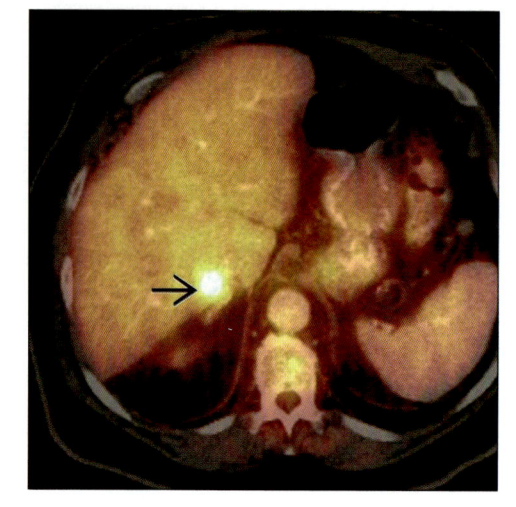

Axial fused PET/CT in same patient as previous image shows focal intense FDG activity ➔, signifying hepatic metastasis not evident on CT.

TERMINOLOGY

Abbreviations and Synonyms
- Liver metastases

Definitions
- Malignant invasion into liver parenchyma from extrahepatic primary tumor

IMAGING FINDINGS

General Features
- Best diagnostic clue
  - Multiple lesions in liver parenchyma in patient with primary malignancy
  - Likelihood of liver metastasis by primary
    - Eye 77.8%
    - Pancreas 75.1%
    - Breast 60.6%
    - Gallbladder, extrahepatic bile ducts 60.5%
    - Colon/rectum 56.8%
    - Stomach 48.9%
  - In children, most common primaries that metastasize to liver
    - Neuroblastoma
    - Wilms tumor
    - Leukemia
  - 30-70% of patients dying of cancer have liver metastases

Nuclear Medicine Findings
- PET
  - PET and PET/CT: Sensitive/specific for hepatic metastases for many primary tumors
    - Colorectal
    - Lung
    - Esophagus
    - Breast
  - Some tumors show variable FDG activity with metastases
    - Sarcomas, neuroendocrine tumors
    - If somatostatin receptor analogue scintigraphy negative in patient with neuroendocrine tumor, FDG PET may detect metastases

DDx: Other CT Enhancing Hepatic Lesions with Variable Uptake on FDG PET

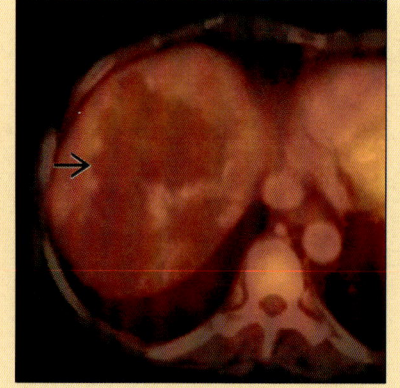

Hemangioma

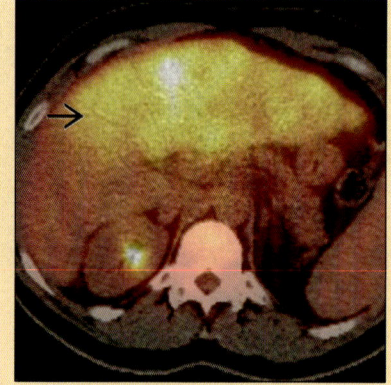

Cholangiocarcinoma

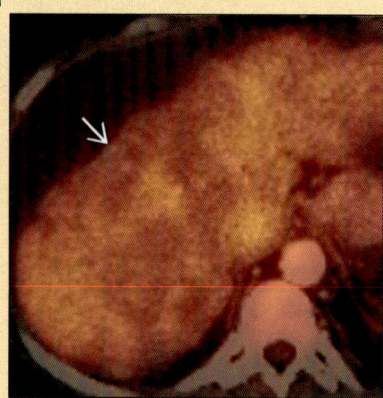

Cirrhosis

HEPATIC METASTASES

Key Facts

Imaging Findings
- Multiple lesions in liver parenchyma in patient with primary malignancy
- PET and PET/CT: Sensitive/specific for hepatic metastases for many primary tumors
- Tc-99m sulfur colloid scintigraphy: Historical use
- Anti-CEA antibody labeled with Tc-99m to detect liver metastases
- Somatostatin receptor scintigraphy detects metastases of tumors that express somatostatin receptor
- MR most sensitive
- CECT ~ 80-90% sensitive

Top Differential Diagnoses
- Cavernous Hemangioma
- Atypical Hemangiomas
- Focal Nodular Hyperplasia (FNH)
- Liver Abscess
- Focal Fat
- Hepatocellular Carcinoma (HCC)
- Granulomatous Disease
- Hydatid Liver Disease

Diagnostic Checklist
- PET/CT most sensitive modality for detecting liver metastases
- FDG PET if anatomic imaging negative and high clinical suspicion of metastases
- In case of negative somatostatin receptor scintigraphy: FDG PET may be useful in patient with neuroendocrine tumor to detect metastases
- Some metastatic lesions may not be FDG-avid (e.g., carcinoid, mucinous adenocarcinoma)

  - Tumors with poor uptake of FDG: Highly mucinous, low grade lymphoma, MALT lymphoma, bronchogenic Ca, lobular or tubular breast cancer
  - Small tumors may be indistinguishable from normal liver on FDG PET
- Tc-99m Sulfur Colloid
  - Tc-99m sulfur colloid scintigraphy: Historical use
  - Metastases appear photopenic; nonspecific
  - Replaced by CT, MR, FDG PET
- Carcinoembryonic antigen (CEA) immunoscintigraphy
  - Anti-CEA antibody labeled with Tc-99m to detect liver metastases
  - CEA expressed in variety of adenocarcinomas, e.g., colorectal cancer
  - Does not provoke immune response
- Somatostatin receptor analogue scintigraphy
  - Somatostatin receptor scintigraphy detects metastases of tumors that express somatostatin receptor
  - Useful for insulinoma, glucagonoma, small-cell lung cancer, thyroid cancer, carcinoid
  - Can detect subcentimeter liver metastases with high signal-to-noise ratio
  - 80-90% sensitivity/specificity for primary and metastatic gastrinoma

Radiographic Findings
- Calcification within metastases may be seen on plain radiographs
  - Tend to be amorphous, unlike solid calcification of granuloma

CT Findings
- Contrast-enhanced CT: Sensitivity 80-90%, specificity 99%
- Portal venous phase
  - Normal parenchyma enhances
  - Relatively hypoattenuating metastases
- Peripheral enhancement may be present (contrast between viable tumor, necrotic center)
- Cystic changes may also cause hypoattenuating center
- Lesion hyperattenuation uncommon for most metastases
- Nonenhanced CT: Differentiates hyperdense cysts from other pathology

Imaging Recommendations
- Best imaging tool
  - MR most sensitive
  - CECT ~ 80-90% sensitive
  - PET/CT less sensitive for tiny or highly mucinous mets

DIFFERENTIAL DIAGNOSIS

Cavernous Hemangioma
- Most common benign hepatic tumors
- Tc-99m pertechnetate-labeled red blood cells (RBC): Initial photon-deficient mass followed by RBC filling from periphery to center
- Typically low FDG uptake on PET

Atypical Hemangiomas
- May coexist with metastases
- Nonenhanced CT: Often well-defined hypoattenuating lesions that mimic vascular metastases
- Contrast enhanced CT: Peripheral enhancement
- Unlike vascular metastases, hemangiomas take several minutes to become completely filled

Focal Nodular Hyperplasia (FNH)
- If lacking prominent central scar, may look like vascular metastases
- Tc-99m sulfur colloid scintigraphy: Best modality for demonstrating Kupffer cells (second most important finding to central scar)
- MR with superparamagnetic contrast also useful
- Most negative on PET: However, case reports of FDG-avid FNH

Liver Abscess
- Pyogenic liver abscess: Ga-67-avid in > 80% of patients with liver abscesses
- Amebic abscesses: Concentrate Ga-67 peripherally
- Usually (+) on FDG PET and indistinguishable from metastatic lesions

HEPATIC METASTASES

Focal Fat
- Focal fatty infiltration/sparing in diffusely fatty liver can mimic metastases
- Tc-99m sulfur colloid scintigraphy usually normal
- Nonenhanced CT: Fatty regions appear nonspherical/geographic; no mass effect or distortion

Hepatocellular Carcinoma (HCC)
- Nonspecific photon-deficient mass on Tc-99m sulfur colloid scintigraphy
- Ga-67: ↑ Activity in 80% of HCC
- HCC variable on FDG PET: Usually similar to normal liver

Granulomatous Disease
- Calcifications common
- Correlate with evidence of granulomatous disease elsewhere
- Metastatic disease can calcify also
- Can be + on FDG PET

Hydatid Liver Disease
- In endemic regions of world

PATHOLOGY

General Features
- General path comments
  - Hepatic metastases supported by
    - Dual blood supply of liver (hepatic artery supplies metastases)
    - Local cell growth factors
    - Fenestrations in sinusoidal endothelium
  - Most metastases hypovascular
  - Hypervascular metastases
    - Carcinoid
    - Leiomyosarcoma
    - Neuroendocrine tumors
    - Renal carcinoma
    - Thyroid carcinomas
    - Choriocarcinoma
  - Blood flow increases relative to normal parenchyma in all metastases, even hypovascular ones
  - Breast and pancreatic metastases incite intense sclerosing reaction leading to fibrous scar formation ± capsular retraction
  - Calcifications common with mucinous primary tumors (e.g., colon, ovary, breast)

CLINICAL ISSUES

Presentation
- Most common signs/symptoms
  - ~ 50% of patients with hepatic metastases demonstrate hepatomegaly or ascites
  - Obstructive jaundice may be present
    - Due to large liver metastases or bile duct involvement
  - Ascites = grave prognostic sign

Treatment
- Surgical resection
  - Usually 1-2 metastases
  - Followed by local, systemic chemotherapy
- Minimally invasive techniques
  - Localized chemotherapy via hepatic arterial infusion pump
  - Transcatheter arterial chemoembolization (TACE)
  - Radiofrequency ablation (RFA)
  - Radiolabeled microspheres (e.g., Y-90) deposited via hepatic arterial catheter
  - Cryoablation
  - Microwave ablation
  - Ethanol ablation
  - Laser ablation
- Chemotherapy
  - Systemic chemotherapy alone often palliative

DIAGNOSTIC CHECKLIST

Consider
- PET/CT most sensitive modality for detecting liver metastases
- FDG PET if anatomic imaging negative and high clinical suspicion of metastases
- In case of negative somatostatin receptor scintigraphy: FDG PET may be useful in patient with neuroendocrine tumor to detect metastases

Image Interpretation Pearls
- Some metastatic lesions may not be FDG-avid (e.g., carcinoid, mucinous adenocarcinoma)

SELECTED REFERENCES

1. Amthauer H et al: Evaluation of patients with liver metastases from colorectal cancer for locally ablative treatment with laser induced thermotherapy. Impact of PET with 18F-fluorodeoxyglucose on therapeutic decisions. Nuklearmedizin. 45(4):177-84, 2006
2. Dimitrakopoulou-Strauss A et al: Quantitative studies using positron emission tomography (PET) for the diagnosis and therapy planning of oncological patients. Hell J Nucl Med. 9(1):10-21, 2006
3. Erturk SM et al: PET imaging for evaluation of metastatic colorectal cancer of the liver. Eur J Radiol. 58(2):229-35, 2006
4. Khan S et al: An audit of fusion CT-PET in the management of colorectal liver metastases. Eur J Surg Oncol. 32(5):564-7, 2006
5. Lim JS et al: CT and PET in stomach cancer: preoperative staging and monitoring of response to therapy. Radiographics. 26(1):143-56, 2006
6. Mackie GC et al: Use of [18F]fluorodeoxyglucose positron emission tomography in evaluating locally recurrent and metastatic adrenocortical carcinoma. J Clin Endocrinol Metab. 91(7):2665-71, 2006
7. Mucha SA et al: Positron emission tomography ((18)FDG-PET) in the detection of medullary thyroid carcinoma metastases. Endokrynol Pol. 57(4):452-5, 2006
8. Watanabe N et al: F-18 FDG PET imaging in gastric neuroendocrine carcinoma. Clin Nucl Med. 31(6):345-6, 2006
9. Wiering B et al: The Role of FDG-PET in the Selection of Patients with Colorectal Liver Metastases. Ann Surg Oncol. 2006

HEPATIC METASTASES

IMAGE GALLERY

Typical

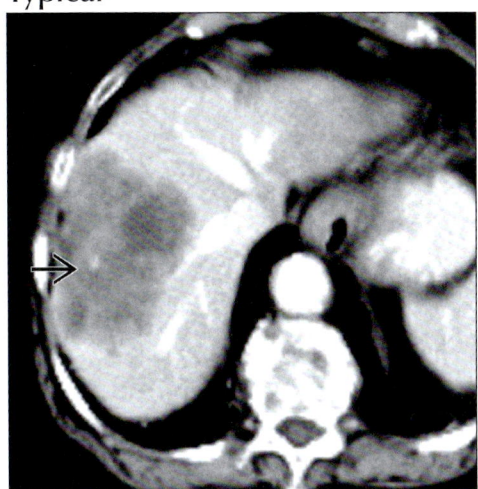

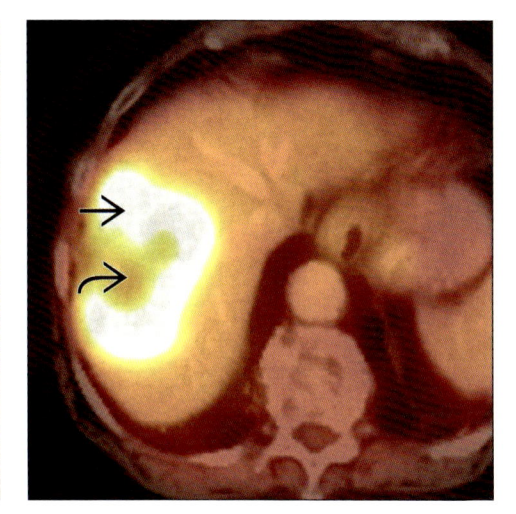

(Left) Axial CECT shows a large low attenuation lesion ➔ in right hepatic lobe, characteristic appearance for metastatic disease. *(Right)* Axial fused PET/CT in same patient as previous image shows intense FDG activity ➔ with central photopenia ➔, signifying central necrosis in colon cancer metastasis.

Typical

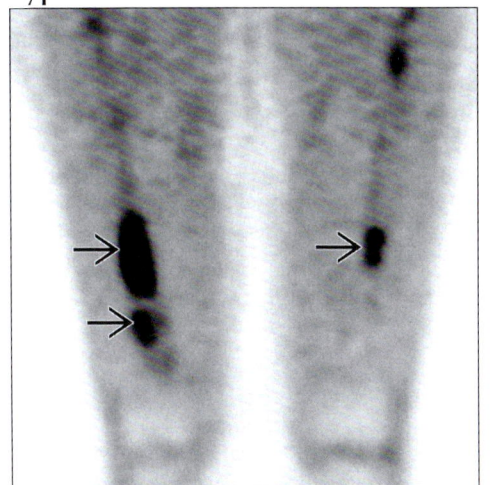

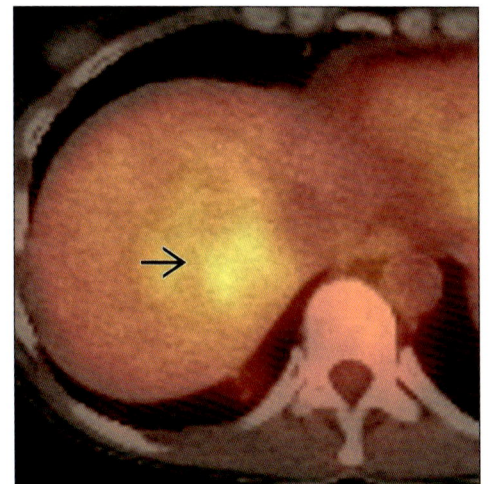

(Left) Coronal PET shows intense FDG activity ➔ in patient with lower limb sarcoma, consistent with metastases. *(Right)* Axial fused PET/CT in same patient as previous image shows only mild-to-moderate FDG activity in a large hepatic metastasis ➔. Variable FDG uptake by sarcomatous metastases is characteristic.

Typical

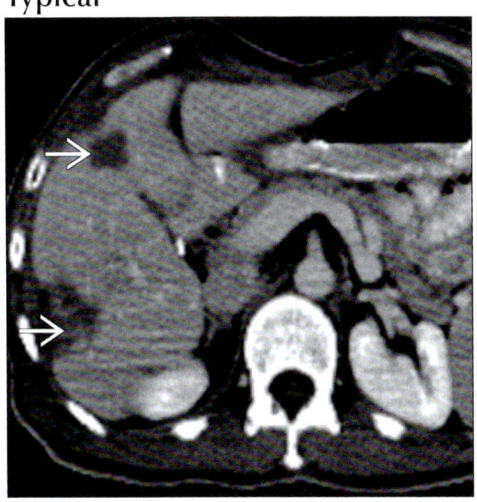

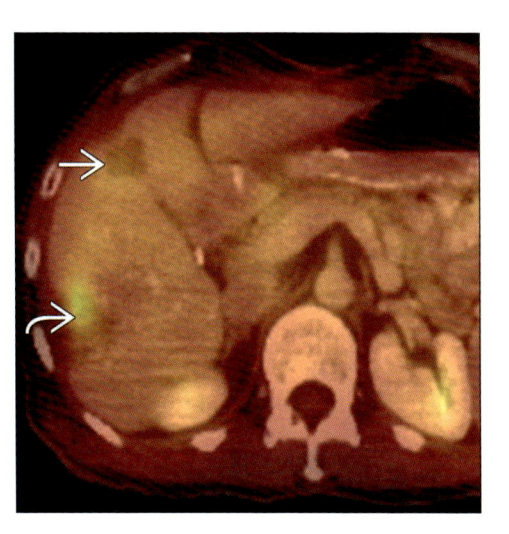

(Left) Axial CECT shows two low attenuation hepatic lesions ➔ in patient with colon cancer metastases post radiofrequency ablation. *(Right)* Axial fused PET/CT in same patient as previous image shows normal FDG activity in anterior lesion ➔ and residual tumor in posterior lesion ➔.

HEPATOBLASTOMA

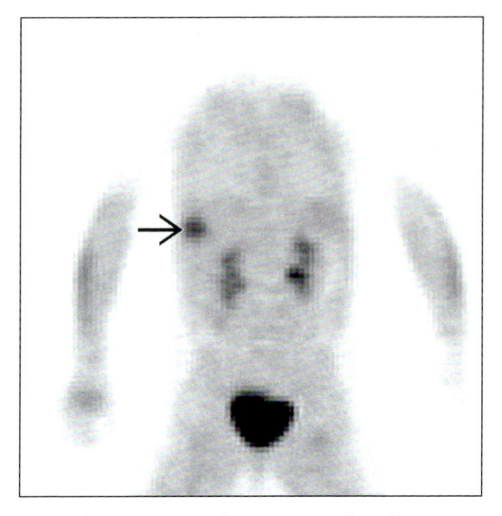

Coronal FDG PET scan shows increased uptake in mass ➔ in right lobe of liver in neonate with small hepatic mass (found incidentally) and elevated α-fetoprotein levels. See next image.

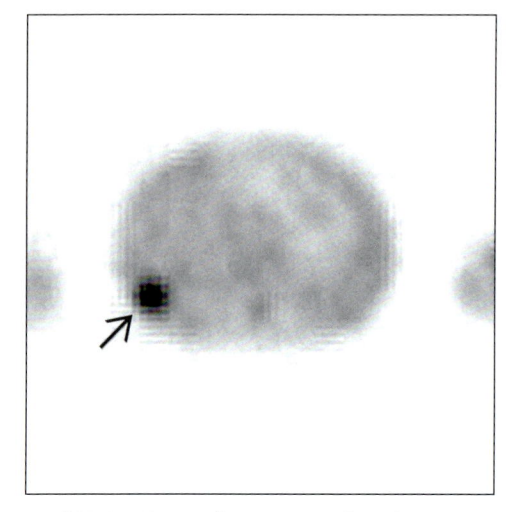

Axial FDG PET scan shows increased uptake in mass ➔ in right lobe of liver in neonate with small hepatic mass (found incidentally) and elevated α-fetoprotein level: Hepatoblastoma at surgery.

TERMINOLOGY

Definitions
- Malignant embryonic hepatic tumor composed of epithelial cells and occasionally a mixture of epithelial and mesenchymal cells

IMAGING FINDINGS

General Features
- Best diagnostic clue: Large, well-defined and heterogeneous liver mass in an infant
- Location: Liver: > 60% right lobe
- Size: Large, 10-12 cm
- Morphology
  - Tend to be well-defined masses; may be lobulated
  - Tend to displace rather than invade adjacent hepatic structures such as falciform ligament
  - Usually single contiguous mass; may be multifocal; rarely diffusely infiltrative
  - May be heterogeneous in consistency secondary to areas of hemorrhage or necrosis
  - In very large masses of questionable origin
  - Calcifications in 50%

Nuclear Medicine Findings
- PET
  - Hepatoblastoma is typically appreciably more hypermetabolic than normal background tissues
    - "Cutoff" standardized uptake value (SUV) has not been established for hepatoblastoma
  - FDG PET currently not approved for reimbursement of FDG PET by Committee on Medicare and Medicaid Services (CMS)
    - PET requires preauthorization for third party payment
  - Uses of FDG PET in hepatoblastoma
    - Initial staging
    - Evaluating response to treatment
    - Restaging for suspected recurrence: α-fetoprotein (+) or (-): Small areas of recurrent tumor may be difficult to evaluate by conventional imaging
  - When using FDG PET in hepatoblastoma, it is critical to understand potential pitfalls
    - Normal duodenal FDG activity: Mimic recurrence in porta hepatis or hepatoduodenal regions

DDx: FDG PET Mimics of Hepatoblastoma

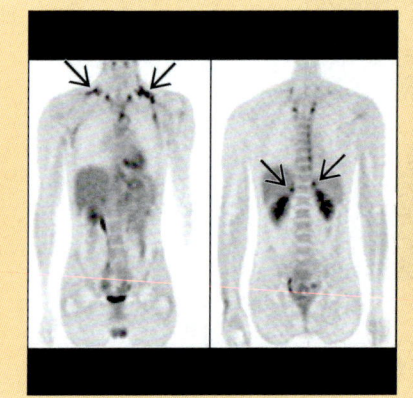

Hypermetabolic Brown Fat 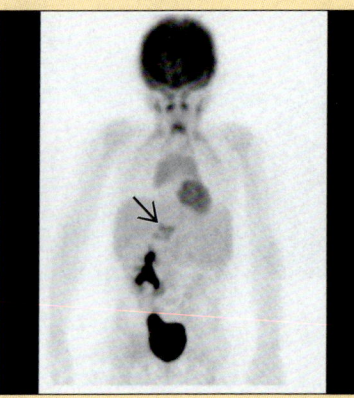 | Lymphoma-Renal Transplant Patient 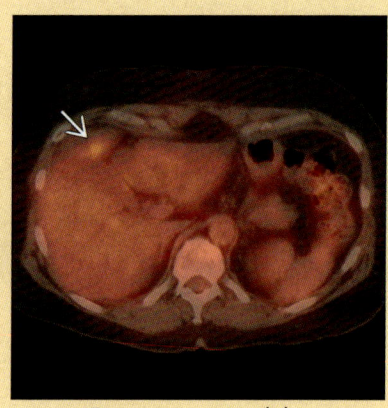 | Regenerating Nodule

HEPATOBLASTOMA

Key Facts

Terminology
- Malignant embryonic hepatic tumor composed of epithelial cells and occasionally a mixture of epithelial and mesenchymal cells

Imaging Findings
- Best diagnostic clue: Large, well-defined and heterogeneous liver mass in an infant
- Tend to be well-defined masses; may be lobulated
- Hepatoblastoma is typically appreciably more hypermetabolic than normal background tissues
- "Cutoff" standardized uptake value (SUV) has not been established for hepatoblastoma
- FDG PET currently not approved for reimbursement of FDG PET by Committee on Medicare and Medicaid Services (CMS)
- PET requires preauthorization for third party payment
- When using FDG PET in hepatoblastoma, it is critical to understand potential pitfalls
- Normal duodenal FDG activity: Mimic recurrence in porta hepatis or hepatoduodenal regions
- Areas of liver regeneration may be hypermetabolic and mimic tumor
- Hypermetabolic brown adipose tissue may surround adrenal glands, mimicking tumor involvement
- FDG PET/CT strongly recommended over conventional FDG PET: Precise anatomic localization of sites of uptake is critical
- CT in conjunction with PET should be high quality, standard CT with oral, IV contrast

---

- Areas of liver regeneration may be hypermetabolic and mimic tumor
- Hypermetabolic brown adipose tissue may surround adrenal glands, mimicking tumor involvement
- Bone Scan: Typically increased uptake in metastases

Radiographic Findings
- Radiography: Homogeneous soft tissue mass in right upper quadrant displacing bowel gas; ± dense, chunky calcification

CT Findings
- NECT
  - Well-defined, heterogeneous lesion predominantly hypoattenuating compared to normal liver parenchyma
  - As many as 50% of lesions have calcification
  - Mass typically large at presentation (10-12 cm)
- CECT
  - Mass typically well-defined, heterogeneous, may be lobulated
  - Enhancement: Nonuniform, < normal liver, occasionally peripheral rim
  - Coarse calcifications common, osseous matrix if mixed type
  - Metastatic disease is common: Lung, periaortic lymph nodes, brain (rare)

Angiographic Findings
- Vascular structures draped over, displaced by mass
- Mass with dense blush due to neovascularity; typically no arteriovenous shunting
- Unresectable if inferior vena cava (IVC) invasion

MR Findings
- T1WI: Low signal intensity; high signal if hemorrhage
- T2WI
  - Signal on T2WI typically high but variable secondary to amounts of hemorrhage and necrosis
  - May have hypointense fibrous bands
- T1 C+: Heterogeneous enhancement

Ultrasonographic Findings
- Grayscale Ultrasound
  - Well-defined, solid mass
  - Spoked-wheel appearance: Fibrous septa
  - Heterogeneous echogenicity: Hemorrhage/necrosis
  - Acoustic shadowing: Calcifications
  - Cystic areas: Necrosis, extramedullary hematopoiesis
- Color Doppler: Mass typically hypervascular on Doppler sonography

Imaging Recommendations
- Best imaging tool
  - Initial evaluation: Ultrasound
  - MR or CT as definitive imaging study: Controversial
  - FDG PET/CT for difficult cases
- Protocol advice
  - Major goal of imaging: To define anatomic extent of disease, relationship to hepatic lobar anatomy for
    - Critical to pre-operative planning/monitor response to chemotherapy
  - FDG PET/CT strongly recommended over conventional FDG PET: Precise anatomic localization of sites of uptake is critical
    - CT in conjunction with PET should be high quality, standard CT with oral, IV contrast
    - Patient should be kept very warm before and after injection of FDG to prevent hypermetabolic brown adipose tissue
    - Every attempt should be made to minimize causes of discomfort and crying to reduce muscle FDG uptake
    - Tc-99m sulfur colloid or Choletec: Uptake in areas of hepatic regeneration helps exclude tumor recurrence

DIFFERENTIAL DIAGNOSIS

Hemangioendothelioma
- Presentation with congestive heart failure or thrombocytopenia; prominent vascular structures; negative serum α-fetoprotein

HEPATOBLASTOMA

Neuroblastoma Metastasis
- Usually multiple liver masses or diffuse liver heterogeneity; adrenal mass typically present

Mesenchymal Hamartoma
- Well-defined, multilobulated, cystic mass

Hepatocellular Carcinoma
- Most common hepatic malignancy in children > 5 yrs of age, rarely < 3 yrs

Hepatic Regeneration
- May mimic recurrent tumor on FDG PET; Tc-99m Choletec or sulfur colloid may show increased uptake

PATHOLOGY

General Features
- General path comments: Well-defined borders with pseudocapsule; usually no history of underlying liver disease; positive serum α-fetoprotein
- Genetics
  - May be familial
  - Short arm chromosome 11: Similar to rhabdomyosarcoma and Wilms tumor
- Etiology: Congenital hepatic malignancy
- Epidemiology
  - Hepatic masses constitute only 5-6% of all intraabdominal masses in children
  - Primary hepatic neoplasms are 0.5-2% of all pediatric malignancies
  - 3rd most common abdominal malignancy: After neuroblastoma and Wilms tumor
  - Most common primary liver tumor of childhood (43% of liver masses)
  - Most common hepatic malignancy in children
- Associated abnormalities: Predisposing conditions: Beckwith-Wiedemann syndrome, hemihypertrophy, familial polyposis coli, Gardner syndrome, fetal alcohol syndrome, Wilms tumor, biliary atresia

Gross Pathologic & Surgical Features
- Fleshy, nodular lesion, fibrous bands throughout (reason for spoked-wheel appearance), areas of necrosis or hemorrhage

Microscopic Features
- Epithelial types: Fetal; embryonal; macrotrabecular; small cell
- Mixed type with epithelial and foci of mesenchymal cells: Cartilage, muscle, fibrous tissue, osteoid may be present

CLINICAL ISSUES

Presentation
- Most common signs/symptoms: Painless abdominal mass; hepatomegaly
- Other signs/symptoms
  - Nonspecific: Weight loss, nausea, vomiting, anemia
  - Usually no history of underlying liver disease
  - May be present at birth; most commonly < 3 yrs
  - ↑ α-fetoprotein in > 90% of patients
  - Precocious puberty

Demographics
- Age
  - Most common in infants
  - Range: Newborn to 15 yrs; peak 1-2 yrs
- Gender: 2:1 = M:F predilection

Natural History & Prognosis
- Overall survival rate 63-67%: Better prognosis for epithelial than mixed type
- Better prognosis than hepatoma
- 60% of lesions resectable

Treatment
- Chemotherapy: Neoadjuvant improves resectability
- Surgical resection
- Boiled Ethiodol and chemotherapy embolization
- Radiofrequency ablation
- Liver transplantation for nonresectable tumor

DIAGNOSTIC CHECKLIST

Consider
- FDG PET for staging, restaging, evaluating response to treatment in difficult cases

Image Interpretation Pearls
- Classic imaging appearance: Large, well-defined and heterogeneous liver mass in an infant
- Include CT of chest for evidence of metastatic disease during initial CT evaluation
- Note if IVC invasion

SELECTED REFERENCES

1. Mody RJ et al: FDG PET for the study of primary hepatic malignancies in children. Pediatr Blood Cancer. 47(1):51-5, 2006
2. Figarola MS et al: Recurrent hepatoblastoma with localization by PET-CT. Pediatr Radiol. 35(12):1254-8, 2005
3. Philip I et al: Positron emission tomography in recurrent hepatoblastoma. Pediatr Surg Int. 21(5):341-5, 2005
4. Woodward PJ et al: From the archives of the AFIP: a comprehensive review of fetal tumors with pathologic correlation. Radiographics. 25(1):215-42, 2005
5. Albrecht S et al: Allelic loss but absence of mutations in the polyspecific transporter gene BWR1A on 11p15.5 in hepatoblastoma. Int J Cancer. 111(4):627-32, 2004
6. Alobaidi M et al: Malignant cystic and necrotic liver lesions: a pattern approach to discrimination. Curr Probl Diagn Radiol. 33(6):254-68, 2004
7. Fiegel HC et al: Stem-like cells in human hepatoblastoma. J Histochem Cytochem. 52(11):1495-501, 2004
8. Hemming AW et al: Combined resection of the liver and inferior vena cava for hepatic malignancy. Ann Surg. 239(5):712-9; discussion 719-21, 2004
9. Wong KK et al: The use of positron emission tomography in detecting hepatoblastoma recurrence--a cautionary tale. J Pediatr Surg. 39(12):1779-81, 2004
10. Donnelly LF et al: Pediatric hepatic imaging. Radiol Clin North Am. 36(2):413-27, 1998
11. Boechat MI et al: Primary liver tumors in children: comparison of CT and MR imaging. Radiology. 169(3):727-32, 1988

HEPATOBLASTOMA

IMAGE GALLERY

Typical

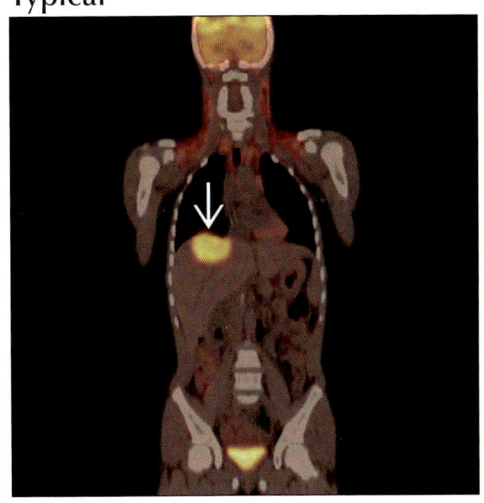

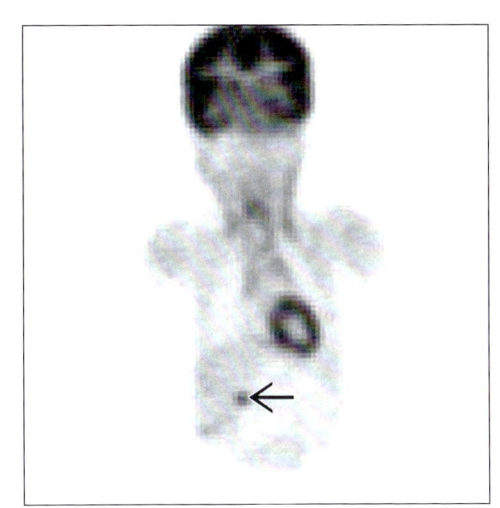

(Left) Coronal FDG PET/CT in 12 year old with hypermetabolic mass ➔ in dome of the liver: Hepatoblastoma found at surgery. *(Right)* Coronal FDG PET in 4 year old s/p resection of lateral segment of left lobe of liver for hepatoblastoma, rising α-fetoprotein level and negative CT. Focal increased uptake ➔ suggests recurrence. See next 2 images.

Typical

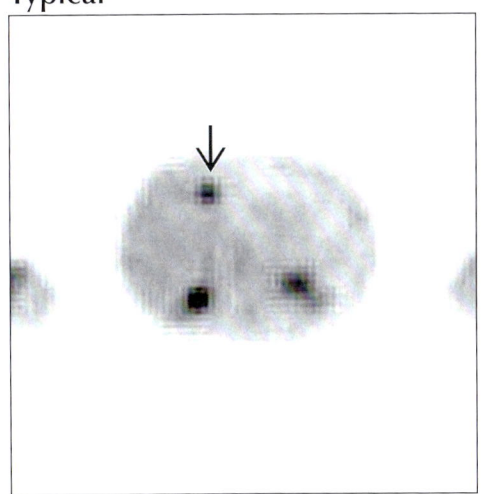

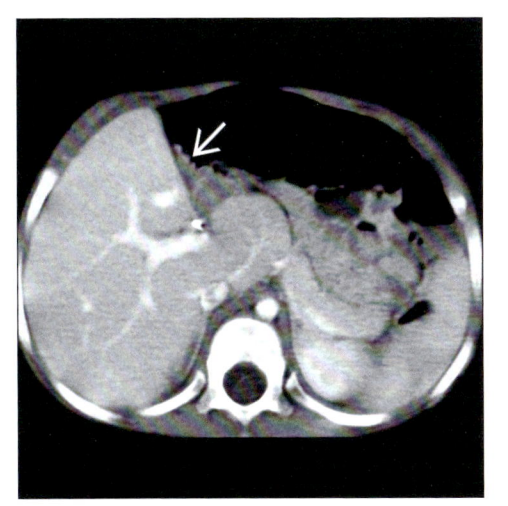

(Left) Axial FDG PET shows focal increased uptake ➔ along left margin of resected liver, suggesting recurrence. See next image. *(Right)* Same as previous 2 images. CT in 4 year old with focal FDG uptake along left margin of resected liver. CT suggested duodenum, but at surgery, small focus of recurrent hepatoblastoma ➔ was identified and removed.

Typical

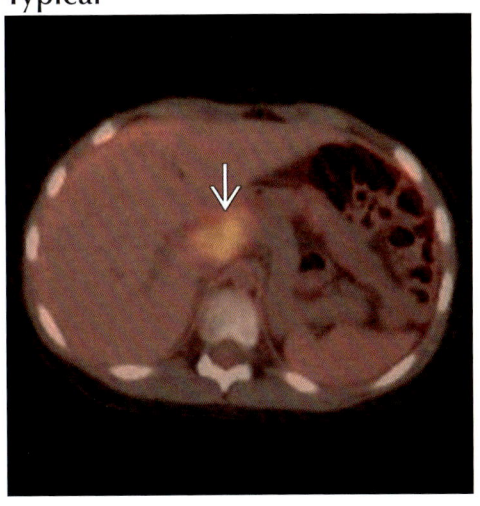

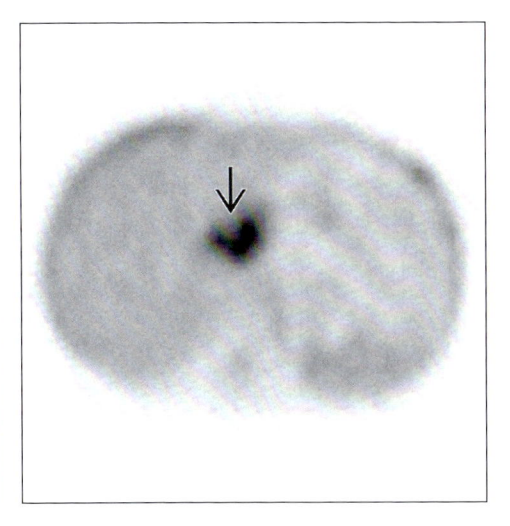

(Left) Axial FDG PET in patient with past history of hepatoblastoma resected from dome of liver shows hypermetabolic mass ➔ in periportal region. See next image. *(Right)* Axial FDG PET in patient with past history of hepatoblastoma resected from dome of liver shows hypermetabolic mass ➔ in periportal region. At surgery, nodal recurrence of hepatoblastoma was found.

HEPATOCELLULAR CARCINOMA

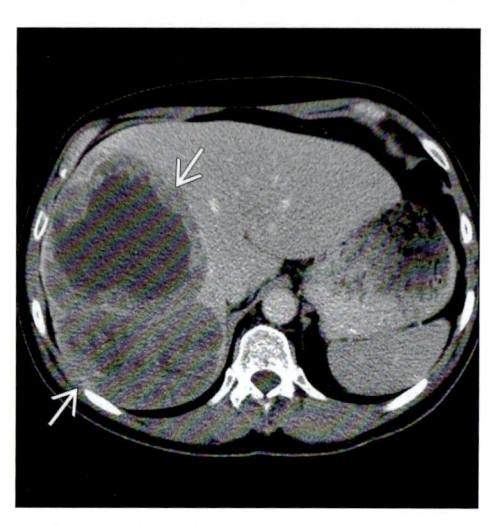

Axial CECT shows large heterogeneously enhancing masses ➡ with central necrosis, proven at biopsy to be hepatocellular carcinoma. See next image.

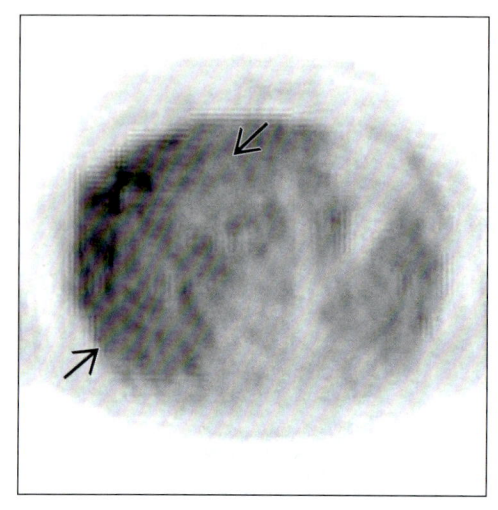

Axial FDG PET in same patient as previous image shows large hepatic masses ➡ to be isometabolic to normal portions of the liver, typical for more clearly-differentiated hepatocellular carcinomas.

TERMINOLOGY

Abbreviations and Synonyms
- Hepatocellular carcinoma (HCC); hepatoma or primary liver cancer; alpha-fetoprotein (AFP); liver transplantation (LT)

Definitions
- Most common primary malignant liver tumor usually arising in cirrhotic liver due to chronic viral hepatitis (HBV/HCV) or alcoholism

IMAGING FINDINGS

General Features
- Best diagnostic clue
  - CECT/MR: Large heterogeneous hypervascular mass with portal vein invasion
  - FDG PET
    - Well-differentiated-iso-/hypometabolic relative to normal liver
    - High grade undifferentiated-hypermetabolic
- Location
  - Most often right lobe of liver (solitary)
  - Both hepatic lobes (multicentric small nodular)
  - Throughout liver in a diffuse manner
- Size
  - Small (< 3 cm) to > 5 cm
  - Diffuse/cirrhotomimetic: < 1 cm to few cm
- Key concepts
  - Most frequent primary visceral malignancy in world
    - Accounts 80-90% of all primary liver malignancies
  - 2nd most common malignant liver tumor in children after hepatoblastoma
  - Growth patterns of HCC: Solitary, multifocal, diffuse
  - Fibrolamellar subtype
    - Typically arises within normal liver
    - Distinct imaging and histologic characteristics from typical HCC

Nuclear Medicine Findings
- PET
  - Variable FDG avidity; low general sensitivity 50% (compared to 90% for CT)
    - Well-differentiated tumors may be similar to normal liver

DDx: Hepatic Lesions

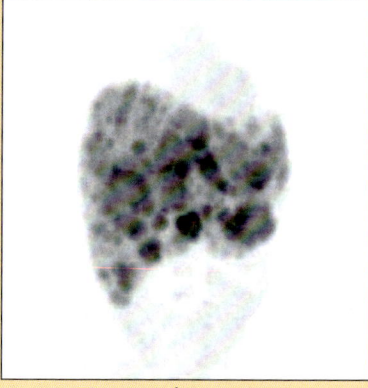

| Carcinoid Tumor PET | Mucinous Adenocarcinoma PET | Hemangiomas PET/CT |

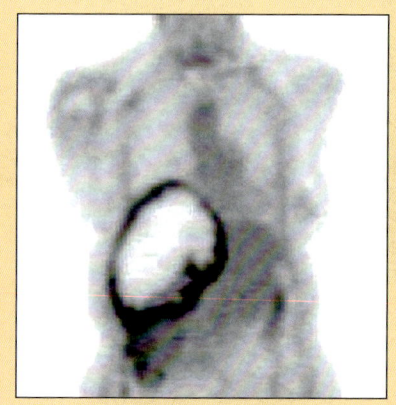

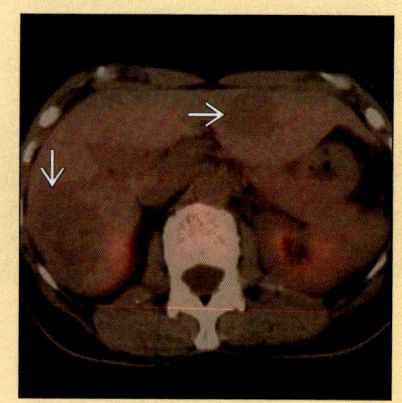

HEPATOCELLULAR CARCINOMA

Key Facts

Terminology
- Most common primary malignant liver tumor usually arising in cirrhotic liver due to chronic viral hepatitis (HBV/HCV) or alcoholism

Imaging Findings
- CECT/MR: Large heterogeneous hypervascular mass with portal vein invasion
- Variable FDG avidity; low general sensitivity 50% (compared to 90% for CT)
- Well-differentiated tumors may be similar to normal liver
- High positive rate FDG accumulation in high grade HCC and markedly elevated AFP

Top Differential Diagnoses
- Cholangiocarcinoma (Peripheral)
- Nodular Regenerative Hyperplasia
- Hypervascular Metastases
- Focal Nodular Hyperplasia
- Small Hepatic Hemangioma

Pathology
- Cirrhosis (60-90%): Chronic viral hepatitis or alcoholism

Clinical Issues
- Clinical Profile: Elderly patient with history of cirrhosis, ascites, weight loss, RUQ pain & ↑ AFP

Diagnostic Checklist
- FDG PET: HCC may be similar to normal liver in appearance
- Regenerating liver may be hypermetabolic on FDG PET

  - Higher grade tumors more metabolically active: Tumor:liver ratio > 2:1
  - FDG metabolism in HCC often less than in areas of regenerating normal liver
 - FDG PET useful for detecting extrahepatic metastases: Pre-operative assessment for LT candidacy
 - High positive rate FDG accumulation in high grade HCC and markedly elevated AFP
   - Potential pre-operative tool for estimating post-LT recurrence
 - C-11 or F-18 choline may show better performance than FDG for HCC: Investigational
- Hepatobiliary scan
 - Uptake of IDA derivatives in 50% of HCC lesions
- Tc-99m sulfur colloid liver-spleen scan
 - HCC in a cirrhotic liver: Seen as a cold defect
 - HCC in a noncirrhotic liver: Heterogeneous uptake
- Ga-67 scan
 - HCC is Ga-67 avid in 80-90% of cases: Lower in diffuse HCC 2° cirrhosis, chronic hepatitis

CT Findings
- NECT
 - In noncirrhotic liver
   - Large hypodense mass; ± necrosis, fat, calcification; solitary or multifocal
   - Encapsulated HCC: Well-defined, rounded, hypodense mass
 - In cirrhotic liver: Iso-/hypodense mass with cirrhotic liver, ascites and varices
- CECT
 - Hepatic arterial phase (HAP) scan: Heterogeneous enhancement
   - Wedge-shaped areas ↑ density on HAP: Perfusion abnormality due to portal vein occlusion by tumor thrombus & increased arterial flow
 - Portal venous phase (PVP) scan: Decreased attenuation with heterogeneous areas of contrast accumulation
 - Delayed scan: Hypodense to surrounding liver
 - Small hypervascular HCC
   - Early & late arterial phases: Hyperattenuating, more on late phase
   - CT during arterial portography: No enhancement

Angiographic Findings
- Conventional: Hypervascular tumor with AV shunting and portal vein invasion

MR Findings
- Variable intensity and enhancement depending on degree of fatty change, fibrosis, necrosis, presence of cirrhosis

Ultrasonographic Findings
- Grayscale Ultrasound
 - Mixed echogenicity due to tumor necrosis, hypervascularity, presence of fat
 - Small hyperechoic HCC simulate hemangioma

Imaging Recommendations
- Best imaging tool: CECT: 90% sensitivity
- Protocol advice: SPECT imaging improves contrast resolution, so that sensitivity for small lesions increased
- Helical triphasic CT (NE, arterial & venous phases) or MR & CEMR; angiography

DIFFERENTIAL DIAGNOSIS

Cholangiocarcinoma (Peripheral)
- May obstruct bile ducts; capsular retraction; volume loss
- Delayed enhancement on CECT; hypermetabolic on FDG PET

Nodular Regenerative Hyperplasia
- Large regenerative nodules: 1-4 cm
- Small nodules: Not detectable
- Large nodules: Homogeneously hypervascular on CECT
- Moderately hypermetabolic on FDG PET

HEPATOCELLULAR CARCINOMA

Hypervascular Metastases
- Mimic small nodular or multifocal HCC
- Less likely to invade portal vein
- Degree of FDG uptake depends on histology of primary lesion

Focal Nodular Hyperplasia
- Homogeneous hypervascular mass with central scar
- On nonenhanced & delayed CECT & CEMR almost isodense/isointense to liver
- Tc99m sulfur colloid: 70% iso- to increased uptake; 30% cold defect
- FDG PET: Variable uptake (↑ to ↓, compared to normal liver)

Small Hepatic Hemangioma
- Well-defined, spherical mass isodense to blood
- CECT: "Flash filling" (isodense to blood); US: Usually hyperechoic
- Angiography: "Cotton wool" appearance
- Tc-99m RBC: ↑ Uptake; FDG PET: Isometabolic to liver

PATHOLOGY

General Features
- General path comments
  - Soft tumor; may have necrosis & hemorrhage
  - Invasion: Vascular (common) & biliary (uncommon)
  - Clear cell carcinoma: HCC with large amounts of fat
- Genetics: HBV DNA integrated into host's genomic DNA in tumor cells
- Etiology
  - Cirrhosis (60-90%): Chronic viral hepatitis or alcoholism
  - Carcinogens: Aflatoxins, siderosis, thorotrast, androgens
  - α-1-antitrypsin deficiency, hemochromatosis
  - Wilson disease, tyrosinosis
- Epidemiology
  - High incidence: Africa & Asia (HBV & aflatoxins)
  - Low incidence: Western hemisphere
  - Worldwide highest incidence is in Japan (4.8%)
  - HCC in cirrhosis due to hepatitis C virus
    - United States: 30-50% of cases of HCC
    - Japan: 70% of cases of HCC
  - North America: 40% of HCC in non-cirrhotic livers

Gross Pathologic & Surgical Features
- Solitary, nodular or multifocal, diffuse, encapsulated
- Soft tumor with or without necrosis, hemorrhage, calcification, fat, vascular invasion

Microscopic Features
- Histologic appearances: Solid (cellular) or acinar
- Increased fat & glycogen in cytoplasm

CLINICAL ISSUES

Presentation
- Clinical Profile: Elderly patient with history of cirrhosis, ascites, weight loss, RUQ pain & ↑ AFP
- Lab data: Increased alpha-fetoprotein (AFP) & LFTs
- Diagnosis: Biopsy & histology

Demographics
- Age
  - Low incidence areas: 6th-7th decade
  - High incidence areas: 30-45 years
- Gender
  - Low incidence areas (M:F = 2.5:1)
  - High incidence areas (M:F = 8:1)

Natural History & Prognosis
- Complications
  - Spontaneous rupture & massive hemoperitoneum
- Prognosis
  - More than 90% mortality rate; 17% resectability rate
  - 6 Months average survival time; 30% 5 year survival

Treatment
- Radiofrequency & alcohol ablation: Small isolated tumors
- Intraarterial chemoembolization: Multifocal unresectable tumor
- Surgical resection: Limited by inadequate hepatic reserve
- Intra hepatic arterial Y-90 microspheres (TheraSphere, SIRSphere)
- Liver transplantation: Lower grade lesions, unresectable, no metastases

DIAGNOSTIC CHECKLIST

Image Interpretation Pearls
- HCC: Hypervascular mass invading portal vein
- Small HCC may mimic hemangioma or metastasis in cirrhosis
- FDG PET: HCC may be similar to normal liver in appearance
- Regenerating liver may be hypermetabolic on FDG PET

SELECTED REFERENCES

1. Yang SH et al: The role of (18)F-FDG-PET imaging for the selection of liver transplantation candidates among hepatocellular carcinoma patients. Liver Transpl, 2006
2. Chen YK et al: Utility of FDG-PET for investigating unexplained serum AFP elevation in patients with suspected hepatocellular carcinoma recurrence. Anticancer Res. 25(6C):4719-25, 2005
3. Carr BI: Hepatic arterial 90Yttrium glass microspheres (Theraphere) for unresectable hepatocellular carcinoma: interim safety and survival data on 65 patients. Liver Transpl. 10(2 Suppl 1):S107-10, 2004
4. Kashiwagi T: FDG-PET and hepatocellular carcinoma. J Gastroenterol. 39(10):1017-8, 2004
5. Laghi A et al: Hepatocellular carcinoma: detection with triple-phase multi-detector row helical CT in patients with chronic hepatitis. Radiology. 226(2):543-9, 2003
6. Murakami T et al: Hypervascular hepatocellular carcinoma: detection with double arterial phase multi-detector row helical CT. Radiology. 218(3):763-7, 2001
7. Peterson MS et al: Pretransplantation surveillance for possible hepatocellular carcinoma in patients with cirrhosis: epidemiology and CT-based tumor detection rate in 430 cases with surgical pathologic correlation. Radiology. 217(3):743-9, 2000

HEPATOCELLULAR CARCINOMA

IMAGE GALLERY

Typical

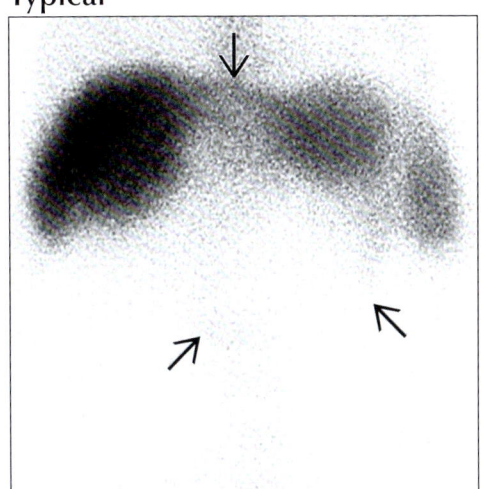

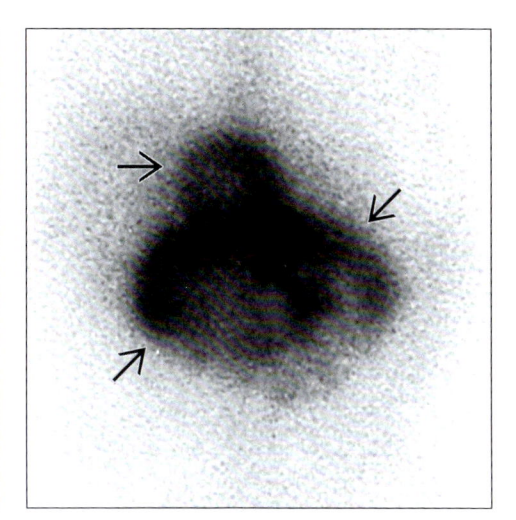

(Left) Anterior Tc-99m sulfur colloid liver spleen scan shows photopenic lesion in left lobe of liver with faint inferior rim of normal tissue ➔. See next image. (Right) Anterior Ga-67 scan of upper abdomen (same patient as previous image) shows hepatic mass ➔ to be intensely gallium-avid, typical in appearance for HCC.

Typical

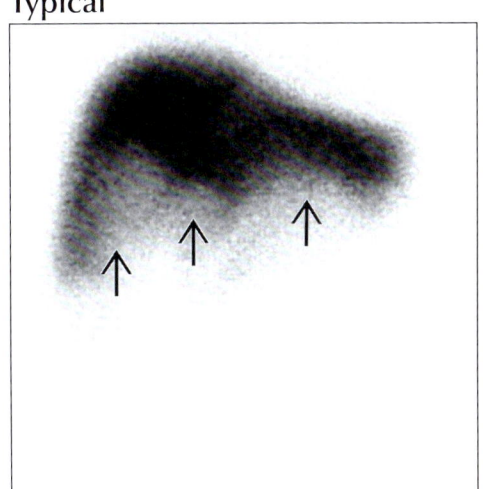

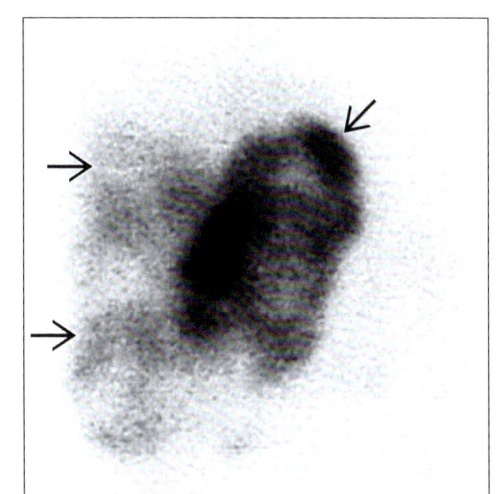

(Left) Anterior Tc-99m sulfur colloid scan of upper abdomen shows notched inferior margin of the liver ➔ in patient with large abdominal mass. See next image. (Right) Anterior Ga-67 scan of upper abdomen in same patient as previous image shows a large heterogeneous gallium-avid mass in the right upper quadrant conforming to the Tc-99m SC defect ➔, consistent with hepatoma.

Typical

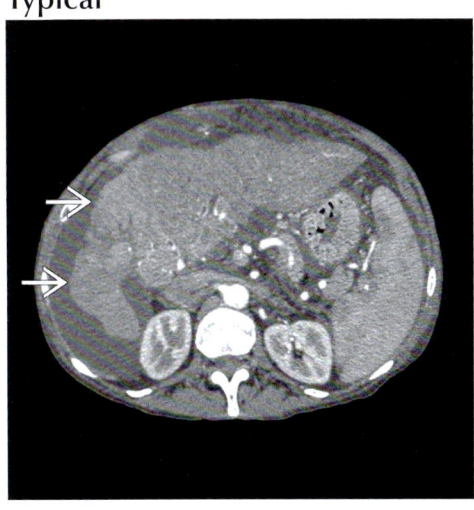

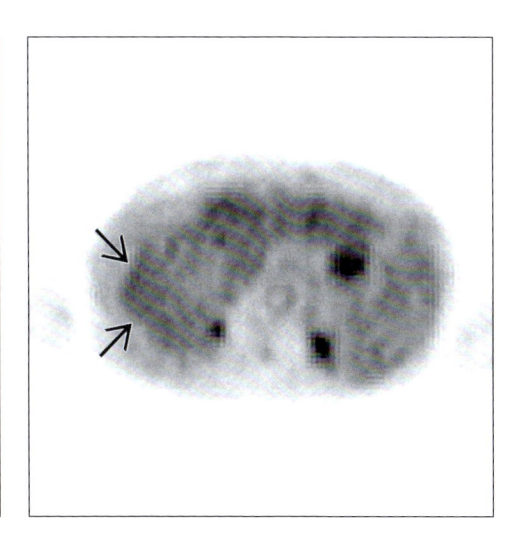

(Left) Axial CECT of the upper abdomen in a patient with severe cirrhosis and ascites shows relative enhancement of right lobe ➔ of liver (autopsy-proven diffuse HCC). (Right) Axial FDG PET at same level as previous CT image shows subtle inhomogeneity in metabolism within the liver but no distinct region of hypermetabolism in patient with diffuse HCC of right lobe of liver ➔.

HEPATOCELLULAR CARCINOMA

(Left) Axial CECT of upper abdomen shows patchy geographic area of enhancement ➡ in patient with moderately well-differentiated HCC. Pretreatment scan. See next 5 images. (Right) Pretreatment axial FDG PET shows only vague hypermetabolism in region of HCC ➡, typical of well differentiated HCC.

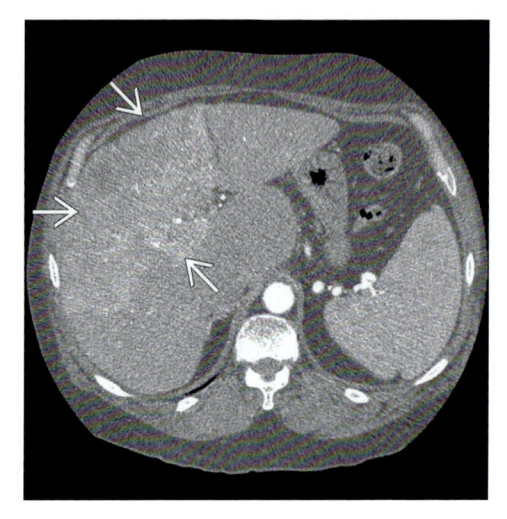

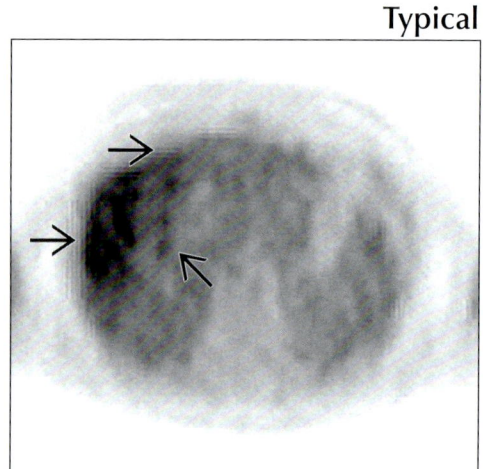

(Left) Pretreatment coronal FDG PET shows only vague hypermetabolism in region of HCC ➡, compared to normal liver ⊳, typical of well differentiated HCC. (Right) Coronal repeat FDG PET, following intra hepatic arterial Y-90 microsphere treatment, shows focal increased uptake in the liver ➡.

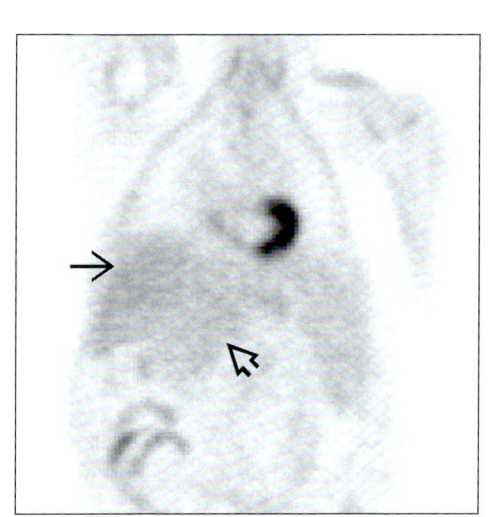

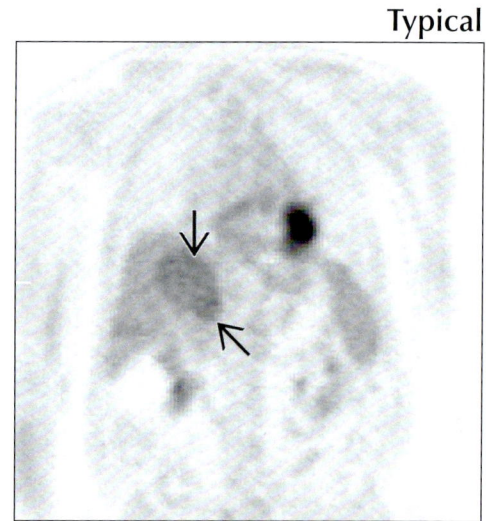

(Left) Post Y-90 FDG PET (axial image) shows focal region of increased uptake in caudate lobe of liver ➡ (previously not involved with HCC). (Right) Post Y-90 microsphere CT of the liver shows enlargement of caudate lobe (increased uptake on FDG PET), biopsy proven regenerating liver. Right and medial segment left lobe smaller with patchy enhancement, biopsy proven fibrosis.

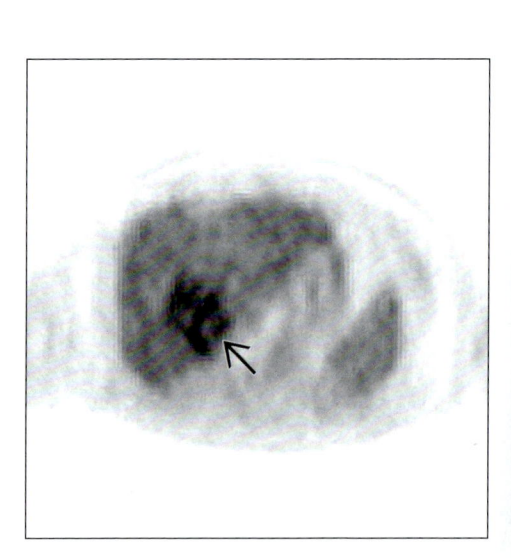

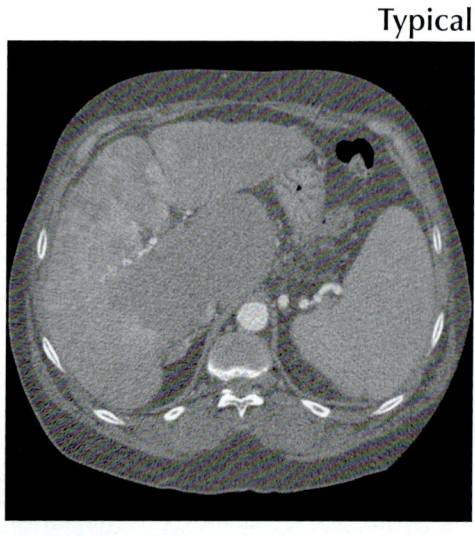

HEPATOCELLULAR CARCINOMA

Variant

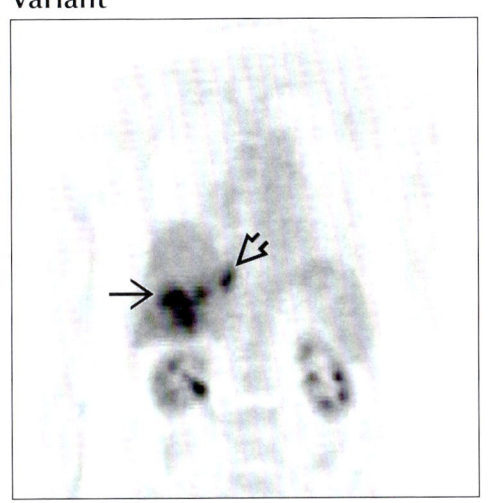

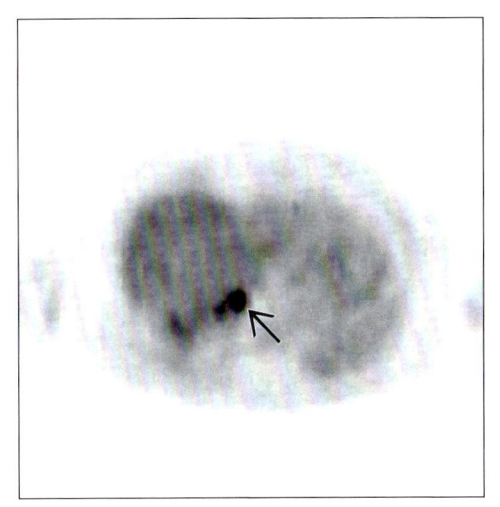

(Left) Coronal FDG PET shows patchy hypermetabolism in liver in patient with moderate-to-poorly differentiated HCC ➔. Superomedial site of uptake was tumor thrombus in IVC ➔. See next image. *(Right)* Same patient as previous image. Axial FDG PET in patient with HCC shows focal uptake along posteromedial aspect of liver, proven to be tumor thrombus in IVC ➔.

Typical

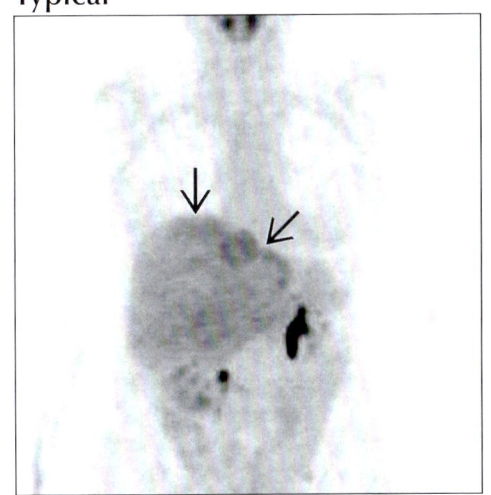

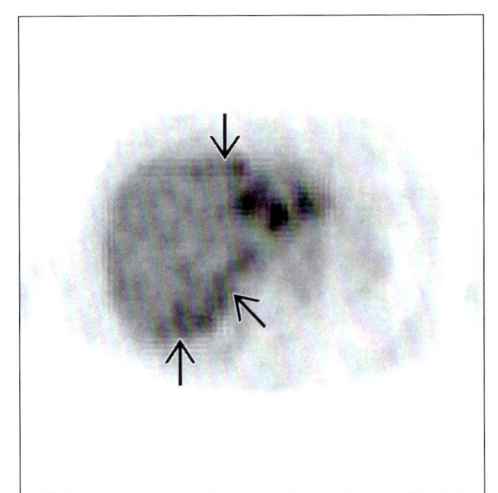

(Left) FDG PET MIP image in patient with well-differentiated HCC replacing right lobe of liver shows rim of increased metabolism ➔ (relative to HCC) in rim of normal liver surrounding mass. See next image. *(Right)* Same patient as previous image. Axial FDG PET shows relative increase in metabolism in rim of normal liver ➔ surrounding large HCC replacing right lobe of liver.

Variant

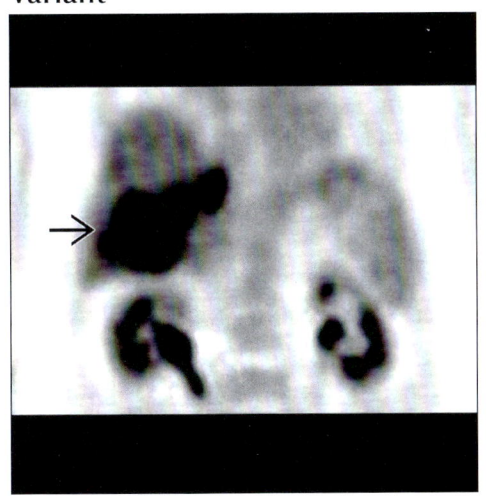

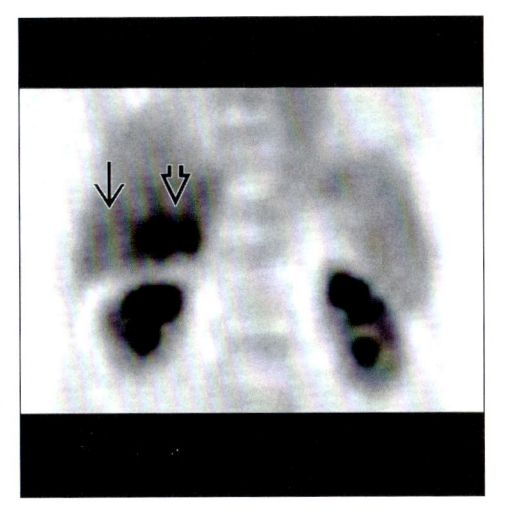

(Left) Coronal FDG PET shows intensely hypermetabolic mass ➔ in liver, consistent with high grade HCC. Scan was performed prior to Y-90 microsphere treatment. See next image. *(Right)* Coronal FDG PET following Y-90 microsphere treatment (same patient as previous image) shows decrease in a large portion of the previous hypermetabolic mass ➔, but one site remains metabolically active ➔, suggesting residual viable tumor.

CAVERNOUS HEMANGIOMAS

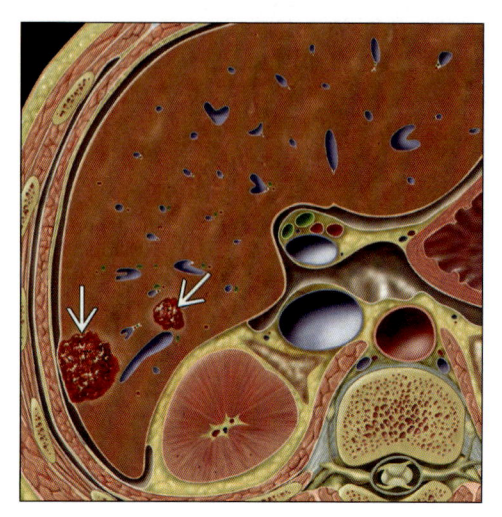

Graphic shows nonencapsulated collections of blood ➔ in enlarged sinusoidal spaces, characteristic of CH.

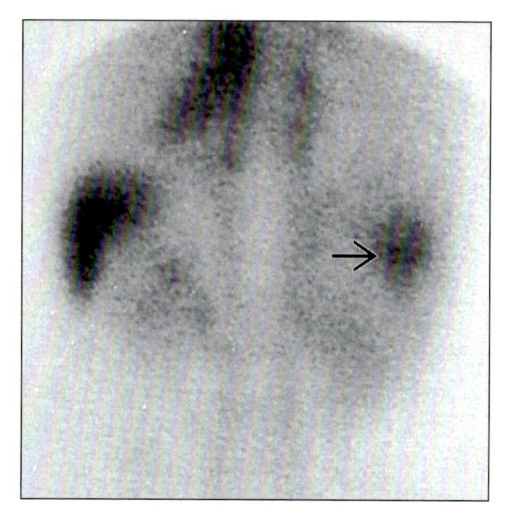

Posterior Tc-99m RBC scintigraphy shows persistent tracer in superior right hepatic lobe ➔ on delayed imaging, consistent with CH.

TERMINOLOGY

Abbreviations and Synonyms
- Cavernous hemangioma (CH)
- Hepatic cavernous hemangioma
- Capillary hemangioma (small lesion)
- Giant hemangioma (large lesion)

Definitions
- Multiple sinusoidal vascular structures lined by single-layer endothelial cells embedded in thin fibrous septations

IMAGING FINDINGS

General Features
- Best diagnostic clue
  - Lesion that displays slow filling on Tc-99m labeled red blood cell (RBC) scan
    - Sluggish blood flow delays visualization
  - CECT/MR: Slow filling by contrast; larger lesions may show "dot-dash" peripheral nodular enhancement with progressive centripetal enhancement
  - Small lesions typically have uniform filling on delayed imaging
- Location: Throughout liver, occasionally pedunculated
- Size
  - < 1 cm to > 20 cm
    - Giant CH variably defined as ≥ 4-10 cm
- Morphology
  - Spherical, ellipsoid, well-circumscribed vascular lesion
  - Up to 50% of patients have multiple lesions
  - Can demonstrate slow growth

Nuclear Medicine Findings
- Tc-99m RBC scan: Most useful nuclear medicine imaging strategy
  - Initially photopenic, slow visualization, with subsequent filling by 2 hrs as RBCs slowly replace pooled blood in dilated sinusoids
  - Filling typically uniform or progressive from peripheral to central but can be opposite

DDx: Hepatic Lesions on Tc-99m RBC Scan

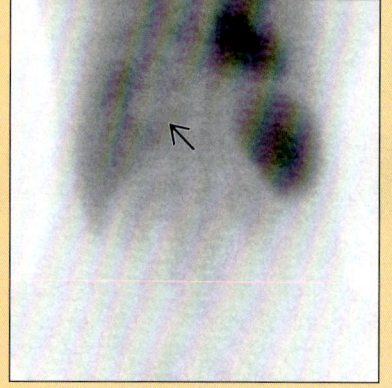

Hepatic Adenoma

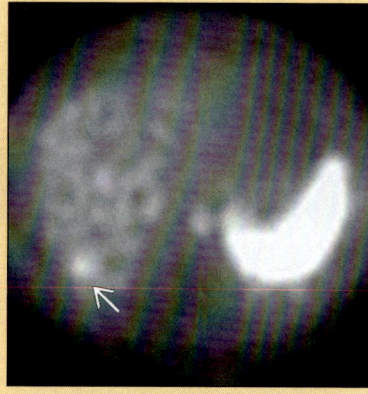

Cavernous Hemangioma

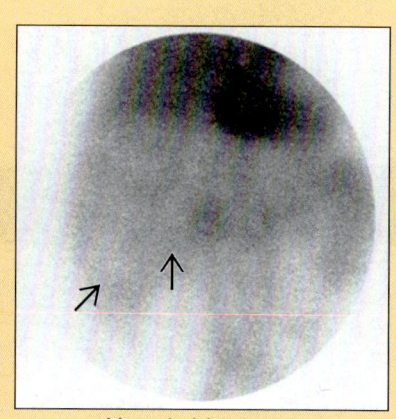

Hepatic Metastases

CAVERNOUS HEMANGIOMAS

Key Facts

Imaging Findings
- Tc-99m RBC scan: Most useful nuclear medicine imaging strategy
- Initially photopenic, slow visualization, with subsequent filling by 2 hrs as RBCs slowly replace pooled blood in dilated sinusoids
- Filling typically uniform or progressive from peripheral to central but can be opposite
- On delayed imaging: Tc-99m RBCs in CH more intense than adjacent hepatic parenchyma
- Limits of resolution on Tc-99m RBC scan 1-2 cm
- Specificity ~ 99% in larger lesions
- False positives very rare
- 20-25 mCi (740-925 MBq) Tc-99m pertechnetate
- Whole blood labeling kit to tag Tc-99m to RBCs in vitro
- SPECT useful for 3D visualization and localization
- Many lesions initially identified incidentally by other modalities: CT, MR, US

Clinical Issues
- Typical appearance requires no further imaging unless clinically indicated
- Important to correctly identify CH with noninvasive imaging to avoid complications of biopsy (hemorrhage)

Diagnostic Checklist
- Tc-99m RBC scan in cases not characteristic of hemangioma by conventional imaging
- Tc-99m RBC scan particularly useful with larger CH: Heterogeneous appearance can confound CECT/MR interpretation

---

  - On delayed imaging: Tc-99m RBCs in CH more intense than adjacent hepatic parenchyma
  - Limits of resolution on Tc-99m RBC scan 1-2 cm
  - Specificity ~ 99% in larger lesions
  - False positives very rare
- Tc-99m sulfur colloid (SC) scan
  - CH is photopenic (nonspecific)
- Tc-99m hepatobiliary scintigraphy
  - CH is photopenic (nonspecific)

Imaging Recommendations
- Best imaging tool
  - Tc-99m RBC scan useful in cases atypical on conventional imaging
  - Ultrasound (US) usually first line modality
    - Limited sensitivity, nonspecific
  - CECT or contrast-enhanced MR with liver mass protocol (3 phase)
    - Strict CT criteria (isodense by 30 min) has limited sensitivity (~ 55%)
    - CECT criteria: Hypodense pre-contrast, peripheral filling early post-contrast, progressive central filling delayed post-contrast, homogeneous isodensity to hepatic parenchyma 15-30 min post-contrast
    - MR: Bright T2WI, not as specific as Tc-99m RBC with SPECT, but better resolution for lesions less than 1-2 cm
- Protocol advice
  - 20-25 mCi (740-925 MBq) Tc-99m pertechnetate
  - Whole blood labeling kit to tag Tc-99m to RBCs in vitro
  - 1-2 second vascular phase planar acquisitions over 1 min coincident with bolus injection, anterior projection
  - Immediate anterior static image, additional projections as needed
  - Imaging to 2 hrs allows hepatic clearance, demonstrates persistent pooling in CH
  - SPECT useful for 3D visualization and localization
- Correlative imaging features
  - Many lesions initially identified incidentally by other modalities: CT, MR, US
  - Larger lesions prone to areas of thrombosis, fibrosis: Causes heterogeneous appearance, confounds CECT or MR interpretation

DIFFERENTIAL DIAGNOSIS

Primary Hepatic Neoplasm, Hepatoma
- Irregular or central scars and radiating septae
- Absent or ↓ accumulation of Tc-99m SC
- Associated with secondary signs of malignancy: Additional lesions, adenopathy, local invasion, calcifications, metastases

Focal Nodular Hyperplasia
- Tc-99m SC scan
  - Iso- to hyperintense relative to normal hepatic parenchyma
- Tc-99m hepatobiliary scan
  - Iso- to hyperintense to normal hepatic parenchyma
  - Delayed clearance in ≤ 80%

Hypervascular Metastatic Disease
- Frequently multiple
- Hypointense to liver parenchyma on portal phase CECT or CEMR
- Known primary lesion or other metastatic foci
- More common with advanced age

Regenerative Nodule
- Cirrhosis: Macroregenerative, degenerative nodule
  - Hemangiomas uncommon in cirrhotic liver

Treated Metastases
- Frequently multiple lesions with clinical history
- Can show central necrosis with peripheral enhancement/tracer accumulation
  - Fail to fill centrally on CECT
  - Do not show delayed hyperintensity relative to adjacent hepatic parenchyma on Tc-99m RBC scan

Hepatic Adenoma
- Absence of dilated sinusoids, therefore no delayed hyperintensity relative to liver

CAVERNOUS HEMANGIOMAS

- Frequently larger, average 8-10 cm
- No central scar
- More inclined to hemorrhage
- Associated with oral contraceptive use in younger women
- Typically photopenic by Tc-99m hepatobiliary scan despite presence of hepatocytes
- Kupffer cells normal or ↓; do not effectively accumulate Tc-99m SC (photopenic)

Intrahepatic Cholangiocarcinoma
- May be locally aggressive or invasive

PATHOLOGY

General Features
- Etiology: Not clearly established
- Epidemiology
  - Most common benign liver tumor
    - Up to 20% of population
    - Increases with multiparity
- Associated abnormalities
  - Focal nodular hyperplasia
  - Osler-Weber-Rendu

Microscopic Features
- Ectatic vascular channels lined by single-layer endothelium interleaved with webs of collagenous fibrous sheets
- Bile ducts absent

CLINICAL ISSUES

Presentation
- Most common signs/symptoms: Usually asymptomatic; typically discovered incidentally
- Other signs/symptoms: Pain (mass effect on adjacent structures), thrombosis, hemorrhage

Demographics
- Age
  - Incidence ↑ with age, especially multiparous, postmenopausal women
  - Rare in children
- Gender: M:F = 1:5

Natural History & Prognosis
- Good, rarely requires further evaluation, usually stable or minimal enlargement
  - Typical appearance requires no further imaging unless clinically indicated
  - Important to correctly identify CH with noninvasive imaging to avoid complications of biopsy (hemorrhage)
- Slow growth, particularly in larger lesions
- Growth accelerated with pregnancy
  - Mechanism of hormonal stimulation not elucidated
- Occasionally more rapid growth
  - Accelerated enlargement should prompt diagnostic imaging evaluation
- Rare complications
  - Hemorrhage or rupture may be catastrophic
  - Kasabach-Merritt syndrome uncommon; however, mortality significant (10-30%)
    - Thrombocytopenia-hemangioma-coagulopathy syndrome: Intravascular coagulation, consumption of coagulation factors, platelet sequestration

Treatment
- Usually no intervention indicated
- No therapy for small, asymptomatic lesions
- Symptomatic or large lesions may benefit from surgical resection or radiofrequency ablation
- Larger lesions more susceptible to rupture, may benefit from intervention
  - Blunt dissection with surgical enucleation
  - Percutaneous transvascular embolization

DIAGNOSTIC CHECKLIST

Consider
- Tc-99m RBC scan in cases not characteristic of hemangioma by conventional imaging
- Tc-99m RBC scan particularly useful with larger CH: Heterogeneous appearance can confound CECT/MR interpretation

Image Interpretation Pearls
- Delayed accumulation of tracer with subsequent increasing pooling and persistence of Tc-99m RBCs on delayed imaging = highly accurate for diagnosis of cavernous hemangioma

SELECTED REFERENCES

1. Choi BY et al: The diagnosis and management of benign hepatic tumors. J Clin Gastroenterol. 39(5):401-12, 2005
2. Ishikawa K et al: Detection of bladder hemangioma in a child by blood-pool scintigraphy. Pediatr Radiol. 33(6):433-5, 2003
3. Ozdemir S et al: Hepatic cavernous hemangioma with atypical peripheral rim activity on hepatic blood pool imaging. Clin Nucl Med. 28(10):834-5, 2003
4. Frevel T et al: Giant cavernous haemangioma with Kasabach-Merritt syndrome: a case report and review. Eur J Pediatr. 161(5):243-6, 2002
5. Tsai CC et al: The value of Tc-99m red blood cell SPECT in differentiating giant cavernous hemangioma of the liver from other liver solid masses. Clin Nucl Med. 27(8):578-81, 2002
6. Lim ST et al: A case of hepatocellular carcinoma mimicking cavernous hemangioma on Tc-99m RBC liver SPECT. Clin Nucl Med. 26(3):253-4, 2001
7. Vu D et al: Pseudohepatic cavernous hemangioma resulting from a prominent left portal vein of a portal systemic shunt collateral on Tc-99m SPECT red blood cell scintigraphy. Clin Nucl Med. 26(4):348-9, 2001
8. Dodd GD 3rd et al: Spectrum of imaging findings of the liver in end-stage cirrhosis: Part I, gross morphology and diffuse abnormalities. AJR. 173(4):1031-6, 1999
9. Dodd GD 3rd et al: Spectrum of imaging findings of the liver in end-stage cirrhosis: Part II, focal abnormalities. AJR. 173(5):1185-92, 1999

CAVERNOUS HEMANGIOMAS

IMAGE GALLERY

Typical

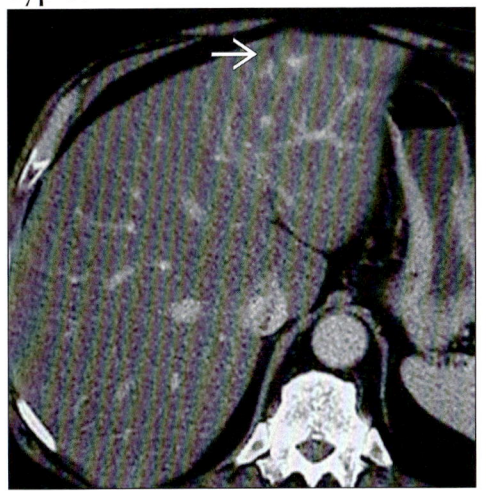

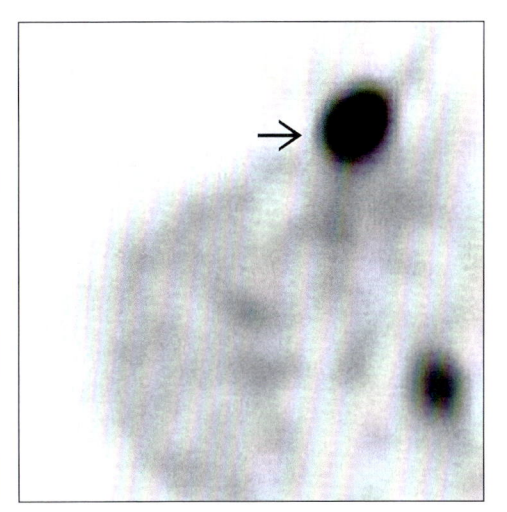

(Left) Axial CECT shows nodular lesion in subcapsular left hepatic lobe ➡. *(Right)* Axial Tc-99m RBC SPECT in same patient as previous image shows marked pooling of RBCs in corresponding region ➡ on delayed imaging, indicating CH.

Typical

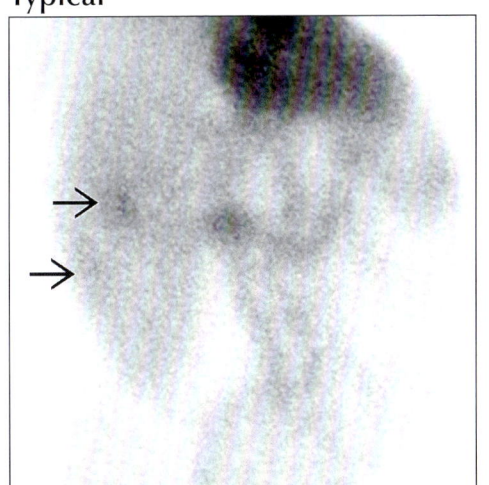

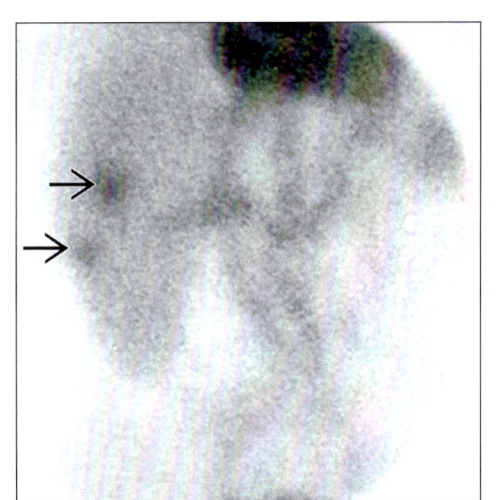

(Left) Anterior Tc-99m RBC scintigraphy immediately after injection shows two areas of early tracer accumulation in right hepatic lobe ➡. *(Right)* Anterior Tc-99m RBC scintigraphy in same patient as previous image shows increased pooling of RBCs ➡ on delayed image, confirming both as CH.

Typical

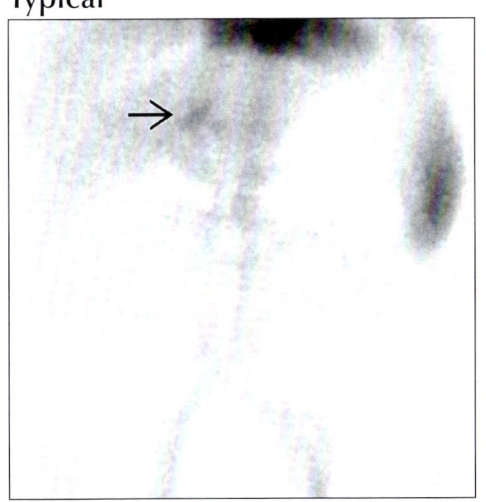

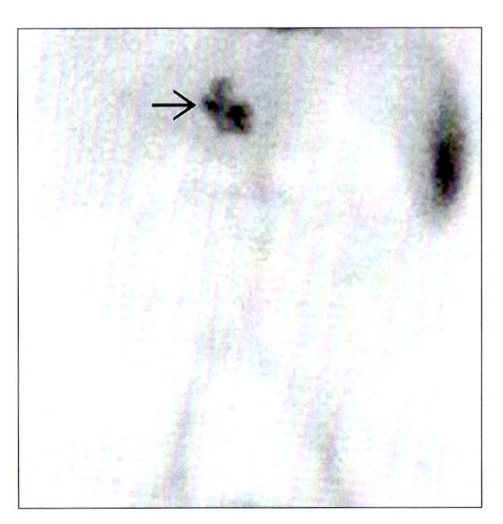

(Left) Anterior Tc-99m RBC scintigraphy immediately after injection shows early, focal Tc-99m RBC accumulation ➡. *(Right)* Anterior Tc-99m RBC scintigraphy in same patient as previous image shows increased pooling of RBCs ➡ on delayed image confirming CH.

ADRENAL MALIGNANCY

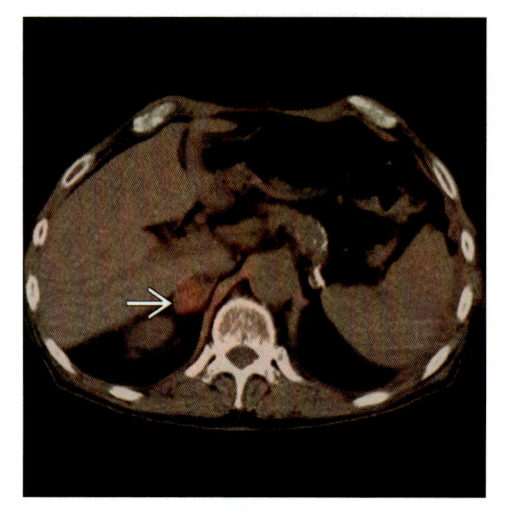

Axial fused PET/CT shows enlarged, hypermetabolic right adrenal ➡ with HU of 66 and adrenal:liver (A:L) SUV ratio of 2.2, consistent with malignancy. See next image.

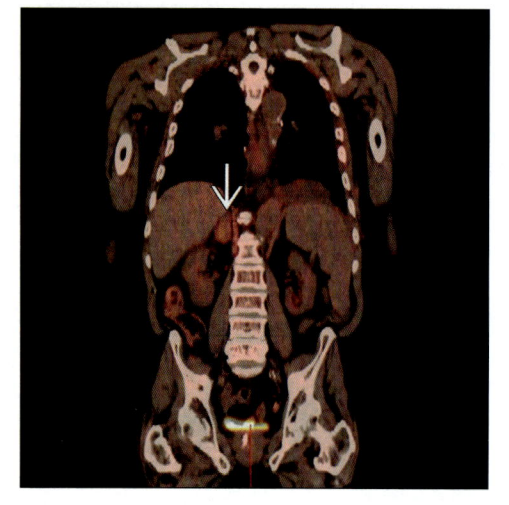

Coronal fused FDG PET/CT in same patient as previous image, shows increased uptake in enlarged right adrenal ➡, biopsy-proven adenocarcinoma metastasis from colorectal primary.

TERMINOLOGY

Definitions
- Adrenal metastases from other primary cancer sites
- Adrenal lymphoma: Malignant tumor of B-lymphocytes

IMAGING FINDINGS

General Features
- Best diagnostic clue: Suprarenal mass of low soft tissue density; hypermetabolic on FDG PET
- Key concepts
  ○ Adrenal metastases
    ▪ Adrenal glands 4th most common site of metastases after lungs, liver & bone
    ▪ Most commonly come from lung, breast, skin (melanoma), kidney, thyroid & colon cancers
    ▪ Indicates stage IV disease
    ▪ 27% of autopsy cases: Epithelial origin
    ▪ May be unilateral or bilateral; small or large
    ▪ Direct contiguous extension into adrenals from surrounding malignancy
    ▪ Malignant melanoma: 50% metastasize to adrenal glands
    ▪ Lung & breast cancers: 30-40% metastasize to adrenal glands
    ▪ Renal & GI tract malignancies: 10-20% metastasize to adrenal glands
    ▪ Most clinically silent; occasionally adrenal insufficiency
  ○ Adrenal lymphoma
    ▪ 25% cases of lymphoma involve adrenals at autopsy
    ▪ Primary lymphoma (rare); secondary (common)
    ▪ 4% of cases of non-Hodgkin lymphoma have adrenal involvement; rare in Hodgkin
    ▪ Diffuse cell type > nodular type
    ▪ Bilateral (50%), usually with retroperitoneal adenopathy

Nuclear Medicine Findings
- FDG PET
  ○ SUV-based distinction of benign vs. malignant: Sensitivity 98%, specificity 92% for SUV ≥ 3.1 as malignancy

DDx: Mimics of Adrenal Malignancy

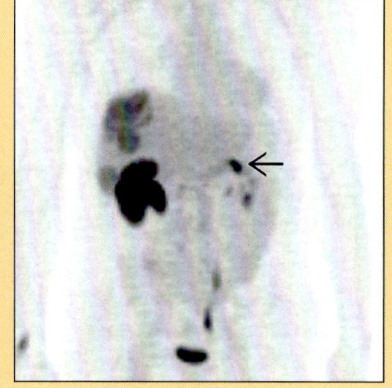

Renal Collecting System

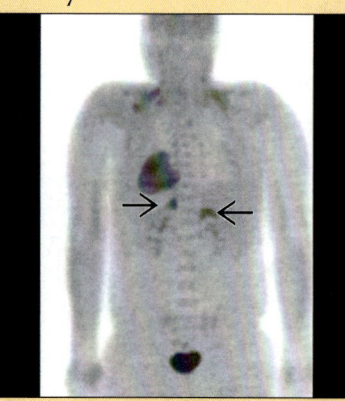

Hypermetabolic Brown Fat

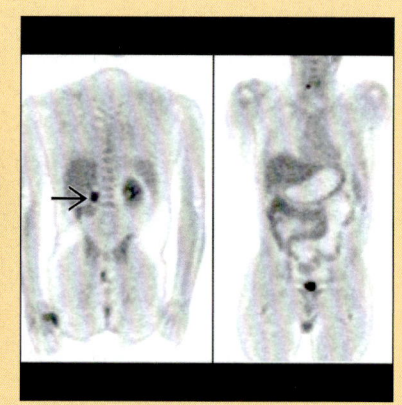

Duodenal Tumor

ADRENAL MALIGNANCY

Key Facts

Imaging Findings
- Best diagnostic clue: Suprarenal mass of low soft tissue density; hypermetabolic on FDG PET
- Adrenal glands 4th most common site of metastases after lungs, liver & bone
- Most commonly come from lung, breast, skin (melanoma), kidney, thyroid & colon cancers
- 25% cases of lymphoma involve adrenals at autopsy
- 4% of cases of non-Hodgkin lymphoma have adrenal involvement; rare in Hodgkin
- SUV-based distinction of benign vs. malignant: Sensitivity 98%, specificity 92% for SUV ≥ 3.1 as malignancy
- Adrenal:liver (A:L) ratio distinction of benign vs. malignant: Sensitivity 100%, specificity 94% for A:L ratio > 1.5 as malignancy

Top Differential Diagnoses
- Lipid-rich adenoma: Low CT attenuation (< 10 HU) diagnostic
- Lipid-poor adenoma: Attenuation varies, 10-30 HU; simulate metastases on NECT
- Lipid-rich & poor adenomas: 10 min post contrast injection, > 50% washout of contrast = adenoma
- Adrenal Carcinoma
- Adrenal Hemorrhage
- Adrenal Pheochromocytoma
- Adrenal Myelolipoma

Diagnostic Checklist
- FDG PET: Adrenal:liver (A:L) SUV ratio > 1.5 likely malignant, < 1.0 likely benign
- FDG PET: Confirmatory CECT, biopsy for A:L SUV ratio of 1.0-1.5 (indeterminate)

- Some overlap between benign and malignant tumors: SUV 1.1-6.0
- Adrenal:liver (A:L) ratio distinction of benign vs. malignant: Sensitivity 100%, specificity 94% for A:L ratio > 1.5 as malignancy
- CECT washout, biopsy confirmation recommended: A:L ratio 1.0-1.5
- [Iodine-131] 6-iodomethyl-19-norcholesterol (NP-59): Not FDA approved, currently not available
  - Malignant lesions (adrenal metastases & lymphoma): Lack of uptake
  - Benign lesion (functioning adrenal adenoma): Unilateral early adrenal visualization before day 5 after injection
  - Normal adrenal glands or normal NP-59: Bilateral adrenal glands on or beyond day 5 after injection (suppressible by dexamethasone)
- Tc-99m diphosphonate bone scan: Uptake in neuroblastoma adrenal tumors, calcified adrenal masses
- In-111 pentetreotide (Octreoscan): Uptake in wide variety of primary, metastatic neuroendocrine adrenal tumors
- I-123, I-131 MIBG: Uptake in neuroblastoma, pheochromocytoma

CT Findings
- Adrenal metastases
  - Small metastases: Well-defined, round or oval; homogeneous soft tissue density, unilateral or bilateral; adrenal gland contour maintained; necrosis, hemorrhage & calcification (rare); may mimic lipid poor adrenal adenoma on NECT
  - Large metastases: Unilateral or bilateral enlarged adrenal glands; lobulated or irregular in shape; heterogeneous density (necrosis, hemorrhage); distortion of normal contour; ± central necrosis, hemorrhage, calcification
  - Hypervascular or hypovascular; may have thick enhancing rims (metastases)
  - Washout value of < 50% after 10-15 min: Indicates either metastases or atypical adenoma
  - Direct contiguous adrenal invasion: From kidney, pancreas, stomach, liver & retroperitoneal sarcoma
- Adrenal lymphoma
  - Discrete or diffuse mass, configuration of adrenal limbs is preserved
  - Homogeneous soft tissue density on NECT; hypovascular, moderate enhancement with contrast (40-60 HU)
  - Unilateral or bilateral; usually associated with retroperitoneal adenopathy
  - Necrosis uncommon without prior therapy unless rapidly growing
  - May mimic lipid-poor adenoma

Angiographic Findings
- Adrenal metastases
  - Hypervascular: Renal cell carcinoma or sarcoma metastases
  - Hypovascular: Squamous cell cancer metastases
- Adrenal lymphoma
  - Hypovascular adrenal mass; palisading of vessels may be seen
  - Infiltration: Encasement & amputation of vessels

MR Findings
- Adrenal metastases
  - Without necrosis & hemorrhage: T1WI usually homogeneous & hypointense; T2WI relatively hyperintense (due to fluid content)
  - With necrosis & hemorrhage: T1 & T2WI heterogeneous signal intensity; exception with metastatic malignant melanoma: Hyperintense on T1WI, occasionally remain hyperintense on T2WI (mimic pheochromocytoma)
  - Hyperintense on T1WI; out of phase & T1WI fat-saturated sequences excludes adenoma
- Adrenal lymphoma: Nonspecific MR findings

Ultrasonographic Findings
- Grayscale Ultrasound
  - Adrenal metastases: Solid lesions with heterogeneous echogenicity; echogenicity usually < surrounding fat

ADRENAL MALIGNANCY

- Adrenal lymphoma: Relatively homogeneous, hypoechoic lesions; ± areas of echogenicity within mass lesion

Imaging Recommendations
- Best imaging tool: Relative value of FDG PET vs. NE/CECT or MR not yet established
- Protocol advice
  - PET/CT preferred over PET
  - CT: 3 mm thick section at 3 mm intervals
  - MR T1WI in & out of phases

DIFFERENTIAL DIAGNOSIS

Adrenal Adenoma
- NECT
  - Lipid-rich adenoma: Low CT attenuation (< 10 HU) diagnostic
  - Lipid-poor adenoma: Attenuation varies, 10-30 HU; simulate metastases on NECT
  - Large adenoma: Heterogeneous due to hemorrhage, cystic degeneration, Ca++
- CECT
  - Lipid-rich & poor adenomas: 10 min post contrast injection, > 50% washout of contrast = adenoma
- T1WI out of phase
  - Lipid-rich adenoma: Marked signal drop-out
  - Lipid-poor adenoma: Minimal signal loss

Adrenal Carcinoma
- Rare, unilateral, invasive & enhancing mass, > 6 cm at diagnosis

Adrenal Hemorrhage
- Acute: High-density fluid collection (40-60 HU)
- Chronic: Low-density collection (clot ~ 20-30 HU); may mimic metastases, lymphoma

Adrenal Pheochromocytoma
- Highly vascular; prone to hemorrhage & necrosis; very hyperintense on T2WI
- Bilateral adrenal tumors in MEN IIA & IIB syndromes, neurofibromatosis type-I

Adrenal Myelolipoma
- Composed of fat & hematopoietic elements; heterogeneous fatty adrenal masses
- MR: Hypointense on fat suppression; marked signal drop-out at fat-soft tissue interface

False-Positive FDG PET
- Hypermetabolic brown fat, high-dose methotrexate, diaphragmatic crus, renal collecting system

PATHOLOGY

General Features
- General path comments: Normal anatomy: Anteromedial ridge & 2 limbs; maximum body width 0.79 mm (Rt), 0.6 mm (Lt); length varies (up to 4 cm); width of limbs < 1 cm (right < left)
- Etiology
  - Adrenal metastases: Lung, breast, skin (melanoma), kidney, thyroid, GI tract primary
  - Adrenal lymphoma: Often secondary, non-Hodgkin
- Associated abnormalities
  - Primary malignant tumor in case of metastases
  - Generalized adenopathy in case of lymphoma
  - Adrenal collision tumor: Metastases & adenoma in same adrenal gland

Gross Pathologic & Surgical Features
- Discrete or diffuse; unilateral or bilateral
- ± Cystic, necrotic, hemorrhagic, calcific areas

Microscopic Features
- Metastases: Varies based on etiology
- Lymphoma: Lymphoepithelial, Reed-Sternberg cells

CLINICAL ISSUES

Presentation
- Most common signs/symptoms
  - Usually clinically silent
  - Adrenocortical insufficiency (Addison disease) when 90% of tissue damaged
    - Weakness, weight loss, anorexia, nausea, vomiting, hypotension, skin pigmentation
    - ↓ Cortisol, aldosterone, androgens & ↑ ACTH; ↓ Na+, Cl & ↑ K+ levels

Demographics
- Gender: M = F

Natural History & Prognosis
- Complications: Adrenocortical insufficiency; prognosis usually poor

DIAGNOSTIC CHECKLIST

Image Interpretation Pearls
- FDG PET: Adrenal:liver (A:L) SUV ratio > 1.5 likely malignant, < 1.0 likely benign
- FDG PET: Confirmatory CECT, biopsy for A:L SUV ratio of 1.0-1.5 (indeterminate)

SELECTED REFERENCES
1. Blake MA et al: Adrenal lesions: characterization with fused PET/CT image in patients with proved or suspected malignancy--initial experience. Radiology. 238(3):970-7, 2006
2. Metser U et al: 18F-FDG PET/CT in the evaluation of adrenal masses. J Nucl Med. 47(1):32-7, 2006
3. Kumar R et al: 18F-FDG PET in evaluation of adrenal lesions in patients with lung cancer. J Nucl Med. 45(12):2058-62, 2004
4. Dunnick NR et al: Imaging of adrenal incidentalomas: current status. AJR Am J Roentgenol. 179(3):559-68, 2002
5. Erasmus JJ et al: Evaluation of adrenal masses in patients with bronchogenic carcinoma using 18F-fluorodeoxyglucose positron emission tomography. AJR Am J Roentgenol. 168(5):1357-60, 1997
6. Dunnick NR et al: Adrenal radiology: distinguishing benign from malignant adrenal masses. AJR Am J Roentgenol. 167(4):861-7, 1996

ADRENAL MALIGNANCY

IMAGE GALLERY

Typical

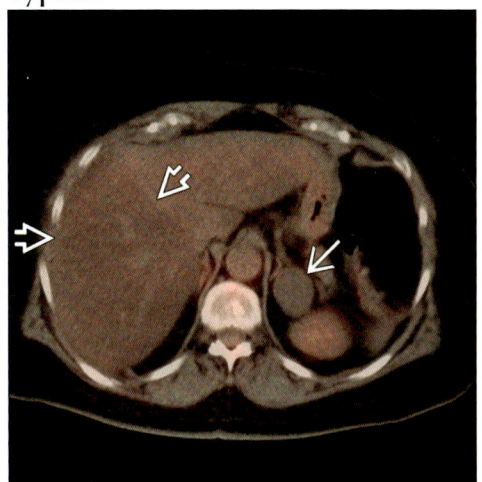

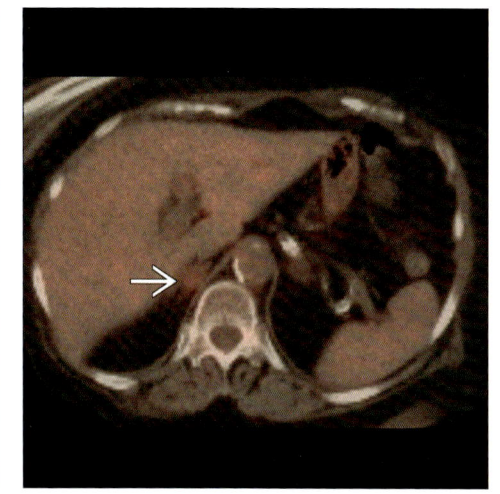

(Left) Axial fused PET/CT shows enlarged, low-attenuating left adrenal mass ➡ with HU = 4 and low A:L SUV ratios of 0.6, favoring benign etiology. Note also fatty right hepatic lobe ➡. **(Right)** Axial fused PET/CT shows small hypermetabolic right adrenal ➡ with HU of 21 and A:L SUV ratio of 1.45. Ratio favors benign etiology but small size may result in partial volume effects, underestimating SUV.

Typical

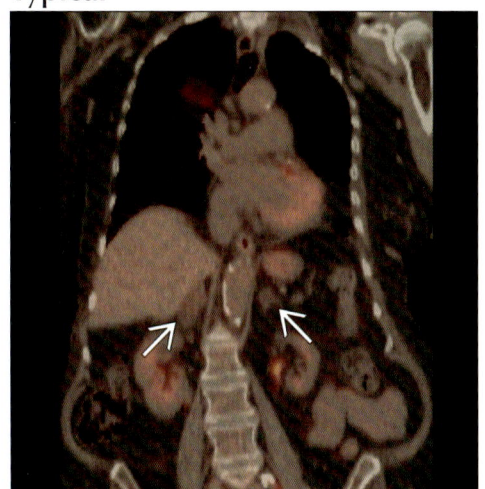

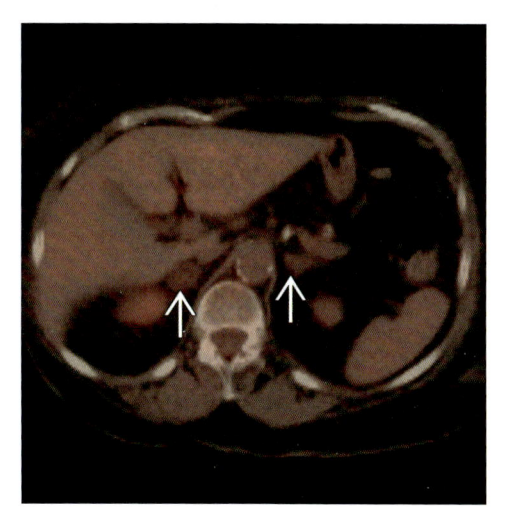

(Left) Coronal fused PET/CT shows bilaterally enlarged adrenals ➡. See next image. **(Right)** Axial fused PET/CT shows bilaterally enlarged adrenals ➡ with A:L SUV ratios ~ 1, HU ~ 15 m, and CECT 10 min washout > 50%, favoring lipid-poor adenomas.

Typical

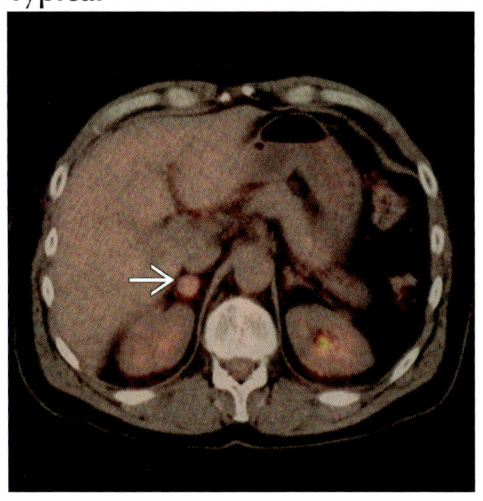

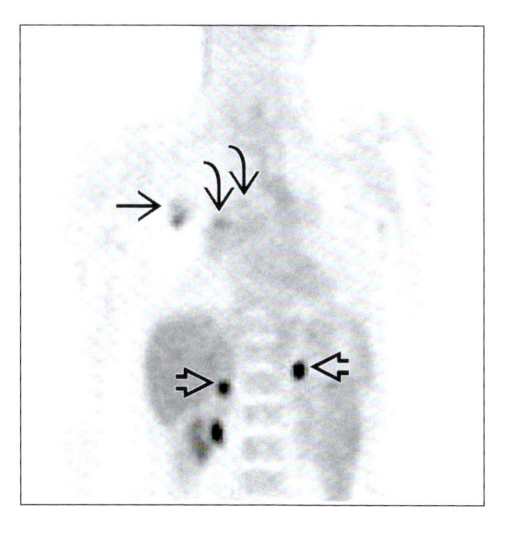

(Left) Axial fused PET/CT shows hypermetabolic right adrenal gland ➡ with A:L ratios of 2.3, consistent with malignancy. **(Right)** Coronal FDG PET shows increased activity in right lung cancer ➡, lymphadenopathy ➡, and adrenal metastases ➡. Adrenal metastases may show greater FDG uptake than primary tumor.

ADRENAL MALIGNANCY

Variant

(Left) Axial MR shows complex increased signal in right adrenal mass ➡, suggesting areas of necrosis, hemorrhage. See next image. (Right) Axial FDG PET in same patient as previous image shows intense activity in right adrenal mass ➡, biopsy-proven primary adrenal carcinoma.

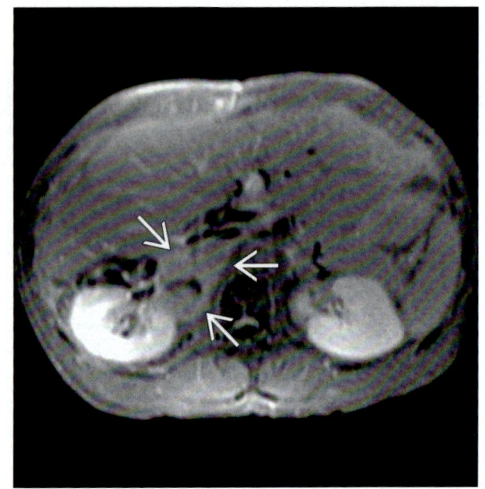

Typical

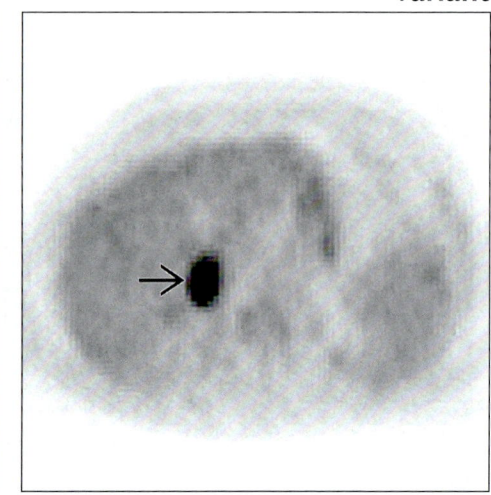

(Left) Coronal MR shows right adrenal mass ➡ in patient with history of lung cancer. Small left adrenal mass was also present (not seen here). See next image. (Right) Coronal FDG PET in same patient as previous image shows marked uptake in right adrenal metastasis ➡, smaller left adrenal metastasis ➡, and metastasis to L-5 vertebral body ➡.

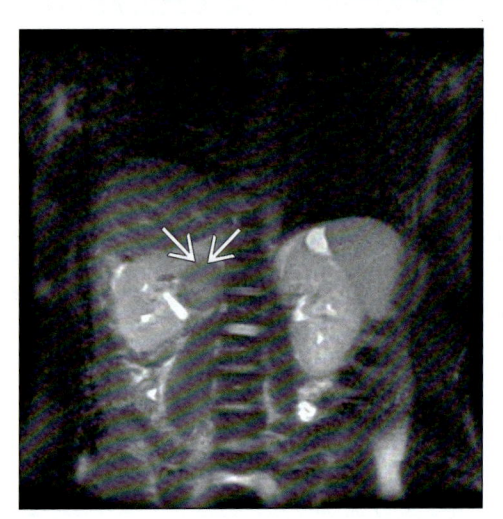

Typical

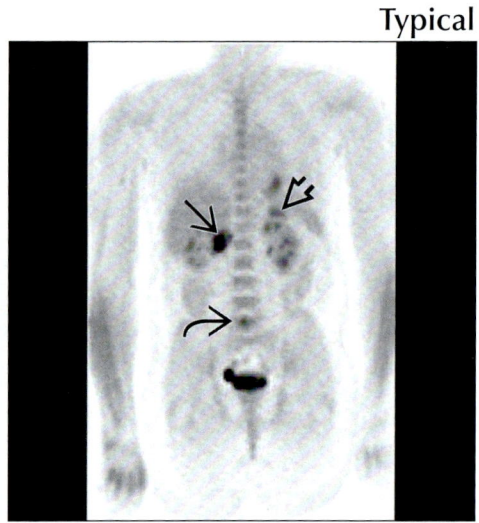

(Left) Pretreatment MIP FDG PET shows increased uptake in hilar bronchogenic carcinoma ➡. See next image. (Right) MIP FDG PET in same patient as previous image 3 months after chemoradiation shows ↑ size and activity in right hilar bronchogenic carcinoma ➡ as well as new right adrenal metastasis ➡.

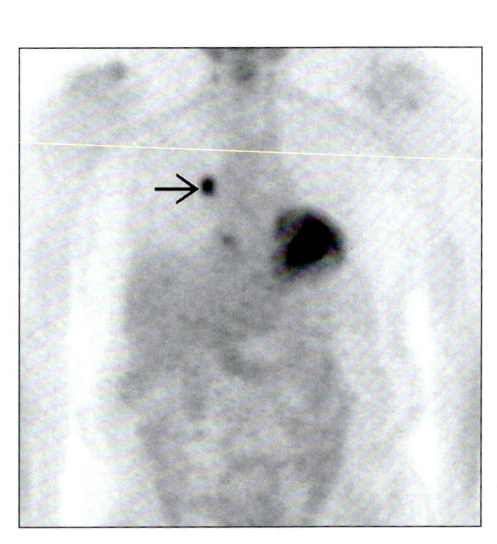

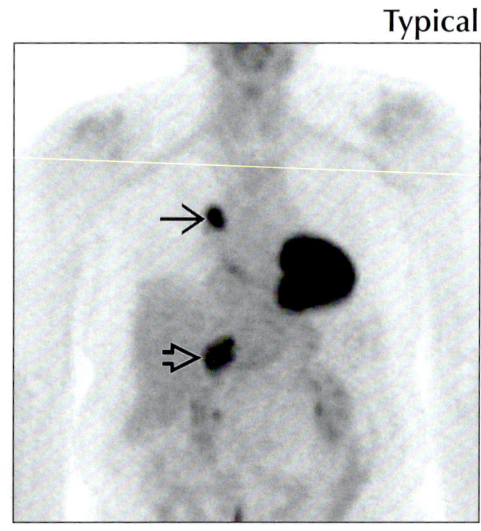

ADRENAL MALIGNANCY

Typical

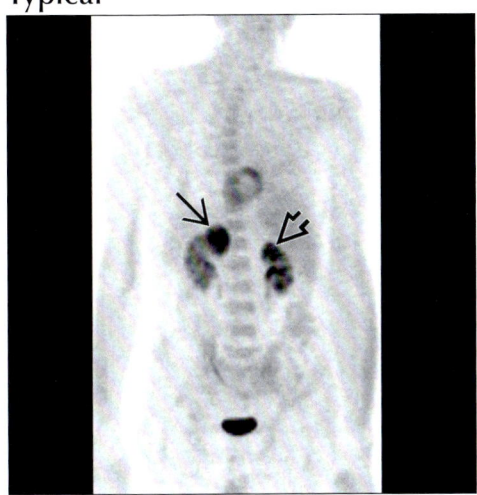

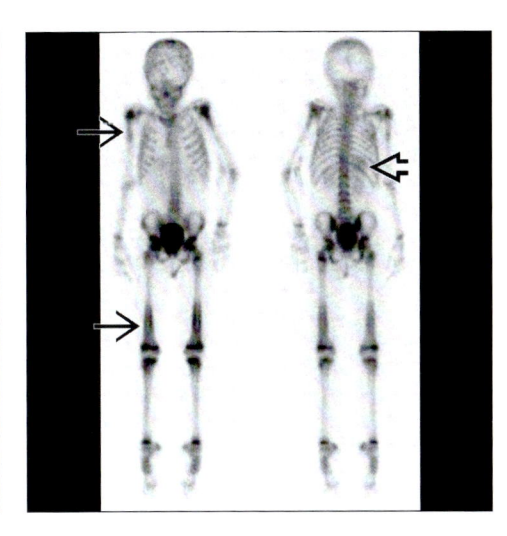

(**Left**) Coronal FDG PET shows hypermetabolic right adrenal metastasis ➡. Note normal collecting system activity in superior pole ➡ of left kidney mimicking adrenal metastasis. (**Right**) Anterior and posterior bone scan shows uptake in right adrenal gland ➡ in child with neuroblastoma. Note widespread metastatic disease to skeleton, most pronounced in metadiaphyses of long bones ➡.

Typical

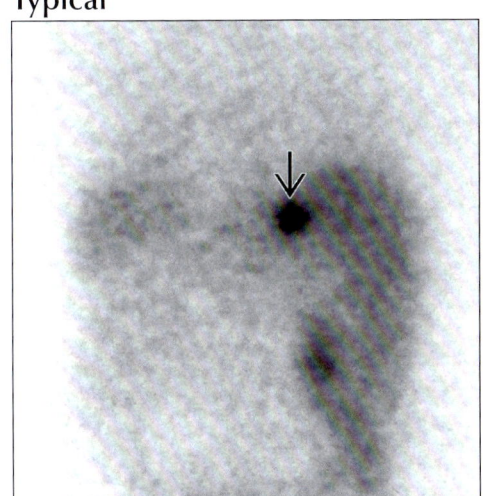

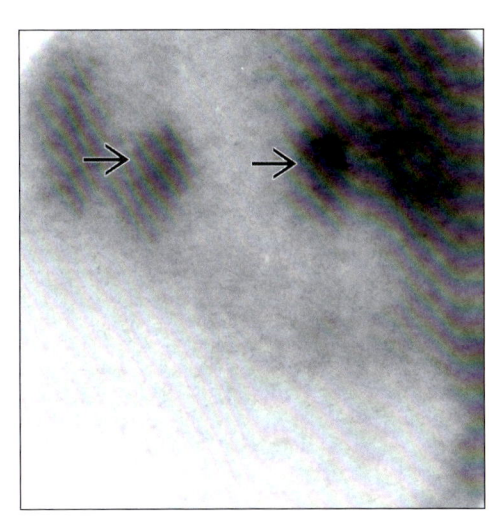

(**Left**) Posterior I-131 NP-59 scan in patient with hypokalemia and hypertension shows uptake in right adrenal gland ➡, biopsy-proven aldosteronoma. (**Right**) Posterior I-131 NP-59 scan shows bilateral adrenal uptake ➡, normal ≥ 5 days post injection and if suppressible by dexamethasone. If seen earlier and nonsuppressible, may indicate bilateral hyperplasia from ACTH-producing tumor.

Typical

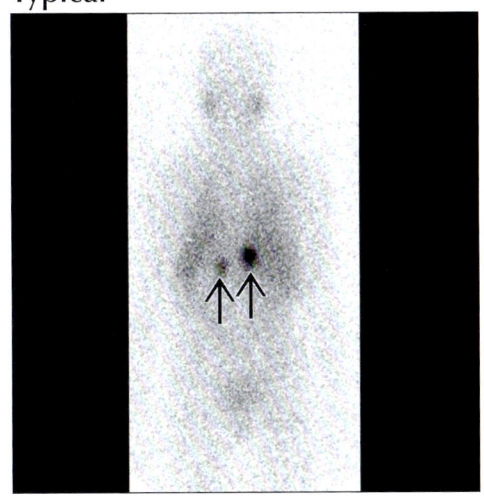

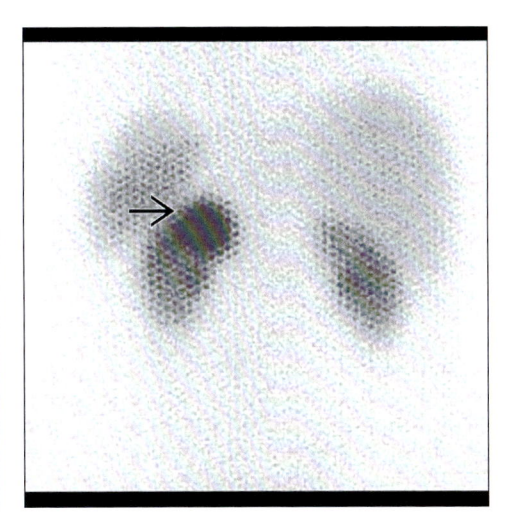

(**Left**) Posterior I-131 MIBG scan in patient with neurofibromatosis type-I shows uptake in bilateral adrenal pheochromocytomas ➡. (**Right**) Posterior In-111 Octreoscan image shows uptake in left adrenal pheochromocytoma ➡. Octreoscan has better imaging characteristics but is less sensitive than MIBG for pheochromocytoma, neuroblastoma.

PHEOCHROMOCYTOMA

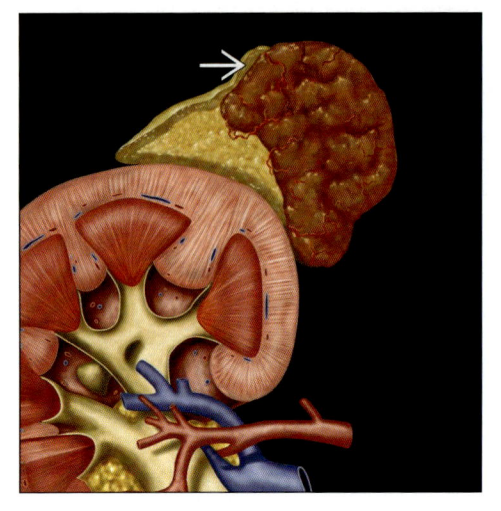

Graphic shows heterogeneous hypervascularity of pheochromocytoma of the adrenal gland ➡.

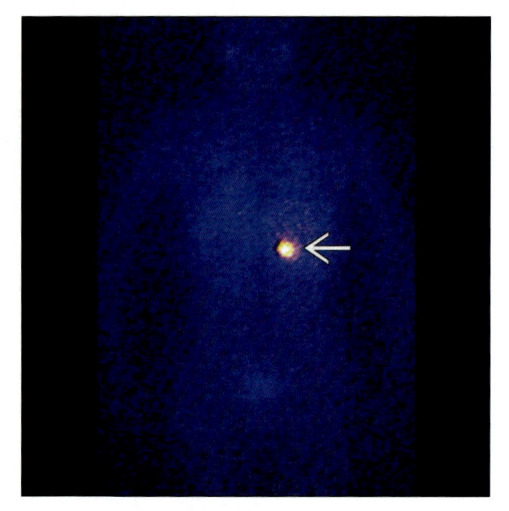

Posterior I-131 MIBG scintigraphy shows uptake in 1.8 cm mass in right adrenal gland ➡ in patient with pheochromocytoma.

TERMINOLOGY

Abbreviations and Synonyms
- Extra-adrenal: Paraganglioma, ganglioneuroma

Definitions
- Tumor arising from chromaffin cells of adrenal medulla or extra-adrenal ectopic tissue

IMAGING FINDINGS

General Features
- Best diagnostic clue
  - I-123 or I-131 MIBG scintigraphy: Mass with focal, intense uptake after 24-72 hr
  - F-18 FDG PET: Mass with increased FDG activity; highest in malignant pheo
  - MR: Very hyperintense mass on T2WI; bright heterogeneous enhancement
- Location: Along sympathetic chain: Neck to urinary bladder; adrenal medulla (90%); extra-adrenal (10%); subdiaphragmatic (98%); thorax (1-2%)
- Size: Usually > 3 cm
- Morphology: Well-circumscribed, encapsulated tumor
- Rule of tens: 10% extra-adrenal (paragangliomas/chemodectomas); 10% bilateral, malignant & extra-abdominal; 10% familial, pediatric, silent; 10% have autosomal dominant transmission & associated with various other dominant conditions
  - 90% patients present with hypertension
  - Difficult to distinguish benign vs. malignant: Benign lesions can locally invade IVC & renal capsule; distant metastases = malignancy
  - Extra-adrenal tumors arise from sympathetic ganglia: Neck, mediastinum, pelvis; urinary bladder; aortic bifurcation (organ of Zuckerkandl)

Nuclear Medicine Findings
- I-131 or I-123 Metaiodobenzylguanidine (MIBG)
  - Norepinephrine analogue: Little pharmacologic effect; incorporated in adrenergic storage granules
  - After 24-72 hr: ↑ Uptake of MIBG in tumor
  - MIBG best for detecting extra-adrenal tumors: Metastatic pheos; recurrent & extra-abdominal tumors
  - MIBG 80-90% sensitivity & 90-100% specificity: Many in these series large, known pheos

DDx: Mimics of Pheochromocytoma

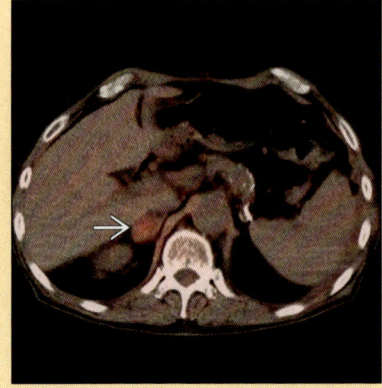

Adrenal Metastases (FDG PET/CT) 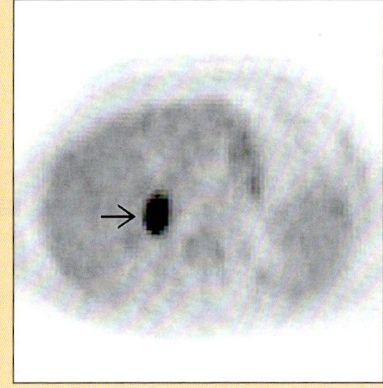 | *Adrenal Carcinoma (FDG PET)* 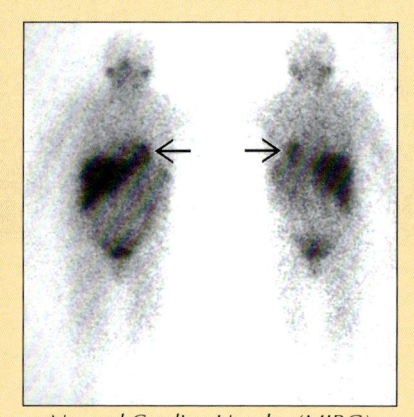 | *Normal Cardiac Uptake (MIBG)*

PHEOCHROMOCYTOMA

Key Facts

Terminology
- Tumor arising from chromaffin cells of adrenal medulla or extra-adrenal ectopic tissue

Imaging Findings
- I-123 or I-131 MIBG scintigraphy: Mass with focal, intense uptake after 24-72 hr
- F-18 FDG PET: Mass with increased FDG activity; highest in malignant pheo
- MIBG 80-90% sensitivity & 90-100% specificity: Many in these series large, known pheos
- Yield of MIBG scan low for finding occult clinically/chemically suspected pheos when all other modalities are negative
- Most pheos FDG-avid: Greatest uptake in malignant pheo
- Somatostatin receptor scintigraphy (In-111 octreotide): Probably ↓ sensitivity compared to I-131 MIBG, but better imaging characteristics

Top Differential Diagnoses
- Adrenal medullary hyperplasia (MIBG + bilaterally)
- Neural crest tumors (MIBG+): Paraganglioma, chemodectoma, glomus jugulare tumors, neuroblastoma, ganglioneuroma
- Occasionally MIBG + tumors: Schwannoma, Merkel cell, retinoblastoma, islet cell, small cell lung cancer, melanoma, peripheral nerve sheath

Diagnostic Checklist
- MIBG scintigraphy for occult, ectopic, recurrent, metastatic tumors
- Most pheos are FDG-PET positive

   - Yield of MIBG scan low for finding occult clinically/chemically suspected pheos when all other modalities are negative
   ○ I-123 MIBG: Better imaging characteristics, dosimetry, photon flux than I-123; not FDA-approved; often not reimbursed
- F-18-FDG PET
   ○ Most pheos FDG-avid: Greatest uptake in malignant pheo
   ○ Helpful in identifying sites of metastatic pheo; cannot distinguish from other mets
- Investigational PET approaches: Promising for future applications
   ○ Synthesis, storage, and release of hormones: (11)C-hydroxyephedrine
   ○ Hormone precursors: (11)C-5-hydroxytryptophan, (11)C- or (18)F-dihydroxyphenylalanine, (18)F-fluorodopamine
   ○ Receptors: Ga-68-labeled somatostatin analogs
- Somatostatin receptor scintigraphy (In-111 octreotide): Probably ↓ sensitivity compared to I-131 MIBG, but better imaging characteristics

CT Findings
- NECT: Well-defined, round, homogeneous (muscle density); variable regions (hemorrhage, necrosis, calcification)
- CECT: Typically marked homogeneous & delayed enhancement; heterogeneity with necrosis, hemorrhage; peripheral enhancement with fluid-levels

Angiographic Findings
- Conventional: Hypervascular tumor

MR Findings
- T1WI: Isointense to muscle; hypointense to liver; heterogeneous with hemorrhage, necrosis
- T1 C+: Salt (enhancing parenchyma) and pepper (flow void of vessels) pattern; ± marked early & prolonged contrast-enhancement
- T2WI: Markedly hyperintense on T2WI (characteristic); long T2 relaxation, heterogeneity with necrosis, hemorrhage

Ultrasonographic Findings
- Grayscale ultrasound: Iso/hypo-echoic (77%) & hyperechoic (23%) compared to renal parenchyma

Imaging Recommendations
- Protocol advice
   ○ I-123 or I-131 MIBG
      - Block free iodine uptake by thyroid gland with Lugol solution (supersaturated potassium iodine, SSKI): 2-3 drops po from 2 days prior through 7 days after MIBG injection
      - Discontinue drugs that may interfere with MIBG uptake for 48-72 h: Tricyclic antidepressants, labetalol, reserpine, tetrabenazine, norepinephrine, serotonin, guanethidine, reserpine, sympathomimetics, calcium channel blockers
      - Alpha and beta blockers in normal doses (with exception of labetalol) can be used
      - 0.5-1.0 mCi (18-37 MBq) I-131 MIBG or 2.0-8.0 mCi (74-296 MBq) I-123 MIBG IV
      - I-131 MIBG: Image at 24, 48 h (72 h rarely necessary); SPECT at 24, 48 h
      - I-123 MIBG: Planar images at 24 h; SPECT abdomen, chest at 24 h
      - Tc-99m renal scan or liver spleen scan subtracted from MIBG image: May help localize site of MIBG uptake
   ○ Helical NE + CECT
      - Hypertensive crisis rare/nonexistent with IV administration of nonionic contrast material
      - Routine premedication (α and β blockade) not recommended

---

DIFFERENTIAL DIAGNOSIS

Other MIBG-Positive Conditions
- Adrenal medullary hyperplasia (MIBG + bilaterally)
- Neural crest tumors (MIBG+): Paraganglioma, chemodectoma, glomus jugulare tumors, neuroblastoma, ganglioneuroma

PHEOCHROMOCYTOMA

- Occasionally MIBG + tumors: Schwannoma, Merkel cell, retinoblastoma, islet cell, small cell lung cancer, melanoma, peripheral nerve sheath

Adrenal Adenoma
- Imaging: NECT (< 10 HU lipid rich, > 10 HU lipid poor), CECT (10 min post injection washout > 50%)

Adrenocortical Carcinoma
- Rare; usually unilateral; rarely bilateral (up to 10%)
- Functioning tumors (small); nonfunctioning (large)
- Large, unilateral, invasive margins; ± necrosis, hemorrhage, variable enhancement, calcification

Adrenal Metastases & Lymphoma
- Adrenal metastases: Unilateral or bilateral; central necrosis ± hemorrhage; e.g., lung, breast, renal cell carcinoma & melanoma
- Adrenal lymphoma: 25% cases of secondary lymphoma; primary (rare); non-Hodgkin most common

Adrenal Myelolipoma
- Rare benign tumor (fat + hematopoietic elements); unilateral fatty adrenal tumor (-100 to -30 HU)
- T1WI: Typically hyperintense; size varies (2-10 cm); out of phase T1WI w/focal areas of signal loss

Adrenal Hemorrhage
- Etiology: Septicemia, burns, trauma, stress, hypotension & hematological abnormalities
- CT findings: Often bilateral; old hemorrhage (soft tissue attenuation); recent hemorrhage ↑ attenuation
- T1 & T2WI MR: Variable

Granulomatous Infection
- Usually bilateral, heterogeneous, poorly enhancing (acute); small & calcified (chronic)

PATHOLOGY

General Features
- General path comments: Neoplasm of chromaffin cells derived from neural crest or neuroectoderm
- Etiology: Chromaffin cells of sympathetic nervous system: Adrenal medulla (pheo); extra-adrenal (paraganglioma)
- Epidemiology: Incidence: 0.13% in autopsy series; 0.1-0.5% with hypertension (HTN)
- Associated abnormalities (10% inherited): Von Hippel-Lindau syndrome, type 1 neurofibromatosis, multiple endocrine neoplasia syndromes (MEN) type IIA & type IIB, tuberous sclerosis, Sturge-Weber syndrome, Carney syndrome (pulmonary chondroma, gastric leiomyosarcoma, pheochromocytoma)

Gross Pathologic & Surgical Features
- Round, tan-pink to violaceous encapsulated mass; ± cystic, mucoid, serosanguineous, hemorrhage

Microscopic Features
- Large cells: Granular cytoplasm & pleomorphic nuclei
- Chromaffin reaction: Cells stained with chromium salt

CLINICAL ISSUES

Presentation
- Most common signs/symptoms
  - Clinical profile: Young patient with paroxysmal/episodic attacks of headache, palpitations, sweating & tremors
  - Crisis: Headaches, HTN, palpitations, sweating, tremors, arrhythmias, pain
  - Classic: Paroxysmal HTN ± visual changes
  - Atypical: Labile HTN, myocardial infarction, CVA
- Lab data: ↑ Levels of vanillylmandelic acid (VMA) 24-h urine

Demographics
- Age: 3rd & 4th decades
- Gender: M = F

Natural History & Prognosis
- Complications: During hypertensive crisis
  - Cerebrovascular accidents (CVA)
  - Pregnancy + pheo: Mortality (48%)
  - Malignancy in 2-14% cases; distant metastases
- Prognosis
  - Noninvasive & nonmetastatic: Good prognosis
  - Malignant & metastatic: Poor prognosis (< 5 yr survival)

Treatment
- Medical therapy: Before, during, after surgery
  - Alpha-adrenergic blockers: Phenoxybenzamine, phentolamine
  - Beta-adrenergic blocker: Propranolol
- Surgical resection: Benign & malignant
- Chemotherapy: Cyclophosphamide + vincristine + dacarbazine

DIAGNOSTIC CHECKLIST

Consider
- Imaging findings + history & labs (usually diagnostic)
- MIBG scintigraphy for occult, ectopic, recurrent, metastatic tumors

Image Interpretation Pearls
- Most pheos are FDG-PET positive

SELECTED REFERENCES

1. Avram AM et al: Adrenal gland scintigraphy. Semin Nucl Med. 36(3):212-27, 2006
2. Esfandiari NH et al: Multimodality imaging of malignant pheochromocytoma. Clin Nucl Med. 31(12):822-5, 2006
3. Rufini V et al: Imaging of neuroendocrine tumors. Semin Nucl Med. 36(3):228-47, 2006

PHEOCHROMOCYTOMA

IMAGE GALLERY

Variant

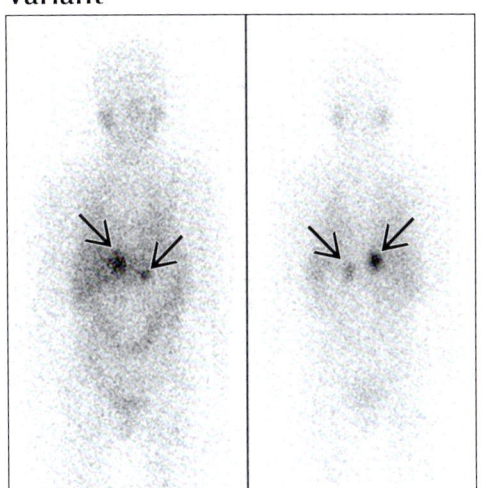

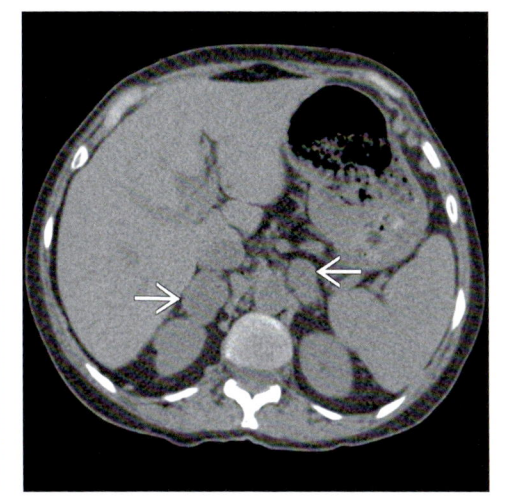

(Left) Anterior (left) and posterior (right) I-131 MIBG scintigraphy in patient with neurofibromatosis type-I shows uptake in bilateral pheochromocytomas ➔. See next image. (Right) Axial NECT in the same patient at left shows bilateral, enlarged adrenal glands ➔. Dx was bilateral adrenal pheochromocytomas, but adrenal hyperplasia can show bilateral uptake on MIBG.

Variant

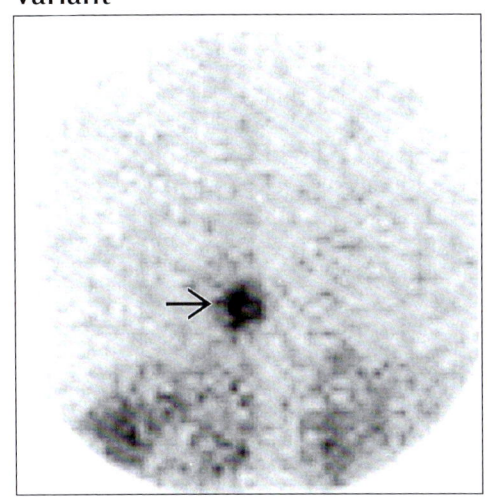

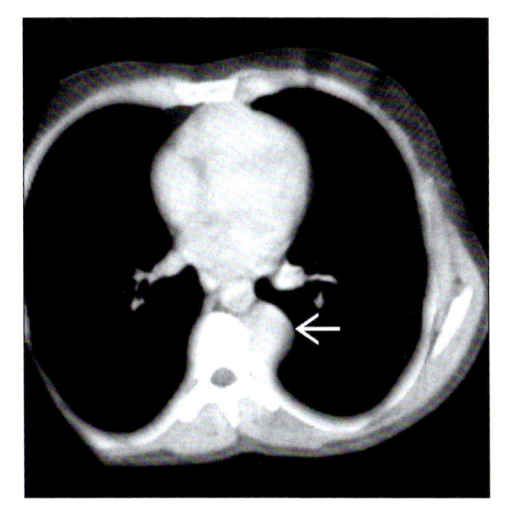

(Left) Posterior I-131 MIBG shows focal uptake left of the thoracic spine ➔ in a patient with extra-adrenal pheochromocytoma. See next image. (Courtesy N. Watson, MD). (Right) Axial CT in same patient at left, shows left paraspinous mass ➔ corresponding to MIBG positive lesion, consistent with extra-adrenal pheochromocytoma.

Typical

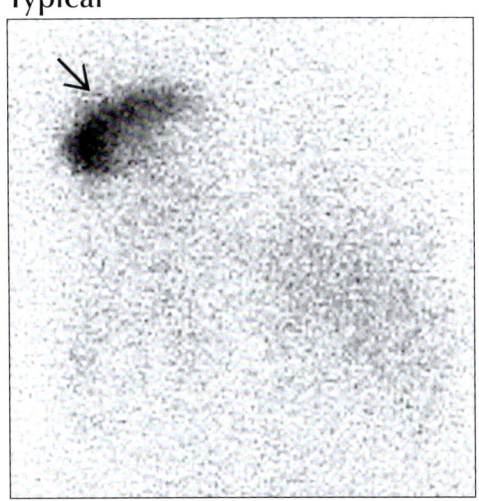

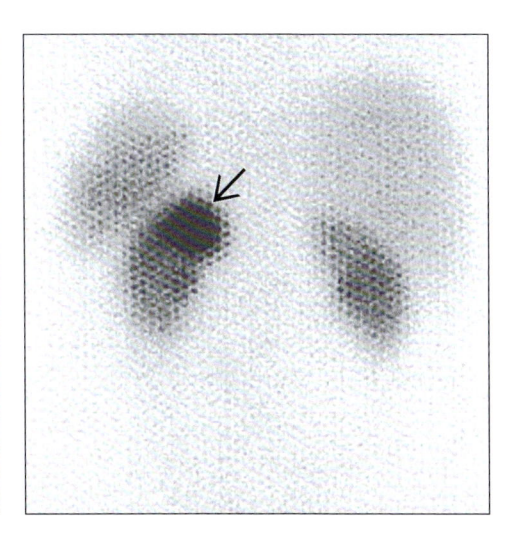

(Left) Posterior I-131 MIBG scintigraphy of lower chest/upper abdomen shows uptake ➔ in a left posterior rib in a patient with metastatic pheochromocytoma. (Right) Posterior In-111 somatostatin receptor scintigraphy shows uptake in left adrenal ➔ in patient with pheochromocytoma. Somatostatin receptor scintigraphy is usually less sensitive than MIBG for pheochromocytoma.

NEUROBLASTOMA

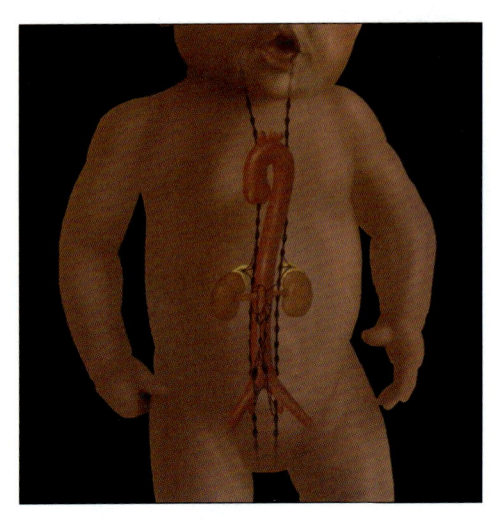

Anterior graphic shows the location of sympathetic nervous tissue in the body.

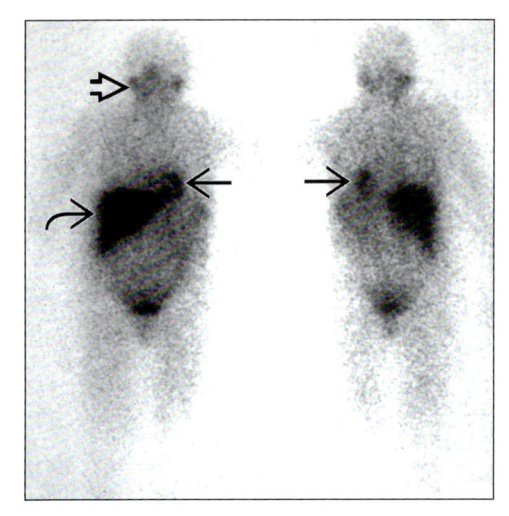

Anterior (left) and posterior (right) I-131 MIBG scintigraphy shows normal distribution including salivary glands ⇨, heart ⇒ liver ⇾ and bladder. Note absence of bone activity.

TERMINOLOGY

Abbreviations and Synonyms
- Metaiodobenzylguanidine (MIBG)

Definitions
- Malignant tumor derived from undifferentiated neural crest cells
- MIBG: Structurally similar to norepinephrine; localizes to catecholamine-storing granules via active transport

IMAGING FINDINGS

General Features
- Best diagnostic clue
  - MIBG avidity on a nuclear scan
  - Suprarenal mass with typical calcifications on anatomic imaging
- Location
  - Correspond to the locations of the sympathetic chain: Adrenal medulla, retroperitoneum, pelvis, mediastinum, extracranial craniofacial space
    - Adrenal medulla (35%)
    - Extraadrenal retroperitoneum (30-35%)
    - Posterior mediastinum (20%)
    - Pelvis (2-3%)
    - Neck (1-5%)
    - Metastatic disease with no primary identified (1%)
  - 60% present with metastases to cortical bone, bone marrow, lymph nodes, and liver; lung and brain metastases are rare
- Size: Variable and depending upon location but most are less than 10 cm in greatest diameter
- Morphology: CT/MR for evaluation of primary mass and its relationship to adjacent structures

Nuclear Medicine Findings
- PET: FDG avidity seen but clinical role not yet defined
- Bone Scan
  - Bone lesions show focal increased activity, often at the metaphysis
  - False negatives and cold bone scan lesions can occur
  - Soft tissue primary labels on bone scan 74% of the time, more often than calcifications are seen
  - Bone scan may be positive when MIBG scan is negative
- MIBG Scintigraphy

DDx: Mimics of Bony Neuroblastoma Metastases

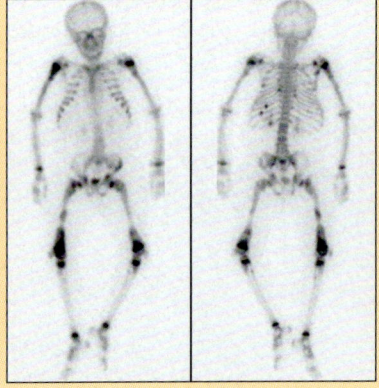

Osteogenesis Imperfecta Fractures

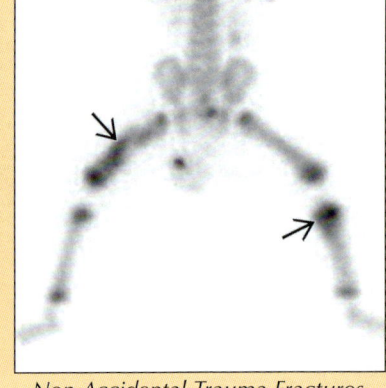

Non-Accidental Trauma Fractures

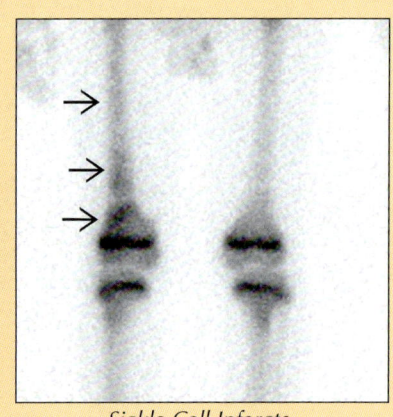

Sickle Cell Infarcts

NEUROBLASTOMA

Key Facts

Terminology
- Malignant tumor derived from undifferentiated neural crest cells
- MIBG: Structurally similar to norepinephrine; localizes to catecholamine-storing granules via active transport

Imaging Findings
- MIBG avidity on a nuclear scan
- Suprarenal mass with typical calcifications on anatomic imaging
- Correspond to the locations of the sympathetic chain: Adrenal medulla, retroperitoneum, pelvis, mediastinum, extracranial craniofacial space
- 60% present with metastases to cortical bone, bone marrow, lymph nodes, and liver; lung and brain metastases are rare
- Bone lesions show focal increased activity, often at the metaphysis
- False negatives and cold bone scan lesions can occur
- Soft tissue primary labels on bone scan 74% of the time, more often than calcifications are seen
- MIBG normal distribution to myocardium, liver, spleen, bladder, less often bowel, rarely normal adrenal glands, not to bone

Pathology
- Most common extracranial solid tumor in children accounting for 8-10% of all childhood cancers

Diagnostic Checklist
- Metastases on bone scan often symmetric and near metaphyses which requires meticulous attention to image quality and careful attention by the reader

---

- Lesions show increased activity
- 90% accurate
  - MIBG false negatives: Small lesions, physiologic uptake masking lesions, variable MIBG uptake, interfering drugs
- MIBG normal distribution to myocardium, liver, spleen, bladder, less often bowel, rarely normal adrenal glands, not to bone
- Additional nuclear medicine imaging options
  - Somatostatin receptor imaging with In-111 pentetreotide: Lower sensitivity than MIBG (64% vs. 94%) but option in MIBG negative patients

Imaging Recommendations
- Best imaging tool: MIBG for evaluating extent of metastatic disease at presentation and restaging following treatment
- Protocol advice
  - SSKI pretreatment mandatory to protect thyroid from free iodide, protocols vary slightly
    - Typical protocol 2-4 drops tid starting 2 days before until 5 days after intravenous injection of MIBG
  - Interfering drugs withdrawn at least 7 days prior to imaging
    - Tricyclic antidepressants, over the counter cough/cold remedies containing pseudoephedrine, labetalol, cocaine, opioids, metoprolol, antipsychotics
  - Typical dose 2 mCi I123 or 200-500 µCi I131 MIBG intravenously - 24, 48, and sometimes 72 hour anterior and posterior planar images
    - I-123 MIBG may offer better dosimetry and image quality than I-131, allows SPECT

DIFFERENTIAL DIAGNOSIS

Other MIBG-Positive Tissues, Lesions
- Ganglioneuroma, pheochromocytoma, paraganglioma, retinoblastoma, medullary thyroid carcinoma, carcinoid, adrenal hyperplasia, unblocked normal thyroid

Other MIBG-Negative Bone Tumors
- Wilms tumor, osteosarcoma, Ewing sarcoma, rhabdomyosarcoma, malignant lymphoma

Leukemia
- Similar appearance on plain film: Symmetrical rarefaction of metaphyses

Sickle Cell Disease with Bone Infarcts, Osteomyelitis
- Uptake on bone scan
- Osteomyelitis may be parametaphyseal in children

PATHOLOGY

General Features
- Genetics: No candidate gene has been identified
- Etiology: Most cases are sporadic with multiple cytogenetic abnormalities with approximately 1-2% inherited in an autosomal dominant pattern
- Epidemiology
  - Most common extracranial solid tumor in children accounting for 8-10% of all childhood cancers
  - Annual incidence of 10-15 per 100,000 infants with approximately 600 cases diagnosed annually in the USA
- Associated abnormalities: Girls with Turner syndrome may be predisposed to the development of neuroblastoma and related tumors

Gross Pathologic & Surgical Features
- Circumscribed or infiltrative mass that typically has a soft consistency with no capsule
  - May have calcified, necrotic or hemorrhagic foci
- 7-15% present with spinal cord involvement

Microscopic Features
- Primary features are neuroblasts (immature, undifferentiated sympathetic cells) and their derivatives (ganglion and Schwann cells) and stroma

NEUROBLASTOMA

Staging, Grading or Classification Criteria
- International Neuroblastoma Staging System (INSS)
  - 1: Localized tumor with complete gross excision and ipsilateral nodes negative
  - 2A: Localized tumor with incomplete gross excision and ipsilateral nodes negative
  - 2B: Localized tumor +/- complete gross excision with ipsilateral nodes positive and contralateral nodes negative
  - 3: Unresectable unilateral tumor infiltrating across the midline +/- nodal involvement, or midline tumor with bilateral extension by infiltration or by nodal involvement
  - 4: Any primary tumor with dissemination to distant lymph nodes, bone, bone marrow, liver, skin, or other organs
  - 4S: Localized primary (as defined for stage 1, 2a, 2b) with dissemination limited to skin, liver, < 10% tumor cells in marrow, and in infants less than 1 year

CLINICAL ISSUES

Presentation
- Most common signs/symptoms
  - Approximately two-thirds have retroperitoneal or abdominal tumors
  - Can present with a painless abdominal mass or symptoms related to mass effect including pain, weight loss, anorexia, and vomiting
- Other signs/symptoms
  - Dependent upon tumor site and size
    - Urinary dysfunction, constipation, fecal incontinence, lower-extremity weakness due to cord compression from paraspinal tumors or mass effect from pelvic tumors
    - Asymptomatic thoracic disease on chest radiography or symptoms including dysphagia and respiratory distress
    - Horner syndrome due to thoracic or neck primary
    - Hypertension, palpitations, flushing, sweating, malaise, and headache due to excess catecholamine production
    - Paraneoplastic syndromes including VIP secreting tumors causing secretory diarrhea
    - Extremity pain secondary to mets to bone and bone marrow (Hutchinson syndrome)
    - "Raccoon eyes" due to mets to retrobulbar and orbital regions
    - "Blueberry muffin syndrome" from skin metastases appearing as dark purple or blue masses

Demographics
- Age
  - Mean age at presentation: 22 months
  - 50% of patients younger than 2 years, and 75% younger than 4 years
- Gender: Slight male preponderance

Natural History & Prognosis
- Broad spectrum of behavior ranging from spontaneous regression, maturation to a benign ganglioneuroma, or aggressive fatal metastatic disease
- 15% of all cancer related deaths in children
- Poor prognostic signs include N-myc amplification (> 10 copies), substantial bone marrow involvement; telomerase expression, low expression of CD 44, high serum levels of lactate dehydrogenase and ferritin, increasing age at presentation

Treatment
- Depends on clinical stage, Shimada histopathology, and resectability
- May consider watchful waiting for stage 4S: Spontaneous regression can occur

DIAGNOSTIC CHECKLIST

Image Interpretation Pearls
- Metastases on bone scan often symmetric and near metaphyses which requires meticulous attention to image quality and careful attention by the reader
- Bone labeling on MIBG scan is not normal and abnormal labeling can be faint and symmetrical

SELECTED REFERENCES
1. Ilias I et al: New functional imaging modalities for chromaffin tumors, neuroblastomas and ganglioneuromas. Trends Endocrinol Metab. 16(2):66-72, 2005
2. Kushner BH: Neuroblastoma: a disease requiring a multitude of imaging studies. J Nucl Med. 45(7):1172-88, 2004
3. Lee KL et al: Neuroblastoma: management, recurrence, and follow-up. Urol Clin North Am. 30(4):881-90, 2003
4. Juweid ME et al: 111In-pentetreotide versus bone scintigraphy in the detection of bony metastases of neuroblastoma. Nucl Med Commun. 23(10):983-9, 2002
5. Lonergan GJ et al: Neuroblastoma, ganglioneuroblastoma, and ganglioneuroma: radiologic-pathologic correlation. Radiographics. 22(4):911-34, 2002
6. Minard V et al: Adverse outcome of infants with metastatic neuroblastoma, MYCN amplification and/or bone lesions: results of the French society of pediatric oncology. Br J Cancer. 83(8):973-9, 2000
7. Hugosson C et al: Imaging of abdominal neuroblastoma in children. Acta Radiol. 40(5):534-42, 1999
8. Perel Y et al: Clinical impact and prognostic value of metaiodobenzylguanidine imaging in children with metastatic neuroblastoma. J Pediatr Hematol Oncol. 21(1):13-8, 1999
9. Shulkin BL et al: Current concepts on the diagnostic use of MIBG in children. J Nucl Med. 39(4):679-88, 1998
10. Blatt J et al: Neuroblastoma and related tumors in Turner's syndrome. J Pediatr. 131(5):666-70, 1997
11. Leung A et al: Specificity of radioiodinated MIBG for neural crest tumors in childhood. J Nucl Med. 38(9):1352-7, 1997
12. Manil L et al: Indium-111-pentetreotide scintigraphy in children with neuroblast-derived tumors. J Nucl Med. 37(6):893-6, 1996
13. Shulkin BL et al: Iodine-131-metaiodobenzylguanidine and bone scintigraphy for the detection of neuroblastoma. J Nucl Med. 33(10):1735-40, 1992

NEUROBLASTOMA

IMAGE GALLERY

Other

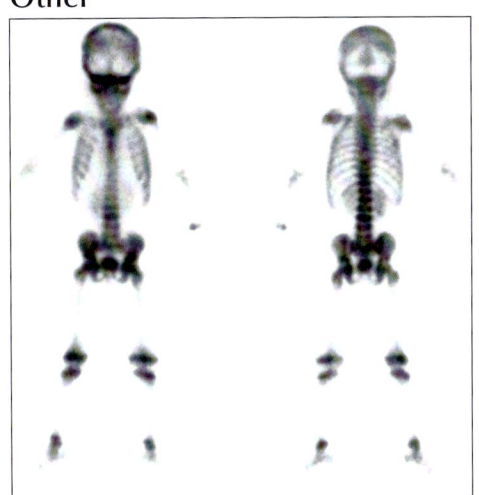

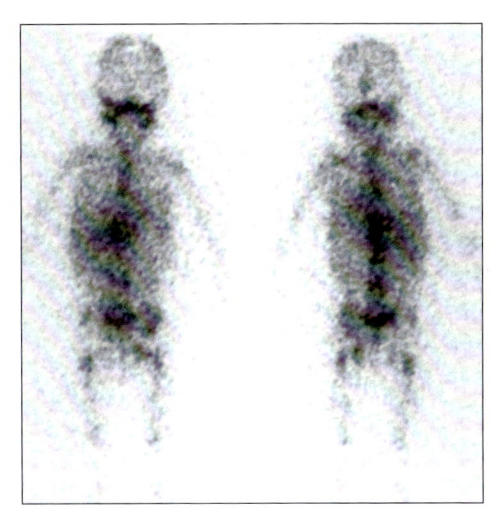

(Left) Anterior and posterior bone scan in child with diffuse skeletal neuroblastoma. Homogeneous intense uptake can be confused with normal scan at increased intensity settings. See MIBG at right. *(Right)* I-131 MIBG scan. Same patient as at left with diffuse skeletal metastases due to neuroblastoma. Note widespread skeletal uptake. There should be no bone uptake on a normal MIBG scan.

Typical

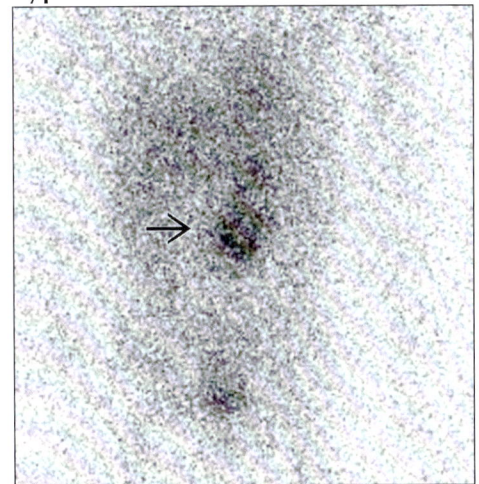

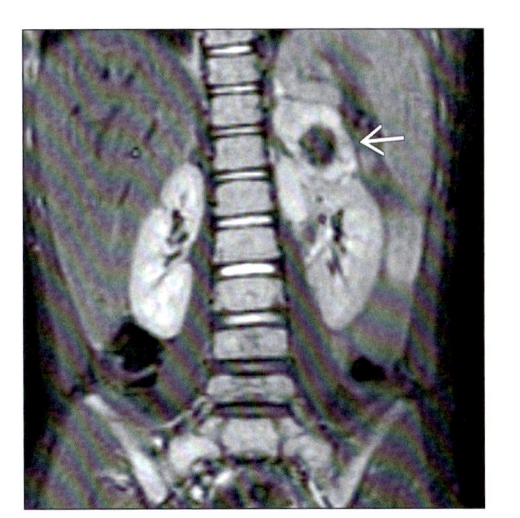

(Left) Anterior I-131 MIBG scan of abdomen and pelvis shows increased activity labeling a primary neuroblastoma ➔. *(Right)* Coronal MR shows the left adrenal neuroblastoma seen on the previous nuclear image ➔.

Typical

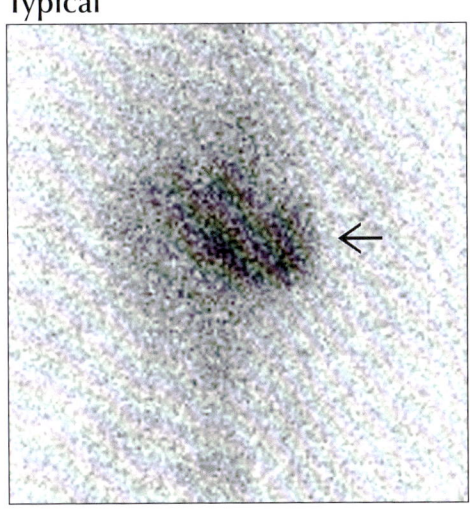

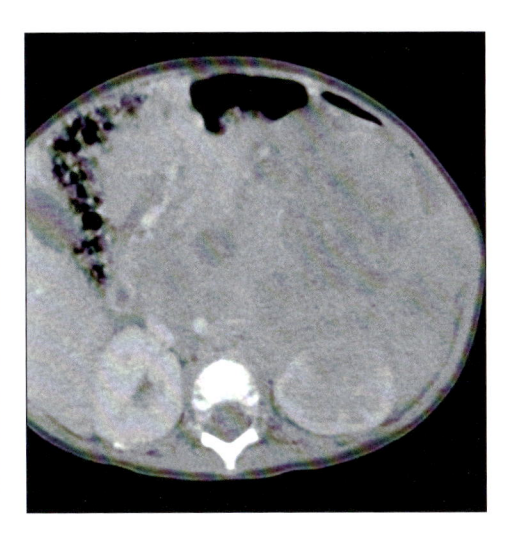

(Left) Anterior I-131 MIBG scan of trunk shows labeling of a large neuroblastoma ➔; see next image. *(Right)* Axial CECT shows the large neuroblastoma seen on the MIBG scan (prior image).

NEUROBLASTOMA

Typical

(Left) Anterior and posterior bone scan shows uptake in right adrenal neuroblastoma ➡, symmetrical diffuse metaphyseal uptake consistent with widespread bony metastases ➣. (Right) Anterior bone scan shows symmetric labeling of all metaphyses ➡ with loss of distinctness of the epiphyseal margins due to metastatic neuroblastoma (see next image).

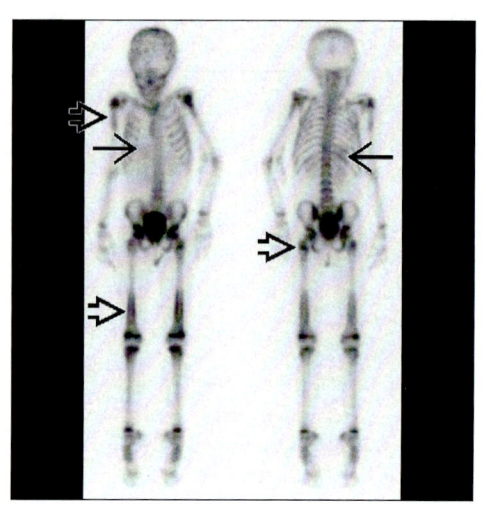

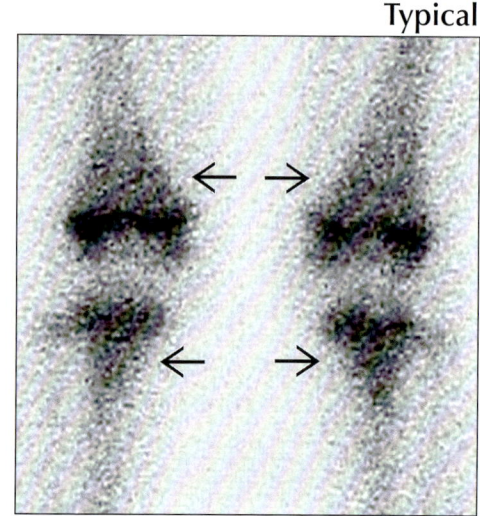

Other

(Left) Anterior bone scan shows prior patient post therapy. The metaphyses are markedly improved but the epiphyseal margins remain subtly indistinct ➣. (Right) Anterior Tc-99m sulfur colloid shows areas of decreased activity over both hips ➡ and left pelvis ➣ from neuroblastoma metastases displacing bone marrow (see next 2 images).

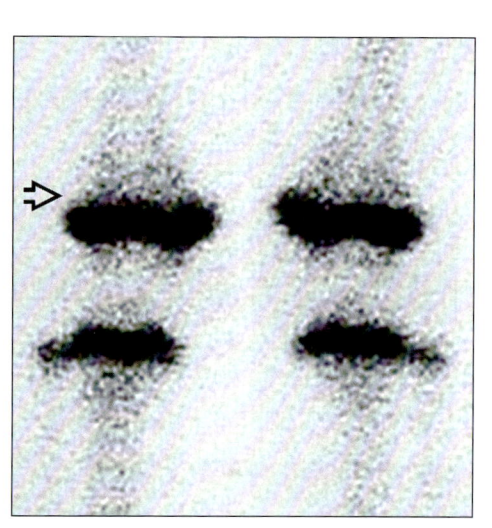

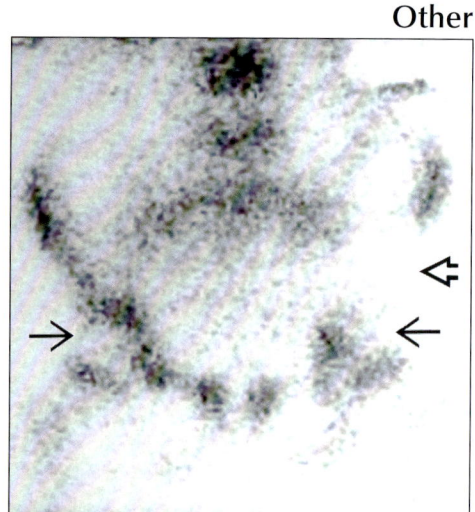

Other

(Left) Anterior bone scan shows on the same patient increased osteoblastic activity in hips ➡ and left iliac crest ➣ where the colloid is being displaced on the prior image. See next image (Right) Same patient as prior 2 images. Anterior MIBG scintigraphy of pelvis shows increased activity at sites of tumor in the proximal femurs ➡ and in the left iliac crest ➣.

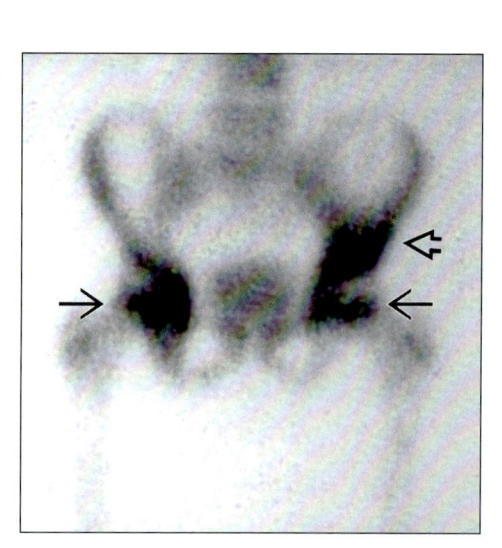

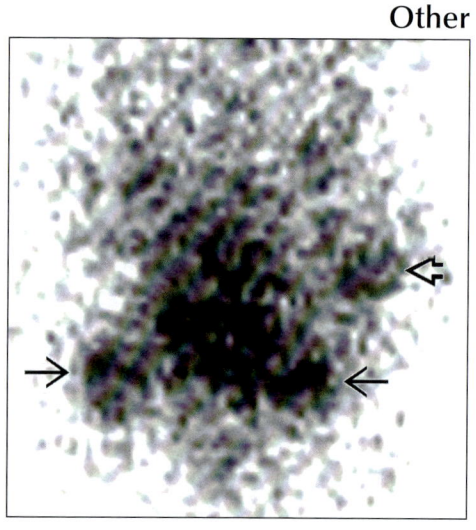

NEUROBLASTOMA

Typical

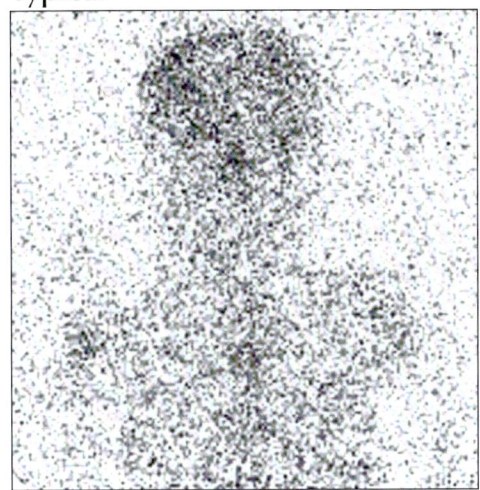

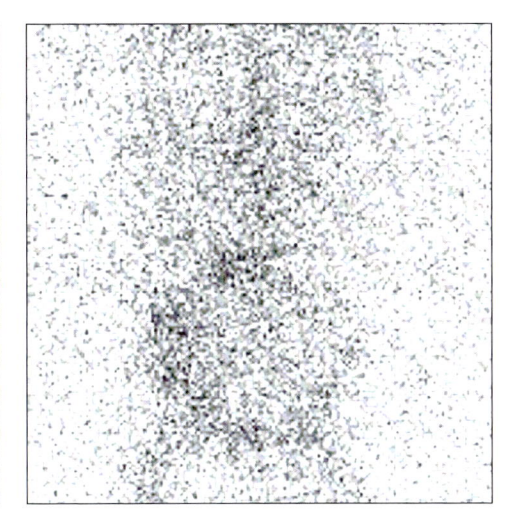

(Left) Anterior I-131 MIBG scan of head and chest shows relatively diffuse skeletal neuroblastoma metastases (see next 2 images), which can look more subtle than this. *(Right)* Anterior I-131 MIBG scan of abdomen and pelvis shows diffuse skeletal neuroblastoma metastases.

Typical

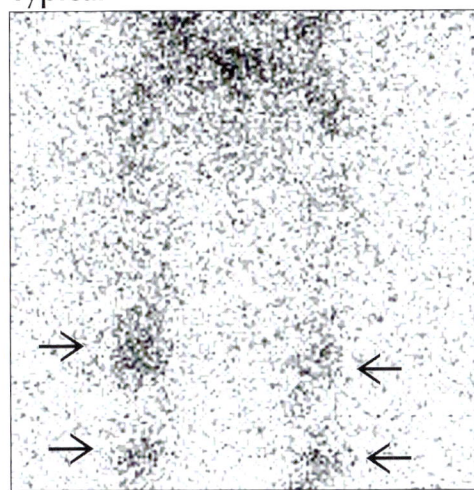

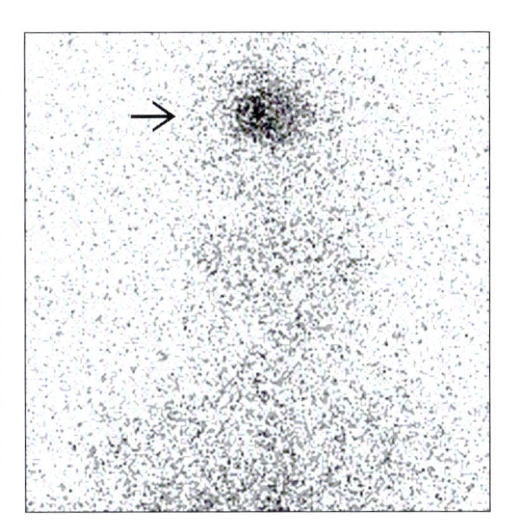

(Left) Anterior I-131 MIBG scan of thighs and knees show relatively diffuse skeletal metastases including symmetric metaphyseal involvement around the knees ➡. *(Right)* Posterior I-131 MIBG of head shows a calvarial neuroblastoma metastasis ➡ (see next 2 images).

Typical

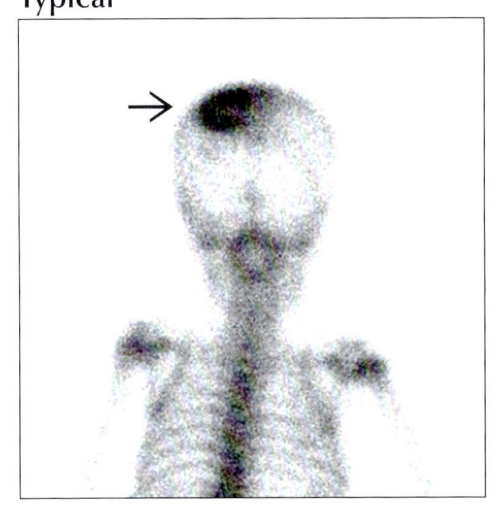

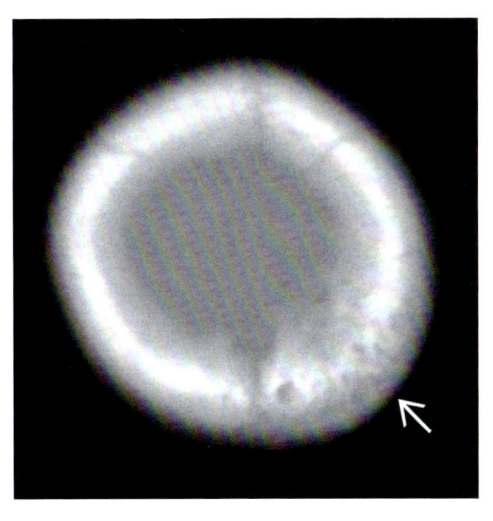

(Left) Posterior bone scan shows the calvarial metastasis seen on the prior nuclear image ➡. *(Right)* Axial NECT shows the calvarial neuroblastoma metastasis seen on the prior 2 images ➡.

ASPLENIA/POLYSPLENIA SYNDROMES

Graphic shows variant position of stomach and spleen. Stomach location defines site of dorsal aspect of mesentery, where spleen should be located, if it exists.

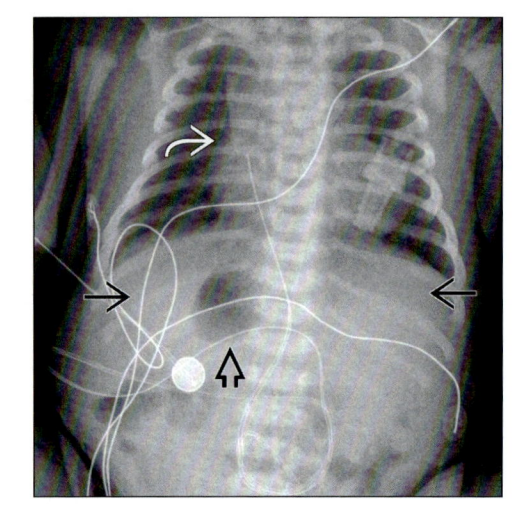

Anterior radiograph shows horizontally oriented liver, abnormal mediastinal contour (descending aorta) and right-sided stomach. If present, the spleen would also be expected on the right.

TERMINOLOGY

Abbreviations and Synonyms
- Asplenia
  - Ivemark syndrome
  - Bilateral right-sidedness
  - Right isomerism
- Polysplenia
  - Bilateral left-sidedness
  - Left isomerism

Definitions
- Heterotaxy syndrome (HS): Embryological mishap of aberrant lateralization of visceral organs and vena cavae, including splenic abnormalities
  - Greek
    - "Heteros" = other
    - "Taxis" = arrangement
- Splenic anomalies associated with heterotaxy
  - Asplenia (53%)
    - Absent spleen
  - Polysplenia (42%)
    - Usually right-sided
    - Clustered small splenules
    - One large spleen with several splenules
    - Multilobed spleen
  - Single right-sided spleen (5%)
    - Right upper quadrant
  - Normal left-sided spleen (rare)
    - Left upper quadrant

IMAGING FINDINGS

General Features
- Best diagnostic clue
  - Tc-99m heat-damaged red blood cell (RBC) scan
    - Activity in splenic tissue ↑ over time due to accumulation of heat-damaged RBCs
- Location
  - Abdominal radiograph
    - Stomach location defines site of dorsal aspect of mesentery
    - Spleen should be located at dorsal aspect of mesentery (if it exists)

Nuclear Medicine Findings
- Tc-99m labeled, heat-damaged RBC scan

DDx: Splenosis, Accessory Splenic Tissue

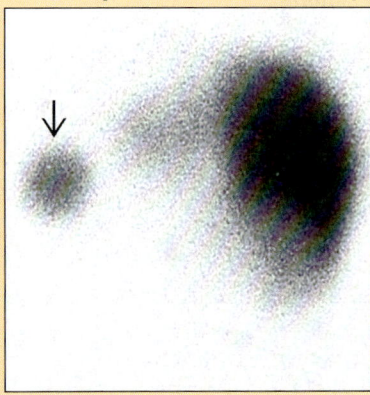

Splenule Post Splenectomy

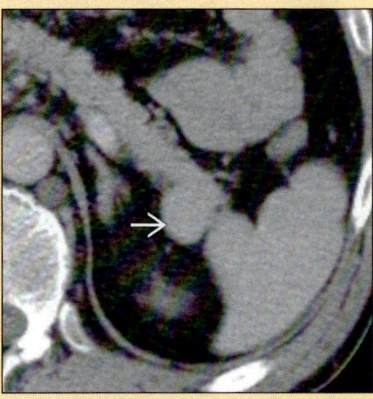

Accessory Spleen (M. Federle, MD)

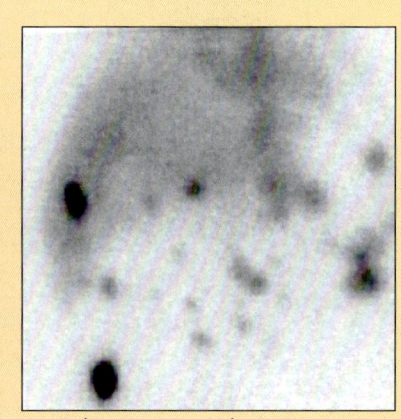

Splenosis Post Splenic Trauma

ASPLENIA/POLYSPLENIA SYNDROMES

Key Facts

Terminology
- Heterotaxy syndrome (HS): Embryological mishap of aberrant lateralization of visceral organs and vena cavae, including splenic abnormalities
- Asplenia (53%)
- Polysplenia (42%)
- Single right-sided spleen (5%)
- Normal left-sided spleen (rare)

Imaging Findings
- Tc-99m heat-damaged red blood cell (RBC) scan
- Activity in splenic tissue ↑ over time due to accumulation of heat-damaged RBCs
- Thermal injury to RBCs ⇒ rigidity, spherocytosis, budding and microspherocytosis
- Spleen culls abnormal RBCs from circulation
- Spleen: Increased radiotracer uptake over time
- Liver: Stable or decreased radiotracer uptake over time
- Evaluate contours of liver and spleen with SPECT
- Confirm separate organs vs. horizontally oriented liver

Clinical Issues
- Asplenia
- Immunologic and hematologic abnormalities
- Up to 80% mortality in first year

Diagnostic Checklist
- Check abdominal radiograph
- If present, spleen should be on same side as stomach due to mesenteric anatomy
- Confirm that spleen is separate from liver
- Determine hepatic contours with hepatobiliary scan
- SPECT often useful

- Thermal injury to RBCs ⇒ rigidity, spherocytosis, budding and microspherocytosis
  - Spleen culls abnormal RBCs from circulation
  - Insufficient damage: Blood pool activity, little spleen accumulation
  - Excessive damage: Hepatic uptake > splenic uptake
- Posterior planar images
  - Spleen: Increased radiotracer uptake over time
  - Liver: Stable or decreased radiotracer uptake over time
- SPECT often useful, especially with hepatic variants
  - Evaluate contours of liver and spleen with SPECT
  - Confirm separate organs vs. horizontally oriented liver

Imaging Recommendations
- Best imaging tool: Tc-99m labeled, heat-damaged RBC scan
- Protocol advice
  - Heat-damaged RBC scan
    - Heat damage RBCs in water bath for 20 min. at 49-50°C
    - Label 3 cc patient's blood with 15-30 mCi (555-1110 MBq) Tc-99m (adult); 0.2-0.4 mCi/kg [(7-15 MBq/kg) children]
    - Parallel hole collimator
    - Posterior planar images at 15, 30, and 45 minutes
    - SPECT to define organ contours
- Additional nuclear medicine imaging options
  - Tc-99m sulfur colloid liver-spleen scan
    - Uptake in liver and spleen
    - Often compared to hepatobiliary scintigraphy
  - Hepatobiliary scintigraphy
    - Defines hepatic contours
    - Early planar or SPECT images
    - Correlate with heat-damaged RBC scan or liver-spleen scan
- Correlative imaging features
  - Radiographs
    - Situs solitus: Aortic arch, cardiac apex, gastric bubble on left
    - Situs inversus: Aortic arch, cardiac apex, gastric bubble on right
    - Situs ambiguous: Unable to classify as situs solitus or inversus; heterotaxy
    - Cardiomegaly
    - Diminished pulmonary blood flow
    - Stomach localization
  - Abdominal ultrasound (US)
    - Can identify spleen
    - Can confuse liver with spleen
    - Determine position of great vessels
  - Echocardiography
    - Define cardiac anomalies
    - Define cardiovascular anatomy
  - MR
    - Surgical planning for cardiac anomalies
  - CT
    - Determine anatomy when other modalities nondiagnostic

DIFFERENTIAL DIAGNOSIS

Wandering Spleen
- Normal spleen
- No ligamentous attachments to keep spleen in normal position

Splenectomy
- Post-surgical absence of spleen
- Splenules may be present

Accessory Spleen
- Congenital focus of splenic tissue in addition to normal spleen
- Functions normally
- Most frequently just outside hilum of normal spleen

Splenosis
- Multiple foci of splenic tissue
- Post-traumatic

ASPLENIA/POLYSPLENIA SYNDROMES

PATHOLOGY

General Features
- Genetics
  - Usually sporadic
  - Familial cases autosomal recessive
- Etiology
  - Early disruption of midline cell signals responsible for left-right lateralization
  - Lateralization of organs begin embryonic day 23 with cardiac tube
- Epidemiology: Incidence: 1 in 6,000 to 20,000 live births
- Associated abnormalities: Diabetes mellitus

Gross Pathologic & Surgical Features
- Asplenia syndrome
  - Bilateral right-sidedness (right isomerism)
    - Bilateral right atria
    - Horizontally oriented liver
    - Three-lobed lungs (bilateral minor fissures)
    - Symmetry of tracheobronchial tree
    - Asplenia
    - Descending aorta and inferior vena cava (IVC) on same side of spine
    - Stomach midline, right or left
    - Bowel malrotation
- Polysplenia syndrome
  - Bilateral left-sidedness (left isomerism)
    - Bilateral left atria
    - Two-lobed lungs
    - Polysplenia
    - IVC may connect with azygous or hemiazygous
    - Stomach midline, right or left
    - Bowel malrotation

Microscopic Features
- Howell-Jolly bodies
  - Asplenic newborns: RBC inclusions in peripheral blood smear (also in normal newborns)

CLINICAL ISSUES

Presentation
- Most common signs/symptoms
  - Asplenia syndrome
    - Cyanosis due to cardiac anomalies
    - Palpable bilobed liver
    - Intestinal obstruction
    - Overwhelming infection
  - Polysplenia syndrome
    - Cardiac anomalies less severe
    - Cyanosis uncommon
    - Intestinal obstruction
    - Overwhelming infection due to functional asplenism

Demographics
- Age: Usually neonatal diagnosis
- Gender
  - Asplenia: M > F
  - Polysplenia: M = F

Natural History & Prognosis
- Normal spleen
  - Red pulp
    - Reticuloendothelial clearance (RBCs, white blood cells, platelets)
  - White pulp
    - B lymphocytes, plasma cells, macrophages
- Asplenia
  - Immunologic and hematologic abnormalities
  - Up to 80% mortality in first year
- Polysplenia
  - Functional asplenia ⇒ immunologic/hematologic abnormalities
  - Up to 60% mortality in first year
  - 10% survive to mid-adolescence

Treatment
- Asplenia
  - Cardiac anomalies
    - Surgery
  - Asplenia
    - Antibiotics (encapsulated organisms)
  - Intestinal malrotation ⇒ obstruction
    - Surgery
- Polysplenia
  - Functional asplenia
    - Antibiotics (encapsulated organisms)

DIAGNOSTIC CHECKLIST

Consider
- Horizontally oriented liver/liver tail can be misconstrued as splenic tissue on US
  - Consider Tc-99m labeled, heat-damaged RBC scintigraphy
    - Increases specificity of US
    - Misdiagnosing asplenia has dire infectious consequences

Image Interpretation Pearls
- Check abdominal radiograph
  - If present, spleen should be on same side as stomach due to mesenteric anatomy
- Splenic activity ↑ over time on heat-damaged RBC scan
- Confirm that spleen is separate from liver
  - Determine hepatic contours with hepatobiliary scan
  - SPECT often useful

SELECTED REFERENCES
1. Applegate KE et al: Situs revisited: imaging of the heterotaxy syndrome. Radiographics. 19(4):837-52; discussion 853-4, 1999
2. Freeman JL et al: CT of congenital and acquired abnormalities of the spleen. Radiographics. 13(3):597-610, 1993
3. Armas RR. Related Articles et al: Clinical studies with spleen-specific radiolabeled agents. Semin Nucl Med. 15(3):260-75, 1985
4. Sty JR et al: The spleen: development and functional evaluation. Semin Nucl Med. 15(3):276-98, 1985

ASPLENIA/POLYSPLENIA SYNDROMES

IMAGE GALLERY

Typical

Typical

Typical

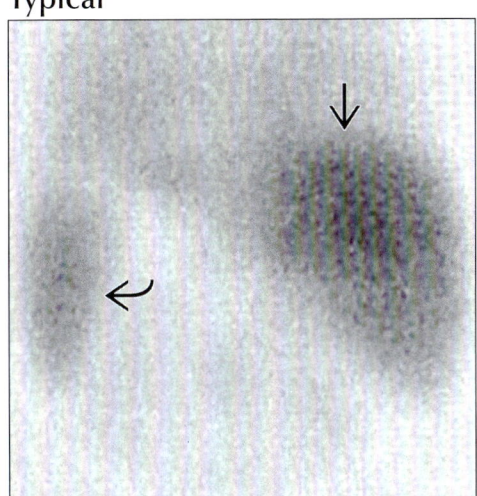

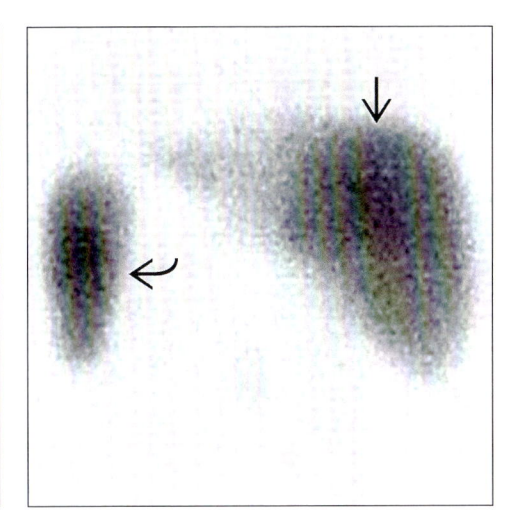

(Left) Posterior heat damaged red cell scan imaged at 15 minutes shows normal hepatic contour ➔ and focal activity in expected location of spleen ➔. (Right) Posterior heat damaged red cell scan in same patient at left imaged at 45 minutes shows normal hepatic contour ➔. Over time, activity has increased in expected location of spleen ➔, signifying progressive accumulation of damaged red cells in patient with normal spleen.

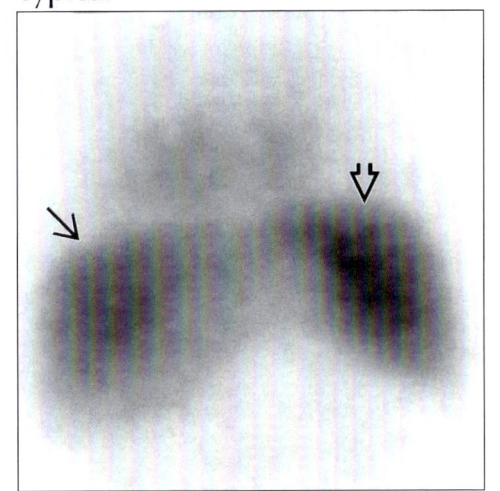

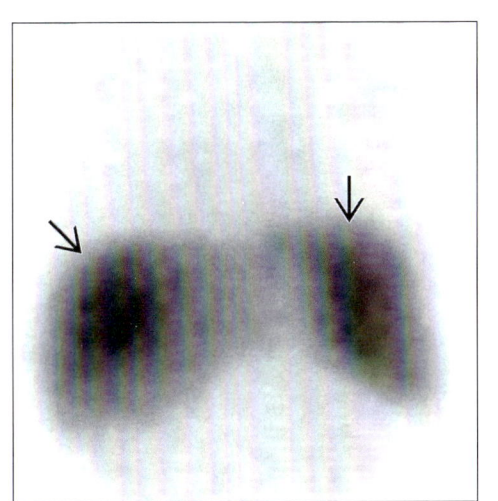

(Left) Anterior heat damaged red cell scan shows uptake in liver ➔ as well as tissue in expected location of spleen ➔. (Right) Anterior hepatobiliary IDA scan in same patient as previous image shows similar appearance to heat damaged red cell scan. Thus, a horizontally oriented liver ➔ is present and asplenia confirmed.

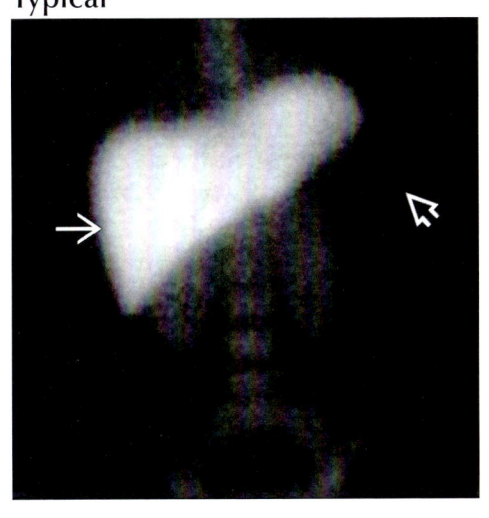

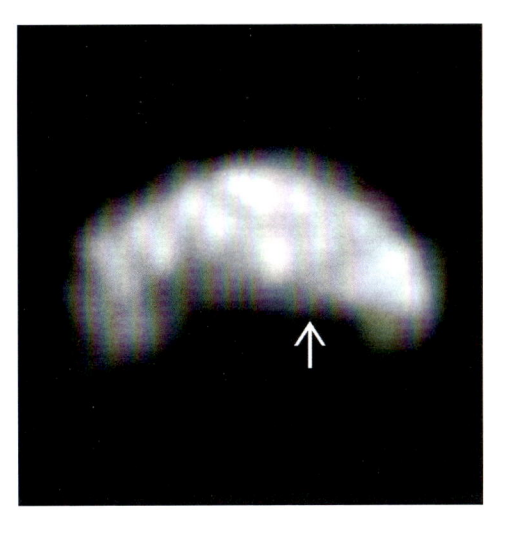

(Left) Anterior Tc-99m sulfur colloid shows normal hepatic contours ➔ with no focal activity expected location of spleen ➔. (Right) Axial Tc-99m sulfur colloid SPECT of same patient at left confirms contiguous left hepatic contour ➔ without photopenic space that would signify separate splenic tissue, confirming asplenia.

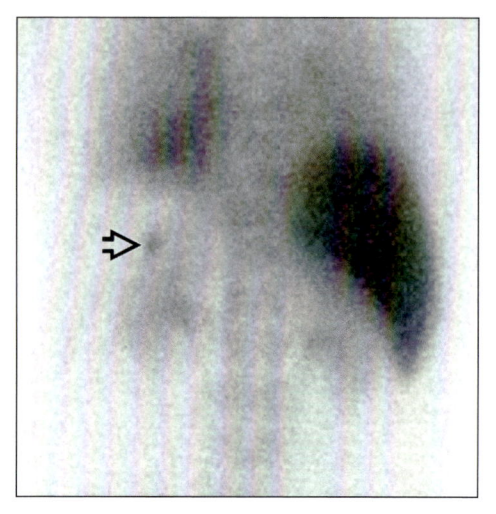

ACCESSORY & ECTOPIC SPLENIC TISSUE

Posterior heat damaged red cell scan 10 minutes post-injection shows moderate labeling of splenic tissue ⇨ projected over left kidney. Damaged red blood cells are also seen in blood pool.

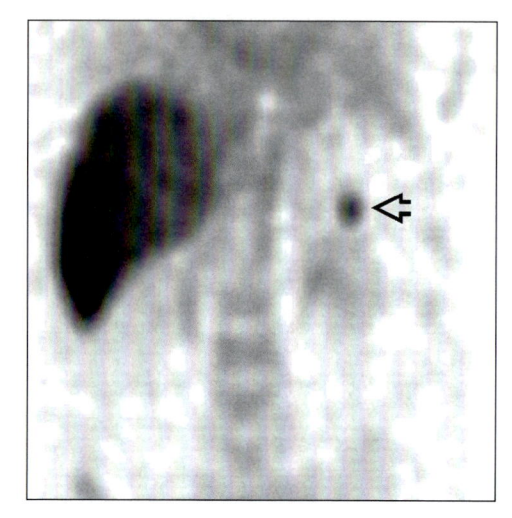

Coronal heat damaged red cell scan delayed SPECT image in same patient as previous image shows the accessory spleen ⇨ to better advantage than the earlier planar image.

TERMINOLOGY

Abbreviations and Synonyms
- Splenosis, spleniculi, splenules, heterotopic splenic transplantation; idiopathic thrombocytopenic purpura (ITP)

Definitions
- Accessory spleen: Ectopic splenic tissue of congenital origin
  - Common anatomic variant
- Splenosis: Fragments of tissue from a ruptured spleen become implanted in peritoneal or thoracic cavity and undergo regeneration and vascularization
  - Typically post-traumatic, less likely post-surgical

IMAGING FINDINGS

General Features
- Best diagnostic clue
  - Accumulation of tracer outside of the expected location of the spleen, bone marrow and liver on denatured RBC scan
- CT SPECT fusion can improve anatomic localization
- Location
  - Accessory spleens most commonly occur near the splenic hilum
    - Approximately 20% occur elsewhere in the abdomen or retroperitoneum, typically in left upper quadrant
    - Rarely can be found embedded in pancreatic tail, intrahepatic, or paratesticular
    - Multiple in approximately 12% of cases and typically clustered in the same location
  - Splenosis secondary to trauma can be widely distributed
    - Thoracic splenosis occurs when there is simultaneous splenic and diaphragmatic injury allowing for distribution of splenic rests into thoracic cavity
- Size: Varies from several mm to several cm diameter
- Morphology: Generally round or ovoid with texture and contrast-enhancement identical to normal spleen

Nuclear Medicine Findings
- Denatured RBC scan

DDx: Splenosis Appearance with Various Nuclear Medicine Modalities

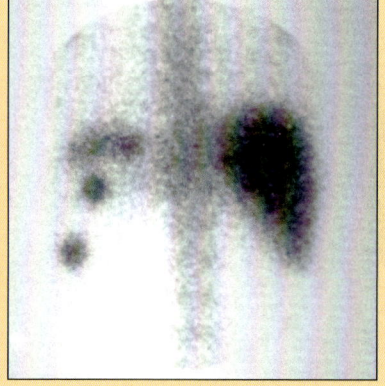

In-111 WBCs 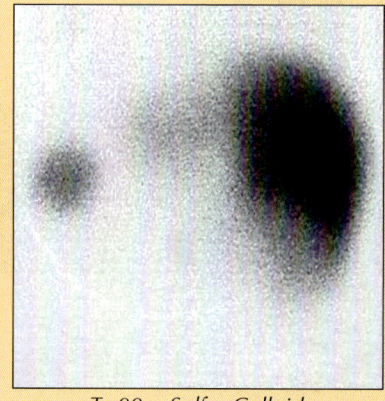 | *Tc-99m Sulfur Colloid* 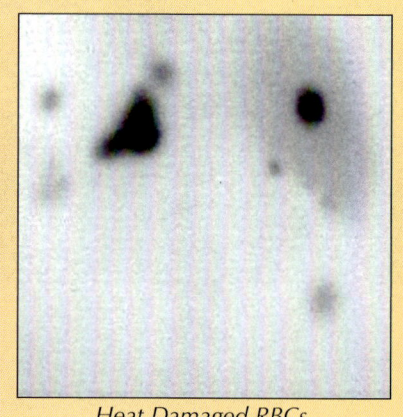 | *Heat Damaged RBCs*

ACCESSORY & ECTOPIC SPLENIC TISSUE

Key Facts

Terminology
- Accessory spleen: Ectopic splenic tissue of congenital origin
- Splenosis: Fragments of tissue from a ruptured spleen become implanted in peritoneal or thoracic cavity and undergo regeneration and vascularization

Imaging Findings
- Accessory spleens most commonly occur near the splenic hilum
- Splenosis secondary to trauma can be widely distributed
- Functional splenic tissue sequesters senescent or denatured RBCs
- Can identify nodules down to 1-2 cm in size
- Tc-99m denatured RBC scan
- CT or MR can be fused to SPECT off-line or can be acquired together with SPECT/CT scanner
- Label cells using in-vitro kit as for radionuclide ventriculogram (e.g. "Ultratag" kit)
- Heat in a 49 degree Celsius water bath for 45 minutes to denature cells
- Let cool and reinject into patient
- Consider SPECT as part of standard protocol

Pathology
- Accessory spleen common and present in 10-30% of population at autopsy
- Splenosis results in 25-66% of patients who require a splenectomy for trauma
- Polysplenia syndrome occurs in approximately 4 per 1 million live births

---

  - Functional splenic tissue sequesters senescent or denatured RBCs
  - Can identify nodules down to 1-2 cm in size
  - Focal labeling not associated with liver or spleen
  - Time course of appearance may parallel normal splenic tissue, if present
- Alternative agents to denatured RBC may be useful if initial study is negative
  - Tc-99m sulfur colloid
    - Localization based on phagocytic function of ectopic splenic tissue
    - Recommended when cannot obtain adequate blood volume for labeling
  - In-111 WBC
    - Localizes based on WBC trapping by splenic tissue
- Case reports of In-111 octreotide uptake in ectopic splenic tissue mimicking tumor

CT Findings
- NECT: Well-marginated, uniform soft tissue mass varying in number and shape
- CECT
  - Same enhancement as normal splenic tissue
    - For accessory spleens, vascularization is typically supplied by branches of splenic artery

Angiographic Findings
- Accessory spleens show blood supply from a branch of splenic artery with drainage into splenic veins
  - No longer used for diagnosis

Ultrasonographic Findings
- Homogeneous round contour typically near splenic hilum with echogenicity identical to normal spleen

Imaging Recommendations
- Best imaging tool
  - Tc-99m denatured RBC scan
  - CT or MR useful in providing anatomic information
    - CT or MR can be fused to SPECT off-line or can be acquired together with SPECT/CT scanner
- Protocol advice
  - Label red cells
    - Label cells using in-vitro kit as for radionuclide ventriculogram (e.g. "Ultratag" kit)
    - Alternative "in-vivtro" method: Intravenous injection of unlabeled pyrophosphate bone kit (stannous chloride is essential reducing agent), wait 20 minutes, withdraw 20 ml blood, centrifuge, labeled with Tc-99m pertechnetate
  - Heat denaturation of red cells
    - Heat in a 49 degree Celsius water bath for 45 minutes to denature cells
    - Let cool and reinject into patient
  - Consider SPECT as part of standard protocol
    - SPECT can be positive when planar images are negative and provides superior localization for positive studies
  - Heat denatured RBC formulation problems
    - Low heating temperature or inadequate heating time results in decreased spleen uptake and persistent blood pool residence
    - High heating temperature or excessive heating time results in decreased spleen uptake and increased liver, bone marrow uptake
    - Recent RBC transfusion may result in excessive denaturing despite conventional protocol

DIFFERENTIAL DIAGNOSIS

Accessory Spleen
- Accessory spleen is congenital and often an incidental finding

Splenosis
- Splenosis may mimic malignancy in the chest, abdomen, and pelvis on anatomic imaging

Polysplenia Syndrome
- Congenital disorder with multiple small spleens associated with variable cardiac and situs anomalies

ACCESSORY & ECTOPIC SPLENIC TISSUE

PATHOLOGY

General Features
- Etiology
  - Accessory spleens
    - Failed fusion of embryonic splenic buds
    - Extreme splenic lobulation with pinching off of splenic tissue
  - Splenosis
    - History of abdominal trauma or splenectomy
  - Polysplenia syndrome
    - Genetics not clearly defined but appears to have familial predisposition
- Epidemiology
  - Accessory spleen common and present in 10-30% of population at autopsy
  - Splenosis results in 25-66% of patients who require a splenectomy for trauma
  - Polysplenia syndrome occurs in approximately 4 per 1 million live births
- Associated abnormalities: Cardiac and situs disorders may be present with polysplenia syndrome

Gross Pathologic & Surgical Features
- Same texture as normal spleen with variable distribution in abdomen but most commonly in splenic hilum or left upper quadrant

Microscopic Features
- Structurally identical to normal splenic tissue

CLINICAL ISSUES

Presentation
- Most common signs/symptoms
  - Accessory spleens are generally asymptomatic
    - Often an incidental finding on imaging for unrelated symptoms
    - May be mistaken for tumor on cross-sectional imaging
  - Ectopic splenic tissue may cause persistent or recurrent anemia or thrombocytopenia following surgical splenectomy for ITP
- Other signs/symptoms: Ectopic splenic tissue can cause abdominal pain from torsion, rupture, or infarction

Natural History & Prognosis
- Ectopic splenic tissue can rupture, infarct, or become torsed
- Recurrence of anemia, thrombocytopenia following therapeutic splenectomy

Treatment
- Generally no treatment for asymptomatic ectopic splenic tissue
- Surgical resection if causing clinical symptoms

DIAGNOSTIC CHECKLIST

Image Interpretation Pearls
- Acquire planar images for preset time
  - Planar images acquired for total counts may be falsely negative due to high uptake in normal organs
- Infants: Relatively large liver more likely to mask the left upper quadrant
  - Consider SPECT and multiple projections
- Window images to optimize intensity and contrast
  - Study may be better viewed on a monitor
- In patients with potential asplenia or poorly defined anatomy, splenic tissue on serial images increases in intensity, blood pool decreases
  - If no hemolysis, the liver will also decrease

SELECTED REFERENCES

1. Mortele KJ et al: CT features of the accessory spleen. AJR Am J Roentgenol. 183(6):1653-7, 2004
2. Phom H et al: Comparative evaluation of Tc-99m-heat-denatured RBC and Tc-99m-anti-D IgG opsonized RBC spleen planar and SPECT scintigraphy in the detection of accessory spleen in postsplenectomy patients with chronic idiopathic thrombocytopenic purpura. Clin Nucl Med. 29(7):403-9, 2004
3. Yammine JN et al: Radionuclide imaging in thoracic splenosis and a review of the literature. Clin Nucl Med. 28(2):121-3, 2003
4. Zuckier LS et al: Selective role of nuclear medicine in evaluating the acute abdomen. Radiol Clin North Am. 41(6):1275-88, 2003
5. Phom H et al: Detection of multiple accessory spleens in a patient with chronic idiopathic thrombocytopenia purpura. Clin Nucl Med. 26(7):593-5, 2001
6. Coventry BJ et al: Intraoperative scintigraphic localization and laparoscopic excision of accessory splenic tissue. Surg Endosc. 12(2):159-61, 1998
7. Normand JP et al: Thoracic splenosis after blunt trauma: frequency and imaging findings. AJR Am J Roentgenol. 161(4):739-41, 1993
8. Cardaci GT et al: Scintigraphic diagnosis and computed tomographic localization of an accessory spleen following relapse of chronic immune thrombocytopaenia. Australas Radiol. 36(3):268-70, 1992
9. Harwood SJ et al: Functional studies of left upper quadrant mass aid management of idiopathic thrombocytopenic purpura. Clin Nucl Med. 17(8):652-5, 1992
10. Massey MD et al: Residual spleen found on denatured red blood cell scan following negative colloid scans. J Nucl Med. 32(12):2286-7, 1991
11. Schiff RG et al: The noninvasive diagnosis of intrathoracic splenosis using technetium-99m heat-damaged red blood cells. Clin Nucl Med. 12(10):785-7, 1987
12. Zwas ST et al: Scintigraphic assessment of ectopic splenic tissue localization and function following splenectomy for trauma. Eur J Nucl Med. 12(3):125-9, 1986
13. Srivastava SC et al: Radionuclide-labeled red blood cells: current status and future prospects. Semin Nucl Med. 14(2):68-82, 1984
14. Moallem AG et al: The roles of scintigraphy in splenic trauma. Clin Nucl Med. 7(6):267-8, 1982
15. Armas RR et al: A simplified method of selective spleen scintigraphy with Tc-99m-labeled erythrocytes: clinical applications. Concise communication. J Nucl Med. 21(5):413-6, 1980

ACCESSORY & ECTOPIC SPLENIC TISSUE

IMAGE GALLERY

Typical

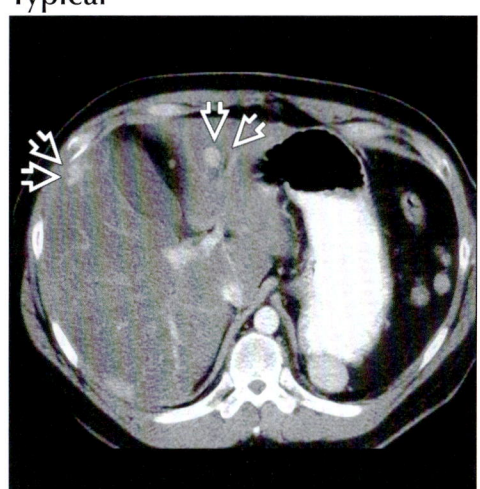

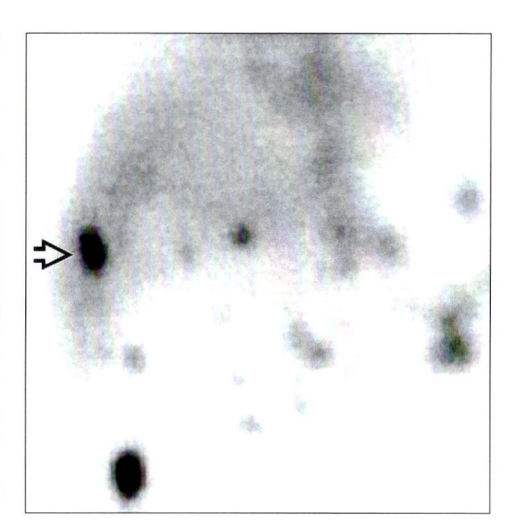

(Left) Axial CECT in patient with prior splenic rupture and surgical removal. Multiple splenules, including in liver ⮕. *(Right)* Anterior heat damaged red cell scan shows widespread splenosis, including a deposit in the liver ⮕.

Variant

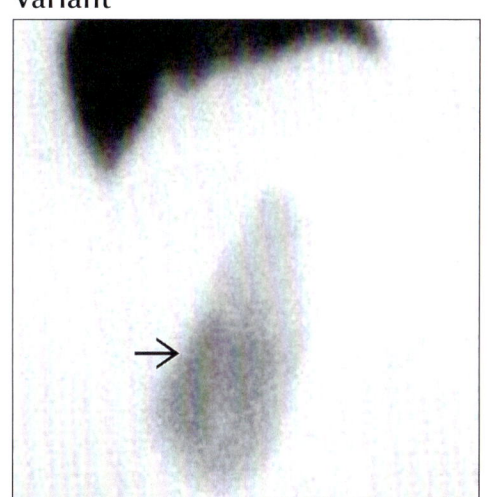

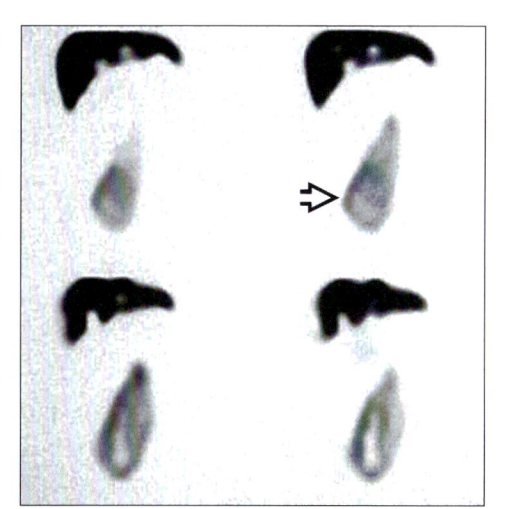

(Left) Anterior planar Tc-99m sulfur colloid shows an ectopic spleen ⮕. *(Right)* Coronal Tc-99m sulfur colloid SPECT in same patient as previous image shows an ectopic spleen ⮕. The photopenic region is the splenic hilum.

Variant

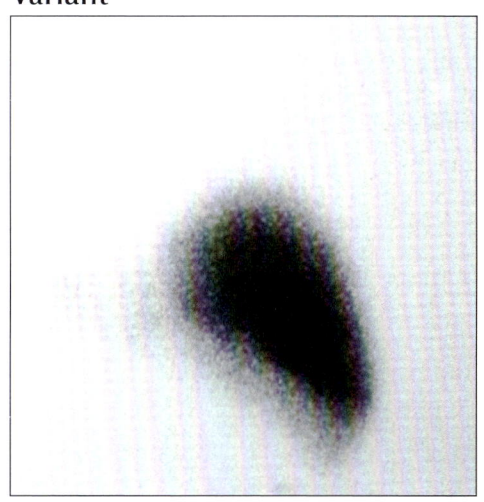

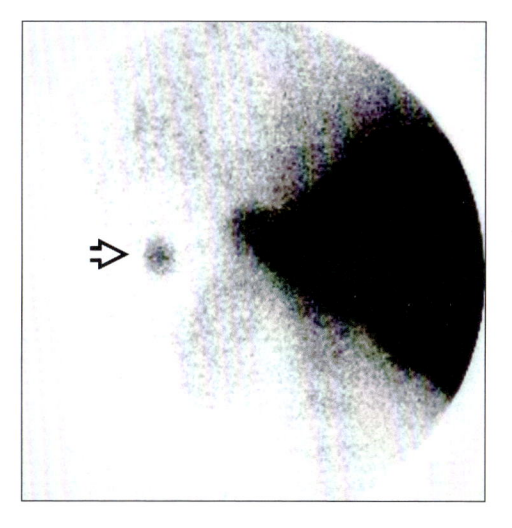

(Left) Posterior Tc-99m sulfur colloid image fails to show accessory splenic tissue and standard intensity settings and acquisition times. See next image. *(Right)* Posterior Tc-99m sulfur colloid image, obtained for additional counts and higher intensity settings show small accessory spleen ⮕. (Same patient as previous image).

ESOPHAGEAL CANCER

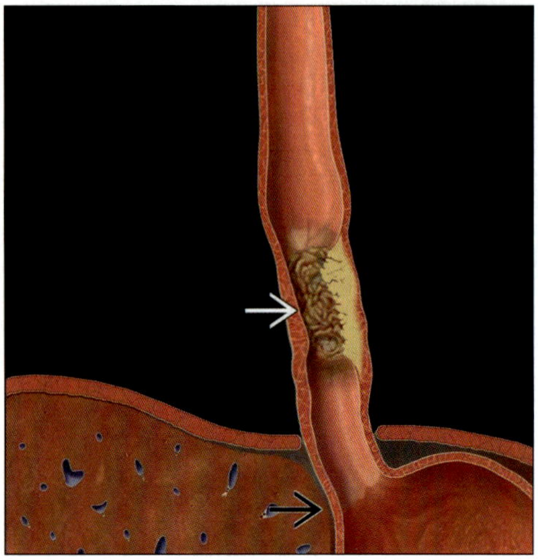

Graphic shows sessile mass ➡ in distal esophagus above gastroesophageal junction ➡, representing esophageal adenocarcinoma.

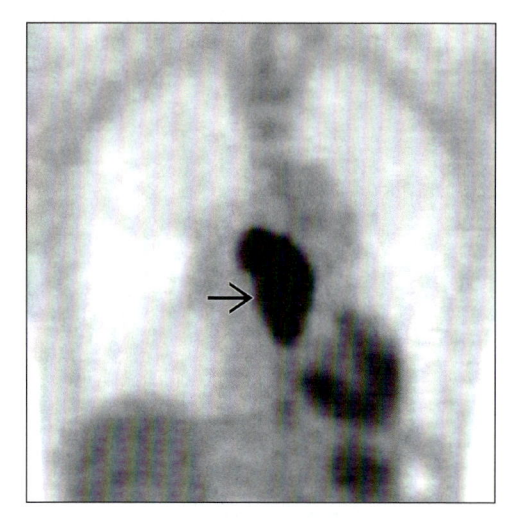

Coronal FDG PET shows bulky hypermetabolic mass in mid-esophagus ➡ in patient with primary esophageal adenocarcinoma.

TERMINOLOGY

Abbreviations and Synonyms
- Esophageal cancer/carcinoma (EC)

Definitions
- Squamous cell carcinoma (SCCA): Malignant transformation of squamous epithelium
- Adenocarcinoma (ACA): Malignant dysplasia in columnar metaplasia (Barrett mucosa)

IMAGING FINDINGS

General Features
- Best diagnostic clue
  - FDG PET: Hypermetabolic esophageal mass, lymphadenopathy, distant metastases
  - CECT: Fixed, irregular narrowing of lumen
- Location: Middle 3rd (50%), lower 3rd (30%), upper 3rd (20%) of esophagus
- Size: Early EC < 3.5 cm; advanced EC > 3.5 cm
- Morphology: Mass that narrows esophageal lumen: Infiltrating, polypoid, ulcerative, varicoid
- Other general features
  - Carcinoma: Most common tumor of esophagus
  - SCCA
    - 50-70% of all ECs
    - 1% of all cancers; 7% of all GI cancers
    - Two major risk factors in US: Tobacco & alcohol abuse
    - Synergistic risk factor in China & South Africa: Human papillomavirus
  - ACA
    - 30-50% of all ECs
    - Barrett mucosa ⇒ 90-100% of cases
    - Increasing in prevalence relative to SCCA

Nuclear Medicine Findings
- PET
  - ACA and SCCA are FDG avid
  - PET indicated for initial staging and to identify surgical candidates
  - Less sensitive than combined CT and EUS for detection of locoregional LN metastases
    - Does not allow reliable differentiation between N0 and N1 disease, frequently due to intense uptake by primary lesion masking adjacent LN metastases

DDx: Benign Mimics of Esophageal Cancer on FDG PET

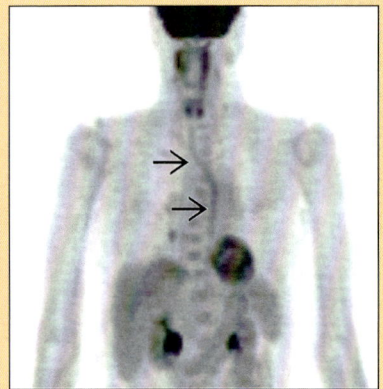

Normal Esophagus 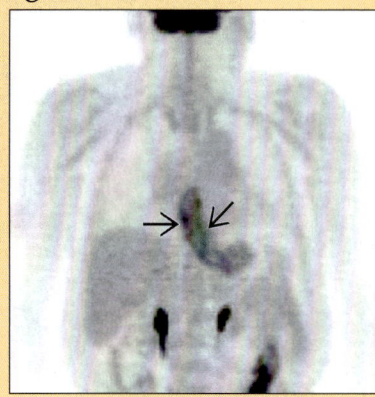 | *Hiatal Hernia* 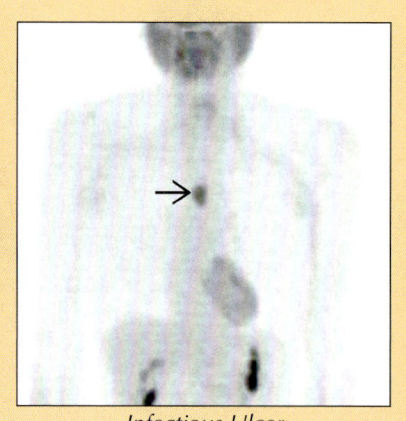 | *Infectious Ulcer*

ESOPHAGEAL CANCER

Key Facts

Terminology
- Squamous cell carcinoma (SCCA): Malignant transformation of squamous epithelium
- Adenocarcinoma (ACA): Malignant dysplasia in columnar metaplasia (Barrett mucosa)

Imaging Findings
- FDG PET: Hypermetabolic esophageal mass, lymphadenopathy, distant metastases
- CECT: Fixed, irregular narrowing of lumen
- Carcinoma: Most common tumor of esophagus
- PET indicated for initial staging and to identify surgical candidates
- More accurate than combined CT and EUS for detection of stage IV disease (69% sens, 93% spec)

Top Differential Diagnoses
- Inflammatory Esophagitis
- Intramural Primary Esophageal Tumor
- Other Thoracic Malignancy

Pathology
- Smoking, alcohol, achalasia, lye strictures
- ACA
- Spread: Local, lymphatic, hematogenous

Clinical Issues
- Clinical Profile: Elderly patient with difficulty swallowing solids & weight loss

Diagnostic Checklist
- Overlap of imaging findings with inflammatory causes of hypermetabolic esophageal lesions

---

  - More accurate than combined CT and EUS for detection of stage IV disease (69% sens, 93% spec)
  - Useful for evaluating response to therapy

Radiographic Findings
- Radiography
  - Chest x-ray (advanced carcinoma)
    - Hilar, retrohilar or retrocardiac mass
    - Anterior bowing of posterior tracheal wall
    - Retrotracheal stripe thickening more than 3 mm
- Double-contrast esophagography
  - Early SCCA
    - Plaque-like lesions; small, sessile polyps or depressed lesions
  - Early ACA in Barrett esophagus
    - Plaque-like lesions; flat, sessile polyps
    - Localized area of flattening/stiffening in wall of peptic stricture (common in distal 1/3)
  - Advanced SCCA
    - Infiltrating lesion (most common): Irregular narrowing/luminal constriction (stricture) with nodular/ulcerated mucosa
    - Polypoid lesion: Lobulated/fungating intraluminal mass
    - Ulcerative lesion: Well-defined meniscoid ulcers with a radiolucent rim of tumor surrounding ulcer in profile view
    - Varicoid lesion: Thickened, tortuous, serpiginous longitudinal folds due to submucosal spread of tumor, mimicking varices (nonpliable)
  - Advanced ACA in Barrett esophagus
    - Radiologically indistinguishable from SCCA
    - Long infiltrating lesion in distal esophagus
  - Stricture in advanced carcinoma
    - Asymmetric contour with abrupt proximal borders of narrowed distal segment (rat-tail appearance)

CT Findings
- CT: Staging of EC
  - Stage I: Localized wall thickening of 3-5 mm or intraluminal tumor
    - CT not as accurate as endoscopic ultrasonography
  - Stage II: Localized wall thickening > 5 mm & no mediastinal extension
  - Stage III: Tumor extends beyond esophagus into mediastinal tissues
    - Tracheobronchial invasion: Posterior wall indentation/bowing & tracheobronchial displacement/compression; ± collapse of lobes
    - Aortic invasion: Uncommon finding (2% of cases)
    - Pericardial invasion: Based on obliteration of fat plane/mass effect
    - Mediastinal adenopathy: Discrete/inseparable from primary tumor
  - Stage IV: Extends into mediastinum & distant areas
    - Liver, lungs, pleura, adrenals, kidneys & lymph nodes (LN)
    - Subdiaphragmatic adenopathy: Seen in more than 2/3 of distal cancers

Ultrasonographic Findings
- Grayscale Ultrasound
  - Endoscopic ultrasonography (EUS)
    - More accurate than CT for T (85% vs. 45%) and N (77% vs. 54%) staging
    - Malignant LN: Hypoechoic & well-defined
    - Benign LN: Hyperechoic; indistinct borders

Imaging Recommendations
- EUS for most accurate T and N staging
- CT useful for detecting locoregional LN metastases
- PET for distant metastases detection

DIFFERENTIAL DIAGNOSIS

Inflammatory Esophagitis
- Radiation esophagitis; vertebral bodies in radiation port may be photopenic
- Reflux esophagitis
- Infectious esophagitis: Fungal (candidiasis), viral (Herpes, CMV, HIV)
- Caustic esophagitis

ESOPHAGEAL CANCER

Intramural Primary Esophageal Tumor
- Examples: Leiomyoma or fibrovascular polyp
- FDG activity variable

Other Thoracic Malignancy
- Extrinsic compression of esophagus by mediastinal lymphadenopathy, adjacent lung cancer, etc.

Normal Variants (FDG PET)
- Hiatal hernia
- Normal diffuse esophageal activity

PATHOLOGY

General Features
- Genetics: Genomic instability in patients with Barrett esophagus may increase risk of ACA
- Etiology
  - SCCA
    - Smoking, alcohol, achalasia, lye strictures
    - Celiac disease, head & neck tumor
    - Plummer-Vinson syndrome, radiation, tylosis
  - ACA
    - Barrett esophagus
    - Risk factors: GERD, reflux esophagitis, motility disorders
  - Spread: Local, lymphatic, hematogenous
- Epidemiology: Increased incidence in Turkey, Iran, India, China, South Africa, France, Saudi Arabia

Gross Pathologic & Surgical Features
- Infiltrating, polypoid, ulcerative or varicoid lesions

Microscopic Features
- Squamous cell atypia
- Columnar glands
- Adeno & squamous components

Staging, Grading or Classification Criteria
- TNM staging
  - Stage 0: Carcinoma in situ
  - Stage I: Lamina propria or submucosa
  - Stage IIA: Muscularis propria & adventitia
  - Stage IIB: Lamina propria, submucosa, muscularis propria and regional LN
  - Stage III: Adventitia, adjacent structures, regional LN and any other LN
  - Stage IV: All layers, adjacent structures, regional LN, any other LN and distant metastases

CLINICAL ISSUES

Presentation
- Most common signs/symptoms
  - Dysphagia (solids)
  - Odynophagia (painful swallowing)
  - Anorexia
  - Weight loss
  - Retrosternal pain
- Clinical Profile: Elderly patient with difficulty swallowing solids & weight loss
- Lab data
  - Hypochromic, microcytic anemia
  - Hemoccult positive stool
  - Decreased albumin
- Diagnosis
  - Endoscopic biopsy & histology

Demographics
- Age: Usually > 50 y
- Gender: M:F = 4:1
- Ethnicity: African-Americans > Caucasians (2:1)

Natural History & Prognosis
- Complications
  - Fistulous tracts to trachea (5-10%), bronchi, pericardium
- Prognosis
  - Early cancer: 5 year survival ~ 90%
  - Advanced cancer: 5 year survival < 10%

Treatment
- Curative
  - Surgery
  - Radiation (pre & post-operative)
- Palliative
  - Surgery
  - Radiation
  - Chemotherapy
  - Laser treatment
  - Esophageal stent

DIAGNOSTIC CHECKLIST

Consider
- Overlap of imaging findings with inflammatory causes of hypermetabolic esophageal lesions
  - Endoscopic biopsy often required

SELECTED REFERENCES

1. Gupta S et al: Usefulness of barium studies for differentiating benign and malignant strictures of the esophagus. AJR Am J Roentgenol. 180(3):737-44, 2003
2. Iyer RB et al: Diagnosis, staging, and follow-up of esophageal cancer. AJR Am. J. Roentgenol. 181:785-93, 2003
3. Kostakoglu L et al: Clinical role of FDG PET in evaluation of cancer patients. Radiographics. 23(2):315-40; quiz 533, 2003
4. Skehan SJ et al: Imaging features of primary and recurrent esophageal cancer at FDG PET. Radiographics. 20(3):713-23, 2000
5. Levine MS et al: Carcinoma of the esophagus and esophagogastric junction: sensitivity of radiographic diagnosis. AJR Am J Roentgenol. 168(6):1423-6, 1997
6. Levine MS: Esophageal cancer. Radiologic diagnosis. Radiol Clin North Am. 35(2):265-79, 1997
7. Levine MS et al: Fibrovascular polyps of the esophagus: clinical, radiographic, and pathologic findings in 16 patients. AJR Am J Roentgenol. 166(4):781-7, 1996
8. Glick SN: Barium studies in patients with Barrett's esophagus: importance of focal areas of esophageal deformity. AJR Am J Roentgenol. 163(1):65-7, 1994
9. Vilgrain V et al: Staging of esophageal carcinoma: comparison of results with endoscopic sonography and CT. AJR. 155:277-81, 1990

ESOPHAGEAL CANCER

IMAGE GALLERY

Typical

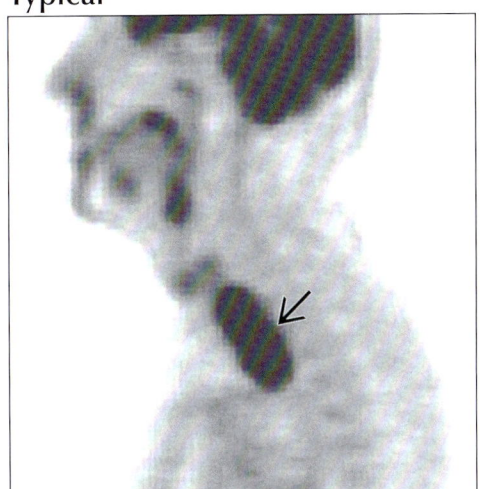

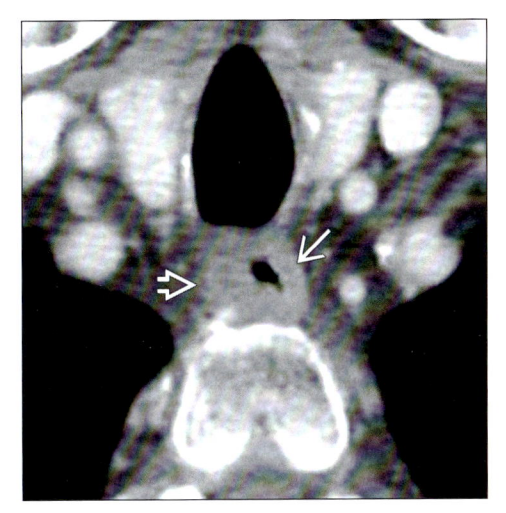

(Left) Sagittal PET shows hypermetabolic carcinoma of upper esophagus ➡. As in this case, carcinomas in upper 1/3 of esophagus are usually squamous cell in origin. See next image. *(Right)* Axial CECT in same patient at left shows circumferential thickening of cervical esophageal wall ➡ with invasion of surrounding fat planes ➡. PET cannot be used to assess local invasion.

Typical

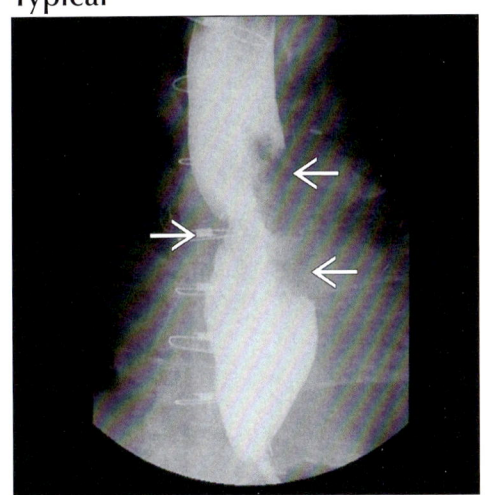

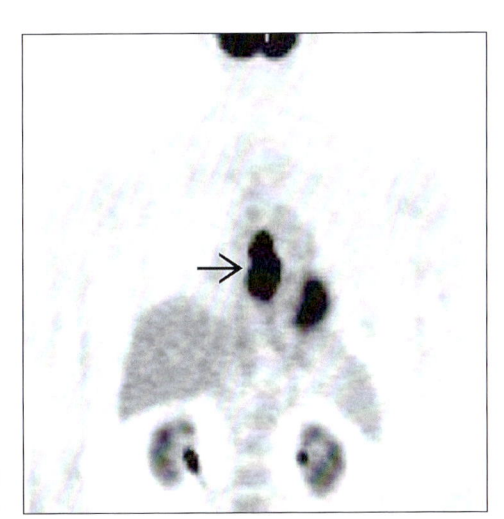

(Left) Anterior barium esophagram shows apple-core lesion in mid esophagus ➡, typical in appearance for esophageal carcinoma. See next image. *(Right)* Coronal FDG PET in same patient at left shows bulky region of hypermetabolism in mid esophagus ➡, typical in appearance for esophageal carcinoma.

Variant

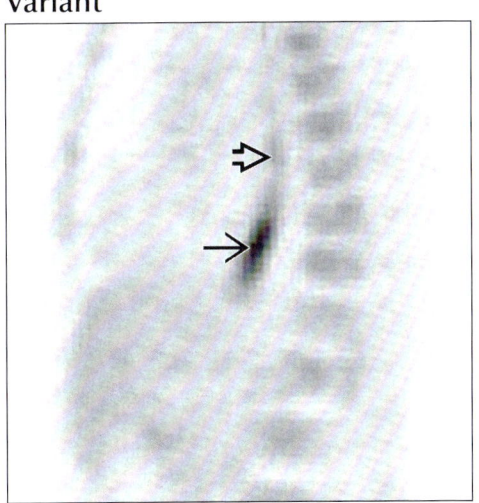

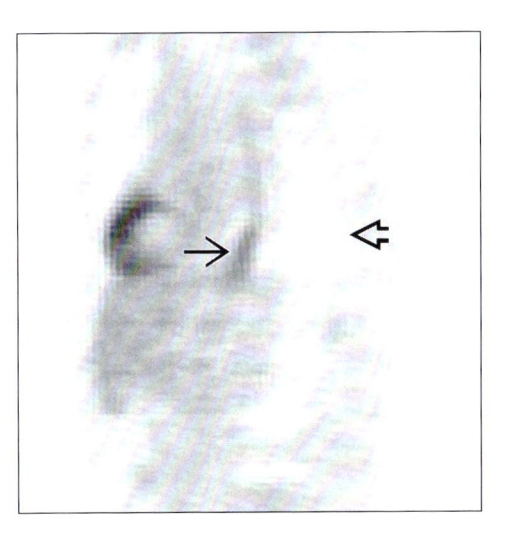

(Left) Sagittal FDG PET prior to chemoradiation shows uptake in distal esophageal adenocarcinoma ➡. Mild uptake more proximally ➡ was biopsy-negative (normal or inflammatory). See next image. *(Right)* Sagittal FDG PET in same patient at left after chemoradiation shows residual activity in distal esophagus ➡, which could be due to inflammation or residual tumor. Note photopenic vertebral bodies ➡ in radiation port.

ESOPHAGEAL DYSMOTILITY

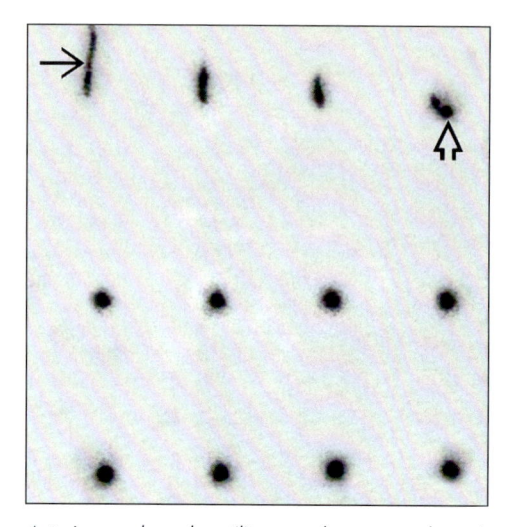

Anterior esophageal motility scan shows normal transit of radiotracer in liquid through the esophagus ➡ and into the stomach ⇨. The normal esophageal transit time is 2 seconds for liquids.

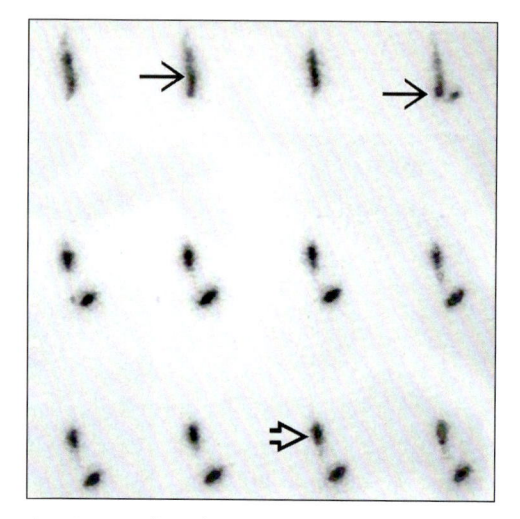

Anterior esophageal motility scan shows delayed esophageal transit ➡ of radiotracer in liquid, as well as gastroesophageal reflux ⇨.

TERMINOLOGY

Definitions
- Esophageal dysphagia
  - Esophageal dysfunction: Difficulty swallowing due to mechanical, motility, functional disorder
    - Solids progressing to liquids: Mechanical disorder
    - Solids and liquids: Motility disorder
    - No apparent cause: Functional disorder
  - Dysphagia in esophageal body or lower esophageal sphincter (LES)
  - Distinguished from oropharyngeal dysphagia and globus sensation
- Esophagus: Hollow tube 2.5 cm in diameter; ~ 25 cm long connecting oropharynx and stomach
- Esophageal motility disorders: Primary and secondary motility disorders of esophageal smooth muscle
  - Achalasia: Idiopathic or neurogenic disorder
    - No primary peristalsis
    - Incomplete or absent lower esophageal sphincter (LES) relaxation on swallowing
  - Spastic motility disorders
    - Diffuse esophageal spasm: Normal LES relaxation
    - Nutcracker esophagus
    - Ineffective esophageal motility disorder
  - Presbyesophagus: Esophageal motility dysfunction associated with aging
  - Systemic sclerosis (scleroderma): Multisystem disorder of small vessels and connective tissue
    - Dilated atonic esophagus (no peristalsis in distal 2/3)
    - Decreased, absent resting LES pressure
  - Sjögren syndrome
    - Autoimmune disease ⇒ ↓ saliva production
- Gastroesophageal reflux (GER): Retrograde flow of gastric contents into esophagus; normally occurs intermittently, particularly after meals
- Gastroesophageal reflux disease (GERD): Symptomatic GER ± esophagitis

IMAGING FINDINGS

General Features
- Best diagnostic clue
  - Esophageal motility disorder: Radiotracer in dilated esophagus ± tapered, narrow esophagus; delayed esophageal transit; disorganized esophageal transit

DDx: Esophageal Dysfunction, Obstructive Etiologies

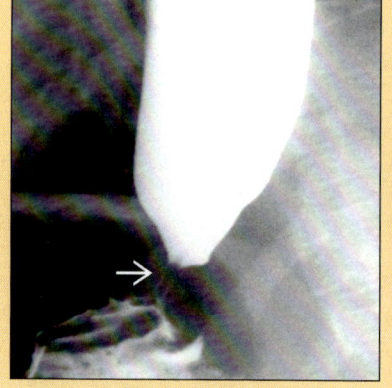

Peptic Stricture

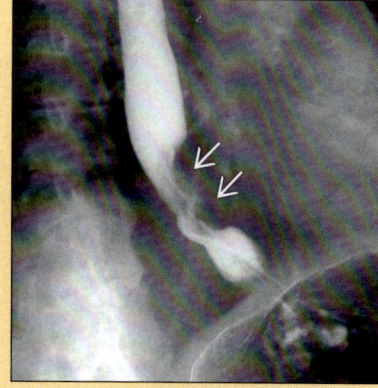

Esophageal Cancer

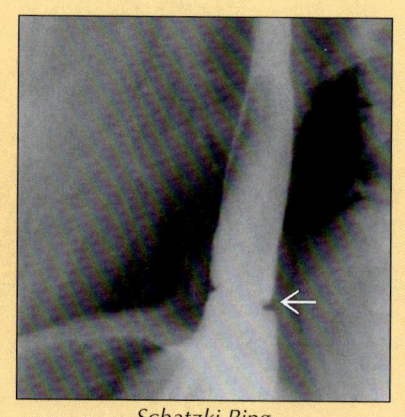

Schatzki Ring

ESOPHAGEAL DYSMOTILITY

Key Facts

Terminology
- Esophageal dysfunction: Difficulty swallowing due to mechanical, motility, functional disorder
- Gastroesophageal reflux (GER): Retrograde flow of gastric contents into esophagus; normally occurs intermittently, particularly after meals

Imaging Findings
- Esophageal motility disorder: Radiotracer in dilated esophagus ± tapered, narrow esophagus; delayed esophageal transit; disorganized esophageal transit
- GER: Retrograde flow of radiopharmaceutical from stomach into esophagus
- Nuclear medicine: Esophageal transit scintigraphy
- Nuclear medicine: Gastric emptying scintigraphy
- Radiography: Esophagram or upper gastrointestinal (UGI) evaluation
- Other: Esophagogastroduodenoscopy (often 1st line study), manometry, pH monitoring

Clinical Issues
- Esophageal motility disorder: Medical Rx, dilatation
- GER: Lifestyle modifications, medical Rx, fundoplication

Diagnostic Checklist
- Adynamic pattern: Craniocaudal, slow (or no) tracer transit; time-activity curve shows retention of radiotracer in region of interest
- Uncoordinated pattern: Disorganized tracer movement throughout proximal and distal esophagus; time-activity curve shows multiple peaks of radiotracer in regions of interest

---

  - GER: Retrograde flow of radiopharmaceutical from stomach into esophagus

Nuclear Medicine Findings
- Esophageal dysfunction: Esophageal transit scintigraphy
  - Normal esophageal transit times
    - Liquid: 2 seconds
    - Solid: 9 seconds
  - Slow rate of esophageal transit, little tracer in stomach
    - Achalasia, scleroderma
    - Time-activity curve shows esophageal retention
  - Disordered movement of esophageal contents (craniocaudal and vice versa)
    - Diffuse esophageal spasm, presbyesophagus
    - Multiple peaks on time activity curves
- GER: Esophageal transit scintigraphy/gastric emptying
  - Reflux of tracer from stomach into esophagus
  - Radiotracer in pulmonary tree 2° to aspiration

Radiographic Findings
- Radiography
  - Achalasia
    - Markedly dilated esophagus
    - Bird-beak deformity: V-shaped conical, smoother tapered narrowing as GEJ
  - Diffuse esophageal spasm
    - Primary peristalsis in cervical esophagus
    - Thoracic esophagus: No primary peristalsis, focally obliterative contractions
    - Repetitive contractions; esophageal lumen may show corkscrew or rosary bead pattern
  - Presbyesophagus
    - Multiple nonperistaltic contractions, disrupted primary peristalsis
  - Scleroderma
    - Mild-moderate dilatation of proximal esophagus
    - Absence of peristalsis in lower 2/3
    - Patulous GE region + reflux → fusiform distal peptic stricture; ± hiatal hernia
    - Erosions & superficial ulcers in distal esophagus
    - ± Wide-mouthed sacculations of esophagus
  - GER
    - Reflux of barium from stomach into esophagus
    - Mucosal edema, ulceration, strictures, wide gastroesophageal junction (GEJ)

Imaging Recommendations
- Best imaging tool
  - Nuclear medicine: Esophageal transit scintigraphy
    - Quantify rate of esophageal transit through visual analysis, region-of-interest analysis, and time-activity curves
    - Evaluate for GER
    - Sensitivity 95%, specificity 96%
  - Nuclear medicine: Gastric emptying scintigraphy
    - Tc-99m labeled sulfur colloid in solid or liquid meal
    - Evaluate for GER
  - Radiography: Esophagram or upper gastrointestinal (UGI) evaluation
    - Evaluate anatomy
    - Identify category of esophageal dysfunction
    - Evaluate for GER
  - Other: Esophagogastroduodenoscopy (often 1st line study), manometry, pH monitoring
- Protocol advice
  - Esophageal transit scintigraphy
    - Patient fasts 4-12 hours before study
    - High resolution collimator, anterior and posterior images
    - High temporal resolution imaging: Dynamic images at 4 to 10 frames/sec for 60 sec
    - If patient upright during imaging, mimics physiologic conditions
    - 200-300 µCi (7-11MBq) Tc-99m sulfur colloid, Tc-99m nanocolloid, Tc-99m diethylenetriaminepentaacetic acid (DTPA)
    - Radiotracer mixed with 10-20 ml water, juice, or semisolid ("thickened") liquid
    - Residual fraction of radiotracer in esophagus: One wet swallow followed by 3 dry swallows within 75 seconds, region-of-interest analysis

ESOPHAGEAL DYSMOTILITY

- Esophageal transit time and retention: 6 wet swallows (3-5 ml 25°C water) at 30 second intervals followed by generation of time-activity curves
- GER: Image over 120 seconds with ~ 4 second per frame dynamic images while patient performs ~ 5 Valsalva maneuvers
- Geometric mean method for calculations
  - GER scintigraphy
    - Patient fasts 4-12 hours before study
    - High resolution collimator
    - Image supine, anterior and posterior, dynamic
    - Abdominal binder to ↑ pressure in 20 mm increments up to 100 mm Hg
    - ~ 300 µCi (11MBq) Tc-99m sulfur colloid suspended in 150 mL of orange juice mixed with 0.1N HCl
    - Static thoracic image at conclusion of study to evaluate for aspiration
    - Also diagnosed with esophageal motility scan

DIFFERENTIAL DIAGNOSIS

Esophageal Motility Disorder
- Esophageal smooth muscle dysfunction

Mechanical Disorders
- Esophageal webs/rings, peptic stricture, cardiovascular anomalies, pyloric stenosis

Esophagitis ± Stricture
- GER, hiatal hernia, immunocompromised, pill-induced, obesity, smoking

Neoplasia
- Esophageal cancer; other thoracic, abdominal cancer

Iatrogenic
- Post-fundoplication

Functional Dysphagia
- Diagnosis of exclusion; no apparent anatomic or motility disorder

PATHOLOGY

General Features
- Etiology
  - Esophageal dysmotility
    - Idiopathic, neurogenic, aging (presbyesophagus), connective tissue disease, functional
  - GER
    - LES abnormality; hiatal hernia; certain foods, medications, hormones; obesity
- Epidemiology
  - Esophageal dysmotility: < 50% of patients without structural abnormality
  - Esophageal dysfunction: 2nd most common functional GI tract disorder (irritable bowel syndrome = 1st)
  - GER: ~ 7% of US has daily symptoms

CLINICAL ISSUES

Presentation
- Most common signs/symptoms
  - Esophageal mechanical obstruction: Dysphagia (solids, later liquids), chest pain
  - Esophageal motility: Dysphagia (liquids and solids), chest pain
  - GER
    - Infants: Effortless regurgitation, vomiting, failure to thrive, irritable, recurrent pulmonary infections
    - Children/adults: Dyspepsia, vomiting, reactive airway disease, hoarseness, cough

Natural History & Prognosis
- Esophageal dysmotility
  - ↓ Quality of life
  - Depends on etiology
- GER
  - Medical therapy heals 80-100% of patients, 30%-60% sustain resolution
  - Most infantile GER resolves by age 1-2
  - Prognosis: ~ 99% improve with medication, nonsurgical therapy

Treatment
- Esophageal motility disorder: Medical Rx, dilatation
  - Medical: Prokinetic agents, antisecretory (GER) agents, calcium channel blockers, antidepressants, anticholinergics, smooth muscle relaxants, nitrates
  - Interventional: Dilatation, myotomy
- GER: Lifestyle modifications, medical Rx, fundoplication
  - Nonsurgical: Elevate head of bed, modify type/timing of meals; prokinetic agents, antacids and proton pump inhibitors
  - Surgical: If failed medical therapy, Barrett esophagus, extraesophageal symptoms
    - Fundoplication: Alleviates symptoms in 94%

DIAGNOSTIC CHECKLIST

Consider
- Static images over thorax prior to conclusion of study to diagnose pulmonary aspiration

Image Interpretation Pearls
- Pattern analysis
  - Adynamic pattern: Craniocaudal, slow (or no) tracer transit; time-activity curve shows retention of radiotracer in region of interest
    - Achalasia, scleroderma
  - Uncoordinated pattern: Disorganized tracer movement throughout proximal and distal esophagus; time-activity curve shows multiple peaks of radiotracer in regions of interest
    - Diffuse esophageal spasm, presbyesophagus

SELECTED REFERENCES

1. Mariani G et al: Radionuclide gastroesophageal motor studies. J Nucl Med. 45(6):1004-28, 2004

ESOPHAGEAL DYSMOTILITY

IMAGE GALLERY

Typical

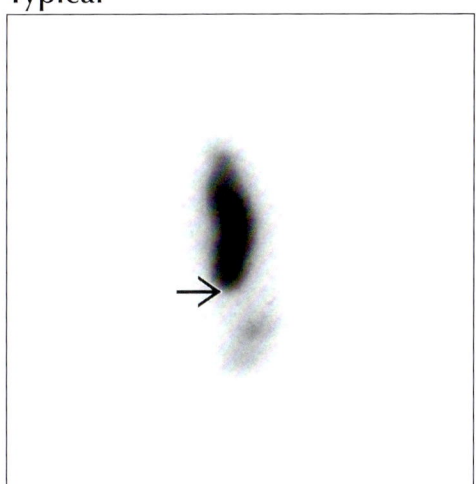

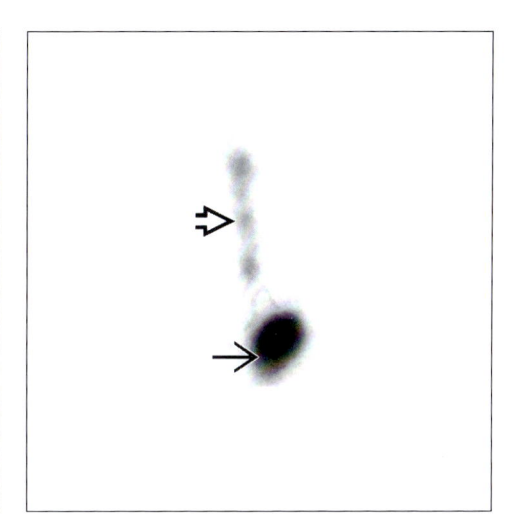

(**Left**) Anterior esophageal transit study in a patient with achalasia shows tracer retention in the esophagus at the lower esophageal sphincter ➔, corresponding to classic bird beak deformity. See next image. (**Right**) Anterior esophageal transit study in a patient with achalasia after dilatation shows majority of radiotracer in the stomach ➔ with a small amount of residual in the esophagus ➔.

Typical

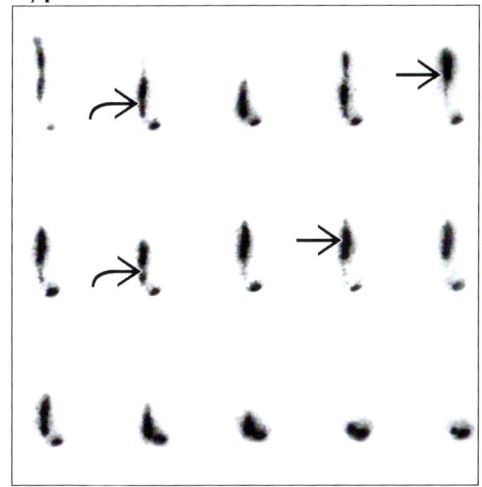

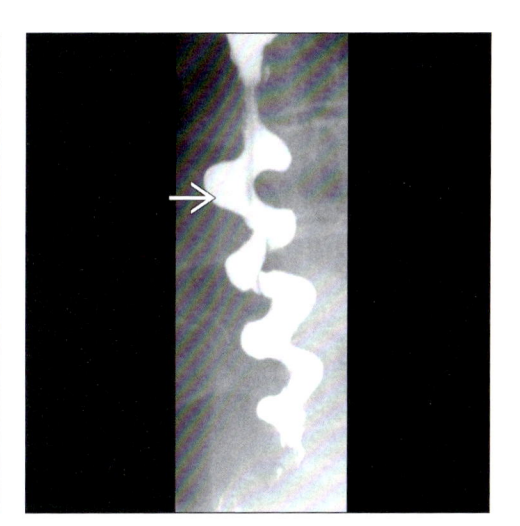

(**Left**) Anterior esophageal motility scan shows irregular movement of radiotracer bolus over time, both proximally ➔ and distally ➔, characteristic of diffuse esophageal spasm. See next image. (**Right**) Anterior radiograph shows corkscrew pattern of barium in the esophagus ➔, typical of a patient with diffuse esophageal spasm.

Typical

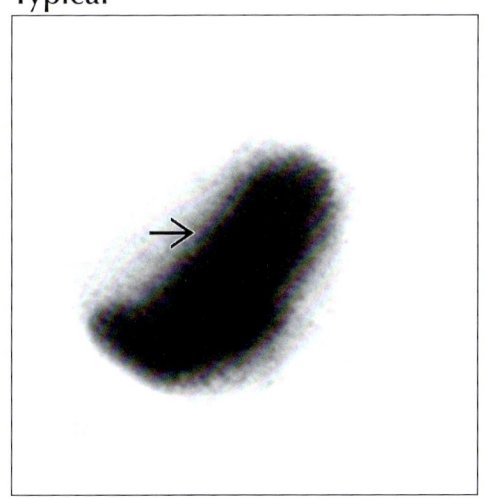

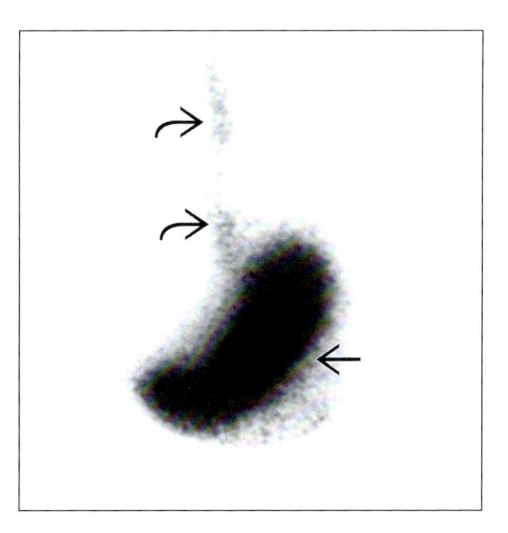

(**Left**) Anterior gastroesophageal reflux scan shows liquid radiotracer in the stomach ➔ of a patient with postprandial dyspepsia. See next image. (**Right**) Anterior gastroesophageal reflux scan in the same patient as previous image, after Valsalva shows reflux of radiotracer into the esophagus ➔ from the stomach ➔.

GASTRITIS

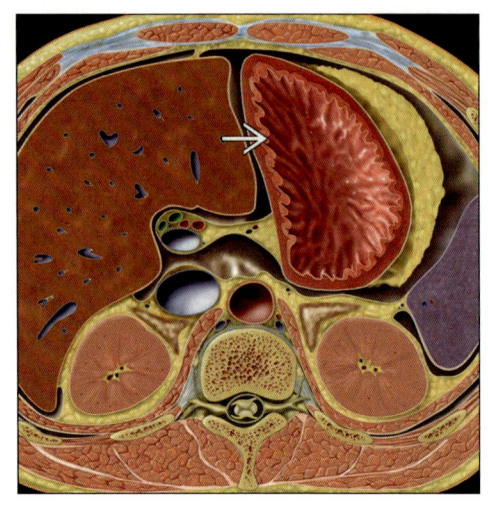

Axial graphic shows circumferential thickening of gastric folds and gastric wall ➡ in patient with gastritis.

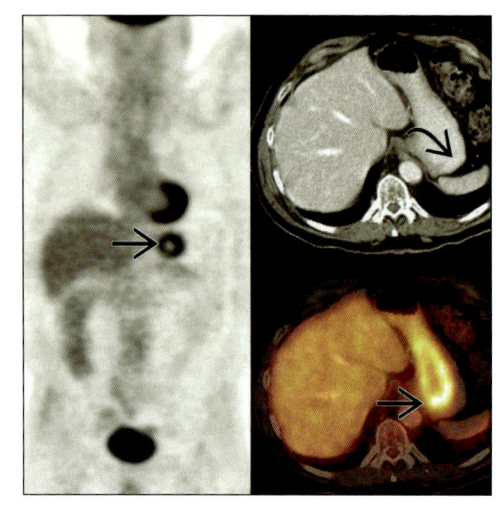

Coronal PET, axial CT, and axial fused PET/CT show hypermetabolic activity ➡ in mildly thickened gastric wall ➡ in patient with gastritis.

TERMINOLOGY

Abbreviations and Synonyms
- Erosive gastritis, atrophic gastritis

Definitions
- Inflammation of gastric mucosa leading to erosion or nonerosive changes

IMAGING FINDINGS

Nuclear Medicine Findings
- PET
  - Diffuse FDG activity within stomach is nonspecific
  - FDG uptake confounded by overlap of physiologic, inflammatory, infectious, neoplastic etiologies

Radiographic Findings
- Barium studies
  - Enlarged areae gastricae
  - Hypertrophied antral-pyloric fold
  - Mucosal nodularity and erosions

CT Findings
- Nonspecific thickening of gastric folds and wall
- H. pylori gastritis can simulate gastric neoplasm due to focal thickening
- Severe gastritis
  - Low-attenuation wall indicates submucosal edema, inflammation
  - Hyperemia may give wall a layered appearance with enhancement

Imaging Recommendations
- Best imaging tool
  - CT often first-line for complaints of abdominal pain
  - Barium upper GI studies and endoscopy most useful for diagnosis
- Protocol advice: Water is an excellent contrast agent

DIFFERENTIAL DIAGNOSIS

Gastric Neoplasm
- Gastric carcinoma
- Lymphoma
- GI stromal tumor (GIST)

DDx: Gastric Hypermetabolic FDG Activity

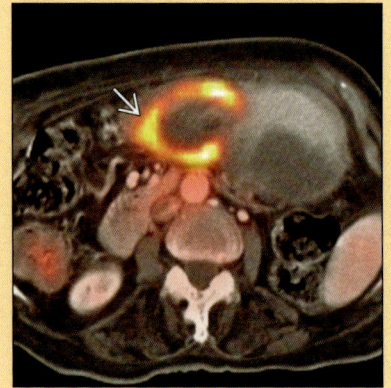

Metastatic Melanoma

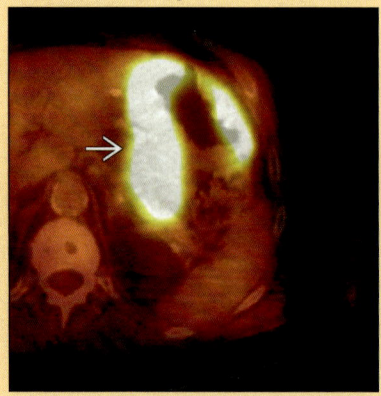

Gastric Lymphoma

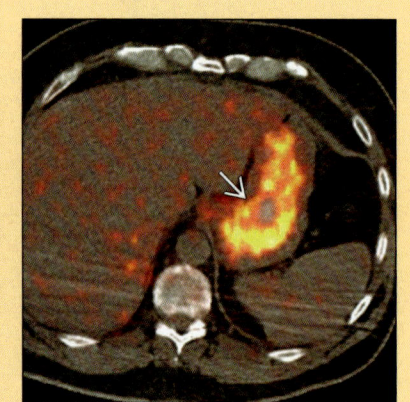

Physiologic FDG Uptake

GASTRITIS

Key Facts

Terminology
- Erosive gastritis, atrophic gastritis
- Inflammation of gastric mucosa leading to erosion or nonerosive changes

Imaging Findings
- Diffuse FDG activity within stomach is nonspecific
- FDG uptake confounded by overlap of physiologic, inflammatory, infectious, neoplastic etiologies

Top Differential Diagnoses
- Gastric Neoplasm
- Physiologic FDG Activity
- Gastric Ulcer
- Crohn Disease

Pathology
- Etiology: NSAID ingestion, alcohol, H. pylori, autoimmune disease, radiation, ischemia, mucosal atrophy

Physiologic FDG Activity
- Usually diffuse, mildly increased activity

Gastric Ulcer
- Focal (vs. diffuse) increased activity in stomach on PET

Crohn Disease
- Rarely affects stomach
- Increased activity on PET in active disease

PATHOLOGY

General Features
- Etiology: NSAID ingestion, alcohol, H. pylori, autoimmune disease, radiation, ischemia, mucosal atrophy
- Epidemiology: 35% of U.S. adults infected with H. pylori

CLINICAL ISSUES

Presentation
- Most common signs/symptoms: Upper abdominal pain, indigestion, loss of appetite

Demographics
- Age: H. pylori: > 60 years: 50% rate of infection; < 40 years: 20% rate of infection
- Gender: Autoimmune gastritis affects men > women (1:3)

Natural History & Prognosis
- Complications of H. pylori: Peptic ulcer or malignancy (MALT lymphoma)
- In general, gastritis improves rapidly with treatment

Treatment
- Proton pump inhibitors (PPI)
- For H. pylori: Three-drug regimen including PPI and two antibiotics
- Ameliorate etiology: Stop NSAID, alcohol, etc.

DIAGNOSTIC CHECKLIST

Image Interpretation Pearls
- Increased activity in stomach on FDG PET highly nonspecific
  - Need upper endoscopy/biopsy for definitive diagnosis

SELECTED REFERENCES

1. Ak I et al: Intense F-18 FDG accumulation in stomach in a patient with Hodgkin lymphoma: Helicobacter pylori infection as a pitfall in oncologic diagnosis with F-18 FDG PET imaging. Clin Nucl Med. 30(1):41, 2005
2. Israel O et al: PET/CT detection of unexpected gastrointestinal foci of 18F-FDG uptake: incidence, localization patterns, and clinical significance. J Nucl Med. 46(5):758-62, 2005

IMAGE GALLERY

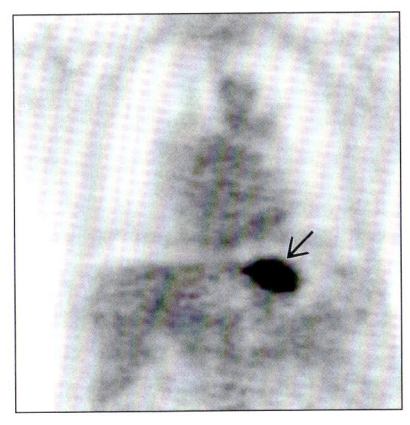

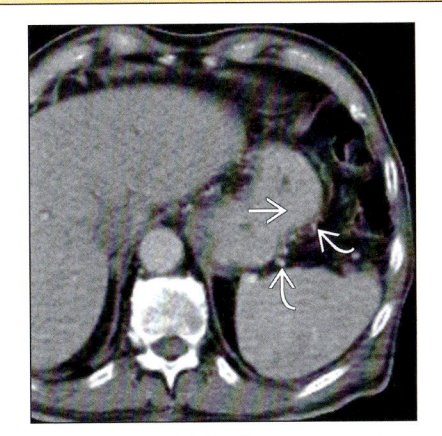

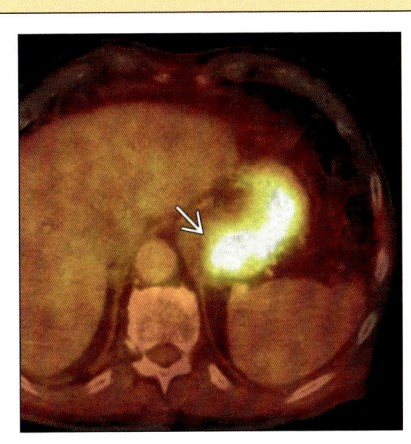

(Left) Coronal PET shows diffuse hypermetabolic activity in stomach ➡. The appearance is compatible with gastritis; however, this finding is non-specific. *(Center)* Axial CECT shows diffuse gastric wall thickening ➡ and mild hyperemia as evidenced by enlarged gastric vessels ➡ in patient with gastritis. *(Right)* Axial fused PET/CT shows diffuse hypermetabolic activity in gastric wall ➡, compatible with, but not diagnostic of, gastritis. This finding on PET/CT should be correlated with endoscopy.

GASTRIC EMPTYING DISORDERS

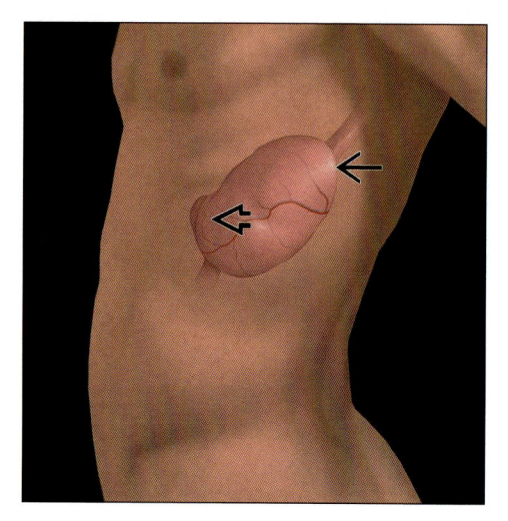

Left lateral graphic of abdomen shows position of stomach. Anterior and posterior imaging over stomach corrects for soft tissue attenuation and normal posterior ➔ to anterior ➔ gastric emptying.

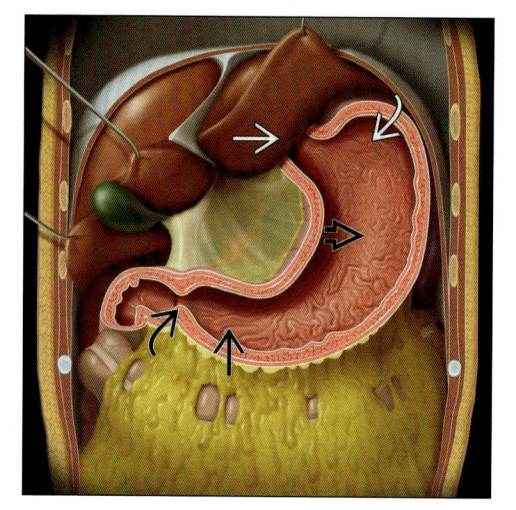

Coronal graphic shows anatomy of normal stomach: Gastroesophageal junction ➔, fundus ➔, body ➔, antrum ➔, pylorus ➔.

TERMINOLOGY

Abbreviations and Synonyms
- Gastric emptying (GE)

Definitions
- Delayed gastric emptying: Reduced clearance of food from the stomach caused by gastroparesis or partial gastric outlet obstruction

IMAGING FINDINGS

General Features
- Best diagnostic clue
  o Partial gastric outlet obstruction (GOO): Delayed emptying of solids on GE scan; liquids less effected unless high grade GOO but may show some delay
  o Gastroparesis: Delayed emptying of both solid and liquid phases on GE scan

Nuclear Medicine Findings
- Normal values for dual labeled meal using fried egg sandwich and water (see protocol)
  o Solid T 1/2 60-105 minutes
  o Liquid T 1/2 10-45 minutes
- Liquids only: Percent emptied at 1 hour on GE scintigraphy
  o Infants: 48 ± 16% emptied (1-23 months)
  o Children: 51 ± 7% emptied (2-14.5 years)
- Delayed GE
  o Gastroparesis: Reduced or absent peristalsis
    ▪ Solid and liquid emptying rates both prolonged
  o Partial GOO: Reduced emptying secondary to narrowing of pylorus, proximal duodenum or gastric antrum
    ▪ Solids emptying typically more prolonged than liquids, although some delay in liquid emptying can occur
- Accelerated GE
  o Dumping syndrome: Accelerated emptying into duodenum producing diarrhea, nausea, cramping
    ▪ Rapid gastric emptying rates must be correlated with symptoms for diagnosis of dumping syndrome

DDx: Associated Findings on GE Scintigraphy

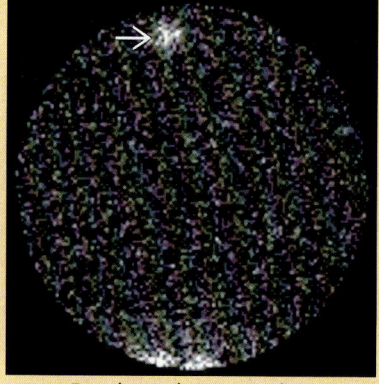

Esophageal Diverticulum 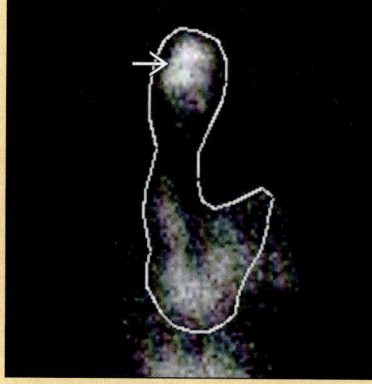 *Hiatal Hernia* 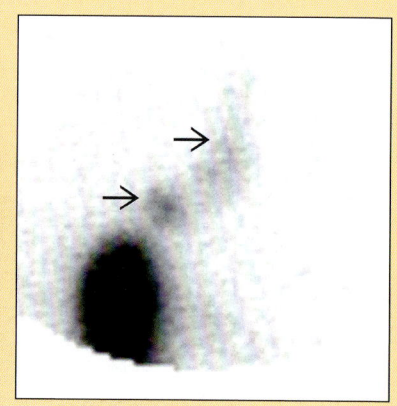 *Gastroesophageal Reflux*

GASTRIC EMPTYING DISORDERS

Key Facts

Imaging Findings
- Gastroparesis: Reduced or absent peristalsis
- Partial GOO: Reduced emptying secondary to narrowing of pylorus, proximal duodenum or gastric antrum
- Dumping syndrome: Accelerated emptying into duodenum producing diarrhea, nausea, cramping
- Rapid gastric emptying rates must be correlated with symptoms for diagnosis of dumping syndrome
- Measurement of both solid and liquid emptying rate may help distinguish partial gastric outlet obstruction from gastroparesis
- Option #1: Label solids first; if abnormal may repeat GE scan with same meal but with liquids labeled
- Option #2: Dual label of solids (Tc-99m) and liquids (In-111) in same meal
- Gastric emptying varies with meal size and composition: Must use published normal emptying rates for each type of meal
- Acquire anterior and posterior 60 second images every 15 min x 120 min: Use geometric mean to determine counts at each time point
- GE dependent on many factors
- Gender: GE faster in men and postmenopausal women than in premenopausal women
- Meal composition: Slower emptying with large meal, high calorie, high fat content

Top Differential Diagnoses
- Peptic Ulcer Disease
- Gastroesophageal Reflux Disease (GERD)
- Malignancy
- Hepatobiliary Disease

Imaging Recommendations
- Best imaging tool: GE scintigraphy with dual label of both solids (Tc-99m) and liquids (In-111)
- Protocol advice
  - Measurement of both solid and liquid emptying rate may help distinguish partial gastric outlet obstruction from gastroparesis
    - Option #1: Label solids first; if abnormal may repeat GE scan with same meal but with liquids labeled
    - Option #2: Dual label of solids (Tc-99m) and liquids (In-111) in same meal
  - Choice of meal: Many options have been published
    - Gastric emptying varies with meal size and composition: Must use published normal emptying rates for each type of meal
    - If non-standard meal is used, must determine emptying rates in normal patients
    - Formula labeled with Tc-99m sulfur colloid can be used for infants but standardization is difficult unless meal introduced by gavage
  - Typical labeled meal: Fried egg sandwich and water
    - Solid label: Two eggs broken into beaker & injected with 500 µCi Tc-99m sulfur colloid; wait 5 minutes; scramble and cook; place between two slices of white bread
    - Liquid label: 125 µCi In-111 diethylenetriamine pentaacetic acid (DTPA) in 300 mL water; 500 µCi Tc-99m sulfur colloid if liquid emptying measured separately
  - Patient preparation: NPO 8 hours
  - Eat in meal 10 min, record any uneaten meal
  - Stand or sit between detectors for imaging sessions (supine for infants)
  - Emptying of food from gastric interposition of esophagus (gastric pull-up) is gravity dependent: Patients must remain upright throughout procedure
  - Can use single left anterior oblique view over stomach, if infant
  - Dual label technique: Camera peaked on Tc-99m and 247 keV, 20% windows
  - Static posterior image over thorax prior to first gastric image to evaluate pulmonary aspiration/GERD
  - Acquire anterior and posterior 60 second images every 15 min x 120 min: Use geometric mean to determine counts at each time point
  - Extended imaging to 4 h: Greatest specificity in diagnosis of delayed gastric emptying
    - Should be performed if abnormal or borderline at 120 min
  - Dynamic image protocol
    - Continuous data with framing rate of 30-60 s per image for ≥ 90 min
    - Advantages: Better represents fundus and antrum, more accurate account of lag phase
    - Disadvantages: More labor intensive, requires imaging equipment for long time periods
  - GE dependent on many factors
    - Body position: Standing, sitting, supine (choose one position for GE scintigraphy)
    - Gender: GE faster in men and postmenopausal women than in premenopausal women
    - Menstrual cycle: Can ↓ GE; menstrual cycle days 1-10 most accurate
    - Time of day: Best if begin fasting before midnight
    - Tobacco and alcohol: Withhold for ≥ 24 hours
    - Drugs that affect gastric motility: Discontinue for testing purposes unless evaluating Rx efficacy
    - Meal composition: Slower emptying with large meal, high calorie, high fat content
- Solids curve analysis
  - Phase 1 = lag phase: Retained in proximal stomach, transported to antrum where diluted, ground (~ 60 min post ingestion)
  - Phase 2: Antropyloric wave-like contractions dilute, empty into duodenum
  - Relatively linear (actually slightly sigmoid) emptying following lag phase: Use linear fit following lag phase quantify emptying
- Liquids curve analysis
  - Empty directly into duodenum, no lag phase

GASTRIC EMPTYING DISORDERS

- Bimodal emptying with dual label technique used: Use linear fit of first phase to quantify liquid emptying
- Liquid meal only: Exponential emptying
- Analysis of shape of emptying curves (not just rates of emptying) has been advocated to better characterize gastric emptying disorders

DIFFERENTIAL DIAGNOSIS

Peptic Ulcer Disease
- Stomach, duodenal epithelium ulcers extend to muscularis mucosae

Gastroesophageal Reflux Disease (GERD)
- Gastroesophageal junction injury, abnormal anatomical features allow gastric reflux

Malignancy
- Tumor infiltration of gastric wall, loss of distensibility

Hepatobiliary Disease
- Cholestasis impedes fat absorption, transport

Iatrogenic
- Medications: Narcotic analgesics, antidepressants, calcium channel blockers, gastric acid suppressants, anticholinergics, aluminum-containing antacids, somatostatin
- Surgeries: Nissen fundoplication, vagotomy, pyloroplasty, gastrojejunostomy

Gastric Obstruction
- Abnormal biologic or foreign obstruction (e.g., bezoar)

PATHOLOGY

General Features
- Etiology
  - Dumping syndrome: Gastric resection, vagotomy
  - Gastroparesis: Diabetes mellitus with poor glycemic control, scleroderma, enteric neuropathy, enteric myopathy, anorexia nervosa, post-vagotomy
  - Partial GOO: Peptic ulcer disease, neoplasm, caustic or inflammatory structure
- Epidemiology
  - Dyspepsia (abdominal discomfort and pain): 30-70% have GE disorder
  - Diabetics: 20-40% have gastroparesis
  - Dumping syndrome: 25-50% patients post gastric surgery
- Associated abnormalities: GERD, aspiration

Gross Pathologic & Surgical Features
- Gastroparesis: Loss of Cajal interstitial cells: GI pacemaker, regulate motility & peristalsis
- GOO: Scarring, stricture, encasing or obstructing mass

CLINICAL ISSUES

Presentation
- Most common signs/symptoms
  - Delayed GE: Nausea (93%), nausea (93%), dyspepsia (90%), early satiety (86%), vomiting (68%)
  - Dumping syndrome: Early satiety, abdominal pain, nausea, vomiting, explosive diarrhea; vasomotor symptoms (diaphoresis, flushing, palpitations, dizziness)
- Other signs/symptoms: Weight loss, depression

Demographics
- Age
  - Pediatrics: GERD in 1/500 infants 1.5-18 months
  - Adults: Mean onset gastroparesis 33.7 yr; 68% ≤ 40 yr
- Gender: Gastroparesis: 82% female

Treatment
- Dumping syndrome: Severe cases may require surgery
- Delayed GE
  - Supportive: Liquified, homogenized meals; replacement of fluids, electrolytes, nutrients; jejunal feeding tube in severe cases; low-fat diet, frequent small meals, no undigestible fiber
  - Medications
    - Prokinetic agents: Erythromycin, metoclopramide
    - Antiemetic agents: Antihistamines, phenothiazines, 5HT3 antagonists
    - Diabetic gastroparesis: 75% resolved with prokinetics
  - Glycemic control in diabetics
  - Pyloroplasty, gastrectomy, gastrojejunal bypass: Indicated for GOO

DIAGNOSTIC CHECKLIST

Consider
- Left anterior oblique images in bedridden patients
- Evidence of pulmonary aspiration/GERD may be present on static image of thorax

SELECTED REFERENCES

1. Maurer AH et al: Update on gastrointestinal scintigraphy. Semin Nucl Med. 36(2):110-8, 2006
2. Forster J et al: Absence of the interstitial cells of Cajal in patients with gastroparesis and correlation with clinical findings. J Gastrointest Surg. 9(1):102-8, 2005
3. Couturier O et al: Gastric scintigraphy with a liquid-solid radiolabelled meal: performances of solid and liquid parameters. Nucl Med Commun. 25(11):1143-50, 2004
4. Savino F et al: Gastric emptying in infants: epigastric impedance versus scintigraphy. Acta Paediatr. 93(5):608-12, 2004
5. Ziessman HA et al: Standardization and quantification of radionuclide solid gastric-emptying studies. J Nucl Med. 45(5):760-4, 2004
6. Tougas G et al: Assessment of gastric emptying using a low fat meal: establishment of international control values. Am J Gastroenterol. 95(6):1456-62, 2000
7. Tougas G et al: Standardization of a simplified scintigraphic methodology for the assessment of gastric emptying in a multicenter setting. Am J Gastroenterol. 95(1):78-86, 2000
8. Donohoe KJ et al: Procedure guideline for gastric emptying and motility. Society of Nuclear Medicine. J Nucl Med. 40(7):1236-9, 1999

GASTRIC EMPTYING DISORDERS

IMAGE GALLERY

Typical

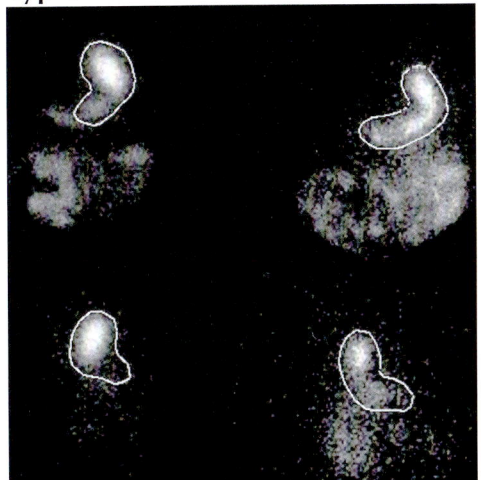

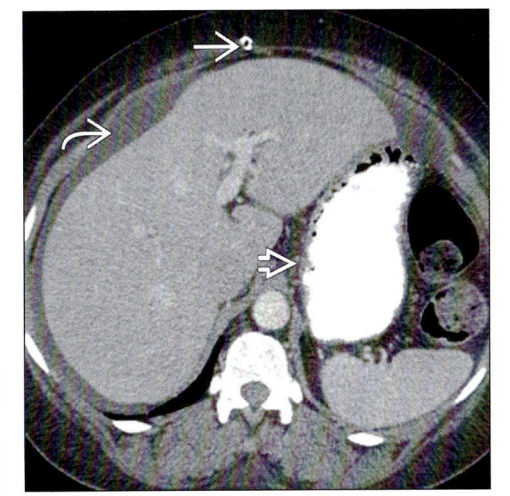

(Left) Gastric emptying scan shows mild to moderate gastric emptying delay of solids (30% emptied at 120 min; 55% emptied at 240 min) in a diabetic patient. Confirmation of prolonged liquid emptying as well would confirm gastroparesis. *(Right)* Axial CECT (same patient as previous image) shows retained contrast in stomach ➡. Peritoneal dialysis catheter ➡ with peritoneal fluid ➡ evident due to end-stage renal disease.

Typical

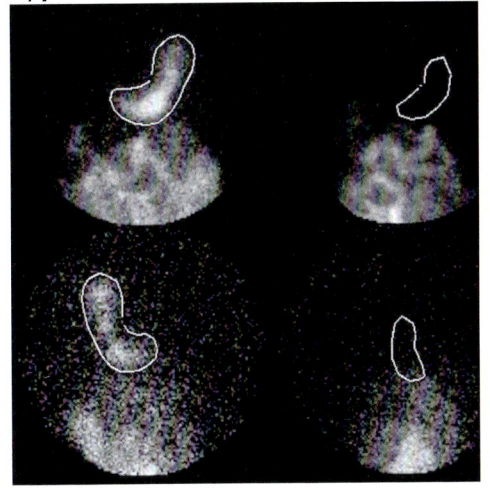

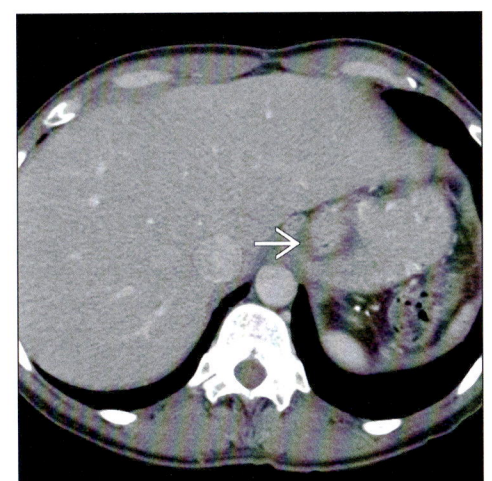

(Left) Gastric emptying scan shows 83% GE at 60 min and 99% GE at 120 min in patient post-vagotomy. This is a normal study. *(Right)* Axial CECT shows Nissen fundoplication ➡ in patient with dumping syndrome.

Typical

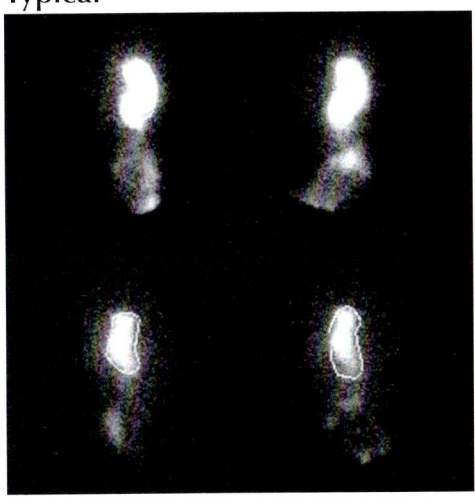

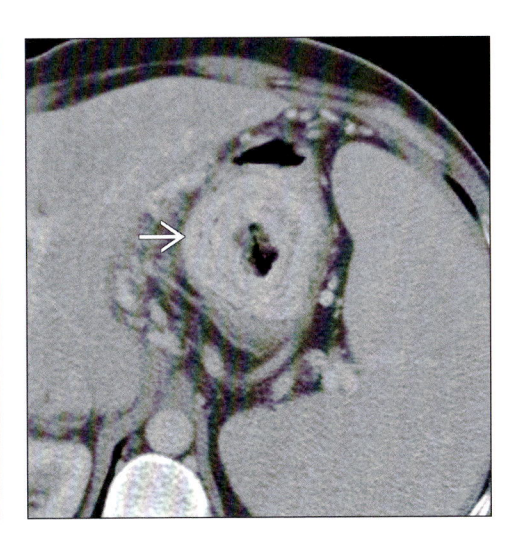

(Left) Gastric emptying scan shows severe delay (32% GE at 120 min) in solid emptying patient post multiple surgeries including partial gastrectomy, vagotomy, Billroth II pyloroplasty. *(Right)* Axial CECT shows laminated mass in stomach ➡ due to phytobezoar, which can be caused by delayed gastric emptying. (Courtesy M. Federle, MD).

GASTRIC CARCINOMA

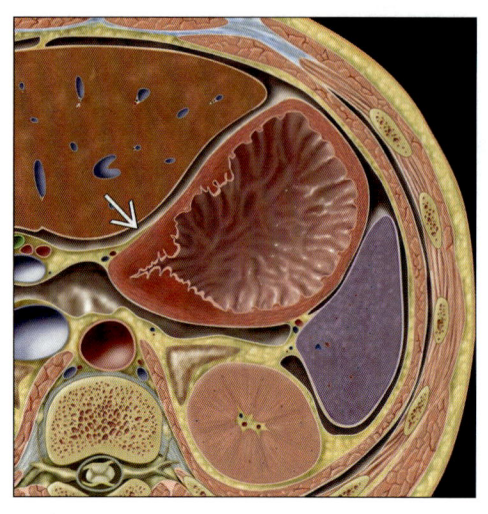

Axial graphic shows asymmetrically thickened gastric mucosa ➡ in medial gastric wall, signifying gastric carcinoma.

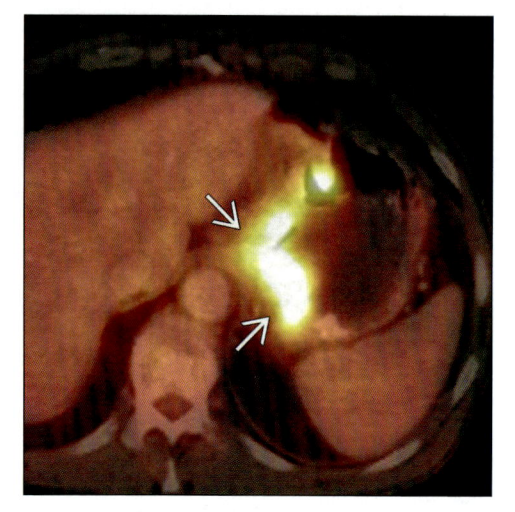

Axial fused PET/CT shows intense FDG activity ➡ corresponding to thickened gastric mucosa in medial gastric wall in patient with gastric carcinoma.

TERMINOLOGY

Abbreviations and Synonyms
- Gastric adenocarcinoma, early/advanced gastric carcinoma (EGC, AGC), gastric cancer, stomach cancer

Definitions
- Adenocarcinoma arising from gastric mucosa
  - Malignant pathway: Gastritis, gastric atrophy, metaplasia, dysplasia, cancer
  - Most common primary tumor to metastasize to ovaries, usually bilaterally (Krukenberg tumors)

IMAGING FINDINGS

General Features
- Best diagnostic clue
  - FDG PET
    - Hypermetabolic FDG activity in primary gastric tumor, regional lymph nodes (LN), peritoneum, distant metastases
  - CT
    - Polypoid mass ± ulceration
    - Focal wall thickening with mucosal irregularity, ulceration
    - Regional LN > 8 mm: Suspicious for metastatic disease
    - Peritoneal dissemination: Peritoneal caking, nodularity, beaded thickening, malignant ascites
- Location
  - Fundus and cardia 40%
  - Body 30%
  - Antrum 30%
- Size
  - Variable
    - Lesions in body usually larger before symptoms develop
- Morphology
  - Type I: Elevated, protrude > 5 mm into lumen
  - Type II: Superficial lesions that are elevated (IIa), flat (IIb), depressed (IIc)
  - Type III: Early gastric cancers that are shallow, irregular ulcers surrounded by nodular, clubbed mucosal folds
  - Tumor depth difficult to assess on CT
  - Perigastric fat invasion seen as soft tissue stranding

DDx: Gastric Hypermetabolic FDG Activity

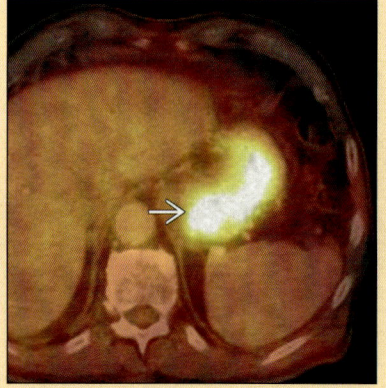

Gastritis 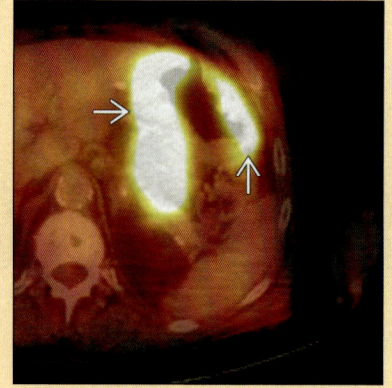 | *Gastric Lymphoma* 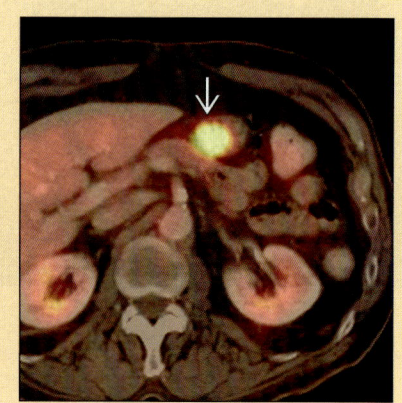 | *Gastrointestinal Stromal Tumor*

GASTRIC CARCINOMA

Key Facts

Imaging Findings
- PET and CT similar sensitivity for primary (94% vs. 93%), PET higher specificity (92% vs. 62%)
- PET similar/slightly higher accuracy as CT for detecting primary tumors, local/distant lymphadenopathy in EGC or AGC
- Peritoneal dissemination: PET low sensitivity and CT low specificity, but similar accuracy overall
- In general, well differentiated gastric adenocarcinomas tend to take up less FDG than poorly differentiated ones
- Change in tumor uptake of FDG after therapy predicts response to therapy, with sensitivity of 77% and specificity of 86%; predictive of survival
- Protocol advice: PET sensitivity for recurrent disease post-gastrectomy may be ↑ by water ingestion (~ 300 cc) to distend remnant stomach

Top Differential Diagnoses
- Gastric Ulcer
- Gastrointestinal Stromal Tumor (GIST)
- Gastric Lymphoma
- Gastritis
- Physiologic FDG Activity
- Crohn Disease

Clinical Issues
- Adjacent organ involvement, peritoneal carcinomatosis, LN metastases, distant metastases: Important factors for determining surgical resectability

---

- o Direct tumor extension common, into pancreas via lesser sac, into transverse colon via gastrocolic ligament, into liver via gastrohepatic ligament
- o 60% of carcinoma of cardia will spread to distal esophagus
- o 5-20% of antral carcinoma will involve duodenum

Nuclear Medicine Findings
- PET
  - o PET sensitivity for primary tumor depends on extent
    - EGC 47%
    - AGC 98%
  - o PET and CT similar sensitivity for primary (94% vs. 93%), PET higher specificity (92% vs. 62%)
  - o PET similar/slightly higher accuracy as CT for detecting primary tumors, local/distant lymphadenopathy in EGC or AGC
  - o Lymphadenopathy: PET insensitive for N1 disease (56%), equally sensitive for N2-3 disease as CT (78%)
  - o Overall lymph node evaluation: PET less sensitive than CT (56% vs. 78%) but more specific (92% vs. 62%)
  - o Peritoneal dissemination: PET low sensitivity and CT low specificity, but similar accuracy overall
  - o In general, well differentiated gastric adenocarcinomas tend to take up less FDG than poorly differentiated ones
  - o Mucinous and signet-ring cell adenocarcinoma: Low FDG avidity 2° to high mucus, lack of Glut-1 transporters
  - o Poorly differentiated tubular adenomas: Widely variable FDG uptake, from low to intensely hypermetabolic
  - o False positives: Normal stomach uptake, gastritis, inflammatory local LN, liver with cholecystitis
    - Especially problematic in remnant stomach post-gastrectomy
    - Water ingestion may decrease false positive from 31% to 8%

CT Findings
- CECT: Focal gastric wall thickening or mass lesion with enhancement

Imaging Recommendations
- Best imaging tool
  - o PET/CT for staging, recurrence, response to therapy
    - Pretreatment staging essential to determine potential curability and to plan optimal therapy
    - Most likely sites of recurrence post-gastrectomy: Gastric bed, peritoneal dissemination, liver
    - Change in tumor uptake of FDG after therapy predicts response to therapy, with sensitivity of 77% and specificity of 86%; predictive of survival
  - o CECT: To determine resectability
- Protocol advice: PET sensitivity for recurrent disease post-gastrectomy may be ↑ by water ingestion (~ 300 cc) to distend remnant stomach

DIFFERENTIAL DIAGNOSIS

Gastric Ulcer
- Benign ulcer: Crater margin sharply defined and smooth en face, symmetric, confluent with healthy mucosa, mucosal folds radiate ulcer edge
- Most benign ulcers located in lesser curve or posterior wall of antrum, body of stomach

Gastrointestinal Stromal Tumor (GIST)
- Well-demarcated, spherical, intramural masses that arise from muscularis propria; often project exophytically, intraluminally
- May have overlying mucosal ulceration
- Larger GISTs often outgrow vascular supply ⇒ necrosis and hemorrhage

Gastric Lymphoma
- Usually correlative gastric wall thickening
- May be diffuse throughout stomach
- Variable PET activity

Gastritis
- Usually mild to moderate FDG activity
- No associated signs of malignancy on CT

GASTRIC CARCINOMA

Physiologic FDG Activity
- Usually mild activity; nonfocal

Crohn Disease
- Rarely affects stomach
- Abscess, fistula, small-bowel disease, mesenteric fibrofatty proliferation
- Hypermetabolic PET activity in active disease

PATHOLOGY

General Features
- General path comments
  - T Classification
    - Tis: Carcinoma in situ, intraepithelial tumor
    - T1: Tumoral extension to submucosa
    - T2: Tumoral extension to the muscularis propria or subserosa
    - T3: Tumoral penetration of the serosa
    - T4: Tumoral invasion of the adjacent organs
  - ~ 95% of all malignant gastric neoplasms are adenocarcinoma
    - Remaining 5%: Lymphoma, leiomyosarcoma, carcinoid, sarcoma
- Genetics: Hereditary factors implicated
- Etiology
  - Dietary nitrates
  - Hypochlorhydria
  - H. pylori (however, infection with H. pylori may be beneficial prognostic factor in patients with EGC)
  - Smoking
  - Food
    - Starch
    - Pickled vegetables
    - Salted fish/meat
    - Smoked foods
- Epidemiology
  - Incidence decreasing
    - 33 cases per 100,000 population in 1930
    - 3.7 cases per 100,000 population in 1990
  - Worldwide, second only to lung cancer for cancer deaths
- Associated abnormalities: Chronic atrophic gastritis, pernicious anemia, previous partial gastrectomy, Ménétrier disease, gastric dysplasia, adenomatous polyps

CLINICAL ISSUES

Presentation
- Most common signs/symptoms
  - Early stage asymptomatic
  - Most patients present with advanced disease
    - Epigastric pain
    - Bloating
    - Early satiety
    - Nausea, vomiting
    - Dysphagia
    - Anorexia
    - Weight loss
- Other signs/symptoms: Signs of upper GI bleeding (hematemesis, melena, iron deficiency anemia, positive fecal occult blood test)

Demographics
- Age: Peak incidence 50-70 years
- Gender: M:F = 2:1
- Ethnicity: 1.5-2.5x more common in African-American, Hispanic, American Indian than Caucasian

Natural History & Prognosis
- Poor prognosis due to advanced disease at presentation
  - Overall 5 year survival rate < 20%
- Prognosis of EGC excellent with radical gastrectomy: 5 year survival > 95%, regardless of lymphadenopathy
- No survival benefit proven for total or subtotal gastrectomy
- When tumor recurs in remnant stomach, any treatment is palliative

Treatment
- Only curative treatment: Surgical resection for localized disease
- Adjacent organ involvement, peritoneal carcinomatosis, LN metastases, distant metastases: Important factors for determining surgical resectability
- Inoperable obstructing gastric carcinomas can be treated with stent to avoid palliative surgery in frail patients

DIAGNOSTIC CHECKLIST

Consider
- PET/CT for most complete pre-operative staging
- PET/CT to evaluate response to therapy
- PET/CT to identify recurrence

Image Interpretation Pearls
- PET may miss LN metastases adjacent to primary tumor
- PET has high accuracy for N2, visceral, distant metastases
- PET has limited sensitivity for peritoneal metastases due to small size, resolution limits of equipment

SELECTED REFERENCES
1. Chen J et al: Improvement in preoperative staging of gastric adenocarcinoma with positron emission tomography. Cancer. 103(11):2383-90, 2005
2. Hong D et al: Value of baseline positron emission tomography for predicting overall survival in patient with nonmetastatic esophageal or gastroesophageal junction carcinoma. Cancer. 104(8):1620-6, 2005
3. Yun M et al: Lymph node staging of gastric cancer using (18)F-FDG PET: a comparison study with CT. J Nucl Med. 46(10):1582-8, 2005
4. Yun M et al: The role of gastric distention in differentiating recurrent tumor from physiologic uptake in the remnant stomach on 18F-FDG PET. J Nucl Med. 46(6):953-7, 2005
5. Drop A et al: The modern methods of gastric imaging. Ann Univ Mariae Curie Sklodowska [Med]. 59(1):373-81, 2004

GASTRIC CARCINOMA

IMAGE GALLERY

Typical

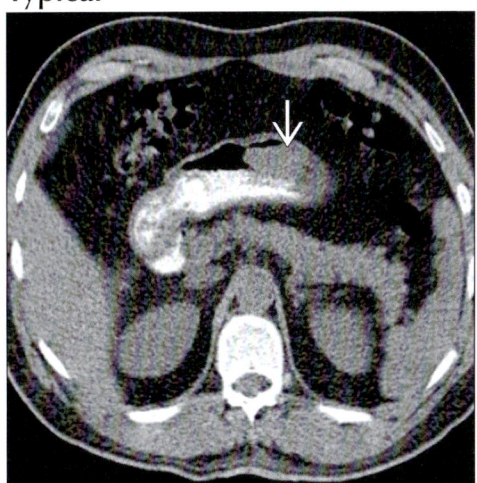

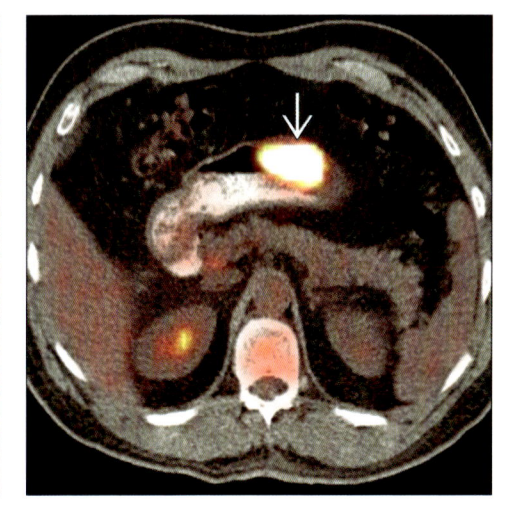

(Left) Axial NECT shows polypoid mass ➡ arising from anterior gastric wall. (Right) Axial fused PET/CT in same patient as previous image shows hypermetabolic activity ➡ corresponding to polypoid gastric carcinoma.

Typical

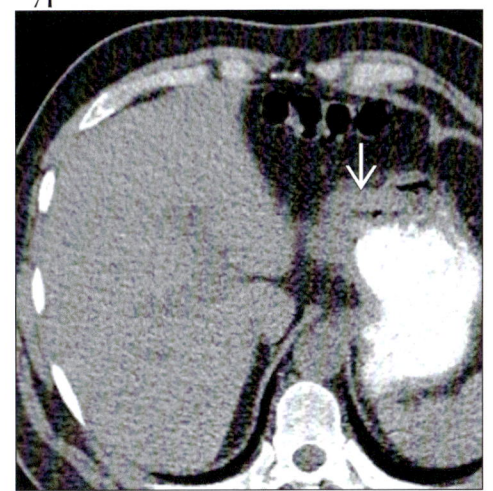

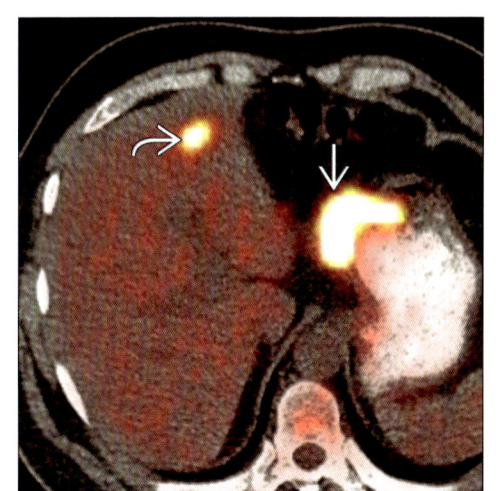

(Left) Axial NECT shows asymmetric gastric wall thickening ➡ in anteromedial gastric mucosa. No other evidence of malignancy on this noncontrast CT. (Right) Axial fused PET/CT in same patient as previous image shows hypermetabolic activity ➡ corresponding to gastric wall thickening. Focal hypermetabolic activity in liver ➡, representing hepatic metastases.

Typical

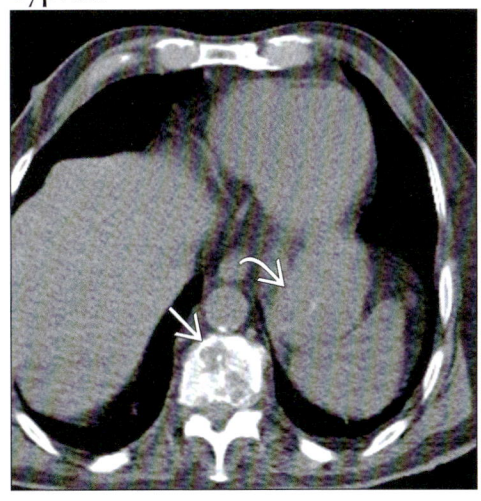

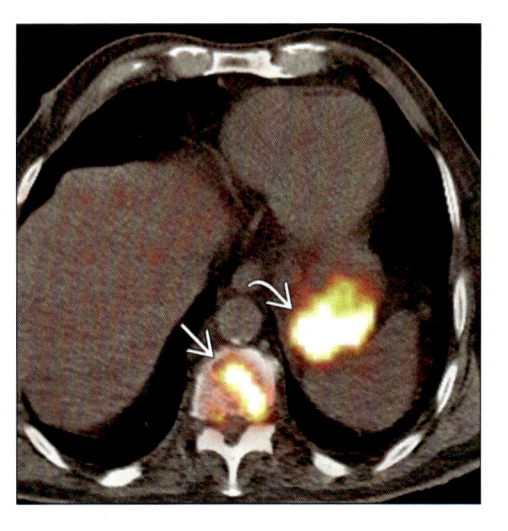

(Left) Axial NECT shows two lytic vertebral lesions ➡. Although the stomach is collapsed, there appears to be diffuse wall thickening ➡. (Right) Axial fused PET/CT in same patient as previous image shows hypermetabolic FDG activity in gastric wall ➡ and vertebral body compatible with metastatic disease ➡, excluding this patient from curative surgery.

INTESTINAL CANCER, PRIMARY AND STAGING

Axial graphic shows intraluminal polypoid mass ➔ in descending colon. Colon cancer is the third most common cancer in the US.

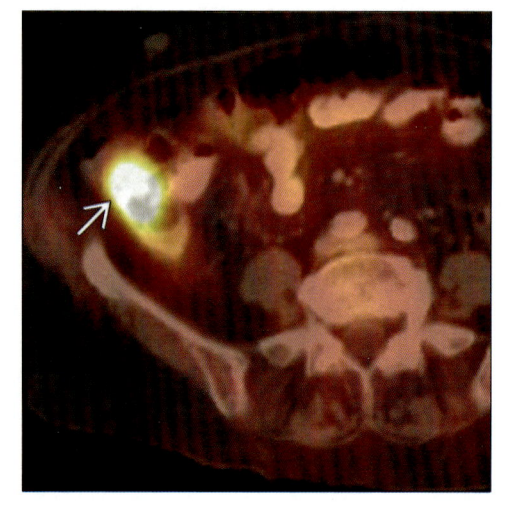

Axial fused PET/CT shows increased activity in a colonic wall mass ➔, confirmed adenocarcinoma at colonoscopy.

TERMINOLOGY

Abbreviations and Synonyms
- Colorectal carcinoma, non-Hodgkin lymphoma (NHL), mucosa-associated lymphoid tissue (MALT) lymphoma, gastrointestinal stromal tumor (GIST), carcinoid

IMAGING FINDINGS

Nuclear Medicine Findings
- PET
  - Colorectal
    - Accuracy of distant staging for colorectal cancer: PET 78%, PET/CT 89%
    - PET poorly sensitive for small (< 1 cm) lesions; high positive predictive value
    - PET limited sensitivity for peritoneal, omental metastases, highly mucinous tumors
    - PET insensitive (29%) for small (< 1 cm) regional lymph nodes
    - Clinical management: PET affects surgical planning in ≤ 30% of colorectal cancer patients
    - Primary colon cancers have been identified with PET as incidental finding
    - Colonic adenoma can take up significant FDG and look similar to carcinoma
    - May be useful for screening in patients with familial polyposis
  - Small bowel lymphoma
    - Focal nodular or diffuse hypermetabolic PET activity in high grade NHL
    - MALT has variable FDG activity and some may not take up significant FDG
  - GIST
    - PET and CT comparable sensitivity at 90% for untreated GIST

Imaging Recommendations
- Best imaging tool
  - Primary colorectal cancer
    - Colonoscopy
    - Double contrast barium enema; low sensitivity for polyps smaller than 1 cm
    - CT: Small lesions harder to identify than larger ("apple core") lesions
    - Can be seen as focal hot spot in colon on PET

DDx: Increased Activity in Colon on FDG PET

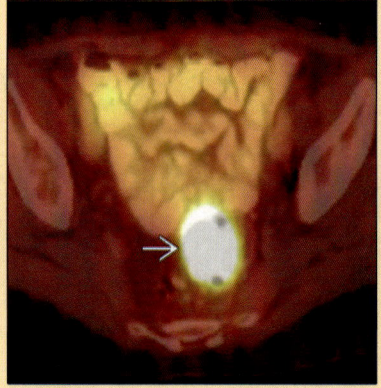

Villous Adenoma

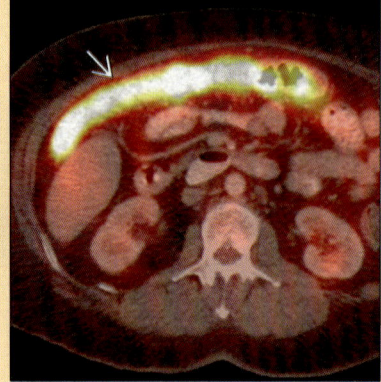

Ulcerative Colitis

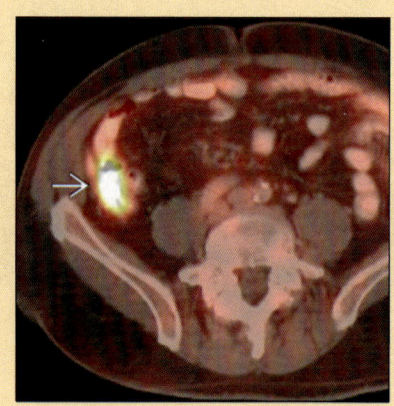

Benign Colon Polyp

INTESTINAL CANCER, PRIMARY AND STAGING

Key Facts

Imaging Findings
- Accuracy of distant staging for colorectal cancer: PET 78%, PET/CT 89%
- PET limited sensitivity for peritoneal, omental metastases, highly mucinous tumors
- PET insensitive (29%) for small (< 1 cm) regional lymph nodes
- Clinical management: PET affects surgical planning in ≤ 30% of colorectal cancer patients
- Primary colon cancers have been identified with PET as incidental finding
- Focal nodular or diffuse hypermetabolic PET activity in high grade NHL

Top Differential Diagnoses
- Adenomas
- Inflammatory Bowel Disease
- Infection
- Physiologic FDG Activity in Bowel

Pathology
- Colorectal cancer staging: Modified Dukes staging system
- Non-Hodgkin lymphoma: May involve intestine
- MALT: May involve intestine
- Carcinoid, GIST, sarcoma: No staging system

Diagnostic Checklist
- Pre-treatment PET for staging, confirmation of FDG-avid disease
- Mucinous adenocarcinoma, MALT, NHL, carcinoid: Variable PET activity
- Correlate focal increased activity in bowel on FDG PET with colonoscopy

---

- Virtual colonography: Gaining acceptance
○ Colorectal staging
  - PET/CT more sensitive for regional/distant metastases than CT alone
  - Colon metastases most commonly go to liver
  - Rectal metastases may bypass liver and go to lung
  - Mucinous adenocarcinoma metastases may show calcification on CT
  - Mucinous adenocarcinoma can be false (-) on PET
○ GIST
  - PET may be helpful for differentiating among benign, low grade, high grade tumors
  - PET for response to therapy
○ Carcinoid
  - Somatostatin receptor imaging (many neuroendocrine tumors contain somatostatin receptors) + CT
  - Carcinoid variable on PET
○ Small bowel lymphoma
  - FDG PET or PET/CT standard clinical staging tool for lymphoma
  - High grade NHL shows intense uptake on PET
  - Low grade NHL also usually takes up FDG, but to a lesser degree than high grade
  - Gallium-67 scintigraphy also useful (however PET imaging characteristics = higher sensitivity)
  - PET at least as sensitive as CT, but more specific
○ MALT
  - 2/3 of cases in stomach (H. pylori-associated)
  - Variable PET activity

DIFFERENTIAL DIAGNOSIS

Adenomas
- Variable PET activity
- Benign adenomas can show intense FDG activity and mimic carcinoma

Inflammatory Bowel Disease
- Ulcerative colitis, Crohn disease
- Increased activity in affected bowel on PET

Infection
- Increased activity in affected segments of bowel
- e.g., pseudomembranous colitis

Physiologic FDG Activity in Bowel
- Diffuse activity in part or all of bowel
- No corresponding bowel thickening on CT

PATHOLOGY

General Features
- General path comments
  ○ Colon polyps
    - 10% of all polyps are adenomatous
    - ↑ Incidence of carcinoma with villous tumors
  ○ GIST: Most common mesenchymal tumors of GI tract
    - Poor prognosis in past; treatment with tyrosine kinase inhibitors promising
  ○ Small bowel tumors
    - 64% malignant; 40% adenocarcinomas
    - Tumors cluster toward proximal small intestine: 50% duodenum, 30% jejunum, 20% ileum
    - 15% of small bowel cancer = GIST
    - 30% of GIST occurs in small bowel; more common in stomach
    - Small bowel GIST = worse prognosis
- Etiology
  ○ Colorectal cancer
    - Arises from pre-existing adenomatous polyps in colonic or rectal mucosa
    - Age, smoking, diet high in fat and cholesterol, inflammatory bowel disease (especially ulcerative colitis), genetic predisposition
  ○ Small bowel cancer
    - Familial adenomatous polyposis (FAP), hereditary nonpolyposis colorectal cancer (HNPCC), animal fat intake, smoking, alcohol, Crohn disease
    - Crohn-related tumors usually begin at ileum, unlike other small bowel tumors
- Epidemiology

INTESTINAL CANCER, PRIMARY AND STAGING

- Colorectal cancer
  - Third most common cancer in US
  - 135,000 new cases per year in US; 55,000 deaths per year
  - Lifetime risk in general US population: 5.9%
  - 2/3 in colon, 1/3 in rectum
- Small bowel cancer
  - 1,100 patients die each year
  - 5 year overall survival 30-35% for adenocarcinoma, 25% for sarcoma
- Small bowel lymphoma (SBL)
  - Primary SBL comprises 25% of small bowel malignancies, virtually all non-Hodgkin lymphoma
  - Great majority of B-cell origin

Staging, Grading or Classification Criteria

- Colorectal cancer staging: Modified Dukes staging system
  - Dukes A: Carcinoma in situ limited to mucosa or submucosa (T1, N0, M0)
  - Dukes B: Cancer that extends into the muscularis (B1), into or through the serosa (B2)
  - Dukes C: Cancer that extends to regional lymph nodes (T1-4, N1, M0)
  - Dukes D: Modified classification; cancer that has metastasized to distant sites (T1-4, N1-3, M1)
- Non-Hodgkin lymphoma: May involve intestine
  - I: Single lymph node region or extralymphatic organ/site
  - II: 2 or more lymph node regions/structures on same side of diaphragm; limited, contiguous extralymphatic organ/tissue
  - III: Malignancy on both sides of diaphragm
  - IV: Diffuse/disseminated involvement (≥ 1 extralymphatic organ/tissue); ± lymphatic involvement
- MALT: May involve intestine
  - Stage: Lymph node (rare), visceral metastases
  - Grade: Low grade (more common); can transform to high grade
- Carcinoid, GIST, sarcoma: No staging system
  - Optimal: Surgical resection of primary

CLINICAL ISSUES

Presentation

- Most common signs/symptoms
  - Colorectal cancer
    - Bleeding in 60% of patients
  - Small bowel cancer
    - Asymptomatic; abdominal pain, weight loss
  - Colon adenoma
    - 50% abdominal pain, 35% bowel habit changes, 30% occult bleeding
  - Carcinoid
    - Flushing, diarrhea, bronchoconstriction, cardiac disease, bowel obstruction

Demographics

- Age
  - Colorectal cancer: Peak 7th decade; risk rises ≥ 40
  - Small bowel cancer: Mean 60 years
  - Carcinoid: Peak 62 years; rare in children
- Gender
  - Colon polyps: Male preponderance
  - Small bowel cancer: M:F = 1.4:1
  - Carcinoid: No gender difference

Natural History & Prognosis

- Colorectal cancer
  - Dukes A: 5 year > 90%
  - Dukes B: 5 year > 70%
  - Dukes C: 5 year < 60%
  - Dukes D: 5 year ~ 5%
- Carcinoid tumors
  - Metastases to mesenteric, para-aortic lymph nodes, liver
  - 5 year survival 67% for metastatic disease

Treatment

- Colorectal cancer
  - Surgically curable if detected early
  - Adjuvant chemotherapy to prolong survival with lymph node + disease
  - Rectal adenocarcinomas are sensitive to radiation
- Small bowel cancer
  - Chemotherapy, wide-excision, radiation
- Carcinoid tumor
  - Optimum: Resection of primary tumor
  - Presence of metastases ⇒ palliative surgery, medical management
  - Medical therapy with somatostatin analogue improved 5 year survival from 18% to 67%

DIAGNOSTIC CHECKLIST

Consider

- Pre-treatment PET for staging, confirmation of FDG-avid disease

Image Interpretation Pearls

- Mucinous adenocarcinoma, MALT, NHL, carcinoid: Variable PET activity
- Correlate focal increased activity in bowel on FDG PET with colonoscopy

SELECTED REFERENCES

1. Dobos N et al: Radiologic imaging modalities in the diagnosis and management of colorectal cancer. Hematol Oncol Clin North Am. 16(4):875-95, 2002
2. Zhuang H et al: The role of positron emission tomography with fluorine-18-deoxyglucose in identifying colorectal cancer metastases to liver. Nucl Med Commun. 21(9):793-8, 2000
3. Yoshioka T et al: FDG PET evaluation of residual masses and regrowth of abdominal lymph node metastases from colon cancer compared with CT during chemotherapy. Clin Nucl Med. 24(4):261-3, 1999
4. Goldberg MA et al: Fluorodeoxyglucose PET of abdominal and pelvic neoplasms: potential role in oncologic imaging. Radiographics. 13(5):1047-62, 1993
5. Gupta NC et al: Pre-operative staging of colorectal carcinoma using positron emission tomography. Nebr Med J. 78(2):30-5, 1993

INTESTINAL CANCER, PRIMARY AND STAGING

IMAGE GALLERY

Typical

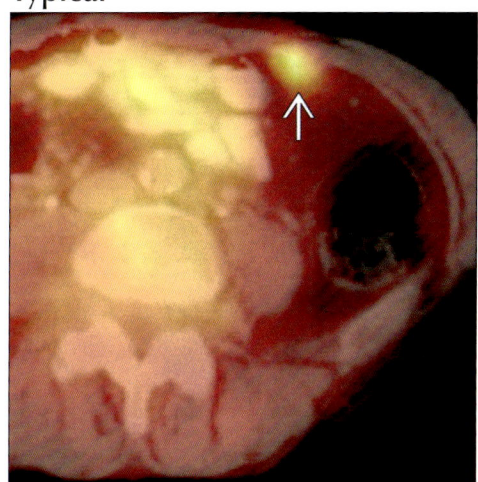

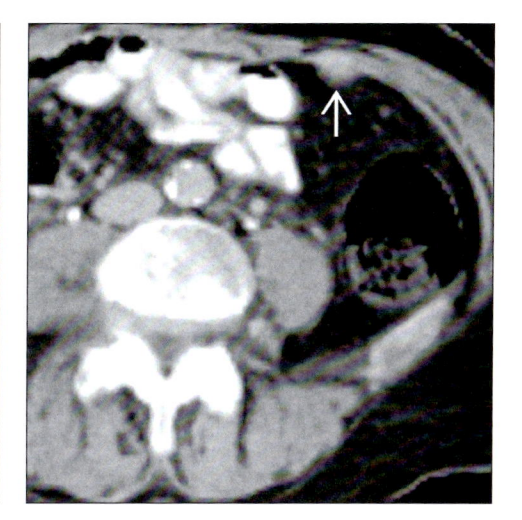

(**Left**) Axial fused PET/CT in patient with colorectal cancer shows increased activity in left anterior abdominal wall ➡, consistent with metastasis. (**Right**) Axial CECT in same patient as previous image shows soft tissue adherent to left anterior abdominal wall ➡, missed prospectively on CT.

Typical

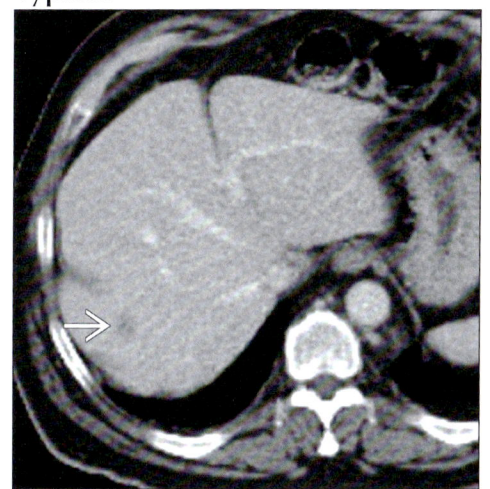

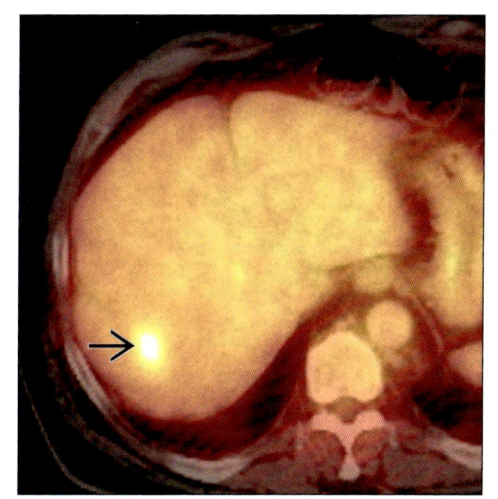

(**Left**) Axial fused PET/CT shows subtle, nonspecific low attenuation hepatic lesion ➡ in patient with colon cancer. The differential diagnosis includes cyst, hemangioma, focal nodular hyperplasia, metastasis, infection. (**Right**) Axial fused PET/CT in same patient as previous image shows focal increased activity corresponding to the hepatic lesion ➡, confirming metastatic disease.

Variant

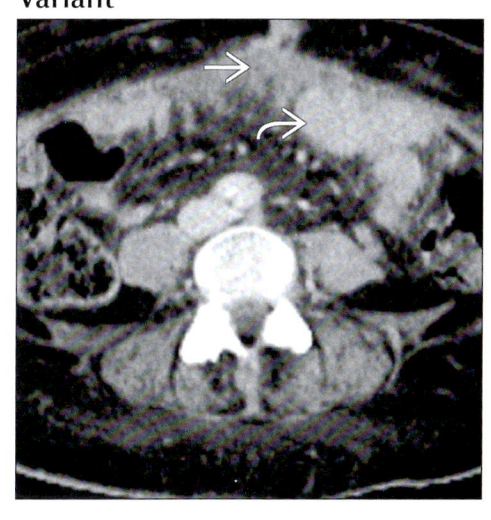

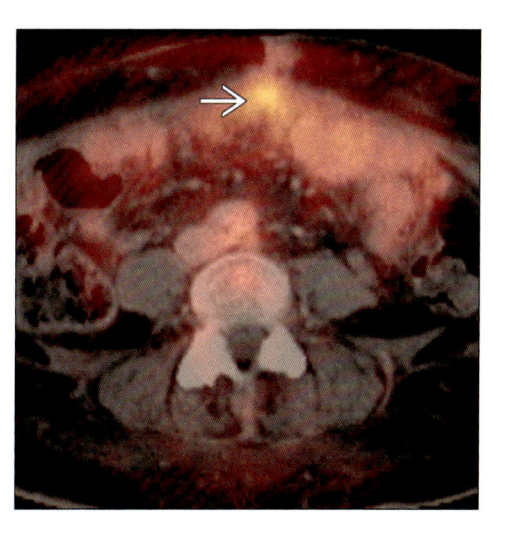

(**Left**) Axial fused PET/CT in patient with colon cancer shows subtle omental nodularity ➡ anterior and superior to bowel ➡, which has higher attenuation. (**Right**) Axial fused PET/CT in same patient as previous image shows increased FDG activity in the nodule ➡, consistent with omental metastases. Note that PET has limited sensitivity for very small omental and peritoneal lesions.

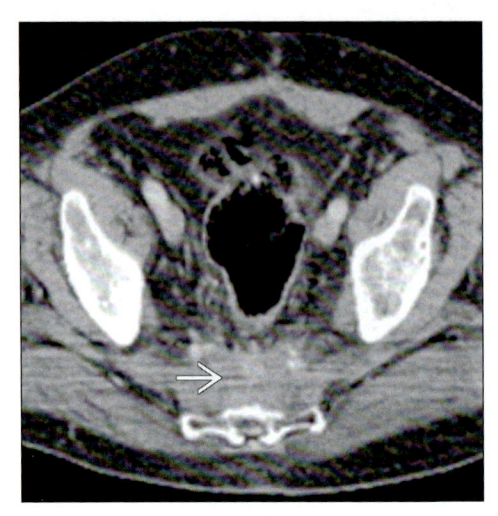

INTESTINAL CANCER, THERAPY EVAL./RESTAGING

Axial CECT in patient with ↑ CEA after surgery for colon cancer shows presacral soft tissue mass ➡ that may represent post-surgical changes or recurrent tumor.

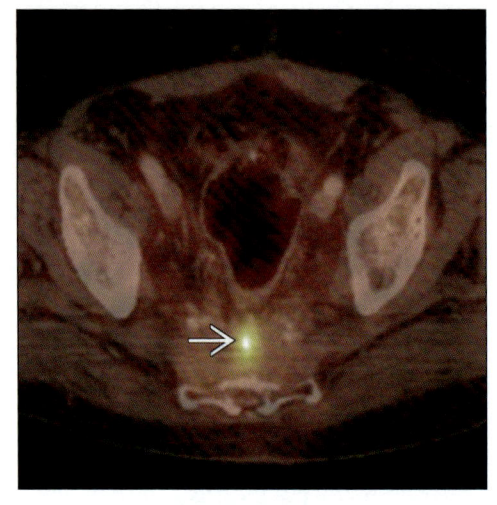

Axial fused PET/CT in same patient as left shows ↑ FDG activity in presacral soft tissue ➡, consistent with recurrence which was confirmed by biopsy.

TERMINOLOGY

Abbreviations and Synonyms
- Colorectal cancer, lymphoma, gastrointestinal stromal tumor (GIST)

IMAGING FINDINGS

General Features
- Best diagnostic clue: ↑ FDG activity on PET

Imaging Recommendations
- Best imaging tool
  - Colorectal cancer
    - ↑ Tumor marker: Carcinoembryonic antigen (CEA)
    - Recurrence: Surgical anastomosis, regional lymph nodes, presacral area
    - FDG PET to localize relapse in patients with ↑ CEA: Sensitivity > 95%, specificity ~ 71%
    - Restage to detect locally recurrent disease, isolated metastatic disease in liver/lung, diffuse metastases
    - FDG PET to differentiate scar/fibrosis after surgery or radiation vs. tumor in rectal cancer
    - Mucinous adenocarcinoma: Often false (-) on FDG PET
  - GIST
    - Recurrence: Primary tumor site, peritoneum, liver
    - ↓ FDG activity 8 days after start of therapy correctly predicts therapy response, longer progression-free survival
    - CT-based evaluation of response lags behind FDG PET by weeks-months
  - Non-Hodgkin lymphoma (NHL)
    - Residual mass on CT post-therapy common: FDG PET evaluates malignant activity
    - FDG PET = CT sensitivity; FDG PET more specific, especially for restaging
    - High grade NHL: FDG PET very sensitive
    - Low grade lymphoma: May be false (-) on FDG PET

DIFFERENTIAL DIAGNOSIS

Post-Surgical Scar/Fibrosis
- Mildly ↑ FDG activity with normal post-surgical healing

DDx: Benign Presacral Masses Post Treatment

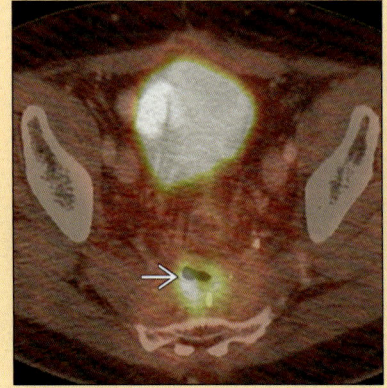

Abscess 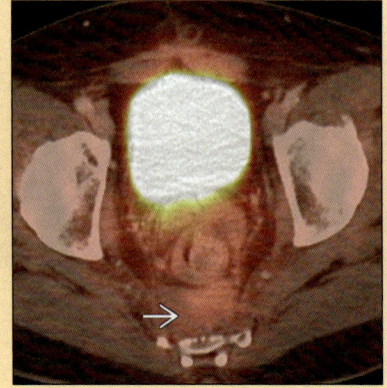   *Scar/Fibrosis* 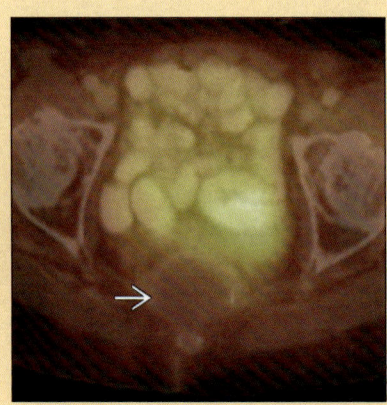   *Seroma*

INTESTINAL CANCER, THERAPY EVAL./RESTAGING

Key Facts

Imaging Findings
- Best diagnostic clue: ↑ FDG activity on PET

Top Differential Diagnoses
- Post-Surgical Scar/Fibrosis
- Abscess
- Seroma
- Post-Radiation Change
- Physiologic FDG Activity in Adjacent Bowel

Diagnostic Checklist
- Rectal cancer: FDG PET to differentiate scar/fibrosis after surgery or radiation vs. tumor
- Mucinous adenocarcinoma: Often false (-) on FDG PET
- Lymphoma: FDG PET to evaluate activity in residual mass post-therapy
- Post-radiation and post-surgical inflammation: Can have ↑ FDG activity; should ↓ over time

- Serial FDG PET: Scar/fibrosis stable or ↓ activity

Abscess
- Abscess and tumor both can show ↑ FDG activity
- ↑ FDG activity surrounding photopenic center: Abscess, necrotic tumor
  - Time course, prior studies useful to differentiate
- Gas + fluid collection more specific for abscess

Seroma
- Photopenia on FDG PET; fluid density on CT

Post-Radiation Change
- Early: Often difficult to assess due to ↑ FDG activity 2° to inflammation
- Typically resolves in 3-6 months

Physiologic FDG Activity in Adjacent Bowel
- Usually linear; corresponds to normal bowel

CLINICAL ISSUES

Presentation
- Most common signs/symptoms
  - Rising CEA level
  - Abdominal pain (obstruction)

Treatment
- Local recurrence: Surgery, chemo ± radiation
- Hepatic recurrence: Resection, radiofrequency ablation, hepatic arterial chemotherapy/radiotherapy

DIAGNOSTIC CHECKLIST

Image Interpretation Pearls
- Rectal cancer: FDG PET to differentiate scar/fibrosis after surgery or radiation vs. tumor
- Mucinous adenocarcinoma: Often false (-) on FDG PET
- Lymphoma: FDG PET to evaluate activity in residual mass post-therapy
- Post-radiation and post-surgical inflammation: Can have ↑ FDG activity; should ↓ over time

SELECTED REFERENCES

1. Chun H et al: The usefulness of a repeat study for differentiating between bowel activity and local tumor recurrence on FDG PET scans. Clin Nucl Med. 28(8):672-3, 2003
2. Libutti SK et al: A prospective study of 2-[18F]fluoro-2-deoxy-D-glucose/positron emission tomography scan, 99mTc-labeled arcitumomab (CEA-scan), and blind second-look laparotomy for detecting colon cancer recurrence in patients with increasing carcinoembryonic antigen levels. Ann Surg Oncol. 8(10):779-86, 2001
3. Kalff V V et al: 29. F-18 FDG PET for Suspected or Confirmed Regional Recurrence of Colon Cancer. A Prospective Study of Impact and Outcome. Clin Positron Imaging. 3(4):183, 2000
4. Whiteford MH et al: Usefulness of FDG-PET scan in the assessment of suspected metastatic or recurrent adenocarcinoma of the colon and rectum. Dis Colon Rectum. 43(6):759-67; discussion 767-70, 2000

IMAGE GALLERY

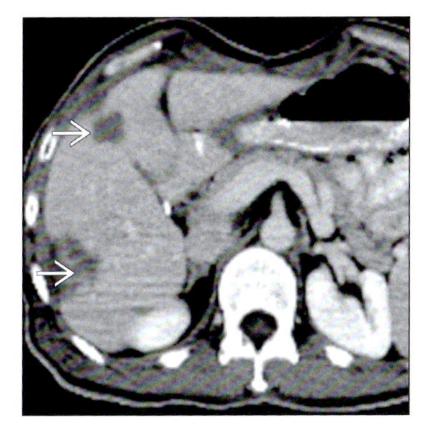

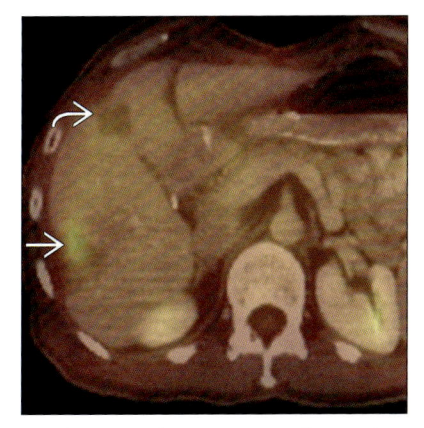

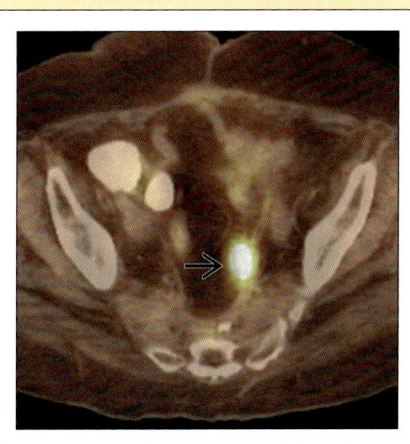

(Left) Axial CECT in patient with colorectal metastases shows two low attenuation hepatic lesions ➔ following radiofrequency ablation, the typical appearance of successful ablation. *(Center)* Axial fused PET/CT in same patient as left shows ↑ FDG activity along anterior margin of posterior lesion ➔, consistent with residual tumor. Normal FDG activity present in anterior lesion ➔. *(Right)* Axial fused PET/CT shows ↑ FDG activity at the colonic anastomosis ➔, consistent with recurrent colon carcinoma.

MECKEL DIVERTICULUM

Anterior Meckel scan shows a focus of activity in the right lower quadrant ➔ whose intensity parallels that of the stomach and remains focal with no nearby bowel or renal activity.

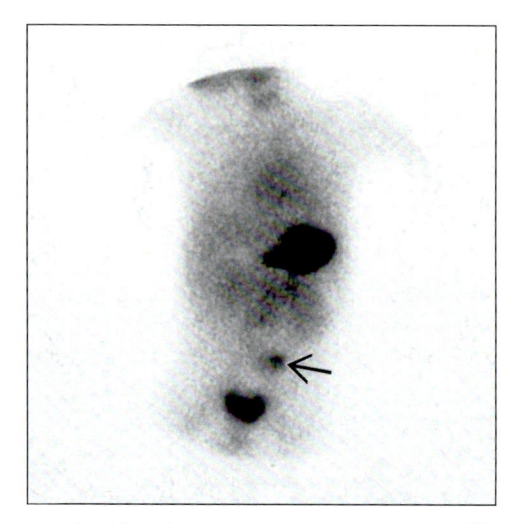

Anterior Meckel scan shows an intense focus ➔ matching that of the stomach. The location is not classic but it is common.

TERMINOLOGY

Abbreviations and Synonyms
- Ectopic gastric mucosa
- Vitelline duct remnant
- Omphalomesenteric duct remnant

Definitions
- The remains of an improperly closed omphalomesenteric or vitelline duct arising from the ileum a short distance above the cecum which may contain ectopic gastric mucosa

IMAGING FINDINGS

General Features
- Best diagnostic clue
  - Imaging of the patient using Tc-99m pertechnetate
    - The pertechnetate visualizes the ectopic mucosa, not the diverticulum
  - Focal increased activity usually but not necessarily in the right lower quadrant appears with a time course matching that of the stomach
- Location: Usually in the right lower quadrant of the abdomen
- Size: Small
- Morphology: Focal

Nuclear Medicine Findings
- Tc-99m Sulfur Colloid
  - This might be performed in a gastrointestinal (GI) bleeder in whom Meckel diverticulum is not in the differential
  - This is an actual GI bleeding scan
    - The scan will be positive for bleeding from any cause including but not limited to a Meckel diverticulum
    - A very sensitive technique for GI or non GI bleeding based on rapid clearance of non bled tracer into the liver and spleen.
    - The images have high target to background ratios in areas of active bleeding
- Tc-99m Labeled Red Cell Scintigraphy
  - This might be performed for a GI bleed where Meckel diverticulum is not in the differential

DDx: Mimics of Meckel Diverticulum

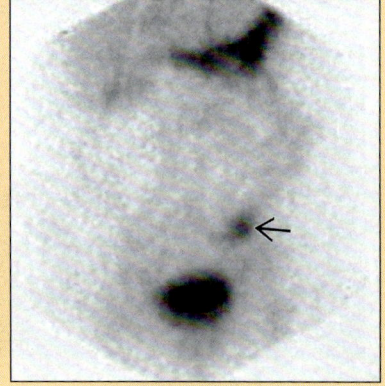

Colonic Bleed

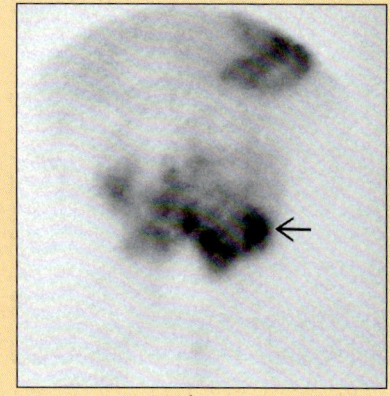

Duplication

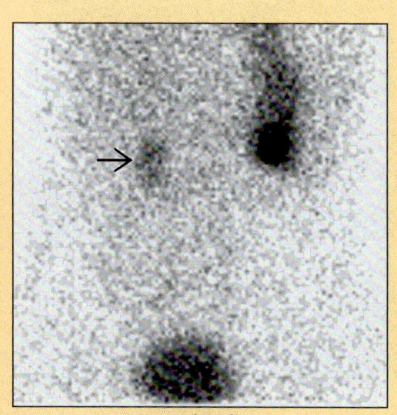

Renal Pelvis

MECKEL DIVERTICULUM

Key Facts

Terminology
- The remains of an improperly closed omphalomesenteric or vitelline duct arising from the ileum a short distance above the cecum which may contain ectopic gastric mucosa

Imaging Findings
- Focal increased activity usually but not necessarily in the right lower quadrant appears with a time course matching that of the stomach
- Location: Usually in the right lower quadrant of the abdomen
- Best imaging tool: Scanning using Tc-99m pertechnetate
- The abnormality usually appears during the first ten minutes after tracer injection
- Continuous imaging may be more helpful than static images
- Stomach secretions passing into bowel should be prevented
- Positioning the patient RPO while still positioning the camera to obtain anterior images is often sufficient to delay gastric emptying
- Pharmacologic preparation is advised

Top Differential Diagnoses
- Gastrointestinal Bleeding from Other Causes
- Intestinal Duplications Containing Gastric Mucosa
- Visualization of Portion of the Right Ureter

Diagnostic Checklist
- Time course of the abnormal activity often parallels that of the stomach

---

- The scan will be positive for bleeding from any cause including but not limited to a Meckel diverticulum
- A sensitive technique for GI or non GI bleeding with lower target to background ratios than sulfur colloid but longer residence time in the vascular system

Imaging Recommendations
- Best imaging tool: Scanning using Tc-99m pertechnetate
- Protocol advice
  - The abnormality usually appears during the first ten minutes after tracer injection
  - Continuous imaging may be more helpful than static images
  - Patient should have nothing by mouth for 6 hours if possible
  - Stomach secretions passing into bowel should be prevented
    - Positioning the patient RPO while still positioning the camera to obtain anterior images is often sufficient to delay gastric emptying
    - Nasogastric intubation can be used but is generally not necessary
    - Glucagon and/or cimetidine are often helpful
  - Pharmacologic preparation is advised
    - Cimetidine 300 mg qid for 24-48 hours prior to the scan traps tracer in gastric mucosa and improves visualization and is strongly advised if feasible
    - Glucagon 50 ug-1mg/kg IV: Helps decrease gastric secretions from reaching the region of interest
    - Pentagastrin 6 ug/kg increases gastric mucosal uptake of tracer
    - Combinations or all of the above may be used
    - RPO positioning if feasible delays gastric emptying of luminal free pertechnetate

DIFFERENTIAL DIAGNOSIS

Gastrointestinal Bleeding from Other Causes
- Location often different from typical Meckel diverticulum in right lower quadrant
- Timing of appearance often different from that of stomach
- Shape will often change
  - Focal abnormalities will become more linear or curvilinear

Intestinal Duplications Containing Gastric Mucosa
- Location and shape often different from typical Meckel diverticulum in right lower quadrant
- Timing of appearance likely to match that of the stomach like a Meckel diverticulum
- May be indistinguishable from a Meckel diverticulum
  - However the treatment will be the same

Intestinal Malrotations
- Timing of appearance likely to be different from that of the stomach
- Shape will often change
  - Initial focal finding will become more linear or curvilinear

Visualization of Portion of the Right Ureter
- A normal variant
- Timing of appearance likely to be different from that of the stomach
- Visualization of right kidney or other portions of the ureter is a helpful clue
- Vertically oriented shape is often helpful
  - However may be focal anywhere, but especially at the iliac vessel level

PATHOLOGY

General Features
- Etiology

MECKEL DIVERTICULUM

- Improper closure of the omphalomesenteric or vitelline duct which arises from the fetal yolk sac
  - Fetal yolk sac connects fetal intestine with the umbilicus
  - Other related vitelline duct anomalies include umbilical cysts and fibrous connections between the ileum and the umbilicus
- Epidemiology
  - The most common congenital GI tract anomaly
  - Occurs in about 3% of the population
- Physiology
  - The mucus cells in ectopic gastric mucosa concentrate Tc-99m pertechnetate
    - The mucus cells in gastric mucosa show similar physiology
  - A Meckel diverticulum not containing gastric mucosa will not be detectable
    - However due to its wide mouth and lack of gastric mucosa it should not cause symptoms except for rare intussusception

Gross Pathologic & Surgical Features
- On the antimesenteric side of the terminal ileum
- Has its own blood supply
- Within 90 cm of the ileocecal valve
- Average length 6 cm

Microscopic Features
- A true diverticulum containing all layers of bowel wall
- Heterotopic gastric mucosa is often found histologically
- Pancreatic mucosa will occasionally be found

CLINICAL ISSUES

Presentation
- Most common signs/symptoms: Painless GI bleeding
- Other signs/symptoms
  - Abdominal pain
    - Most Meckel diverticula are asymptomatic
    - Occasionally intussusception
    - Occasionally intestinal obstruction
    - Occasionally diverticulitis

Demographics
- Age
  - More than half present by age 2
    - Many of the rest present by age 10
  - Some may not present until adulthood
    - These may present as diverticulitis or intestinal obstruction
- Gender
  - No gender predisposition for presence of the anomaly
  - Symptoms are more common in males

Natural History & Prognosis
- Complications are uncommon
  - Meckel diverticula usually have a wide mouth and are not likely to become obstructed or inflamed
- Complications arise when there is abnormal gastric mucosa which causes bleeding of the adjacent non gastric mucosa
- Prognosis is good after surgery

Treatment
- Asymptomatic
  - No treatment
- Symptomatic
  - Surgery

DIAGNOSTIC CHECKLIST

Image Interpretation Pearls
- Time course of the abnormal activity often parallels that of the stomach
  - This is because it is gastric mucosal activity that is being visualized

SELECTED REFERENCES

1. Levy AD et al: From the archives of the AFIP. Meckel diverticulum: radiologic features with pathologic Correlation. Radiographics. 24(2):565-87, 2004
2. Singh MV et al: A fading Meckel's diverticulum: an unusual scintigraphic appearance in a child. Pediatr Radiol. 34(3):274-6, 2004
3. Adams BK et al: A moving Meckel's diverticulum on Tc-99m pertechnetate imaging in a patient with lower gastrointestinal bleeding. Clin Nucl Med. 28(11):908-10, 2003
4. Howarth DM et al: The clinical utility of nuclear medicine imaging for the detection of occult gastrointestinal haemorrhage. Nucl Med Commun. 23(6):591-4, 2002
5. Lin S et al: Gastrointestinal bleeding in adult patients with Meckel's diverticulum: the role of technetium 99m pertechnetate scan. South Med J. 95(11):1338-41, 2002
6. Ponzo F et al: Tc-99m sulfur colloid and Tc-99m tagged red blood cell methods are comparable for detecting lower gastrointestinal bleeding in clinical practice. Clin Nucl Med. 27(6):405-9, 2002
7. Emamian SA et al: The spectrum of heterotopic gastric mucosa in children detected by Tc-99m pertechnetate scintigraphy. Clin Nucl Med. 26(6):529-35, 2001
8. Swaniker F et al: The utility of technetium 99m pertechnetate scintigraphy in the evaluation of patients with Meckel's diverticulum. J Pediatr Surg. 34(5):760-4; discussion 765, 1999
9. Connolly LP et al: Meckel's diverticulum: demonstration of heterotopic gastric mucosa with technetium-99m-pertechnetate SPECT. J Nucl Med. 39(8):1458-60, 1998
10. Lotfi K et al: Bleeding Meckel's diverticulum presenting as focal extravasation on pertechnetate scintigraphy. Clin Nucl Med. 21(1):1-3, 1996
11. Rossi P et al: Meckel's diverticulum: imaging diagnosis. AJR Am J Roentgenol. 166(3):567-73, 1996
12. Kwok CG et al: Feasibility of Meckel's scan after RBC gastrointestinal bleeding study using in-vitro labeling technique. Clin Nucl Med. 20(11):959-61, 1995
13. Heyman S: Meckel's diverticulum: possible detection by combining pentagastrin with histamine H2 receptor blocker. J Nucl Med. 35(10):1656-8, 1994
14. Yen CK et al: Effect of stannous pyrophosphate red blood cell gastrointestinal bleeding scan on subsequent Meckel's scan. Clin Nucl Med. 17(6):454-6, 1992
15. St-Vil D et al: Meckel's diverticulum in children: a 20-year review. J Pediatr Surg. 26(11):1289-92, 1991
16. Dixon PM et al: The diagnosis of Meckel's diverticulum: a continuing challenge. Clin Radiol. 38(6):615-9, 1987

MECKEL DIVERTICULUM

IMAGE GALLERY

Typical

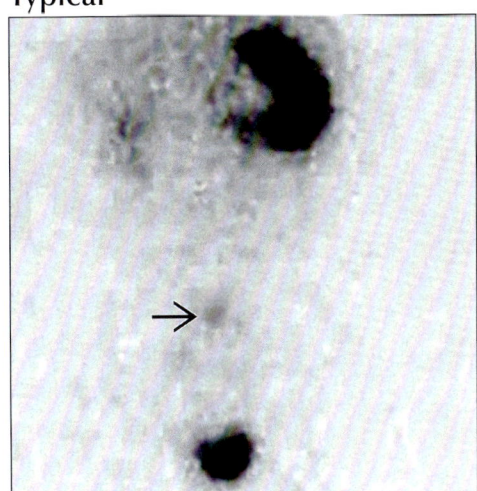

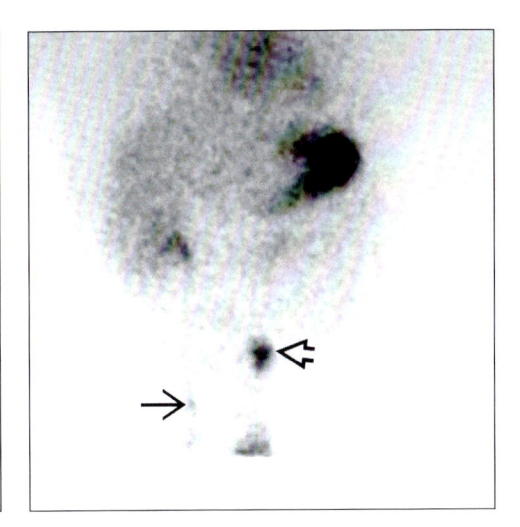

(Left) Anterior Meckel scan shows a faint but definite focus ➡ which persisted on multiple images (not shown). *(Right)* Anterior Meckel scan shows an elongated shape suggesting ureter, but the intensity matches that of the stomach ⇨, confirming Meckel diverticulum. Ureteric activity ➡ is present in the right abdomen, which can mimic diverticulum.

Typical

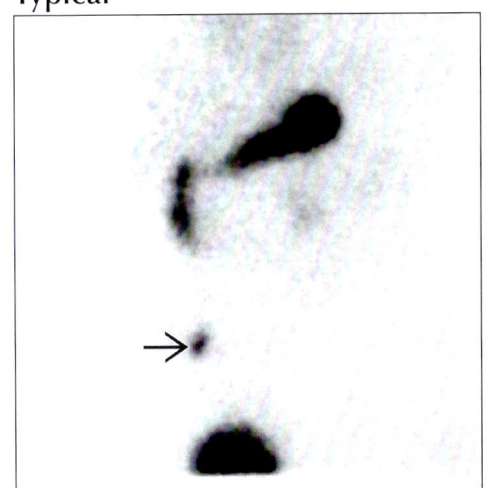

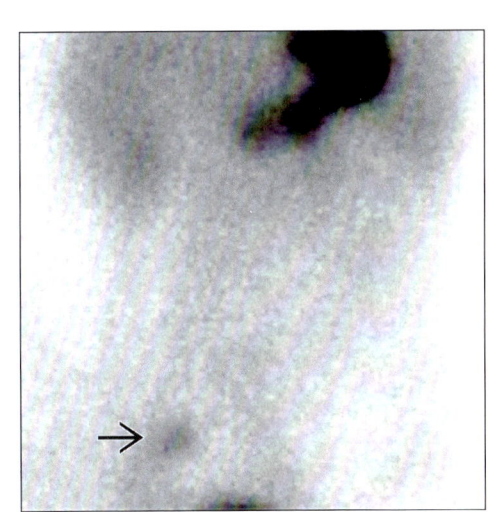

(Left) Anterior Meckel scan Shows a focus of increased activity ➡ typical in appearance and location for a Meckel diverticulum. *(Right)* Anterior Meckel scan Shows a focus of increased activity ➡ typical in appearance and location for a Meckel diverticulum.

Typical

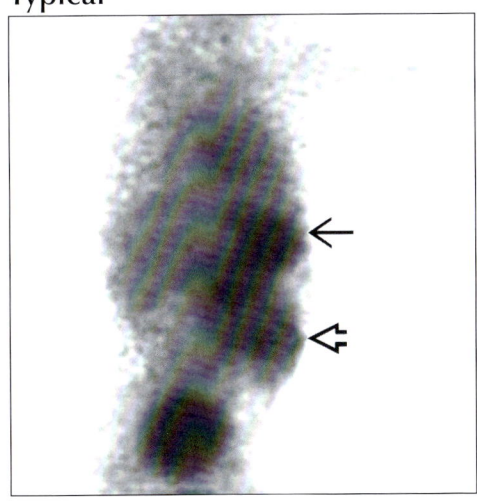

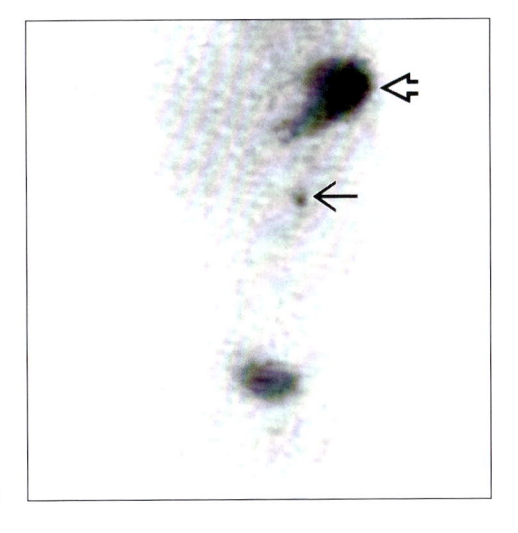

(Left) Anterior Meckel scan shows uptake throughout the abdomen, primarily in stomach ➡ and small bowel ⇨. Patient underwent scan without pretreatment with H2 blockers. See next image. *(Right)* Repeat Meckel scan 24 h after maximum dose of cimetidine, resulting in retention of free pertechnetate by the stomach wall ⇨ without excretion into bowel. Meckel diverticulum ➡ in mid abdomen now clearly seen.

GI BLEEDING LOCALIZATION

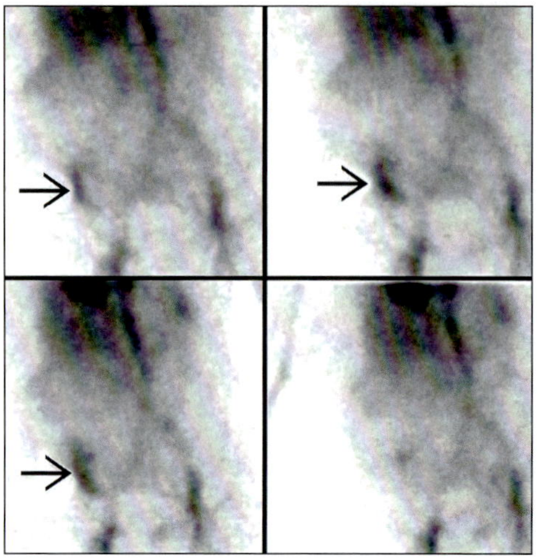

Tc-99m tagged RBC scan (selected sequential images) shows accumulation of radiotracer within the cecum and ascending colon ➡ indicating active bleeding.

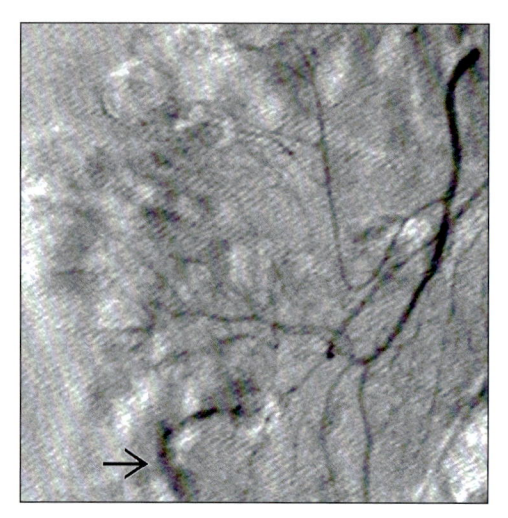

Selective ileocolic arteriogram shows active bleeding in the cecum ➡. Bleeding diverticulum.

TERMINOLOGY

Definitions
- Bleeding from gastrointestinal tract; may be acute, subacute, or chronic

IMAGING FINDINGS

General Features
- Best diagnostic clue: Technetium (Tc) labeled red blood cells (RBC) appearing in tubular structure distinct from normal vascular or organ structure; moves in relatively short time intervals (min)
- Location
  - Upper GI bleed: Proximal to ligament of Treitz
    - Mouth (tumor, trauma)
    - Esophagus (varices, tumor, Mallory-Weiss tear, esophagitis)
    - Stomach (peptic ulcer, gastritis, tumor)
    - Duodenum (ulcer, tumor)
  - Lower GI bleed: Distal to ligament of Treitz
    - Small bowel (inflammatory i.e., Crohn disease, tumor, infection, in pediatric population consider Meckel diverticulum, intussusception)
    - Colon (diverticular disease, angiodysplasia, benign polyps, malignancies, inflammatory bowel disease, arteriovenous malformations)
    - Anorectal (tumor, infection, hemorrhoids, fissures)
  - Bleeding characteristics
    - Upper GI (75%): Hematemesis, melena, rapid bleeding will often result in hematochezia
    - Lower GI (25%): Hematochezia or melena

Nuclear Medicine Findings
- Tc-99m Labeled Red Cell Scintigraphy
  - Sensitivity considerably higher than Tc-99m sulfur colloid (Tc-99m SC) due to intermittent nature of GI bleeding
    - Can perform 24 hour delayed views to assess interval bleeding status
    - May confirm bleeding site by outlining large bowel location and configuration
  - Positive study: Accumulation of activity unrelated to normal organ uptake or vascular structures

DDx: Mimics of GI Bleeding on Tc-99m RBC Scan

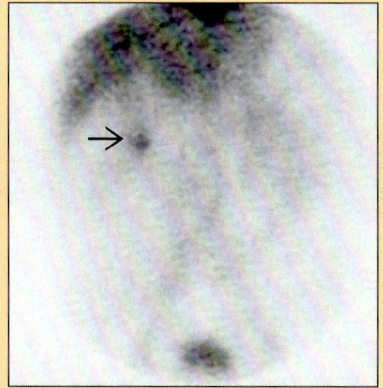

Renal Collecting System 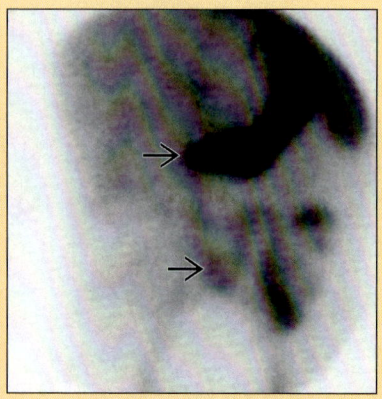 | *Free Pertechnetate* 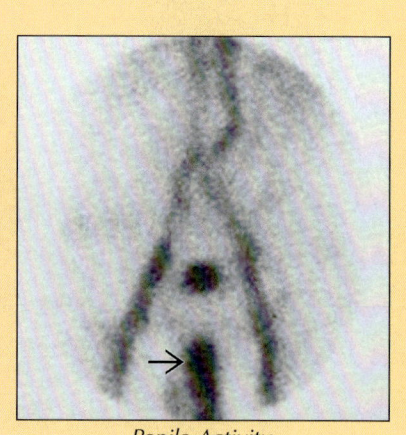 | *Penile Activity*

GI BLEEDING LOCALIZATION

Key Facts

Imaging Findings
- Best diagnostic clue: Technetium (Tc) labeled red blood cells (RBC) appearing in tubular structure distinct from normal vascular or organ structure; moves in relatively short time intervals (min)
- Upper GI bleed: Proximal to ligament of Treitz
- Lower GI bleed: Distal to ligament of Treitz
- Display: Frame by frame hard copy or computer monitor; cine loop for continuous viewing

Top Differential Diagnoses
- Peptic Ulceration and Erosive Gastritis
- Esophageal Varices
- Small Bowel Bleed
- Diverticulosis and Colonic Angiodysplasia (AVM)

Pathology
- Duodenal ulcer (24%), gastric erosions (23%)
- Gastric ulcer (21%), varices (10%)
- Diverticulosis (43%), vascular ectasia (20%)

Clinical Issues
- Hematemesis: Bloody vomitus; red, coffee grounds
- Melena: Black, tarry stools (100-200 mL of blood in upper GI tract is required to produce melena)
- Hematochezia: Red blood per rectum
- Occult blood detected by stool chemical testing

Diagnostic Checklist
- Tc-99m RBC for hemodynamically stable cases
- Angiography for hemodynamically unstable cases

- Minimum of 5cc blood localized; positive when bleeding rate exceeds 0.2-0.5cc/min
- Tc-99m SC may detect lower bleeding rates (≥ 0.05 cc/min) but window for detection following injection is extremely limited
  - Upper GI bleeding: Usually presents in dynamic phase in upper-mid abdomen
    - Look for small bowel pattern
    - 6 or 24 hour views useful; may identify large bowel to enable differentiation from upper GI
  - Small bowel bleeding: May initially appear at any location in abdomen or pelvis
    - Dynamic phase demonstrates small bowel pattern
    - Anterograde or retrograde transit possible
  - Large bowel bleeding: May appear at any location
    - Dynamic phase = large bowel pattern; rectal bleeding pattern atypical
    - Localization may be difficult due to antegrade or retrograde transit; use cine loop display
  - Advantages
    - Tc-99m RBC more sensitive in clinical setting than Tc-99m SC, CT, or angiography
    - One injection can monitor patient bleeding status for 24 hours
    - Often useful in intermittent bleeding
  - Disadvantages
    - May require lengthy protocol
    - No guarantee of localization, especially if bleeding rate is low or intermittent
    - Not useful in chronic GI blood loss
  - Pitfalls
    - Poor label of RBC with Tc-O4- will result in activity in bowel or genitourinary collecting system
    - Failure to recognize normal accumulation of Tc-99m RBC in organs and blood pool of abdominal pelvic vessels, ptotic or pelvic kidney
    - Accumulation in genitalia (especially male) or bladder may be confused with rectal bleeding
    - Accumulation in enlarged uterus or uterine fibroid
    - Attempt to localize bleeding site based on delayed imaging

Imaging Recommendations
- Best imaging tool
  - Tc-99m RBC: Procedure of choice when patient is actively bleeding and hemodynamically stable
    - Superior to Tc-99m SC due to longer window for detection following injection if patient is bleeding intermittently
    - Best guide to bleeding site prior to endoscopy or angiography
    - Best indicator of bleeding over 24 hour period; location may not be possible with delayed views
    - Sensitivity depends on bleeding rate at time of study (> 0.5 cc/min Tc-99m RBC)
    - Specificity depends on study quality and completeness
  - Angiography: Procedure of choice when patient is hemodynamically unstable
    - Successful if patient is actively bleeding at time of study (brisk bleed > 0.5 mL/min for mesenteric angiography and > 5-7 mL/min for non-selective aortic angiography
    - When positive, localization is more precise than scintigraphy
    - Best used when endoscopy is inconclusive, especially when nuclear study is positive but localization difficult
- Protocol advice
  - Tc-99m RBC
    - Flow phase acquisition for 1 min (3 sec/frame x 20): Main utility to delineate vascular structures of abdomen and pelvis; occasional detection of bleeding site
    - Dynamic phase acquisition for 90-120 min: Usually displayed at 2 min/frame (acquired on computer at 30 sec/frame)
    - Display: Frame by frame hard copy or computer monitor; cine loop for continuous viewing
    - Delayed imaging at 4-6 and 24 hr post-injection: Dynamic acquisition for 60 min at 2 min/frame; occasionally helpful for localization; main use to assess bleeding status

GI BLEEDING LOCALIZATION

DIFFERENTIAL DIAGNOSIS

Peptic Ulceration and Erosive Gastritis
- Crescent-shaped collection of Tc-99m RBC in left upper abdomen
- Dx usually made by endoscopy

Esophageal Varices
- Usually rapid collection of Tc-99m RBC in left upper quadrant within stomach
- May see origin above GE junction

Small Bowel Bleed
- Typically small bowel loop is seen early
- Delayed views may demonstrate large bowel pattern

Diverticulosis and Colonic Angiodysplasia (AVM)
- Large bowel pattern
- Angiography helpful with brisk bleed

PATHOLOGY

General Features
- Etiology
  - Upper GI bleeding
    - Duodenal ulcer (24%), gastric erosions (23%)
    - Gastric ulcer (21%), varices (10%)
    - Mallory-Weiss tear (7%), esophagitis (6%)
    - Neoplasm (3%), other causes (11%)
  - Lower GI bleeding
    - Diverticulosis (43%), vascular ectasia (20%)
    - Idiopathic (12%), neoplasia (9%)
    - Colitis: Radiation (6%), ischemic (2%), ulcerative (1%)
  - Risk factors of upper GI bleeding
    - Alcohol, tobacco, anticoagulants
    - Aspirin, non-steroidal anti-inflammatory drugs
- Epidemiology
  - More than 400,000 hospitalizations annually in U.S.
  - Lower GI bleeding
    - Accounts for < 1% of all hospital admissions in U.S.
    - Annual incidence: 20.5/100,000

Gross Pathologic & Surgical Features
- Varies based on underlying pathology

Microscopic Features
- Varies depending on underlying cause

CLINICAL ISSUES

Presentation
- Most common signs/symptoms
  - Upper GI bleeding
    - Hematemesis: Bloody vomitus; red, coffee grounds
    - Melena: Black, tarry stools (100-200 mL of blood in upper GI tract is required to produce melena)
  - Lower GI bleeding
    - Hematochezia: Red blood per rectum
    - May also result from upper GI bleed (> 1,000 cc)
  - Bleed anywhere in GI tract
    - Occult blood detected by stool chemical testing
  - Symptoms & signs of blood loss
    - Dizziness, tachycardia, hypotension, shock
  - Symptoms & signs of underlying pathology
- Lab data
  - Fresh blood in vomitus or stool
  - Occult blood in stool, iron deficiency anemia
  - ↓ CBC count, hematocrit, serum electrolytes
  - Abnormal coagulation profile (aPTT, PT, platelet count, bleeding time)
  - Serum blood urea nitrogen to creatine ratio > 25
    - Suggests upper GI hemorrhage

Demographics
- Age: More common in older age group
- Gender: M > F

Natural History & Prognosis
- Complications
  - Acute massive GI bleeding: Shock & death
  - Complications of underlying cause
- Prognosis
  - Early detection, resuscitation & treatment: Good
  - Delayed detection, resuscitation & treatment: Poor
  - Mortality rate
    - Upper GI bleeding: Esophageal varices (30-50%) & varies based on Rockall risk score
    - Lower GI bleeding: Ranges from 0-21%

Treatment
- Medical: Resuscitation (fluids, electrolytes, blood)
- Endoscopic therapy
  - Topical: Tissue adhesives, collagen, clotting factors
  - Injection: Sclerosant agents & vasoconstrictors
  - Mechanical: Clips, balloons, sutures
  - Thermal: Laser photo & electrocoagulation
- Transjugular intrahepatic portosystemic shunt (TIPS)
- Interventional: Embolotherapy (gelfoam & coils)
- Surgical treatment

DIAGNOSTIC CHECKLIST

Consider
- Tc-99m RBC for hemodynamically stable cases
- Angiography for hemodynamically unstable cases

SELECTED REFERENCES

1. Maurer AH et al: Gastrointestinal bleeding: improved localization with cine scintigraphy. Radiology. 185(1):187-92, 1992
2. Bentley DE et al: The role of tagged red blood cell imaging in the localization of gastrointestinal bleeding. Arch Surg. 126(7):821-4, 1991
3. Bunker SR et al: Scintigraphy of gastrointestinal hemorrhage: superiority of 99mTc red blood cells over 99mTc sulfur colloid. AJR Am J Roentgenol. 143(3):543-8, 1984
4. Winzelberg GG et al: Detection of gastrointestinal bleeding with 99mTc-labeled red blood cells. Semin Nucl Med. 12(2):139-46, 1982
5. Alavi A et al: Scintigraphic detection of acute gastrointestinal bleeding. Radiology. 124(3):753-6, 1977

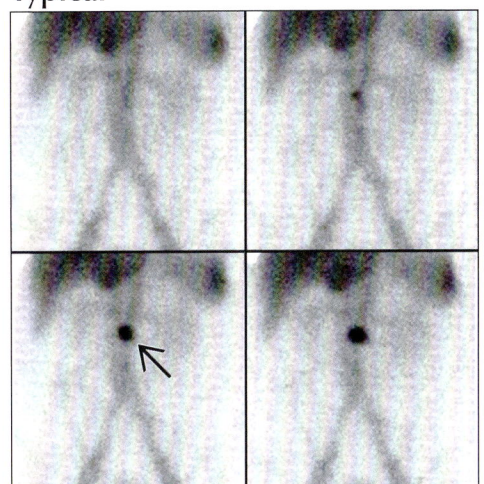

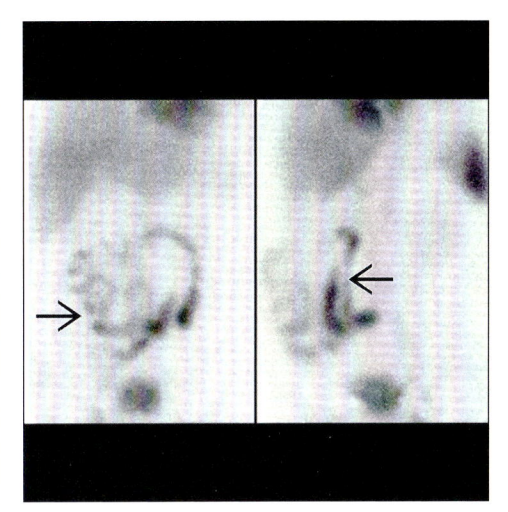

GI BLEEDING LOCALIZATION

IMAGE GALLERY

Typical

(Left) Small bowel bleed. Anterior Tc-99m RBC early views (4-12 min post injection) at 2 min/frame. Note expanding mid abdominal focus ➔. See next image. *(Right)* 4 hour delayed imaging in RAO and LAO views demonstrate small bowel pattern ➔. Delayed views often important in inferring bleeding site origin.

Typical

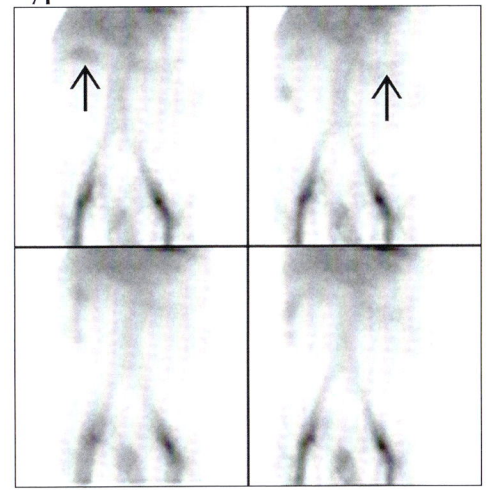

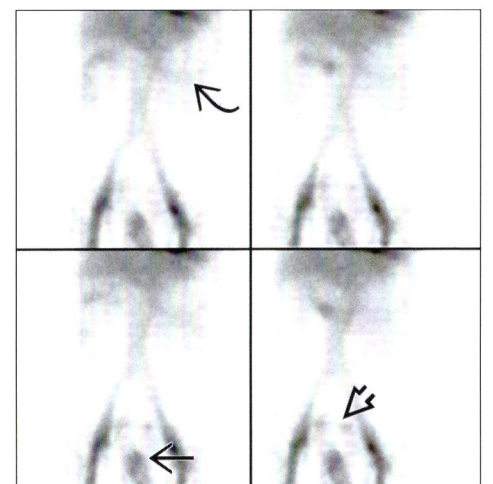

(Left) Large bowel bleed. Anterior Tc-99m RBC early views at 2 min/frame. Ascending colon/hepatic flexure origin from diverticulum ➔. Note Tc-99m RBC moving antegrade and retrograde. See next image. *(Right)* Anterior Tc-99m RBC delayed views more clearly demonstrate transverse colon ➔. Note also male genitalia ➔, and bladder ➔.

Variant

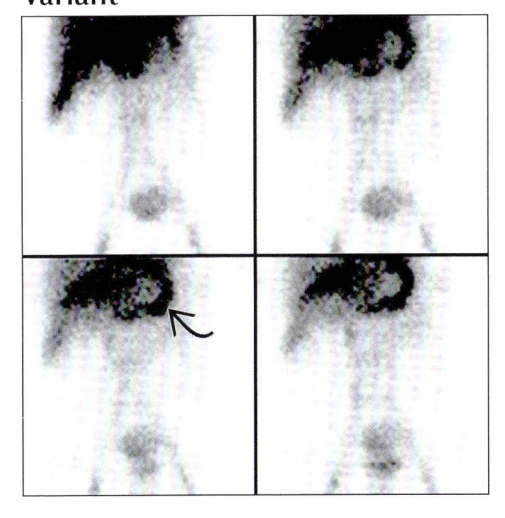

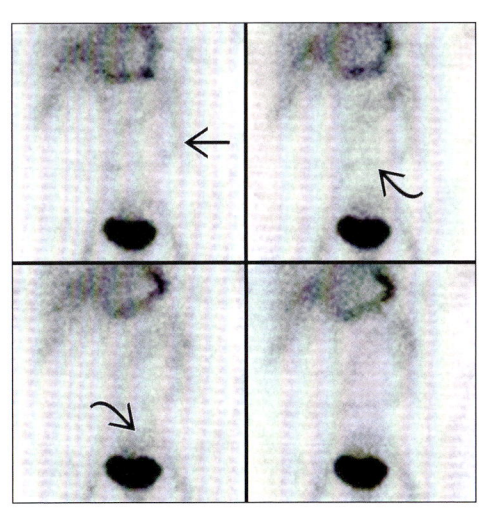

(Left) Anterior Tc-99m RBC early views. Splenic flexure bleed from diverticulum. Note crescent-like activity in left upper abdomen indicating brisk bleeding ➔. Pattern mimics gastric bleeding, but no small bowel evident. Activity travels to descending & sigmoid colon. See next. *(Right)* Anterior Tc-99m RBC delayed views. Accumulation in bladder & kidneys is normal over time. Activity is noted in descending colon ➔ & sigmoid ➔.

INFLAMMATORY BOWEL DISEASE

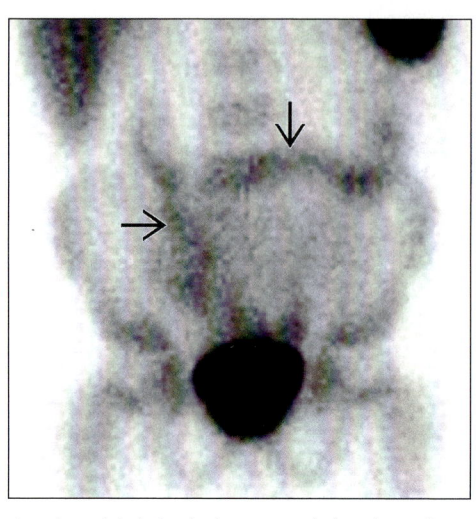

Anterior labeled leukocyte scintigraphy shows accumulation of activity in the small bowel ➡, consistent with acute exacerbation in patient with Crohn disease.

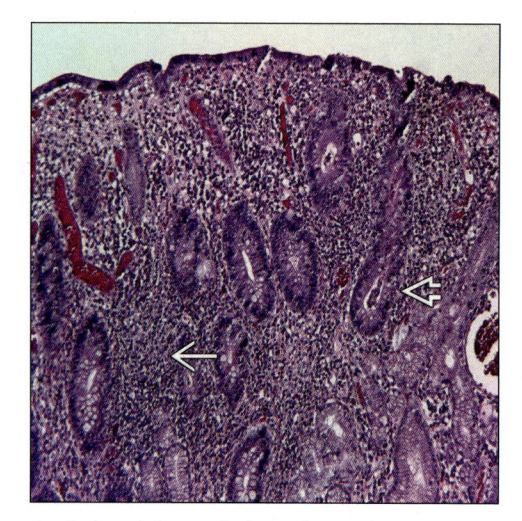

Small bowel histopathology shows dense areas of lymphoplasmacytic infiltrates and neutrophils in the lamina propria ➡, focal crypt abscesses and glandular architectural distortion ➡.

TERMINOLOGY

Abbreviations and Synonyms
- Inflammatory bowel disease (IBD), Crohn disease (CD), ulcerative colitis (UC), indeterminate colitis

Definitions
- Chronic inflammatory disease of gastrointestinal (GI) tract

IMAGING FINDINGS

Nuclear Medicine Findings
- Focal, fixed accumulation of radiolabeled leukocytes at sites of inflammation in GI tract wall
- Initial diagnosis
  - CD: Activity in any part of GI tract (mouth to anus); terminal ileum (65-75%) > right colon > colon only (20-30%) > perianal; skip lesions
  - UC: Contiguous activity distally; rectum (almost always) > rectosigmoid (16%) > left colon (7%) > entire colon (4%); also backwash ileitis
  - Indeterminate colitis: Disease of colon, clinically and pathologically indistinguishable between CD and UC
- Confirmation of disease activity or resolution
  - Degree of accumulation of radiolabeled leukocytes
- Interpretation advice
  - Think CD if skip lesions, right colon predominance, rectal sparing, perianal disease
  - Think UC if rectal involvement with or without contiguous proximal activity
  - Normal distribution in reticuloendothelial system (bone marrow, spleen, liver)
  - Tc-99m based agents show nonspecific activity in lungs, bowel, gallbladder, urine

Imaging Recommendations
- Best imaging tool
  - Tc-99m HMPAO-labeled leukocyte scintigraphy
    - Lipophilic
    - Crosses leukocyte cell membrane then retained intracellularly
    - Sensitivity/specificity for active IBD ~ 98/100% at 1 hour, ~ 98/83% at 3 hours
  - Disadvantages

DDx: Mimics of Inflammatory Bowel Disease on WBC Scan

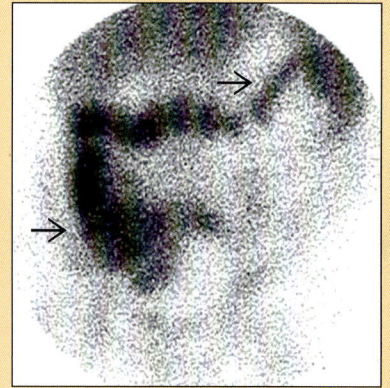

Bleeding into GI Tract 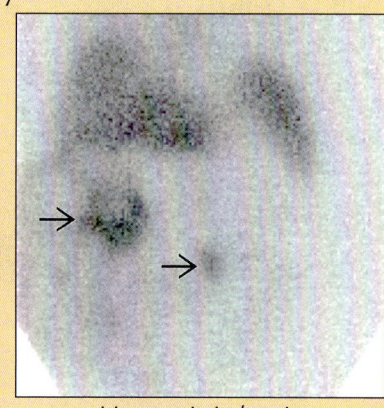 | *Mesenteric Ischemia* 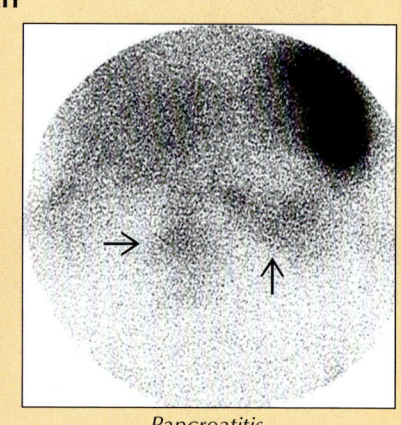 | *Pancreatitis*

INFLAMMATORY BOWEL DISEASE

Key Facts

Terminology
- Inflammatory bowel disease (IBD), Crohn disease (CD), ulcerative colitis (UC), indeterminate colitis
- Chronic inflammatory disease of gastrointestinal (GI) tract

Imaging Findings
- Focal, fixed accumulation of radiolabeled leukocytes at sites of inflammation in GI tract wall
- CD: Activity in any part of GI tract (mouth to anus); terminal ileum (65-75%) > right colon > colon only (20-30%) > perianal; skip lesions
- UC: Contiguous activity distally; rectum (almost always) > rectosigmoid (16%) > left colon (7%) > entire colon (4%); also backwash ileitis
- Normal distribution in reticuloendothelial system (bone marrow, spleen, liver)
- Tc-99m based agents show nonspecific activity in lungs, bowel, gallbladder, urine

Top Differential Diagnoses
- Infection
- Vasculitis
- Malignancy
- Mesenteric Ischemia
- GI Bleeding
- Pancreatitis
- Graft vs. Host Disease
- Epistaxis
- Infectious Colitides

Diagnostic Checklist
- Labeled leukocyte scintigraphy very sensitive but nonspecific for inflammation

---

- Intestinal luminal activity by 3-4 hours due to unbound Tc-99m excretion
- Activity in bladder can obscure pelvic disease
- Protocol advice
  - 5-10 mCi Tc-99m HMPAO (adult); 0.1-0.2 mCi/kg Tc-99m HMPAO (pediatric)
  - Unstabilized form of HMPAO used for labeling
  - Two static anterior planar images at 1 and 3 hours increases specificity and localization
  - Delayed images (> 4 hours) complicated by nonspecific bowel activity
  - SPECT images can increase sensitivity and improve localization
  - Pelvic outlet views to image rectal disease
- Additional nuclear medicine imaging options
  - In-111 labeled leukocyte scintigraphy
    - Drawbacks: Higher absorbed radiation dose, early enhancement of bone marrow may obscure findings, inferior imaging characteristics compared to Tc-99m agents
  - Tc-99m labeled monoclonal antibodies
    - Reports of poor sensitivity and specificity
    - Tc-99m fanolesomab: Monoclonal anti-CD15 IgM may play a future role in IBD detection
- Correlative imaging features
  - Endoscopy
    - Direct visualization and biopsy to confirm diagnosis
  - Radiography (follow-through, enteroclysis, barium enema)
    - Luminal narrowing, cobblestoning, edematous mucosa, ulcerations, fistulas, strictures (string sign), skip lesions, abnormal haustra on contrast radiographs
  - MR/CT
    - Bowel wall thickening, increased vascularity, fat stranding, abscess, phlegmon, lymphadenopathy
  - Ultrasound
    - Bowel wall thickening, no intraluminal content

DIFFERENTIAL DIAGNOSIS

Infection
- Swallowed activity from gingival, upper respiratory, pulmonary infections
- Acute gastroenteritis

Vasculitis
- Leukocyte infiltration into vasa vasorum of GI tract

Malignancy
- Inflammatory reaction to cancer and necrosis
- Substantially higher risk of colorectal cancer in patients with IBD

Mesenteric Ischemia
- Inflammatory response to ischemic tissue

GI Bleeding
- Intraluminal blood containing radiolabeled leukocytes moving through bowel

Pancreatitis
- Epigastric activity resembling disease of small bowel or stomach

Graft vs. Host Disease
- Enteritis usually within first 100 days after bone marrow transplant

Epistaxis
- Intraluminal blood containing radiolabeled leukocytes swallowed during nosebleed

Infectious Colitides
- Pseudomembranous, toxic megacolon, typhilitis, appendicitis: All result in focal uptake of labeled WBC's is areas of involvement

PATHOLOGY

General Features
- Etiology

INFLAMMATORY BOWEL DISEASE

- Likely genetic, environmental, and other unknown causes
- Tobacco use protects against developing UC, increases risk of CD
• Epidemiology
    - CD: Incidence 3.1-14.6 per 100,000; prevalence 26-198 per 100,000
    - UC: Incidence 3-15 per 100,000; prevalence 50-80 per 100,000
    - Highest incidence in developed nations and northern latitudes

Gross Pathologic & Surgical Features
• CD: Noncontiguous distribution (skip lesions), cobblestoning, pseudopolyps, deep ulcerations surrounded by normal mucosa, aphthous ulcers
• UC: Contiguous bowel involvement, granular and friable mucosa, superficial ulcerations, pseudopolyps

Microscopic Features
• CD: Noncaseating granulomas, chronic inflammation in all bowel layers, mucosal fissures, sinus tracts, mucin within goblet cells, aphthous ulcers (superficial ulcerations overlying Peyer patches)
• UC: Mucosal infiltration by neutrophils and monocytes, crypt abscesses, no mucin within goblet cells

CLINICAL ISSUES

Presentation
• Most common signs/symptoms: Abdominal pain, anorexia, diarrhea, tenesmus, weight loss, fatigue, low grade fever, arthralgias
• Other signs/symptoms
    - Perianal disease (CD), clubbing, arthritis, uveitis, hepatobiliary disease, osteopenia, skin lesions, delayed growth in children
    - Extraintestinal manifestations may precede symptoms of IBD by years

Demographics
• Age: Bimodal distribution with highest peak 10-20 years, second peak 55-65 years
• Gender: Roughly equal distribution
• Ethnicity
    - Jewish population at highest risk
    - Higher prevalence in Caucasian and African-American than Asian and Hispanic

Natural History & Prognosis
• Highly variable disease course: Chronic intermittent, unremitting, prolonged remission
    - CD: Unremitting course (13%); chronic intermittent (73%); cured (10%)
    - UC: Intermittent exacerbations; proximal progression in 15% within first 5 years; ~ 30% undergo colectomy
• Higher risk of adenocarcinoma (especially in UC) leads to frequent surveillance colonoscopy

Treatment
• Antidiarrheals for symptomatic relief
• Easily digestible liquid diet containing all necessary nutrients (elemental diet) allows for bowel rest
• Anti-inflammatory and immunosuppressive agents
• Surgery indicated if refractory to medical management

DIAGNOSTIC CHECKLIST

Consider
• Labeled leukocyte scintigraphy very sensitive but nonspecific for inflammation
• To increase specificity when diagnosing IBD, important to rule out infectious colitis

Image Interpretation Pearls
• Fixed GI tract activity on 1 and 3 hour images
• Correlation with anatomic imaging enhances specificity when diagnosis not clear

SELECTED REFERENCES

1. Biancone L et al: Technetium-99m-HMPAO labeled leukocyte single photon emission computerized tomography (SPECT) for assessing Crohn's disease extent and intestinal infiltration. Am J Gastroenterol. 100(2):344-54, 2005
2. Kerry JE et al: Comparison between Tc-HMPAO labelled white cells and Tc LeukoScan in the investigation of inflammatory bowel disease. Nucl Med Commun. 26(3):245-51, 2005
3. Furukawa A et al: Cross-sectional imaging in Crohn disease. Radiographics. 24(3):689-702, 2004
4. Peters MA et al: Nuclear Medicine in Clinical Diagnosis and Treatment: Inflammatory Bowel Disease. 3rd ed. San Francisco, Churchill Livingstone. vol 1. 971-9, 2004
5. Hendrickson BA et al: Clinical aspects and pathophysiology of inflammatory bowel disease. Clin Microbiol Rev. 15(1):79-94, 2002
6. Podolsky DK: Inflammatory bowel disease. N Engl J Med. 347(6):417-29, 2002
7. Gyorke T et al: The role of nuclear medicine in inflammatory bowel disease. A review with experiences of aspecific bowel activity using immunoscintigraphy with 99mTc anti-granulocyte antibodies. Eur J Radiol. 35(3):183-92, 2000
8. Sans M et al: Optimization of technetium-99m-HMPAO leukocyte scintigraphy in evaluation of active inflammatory bowel disease. Dig Dis Sci. 45(9):1828-35, 2000
9. Charron M. Related Articles et al: Technetium leukocyte imaging in inflammatory bowel disease. Curr Gastroenterol Rep. 1(3):245-52, 1999
10. Hyun H et al: Ischemic colitis: Tc-99m HMPAO leukocyte scintigraphy and correlative imaging. Clin Nucl Med. 23(3):165-7, 1998
11. Arndt JW et al: Inflammatory bowel disease activity assessment using technetium-99m-HMPAO leukocytes. Dig Dis Sci. 42(2):387-93, 1997
12. Datz FL et al: Procedure guideline for technetium-99m-HMPAO-labeled leukocyte scintigraphy for suspected infection/inflammation. Society of Nuclear Medicine. J Nucl Med. 38(6):987-90, 1997
13. Ogorek CP et al: Differentiation between Crohn's disease and ulcerative colitis. Med Clin North Am. 78(6):1249-58, 1994

INFLAMMATORY BOWEL DISEASE

IMAGE GALLERY

Typical

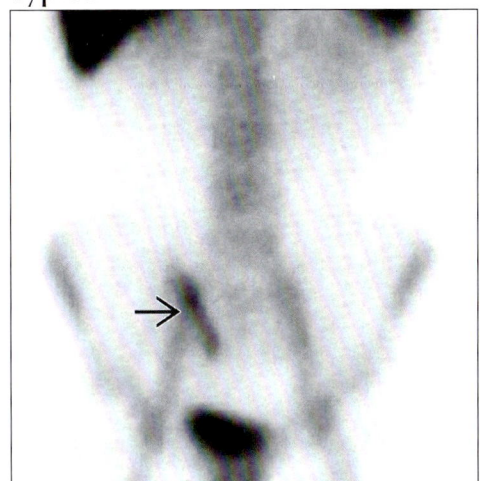

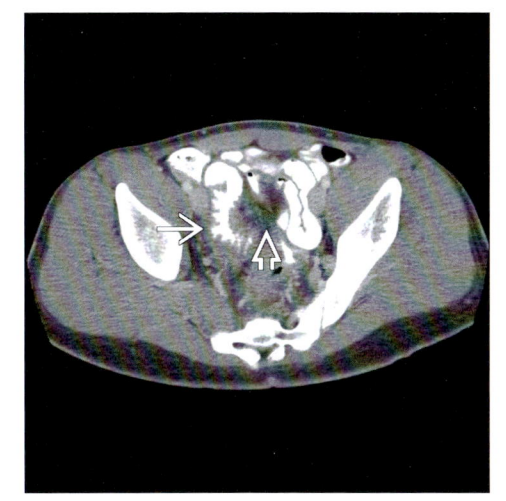

(Left) Anterior labeled leukocyte scintigraphy shows a linear focus of increased activity in the terminal ileum ➔ in patient with Crohn disease. *(Right)* Axial CECT shows bowel wall thickening in the terminal ileum ➔ with adjacent fat stranding ➔.

Typical

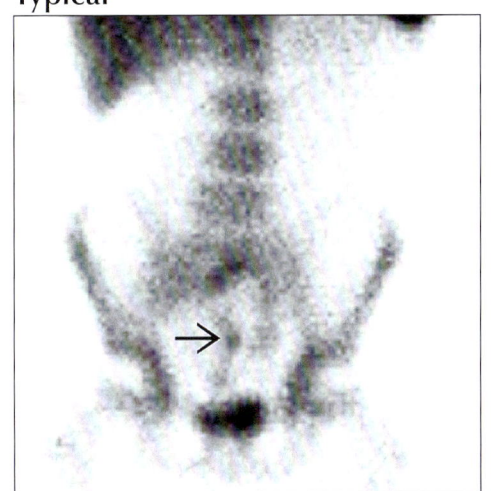

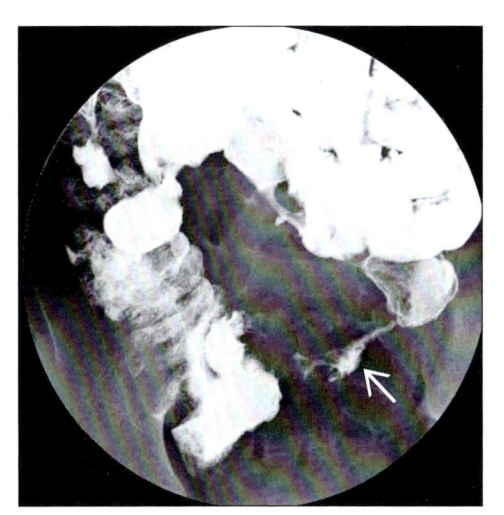

(Left) Anterior labeled leukocyte scintigraphy shows increased activity in the distal ileum ➔ in patient with Crohn disease. *(Right)* Anterior small bowel follow-through radiograph shows small amount of oral contrast ➔ in a narrowed, inflamed distal ileum (string sign).

Typical

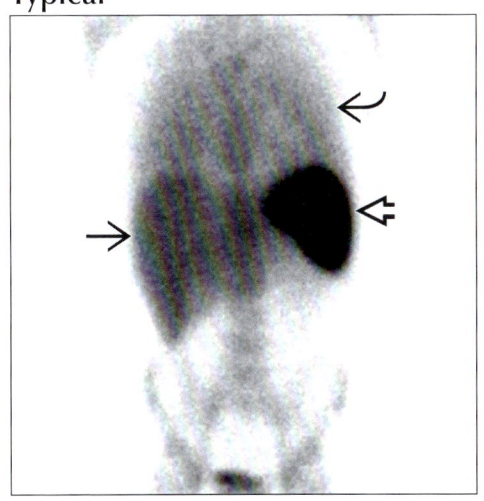

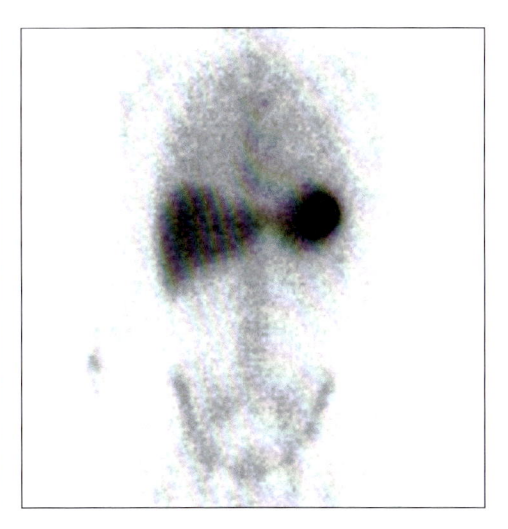

(Left) Anterior Tc-99m HMPAO labeled leukocyte scintigraphy shows normal distribution in liver ➔, spleen ➔, and bone marrow. Diffuse, low level activity in normal lungs is common ➔ < 18 h post injection. *(Right)* Note grainy appearance, decreased counts and resolution of images from higher-energy In-111 labeled leukocyte scintigraphy compared with Tc-99m HMPAO labeled leukocyte scintigraphy at left.

PANCREATITIS

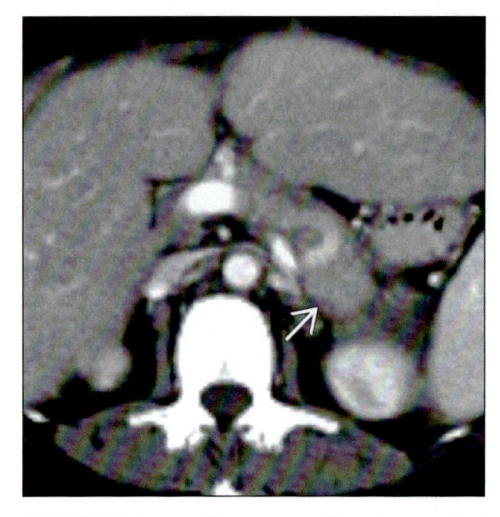

Axial CECT shows diffuse nonspecific enlargement of the pancreas ➡ without any peripancreatic infiltrative changes. Findings are compatible with acute pancreatitis. See next image.

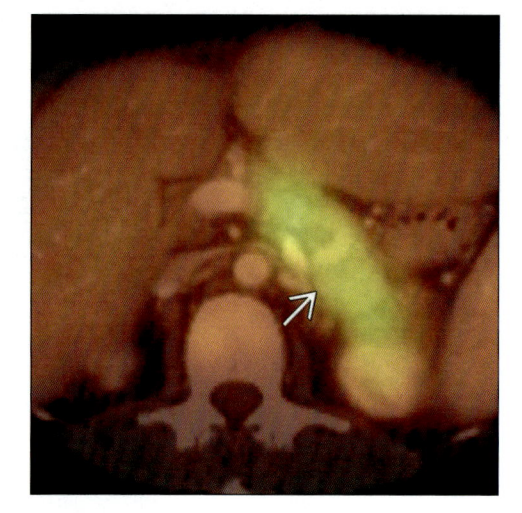

Axial fused PET/CT in same patient as left shows diffuse ↑ FDG activity in pancreas ➡ compatible with acute pancreatitis. This was an incidental finding in a patient with solitary pulmonary nodule.

TERMINOLOGY

Definitions
- Acute pancreatitis (AP): Active pancreatic inflammation
- Chronic pancreatitis (CP): Long-term pancreatic damage due to repeated bouts of acute pancreatitis

IMAGING FINDINGS

General Features
- Best diagnostic clue
  - AP: Pancreatic enlargement with peripancreatic inflammatory change on CT; diffuse hypermetabolism on FDG PET
  - CP: Pancreatic calcification on CT

Nuclear Medicine Findings
- PET
  - AP: Diffuse hypermetabolism most common on PET; focal hypermetabolism less typical (carcinoma needs to be considered in differential)
  - CP: FDG lower uptake than AP; focal uptake in areas of fatty necrosis, granulation tissue

CT Findings
- AP: Pancreatic enlargement on CT with peripancreatic inflammatory change; pancreatic necrosis, fluid collections, pseudocyst, pancreatic abscess; focal enlargement and inflammatory change less typical (difficult to distinguish from carcinoma)
- CP: Pancreatic atrophy on CT or focal enlargement in 40% of cases; calcifications

Imaging Recommendations
- Best imaging tool: FDG PET: Differentiate CP from pancreatic carcinoma; MRCP also useful

DIFFERENTIAL DIAGNOSIS

Pancreatic Adenocarcinoma
- Variable FDG activity, but high positive predictive value if ↑
- PET sensitivity for malignancy with pancreatic mass 81-100%

DDx: Pancreatic Malignant Tumors

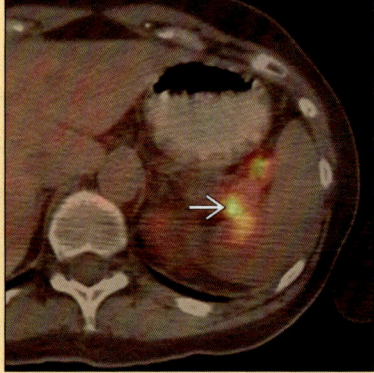

Pancreatic Adenocarcinoma

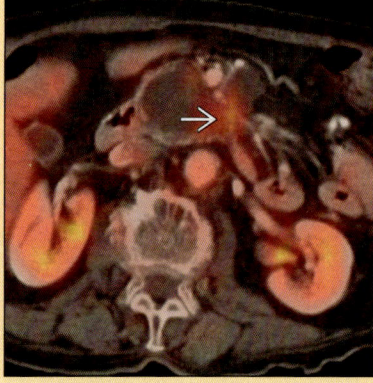

Mucinous Cystic Tumor

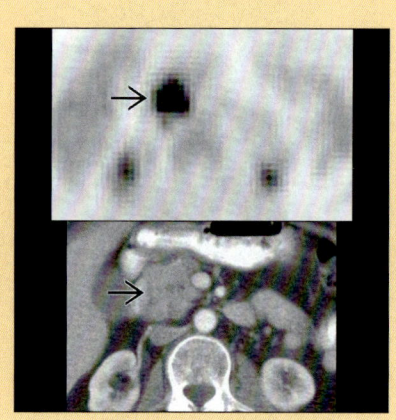

Pancreatic Cancer

PANCREATITIS

Key Facts

Imaging Findings
- AP: Pancreatic enlargement on CT with peripancreatic inflammatory change; pancreatic necrosis, fluid collections, pseudocyst, pancreatic abscess; focal enlargement and inflammatory change less typical (difficult to distinguish from carcinoma)
- CP: Pancreatic atrophy on CT or focal enlargement in 40% of cases; calcifications

- AP: Diffuse hypermetabolism most common on PET; focal hypermetabolism less typical (carcinoma needs to be considered in differential)
- CP: FDG lower uptake than AP; focal uptake in areas of fatty necrosis, granulation tissue

Top Differential Diagnoses
- Pancreatic Adenocarcinoma
- Islet Cell Tumor
- Mucinous Cystic Neoplasm

Islet Cell Tumor
- Hyper- or isodense mass with intense arterial phase enhancement; variable on FDG PET

Mucinous Cystic Neoplasm
- CT shows well-defined, uni/multilocular, cystic mass
- FDG activity variable (↓ with ↓ cellularity)

PATHOLOGY

General Features
- General path comments
  - Repeated episodes of AP ⇒ CP
  - Pseudocyst present in 40% of AP, 30% of CP
- Genetics: Hereditary CP has ↑ risk of pancreatic cancer compared with nonhereditary CP
- Etiology
  - Common causes (70%): Alcohol abuse, cholelithiasis, idiopathic
  - Other causes: Abdominal trauma, hyperlipidemia/calcemia, drugs, genetics

CLINICAL ISSUES

Presentation
- Most common signs/symptoms
  - Mild cases present with pain, vomiting, abdominal tenderness
  - Elevated serum amylase, lipase, white blood cells

Demographics
- Age: 40-50 years
- Gender: Slight male predominance

Natural History & Prognosis
- CP: ↑ Risk of pancreatic carcinoma

Treatment
- Supportive care
- Needle aspiration to determine infected fluid collection; drainage for infected fluid collection and pseudocysts > 5 cm

DIAGNOSTIC CHECKLIST

Consider
- Focal ↑ uptake on PET more likely tumor than infection, but focal necrosis/granulation tissue can show uptake

SELECTED REFERENCES
1. van Kouwen MC et al: FDG-PET is able to detect pancreatic carcinoma in chronic pancreatitis. Eur J Nucl Med Mol Imaging. 32(4):399-404, 2005
2. Imdahl A et al: Evaluation of positron emission tomography with 2-[18F]fluoro-2-deoxy-D-glucose for the differentiation of chronic pancreatitis and pancreatic cancer. Br J Surg. 86(2):194-9, 1999

IMAGE GALLERY

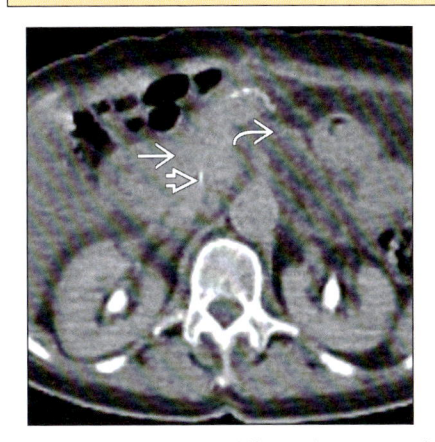

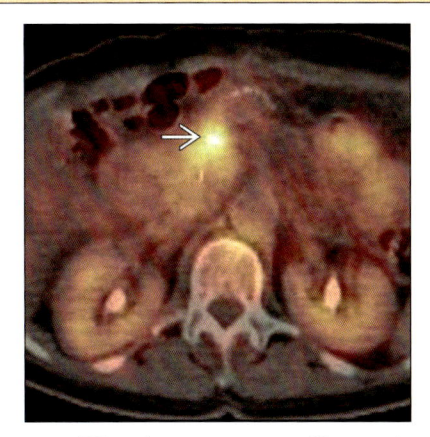

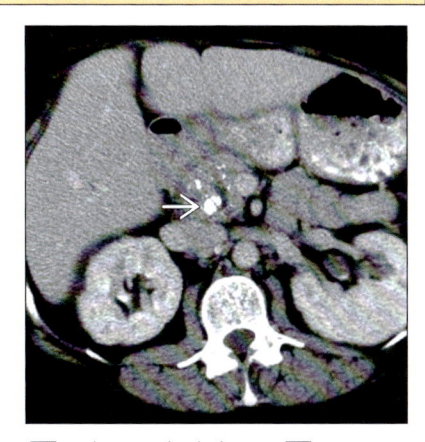

(Left) Axial CECT shows diffuse enlargement of pancreas ➔ with peripancreatic infiltrative changes ➔ and areas of calcification ➔, suggestive of acute or chronic pancreatitis. See next image. *(Center)* Axial fused PET/CT shows focal intense FDG activity within pancreatic body ➔ worrisome for carcinoma. Follow-up endoscopic ultrasound with biopsy showed adenocarcinoma arising within chronic pancreatitis. *(Right)* Axial CECT shows multiple calcifications within pancreatic head ➔ compatible with chronic pancreatitis.

PANCREATIC ADENOCARCINOMA

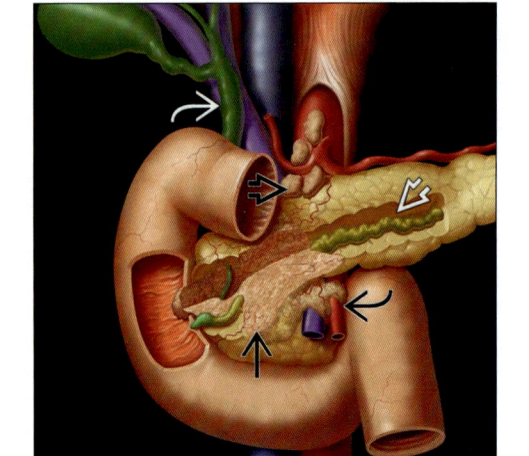

Carcinoma in pancreatic head often encases vessels, invades regional nodes, and causes pancreatic duct and common bile duct obstruction.

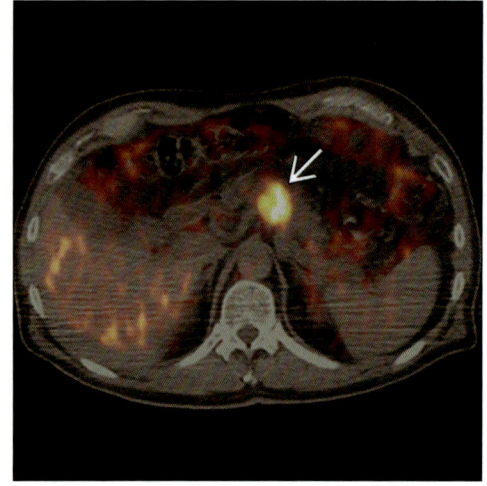

Axial fused PET/CT performed for staging shows primary pancreatic adenocarcinoma in body of pancreas.

TERMINOLOGY

Abbreviations and Synonyms
- Pancreatic cancer, pancreatic ductal carcinoma

Definitions
- Malignant tumor arising from exocrine pancreas
- 2 broad categories of pancreatic neoplasms: Epithelial and nonepithelial (less common; e.g., lymphoma, metastases, sarcomas)
  - Epithelial tumors: Exocrine and endocrine (uncommon; islet cell)
    - 99% of exocrine tumors arise from ductal epithelium, 1% acinar origin
    - 90-95% primary pancreatic tumors = adenocarcinomas

IMAGING FINDINGS

General Features
- Best diagnostic clue
  - Poorly enhancing pancreatic mass with increased FDG uptake
  - Hypermetabolic activity in regional lymph nodes, metastatic sites
- Location: 60-65% head, 20% body, 15% tail, 5-10% diffuse
- Size
  - Variable, averaging 2-3 cm
    - Masses in tail often present late, may reach 10 cm
    - Mass in head obstructing pancreatic or common bile ducts present earlier, may be < 1 cm
- Morphology
  - Typically ill-defined with extensive local invasion
  - Metastasis to regional lymph nodes, then liver

Nuclear Medicine Findings
- PET
  - Moderate to marked increased FDG uptake in pancreatic mass
    - PET tumor diagnosis: Sens 90-95%, spec 82-100%
    - PET changes staging 11-20%, alters patient management 15-50%
    - Useful to identify metastases, especially unenlarged nodes and distant metastasis
    - Detection of recurrent tumor, therapy response promising in early studies

DDx: Mimics of Pancreatic Adenocarcinoma

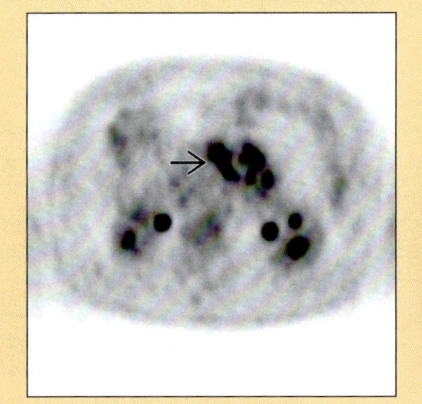

Acute Pancreatitis

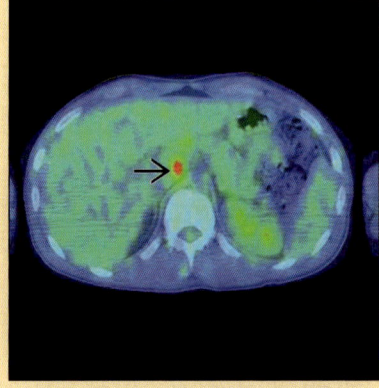

Peripancreatic Metastases

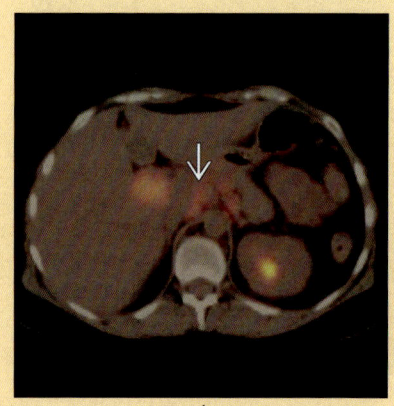

Lymphoma

PANCREATIC ADENOCARCINOMA

Key Facts

Terminology
- Malignant tumor arising from exocrine pancreas
- 90-95% primary pancreatic tumors = adenocarcinomas

Imaging Findings
- Moderate to marked increased FDG uptake in pancreatic mass
- PET tumor diagnosis: Sens 90-95%, spec 82-100%
- PET changes staging 11-20%, alters patient management 15-50%
- Useful to identify metastases, especially unenlarged nodes and distant metastasis
- Detection of recurrent tumor, therapy response promising in early studies
- PET/CT correlated with CECT = most sens/spec (complex anatomy, normal bowel FDG activity)
- SUV: > 2.5 suspicious for malignancy, although most tumors show higher uptake
- Mucinous adenocarcinoma variable due to little FDG uptake in mucin produced by tumor

Top Differential Diagnoses
- Pancreatitis
- Islet Cell Tumor
- Cystic Pancreatic Neoplasm
- Periampullary Tumors
- Nonepithelial Tumors

Diagnostic Checklist
- PET/CT for optimal staging
- PET/CT to determine response to therapy
- CECT to determine resectability

- PET/CT correlated with CECT = most sens/spec (complex anatomy, normal bowel FDG activity)
- SUV: > 2.5 suspicious for malignancy, although most tumors show higher uptake
- Mucinous adenocarcinoma variable due to little FDG uptake in mucin produced by tumor

CT Findings
- NECT
  - Normal gland or isodense mass infiltrating surrounding fat
  - Dilation of pancreatic duct distal to mass
  - Cystic or necrotic areas in benign or malignant disease & calcifications may occur when associated with chronic pancreatitis
- CECT
  - Variable appearance, may only see contour deformity or area of enlargement
  - Requires excellent contrast administration dynamics and CT technique
    - Arterial phase to assess vascular involvement
    - Poorly enhancing, heterogeneous mass after arterial phase during parenchymal enhancement
  - Ductal dilation often present in benign (e.g., obstructing stone) as well as malignant disease
    - Local invasion into porta hepatis or mass in head may also obstruct CBD, producing "double duct sign" seen on ERCP
    - Interrupted duct sign or abrupt termination of pancreatic duct or CBD rather than smooth taper favors malignancy
  - Vascular encasement key to determining resectability
    - Vascular invasion of mesenteric root or encasement of branches with vessel narrowing
    - General rule: Any vessel contiguous with tumor for 180° or > 50% circumference will mean unresectable tumor
    - Venous involvement may show altered shape or thrombosis not encasement
    - Collateral mesenteric veins may form & dilated small splanchnic veins indicates unresectability
  - Direct invasion of adjacent organs, commonly duodenum or stomach

MR Findings
- T1WI: Low signal relative to normal pancreatic tissue
- T1WI FS: Hypointense compared to normal parenchymal high signal
- T2WI: Variable signal intensity
- T2* GRE
  - Breath-hold with fat sat may best show tumor mass
  - May detect vascular invasion but possibly superior to CECT
- T1 C+ FS: Little or no enhancement on dynamic breath-hold acquisition
- MRA: Identify vascular involvement
- MRCP
  - May define level, degree of obstruction
  - Pancreatic duct with smooth dilation often due to benign disease while beaded/irregular duct characteristic for malignancy

Other Modality Findings
- Endoscopic ultrasound
  - Superior to CT for detecting tumors near pancreatic head, CT better for distal lesions
  - Identify regional nodal involvement
  - Allows nonsurgical biopsy of many nodes and masses, usually near pancreatic head or body

Ultrasonographic Findings
- Grayscale Ultrasound: Hypoechoic mass, possibly with ductal dilation

Imaging Recommendations
- Best imaging tool
  - Initial diagnosis: Endoscopic ultrasound for pancreatic head; CECT for body and tail
  - Staging: PET/CT with CECT correlation; current reimbursement limitations
    - CECT Predicts resectability with ~ 70-80% accuracy; many patients later found unresectable at surgery
- Protocol advice

PANCREATIC ADENOCARCINOMA

- PET
  - Patient fast 6-8 hrs, serum glucose < 180-200 U/dL, no insulin administration < 2 hrs before scan, limit strenuous exercise for a few days prior
  - Dose 10-15 mCi (370-555 MBq) F-18 FDG IV, patient relaxed in quiet, warm, dimly lit room; wait 45-60 minutes, image after patient voids
  - Consider water, negative bowel contrast agent

DIFFERENTIAL DIAGNOSIS

Pancreatitis
- Acute pancreatitis: ↑ FDG activity, known cause of false positive PET
- Chronic pancreatitis: Appearance overlaps cancer by conventional imaging; PET reliably differentiates: Sens 85-98%, spec 55-93%
  - Typical findings: Ductal & glandular calcifications, ductal dilation, atrophic gland, pseudocyst, intraglandular vessels alternating narrowed/dilated
  - Focal mass, enlarged gland may not be distinguishable from cancer on anatomic imaging

Islet Cell Tumor
- Endocrine pancreas origin
- FDG PET often negative or mild uptake, In-111 Octreotide imaging useful
- CECT: Hypervascular enhancement with vascular encasement rare

Cystic Pancreatic Neoplasm
- May show little FDG accumulation even in malignant lesion due to hypocellularity
- Intraductal papillary mucinous tumor (IPMT)
- Mucinous cystic neoplasm
  - Formerly known as macrocystic adenoma, mucinous cystadenoma, cystadenocarcinoma
- Microcystic adenoma (serous cystadenoma); benign lesion w/o malignant potential common in von Hippel-Lindau (VHL)

Periampullary Tumors
- Ampullary & duodenal adenocarcinoma; often treated by Whipple; more favorable prognosis than pancreatic adenocarcinoma

Nonepithelial Tumors
- Metastases: Direct invasion or involvement of adjacent lymph node by many tumors including breast, melanoma, lung, GI tumors
- Primary pancreatic lymphoma and sarcoma rare, usually evidence of disease elsewhere

PATHOLOGY

General Features
- General path comments
  - Most common exocrine pancreas primary malignancy
  - Often produces mucin and fibrosis: Reduce sensitivity of PET
- Genetics
  - Usually sporadic
  - Multiple genetic mutations identified including K-ras
- Etiology: Diabetes, cigarette use, high-fat diet
- Epidemiology: In US, 11th most common cancer, 4th leading cause of cancer death

CLINICAL ISSUES

Presentation
- Most common signs/symptoms
  - Usually asymptomatic until late
  - Only 26% resectable: 14% confined to pancreas; 21% with regional node involvement
  - Pancreatic head mass may cause pancreatitis or obstructive jaundice
    - Courvoisier sign: Palpable gallbladder with painless jaundice
  - Body or tail mass may present with weight loss, widely metastatic disease
- Clinical Profile: Laboratory markers: CA19-9 and CEA may be ↑

Demographics
- Age: Peak presentation: 7th decade; mean age at presentation 55 yrs
- Gender: Previously M:F = 2:1 (incidence ↑ in females)
- Ethnicity: African Americans > Caucasians

Natural History & Prognosis
- Post pancreatoduodenectomy: 5 yr survival 20%
- Unresectable tumor 5 yr survival < 5%

Treatment
- Whipple procedure pancreatoduodenectomy: Excision only option for cure
- External beam radiation; chemotherapy

DIAGNOSTIC CHECKLIST

Consider
- PET/CT for optimal staging
- PET/CT to determine response to therapy
- CECT to determine resectability

SELECTED REFERENCES

1. Heinrich S et al: Positron emission tomography/computed tomography influences on the management of resectable pancreatic cancer and its cost-effectiveness. Ann Surg. 242(2):235-43, 2005
2. Lygidakis NJ et al: Adenocarcinoma of the pancreas--past, present and future. Hepatogastroenterology. 52(64):1281-92, 2005
3. van Kouwen MC et al: FDG-PET is able to detect pancreatic carcinoma in chronic pancreatitis. Eur J Nucl Med Mol Imaging. 32(4):399-404, 2005
4. Delbeke D et al: Pancreatic tumors: role of imaging in the diagnosis, staging, and treatment. J Hepatobiliary Pancreat Surg. 11(1):4-10, 2004
5. van Kouwen MC et al: FDG-PET scanning in the diagnosis of gastrointestinal cancers. Scand J Gastroenterol Suppl. (241):85-92, 2004

PANCREATIC ADENOCARCINOMA

IMAGE GALLERY

Typical

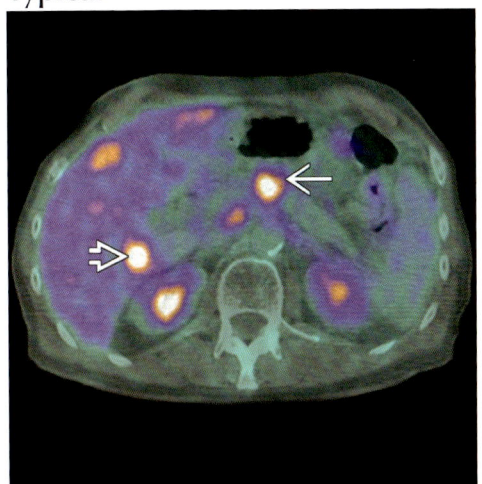

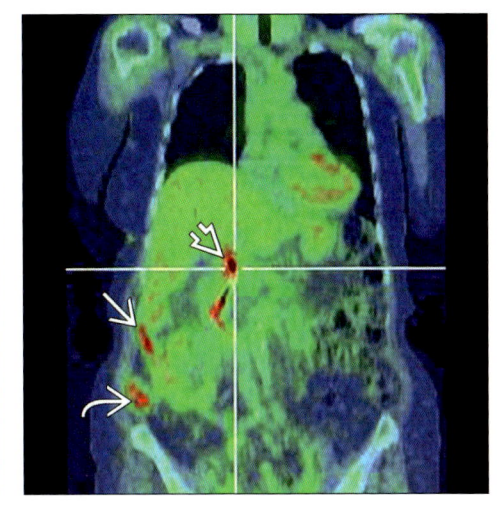

(Left) Axial fused PET/CT performed for staging shows primary pancreatic adenocarcinoma ➡ and liver metastasis ➡. (Right) Coronal fused PET/CT demonstrates benign FDG activity around a common bile duct stent ➡. Normal activity in bowel ➡ is difficult to tell from peritoneal metastases ➡ on this single image.

Typical

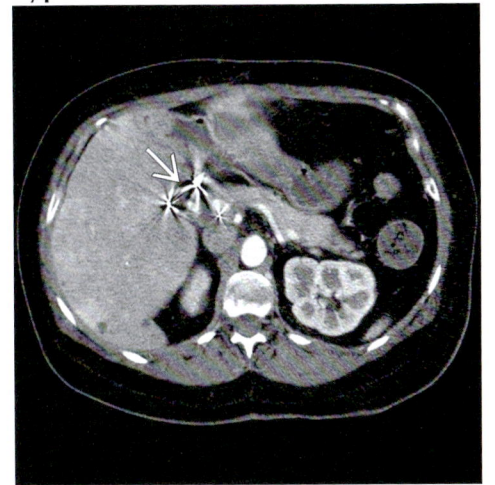

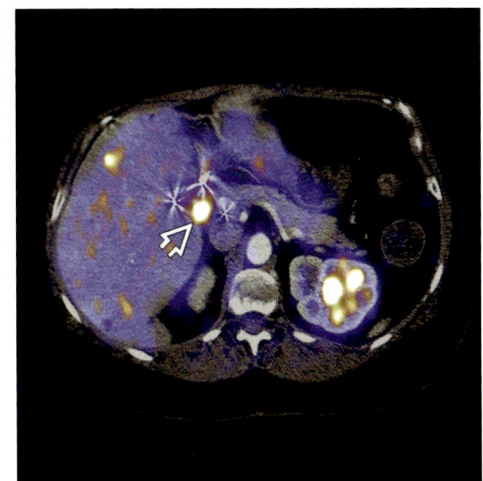

(Left) Axial CECT in patient post Whipple procedure for pancreatic cancer shows operative clips ➡ but no definite recurrence. (Right) Axial fused PET/CT in same patient as previous image shows intense activity in a lymph node metastasis ➡, not identified prospectively on CECT.

Typical

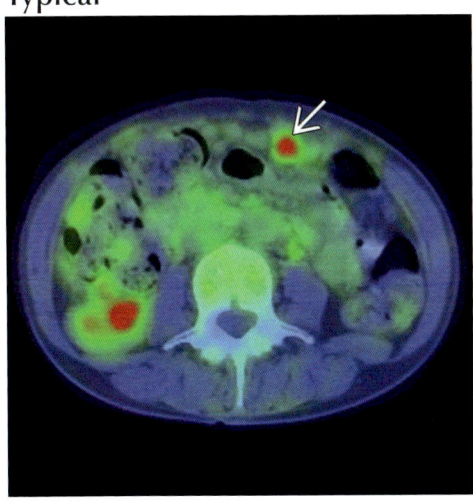

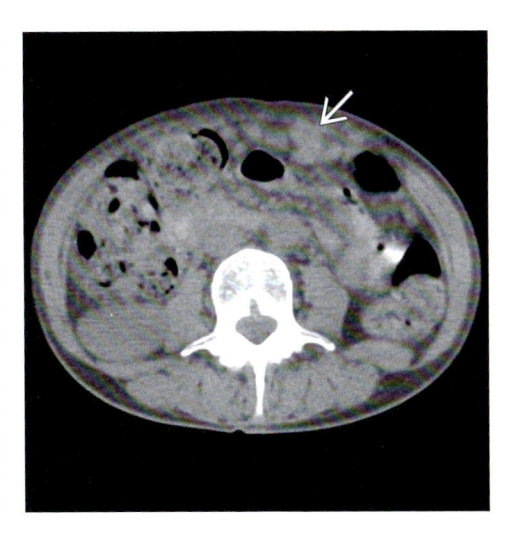

(Left) Axial fused PET/CT in patient with pancreatic cancer and CECT negative for metastases. Note peritoneal metastasis ➡ evident on PET/CT. (Right) Axial NECT in same patient as previous image shows bowel loops anterior to colon and the peritoneal soft tissue mass ➡.

ISLET CELL TUMORS

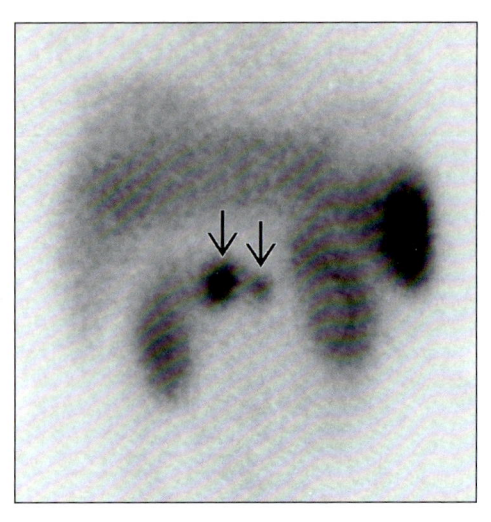

Anterior planar SRS shows two foci of increased uptake in pancreatic head ➡, consistent with pancreatic islet cell tumors.

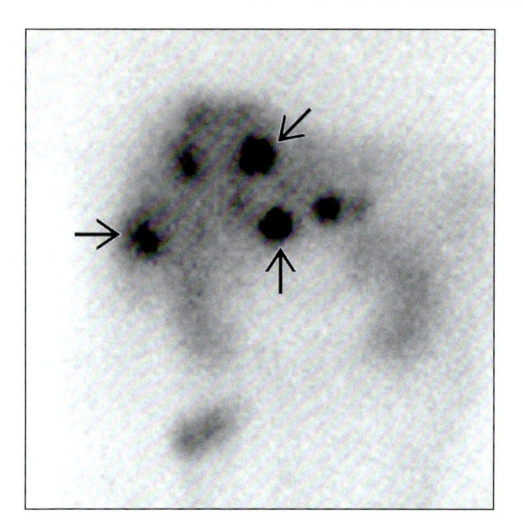

Anterior planar SRS shows multiple foci of increased activity ➡ in liver of patient with metastatic pancreatic islet cell tumor.

TERMINOLOGY

Abbreviations and Synonyms
- Pancreatic or gastroenteropancreatic neuroendocrine tumor (NET)

Definitions
- Tumors arising from pancreatic endocrine cells (islets of Langerhans)

IMAGING FINDINGS

General Features
- Best diagnostic clue: Hypervascular mass(es) in pancreas (primary) & liver (metastases)
- Location
  - Pancreas (85%); ectopic (15%) in duodenum, stomach, lymph nodes (LN), ovary
  - Gastrinoma triangle: Superiorly cystic & common bile duct (CBD), inferiorly 2nd & 3rd parts of duodenum, medially pancreatic neck & body
- Size: Up to 10 cm
- Morphology
  - Rare compared to tumors of exocrine pancreas
  - Benign or malignant, single or multiple (with different cell types)
  - May be hormonally functional (85%) or nonfunctional
  - Functioning tumors often secrete multiple pancreatic hormones, with dominant single defining clinical presentation
    - Insulinoma, glucagonoma, gastrinoma, somatostatinoma, VIPoma (vasoactive intestinal polypeptide), PPoma (pancreatic polypeptide), APUDoma (carcinoid clinical syndromes)
  - Nonfunctioning tumors
    - Hypofunctioning or clinically silent large tumors; larger than functioning tumors at diagnosis; cystic islet cell tumor usually non-insulin producing & nonfunctioning

Nuclear Medicine Findings
- Somatostatin receptor scintigraphy (SRS)
  - In-111-DTPA-D-Phe octreotide (Octreoscan™): Radiolabeled derivative of octreotide, binds to somatostatin receptor (subtypes 2, 5 and to less extent 3)

DDx: Other SRS-Avid Tumors

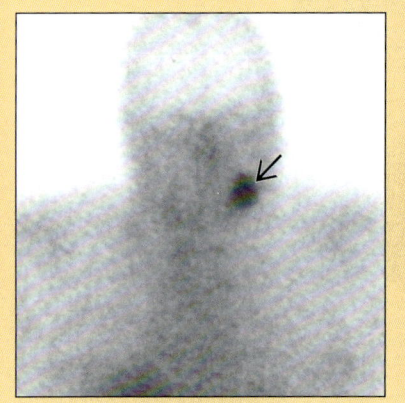

Paraganglioma 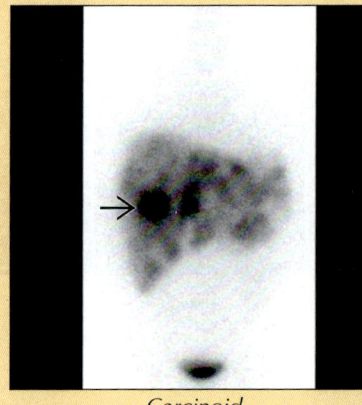 | *Carcinoid* 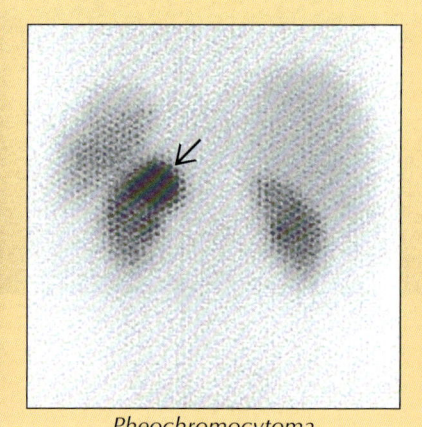 | *Pheochromocytoma*

ISLET CELL TUMORS

Key Facts

Terminology
- Tumors arising from pancreatic endocrine cells (islets of Langerhans)

Imaging Findings
- Best diagnostic clue: Hypervascular mass(es) in pancreas (primary) & liver (metastases)
- Pancreas (85%); ectopic (15%) in duodenum, stomach, lymph nodes (LN), ovary
- In-111-DTPA-D-Phe octreotide (Octreoscan™): Radiolabeled derivative of octreotide, binds to somatostatin receptor (subtypes 2, 5 and to less extent 3)
- SRS sensitivity in detection of pancreatic islet cell tumors: ~ 65%

Top Differential Diagnoses
- Pancreatic Ductal Adenocarcinoma
- Mucinous Cystic Tumor of Pancreas
- Metastases
- Serous Cystadenoma of Pancreas

Pathology
- Insulinoma: Most common islet cell tumor; solitary benign (90%); malignant (10%)
- Gastrinoma: 2nd common; multiple & malignant (60%); MEN I (20-60%)
- Nonfunctioning: 3rd common; 20-45% of islet cell tumors; malignant (80-100%)

Diagnostic Checklist
- SRS for problem cases or where CT, MR negative or equivocal

---

- SRS sensitivity in detection of pancreatic islet cell tumors: ~ 65%
  - Wide variability in sensitivity by cell type: Gastrinomas typically high, insulinomas often low
- Many types of tumors positive on SRS: Not specific for islet cell tumors
- Other SRS-avid conditions
  - Pituitary adenoma; adrenal medullary tumors; paraganglioma; benign and malignant thyroid tissue; Merkel cell and melanoma; carcinoid tumor; small cell lung cancer; non-pancreatic neuroendocrine carcinoma; meningioma; well-differentiated glial-derived tumor; lymphoma, granuloma, infection

CT Findings
- Functioning tumors
  - NECT: Small or large in size; calcification may be seen; small lesions usually undetectable; cystic & necrotic areas (usually non-insulin tumors)
  - CECT: Perform arterial phase (AP) & portal venous phase; most are hypervascular (on AP); delayed solid/ring-enhancement (insulinoma); enhancing metastases (AP) in liver & LN
- Nonfunctioning tumors
  - NECT: Mixed density; usually large & complex; cystic & necrotic areas (large tumors); calcification
  - CECT: Usually hypervascular; nonenhancing cystic or necrotic areas; enhancing viable tumor and metastases; liver metastases often extensive even in relatively healthy patient
- Large functional & nonfunctional tumors: Highly malignant; calcification; local invasion; early invasion of portal vein ⇒ liver metastases

Angiographic Findings
- Hypervascular (primary & secondary); hepatic venous sampling with intra-arterial stimulation → elevated hormones with functioning tumors

MR Findings
- Functional tumors
  - Fat-saturated T1: Hypointense
  - T2: SE & STIR sequences: Hyperintense (both primary & secondaries)
  - T1 C+: Solid or ring-enhancement (insulinoma) on T1; hyperintense (solid enhancing lesions) on fat-saturates delayed enhanced T1 SE
- Nonfunctioning tumors
  - T1 SE: Small tumors isointense; large tumors heterogeneous (cystic & necrotic)
  - T2 SE: Small tumors isointense; large tumors hyperintense (cystic & necrotic)
  - T1 C+: Small tumors hyperintense on fat-saturated delayed enhanced T1WI SE; large tumors nonenhancing cystic + necrotic areas

Ultrasonographic Findings
- Endoscopic ultrasound (EUS): Detects small islet cell tumors; homogeneously hypoechoic, permits transgastric biopsy
- Intra-operative US: Detects very small lesions; sensitivity (75-100%)

Imaging Recommendations
- Best imaging tool
  - CECT with early arterial phase & delayed imaging
  - T1 C+ MR, including fat suppression
  - SRS: Problem or equivocal cases where tumor suspected but CT, MR negative or equivocal
- Protocol advice
  - Somatostatin receptor scintigraphy (SRS)
    - Adult dose 6 mCi In-111 Octreoscan slow IV push under close clinical observation: Hypotension may occur with neurosecretory tumors
    - 4 h SPECT/planar images of abdomen: Visualization of sites of uptake before normal bowel uptake accumulates
    - 24 h SPECT/planar images of neck, chest, abdomen, pelvis: Greater sensitivity than at 4 h, but expect bowel, bladder, gallbladder activity
    - 48 h planar/SPECT after bowel prep if gut activity is complicating interpretation
    - Use of dedicated SPECT/CT camera or off-line fusion of SPECT images to CT or MR highly recommended

ISLET CELL TUMORS

DIFFERENTIAL DIAGNOSIS

Pancreatic Ductal Adenocarcinoma
- Hypovascular tumor; pancreatic ductal obstruction; pancreatic head (60%); obliteration or retropancreatic fat; extensive local invasion, regional mets; irregular, nodular, rat-tailed eccentric obstruction on ERCP

Mucinous Cystic Tumor of Pancreas
- Similar to cystic/necrotic islet cell tumor; more common in tail of pancreas; multiloculated hypodense mass on NECT; enhancement of thin internal septa & wall on CECT; cysts (hyperintense) & septations (hypointense) on T2 MR; predominantly vascular on angiography

Metastases
- Indistinguishable from islet cell tumor metastases on CT, MR

Serous Cystadenoma of Pancreas
- Benign, glycogen-rich cystadenoma; honeycomb or sponge appearance; head of pancreas more common; enhancing septa delineating small cysts; highly vascular on angiography; macrocystic type with thinner wall/septa than islet cell tumors

PATHOLOGY

General Features
- General path comments: Originate from embryonic neuroectoderm
- Etiology
  - Arise from APUD (amine precursor uptake & decarboxylation) cells
  - Nonfunctioning: Derived from α & β cells
  - Functioning tumor: Glucagonoma (α-cell); gastrinoma (islet cell); insulinoma (β-cell)
- Epidemiology
  - Insulinoma: Most common islet cell tumor; solitary benign (90%); malignant (10%)
  - Gastrinoma: 2nd common; multiple & malignant (60%); MEN I (20-60%)
  - Nonfunctioning: 3rd common; 20-45% of islet cell tumors; malignant (80-100%)
- Associated abnormalities: Gastrinoma (Zollinger-Ellison syndrome); MEN type I

Gross Pathologic & Surgical Features
- Small tumor (encapsulated & firm); large tumor, cystic, necrotic, calcified

Microscopic Features
- Sheets of small round cells, uniform nuclei/cytoplasm: Neuron specific enolase on electron microscopy

CLINICAL ISSUES

Presentation
- Most common signs/symptoms
  - Insulinoma: Whipple triad (hypoglycemia + low fasting glucose + relief by IV glucose); palpitations, sweating, tremors, headache, coma
  - Gastrinoma (Zollinger-Ellison syndrome): Peptic ulcer, increased acidity & diarrhea
  - Glucagonoma: Necrolytic erythema migrans, diarrhea, diabetes, weight loss
  - Nonfunctional: Mostly asymptomatic; pain, jaundice, variceal bleeding

Demographics
- Age: 4th-6th decade
- Gender: Insulinoma (M < F); gastrinoma (M > F)

Natural History & Prognosis
- Prognosis: Insulinoma (good); gastrinoma (poor)
- Nonfunctional: 3 year survival (60%), 5 year survival (44%); can live with metastases for many years

Treatment
- Acute phase: Octreotide (potent hormonal inhibitor)
- Insulinoma: Surgery curative
- Gastrinoma: Medical management with omeprazole, 5-fluorouracil; surgery curative in 30% cases
- Nonfunctional: Resection/embolization
- Liver metastases: Transarterial chemoembolization, radioembolization

DIAGNOSTIC CHECKLIST

Consider
- Differentiate from other solid, cystic, vascular tumors
- Correlate with clinical & biochemical information
- SRS for problem cases or where CT, MR negative or equivocal

Image Interpretation Pearls
- Hypervascular pancreatic tumor & liver metastases suggests islet cell/neuroendocrine tumor
- Solid/ring-enhancement (insulinoma): Delayed scans
- Large functioning & nonfunctioning tumors: Hypervascular, complex & highly malignant
- SPECT fusion to CT or MR highly recommended for SRS

SELECTED REFERENCES

1. Herwick S et al: MRI of islet cell tumors of the pancreas. AJR Am J Roentgenol. 187(5):W472-80, 2006
2. Noone TC et al: Imaging and localization of islet-cell tumours of the pancreas on CT and MRI. Best Pract Res Clin Endocrinol Metab. 19(2):195-211, 2005
3. Dromain C et al: MR imaging of hepatic metastases caused by neuroendocrine tumors: comparing four techniques. AJR Am J Roentgenol. 180(1):121-8, 2003
4. Krausz Y et al: Somatostatin-receptor scintigraphy in the management of gastroenteropancreatic tumors. Am J Gastroenterol. 93(1):66-70, 1998
5. van Eijck CH et al: The use of somatostatin receptor scintigraphy in the differential diagnosis of pancreatic duct cancers and islet cell tumors. Ann Surg. 224(2):119-24, 1996
6. Becker W et al: Octreotide scintigraphy localizes somatostatin receptor-positive islet cell carcinomas. Eur J Nucl Med. 18(11):924-7, 1991

ISLET CELL TUMORS

IMAGE GALLERY

Typical

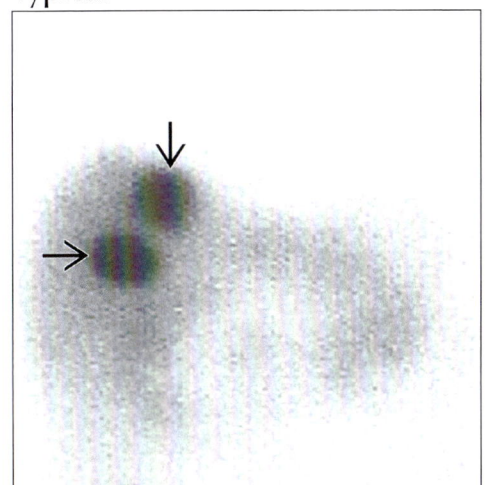

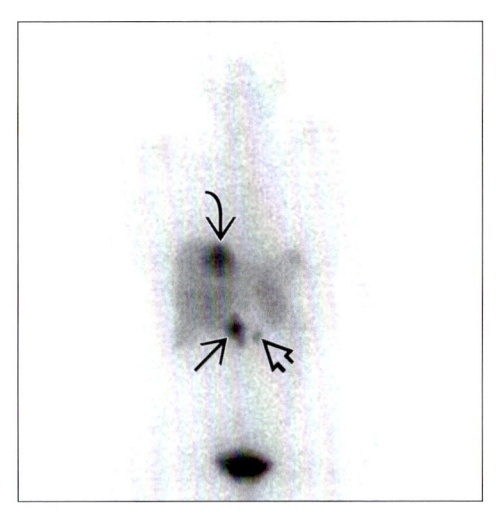

(**Left**) Anterior planar SRS shows two intense foci of increased activity in liver ➡ in patient with metastatic insulinoma. This case is somewhat unusual in that insulinomas are typically less SRS-avid. (**Right**) Anterior planar SRS shows a large focus in pancreatic head ➡, a small focus in pancreatic body ▷, as well as hepatic mass ➡ in patient with metastatic gastrinoma. See next 4 images.

Typical

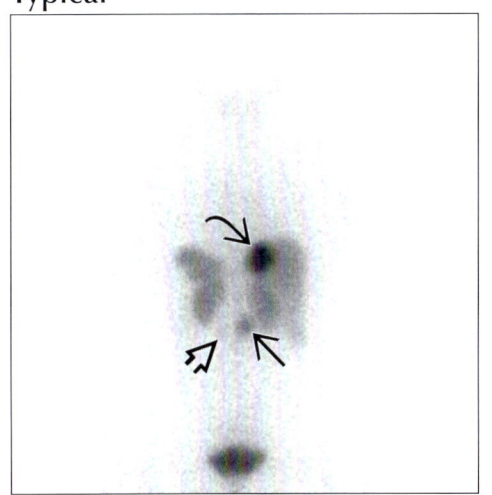

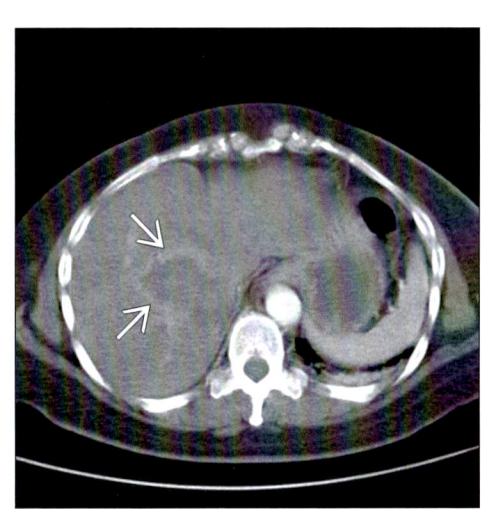

(**Left**) Posterior planar SRS in same patient at left shows uptake in hepatic mass ➡ & pancreatic head mass ➡. A mass in body of pancreas ▷ is better appreciated on the preceding anterior image. (**Right**) Axial CECT in same patient as previous image shows hypoattenuating hepatic mass with peripheral enhancement ➡ corresponding to intensely SRS-avid lesion shown on preceding two images.

Typical

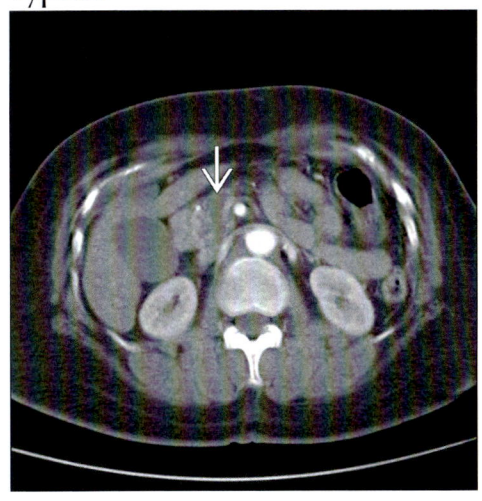

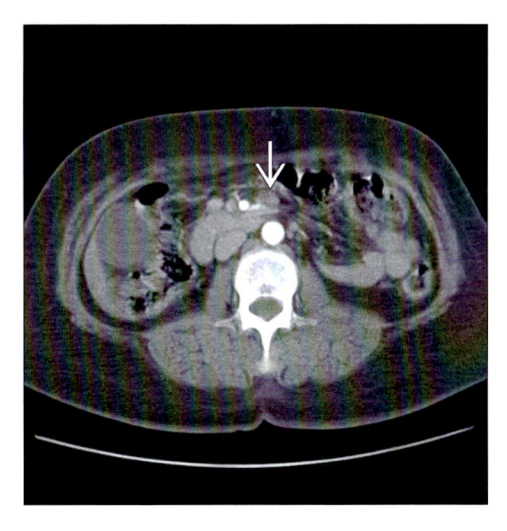

(**Left**) Axial CECT in same patient at left shows hypoattenuating mass in pancreatic head ➡, corresponding to a gastrinoma that was intensely SRS-avid. (**Right**) CECT shows enhancing mass ➡ inferior to body of pancreas in patient with gastrinoma. Islet cell tumors typically show avid enhancement on early arterial phase, but become less conspicuous by portal venous phase.

INTRAABDOMINAL INFECTION

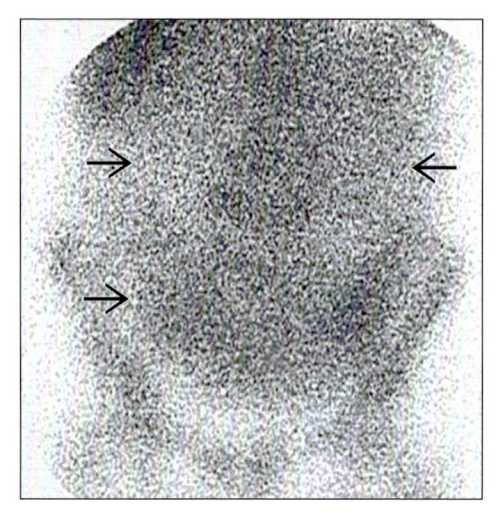

In-111 leukocyte scan shows diffuse uptake in lower abdomen and pelvis ➡, not conforming to shape of bowel. Paracentesis confirmed bacterial peritonitis.

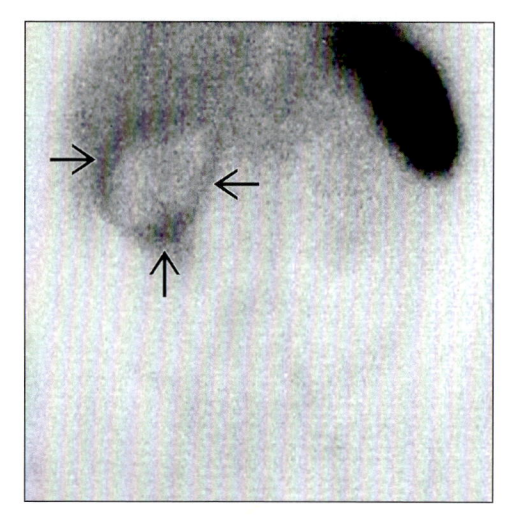

Anterior Tc-99m HMPAO leukocyte scan shows uptake in gallbladder wall ➡ in patient with acalculous cholecystitis. Scan performed 1 h post injection; 4 & 24 h images may demonstrate more sites.

TERMINOLOGY

Abbreviations and Synonyms
- WBC scan: Scintigraphic localization of autologous leukocytes (white blood cells) labeled with In-111 oxine or Tc-99m HMPAO

Definitions
- Infection within peritoneum or retroperitoneum

IMAGING FINDINGS

General Features
- Best diagnostic clue
  - CECT in febrile or septic patient: Phlegmon or fluid collection, peripheral enhancement, air within collection highly specific
  - In-111 WBC scan: Persistent nonphysiologic activity = suspicious for intraabdominal infection
  - In-111 WBC scan: Activity may be focal (e.g., abscess, appendicitis) or diffuse (e.g., peritonitis)
- Location: Peritoneal cavity or retroperitoneum
- Size: Lower limit of detection on scintigraphy: Depends on lesion:background activity; 1-2 cm most cases
- Morphology: May be diffuse or focal, depending on site of infection
- Abdominal abscess
  - CECT: Fluid collection, mass, enhancing rim, ± gas
  - US: Complex fluid collection, low internal echoes, septations, dependent echoes
  - WBC scan: Focal, non-physiologic region of increased uptake, not moving through bowel
- Peritonitis
  - CECT: Ascites, enhancing peritoneum, ± gas
  - WBC scan: Diffuse uptake in ascitic fluid, helpful in identifying loculated site of infection
- Hepatic abscess
  - CECT: Hypodense mass, rim-enhancement, "cluster sign" of coalesced abscesses, air bubbles (< 20%)
  - MR: T1WI hypo-, T2WI hyper-intense, peripheral enhancement, < 1 cm lesions uniform enhancement
  - In-111 WBC, Ga-67: May be similar to normal liver, Tc-99m sulfur colloid shows "cold" lesion
    - Lesions hotter than liver highly specific for pyogenic abscess

DDx: Non-Infectious Causes of Bowel Uptake on In-111 WBC Scan

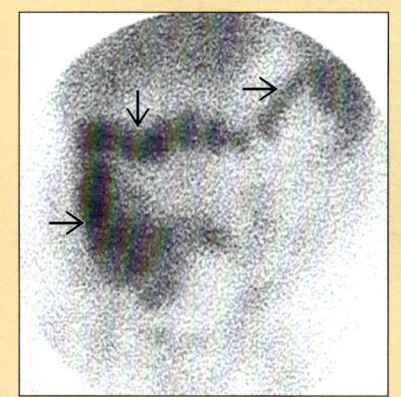

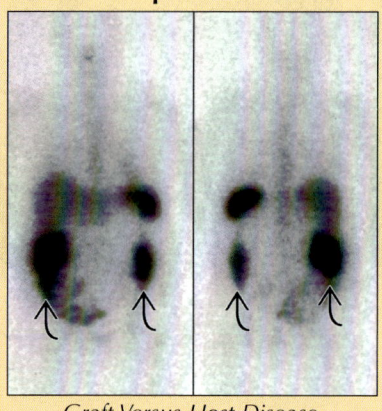

Epistaxis   *Graft-Versus-Host Disease*   *Crohn Disease*

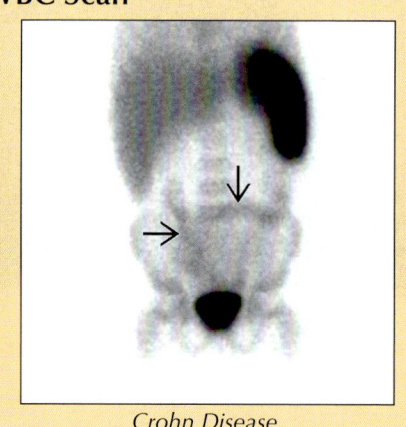

INTRAABDOMINAL INFECTION

Key Facts

Imaging Findings
- CECT in febrile or septic patient: Phlegmon or fluid collection, peripheral enhancement, air within collection highly specific
- In-111 WBC scan: Persistent nonphysiologic activity = suspicious for intraabdominal infection
- In-111 WBC scan: Activity may be focal (e.g., abscess, appendicitis) or diffuse (e.g., peritonitis)
- Size: Lower limit of detection on scintigraphy: Depends on lesion:background activity; 1-2 cm most cases
- Ga-67: Limited use due to normal colonic uptake
- Tc-99m WBCs: Often preferred in pediatric patients because < splenic & marrow dose than In-111 WBC
- Tc-99m WBCs: Most common use for active inflammatory bowel disease, image at 1 h, 4 h

Top Differential Diagnoses
- Pancreatitis
- Splenic/Hepatic Infarct, Hematoma
- Tumor
- Hematoma
- Uninfected Surgical Incision
- Ostomy Sites
- Renal Transplants
- Non-Infectious and Ischemic Colitis

Clinical Issues
- Most common signs/symptoms: Highly variable: Focal pain, no pain, fever, leukocytosis

Diagnostic Checklist
- WBC scan: Complicated cases; In-111 preferred, except Tc-99m for inflammatory bowel disease, peds

---

- Chronic pyogenic abscess: May be cold centrally
- Hepatic amebic abscesses: Cold center & hot rim on WBC scan, Ga-67, Tc-99m DISIDA
  - Hepatic candidiasis: Tiny lesions difficult to DX; peripheral enhancement helpful; "bullseye" or "wheel within wheel" by ultrasound
    - Ga-67 more sensitive than WBC scan for atypical & fungal infection
- Infectious colitis
  - Similar to non-infectious and ischemic colitis on CECT, In-111 WBC scan, BE
    - Tc-99m WBC scan useful only if image at 1-4 h: Thereafter ↑ normal bowel uptake
    - Ga-67: Limited use due to normal colonic uptake
- Diverticulitis
  - CT, CECT: Colonic focal outpouching or small exophytic mass with pericolic fat stranding
  - WBC scan: May show focal uptake, limited if very small
- Appendicitis
  - CECT: Dilated appendix ≥ 7 mm, periappendiceal fat stranding, enhancement of appendix wall (sensitivity & specificity 95%)
  - US: Non-compressible appendix ≥ 7 mm, focal pain with compression, increase color flow
  - WBC: Focal uptake RLQ
- Pyelonephritis
  - CECT: Swollen kidney with striated nephrogram
  - In-111 WBC: Increased uptake in kidney, usually focal or asymmetrical
  - Tc-99m WBC: Normal renal uptake obscures
  - Ga-67: Focal or asymmetrical renal uptake
    - Normal renal uptake to 48 h, longer if renal failure
    - Interstitial nephritis, infiltrative malignancy also +
- Cystitis
  - CECT: Bladder wall thickening, fat stranding
  - In-111 WBC scan: Increased uptake in bladder (pre → post void shows ↓ activity)
- Acalculous cholecystitis
  - CT: Gallbladder wall thickening (± air), pericholecystic fat stranding/fluid
  - WBC scan: Sensitive & specific; uptake in gallbladder wall; Tc-99m WBC at 1-2h often positive
  - Tc-99m DISIDA: "Rim sign", gallbladder may visualize in 15%
- Calculous cholecystitis
  - US, CT: Impacted stone in gallbladder neck, gallbladder wall-thickening, pericholecystic fluid
  - Tc-99m DISIDA: Non-visualization of gallbladder
  - WBC scan, Ga-67 scan: Luminal increased uptake, may not see acutely

Nuclear Medicine Findings
- In-111 WBC scan: Normal patterns and pitfalls
  - In-111 WBC normal biodistribution: Red marrow, liver, spleen ("hottest" organ)
  - Bowel activity
    - In-111 WBC: Faint bowel activity normal finding in 1/3 of patients
    - Moderate bowel activity (moves) on In-111 WBC scan: Common with endotracheal or nasoenteric tubes, sinusitis, pneumonia (swallowed leukocytes)
    - Intense bowel activity (moves) on In-111 WBC scan: Epistaxis or GI bleed; abscess communicating with bowel
    - Fixed bowel activity (doesn't move) on In-111 WBC scan: Active infectious or noninfectious inflammatory bowel disease
  - Lung activity
    - Early diffuse lung activity on WBC scan: Normal finding after injection due to marginated leukocytes; fades by 6-18 h
    - Diffuse lung activity > 18 h: Mild is nonspecific; intense usually diffuse injury (i.e., ARDS)
    - Lung infection is usually focal on WBC scan, false (-) in fungal, atypical, viral pneumonias
    - Tiny foci of intense activity in lungs on WBC scan: Embolized "clumped" WBCs
  - Blood pool activity on In-111 WBC scan: Should be minimal if cells properly labeled
    - Focal increased vascular activity: Recent line placement, infected grafts, aneurysms
- Tc-99m HMPAO leukocytes

INTRAABDOMINAL INFECTION

- ○ Tc-99m WBCs: Marked blood pool, ↑ bowel activity (> 2-4 h), kidney, bladder
- ○ Tc-99m WBCs: Often preferred in pediatric patients because < splenic & marrow dose than In-111 WBC
- ○ Tc-99m WBCs: Most common use for active inflammatory bowel disease, image at 1 h, 4 h
- Ga-67 citrate: Normal patterns and pitfalls
  - ○ Ga-67 scan normal uptake: Skeleton, liver > spleen, large intestine, lacrimal glands, nose, kidneys (≤ 48 h unless renal failure)
  - ○ Ga-67: Sensitive for kidney infection but non-specific (renal failure, interstitial nephritis)
- FDG PET: Sensitive for viral, fungal, bacterial infection, even in neutropenic patients

Imaging Recommendations

- Protocol advice
  - ○ Labeled WBCs: In-111 preferred over Tc-99m HMPAO WBC for all except active inflammatory bowel disease (early imaging), pediatric imaging
  - ○ Ga-67 scan: Infection may be detected by 24 h post injection but images best at 48-72 h
- Additional nuclear medicine imaging options
  - ○ Tc-99m sulfur colloid: Liver, spleen, bone infections often "isointense" to background tissues, cold on colloid improves sensitivity

DIFFERENTIAL DIAGNOSIS

Pancreatitis
- Infected & noninfected: Both ↑ on WBC scan

Splenic/Hepatic Infarct, Hematoma
- Acutely, can show uptake on WBC scan

Tumor
- May be hot on WBC scan; inflammatory component
- Ga-67: Many tumors positive

Hematoma
- May be hot on WBC for > 1 week, depending on size

Uninfected Surgical Incision
- Hot ≤ 10 days on WBC scan; > 10 d ≈ infected

Ostomy Sites
- Typically show uptake on WBC scan

Renal Transplants
- Typically diffuse uptake on In-111 WBC, Ga-67

Non-Infectious and Ischemic Colitis
- May mimic infectious colitis by CECT, In-111 WBC scan, BE

PATHOLOGY

General Features
- Etiology
  - ○ Peritonitis
    - Spontaneous: Chronic ascites, bacterial infection
    - Bacterial: Diverticulitis, appendicitis, ruptured viscus, pelvic inflammatory disease
  - ○ Hepatic abscess
    - Pyogenic/bacterial (88%)
    - Amebic (10%): Entamoeba histolytica; foreign visitors or travelers, poverty
    - Fungal (2%): Candida; immunosuppressed; severely neutropenic
  - ○ Diverticulitis: Fecal impaction of diverticulum mouth
  - ○ Abdominal abscess: Bacterial, fungal, amebic
    - Post-operative: Abdominal surgery
    - Non-surgical patient: Diverticulitis, appendicitis, ruptured viscus, pelvic inflammatory, Crohn disease, pyelonephritis
  - ○ Appendicitis: Obstructing appendicolith, Peyer patches
  - ○ Cholecystitis
    - Acalculous: Immune compromise, sepsis, diabetes, multiple lines, intubation
    - Calculous: Cystic duct obstruction
  - ○ Urinary tract infections: Typically gram negatives

CLINICAL ISSUES

Presentation
- Most common signs/symptoms: Highly variable: Focal pain, no pain, fever, leukocytosis

DIAGNOSTIC CHECKLIST

Consider
- WBC scan: Complicated cases; In-111 preferred, except Tc-99m for inflammatory bowel disease, peds

SELECTED REFERENCES

1. Bartolozzi C: Imaging and invasive techniques for diagnosis and treatment of surgical infections. Surg Infect (Larchmt). 7 Suppl 2:S97-9, 2006
2. Blot S et al: Critical issues in the clinical management of complicated intra-abdominal infections. Drugs. 65(12):1611-20, 2005
3. Brook I: Intra-abdominal, retroperitoneal, and visceral abscesses in children. Eur J Pediatr Surg. 14(4):265-73, 2004
4. Brook I: Microbiology and management of intra-abdominal infections in children. Pediatr Int. 45(2):123-9, 2003
5. Rypins EB et al: Scintigraphic determination of equivocal appendicitis. Am Surg. 66(9):891-5, 2000
6. Sirinek KR: Diagnosis and treatment of intra-abdominal abscesses. Surg Infect (Larchmt). 1(1):31-8, 2000
7. Bearcroft PW et al: Leucocyte scintigraphy or computed tomography for the febrile post-operative patient? Eur J Radiol. 23(2):126-9, 1996
8. Carter CR et al: Indium-111 leucocyte scintigraphy and ultrasound scanning in the detection of intra-abdominal abscesses in patients without localizing signs. J R Coll Surg Edinb. 40(6):380-2, 1995
9. Fry DE: Noninvasive imaging tests in the diagnosis and treatment of intra-abdominal abscesses in the postoperative patient. Surg Clin North Am. 74(3):693-709, 1994
10. Lantto E: Investigation of suspected intra-abdominal sepsis: the contribution of nuclear medicine. Scand J Gastroenterol Suppl. 203:11-4, 1994

INTRAABDOMINAL INFECTION

IMAGE GALLERY

Variant

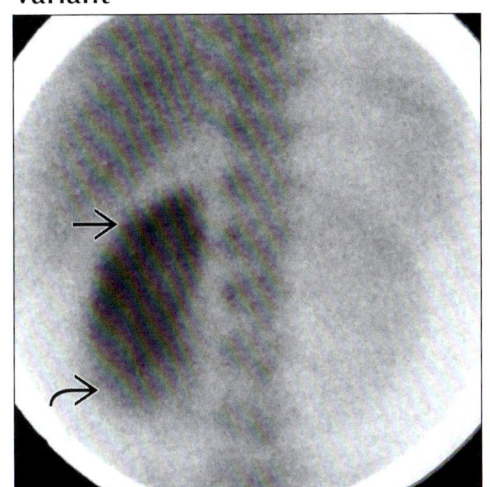

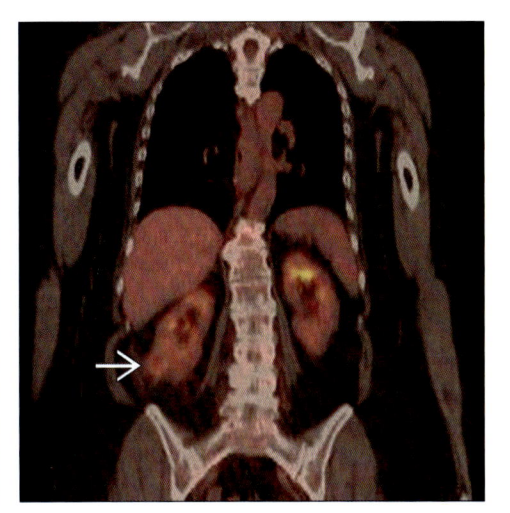

(Left) Posterior planar Ga-67 scan shows increased uptake ➡, indistinct inferior margins ➡ in left kidney in patient with pyelonephritis and inferior perinephric abscess. *(Right)* Coronal FDG PET/CT in neutropenic patient shows focal uptake in region of perinephric stranding ➡: Biopsy proven perinephric abscess.

Typical

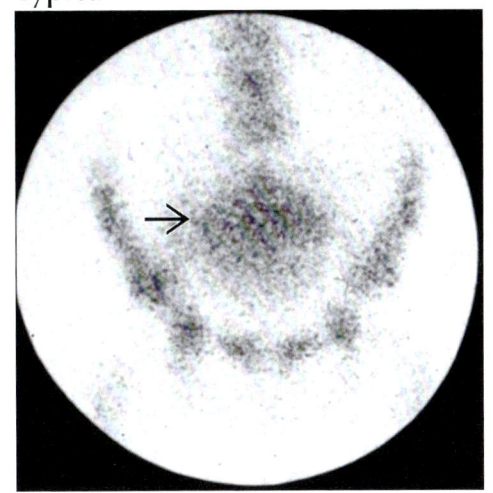

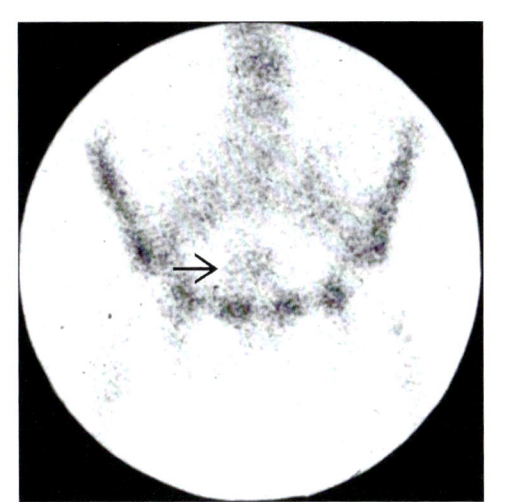

(Left) Anterior pelvis In-111 WBC scan: Pre void image. Ovoid region of uptake ➡ in patient with E. Coli cystitis. See next image. *(Right)* Anterior pelvis In-111 WBC scan: Post void image. Small ovoid region of increased activity ➡ decreased in size and intensity compared to pre-void image, confirming presence of cystitis.

Typical

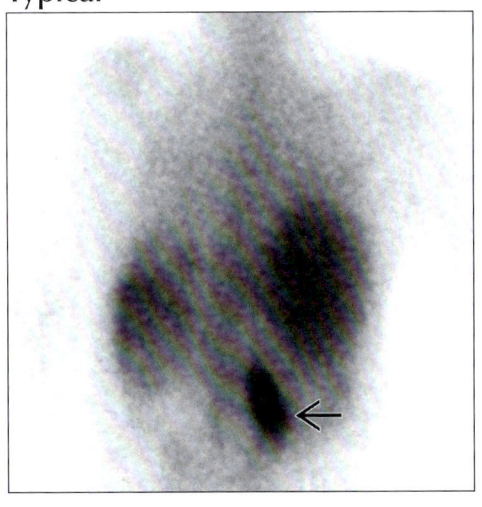

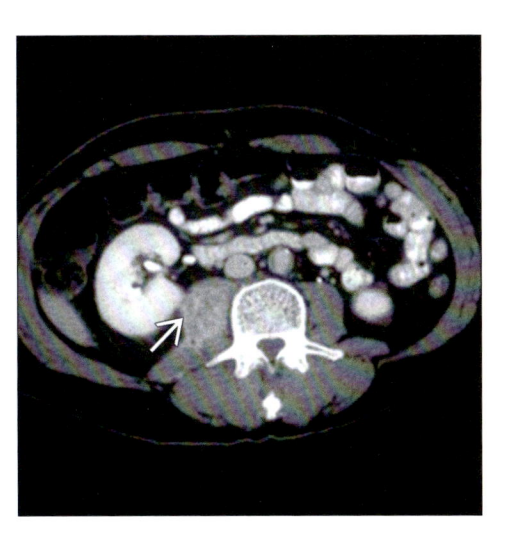

(Left) Posterior planar Ga-67 scan shows focal region of uptake over posterior abdomen in patient with psoas abscess ➡. See CT next image. (Courtesy N. Watson, MD). *(Right)* Same as previous Ga-67 scan. Enhancing psoas mass ➡ was confirmed at biopsy to be abscess. (Courtesy N. Watson, MD).

INTRAABDOMINAL INFECTION

(Left) Anterior In-111 WBC scan of abdomen shows focal collection in right abdomen ➡ in patient with right pyelonephritis. Note normal magnitude of uptake in liver ➡ and spleen ➡. **(Right)** Anterior FDG PET/CT demonstrates small focus of uptake in left abdomen ➡, adjacent to descending colon. Finding is consistent in appearance with diverticulitis.

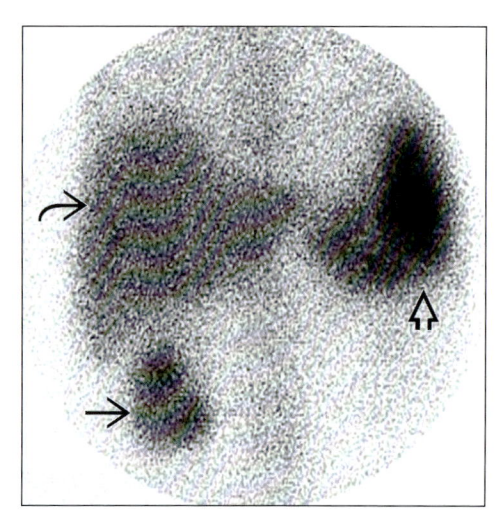

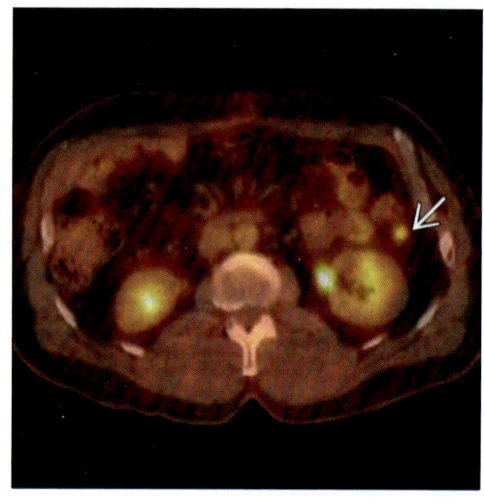

(Left) Anterior In-111 WBC scan of abdomen shows increased uptake in dilated ascending and transverse colon ➡ in patient with amebic colitis. (Courtesy N. Watson, MD). **(Right)** Anterior In-111 WBC scan of abdomen shows increased uptake throughout body ➡ and uncinate process ➡ of pancreas in patient with alcoholic pancreatitis.

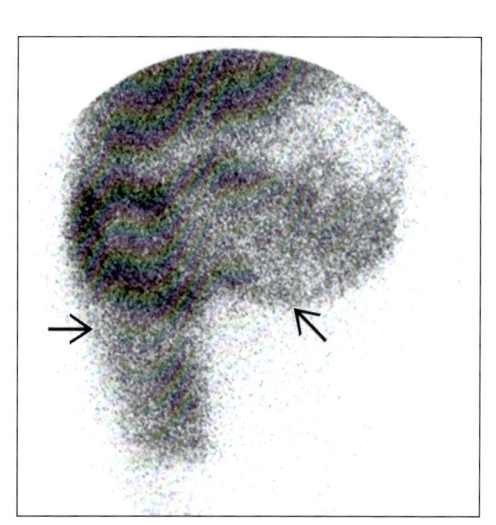

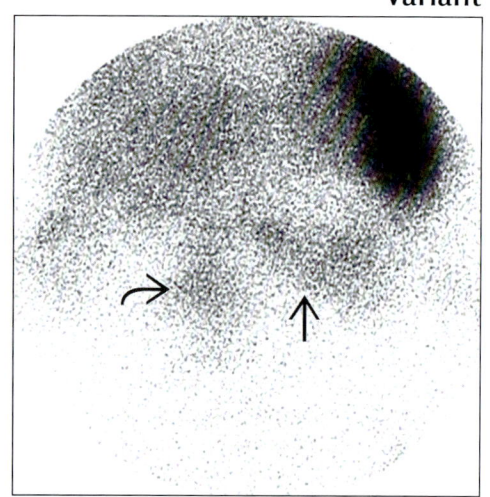

(Left) Posterior planar In-111 WBC scan of the abdomen demonstrates very subtle increased uptake in regions of hepatic abscess ➡, shown as cold defects on companion Tc-99m sulfur colloid scan (next image). Hepatic abscesses may be similar to normal liver in uptake. **(Right)** Posterior Tc-99m sulfur colloid scan of the abdomen shows cold defects in liver ➡, corresponding to sites of uptake on In-111 WBC scan (previous image).

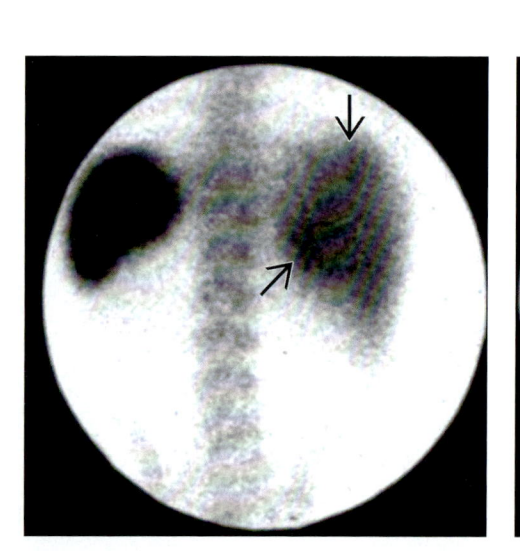

INTRAABDOMINAL INFECTION

Typical

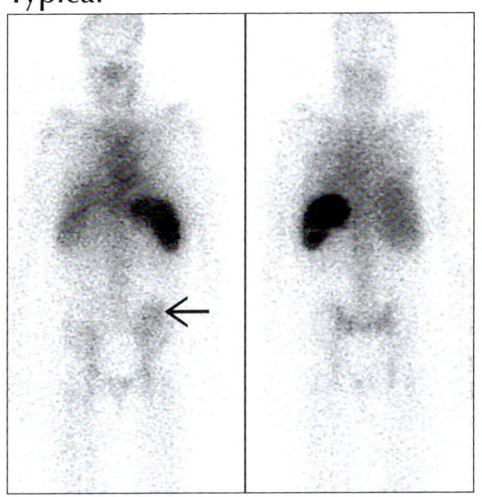

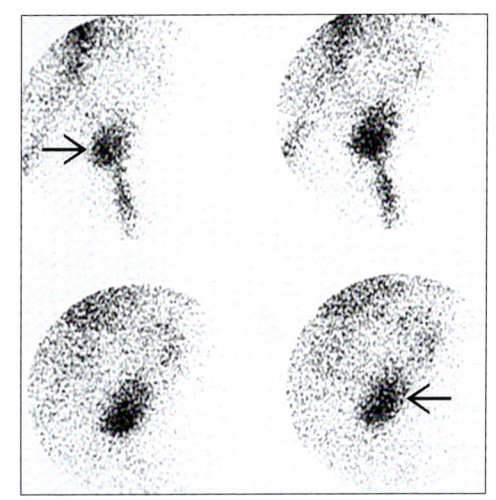

(Left) Anterior and posterior whole body In-111 WBC scan shows increased uptake in left pelvic renal transplant ➔, a normal finding on In-111 WBC scans. Focal or intense uptake may signify rejection or infection. See next image. *(Right)* Angiographic sequence from Tc-99m MAG-3 renal scan confirms good blood flow to, and concentration by, transplanted kidney ➔ (same as left).

Typical

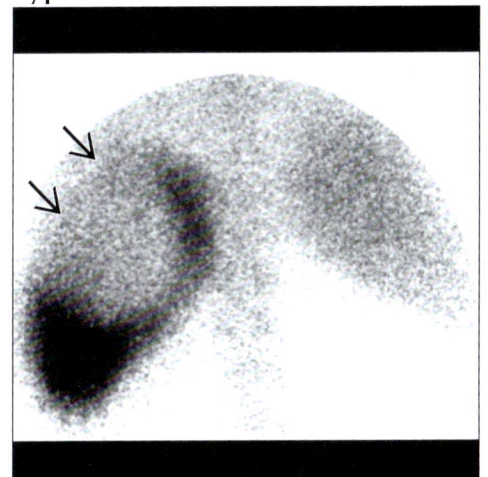

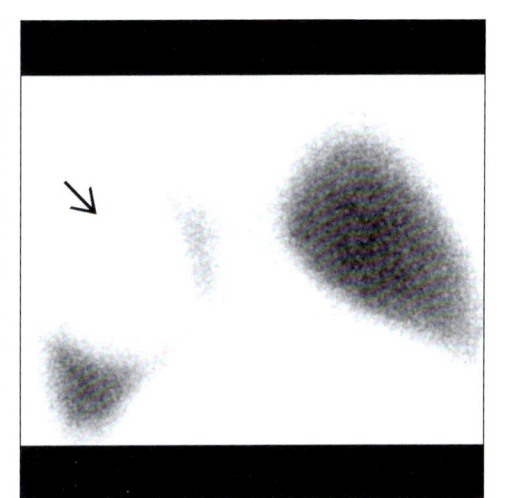

(Left) Posterior In-111 WBC scan of liver and spleen shows uptake in splenic mass ➔. Uptake in splenic mass is worrisome for infection, but mass was hemorrhage into acute splenic infarct. See companion Tc-99m sulfur colloid (next image). *(Right)* Same patient as previous scan. Tc-99m sulfur colloid scan shows large cold defect ➔ in spleen, proved to be hemorrhage into an acute splenic infarct.

Typical

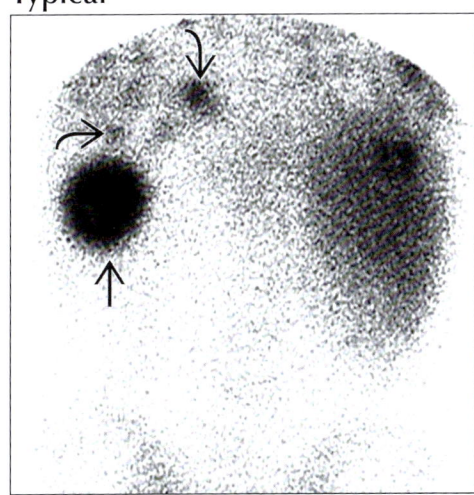

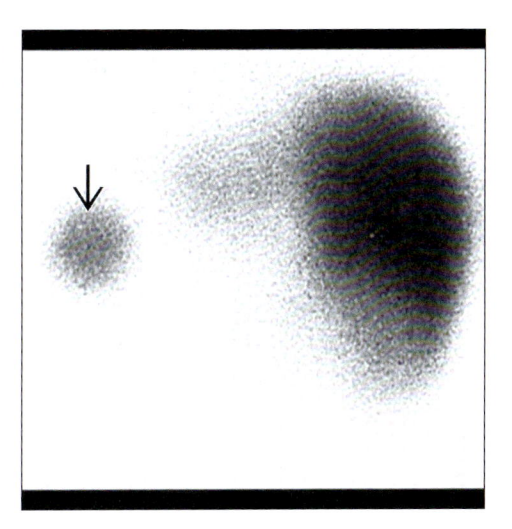

(Left) Posterior In-111 WBC scan of the abdomen in a patient with a prior splenectomy shows multiple focal sites of uptake in lung bases ➔ (embolized "clumped" leukocytes) and a focal area of intense uptake in the splenic bed ➔ (splenule). See next image. *(Right)* Same patient as previous image. Posterior Tc-99m sulfur colloid scan of the abdomen confirms uptake in splenic bed ➔ (splenule).

CARCINOID TUMOR

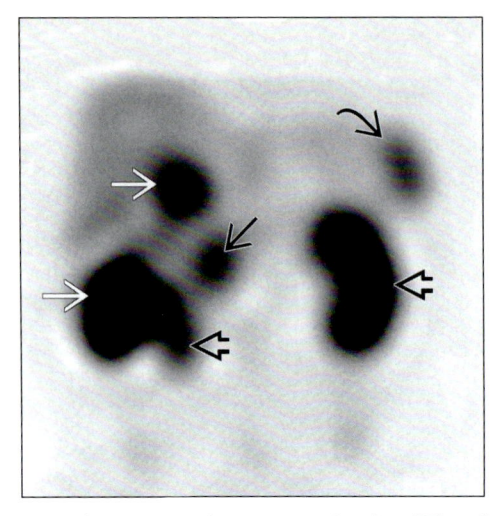

Coronal SRI SPECT shows carcinoid in liver and pancreatic head. Note normal uptake in the kidney and spleen. See next image.

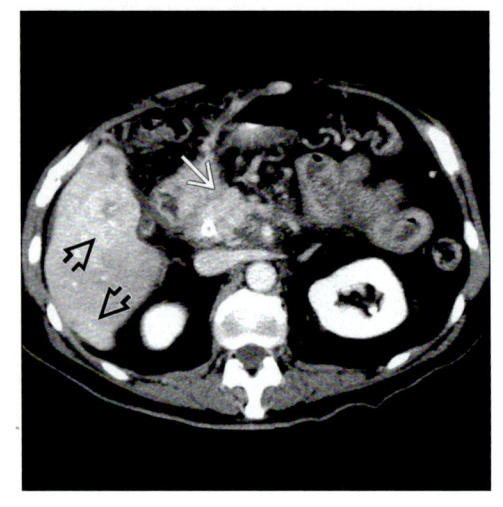

CECT shows enhancing carcinoid tumors in the right lobe of the liver. Carcinoid in pancreatic head also evident.

TERMINOLOGY

Definitions
- Carcinoid
  - Neuroendocrine tumor derived from enterochromaffin cells
  - Secretes serotonin, which is metabolized to 5-hydroxyindoleacetic acid (5-HIAA)
  - Malignant or benign
- Carcinoid syndrome (CS)
  - Common carcinoid tumor presentation
  - Syndrome symptoms: Flushing, diarrhea, asthma, bowel obstruction, gastrointestinal bleed

IMAGING FINDINGS

General Features
- Best diagnostic clue
  - Soft tissue mass in abdomen, hepatic or lung tumors in patient with CS
  - Soft tissue masses in abdomen alone often asymptomatic, found incidentally
  - Chest mass could give post-obstructive pneumonia
  - Appendix most likely site in bowel
- Location
  - Symptomatic
    - Liver, lung
  - Asymptomatic
    - Incidental finding on CT adjacent to bowel or mesentery
    - Incidental finding post-appendectomy
- Size
  - 1 mm to 15 cm
  - ≤ 2 cm = less likely malignant
  - Larger tumors may need wider excision, metastatic survey
- Morphology: Usually ovoid, but will conform to adjacent structures

Nuclear Medicine Findings
- Increased activity in soft tissue masses in bowel, liver, lung by several radionuclides
  - In-111 pentreotide (Octreoscan)
  - I-123 or I-131 MIBG
  - FDG PET

Imaging Recommendations
- Best imaging tool

DDx: Other Octreotide-Avid Tumors and Tissues

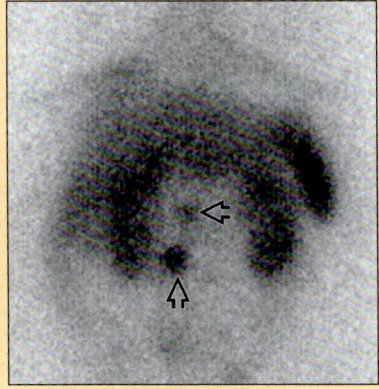

Gastrinoma

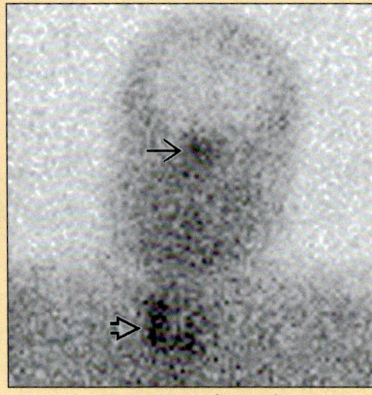

Pituitary, Thyroid

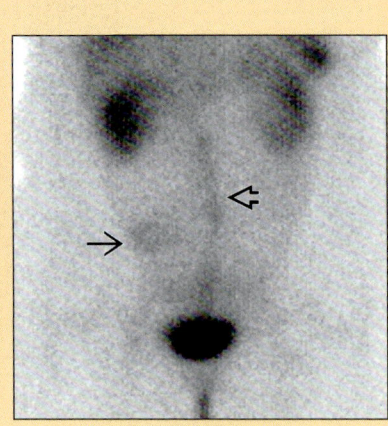

Ileostomy, Surgical Scar

CARCINOID TUMOR

Key Facts

Terminology
- Neuroendocrine tumor derived from enterochromaffin cells
- Secretes serotonin, which is metabolized to 5-hydroxyindoleacetic acid (5-HIAA)
- Malignant or benign
- Syndrome symptoms: Flushing, diarrhea, asthma, bowel obstruction, gastrointestinal bleed

Imaging Findings
- Soft tissue mass in abdomen, hepatic or lung tumors in patient with CS
- Soft tissue masses in abdomen alone often asymptomatic, found incidentally
- ≤ 2 cm = less likely malignant
- Somatostatin receptor imaging (SRI)
- Sensitivity 88-96%; specificity 80-95%

Clinical Issues
- Asymptomatic massive hepatomegaly
- Flushing: 85-90%
- Diarrhea: 70%
- Elevated urinary 5-HIAA
- Elevated serum chromogranin A (sensitivity 80%)

Diagnostic Checklist
- Normal In-111 pentreotide localization in kidneys, bladder, liver, bowel, spleen (usually hottest organ)
- Low uptake in normal thyroid
- Moderate to high uptake in medullary carcinoma of the thyroid
- Low uptake in normal pituitary
- Increased uptake also in pituitary adenomas

- ○ Somatostatin receptor imaging (SRI)
  - In-111 pentreotide (Octreoscan)
  - Sensitivity 88-96%; specificity 80-95%
  - Resolution limit ~ 1.0-1.5 cm
  - High percentage of lesions > 1.5 cm positive
  - Smaller masses less easily located, especially if in organs with normal, mild activity (e.g., liver)
- ○ CECT, MR
  - Sensitivity 50%, specificity 12%
  - Soft tissue mass density > water
  - Liver: Slightly hypo- or hyperintense
- Protocol advice
  - ○ SRI
    - 6 mCi (222 MBq) In-111 pentreotide IV
  - ○ Images
    - ↑ Tumor:background ratio with time
    - 4 hr: Whole body anterior/posterior planar; SPECT abdomen/pelvis (low bowel excretion at this time)
    - 24 hr: Whole body anterior/posterior planar; consider SPECT chest/abdomen/pelvis
    - Optional 48 hr: Whole body anterior/posterior planar; consider SPECT chest/abdomen/pelvis
    - Image with 173 keV and 247 keV photopeaks of In-111
  - ○ If patient not experiencing diarrhea, mild bowel cathartic may decrease colon accumulation
  - ○ Empty bladder completely prior to imaging
    - Bladder accumulation can obscure pelvic findings
- Additional nuclear medicine imaging options
  - ○ I-131 or I-123 metaiodobenzylguanidine (MIBG)
    - Sensitivity 55-75%, specificity 95%
    - Resolution limit ~ 1.0-1.5 cm
    - In most series no lesions added to SRI- or PET-evident ones
  - ○ I-123 or I-131 MIBG
    - 5-10 mCi (180-370 MBq) I-123 MIBG IV: Image with planar/SPECT at 4 or 24 hrs
    - 0.5 mCi (18 MBq) I-131 MIBG IV: Imaging with planar/SPECT at 24 or 48 hrs
    - If using I-131 MIBG: Pretreat with SSKI (3-10 drops/day), Lugol solution (~ 5-20 drops/day) to block thyroid accumulation of radioactive iodine
  - ○ FDG PET
    - Sensitivity 75%
    - Resolution limit ~ 0.6 cm
    - Most helpful in chest
    - Specificity very low, unless classic CS present
  - ○ FDG PET
    - 10-12 mCi (370-450 MBq) FDG IV
    - Whole body images at 60-90 min post-injection

DIFFERENTIAL DIAGNOSIS

Lymphoma
- Nodal disease in addition to bowel, liver, lung masses
- Biopsy, lab tests distinguish
- SRI imaging can also be positive in lymphoma

Other Neuroendocrine Tumors
- Gastrinoma
- Vasoactive intestinal polypeptide-secreting tumors (VIPomas)
- Insulinoma
- Pheochromocytoma
- Medullary carcinoma of thyroid

PATHOLOGY

General Features
- Epidemiology
  - ○ Incidence 1-2 per 100,000
  - ○ Autopsy series of carcinoid in small bowel of asymptomatic individuals: 97 in 14,852 (0.7%)
  - ○ Weak association with MEN-1 syndrome (< 1%)
  - ○ Stronger association with first-degree family member
    - 3.6 relative risk (95% confidence interval of 3.3-4.1)
  - ○ Symptomatic individuals increase with age
- Associated abnormalities
  - ○ Carcinoid heart disease
    - Right heart problems more common than left
    - Right heart failure 2° to severe tricuspid, pulmonary valvular dysfunction

CARCINOID TUMOR

- Left heart symptoms may predominate with pulmonary carcinoid

Gross Pathologic & Surgical Features
- Usually ovoid soft tissue masses
  - Appendix
  - Small and large bowel
  - Metastases
    - Liver
    - Lung
  - Lung primary (rare)

Microscopic Features
- Small cells with uniform round nuclei and stippled chromatin, without prominent nucleoli
- Growth pattern insular, trabecular, glandular, diffuse
- Silver stain, immunohistochemical analysis improve specificity

CLINICAL ISSUES

Presentation
- Most common signs/symptoms
  - Asymptomatic massive hepatomegaly
  - Flushing: 85-90%
  - Diarrhea: 70%
  - Cardiac symptoms: 35-40% (right 30%, left 10%)
  - Bowel obstruction
- Other signs/symptoms
  - Elevated urinary 5-HIAA
    - Sensitivity 73%, specificity ~ 100%
  - Elevated serum chromogranin A (sensitivity 80%)
  - GI bleeding
  - Incidental finding of pulmonary, abdominal mass

Demographics
- Age: Adults
- Gender: No known gender predilection

Natural History & Prognosis
- Larger tumors have greater metastatic potential
- Worse prognosis with severe carcinoid syndrome
- Untreated full-blown carcinoid syndrome has poor 5-year survival (20-50%)

Treatment
- Surgery
  - Excision of smaller masses
    - Usually curative, if full extent of disease
  - Debulk larger masses
    - ↓ Symptoms
    - ↓ Complications
- Angiographic embolization
  - ↓ Tumor mass
- Sandostatin
  - Therapeutic blocking agent for somatostatin receptors
  - In-111 pentreotide-avid tumors likely to respond
  - Blunts symptoms
  - Decrease tumor growth rate
- Limited trials of I-131 or Y-90 therapy with SRI-related agents underway

DIAGNOSTIC CHECKLIST

Consider
- If patient not experiencing frequent (at least QD) bowel movements
  - Obtain early abdominal imaging prior to bowel localization
  - Mild laxative can increase bowel excretion
- SPECT
  - Increases contrast in smaller lesions that may not be apparent on planar images
- Normal excretory bladder activity can obscure findings

Image Interpretation Pearls
- Normal In-111 pentreotide localization in kidneys, bladder, liver, bowel, spleen (usually hottest organ)
- Thyroid uptake of In-111 pentreotide
  - Low uptake in normal thyroid
  - Moderate to high uptake in medullary carcinoma of the thyroid
- Pituitary uptake of In-111 pentreotide
  - Low uptake in normal pituitary
  - Increased uptake also in pituitary adenomas

SELECTED REFERENCES

1. Gunn SH et al: In Vitro Modeling of the Clinical Interactions Between Octreotide and 111In-Pentreotide: Is There Evidence of Somatostatin Receptor Downregulation? J Nucl Med. 47(2):354-359, 2006
2. Mulkeen AL et al: Less common neoplasms of the pancreas. World J Gastroenterol. 12(20):3180-5, 2006
3. Panzuto F et al: Long-term clinical outcome of somatostatin analogues for treatment of progressive, metastatic, well-differentiated entero-pancreatic endocrine carcinoma. Ann Oncol. 17(3):461-6, 2006
4. Dromain C et al: Detection of liver metastases from endocrine tumors: a prospective comparison of somatostatin receptor scintigraphy, computed tomography, and magnetic resonance imaging. J Clin Oncol. 23(1):70-8, 2005
5. Kwekkeboom DJ et al: Radiolabeled somatostatin analog [177Lu-DOTA0,Tyr3]octreotate in patients with endocrine gastroenteropancreatic tumors. J Clin Oncol. 23(12):2754-62, 2005
6. Mulkeen A et al: Gastric carcinoid. Curr Opin Oncol. 17(1):1-6, 2005
7. Teunissen JJ et al: Peptide receptor radionuclide therapy for non-radioiodine-avid differentiated thyroid carcinoma. J Nucl Med. 46 Suppl 1:107S-14S, 2005
8. Belhocine T et al: Fluorodeoxyglucose positron emission tomography and somatostatin receptor scintigraphy for diagnosing and staging carcinoid tumours: correlations with the pathological indexes p53 and Ki-67. Nucl Med Commun. 23(8):727-34, 2002
9. Chatal JF et al: Nuclear medicine applications for neuroendocrine tumors. World J Surg. 24(11):1285-9, 2000
10. Halford S et al: The management of carcinoid tumours. QJM. 91(12):795-8, 1998

CARCINOID TUMOR

IMAGE GALLERY

Other

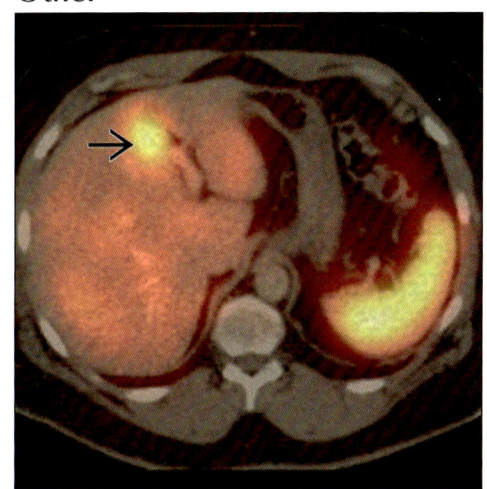

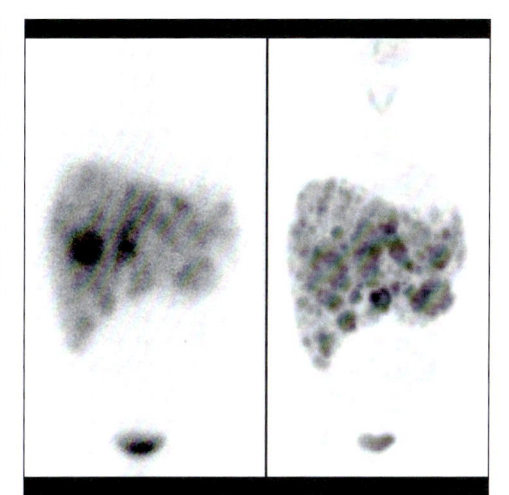

(Left) Axial fused PET/CT shows focus of increased activity ➡ in the medial segment of the left lobe of the liver, representing carcinoid tumor. *(Right)* Anterior planar SRI (Lt) and anterior MIP FDG PET (Rt) images of same patient with carcinoid tumor of the liver. Although PET performance is similar, and image quality better than SRI, PET reimbursement limits utilization.

Typical

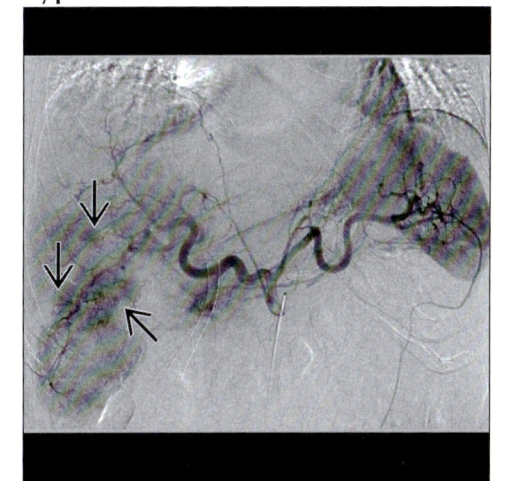

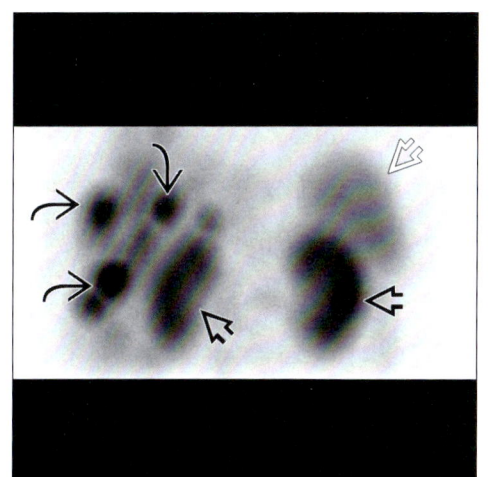

(Left) Angiogram in early capillary phase shows markedly hyperemic carcinoids ➡ in liver. *(Right)* MIP SPECT SRI in same patient as previous image shows multiple hepatic lesions ➡ with normal renal ▷ and splenic ⇨ uptake.

Typical

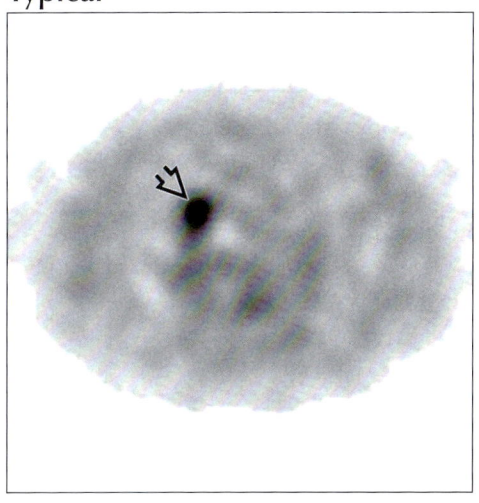

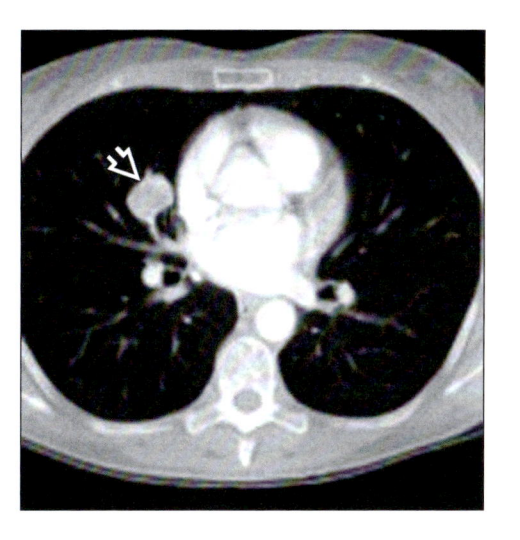

(Left) Axial SPECT SRI shows focus of increased activity ▷ in a carcinoid tumor in the right hilum. Small cell lung cancer can also demonstrate In-111 octreotide uptake. See next image. *(Right)* CECT in same patient as previous image shows corresponding right anterior hilar mass ⇨, biopsy-proven carcinoid.

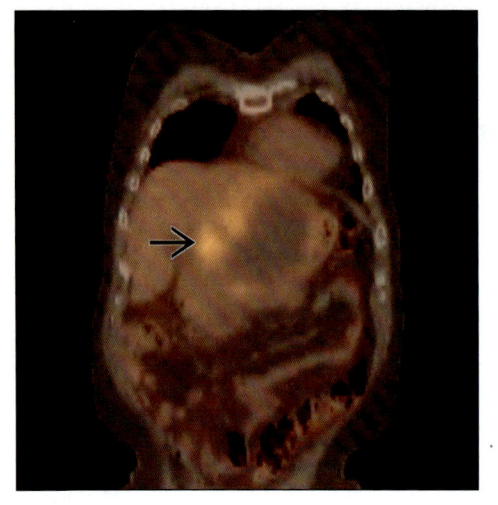

GI STROMAL TUMORS

Coronal fused PET CT shows large necrotic tumor in upper abdomen ➔ with nodular FDG uptake compatible viable tumor in patient with GIST.

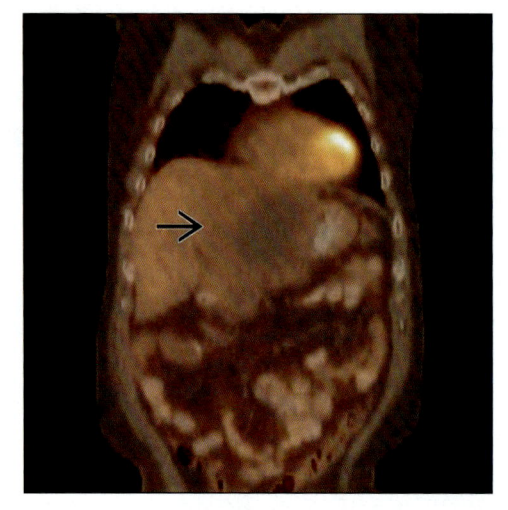

Coronal fused PET/CT (same as prior) after one month of chemotherapy shows areas of peripheral FDG uptake ➔ have resolved consistent with response to therapy. Overall tumor size not significantly changed.

TERMINOLOGY

Abbreviations and Synonyms
- Gastrointestinal stromal tumor (GIST)

Definitions
- Most common mesenchymal tumors of gastrointestinal (GI) tract
- All GISTs potentially malignant
  - If < 2 cm usually considered benign
  - Even small lesions should be resected

IMAGING FINDINGS

General Features
- Best diagnostic clue
  - Large mass outside organ of origin
  - Usually markedly FDG avid
- Location
  - Primary tumor
    - Stomach primary: 60-70%
    - Small intestine primary: 20-25%
    - Colon/rectal primary: 5%
    - Esophageal primary: < 5%
  - Metastases
    - Common metastatic sites: Liver and peritoneum
    - Uncommon metastatic sites: Lymphadenopathy, pulmonary and pleural metastases
- Size
  - Varies, but often large on presentation
    - Can be massive (> 30 cm)
- Morphology
  - Exophytic and outside organ of origin
    - Usually arising from organ periphery
    - Sometimes pedunculated
  - Central necrosis or hemorrhage common
  - Smooth margins
  - Recurrence
    - Nodule within a mass is a sign of recurrence
    - One study reported nodule as first sign of disease progression in 17 of 21 patients

Nuclear Medicine Findings
- FDG PET
  - Primary staging
    - Uptake not corresponding to normal anatomic structure

DDx: Mimics of GIST: Other FDG Avid Abdominal Tumors

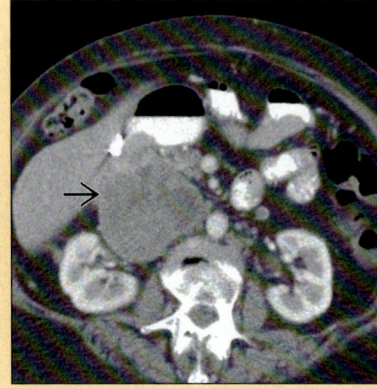

Leiomyosarcoma 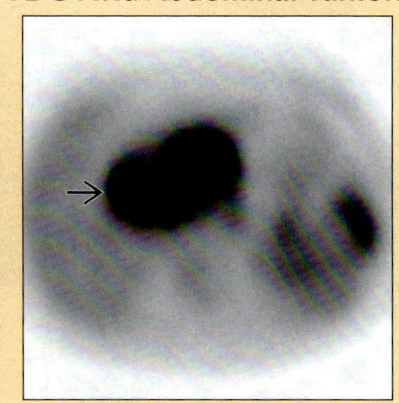   *Lymphoma* 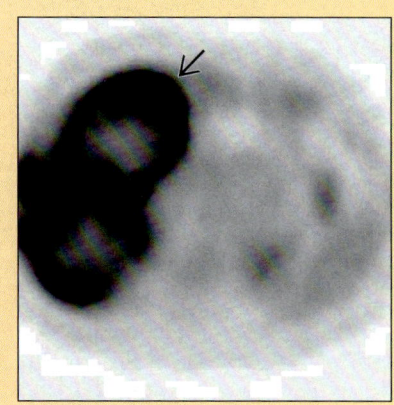   *Colon Cancer Metastases*

GI STROMAL TUMORS

Key Facts

Terminology
- Most common mesenchymal tumors of gastrointestinal (GI) tract
- All GISTs potentially malignant

Imaging Findings
- Stomach primary: 60-70%
- Small intestine primary: 20-25%
- Colon/rectal primary: 5%
- Esophageal primary: < 5%
- Common metastatic sites: Liver and peritoneum
- Uncommon metastatic sites: Lymphadenopathy, pulmonary and pleural metastases

Top Differential Diagnoses
- Leiomyosarcoma, Other Gastric Wall Tumors
- Lymphoma
- Metastases

Clinical Issues
- Prognosis for localized tumors based on size and mitotic rate
- Metastatic GIST: Median survival 19 months
- Local GIST recurrence: Median survival 9-12 months

Diagnostic Checklist
- Bulky abdominal soft tissue mass without lymphadenopathy = common GIST presentation
- Mass usually exophytic (sometimes pedunculated), outside organ of origin
- Central necrosis/hemorrhage common
- Look for small nodular areas of viable tumor in areas of necrosis on F-18 FDG PET

- If small, primary tumor may be difficult to separate from adjacent bowel or stomach which may have normal physiologic activity
- Look carefully at liver for metastatic deposits which could be missed on CT scan
- PET/CT recommended with oral contrast media
  - Response to treatment
    - FDG PET can detect early responders to systemic therapy
    - Prompt decrease in FDG uptake in tumor, before anatomic changes
    - Changes can occur in < one week
    - Sometimes more useful than CT for assessment after therapy

Imaging Recommendations
- Best imaging tool
  - FDG PET and CECT scan
    - Combination of functional and anatomic imaging most accurate
    - Either with concurrent PET and CT or PET/CT
  - MR
    - Sometimes more useful than CT for detecting organ of origin and pre-operative planning
    - Dependent on local expertise
  - Endoscopic ultrasound
    - Especially useful for evaluation of small tumor found incidentally during endoscopy
    - Allows assessment of local extent
    - Also amenable to biopsy
- Protocol advice
  - If performed for staging, obtain FDG PET prior to therapy
  - If scan obtained on PET/CT, oral contrast prior to acquisition helps delineate bowel from tumor
- Additional nuclear medicine imaging options
  - No standard role for bone scan
    - Bone metastases uncommon
- Correlative imaging features
  - Recurrence
    - CECT: Enhancing nodule in a nonenhanced tumor mass
    - Corresponding new FDG PET uptake reported 86% of the time
    - FDG PET may be false negative if < 1 cm

DIFFERENTIAL DIAGNOSIS

Leiomyosarcoma, Other Gastric Wall Tumors
- Expression of KIT an important distinguishing factor
- Leiomyosarcoma especially may occur in same area and also be very FDG avid

Lymphoma
- Can cause bulky abdominal soft tissue mass
- Lymphadenopathy (not seen with GIST)

Metastases
- Including melanoma which can cause cavitary small bowel lesions similar to GIST

PATHOLOGY

General Features
- Genetics
  - Familial
    - Rare autosomal dominant disorder
    - Due to KIT germline mutations
- Etiology
  - Sporadic
    - Mutations of cellular enzyme KIT (CD117) or PDGFR
    - Tyrosine kinase growth factor receptor
    - Mutated enzyme allows cells to uncontrollably grow and proliferate
  - Different mechanism when associated with neurofibromatosis type 1
- Epidemiology: 5,000-10,000 new cases/year in United States
- Associated abnormalities
  - More common in patients with neurofibromatosis type 1

GI STROMAL TUMORS

- Multiple small intestinal GISTs

Gross Pathologic & Surgical Features
- May extend to mucosal surface of involved organ
- ± Mucosal ulceration

Microscopic Features
- Cell types
  - Spindle cell (70%)
  - Epithelioid (20%)
  - Mixed epithelioid and spindle cell (10%)
- Immunohistochemical
  - 95% CD117+

CLINICAL ISSUES

Presentation
- Most common signs/symptoms: Nonspecific
- Other signs/symptoms
  - Depends on tumor size, location
    - Hemorrhage
    - Early satiety
    - Abdominal pain
    - Nausea
    - Vomiting

Demographics
- Age: Middle age or older
- Gender: Possible slight male predominance

Natural History & Prognosis
- Prognosis for localized tumors based on size and mitotic rate
- Metastatic GIST: Median survival 19 months
- Local GIST recurrence: Median survival 9-12 months
- Survival rates improved with new therapies
  - Imatinib mesylate (Gleevec; Novartis, New York, NY)

Treatment
- Aggressive surgical resection
  - Mainstay of treatment
  - High recurrence rates: Extensive re-resection indicated
- Chemotherapy
  - Does not respond well to standard chemotherapy regimens
  - Imatinib mesylate (Gleevec)
    - Tyrosine kinase inhibitor selectively inhibits KIT
    - Used in nonresectable, metastatic GIST
    - More serious events reported in 21% in one study, includes tumoral or gastrointestinal hemorrhage
    - Orally administered
  - Sunitinib malate (Sutent)
    - Multikinase inhibitor
    - Can be used after progression or intolerance to Imatinab
    - Hemorrhage a complication
- External beam radiation
  - Typically refractory

DIAGNOSTIC CHECKLIST

Consider
- Bulky abdominal soft tissue mass without lymphadenopathy = common GIST presentation

Image Interpretation Pearls
- Mass usually exophytic (sometimes pedunculated), outside organ of origin
- Central necrosis/hemorrhage common
- Look for small nodular areas of viable tumor in areas of necrosis on F-18 FDG PET
- Usually highly FDG-avid tumor
- Decreased activity on PET after therapy suggests response

SELECTED REFERENCES

1. Blackstein ME et al: Gastrointestinal stromal tumours: consensus statement on diagnosis and treatment. Can J Gastroenterol. 20(3):157-63, 2006
2. Esteves FP et al: Gastrointestinal tract malignancies and positron emission tomography: an overview. Semin Nucl Med. 36(2):169-81, 2006
3. Hong X et al: Gastrointestinal stromal tumor: role of CT in diagnosis and in response evaluation and surveillance after treatment with imatinib. Radiographics. 26(2):481-95, 2006
4. Maertens O et al: Molecular pathogenesis of multiple gastrointestinal stromal tumors in NF1 patients. Hum Mol Genet. 15(6):1015-23, 2006
5. Blay JY et al: Consensus meeting for the management of gastrointestinal stromal tumors. Report of the GIST Consensus Conference of 20-21 March 2004, under the auspices of ESMO. Ann Oncol. 16(4):566-78, 2005
6. Coindre JM et al: [Gastrointestinal stromal tumors: definition, histological, immunohistochemical, and molecular features, and diagnostic strategy] Ann Pathol. 25(5):358-85; quiz 357, 2005
7. Heinicke T et al: Very early detection of response to imatinib mesylate therapy of gastrointestinal stromal tumours using 18fluoro-deoxyglucose-positron emission tomography. Anticancer Res. 25(6C):4591-4, 2005
8. Sanborn RE et al: Gastrointestinal stromal tumors and the evolution of targeted therapy. Clin Adv Hematol Oncol. 3(8):647-57, 2005
9. Shankar S et al: Gastrointestinal stromal tumor: new nodule-within-a-mass pattern of recurrence after partial response to imatinib mesylate. Radiology. 235(3):892-8, 2005
10. Antoch G et al: Comparison of PET, CT, and dual-modality PET/CT imaging for monitoring of imatinib (STI571) therapy in patients with gastrointestinal stromal tumors. J Nucl Med. 45(3):357-65, 2004
11. Chompret A et al: PDGFRA germline mutation in a family with multiple cases of gastrointestinal stromal tumor. Gastroenterology. 126(1):318-21, 2004
12. Levy AD et al: Gastrointestinal stromal tumors: radiologic features with pathologic correlation. Radiographics. 23(2):283-304, 456; quiz 532, 2003

GI STROMAL TUMORS

IMAGE GALLERY

Typical

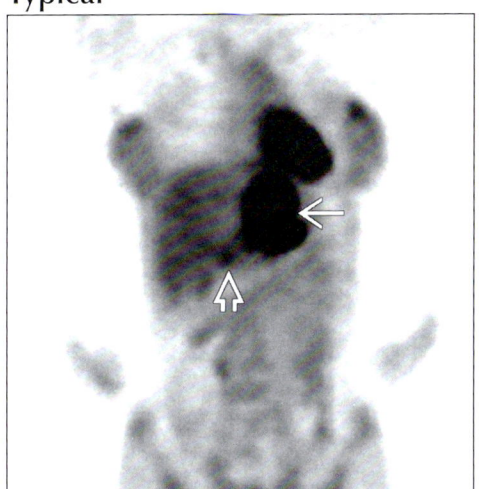

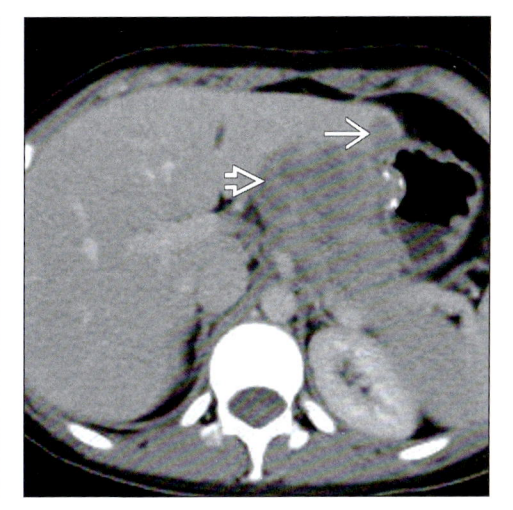

(**Left**) Coronal PET shows marked uptake ➡ in a left upper quadrant mass compatible with GIST. The smaller focus ➡ is a liver metastasis. Lymphadenopathy is uncommon with GIST. (**Right**) Axial CECT shows large mass ➡ with exophytic extension from the stomach. A metastasis ➡ is evident in lateral left hepatic lobe.

Typical

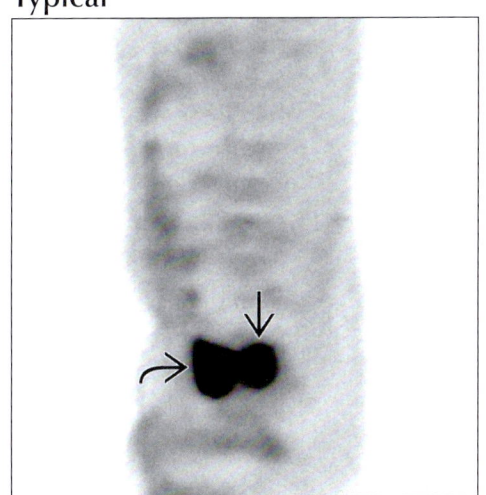

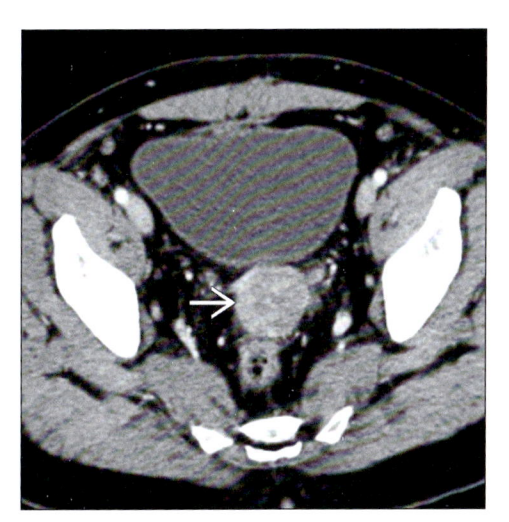

(**Left**) Sagittal PET shows increased uptake in a pelvic mass ➡ posterior to the bladder ➡ in patient with metastatic GIST. See next image. (**Right**) Axial CECT shows the mass identified on PET scan located between the rectum and bladder ➡. Note peripheral enhancement pattern and central areas of decreased attenuation.

Typical

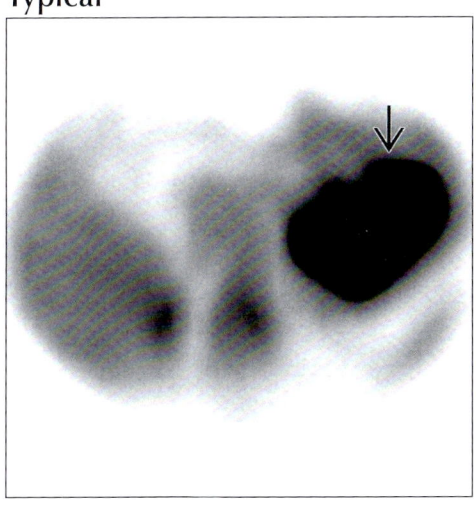

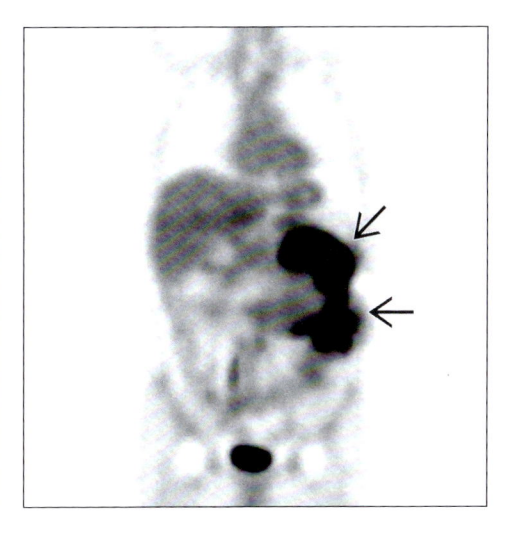

(**Left**) Axial PET shows marked uptake in a mass in the left abdomen ➡ in patient who originally presented with a gastrointestinal bleed. CT demonstrated an 18 cm GIST. See next image. (**Right**) Coronal PET (same patient as previous image) shows large left upper quadrant mass ➡ which originated from jejunum. On laparotomy, tumor invaded the retroperitoneum.

PERITONEAL SYSTEMIC SHUNT EVALUATION

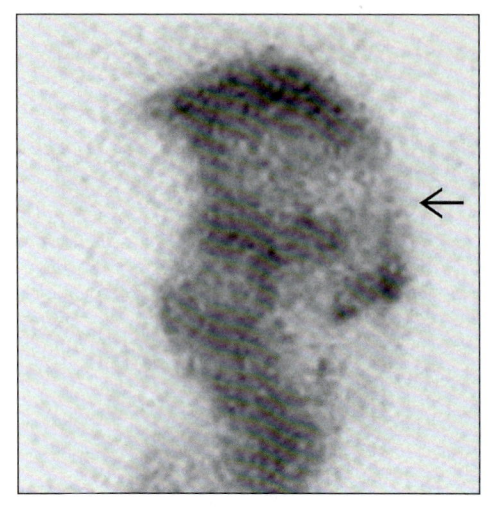

Right lateral image immediately after intraperitoneal injection of Tc-99m MAA shows free flow of radiotracer in peritoneal space ⇨.

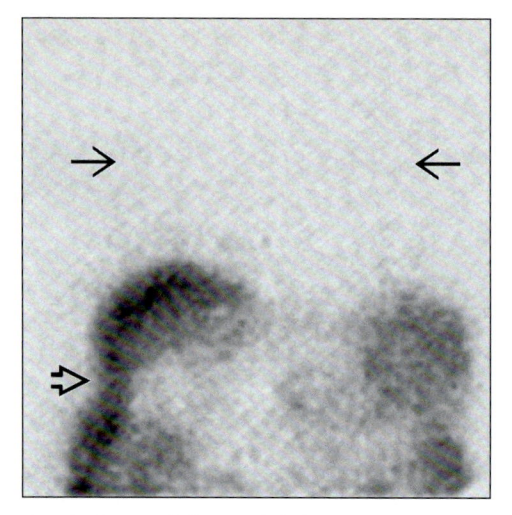

Anterior image of chest and abdomen in same patient as previous image shows Tc-99m MAA in peritoneal space ⇨ and no uptake in lungs ⇨ at 60 minutes, compatible with nonfunctioning shunt.

TERMINOLOGY

Definitions
- Medically refractory ascites
  - Ascites unresponsive to 400 mg spironolactone, 30 mg amiloride, ≤ 160 mg furosemide daily for two weeks
- Peritoneovenous shunt
  - Returns ascitic fluid from peritoneum into systemic circulation
  - Usually shunt from peritoneal cavity to superior vena cava
  - Denver shunt
    - Subcutaneous valve chamber
    - Manual compression to ↑ flow
    - Possibly less prone to blockage
  - LeVeen shunt
    - Pressure-sensitive unidirectional valve
    - Valve pressure typically 3 cm H₂O
  - Saphenous-peritoneal shunt
    - Surgical anastomosis of greater saphenous vein to peritoneal cavity
  - Hyde shunt
    - No longer commonly used

IMAGING FINDINGS

General Features
- Best diagnostic clue: Activity in lungs or heart on Tc-99m MAA study = patent shunt
- Location: Activity above diaphragm

Nuclear Medicine Findings
- Free tracer flow in peritoneal cavity confirms intraperitoneal injection
- Tc-99m MAA in lungs within 60 minutes of injection confirms shunt patency
- Identification of shunt tubing alone not reliable indicator of patency
  - Can have occlusion of distal tubing
  - Continue imaging to document movement into heart and lungs
- Obstruction can occur at venous or peritoneal end of tubing

Imaging Recommendations
- Best imaging tool
  - Tc-99m MAA scan for shunt patency
    - 100% sensitivity

DDx: Other Radiotracer Accumulation in Peritoneal Space

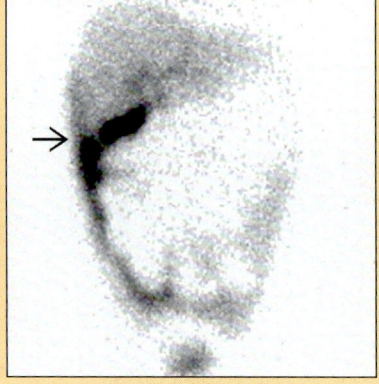

Bile Leak (Choletec)

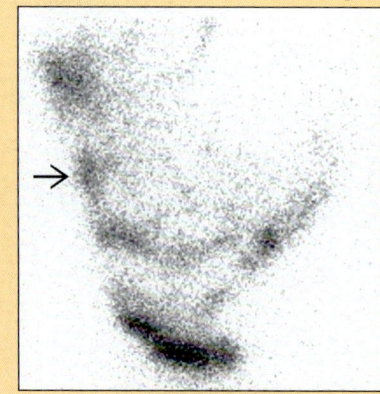

Ventriculoperitoneal Shunt (DTPA)

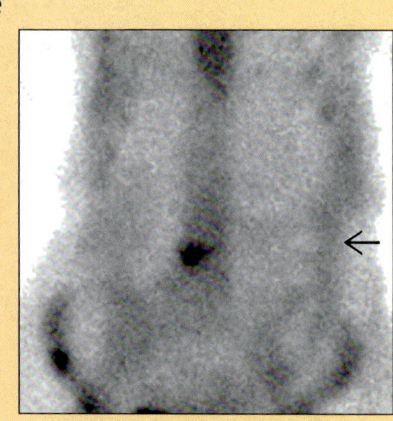

Peritoneal Metastases (MDP)

PERITONEAL SYSTEMIC SHUNT EVALUATION

Key Facts

Imaging Findings
- Best diagnostic clue: Activity in lungs or heart on Tc-99m MAA study = patent shunt
- Free tracer flow in peritoneal cavity confirms intraperitoneal injection
- Identification of shunt tubing alone not reliable indicator of patency
- Continue imaging to document movement into heart and lungs
- If obvious ascites identify injection site via percussion
- If cannot identify injection site via percussion, ultrasound helpful
- If performed correctly, rate of major or minor complication ≤ 1%
- Instead of lung uptake, look for uptake in liver or spleen

Clinical Issues
- Mortality similar in patients with a peritoneovenous shunt compared to medical therapy
- Properly functioning shunt can improve quality of life

Diagnostic Checklist
- Subcutaneous injection if no free flow of tracer peritoneal cavity
- "Z-track" injection needle to reduce risk of persistent leak from puncture site
- If subcutaneous pump, be sure to pump after Tc-99m MAA injection
- Tracer in pleural space can cause false positive lung activity
- Peritoneal and pleural spaces can communicate through diaphragm

---

- 92.2% specificity
- 98.5% accuracy
- Protocol advice
  - Contraindications
    - Severe coagulopathy
    - Patient cooperation
  - 5 mCi (185 MBq) Tc-99m MAA intraperitoneal injection
    - Empty bladder prior to injection
    - If obvious ascites identify injection site via percussion
    - Usually lower flank or midline inferior to umbilicus
    - If cannot identify injection site via percussion, ultrasound helpful
    - Sterile procedure: Prep skin in sterile fashion, sterile gloves, sterile equipment
    - "Z-track" during insertion of needle to minimize risk of persistent ascitic fluid leak from injection site
  - Rock patient side to side to distribute radioisotope
  - Patient takes 10 deep breaths prior to imaging and remains supine
  - Anterior image of abdomen confirms tracer distribution in peritoneal fluid
  - First image of chest obtained immediately after injection, then every 15 minutes to 1 hour
  - If manual valve (Denver shunt), pump valve between images
  - Tracer in pleural space can cause false positive lung activity
    - Peritoneal and pleural spaces can communicate through diaphragm
    - Lateral image helpful to distinguish
  - Complications
    - If performed correctly, rate of major or minor complication ≤ 1%
    - Persistent leak of ascitic fluid from injection site
    - Infection (rare)
    - Bowel injury
    - Solid organ (liver, spleen) injury
    - Intraperitoneal, abdominal wall bleeding
    - Abdominal wall hematoma
    - Pseudoaneurysm of inferior epigastric artery (US guidance helpful)
  - Additional nuclear medicine imaging options
    - Conceivably any radiopharmaceutical which goes outside peritoneal cavity would work
    - Tc-99m sulfur colloid
      - Instead of lung uptake, look for uptake in liver or spleen
      - Liver and spleen sometimes difficult to recognize with imaging secondary to tracer in adjacent ascites
- Correlative imaging features
  - Ultrasound
    - Confirm ascites
    - Doppler ultrasound can assess for flow in tubing
  - Shuntography
    - Inject iodinated contrast directly into shunt chamber
    - Especially useful if obstruction at venous end
  - Radiographs
    - Chest and abdomen
    - Evaluate for shunt disruption, tube displacement, kinking

DIFFERENTIAL DIAGNOSIS

Biliary Leak
- Free flow of tracer within peritoneal cavity
- Either following cholecystectomy or trauma

Ventriculoperitoneal Shunt
- Normally functioning shunt: Free flow of radiotracer from ventricles in brain into peritoneal cavity
- Reduce hydrocephalus

Peritoneal Metastases
- Can be seen incidentally on bone scan
- Mild, diffuse accumulation of radiotracer

PERITONEAL SYSTEMIC SHUNT EVALUATION

PATHOLOGY

General Features
- Etiology
  - Fibrin deposition
  - Catheter displacement, kinking
  - Tumor thromboembolism has been reported
- Epidemiology
  - Reported incidence of shunt obstruction varies
  - Group of 56 cirrhotic patients had 1 year LeVeen shunt blockage rate of 5.6%, 2 year rate of 12%
- Associated abnormalities: Superior vena cava obstruction

CLINICAL ISSUES

Presentation
- Most common signs/symptoms
  - Malfunctioning shunt ⇒ increase in ascites
    - Enlarging waistline
    - Weight gain
    - Abdominal pain
    - ↑ Inguinal or umbilical hernia protrusion
- Other signs/symptoms
  - Anorexia
  - Dyspnea
    - Associated with enlarging pleural effusions
  - ↓ Urine output
    - Due to third-spacing of fluid into peritoneum
- Clinical Profile
  - Peritoneal systemic shunt most valuable in refractory ascites
    - Chronic liver disease
    - Renal disease
    - Chylous ascites
    - Ascites of undetermined etiology
    - Also with any contraindication to repeated paracentesis (e.g., bleeding diathesis, infections)

Demographics
- Age: Peritoneovenous shunting safely performed in children ≥ 3 months and adults

Natural History & Prognosis
- Mortality similar in patients with a peritoneovenous shunt compared to medical therapy
- Properly functioning shunt can improve quality of life
  - ↓ Abdominal girth
  - ↓ Abdominal pain
  - ↓ Body weight

Treatment
- If occluded with fibrin sheath may be able to dissolve with enzyme administration
- Surgical revision of shunt if medical management unsuccessful

DIAGNOSTIC CHECKLIST

Consider
- Subcutaneous injection if no free flow of tracer peritoneal cavity
- "Z-track" injection needle to reduce risk of persistent leak from puncture site
- Ultrasound guidance if difficult to identify intraperitoneal ascitic fluid by percussion prior to injection
- If subcutaneous pump, be sure to pump after Tc-99m MAA injection

Image Interpretation Pearls
- Free tracer flow in peritoneal cavity confirms intraperitoneal injection
- Obstruction can occur at venous or peritoneal end of tubing
- Tracer in pleural space can cause false positive lung activity
  - Peritoneal and pleural spaces can communicate through diaphragm
  - Lateral view helpful to distinguish
- Identification of shunt tubing alone not reliable indicator of patency

SELECTED REFERENCES

1. Tomiyama K et al: Improved quality of life for malignant ascites patients by Denver peritoneovenous shunts. Anticancer Res. 26(3B):2393-5, 2006
2. Chen JH et al: Modified saphenous-peritoneal shunt in refractory ascites: new technique. ANZ J Surg. 75(3):128-31, 2005
3. Sooriakumaran P et al: Peritoneovenous shunting is an effective treatment for intractable ascites. Postgrad Med J. 81(954):259-61, 2005
4. Hussain FF et al: Peritoneovenous shunt insertion for intractable ascites: a district general hospital experience. Cardiovasc Intervent Radiol. 27(4):325-8, 2004
5. Suzuki H et al: Current management and novel therapeutic strategies for refractory ascites and hepatorenal syndrome. QJM. 94(6):293-300, 2001
6. Hillaire S et al: Peritoneovenous shunting of intractable ascites in patients with cirrhosis: improving results and predictive factors of failure. Surgery. 113(4):373-9, 1993
7. Stanley MM et al: Peritoneovenous shunting as compared with medical treatment in patients with alcoholic cirrhosis and massive ascites. Veterans Administration Cooperative Study on Treatment of Alcoholic Cirrhosis with Ascites. N Engl J Med. 321(24):1632-8, 1989
8. Algeo JH Jr et al: Leveen shunt visualization without function using technetium-99m macroaggregated albumin. Clin Nucl Med. 12(9):741-3, 1987
9. Runyon BA: Paracentesis of ascitic fluid. A safe procedure. Arch Intern Med. 146(11):2259-61, 1986
10. Smadja C et al: Recurrent ascites due to central venous thrombosis after peritoneojugular (LeVeen) shunt. Surgery. 100(3):535-41, 1986
11. Stewart CA et al: Evaluation of peritoneovenous shunt patency by intraperitoneal Tc-99m macroaggregated albumin: clinical experience. AJR Am J Roentgenol. 147(1):177-80, 1986
12. Paschold EH et al: Arterial thromboembolic complications of peritoneovenous shunting for malignant ascites. J Surg Oncol. 27(2):71-2, 1984
13. Hyde GL et al: Peritoneal venous shunting for ascites: a 15-year perspective. Am Surg. 48(3):123-7, 1982
14. Gorten RJ: A test for evaluation of peritoneo-venous shunt function: concise communication. J Nucl Med. 18(1):29-31, 1977

PERITONEAL SYSTEMIC SHUNT EVALUATION

IMAGE GALLERY

Typical

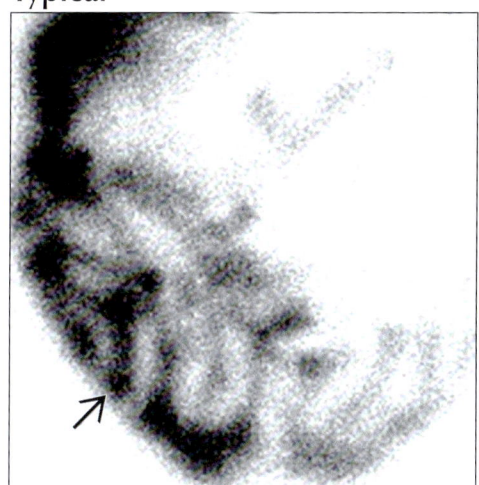

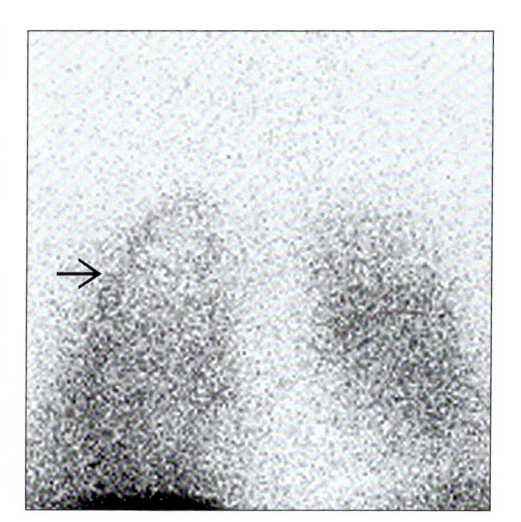

(**Left**) Anterior image of the abdomen shows free flow of Tc-99m MAA between loops of bowel ➡ in peritoneal space. See next image. (**Right**) Anterior image of chest after intraperitoneal Tc-99m MAA injection shows diffuse lung uptake ➡ within 30 minutes, compatible with functioning shunt.

Typical

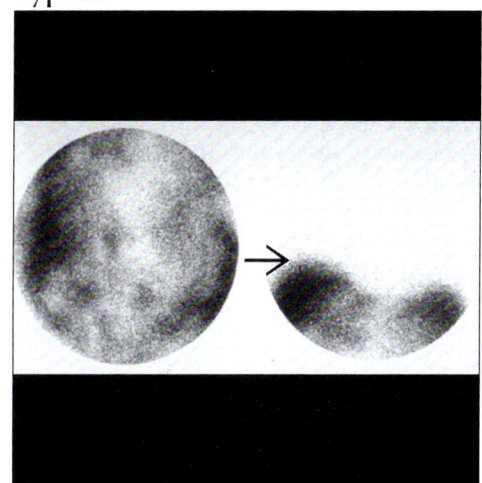

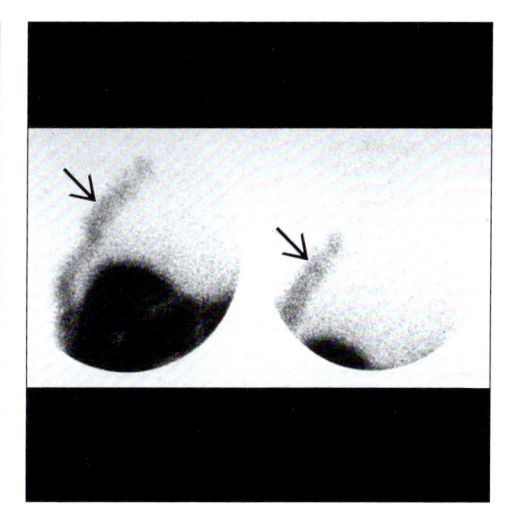

(**Left**) Tc-99m MAA injected intraperitoneally shows diffuse distribution at 15 min post injection (Lt). Anterior chest image (Rt) at 60 min shows no activity above the level of the diaphragm ➡, consistent with non-functioning shunt. See next image. (**Right**) Repeat images of the chest at 3.5 h shows activity tracking outside shunt tubing in over left chest wall ➡, but no activity within lungs. Tube was fractured along left chest wall.

Variant

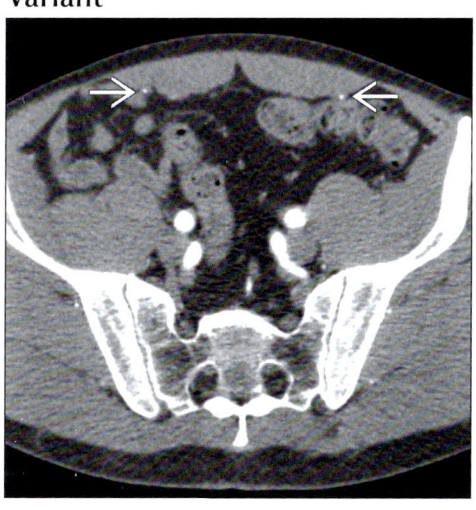

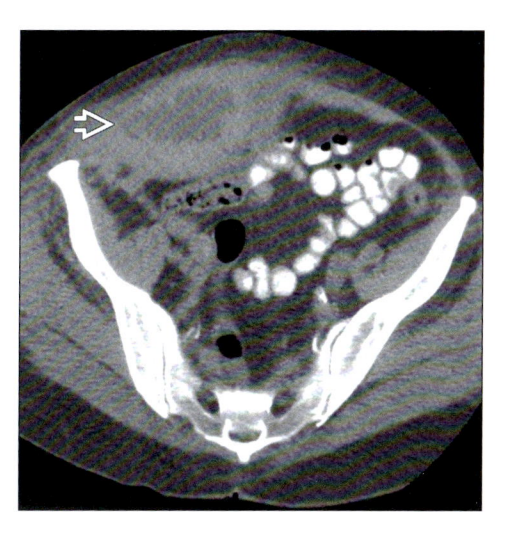

(**Left**) Axial CECT shows inferior epigastric arteries ➡, located in rectus sheath in anterior abdominal wall. Injury of these arteries during paracentesis is a rare but potentially life-threatening complication. (**Right**) Axial NECT shows a large rectus sheath hematoma ➡ in patient after paracentesis. After the procedure, the patient had palpable right abdominal mass with falling hematocrit.

DIAPHRAGMATIC PATENCY DETERMINATION

Posterior Tc-99m MAA intraperitoneal injection in patient with large left pleural effusion. Image at 1 hour prior to thoracentesis. All activity is below diaphragm.

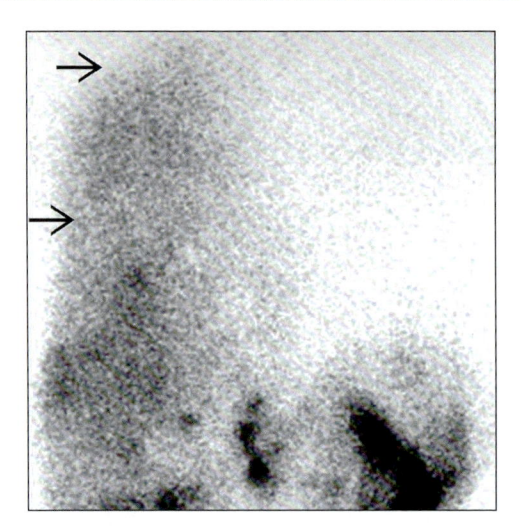

Posterior image in same patient as left with large left pleural effusion. Image obtained post thoracentesis, which creates a pressure gradient allowing flow of fluid into pleural space.

TERMINOLOGY

Abbreviations and Synonyms
- Hepatic hydrothorax, peritoneal pleural shunt, transdiaphragmatic movement of ascites

Definitions
- Accumulation of pleural fluid without primary chest or heart disease

IMAGING FINDINGS

General Features
- Best diagnostic clue: Tracer introduced into peritoneal cavity migrates to the chest
- Location: Fluid in pleural space most commonly on right but can be left or bilateral
- Morphology: Conforms to expected size and location of the pleural space

Imaging Recommendations
- Best imaging tool
  - Chest imaging following intraperitoneal administration of tracer
    - Tc-99m DTPA, sulfur colloid, or macroaggregated albumin (MAA) 1 mCi may be used
    - MAA is often preferred as it does not as easily enter lymphatics or diffuse into third space
- Protocol advice
  - If no ascites present, intraperitoneal saline (not water) may need to be administered
    - Infuse 50 cc saline first, then tracer, then 300-500 cc saline
  - Large effusion may require thoracentesis to facilitate flow across diaphragm
  - Pleural activity may appear in minutes to 24 hours
  - If chest tube present, image chest tube and drainage bag if the chest looks negative
- Additional nuclear medicine imaging options
  - Tc-99m sulfur colloid may demonstrate dilated lymphatics from peritoneum as cause of pleural effusion

DDx: Mimics of Diaphragmatic Leak, Various Tc-99m Agents

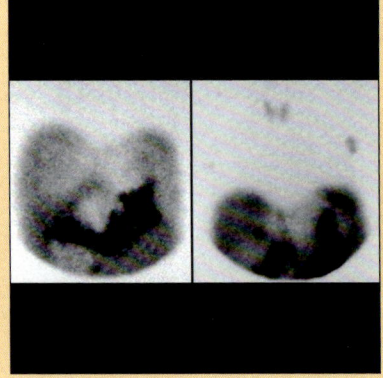

MAA: No Leak

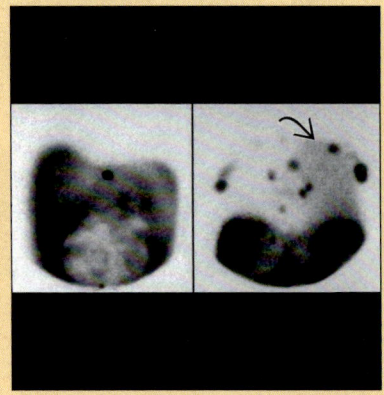

Sulfur Colloid (Dilated Lymphatics)

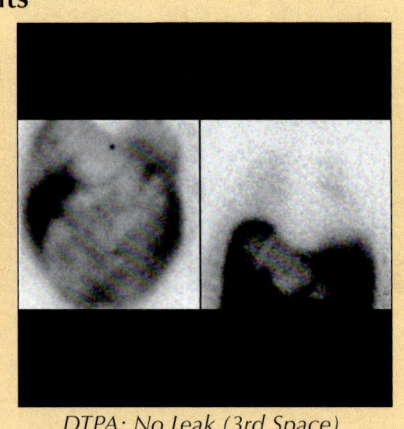

DTPA: No Leak (3rd Space)

DIAPHRAGMATIC PATENCY DETERMINATION

Key Facts

Terminology
- Hepatic hydrothorax, peritoneal pleural shunt, transdiaphragmatic movement of ascites
- Accumulation of pleural fluid without primary chest or heart disease

Imaging Findings
- Best diagnostic clue: Tracer introduced into peritoneal cavity migrates to the chest
- Chest imaging following intraperitoneal administration of tracer
- If no ascites present, intraperitoneal saline (not water) may need to be administered
- Large effusion may require thoracentesis to facilitate flow across diaphragm

Top Differential Diagnoses
- Pleural Effusion with an Intact Diaphragm

DIFFERENTIAL DIAGNOSIS

Pleural Effusion with an Intact Diaphragm
- Diffusable tracer such as Tc-99m DTPA may show false positive

Dilated Lymphatics from Peritoneum
- Positive on Tc-99m sulfur colloid but not on Tc-99m MAA

PATHOLOGY

General Features
- Etiology
  - Anatomic defect in diaphragm: Congenital or acquired (trauma, cirrhosis)
  - Peritoneal dialysis
    - Multiple proposed mechanisms: Lymphatic leak, dilated lymphatic connections, small diaphragmatic defects
- Associated abnormalities
  - Cirrhosis is generally present
  - Ascites usually present, not always

CLINICAL ISSUES

Presentation
- Most common signs/symptoms: Fluid in the chest with attendant symptoms
- Other signs/symptoms: Patient is often cirrhotic

Natural History & Prognosis
- Patients with leaks usually have advanced liver disease and will decompensate further without treatment

Treatment
- Increase pleural pressure: Upright position, IPPB, decrease pleural suction or tube drainage
- Decrease intraabdominal pressure: Remove ascitic fluid
- Thoracentesis, pleurodesis, pleurectomy, pleural/peritoneal venous shunt
- Surgical repair of diaphragmatic defect

DIAGNOSTIC CHECKLIST

Image Interpretation Pearls
- Determine location of diaphragm to distinguish abdominal versus thoracic location of tracer

SELECTED REFERENCES

1. Bhattacharya A et al: Radioisotope scintigraphy in the diagnosis of hepatic hydrothorax. J Gastroenterol Hepatol. 16(3):317-21, 2001
2. Schuster DM et al: The use of the diagnostic radionuclide ascites scan to facilitate treatment decisions for hepatic hydrothorax. Clin Nucl Med. 23(1):16-8, 1998
3. Giacobbe A et al: Hepatic hydrothorax. Diagnosis and management. Clin Nucl Med. 21(1):56-60, 1996
4. LeVeen HH et al: Management of ascites with hydrothorax. Am J Surg. 148(2):210-3, 1984

IMAGE GALLERY

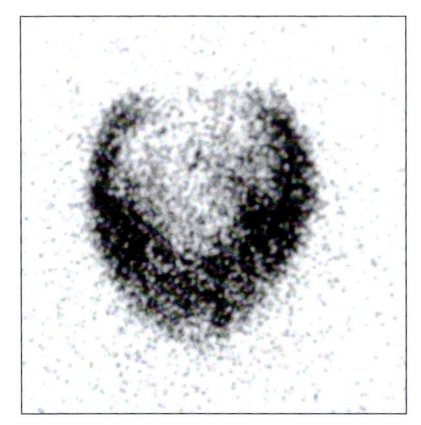

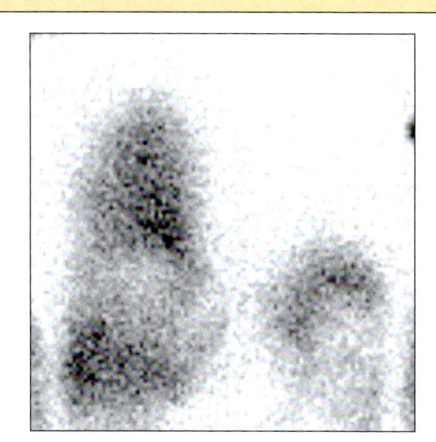

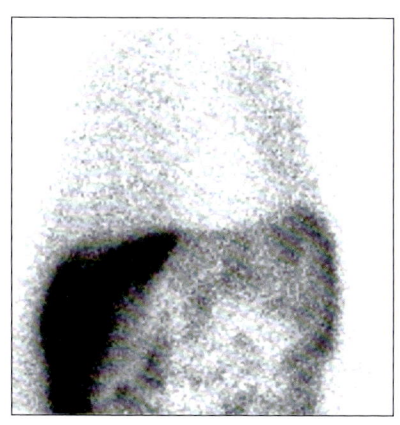

(Left) Posterior 24 hour (abdomen) image with intraperitoneal injection of Tc-99m MAA in patient with large left pleural effusion. No leak is identified. (Center) Posterior repeat study in same patient as left, following left thoracentesis (2 L removed). Activity immediately enters pleural space, confirming leak. (Right) 24 hour anterior abdomen following intraperitoneal injection of Tc-99m DTPA in patient with bilateral pleural effusions. DTPA diffuses into third space (pleural effusion). No leak.

INTRAARTERIAL HEPATIC PUMP EVALUATION

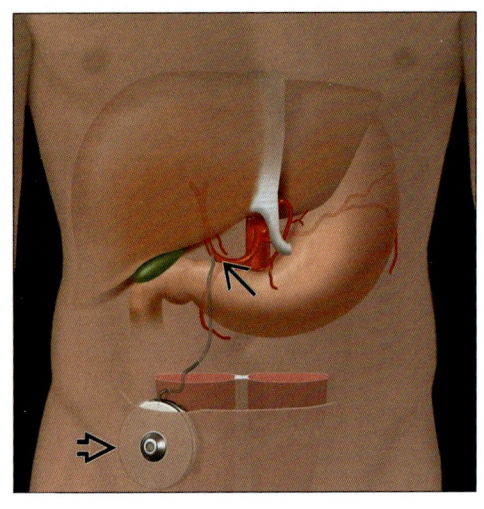

Coronal graphic shows normal placement of intraarterial hepatic infusion pump ⇨ with catheter in hepatic artery ⇨.

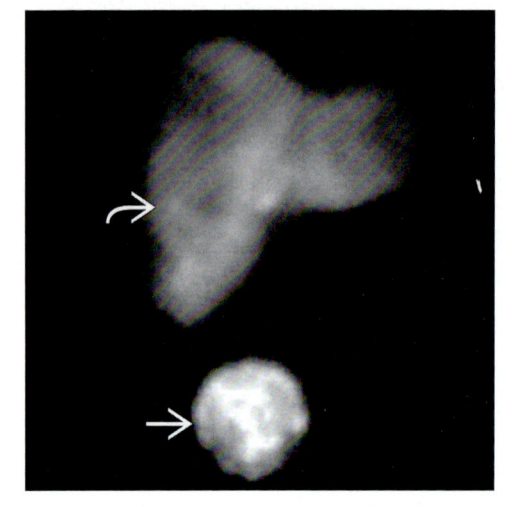

Anterior HAPS shows Tc-99m MAA in hepatic arterial infusion pump ⇨ and liver ⇨, evidence of patent system with appropriate tracer delivery to liver.

TERMINOLOGY

Synonyms
- Hepatic arterial pump scintigraphy (HAPS)

Definitions
- Radiotracer-based evaluation of placement, patency and function of hepatic arterial chemotherapy infusion pump/catheter
- Hepatic arterial infusion pump placed in abdomen surgically, accessed transdermally

PRE-PROCEDURE

Indications
- To evaluate hepatic arterial infusion pump before intraarterial hepatic chemotherapy

Contraindications
- Large hematoma or soft tissue swelling over infusion pump site
- Inability to tolerate procedure (e.g., severe pain, fever, chills, hemodynamic instability, bleeding diathesis)

Getting Started
- Things to Check
  - Check configuration of pump from manufacturer instructions (single central access port vs. side port for HAPS)
  - Placement of hepatic arterial infusion pump on plain radiograph or axial imaging, if available
- Medications: Lidocaine in syringe
- Equipment List
  - Sterile gloves
  - Antiseptic liquid: Chlorhexidine, Betadine
  - Sterile drapes
  - Syringe/needle for lidocaine
  - Bolus needle specific to pump manufacturer
  - 2-way stopcock
  - Connecting tubing
  - Two 10 ml syringes with heparinized saline (100 IU/ml)
  - 1-4 mCi (37-148 MBq) Tc-99m macroaggregated albumin (MAA) in 1-5 ml normal saline

PROCEDURE

Patient Position/Location
- Best procedure approach: Patient supine with lower abdomen exposed

Equipment Preparation
- General purpose collimator
- Anterior, posterior and right lateral images (500K) over abdomen

Procedure Steps
- Locate pump site
- Use sterile technique
- Connect needle, stopcock, connecting tubing, and heparinized saline
- Prime connecting tubing and needle with heparinized saline
- Prepare skin over pump site with antiseptic liquid
- Using sterile gloves, palpate appropriate septum (single central or side, depending on manufacturer)
- Inject lidocaine into skin and soft tissues overlying pump septum
- Insert bolus needle perpendicular to pump septum
- Inject 5 ml heparinized saline very slowly (1-5 ml/min) to confirm needle placement into port
- Inject Tc-99m MAA very slowly (1-5 ml/min)
- Inject 10 ml heparinized saline as flush very slowly (1-5 ml/min)

INTRAARTERIAL HEPATIC PUMP EVALUATION

Key Facts

Terminology
- Radiotracer-based valuation of placement, patency and function of hepatic arterial chemotherapy infusion pump/catheter

Pre-procedure
- Check configuration of pump from manufacturer instructions (single central access port vs. side port for HAPS)
- Antiseptic liquid: Chlorhexidine, Betadine

Procedure
- Confirm correct administration of radiopharmaceutical into pump
- Check for activity at injection site, in hepatic lobes
- Extrahepatic activity is abnormal: Stomach, lungs, spleen, peritoneum

Problems & Complications
- Accessing wrong port or using wrong needle can irreversibly damage hepatic arterial perfusion pump

Findings and Reporting
- Confirm correct administration of radiopharmaceutical into pump
- Check for activity at injection site, in hepatic lobes
- Extrahepatic activity is abnormal: Stomach, lungs, spleen, peritoneum

POST-PROCEDURE

Things To Do
- Confirm correct needle placement into port by injection of heparinized saline prior to radiopharmaceutical injection
  - Should not have resistance if properly placed

Things To Avoid
- Do not aspirate blood from pump into syringe
  - Occlusion may result

PROBLEMS & COMPLICATIONS

Problems
- Inability to access port
  - Overlying seroma, soft tissue
  - Malrotation of pump
  - Fluoroscopy guidance may be necessary
- Injection of tracer outside pump septum
- Inappropriate needle used for tracer injection
- Tracer injected too quickly
  - Can cause false + gastrointestinal activity

Complications
- Most feared complication(s)
  - Accessing wrong port or using wrong needle can irreversibly damage hepatic arterial perfusion pump
  - On pumps with side port for HAPS: Do not inject into central pump reservoir intended for chemotherapy; can ⇒ irreversible pump damage
  - On pumps with single central port for HAPS: Inject tracer into chemotherapy pump reservoir using only special needle per manufacturer
- Other complications: Infection, bleeding

SELECTED REFERENCES
1. Liu DM et al: Angiographic considerations in patients undergoing liver-directed therapy. J Vasc Interv Radiol. 16(7):911-35, 2005
2. Savolaine ER et al: Role of scintigraphy in establishing optimal perfusion in hepatic arterial infusion pump chemotherapy. Am J Clin Oncol. 12(1):68-74, 1989
3. Ensminger WD et al: Regional cancer chemotherapy. Cancer Treat Rep. 68(1):101-15, 1984
4. Kaplan WD et al: Pulmonary uptake of technetium 99m macroaggregated albumin: a predictor of gastrointestinal toxicity during hepatic artery perfusion. J Clin Oncol. 2(11):1266-9, 1984
5. Buchwald H et al: Intraarterial infusion chemotherapy for hepatic carcinoma using a totally implantable infusion pump. Cancer. 45(5):866-9, 1980

IMAGE GALLERY

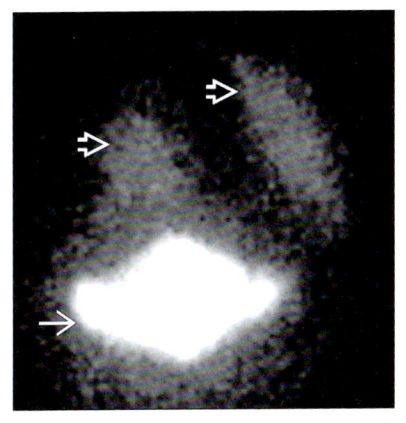

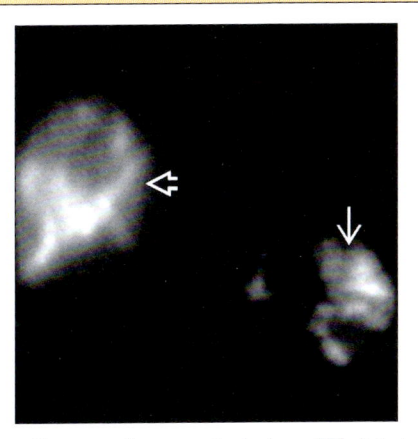

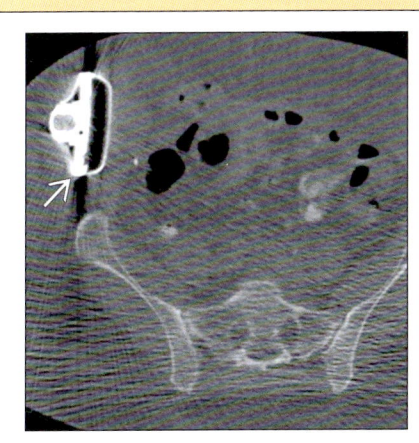

(Left) Anterior HAPS shows activity in liver ➡ as well as a small amount in the lungs ➡. Arteriovenous malformations in hepatic tumor may result in MAA shunting to the lungs. This does not indicate malpositioned catheter. (Center) Anterior HAPS shows deposition of radiotracer in the peritoneum ➡, indicating tracer administered outside pump. Hepatic activity ➡ evident after proper administration of tracer. (Right) Axial CT shows malposition of hepatic arterial infusion pump ➡, which had to be repositioned surgically.

Dr. med. Doris Kirschstein
FACHARZT FÜR NUKLEARMEDIZIN
FACHARZT FÜR DIAGNOSTISCHE RADIOLOGIE

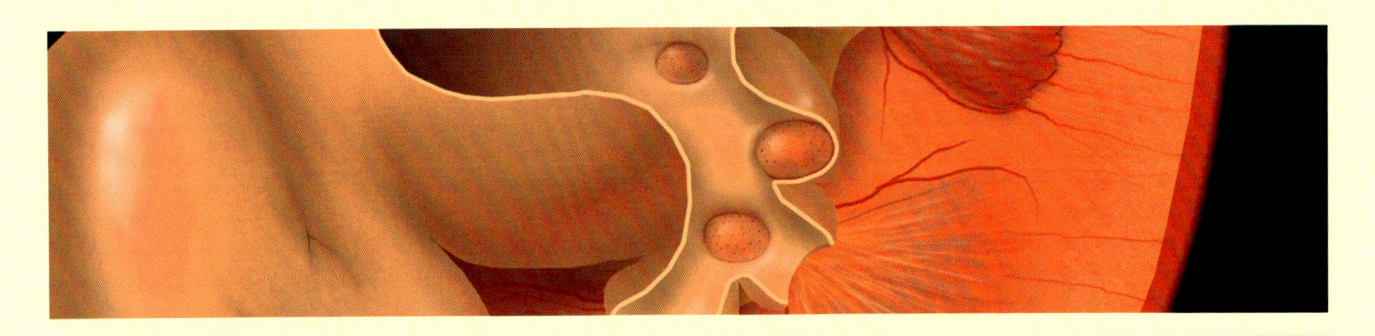

SECTION 9: Genitourinary

Kidney

Renal Cortical Scar	9-2
Renal Ectopy	9-6
Renovascular Hypertension	9-10
Acute Renal Failure	9-14
Renal Masses	9-20
Renal Cell Carcinoma	9-22
Pyelonephritis	9-26
Renal Transplant	9-30
Renal Function Quantification	9-36

Collecting System

Obstructive Uropathy	9-40
Reflux Uropathy	9-44
Urinary Bladder & Epithelial Cancer	9-48

Testes

Testicular Torsion	9-52
Testicular Cancer	9-56

Ovaries

Ovaries, Normal & Benign Pathology	9-60
Ovarian Cancer	9-62

Uterus

Uterus, Normal & Benign Pathology	9-66
Cervical Cancer	9-68
Endometrial Cancer	9-72

Prostate

Prostate Cancer, Antibody Scan	9-76

RENAL CORTICAL SCAR

Coronal SPECT DMSA renal scan shows enlarged central photopenia due to reflux-induced hydronephrosis ➔, and a focal defect in the superolateral cortex ➔, consistent with scar.

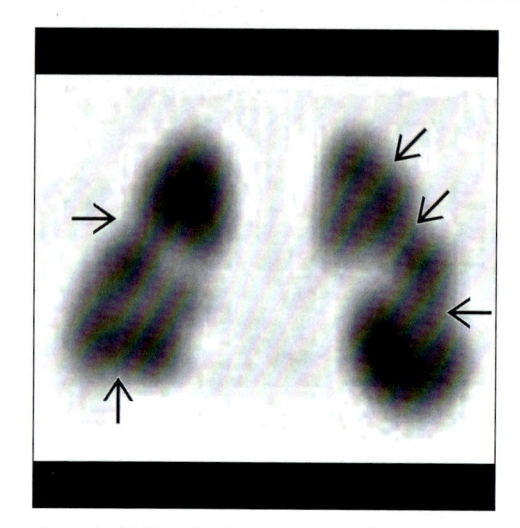

Coronal DMSA SPECT renal scan shows multiple bilateral cortical defects ➔ consistent with multiple scars in a patient with bilateral high grade reflux and multiple previous urinary tract infections.

TERMINOLOGY

Abbreviations and Synonyms
- Renal cortical scar; renal cortical infarct

Definitions
- Infarction or scarring of the renal cortex

IMAGING FINDINGS

General Features
- Best diagnostic clue: Focal absence of DMSA uptake in renal cortex; not due to mass or acute inflammation
- Location: Upper > lower > mid pole for pyelonephritis, vesicoureteral reflux (VUR) induced
- Size: All or part of kidney

Nuclear Medicine Findings
- Tc-99m dimercaptosuccinic acid (DMSA) scan
  - DMSA scan: Gold standard for renal cortical scar/infarct
  - Main cause of renal scar: Acute pyelonephritis, VUR
  - VUR induced renal scarring
    - VUR: Found in > 58% of children with 1st time acute pyelonephritis & scars on DMSA
    - Male patients with high grade reflux presenting with first UTI: Nearly half have renal parenchymal damaged as shown by DMSA scars
    - DMSA scars correlate with ↑ grade VUR: Indication for surgical correction rather than watchful waiting, prophylactic antibiotics
    - New DMSA scars with UTI despite antibiotic prophylaxis: Indication for surgical correction
    - High grade VUR without UTI: DMSA scars in 65%
    - Recommendations for DMSA scan in VUR: ↑ Grade reflux (grade ≥ 3); reflux with recurrent UTI
  - Pyelonephritis induced renal scarring
    - Acute pyelonephritis: Striated appearance on DMSA; deep lesions extending to hilum (scarring tends to be more superficial)
    - Acute 1st time pyelonephritis (< 1 week): DMSA imaging demonstrates cortical abnormalities in 50-79% (US misses 61% of these)
    - Acute pyelonephritis DMSA defects: Many resolve by 6 weeks

DDx: Mimics of Renal Cortical Scar

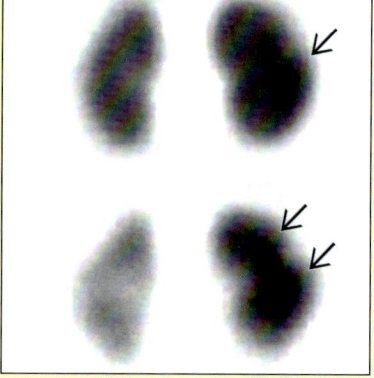

Persistent Fetal Lobulation

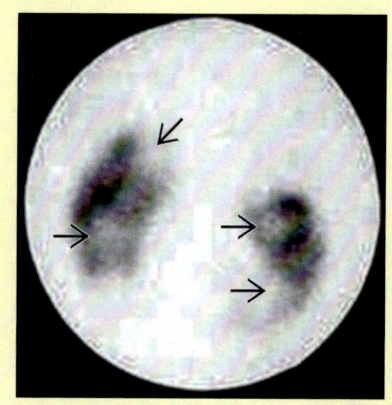

Renal Cysts

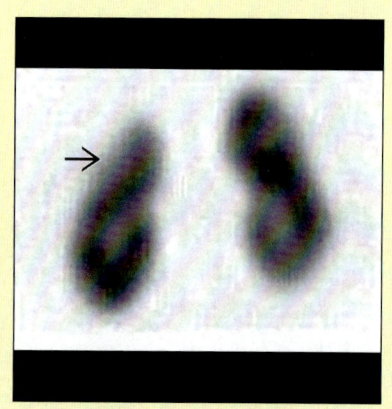

Splenic Impression (Lt)

RENAL CORTICAL SCAR

Key Facts

Terminology
- Infarction or scarring of the renal cortex

Imaging Findings
- Location: Upper > lower > mid pole for pyelonephritis, vesicoureteral reflux (VUR) induced
- DMSA scan: Gold standard for renal cortical scar/infarct
- Main cause of renal scar: Acute pyelonephritis, VUR
- High grade VUR without UTI: DMSA scars in 65%
- Recommendations for DMSA scan in VUR: ↑ Grade reflux (grade ≥ 3); reflux with recurrent UTI
- Acute pyelonephritis: Striated appearance on DMSA; deep lesions extending to hilum (scarring tends to be more superficial)
- Acute pyelonephritis DMSA defects: Many resolve by 6 weeks
- SPECT: Employ conscious sedation of children if necessary to insure lack of motion

Top Differential Diagnoses
- Pyelonephritis
- Renal Masses
- Renal Cyst
- Splenic Impression
- Polyarteritis Nodosa
- Fetal Lobulation

Clinical Issues
- Gender: Pyelonephritis & VUR: M:F (1:2)
- Pyelonephritis and reflux induced renal scarring: Major predisposing factor for proteinuria, hypertension, ultimate renal failure

---

- Late post-pyelonephritis (12-24 months): Resolution of 50% of DMSA defects apparent at ≤ 6 months
- Persistent DMSA scars after acute pyelonephritis: Justifies evaluation for identification, correction of underlying structural abnormalities
- Pyelonephritis-induced renal scarring in absence of VUR: Many children may have abnormal bladder dynamics
- Vascular insult, embolization, trauma: DMSA useful in assessing extent of damage, residual functioning renal mass
- Labeled WBC scan: Identification of acute pyelonephritis in complicated cases
  - In-111 WBC scan: No normal uptake in kidneys; ↑ uptake sensitive & specific for pyelonephritis
  - Tc-99m HMPAO WBC scan: Normal uptake in kidneys & bladder; ↓ sensitivity, specificity for pyelonephritis
- Ga-67 citrate scan: Incidental identification of renal infection when patient scanned for other reasons
  - Sensitive but not specific for acute pyelonephritis
  - Normal symmetrical Ga-67 renal uptake up to 48 h post injection
  - Bilateral renal Ga-67 uptake > 48 h post injection: Renal insufficiency & interstitial nephritis; mimic diffuse acute pyelonephritis
  - Focal increased Ga-67 uptake: Acute pyelonephritis, lymphoma, leukemia, mets

Imaging Recommendations
- Best imaging tool
  - DMSA renal scan with SPECT
    - Identifying renal parenchymal lesions following acute pyelonephritis
    - Identify renal parenchymal scarring in patients with VUR, esp. with "breakthrough UTI"
    - Evaluation of renal function post VUR surgical correction: Differential renal DMSA uptake, scar assessment
    - Identify cortical infarction following trauma, embolic event, vascular injury
- Protocol advice
  - Tc-99m DMSA scan
    - DMSA: 40-65% injected dose bound to proximal convoluted tubule 2 h post injection
    - Careful review of history, correlative imaging
    - 40-50 µCi/kg (children), minimum activity 350 µCi; 5 mCi (adults); IV
    - Posterior & anterior supine planar image at 2 h post injection: Differential renal function by geometric mean
    - High or ultra-high resolution collimator; 300-500 K/image
    - SPECT: Employ conscious sedation of children if necessary to insure lack of motion
    - Bilateral posterior oblique pinhole images: If SPECT cannot be performed
    - Renal tubular acidosis: ↓ DMSA concentration in cortex, ↑ urinary excretion
    - Renal failure: ↑ Hepatic clearance
  - Tc-99m glucoheptonate scan
    - Glucoheptonate: 10-20% bound to proximal convoluted tubule at 2 h, remainder excreted glomerular filtration
    - 80-120 µCi/kg (children), minimum activity 500 µCi; 8.0 mCi (adults); IV
    - Initial renal scan to evaluation flow, function
    - Delayed planar/SPECT at 2-4 h post injection
- Correlative imaging features
  - CECT
    - Acute focal renal injury (pyelonephritis): Absent contrast enhancement
    - Chronic scarring: Focal region of cortical thinning
    - CECT shows similar sensitivity, specificity to DMSA scan: Higher radiation, risk from intravenous contrast
  - US
    - Focal region of cortical thinning or echogenic cortex on grayscale
    - Absent signal on power Doppler ultrasound (PDU)
    - Acute pyelonephritis: US negative in 61% of renal units abnormal by DMSA
    - Post pyelonephritis: DMSA detects scars in 35% of kidneys reported as normal by US

RENAL CORTICAL SCAR

- MR
  - Coronal T1WI FS MR: Best sequence for detecting renal scars
  - Sensitivity 77%, specificity 87% for renal scars using DMSA as gold standard
- IVP
  - DMSA detects 4x as many renal lesions as IVP

DIFFERENTIAL DIAGNOSIS

Pyelonephritis
- Cortical scarring: Defects more superficial
- Pyelonephritis: Defects extend to hilum

Renal Masses
- Focal region of absent DMSA uptake ± mass effect

Renal Cyst
- Rounded region of absent DMSA

Splenic Impression
- Smooth indentation along anterior aspect of left renal upper pole may mimic scar

Polyarteritis Nodosa
- Striated appearance: Mimic acute pyelonephritis

Fetal Lobulation
- Focal indentation between lobules may mimic scar

Interstitial Nephritis
- May mimic diffuse bilateral pyelonephritis on Ga-67

PATHOLOGY

General Features
- Etiology
  - Pyelonephritis
    - Underlying reflux in 1/3 of pediatric patients
    - E. Coli > Klebsiella

CLINICAL ISSUES

Presentation
- Most common signs/symptoms: Acute pyelonephritis: Fever, abdominal pain, irritability (infants), frequency, strong smelling urine
- Other signs/symptoms: Renal cortical scarring silent until renal insufficiency

Demographics
- Gender: Pyelonephritis & VUR: M:F (1:2)

Natural History & Prognosis
- Pyelonephritis and reflux induced renal scarring: Major predisposing factor for proteinuria, hypertension, ultimate renal failure
- High risk variables for renal parenchymal damage with VUR: History of UTIs, reflux grade, age at diagnosis

Treatment
- Acute pyelonephritis: 7-14 d course of antibiotics; may start IV and switch to oral (prophylactic with documented VUR)
- VUR: Watchful waiting in ↓ grade (80% of patients "outgrow"); surgical/endoscopic correction in ↑ grade

DIAGNOSTIC CHECKLIST

Image Interpretation Pearls
- DMSA scan: Gold standard for renal scar detection

SELECTED REFERENCES

1. Agras K et al: Resolution of cortical lesions on serial renal scans in children with acute pyelonephritis. Pediatr Radiol. 37(2):153-8, 2007
2. Basiratnia M et al: Power Doppler sonographic evaluation of acute childhood pyelonephritis. Pediatr Nephrol. 21(12):1854-7, 2006
3. Temiz Y et al: The efficacy of Tc99m dimercaptosuccinic acid (Tc-DMSA) scintigraphy and ultrasonography in detecting renal scars in children with primary vesicoureteral reflux (VUR). Int Urol Nephrol. 38(1):149-52, 2006
4. Ataei N et al: Evaluation of acute pyelonephritis with DMSA scans in children presenting after the age of 5 years. Pediatr Nephrol. 20(10):1439-44, 2005
5. Kavanagh EC et al: Can MRI replace DMSA in the detection of renal parenchymal defects in children with urinary tract infections? Pediatr Radiol. 35(3):275-81, 2005
6. Taskinen S et al: Post-pyelonephritic renal scars are not associated with vesicoureteral reflux in children. J Urol. 173(4):1345-8, 2005
7. Ataei N et al: Screening for vesicoureteral reflux and renal scars in siblings of children with known reflux. Pediatr Nephrol. 19(10):1127-31, 2004
8. Lin KY et al: Acute pyelonephritis and sequelae of renal scar in pediatric first febrile urinary tract infection. Pediatr Nephrol. 18(4):362-5, 2003
9. Szlyk GR et al: Incidence of new renal parenchymal inflammatory changes following breakthrough urinary tract infection in patients with vesicoureteral reflux treated with antibiotic prophylaxis: evaluation by 99MTechnetium dimercapto-succinic acid renal scan. J Urol. 170(4 Pt 2):1566-8; discussion 1568-9, 2003
10. Cascio S et al: Renal parenchymal damage in male infants with high grade vesicoureteral reflux diagnosed after the first urinary tract infection. J Urol. 168(4 Pt 2):1708-10; discussion 1710, 2002
11. McLaren CJ et al: Vesico-ureteric reflux in the young infant with follow-up direct radionuclide cystograms: the medical and surgical outcome at 5 years old. BJU Int. 90(7):721-4, 2002
12. Schiepers C et al: Surgical correction of vesicoureteral reflux: 5-year follow-up with 99Tcm-DMSA scintigraphy. Nucl Med Commun. 22(2):217-24, 2001
13. Vega-P JM et al: High-pressure bladder: an underlying factor mediating renal damage in the absence of reflux? BJU Int. 87(6):581-4, 2001
14. Goldman M et al: The etiology of renal scars in infants with pyelonephritis and vesicoureteral reflux. Pediatr Nephrol. 14(5):385-8, 2000
15. Nguyen HT et al: 99m Technetium dimercapto-succinic acid renal scintigraphy abnormalities in infants with sterile high grade vesicoureteral reflux. J Urol. 164(5):1674-8; discussion 1678-9, 2000

RENAL CORTICAL SCAR

IMAGE GALLERY

Typical

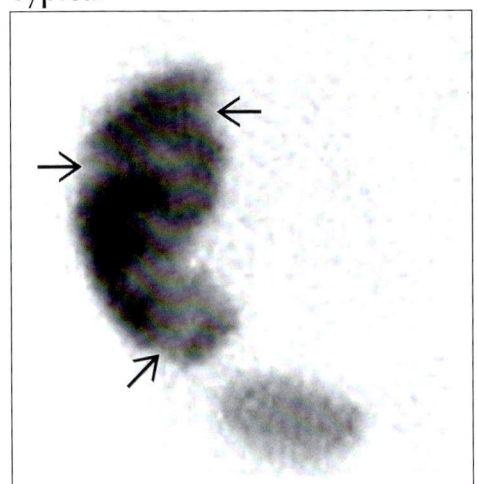

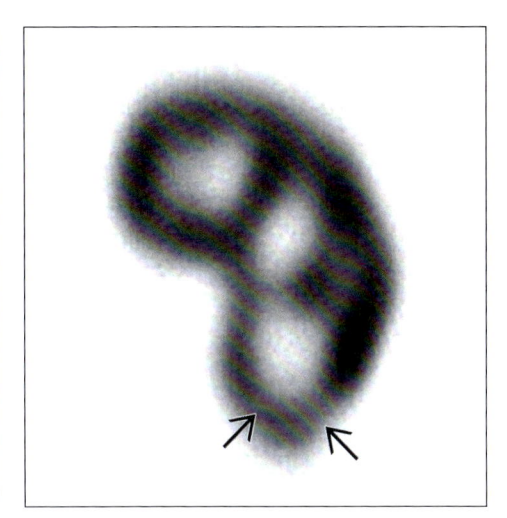

(Left) Anterior planar glucoheptonate renal scan in a transplant shows multiple cortical defects ➔ consistent with chronic rejection & renal scarring. (Right) Coronal DMSA renal scan in a left renal transplant shows thinning of cortex in the inferior pole ➔, but no frank areas of cortical scarring.

Variant

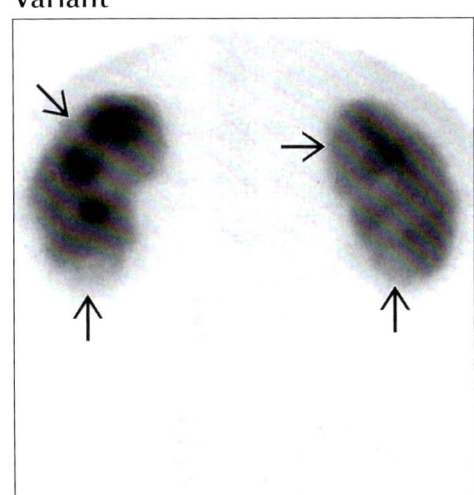

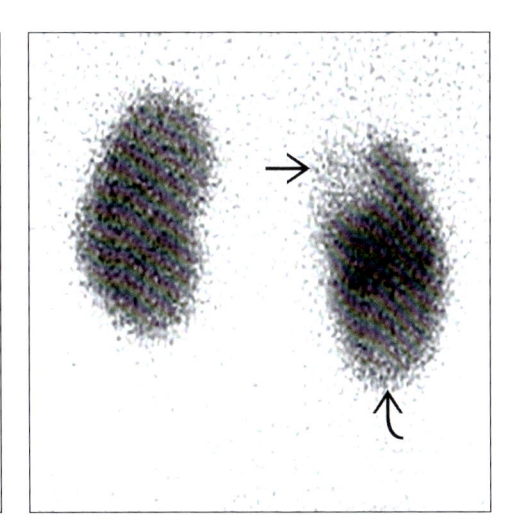

(Left) Coronal SPECT DMSA renal scan shows bilateral striated nephrogram in a patient with bilateral acute diffuse pyelonephritis. Areas of decreased uptake ➔ correspond to sites of severe inflammation. (Right) Posterior planar glucoheptonate renal scan shows focal absence of activity in the superior pole of the right kidney ➔ due to renal abscess, decreased activity in lower pole ➔ due to inflammation.

Other

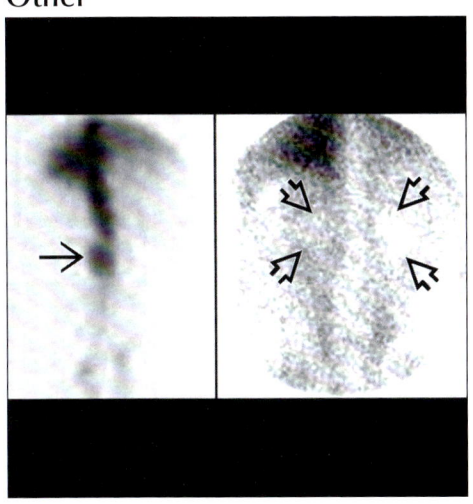

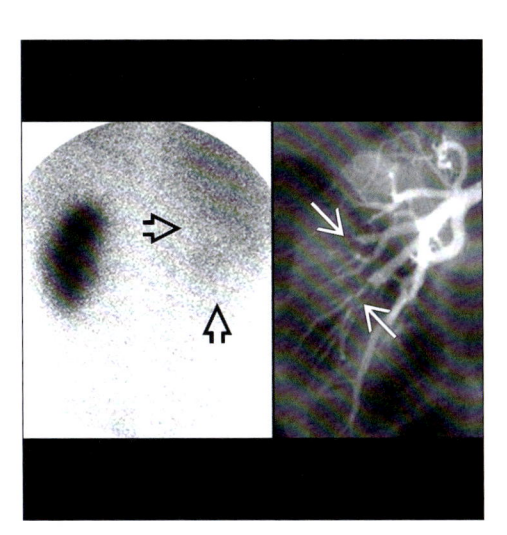

(Left) Posterior angiographic image (left) and delayed nephrogram phase (right) DTPA renal scan shows abdominal aortic aneurysm ➔ which has dissected, infarcting both kidneys, which are photopenic ➔. (Right) Posterior DMSA renal scan of the kidneys shows infarcted right kidney ➔. Angiogram shows vascular truncation, multiple vascular filling defects ➔ (emboli due to atrial fibrillation).

RENAL ECTOPY

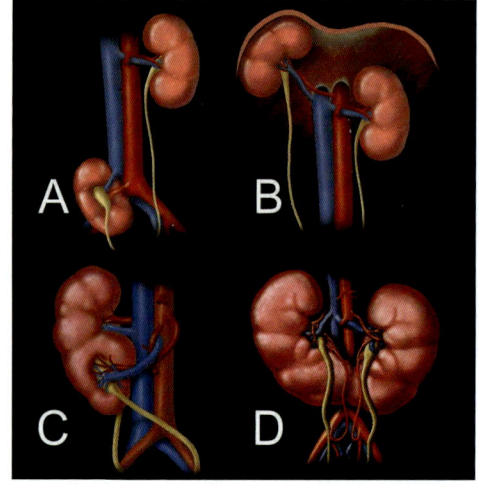

Graphic shows examples of the most common anomalies of renal ectopy and fusion. (A) pelvic kidney, (B) thoracic kidney, (C) crossed fused ectopia, and (D) horseshoe kidney.

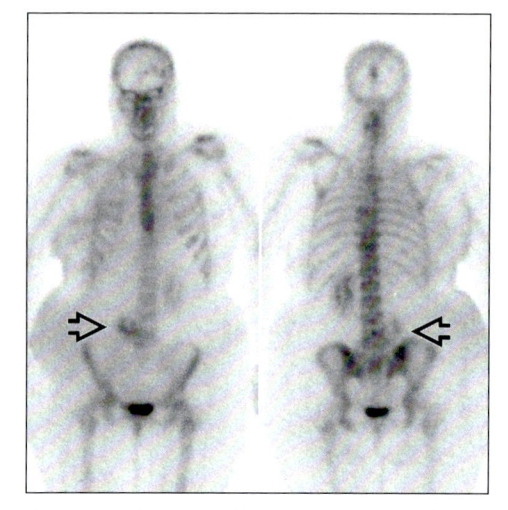

Anterior and posterior bone scan shows a lumbar kidney. Renal ectopias are frequently incidental findings as in this patient in whom metastatic disease was the indication for the study.

TERMINOLOGY

Abbreviations and Synonyms
- Horseshoe kidney, crossed (with or without fusion) ectopia, simple renal ectopia, thoracic kidney

Definitions
- Normal renal tissue outside of the expected location in the retroperitoneum
  - Often asymptomatic with diagnosis being incidental
- Horseshoe kidney
  - Fusion of the inferior poles by a parenchymal or fibrous isthmus
    - 5% of horseshoe kidneys have fused superior poles
    - During development, the isthmus is trapped under the inferior mesenteric artery halting ascent
- Crossed ectopia (with or without fusion)
  - Kidney is located on the side opposite from which its ureter inserts into bladder
  - 90% are fused to the contralateral kidney
- Simple renal ectopia (or caudad renal ectopia)
  - Due to failure of embryonic renal ascent
  - Often categorized by location (pelvic, lumbar, abdominal)
- Thoracic kidney (or cephalad renal ectopia)
  - Partial or complete protrusion of the kidney above the level of the diaphragm into the posterior mediastinum but not in pleural space

IMAGING FINDINGS

General Features
- Best diagnostic clue: Normal kidney seen outside of the expected location and/or abnormally oriented on any imaging modality
- Location: Variable, from pelvis to thorax, and may cross the midline
- Size: Size and shape often normal but may vary with location
- Morphology
  - Identical to functional homotopic renal parenchyma
  - Variable and unpredictable vascular supply

Nuclear Medicine Findings
- Frequently an incidental finding on bone scan or renal imaging
  - Abnormally located or oriented functional renal parenchyma

DDx: Mimics of Renal Ectopia

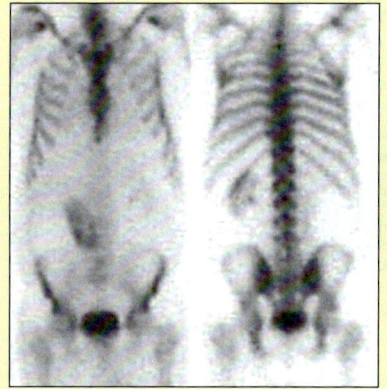

Retroperitoneal Hematoma 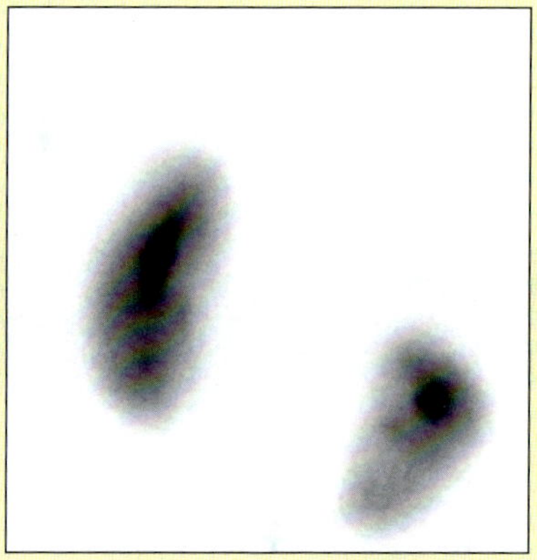 *Ptotic Kidney Upright* 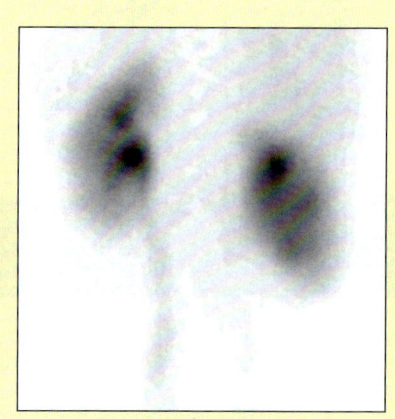 *Ptotic Kidney Supine*

RENAL ECTOPY

Key Facts

Terminology
- Horseshoe kidney, crossed (with or without fusion) ectopia, simple renal ectopia, thoracic kidney
- Normal renal tissue outside of the expected location in the retroperitoneum
- Often asymptomatic with diagnosis being incidental

Imaging Findings
- Best diagnostic clue: Normal kidney seen outside of the expected location and/or abnormally oriented on any imaging modality
- Frequently an incidental finding on bone scan or renal imaging
- Abnormally located or oriented functional renal parenchyma

Pathology
- > 50% of ectopic kidneys have a hydronephrotic collecting system
- Vesicoureteral reflux incidence reported to be as high as 70% and varies with type of ectopy
- Blood supply can be anomalous for all types of renal ectopy

Clinical Issues
- Most are incidental findings at autopsy, on routine perinatal screenings, or on other diagnostic imaging

Diagnostic Checklist
- Horseshoe kidneys may be subtle if isthmus is fibrous
- Ectopic renal tissue overlying an osseous structure on a bone scan may mimic a bone lesion

---

- MAG-3, DTPA, or glucoheptonate renal studies may show obstruction if present in addition to localizing the renal tissue
- DMSA or glucoheptonate studies to evaluate for infection or scarring will also localize renal tissue
- Bone scans may show secondary evidence of hydronephrosis or obstruction

Radiographic Findings
- Radiography
  o Ectopic kidney may mimic an abdominal or pelvic mass or alter bowel gas pattern
  o Thoracic kidneys can be mistaken for tumors
- IVP: Characterize ureteral abnormalities

CT Findings
- NECT
  o Soft tissue mass similar to normal renal tissue
  o May see associated hydronephrosis or stone disease
- CECT: Normal renal enhancement and contrast excretion unless complicated by obstruction

Angiographic Findings
- Characterizes variant arterial supply

Ultrasonographic Findings
- Normal renal echo texture
  o Appearance can be altered by scarring or hydronephrosis
  o Pelvic kidneys may be difficult to identify due to overlying bowel gas

Imaging Recommendations
- Best imaging tool
  o If renal ectopy is an incidental finding, the initial study may have already provided definitive diagnostic information
    ■ Additional functional information can be provided by nuclear medicine (MAG-3, DMSA, glucoheptonate, or DTPA)
    ■ Additional anatomic information can be provided by various anatomic imaging modalities
- Protocol advice
  o Posterior planar images are the preferred orientation for most renal imaging
    ■ Ectopic kidneys may lie more anteriorly in abdomen or be located in front of spine or pelvis necessitating additional anterior and/or oblique planar imaging or SPECT

DIFFERENTIAL DIAGNOSIS

Renal Transplant
- Typically placed in the right or left iliac fossa

Nephroptosis
- Downward displacement of kidney by more than two vertebral bodies or 5 cm when patient changes position from supine to erect

Kidney Displaced by a Space Occupying Lesion
- Adrenal masses, hematoma

PATHOLOGY

General Features
- Genetics
  o Case reports of dominant familial inheritance of cross-fused ectopia
  o Horseshoe kidney is associated with numerous genetic diseases
- Etiology
  o Horseshoe kidney and crossed ectopia
    ■ Mechanism unknown
  o Simple renal ectopy
    ■ Failure of renal ascent
  o Thoracic kidney
    ■ Possibly due to delayed closure of the diaphragm allowing for protracted renal ascent or due to accelerated ascent
- Epidemiology
  o Horseshoe kidney: 1 in 500 births
  o Crossed ectopia: 1 in 1300 to 7500

RENAL ECTOPY

- Simple renal ectopia: 1 in 900 in autopsy studies
  - Pelvic kidney: 1 in 2100 to 3000 in autopsy studies
- Thoracic kidney
  - Fewer than 5% of renal ectopias
- Associated abnormalities
  - Increased incidence of genital abnormalities in most varieties of renal ectopy
    - Hypospadias, cryptorchidism, agenesis of uterus and vagina, unicornuate uterus, imperforate anus
  - > 50% of ectopic kidneys have a hydronephrotic collecting system
  - Vesicoureteral reflux incidence reported to be as high as 70% and varies with type of ectopy
    - Crossed ectopia: Reflux frequently occurs in the collecting system of the ectopic kidney
  - Horseshoe kidney
    - Up to 1/3 of patients have at least one other abnormality, most commonly skeletal anomalies, cardiovascular defects (primarily ventriculoseptal defects), and central nervous defects (neural tube defects)
    - Found in as many as 60% of females with Turner syndrome

Gross Pathologic & Surgical Features
- Blood supply can be anomalous for all types of renal ectopy
- In crossed ectopia, left kidney more commonly (2:1) crosses midline and fuses with inferior pole of right kidney
  - Normal ureter insertion is maintained

Microscopic Features
- Ectopic kidney is histologically identical to the normally located kidney

CLINICAL ISSUES

Presentation
- Most common signs/symptoms
  - Most are incidental findings at autopsy, on routine perinatal screenings, or on other diagnostic imaging
  - If symptomatic, most commonly present with UTI, abdominal pain, or fever
- Other signs/symptoms
  - Palpable abdominal mass, hematuria, incontinence, renal insufficiency, hypertension
  - Simple ectopy can be at increased risk for trauma as the ectopic kidney is not protected by rib cage

Demographics
- Age
  - Variable age at presentation
  - Horseshoe kidneys are more prevalent in children
    - May be due to high incidence of associated congenital anomalies, some of which are incompatible with long term survival
- Gender
  - Simple renal ectopy shows no sex difference in autopsy studies
  - Horseshoe and crossed ectopia 2:1 male

Natural History & Prognosis
- Wilms tumors 2-4x more frequent in children with horseshoe kidneys
  - More frequently in isthmus leading some to suggest fusion is due to teratogenic factors
- No clinical reports of serious urinary or pulmonary complications associated with thoracic kidneys

Treatment
- None required for the majority of patients, otherwise symptomatic treatment as necessary

DIAGNOSTIC CHECKLIST

Image Interpretation Pearls
- Horseshoe kidneys may be subtle if isthmus is fibrous
  - Only clue might be abnormal orientation of collecting systems and kidneys (lower poles closer than upper poles)
- Fused portion of a horseshoe kidney is usually anterior to the vessels and spine and is often better seen on anterior planar images
- Ectopic renal tissue overlying an osseous structure on a bone scan may mimic a bone lesion
- Nephroptosis can be differentiated from renal ectopia by imaging upright and supine
  - Ptotic kidney will be located more caudad, more ventral, and often with lower pole rotated more medial on the upright image and in near normal position on the supine image

SELECTED REFERENCES

1. Guarino N et al: Natural history of vesicoureteral reflux associated with kidney anomalies. Urology. 65(6):1208-11, 2005
2. Guarino N et al: The incidence of associated urological abnormalities in children with renal ectopia. J Urol. 172(4 Pt 2):1757-9; discussion 1759, 2004
3. Kao PF et al: The 99mTc-DMSA renal scan and 99mTc-DTPA diuretic renogram in children and adolescents with incidental diagnosis of horseshoe kidney. Nucl Med Commun. 24(5):525-30, 2003
4. Glassberg KI: Normal and abnormal development of the kidney: a clinician's interpretation of current knowledge. J Urol. 167(6):2339-50; discussion 2350-1, 2002
5. Walsh PC: Campbell's Urology. 8th ed. Philadelphia, Saunders. 1894-1906, 2002
6. Rinat C et al: Familial inheritance of crossed fused renal ectopia. Pediatr Nephrol. 16(3):269-70, 2001
7. Kumar R et al: Nephroptosis: the Tc-99m glucoheptonate scan as a diagnostic method. Clin Nucl Med. 25(6):473, 2000
8. Decter RM: Renal duplication and fusion anomalies. Pediatr Clin North Am. 44(5):1323-41, 1997
9. Gleason PE et al: Hydronephrosis in renal ectopia: incidence, etiology and significance. J Urol. 151(6):1660-1, 1994
10. Jolles PR et al: Crossed renal ectopia. Correlative imaging. Clin Nucl Med. 17(4):306-7, 1992
11. Gordon I: Indications for 99mtechnetium dimercapto-succinic acid scan in children. J Urol. 137(3):464-7, 1987
12. LaManna MM et al: The radionuclide diagnosis of horseshoe kidney. Clin Nucl Med. 10(11):799-803, 1985

RENAL ECTOPY

IMAGE GALLERY

Typical

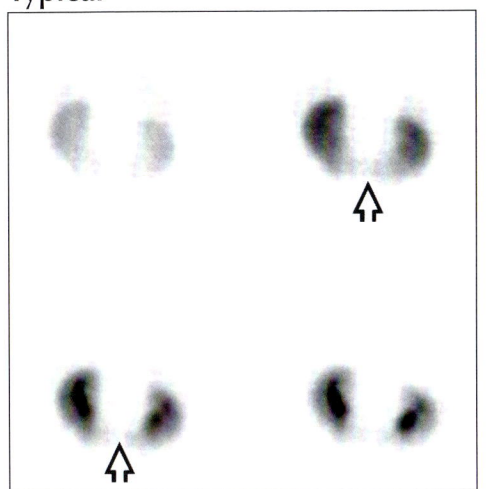

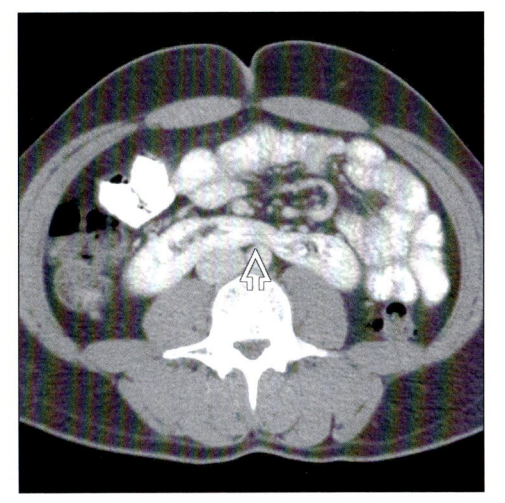

(Left) Anterior renal scan using MAG-3 shows abnormally oriented kidneys connected by an isthmus of functional parenchyma ⇨, characteristic for a horseshoe fusion anomaly. *(Right)* Axial CECT of the same patient as previous image shows normal renal parenchymal enhancement ⇨ in the horseshoe isthmus. Attenuation from the vertebra can mask the isthmus on posterior nuclear imaging.

Typical

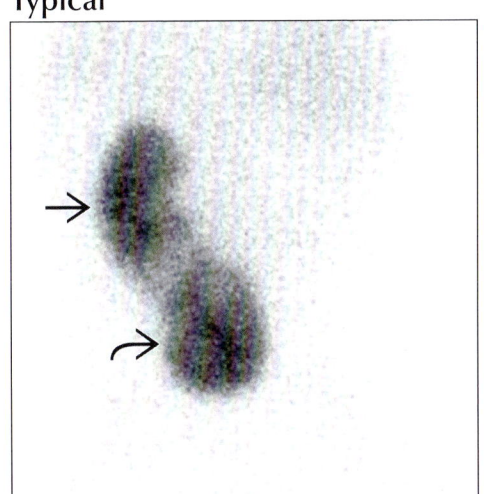

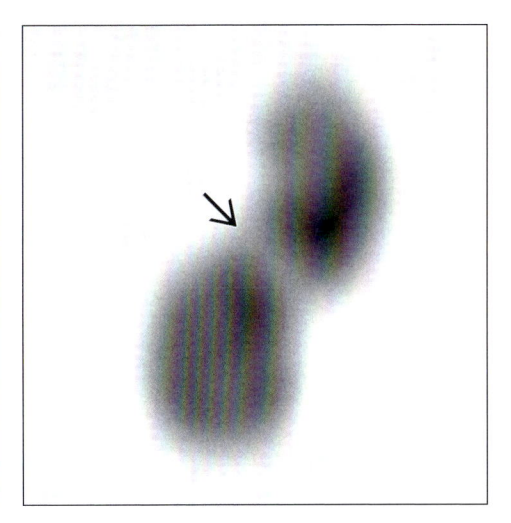

(Left) Posterior Tc-99m DMSA renal scan demonstrates cross-fused ectopia in left abdomen. Left kidney ⇨. Crossed-fused right kidney is inferior ⇨. *(Right)* Coronal SPECT image of a Tc-99m DMSA scan (same patient as previous image) demonstrates crossed fused ectopia. There is a thin rim of functioning tissue connecting the two kidneys ⇨.

Typical

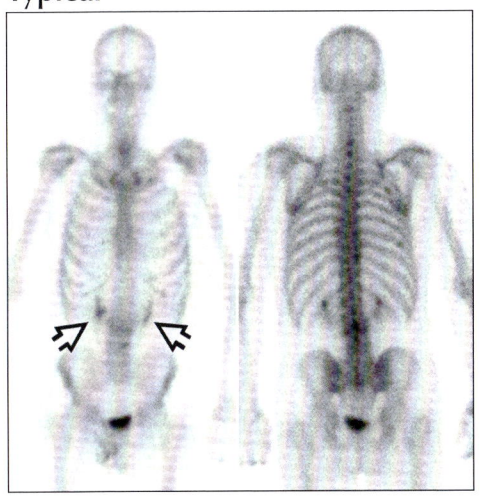

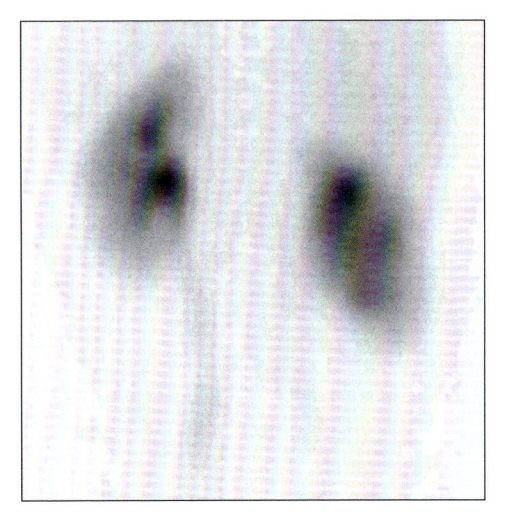

(Left) Bone scan shows abnormal orientation of the renal collecting systems and approximation of the lower poles ⇨. This can be the only clue to horseshoe kidney when the isthmus is not seen. *(Right)* Posterior renal scan with MAG-3 on the same patient, now imaged supine. Note the more normal orientation of the right kidney. This is characteristic of nephroptosis.

RENOVASCULAR HYPERTENSION

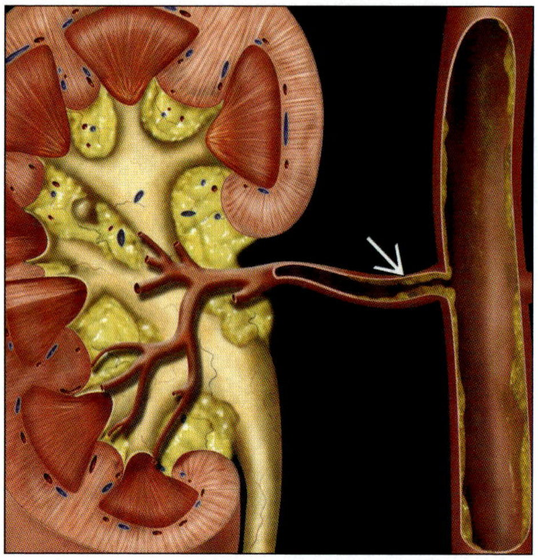

Graphic shows luminal renal artery narrowing ➡ from atherosclerosis, the most common cause of RAS, a condition which may result in RVHT.

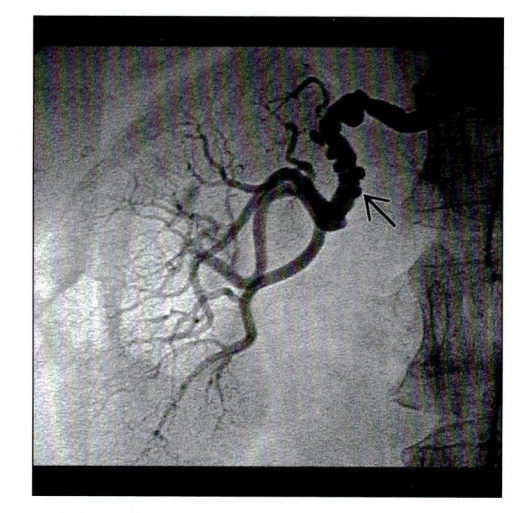

Right renal arteriogram of medial fibroplasia, a less common cause of RVHT, shows classic string of beads appearance ➡. (Courtesy S. Saddekni, MD).

TERMINOLOGY

Abbreviations and Synonyms
- Renovascular hypertension (RVHT), renal artery stenosis (RAS)

Definitions
- Hypertension (HTN) caused by hemodynamically significant RAS activating renin-angiotensin system
- Renin-angiotensin system increases renal blood flow when renal hypoperfusion detected
  - Diminished renal blood flow causes ↑ renin secretion by renal juxtaglomerular cells
  - Renin converts angiotensin I from liver to active enzyme angiotensin II
  - Angiotensin II raises systemic blood pressure by ↑ vascular tone & ↑ aldosterone secretion which ↑ water retention
    - ↑ Blood pressure maintains renal perfusion and glomerular filtration rate (GFR)
- Angiotensin-converting enzyme inhibitor (ACE-I) drugs prevent formation of angiotensin II causing renal function to fall in patients with RVHT
  - ACE-I antihypertensive medications (e.g., captopril & enalapril) are used to identify RVHT on renogram
- Renovascular disease left untreated can result in RVHT, renal failure, end-stage renal disease
  - Not all RAS leads to RVHT & treating RAS does not always reverse HTN

IMAGING FINDINGS

General Features
- Best diagnostic clue: ACE-I renogram showing functional deterioration after ACE-I administration when compared to baseline renogram
- Morphology
  - Renal artery luminal narrowing > 50% for anatomical significance
  - ≥ 75% luminal narrowing usually required for hemodynamic effect; may not cause clinical symptoms until narrowing much more severe

Nuclear Medicine Findings
- Baseline renogram (without ACE-I)

DDx: Retention of Radiotracer on Renogram

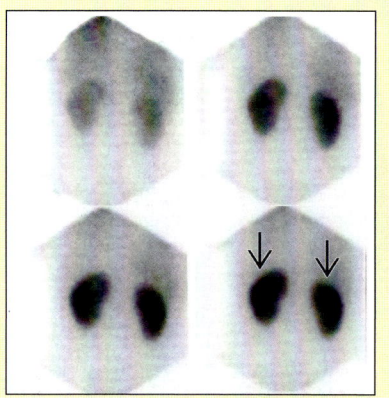

Acute Tubular Necrosis 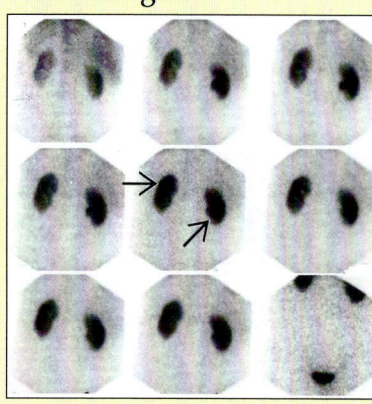 | Dehydration 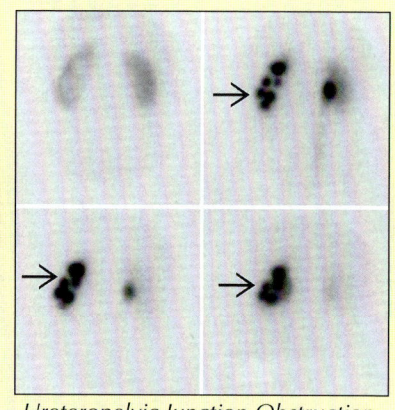 | Ureteropelvic Junction Obstruction

RENOVASCULAR HYPERTENSION

Key Facts

Terminology
- Renin-angiotensin system increases renal blood flow when renal hypoperfusion detected
- ↑ Blood pressure maintains renal perfusion and glomerular filtration rate (GFR)
- Angiotensin-converting enzyme inhibitor (ACE-I) drugs prevent formation of angiotensin II causing renal function to fall in patients with RVHT
- ACE-I antihypertensive medications (e.g., captopril & enalapril) are used to identify RVHT on renogram

Imaging Findings
- Best diagnostic clue: ACE-I renogram showing functional deterioration after ACE-I administration when compared to baseline renogram
- ACE-I renogram: Excellent detection of clinically significant RAS; sens > 90% & spec 95% in those with good renal function
- Renogram using Tc-99m DTPA: Shows an overall decrease in uptake and function of kidney with RAS after ACE-I
- Renogram using Tc-99m MAG3: Shows significant cortical retention of radiotracer in kidney with RAS after ACE-I

Diagnostic Checklist
- 2-day protocol: If ACE-I renogram performed first is normal, no need to perform baseline renogram = no RVHT
- Protocol pitfalls: Poor absorption of ACE-I, dehydration, hypotension, effects of full bladder

---

- ○ Blood flow usually not perceptibly altered; nonspecific small kidney or ↓ function could be seen but scan often normal
- ○ Nonspecific: Any abnormality could be caused by numerous etiologies (e.g., obstruction)
- ACE-I renogram: Excellent detection of clinically significant RAS; sens > 90% & spec 95% in those with good renal function
  - ○ Patients w/o RVHT show no significant change from baseline
  - ○ Functional deterioration after ACE-I compared to baseline identifies patients with reversible RVHT with high accuracy
  - ○ Angiographic phase unreliable: Technically difficult to perform, flow often normal or ↓ due to low tissue volume in small kidneys
- Time activity curves (TAC) and renal function images will vary depending on radiopharmaceutical
- Renogram using Tc-99m DTPA: Shows an overall decrease in uptake and function of kidney with RAS after ACE-I
  - ○ Renal excretion of DTPA exclusively by glomerular filtration & directly reflects GFR
- Renogram using Tc-99m MAG3: Shows significant cortical retention of radiotracer in kidney with RAS after ACE-I
  - ○ MAG3 excreted by tubular secretion so drop in GFR does not affect uptake

CT Findings
- CTA
  - ○ Vessel narrowing/calcification
  - ○ May delineate accessory renal arteries
  - ○ Technical limitations from motion or poor contrast bolus not infrequent
  - ○ Contraindicated when creatinine elevated
  - ○ Limited functional information

Angiographic Findings
- Arteriogram: "Gold standard" to identify RAS; clinical symptoms, successful therapy may not correlate with anatomic finding
- Angioplasty or stenting can be attempted during same session as diagnostic procedure
- Pressure gradients measured across stenosis useful for accurate diagnosis
- Renal artery angiography generally reserved for cases with high clinical suspicion for HTN caused by RAS
  - ○ Potential side effects may be serious including hematoma, contrast reactions (allergic, renal failure), dissection

MR Findings
- MRA
  - ○ Renal artery visualization without ionizing radiation or iodinated contrast risks
  - ○ Caution must be exercised utilizing gadolinium contrast in patients with renal failure

Ultrasonographic Findings
- Doppler peak systolic velocity > 1.8-2.0 m/s or kidney/aortic ratio > 3.5 suggests RAS

Imaging Recommendations
- Protocol advice
  - ○ Patient preparation
    - All ACE-I should be stopped 3-7 days prior to exam; if medications not terminated, sensitivity decreases (~ 15-17%)
    - Stopping diuretics and calcium channel blockers preferable, if safe
    - Hydrate patient orally
    - IV access throughout exam useful, particularly for patients with cardiovascular disease or concern for hypotension post ACE-I
    - Empty bladder immediately before exam
    - Position patient supine with camera posterior for native kidneys & anterior for renal transplant
  - ○ Radiotracer: MAG3 adults 3-5 mCi (110-185 MBq), child 100 μCi/kg (1 mCi min); DTPA 15 mCi (555 MBq), child 200 μCi/kg
  - ○ Choose 1-day or 2-day protocol depending on clinical suspicion or patient population

RENOVASCULAR HYPERTENSION

- 2-day protocol (low probability of disease): ACE-I scan 1st; if abnormal, baseline scan 1-2 days later; routine radiotracer dose used for each exam
- 1-day protocol (high probability of disease): 1-2 mCi (37-74 MBq) low-dose baseline followed by 5-10 mCi (185-370 MBq) high dose ACE-I scan
- ACE-I
  - Captopril: 25-50 mg PO (may crush tablets), monitor blood pressure at least Q15 min for 1 hr; patient should be NPO 4-6 hr for best absorption
  - Enalapril: 40 µg/kg IV up to 2.5 mg given over 3-5 min beginning 15 min before exam
- Diuretic: Furosemide (40 mg) during imaging may improve accuracy of exam
- Acquisition
  - Camera: Low-energy, parallel hole collimator; 15-20% photopeak centered at 140 keV
  - Computer: Blood flow 1-2 sec frames/60 seconds & dynamic 30 sec frames for 25-30 min; prevoid, postvoid static images
- Processing: Regions of interest over closest adjacent vessel (iliac artery) & around kidney with background area near/around kidney
- Interpretation: Probability of RVHT caused by RAS graded as low, intermediate, or high
  - Low probability (< 10%): Pre & post-renograms normal or no change in mildly abnormal curve
  - Intermediate (indeterminate) probability: No change in scan appearance from abnormal baseline
    - ↓ Relative function 5-9%, usually with DTPA
    - Small poorly functioning kidney (< 30%) may not respond appropriately
    - Symmetric bilateral abnormalities most often due to factors such as dehydration
    - Cortical retention, ratio counts at 20 to 3 minutes (20/3 ratio) ~ 0.1-0.5
  - High probability (> 90%)
    - MAG3: ↑ Peak time (by 2-3 min or at least 40%); ↑ ratio of maximum counts over 20 min (max/20) or 20/3 ratio ≥ 0.15
    - DTPA: ↓ Peak and ↓ relative uptake/GFR ≥ 10%,
    - Significant change in differential rarely seen with MAG3 compared to DTPA

DIFFERENTIAL DIAGNOSIS

Hypertension
- Essential (idiopathic) hypertension, most common cause of HTN
- RVHT: Incidence ~ 3-5%; 0.5% of general population, ~ 45% of selected hypertensive populations

Renal Failure
- Acute renal failure: Acute tubular necrosis (ATN), obstruction, trauma
- Chronic renal failure: End result of renal insult with irreversible loss of function

PATHOLOGY

General Features
- Etiology
  - RVHT due to atherosclerosis: 70-90% of cases, variable response to therapy with angioplasty
  - RVHT due to medial fibroplasia (fibromuscular dysplasia): Accounts for most remaining cases of RVHT
    - Noninflammatory arterial disease more common in women; "string of beads" on angiogram; often responds well to angioplasty

CLINICAL ISSUES

Presentation
- Most common signs/symptoms
  - Diagnosis based on clinical presentation difficult
  - HTN presenting at an early age, malignant or resistant to therapy
  - Severe renal dysfunction, azotemia, hypokalemia, atrophic kidney
  - Unexplained CHF, sudden pulmonary edema
- Other signs/symptoms: Angina, multivessel coronary artery disease, peripheral vascular disease

Demographics
- 30-50% normotensive patients may have moderate to severe RAS
- 7% population > 65 years have RAS

Natural History & Prognosis
- Untreated RVHT leads to irreversible renal damage, may cause chronic renal failure
- Rapid identification and therapy required to prevent irreversible damage

Treatment
- Vascular stent and angioplasty most common treatment options
- Trials comparing medical therapy with stenting & angioplasty under way

DIAGNOSTIC CHECKLIST

Consider
- 2-day protocol: If ACE-I renogram performed first is normal, no need to perform baseline renogram = no RVHT
- Protocol pitfalls: Poor absorption of ACE-I, dehydration, hypotension, effects of full bladder

SELECTED REFERENCES

1. Cooper CJ et al: Stent revascularization for the prevention of cardiovascular and renal events among patients with renal artery stenosis and systolic hypertension: rationale and design of the CORAL trial. Am Heart J. 152(1):59-66, 2006
2. Taylor AT Jr et al: Procedure guideline for diagnosis of renovascular hypertension. Society of Nuclear Medicine. J Nucl Med. 39(7):1297-302, 1998
3. Taylor A et al: Consensus report on ACE inhibitor renography for detecting renovascular hypertension. Radionuclides in Nephrourology Group. Consensus Group on ACEI Renography. J Nucl Med. 37(11):1876-82, 1996

RENOVASCULAR HYPERTENSION

IMAGE GALLERY

Typical

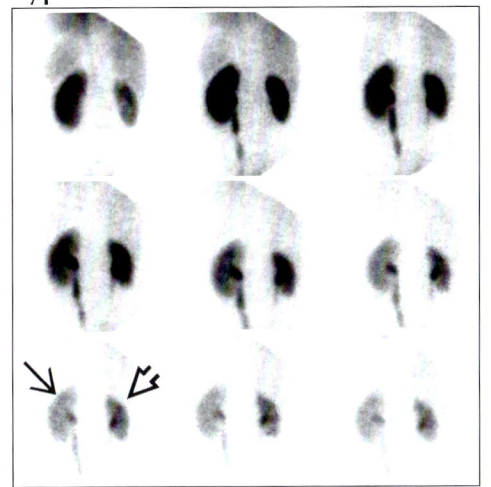

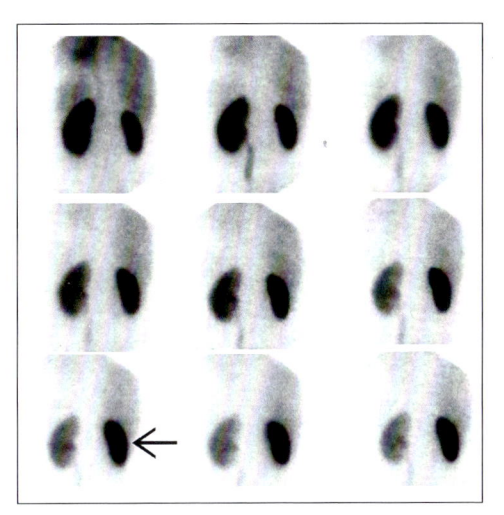

(Left) Baseline renogram shows a nonspecific finding: Smaller right kidney ⇨ with lower overall function when compared to left ⇨. See next image. (Right) Following captopril, renogram (same patient as previous image) shows smaller right kidney ⇨ with functional deterioration characterized by severe cortical retention, indicating RVHT.

Typical

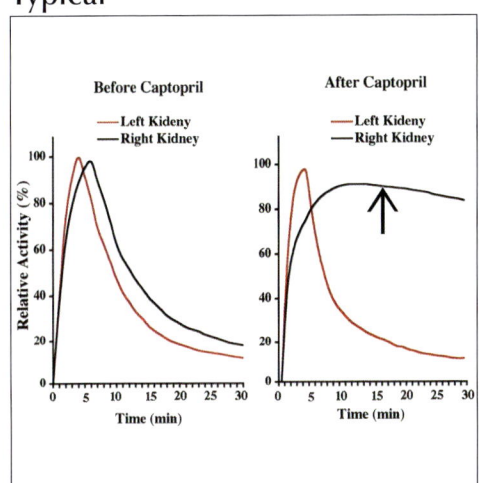

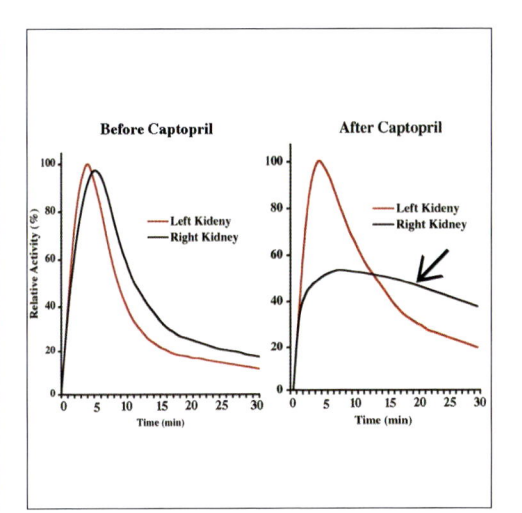

(Left) Tc-99m MAG3 time activity curves (TAC) show typical cortical retention ⇨ seen after ACE-I administration in a patient with RVHT from right RAS. See next image. (Right) In contrast with pattern seen using MAG3, TACs reveal decreased peak activity and overall function ⇨ that occurs on Tc-99m DTPA during ACE-I renogram in a patient with RVHT due to right RAS.

Typical

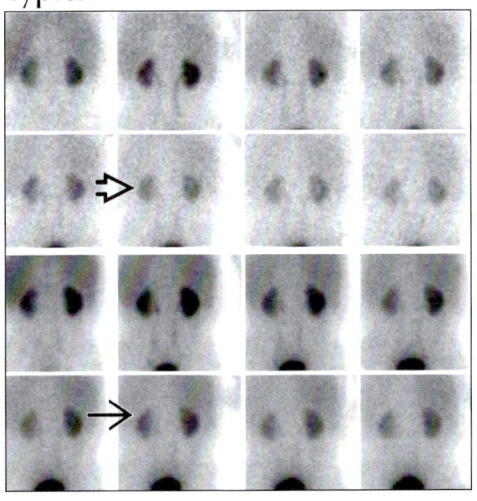

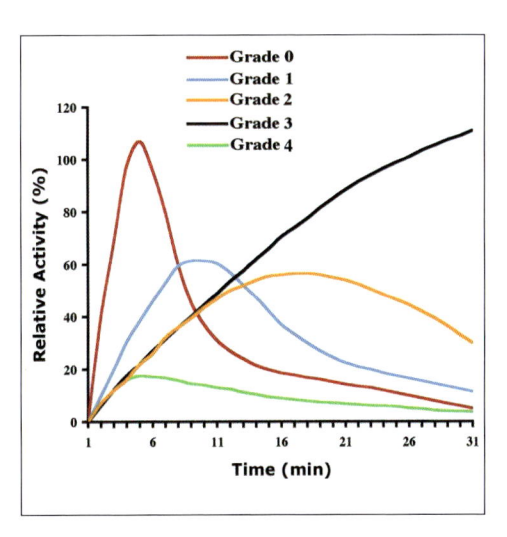

(Left) Renogram shows small left kidney ⇨ on baseline renogram with no difference on ACE-I renogram ⇨, indicating chronic ischemia without reversible RVHT. (Right) TAC patterns in ACE-I renography depend on level of function levels and disease presence. Grade 0 is normal; grade 1-3 show progressively prolonged renal transit; grade 4 indicates some perfusion but no excretion.

ACUTE RENAL FAILURE

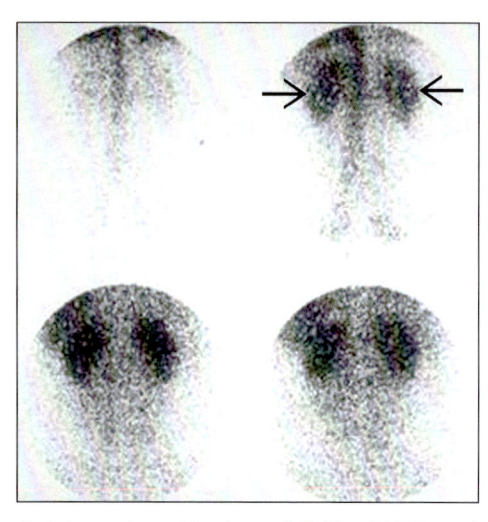

Posterior angiographic phase of Tc-99m MAG3 renal scan shows prompt, symmetrical blood flow to both kidneys ➔ in a patient with mild-moderate ATN from chemotherapy. See next image for nephrogram phase.

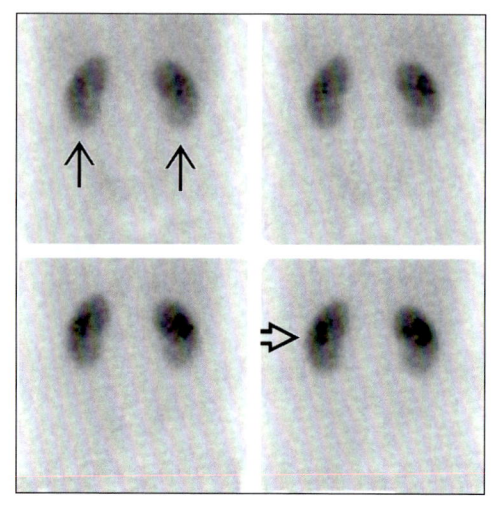

Posterior renographic phase of Tc-99m MAG3 shows symmetric, bilateral delayed uptake ➔ but reduced excretion ⇨ (rising nephrogram pattern) in a patient with mild-moderate ATN from chemotherapy.

TERMINOLOGY

Definitions
- Acute renal failure (ARF)
  - Acutely ↓ renal function; recovery possible
  - Measured by serum creatinine, serum urea, or glomerular filtration rate (GFR)
  - Causes: Prerenal (perfusion), intrinsic renal, postrenal (obstructive)
- Chronic renal failure (CRF)
  - Long-term renal disease, generally irreversible

IMAGING FINDINGS

Imaging Recommendations
- Best imaging tool
  - Renal scan with glomerular filtration rate (GFR) or effective renal plasma flow (ERPF)
    - Useful in ARF for diagnosis and prognosis
    - Tc-99m DTPA: Glomerular filtration, < clearance than tubular agents; used to calculate GFR
    - Tc-99m MAG3: Tubular secretion; better images than Tc-99m DTPA; estimate ERPF
- Protocol advice
  - Patient preparation
    - Hydration: Patient should be well-hydrated (500 ml oral or 7-10 mL/kg over 30-60 min IV)
    - Empty bladder: Patient voids immediately prior to injection, bladder catheter if necessary
    - Position: Supine with camera posterior; anterior for transplanted, horseshoe kidneys
  - Consider diuretics when concern for obstruction (furosemide dose based on creatinine level)
  - Consider ACE inhibitor scan when concern for renal artery stenosis (RAS) as a cause for renovascular hypertension (RVHT)
    - Captopril 25-50 mg oral; enalaprilat 40 µg/kg IV
  - Radiopharmaceutical: Tc-99m MAG3 3-5 mCi (110-185 MBq) IV or Tc-99m DTPA 10-15 mCi (370-555 MBq) IV
    - MAG-3 preferred in face of severe renal insufficiency: DTPA extraction efficiency poor
  - Camera: Low energy collimator, wide field of view camera to include kidneys, at least some bladder
  - Acquisition: 1-2 sec frames for 60 sec then 30 sec frames for 25-30 min, obtain pre- and post-void images of kidneys and bladder

DDx: Chronic Renal Disease Mimicking Acute Renal Failure

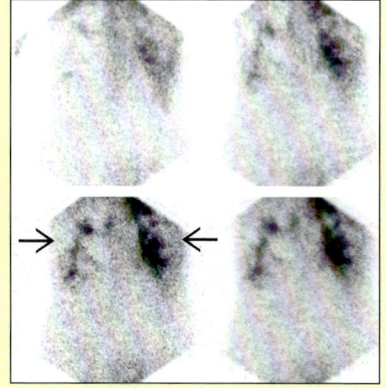

Polycystic Kidneys 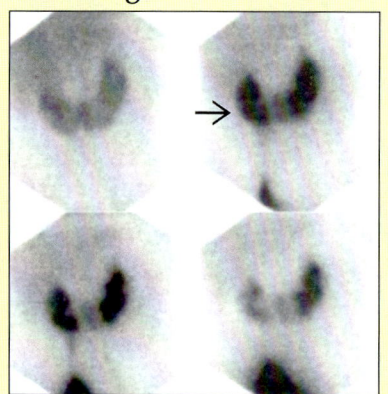 | *Horseshoe Kidney* 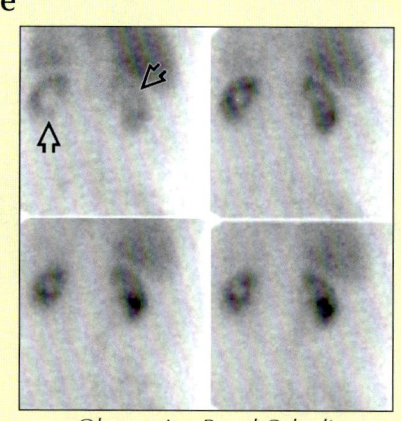 | *Obstructing Renal Calculi*

ACUTE RENAL FAILURE

Key Facts

Terminology
- Causes: Prerenal (perfusion), intrinsic renal, postrenal (obstructive)

Imaging Findings
- Tc-99m DTPA: Glomerular filtration, < clearance than tubular agents; used to calculate GFR
- Tc-99m MAG3: Tubular secretion; better images than Tc-99m DTPA; estimate ERPF
- Prerenal failure: Heart failure, hypovolemia, hypotension, dehydration
- Most intrinsic renal diseases: Non-specific decreased flow/function on renal scan
- Mild-moderate ATN: Blood flow relatively normal, rising (delayed) nephrogram phase
- Severe ATN, frank cortical necrosis: Poor blood flow; decreased or absent cortical uptake
- Pyelonephritis: Patchy striated scintigraphic nephrogram, poor clearance
- Catastrophic vascular occlusion: Lack of flow/function to involved kidney
- Renal vein thrombosis: Asymmetrically enlarged "hot" kidney; may mimic obstruction
- Over time, radiotracer & cortical uptake falls
- Acute complete obstruction: May not visualize collecting system
- Bladder outlet obstruction: Often non-specific ↓ flow, function

Top Differential Diagnoses
- Urine Leak
- Chronic Renal Failure

- Processing
  - Region of interest (ROI) around kidneys & on aorta, place background ROI around kidneys to generate time activity curves (TAC)
  - Calculate kidney to aorta blood flow ratio (K/A ratio), time to peak (Tmax), ratio of activity at 20 min to 3 min (20/3) or 20 min: Peak
  - Calculate split renal function at 1-3 min
- Quantitative nuclear medicine imaging options
  - Quantitative renal analysis (ERPF/GFR)
    - Perform radiopharmaceutical quality control & use only high quality agent (> 95% purity) to ensure accurate results
    - Calibrate dose and count post-injection syringe to determine the correct injected dose for counting
    - Correct pediatric results for body surface area
    - Blood sample method: Draw blood from arm opposite injection, measure activity using scintillation counter, results vary ~ 10%
    - External counting (camera) methods: Count calibrated dose at some distance from camera surface (30 cm), results vary ~ 20%
  - ERPF: Tc-99m MAG3
    - Blood sample at 44 min or determine renal uptake with camera at 1-2 min
  - GFR: Tc-99m DTPA
    - Blood sample at 3 hr (2-4 hr) or determine renal uptake with camera at 2-3 min
    - GFR more widely used by nephrologists than ERPF
- Interpretation
  - ARF: Various patterns may be seen, but ↓ uptake or delayed cortical clearance common
  - Blood flow: Changes on angiogram phase may be difficult to document, generally nonspecific, highly technically dependent (bolus)
  - Peak uptake: Peak activity may be ↓ in ARF particularly with DTPA or if underlying chronic renal disease has caused cortical loss
  - Cortical clearance: ↓ Output seen with both DTPA & MAG3; retention may be very prominent with MAG3 in ARF
  - Output: Obstructive causes will lead to collecting system retention that does not respond to diuretic administration
  - Bladder emptying: Distended bladder on postvoid image suggests bladder outlet obstruction/neurogenic bladder
    - Repeat exam with bladder catheter to confirm impact on kidneys
  - CRF: Generally associated with diminished uptake in a small, scarred kidney
- Specific patterns: Specific cause of ARF usually not identifiable by renal scan
  - Prerenal failure: Heart failure, hypovolemia, hypotension, dehydration
    - Prolonged or severe ↓ prerenal insult may lead to ischemia and cell death
    - Renal scan shows ↓ flow, delayed nephrogram due to ↓ radiotracer delivery & clearance
    - Concentration by kidney variable: Good concentration portends chance for recovery
  - Intrinsic renal disease: May involve glomeruli, tubules, or interstitium
    - Examples: Hemolytic uremic syndrome, acute glomerulonephritis, acute interstitial nephritis
    - Biopsy generally needed for glomerular processes, little role for imaging
    - Most intrinsic renal diseases: Non-specific decreased flow/function on renal scan
  - Acute tubular necrosis (ATN): Perfusion maintained initially and imaging pattern depends on choice of radiotracer; may recover after 1-2 weeks
    - DTPA: Early vascular blush creating an artificially early peak but no true accumulation or excretion
    - MAG3: Cortical retention with increasing activity over time
    - Risk factors: ↑ Age, underlying renovascular disease with ↑ creatinine, diuretics, vasoconstrictors (NSAIDs, COX-2 inhibitors)
    - Mild-moderate ATN: Blood flow relatively normal, rising (delayed) nephrogram phase
    - Severe ATN, frank cortical necrosis: Poor blood flow; decreased or absent cortical uptake

ACUTE RENAL FAILURE

- ○ Rhabdomyolysis: Myoglobin deposition may lead to renal failure with ↓ perfusion
  - ■ May show symmetrically "hot" kidneys on Tc-99m diphosphonate bone scan
- ○ Pyelonephritis: Patchy striated scintigraphic nephrogram, poor clearance
- Vascular causes of acute renal failure
  - ○ Catastrophic vascular occlusion: Lack of flow/function to involved kidney
  - ○ RAS: Atherosclerosis (90-95%); medial dysplasia/fibromuscular dysplasia (5-10%)
    - ■ Early identification & therapy can prevent irreversible damage
    - ■ Chronic ischemia leads to nephron loss & a small, shrunken kidney, ↓ overall function
    - ■ ACE-I renography (captopril scan) can identify renovascular hypertension (RVHT) 2° to RAS
    - ■ ACE-I renography: RVHT shows ↓ uptake/clearance on DTPA, ↓ clearance on MAG3
  - ○ Renal artery embolism, thrombosis
    - ■ Renal artery embolism: Typically unilateral or bilateral diffuse ↓ flow/function; wedge-shaped perfusion defects uncommon
  - ○ Renal vein thrombosis (RV)
    - ■ Renal vein thrombosis: Asymmetrically enlarged "hot" kidney; may mimic obstruction
    - ■ Causes include: Dehydration, malignancy, trauma, steroid use, systemic lupus erythematosus (SLE), nephrotic syndrome
    - ■ RV in renal transplant appears differently, lack of draining collaterals leads to absent perfusion and function
- Post renal obstruction
  - ○ Calculi, ureteropelvic junction (UPJ) obstruction, pelvic mass, pelvic radiation fibrosis, bladder outlet obstruction, neurogenic bladder
  - ○ Obstruction: Activity fills the dilated collecting system, poor clearance, even with diuretic
  - ○ Over time, radiotracer & cortical uptake falls
  - ○ Acute complete obstruction: May not visualize collecting system
  - ○ Marked hydronephrosis without obstruction: May not clear tracer even with diuretic; postural drainage maneuver helpful
  - ○ Bladder outlet obstruction: Often non-specific ↓ flow, function
  - ○ Ultrasound, IVP, or radiographs: Identify calculi, hydronephrosis, masses
  - ○ Repeat imaging helpful to monitor effects of therapy

DIFFERENTIAL DIAGNOSIS

Technical Factors
- May mimic ARF on renal scan: Poor bolus, extravasation of dose, radiopharmaceutical impurity

Urine Leak
- May mimic ARF: ↑ BUN, creatinine due to reabsorbed "recycled" creatinine; ↓ urine output

Ectopic or Ptotic Kidney
- May mimic unilateral renal failure if imaged only posteriorly

Chronic Renal Failure
- Poor flow & function, small kidneys

CLINICAL ISSUES

Presentation
- Most common signs/symptoms
  - ○ Hypovolemia: Thirst, dizziness, orthostatic hypotension, tachycardia, ↓ urine output
  - ○ Cardiac failure: Fluid retention, orthopnea, paroxysmal nocturnal dyspnea
  - ○ Fluid loss: Hemorrhage, GI losses, sweating, renal sources
  - ○ Intrinsic renal failure: Hematuria, edema, HTN, nephrotoxic medication/iodinated contrast
  - ○ Rhabdomyolysis: Tender muscles, recent coma, seizure
- Clinical Profile: Uremia: Pericarditis, encephalopathy, bleeding dyscrasia, nausea/vomiting, pruritus

Demographics
- Incidence: ~ 1% hospital admissions are for community-acquired ARF; up to 20% of critical care admissions develop hospital acquired ARF

Natural History & Prognosis
- Prognosis varies: Mortality may be as high as 50-70%, although prerenal etiologies are most often reversible (only ~ 7% mortality)

Treatment
- Hydration, critical care support, bladder catheter to relieve potential obstruction & measure urine output
- Dialysis for fluid overload, uremia, hyperkalemia/sodium imbalance
- Diuretics, vasodilators, and other medications may be utilized

DIAGNOSTIC CHECKLIST

Consider
- Renal vein thrombosis mimics acute high grade renal obstruction
- Mild-moderate ATN shows relatively normal blood flow, rising nephrogram phase on renal scan

Image Interpretation Pearls
- Hydration and bladder emptying maximizes accuracy of renal scan
- Most intrinsic renal diseases non-specific on renal scan

SELECTED REFERENCES

1. Taylor A: Radionuclide renography: a personal approach. Semin Nucl Med. 29(2):102-27, 1999
2. Taylor AT Jr et al: Procedure guideline for diagnosis of renovascular hypertension. Society of Nuclear Medicine. J Nucl Med. 39(7):1297-302, 1998
3. O'Reilly P et al: Consensus on diuresis renography for investigating the dilated upper urinary tract. Radionuclides in Nephrourology Group. Consensus Committee on Diuresis Renography. J Nucl Med. 37(11):1872-6, 1996

ACUTE RENAL FAILURE

IMAGE GALLERY

Typical

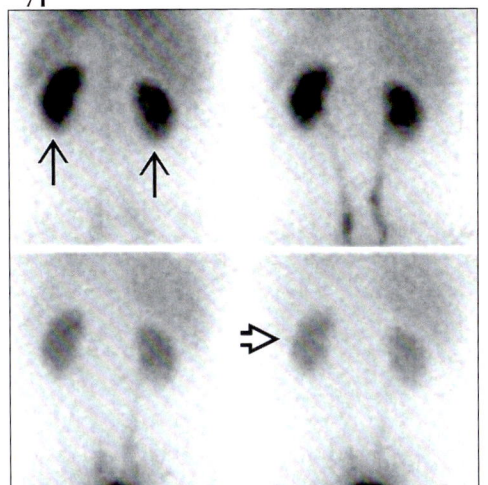

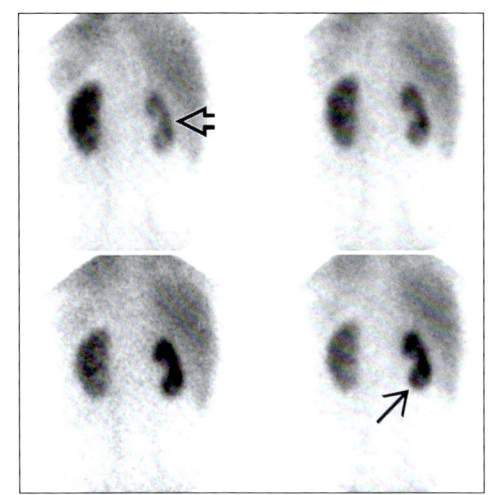

(Left) Normal posterior Tc-99m MAG3 renogram shows prompt symmetric uptake ➙ and clearance ▷ from the kidneys. The 20 minute:3 minute ratio was 0.25 (normal ≤ 0.3). (Right) Posterior captopril DTPA renogram of RAS causing RVHT. Notice delayed uptake ▷ & marked cortical retention ➙ in the affected right kidney.

Typical

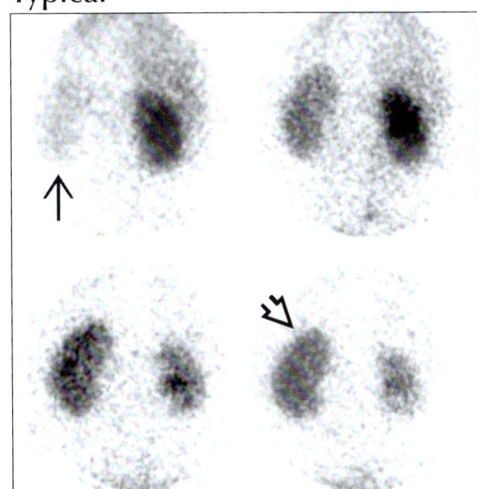

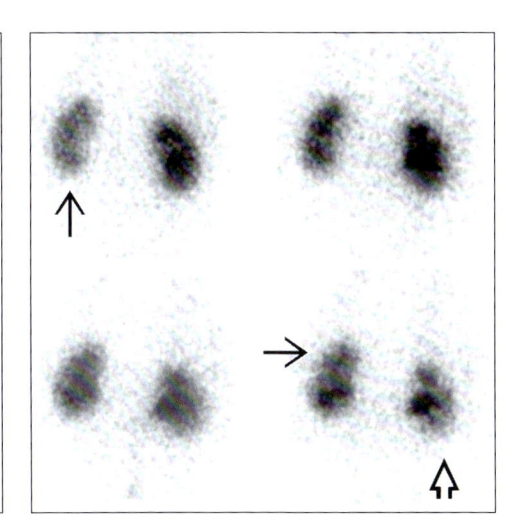

(Left) Posterior renogram shows enlarged left kidney with delayed uptake ➙ and no appreciable clearance ▷ in a patient with nephrotic syndrome and left renal vein thrombosis. See next image. (Right) Posterior renogram in same patient as previous, 4 months later, shows resolution of renal vein thrombosis and more normal function of left kidney ➙ compared to right kidney ▷.

Typical

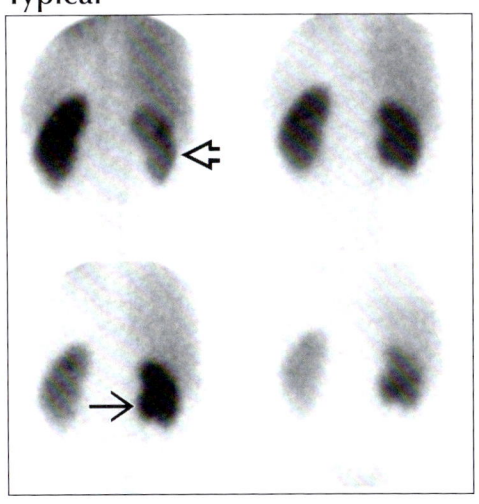

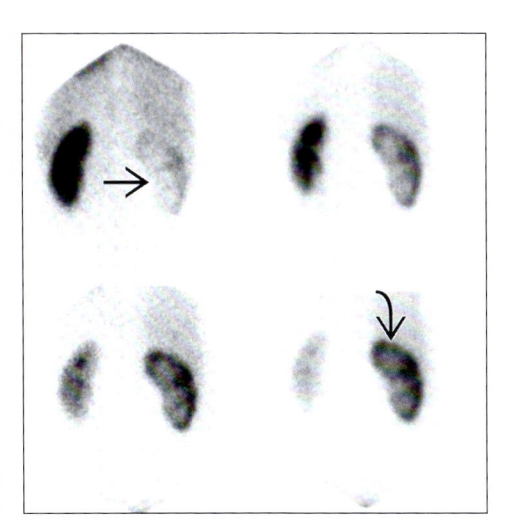

(Left) Posterior renogram shows small right kidney ▷, hydronephrosis, and delayed washout from cortex and collecting system due to chronic recurrent UPJ obstruction ➙. (Right) Posterior renogram shows enlarged right kidney, central photopenic defect ➙ due to hydronephrosis, and decreased cortical uptake and excretion ➙ due to acute obstruction.

ACUTE RENAL FAILURE

(Left) Posterior angiographic phase of renal scan shows abrupt cut-off of aorta ➡, and no obvious renal uptake in a patient with acute aortic occlusion due to atherosclerotic disease. See next image. (Right) Delayed nephrogram phase of renal scan shows only faint suggestion of renal activity ➡ in a patient with acute aortic occlusion due to atherosclerotic disease.

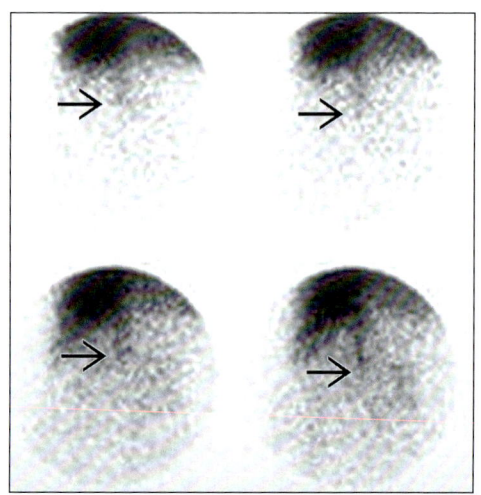

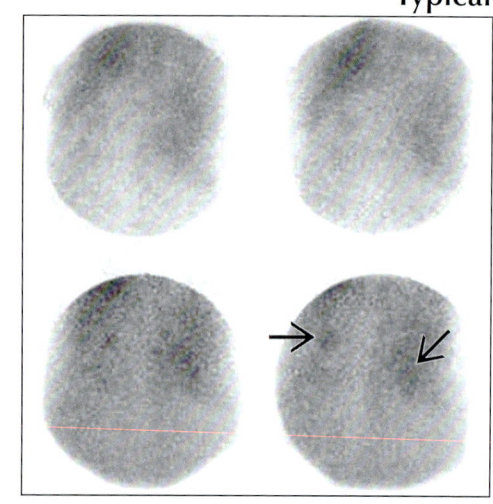

(Left) Posterior angiographic phase of renal scan in a patient with atrial fibrillation and acute thromboembolism of the right renal artery shows no appreciable flow to the right kidney. See next two images. (Right) Single posterior frame of renal scan at 15 min shows virtually no uptake in the right kidney ➡ due to acute thromboembolism of the right renal artery.

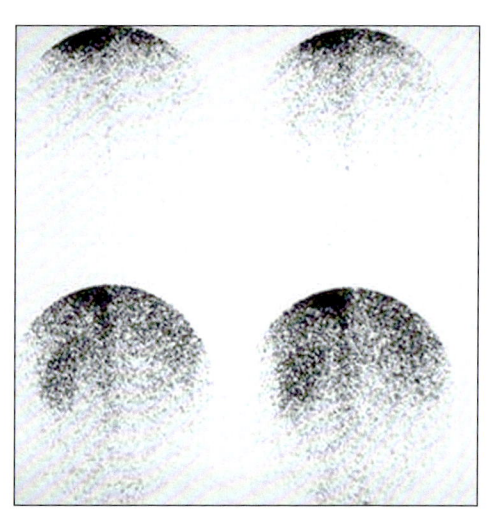

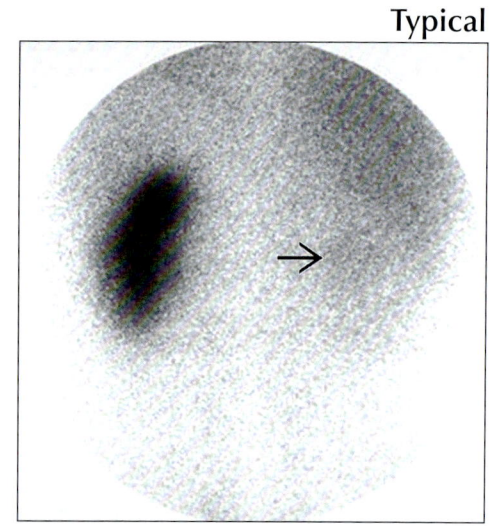

(Left) Right renal arteriogram shows filling defects ➡ and truncation ➡ of subsegmental branches of renal arteries in a patient with thromboembolism of the right renal artery due to atrial fibrillation. (Right) Posterior Tc-99m diphosphonate bone scan shows symmetrical increased uptake in renal parenchyma in a pattern typical of myoglobin deposition in tubules due to rhabdomyolysis.

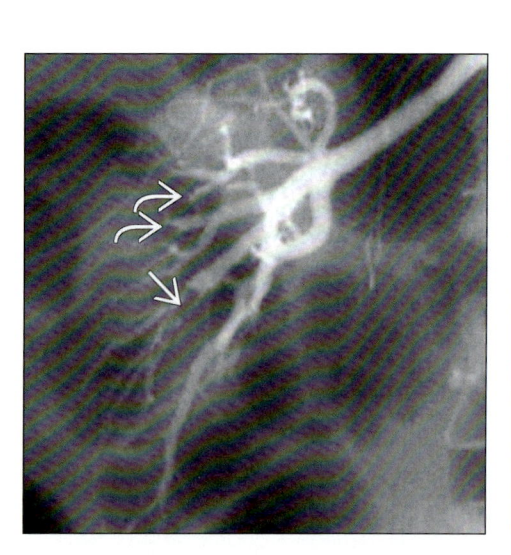

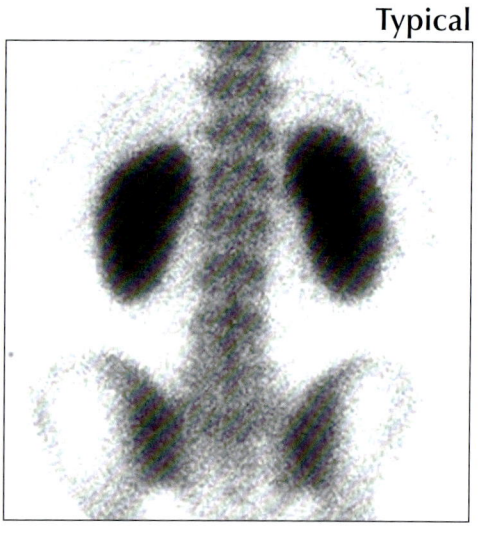

ACUTE RENAL FAILURE

Typical

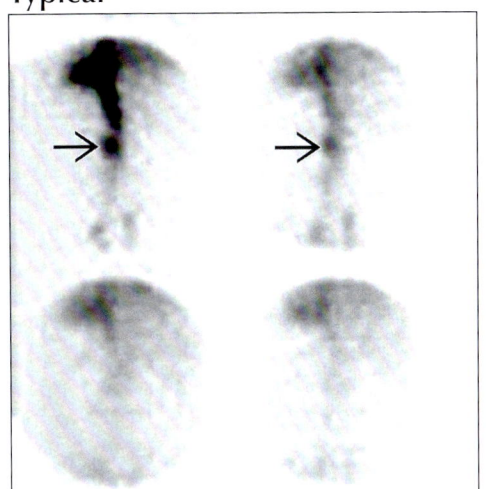

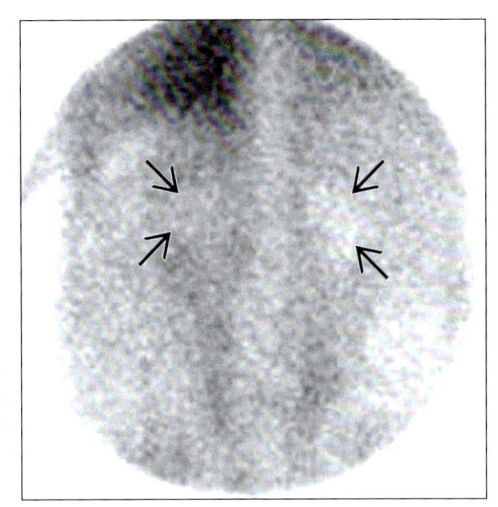

(Left) Posterior angiographic phase of a renal scan in a patient with acute renal failure shows absent renal blood flow due to dissection of an aortic aneurysm ➡ through both renal arteries. See next image. (Right) Nephrographic phase of the same renal scan shows photopenic defects ➡ due to bilateral renal infarction from dissection of an abdominal aortic aneurysm.

Typical

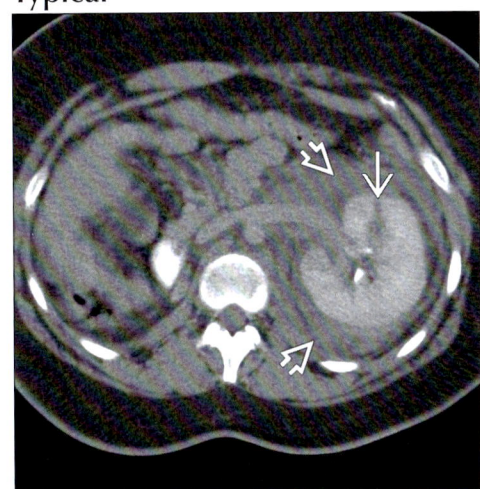

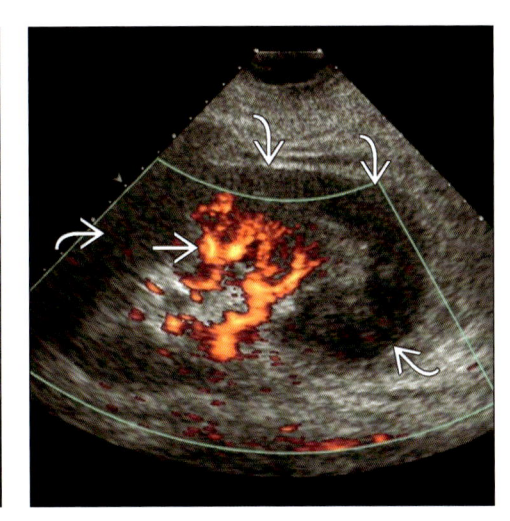

(Left) CECT of the abdomen in a hemodynamically stable trauma patient with a rising creatinine shows a fluid collection ➡ around a fractured ➡ but perfused left kidney. The right kidney was remotely removed surgically. Same as next three images. (Right) Color flow Doppler of the left kidney shows prominent perfusion ➡ of renal parenchyma and a hypoechoic perinephric fluid collection ➡.

Typical

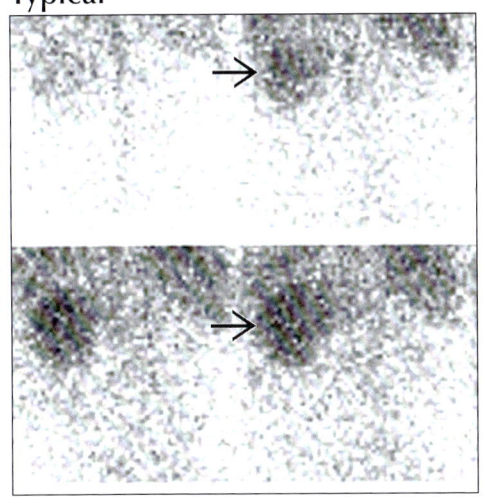

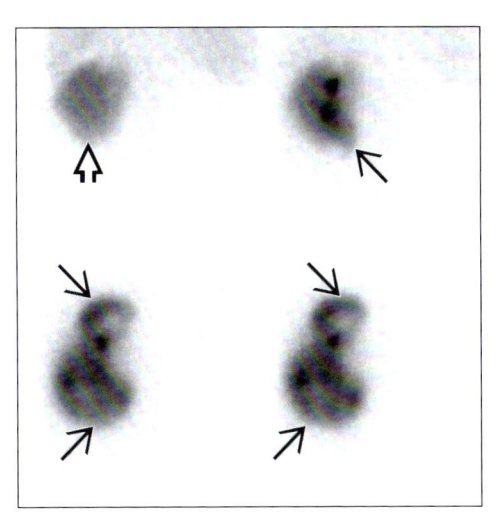

(Left) Posterior angiographic phase of renal scan in the same trauma patient as previous shows prompt blood flow to the left kidney ➡. (Right) The first image of the nephrogram phase of the renal scan shows the shape of the left kidney ➡. Subsequent images show progressive extravasation of tracer ➡ around the kidney, confirming that the perinephric fluid collection is a urinoma.

RENAL MASSES

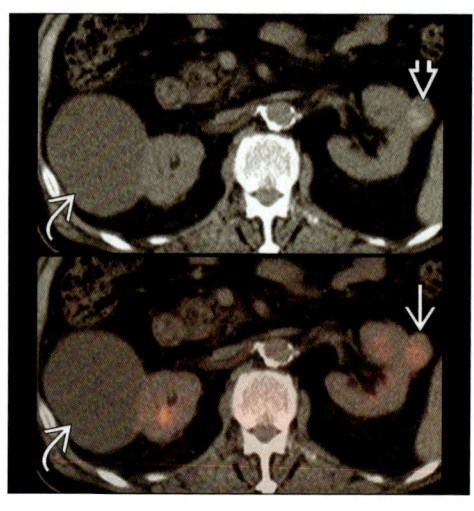

Axial NECT (upper) and fused FDG PET/CT (lower) show left hypermetabolic exophytic renal mass ➡ with subtly increased CT attenuation ⮕, a surgically proven oncocytoma, and right renal cyst ➢.

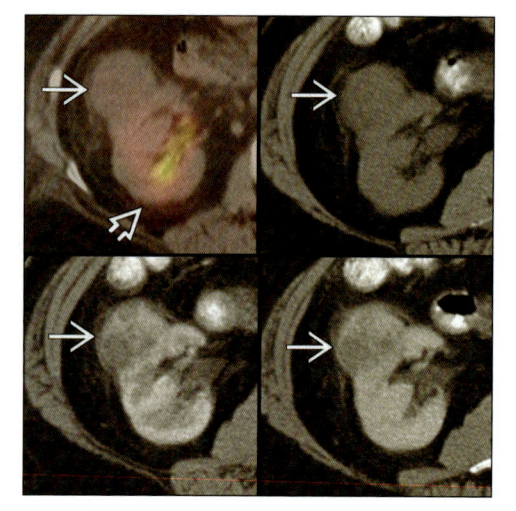

PET/CT (1), NECT (2), early (3) and late (4) CECT show heterogeneously enhancing right renal mass ➡ with FDG uptake less than renal cortex ⮕, pathologically proven clear cell renal carcinoma.

TERMINOLOGY

Definitions
- Benign or malignant mass lesion in kidney

IMAGING FINDINGS

General Features
- Renal cell carcinoma (RCC): Malignant tumor arising from tubular epithelium
  - FDG PET
    - RCC: May show lower, equal or greater FDG uptake than renal cortex
    - FDG PET: Problem solving role in evaluating RCC metastases, not optimal for staging
  - Best imaging tool: Multiphase CT (nephrographic phase); CECT, MR for identifying tumor thrombus
  - MR: Equal or better than CT in staging
- Transitional cell carcinoma (TCC): Malignant uroepithelial tumor of collecting system or urinary bladder
  - TCC: FDG uptake in TCC ≥ renal cortex, often obscured by urine activity
  - Best imaging tool: Retrograde pyelogram, CT urography (minimally enhancing mass in collecting system)
  - MR: Similar to normal renal parenchyma (with or without contrast)
- Renal metastases and lymphoma: Typically multiple, bilateral, infiltrative around kidney
  - Metastases and lymphoma: FDG uptake > renal parenchyma (≤ in MALT lymphoma)
  - CECT: Hypoattenuating, homogeneous, minimally enhancing
  - Best imaging tool: CECT (nephrographic phase)
- Renal medullary carcinoma (RCC): Rare aggressive malignancy of calyceal transitional epithelium; increased risk in sickle cell disease
  - Findings on FDG PET not reported
  - Best imaging tool: CECT, central infiltrative tumor, caliectasis without pelviectasis, necrosis, tumor thrombus, peritoneal extension
- Wilms tumor: Malignant tumor of metanephric blastema; malignant nephroblastoma
  - FDG PET: Problem solving modality; differentiating residual tumor vs. scar

DDx: Mimics of Renal Masses on FDG PET

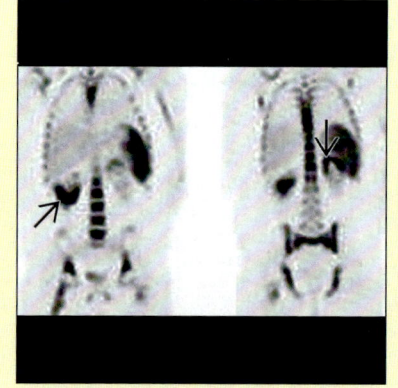

Extramedullary Hematopoiesis 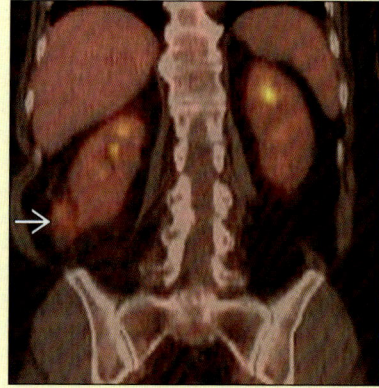 | Perirenal Abscess 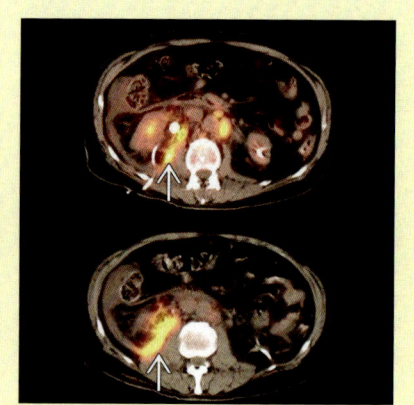 | Urine Leak

RENAL MASSES

Key Facts

Imaging Findings
- RCC: May show lower, equal or greater FDG uptake than renal cortex
- TCC: FDG uptake in TCC ≥ renal cortex, often obscured by urine activity
- Metastases and lymphoma: FDG uptake > renal parenchyma (≤ in MALT lymphoma)
- AML: Heterogeneous FDG uptake

Diagnostic Checklist
- FDG PET cannot distinguish between benign and malignant solid renal masses
- Intense FDG uptake on PET in renal mass: More typical of lymphoma or metastases than primary renal neoplasms
- FDG uptake in primary renal tumor: May be hypo-, iso-, or hypermetabolic relative to normal kidney, may be obscured by FDG in collecting system

---

- Best imaging tool: US screening; CT or MR per national protocols; CT for staging
- Angiomyolipoma (AML): Benign tumor composed of blood vessels, smooth muscle and fat
  - AML: Heterogeneous FDG uptake
  - Best imaging tool: Thin section (< 3 mm) NECT/CECT; fatty elements, variable enhancement
    - Calcification suggests RCC
- Oncocytoma: Benign tumor of eosinophilic epithelial cells, arising from intercalated collecting duct cells
  - FDG PET: FDG uptake > renal cortex, findings nonspecific, few published reports
  - Best imaging tool: MR (spoke-wheel pattern on T2WI), homogeneous enhancement, central scar
  - NECT: Iso- or slightly hyperdense, central stellate scar (CECT HU < renal cortex)
- Multilocular cystic nephroma (MLCN): Rare nonhereditary benign tumor arising from metanephric blastema; differentiated nephroblastoma
  - Best imaging tool: Multiloculated cyst on NECT, capsule enhances on CECT
  - Findings on FDG PET not reported
- Renal cysts
  - FDG PET: Solitary, multiple photopenic (usually benign) or iso-/hyperintense to renal parenchyma (indeterminate, more likely malignant)
  - CECT: Range from uniform density, < 20 HU (Bosniak I) to malignant cystic masses (Bosniak IV)

Imaging Recommendations
- Best imaging tool: Dynamic CT, CEMR

DIFFERENTIAL DIAGNOSIS

Infection
- Appearance on FDG PET mimics hypermetabolic tumor (↑ uptake)

Perinephric Benign Conditions
- Urine leak, extramedullary hematopoiesis, hypermetabolic brown fat ⇒ increased FDG uptake

DIAGNOSTIC CHECKLIST

Image Interpretation Pearls
- FDG PET cannot distinguish between benign and malignant solid renal masses
- Intense FDG uptake on PET in renal mass: More typical of lymphoma or metastases than primary renal neoplasms
- FDG uptake in primary renal tumor: May be hypo-, iso-, or hypermetabolic relative to normal kidney, may be obscured by FDG in collecting system

SELECTED REFERENCES
1. Kaneta T et al: FDG PET in solitary metastastic/secondary tumor of the kidney: a report of three cases and a review of the relevant literature. Ann Nucl Med. 20(1):79-82, 2006
2. Schoder H et al: Positron emission tomography for prostate, bladder, and renal cancer. Semin Nucl Med. 34(4):274-92, 2004

IMAGE GALLERY

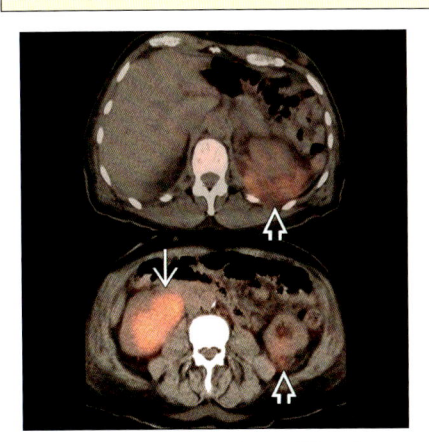

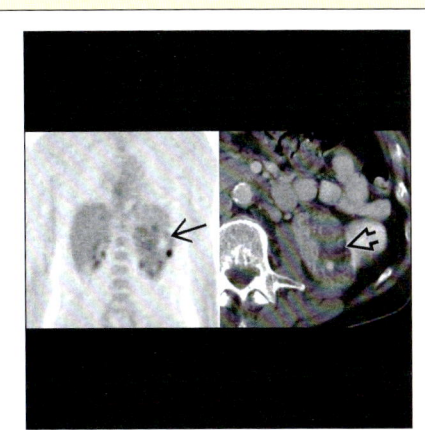

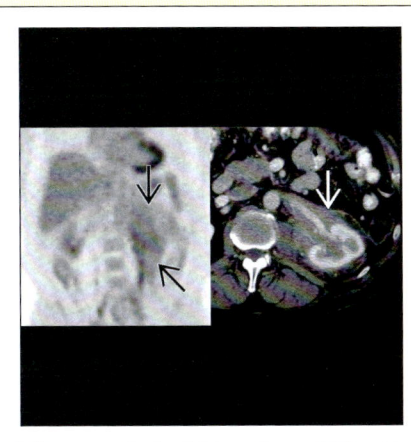

(Left) Axial FDG PET/CT shows diffuse large B-cell non-Hodgkin lymphoma involvement in intensely hypermetabolic right renal mass ➡ and left posterior perirenal mass ➡. *(Center)* Coronal FDG PET shows heterogeneous, moderately hypermetabolic left renal mass ➡. Axial CECT shows regions of fatty attenuation ➡, consistent with angiomyolipoma. *(Right)* Coronal FDG PET shows hypermetabolic activity ➡ and axial CECT shows infiltrative mass ➡ around left kidney in patient with MALT lymphoma (typically low to moderate FDG uptake).

RENAL CELL CARCINOMA

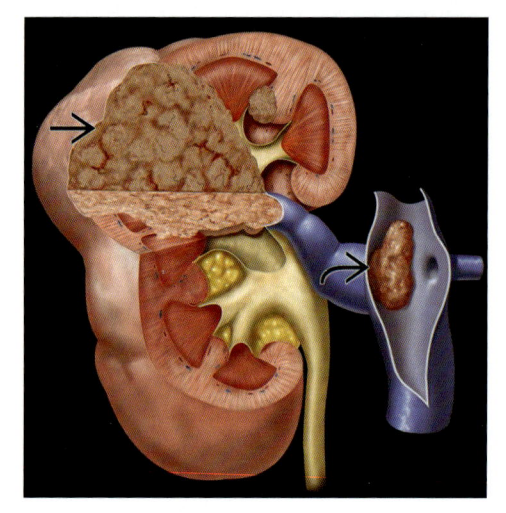

Graphic shows large renal cell carcinoma in renal parenchyma ➔ with tumor in inferior vena cava ➔.

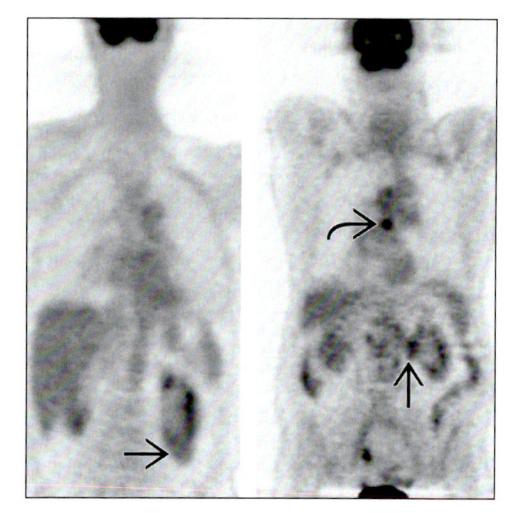

Coronal FDG PET from two patients shows mild activity ➔ in renal cell carcinoma. Note mediastinal metastasis ➔ in patient at right.

TERMINOLOGY

Abbreviations and Synonyms
- Renal cell carcinoma (RCC), clear cell carcinoma, hypernephroma, renal cancer

Definitions
- Carcinoma of renal tubular epithelium

IMAGING FINDINGS

General Features
- Best diagnostic clue
  - Iso- or hypermetabolic renal mass ± lymphadenopathy, metastases on FDG PET
  - Presents most commonly as incidental solid tumor on imaging
  - Enhancing solitary mass on CT highly suspicious for RCC
    - Necrosis, hemorrhage, septae more likely in large masses
- Location
  - Usually renal cortex
  - Often exophytic
  - Rarely bilateral (2%) or multicentric (more common in Von-Hippel Lindau)
- Size: Variable depending on time of diagnosis
- Morphology
  - 10% calcified, often irregular
  - 2-5% cystic

Nuclear Medicine Findings
- **FDG PET and RCC**
  - Iso- or hypermetabolic renal mass ± lymphadenopathy, metastases
  - FDG uptake by RCC, metastases variable
  - Sensitivity 60%, specificity ~ 100% for evaluating primary RCC
  - Excretory FDG in collecting system can mask small RCCs adjacent to collecting system
  - 80-100% specific for bony metastases

CT Findings
- NECT
  - Can be hyperdense, isodense or hypodense to surrounding normal kidney
  - Heterogeneous mass with areas of calcification (~ 10%)

DDx: Other Renal Masses

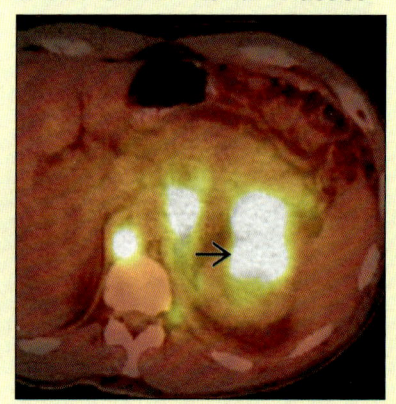

Renal Lymphoma 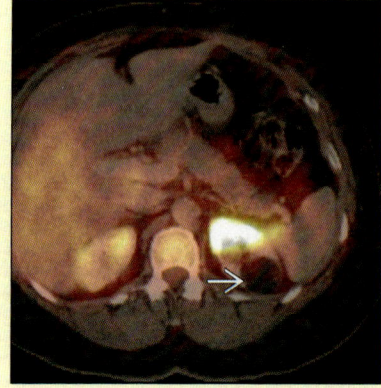 | Angiomyolipoma 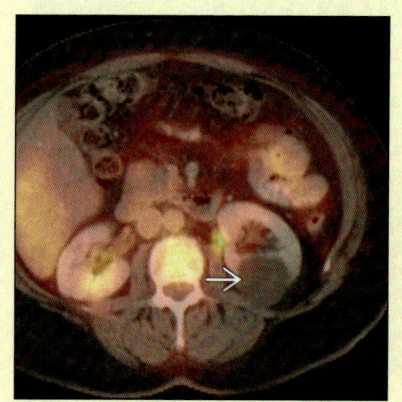 | Renal Cyst

RENAL CELL CARCINOMA

Key Facts

Terminology
- Renal cell carcinoma (RCC), clear cell carcinoma, hypernephroma, renal cancer
- Carcinoma of renal tubular epithelium

Imaging Findings
- FDG PET and RCC
- Iso- or hypermetabolic renal mass ± lymphadenopathy, metastases
- FDG uptake by RCC, metastases variable
- Sensitivity 60%, specificity ~ 100% for evaluating primary RCC
- Excretory FDG in collecting system can mask small RCCs adjacent to collecting system
- 80-100% specific for bony metastases
- CECT often shows enhancing lesion, hyperdense benign cysts will not enhance

Top Differential Diagnoses
- Angiomyolipoma (AML)
- Renal Oncocytoma
- Hemorrhagic Renal Cyst
- Transitional Cell Carcinoma (TCC)
- Lymphoma
- Renal Infection or Abscess
- Metastatic Disease

Clinical Issues
- Complete surgical resection only curative treatment

Diagnostic Checklist
- RCC has variable uptake on FDG PET
- Excretory FDG in collecting system can mask small RCCs adjacent to collecting system

---

   - Rarely contains small areas of fat (-50 to -150 HU)
- CECT
   - Hypervascular mass with enhancement (HU increase by > 20) compared to non-contrast
   - Enhancement often heterogeneous, particularly larger lesions
   - Tumor extension or thrombus in renal vein (23%), inferior vena cava (7%)
   - Local extension common
   - Nodal spread typically to para-aortic or aortocaval lymph nodes
   - Most common metastatic locations include lung, liver, bone, adrenal and opposite kidney

Ultrasonographic Findings
- RCC can be hypo-, hyper-, isoechoic
- US most useful to identify simple renal cyst

Imaging Recommendations
- Best imaging tool
   - FDG PET
      - Helpful in staging known primary RCC
   - Combination of CT, ultrasound
      - CECT often shows enhancing lesion, hyperdense benign cysts will not enhance
      - US indicated in patients with non-enhancing hyperdense renal lesions to differentiate cyst from mass
      - If contraindication to contrast, MR superior to CT
- Protocol advice
   - For CT: Non-contrast and CECT, thin-sections (2.5-5.0 mm), during both corticomedullary and nephrographic phases
      - For PET CT: If only single phase obtained, use later nephrographic phase of contrast enhancement
   - Corticomedullary phase (25-70 seconds post-injection)
      - Better visualization of renal vessels; evaluate for renal vein/IVC thrombosis or tumor extension
      - Limited detection of small renal lesions
      - Centrally located tumors commonly mistaken for normal, hypoattenuating medulla
   - Nephrographic phase (80-180 seconds post-injection)
      - Best imaging of renal medulla masses

DIFFERENTIAL DIAGNOSIS

Angiomyolipoma (AML)
- Fat attenuation (-30 to -150 HU) fairly specific for this neoplasm
- Low FDG uptake
- Reliably distinguished from malignancy by CT characteristics

Renal Oncocytoma
- Central scar on CT/MR and spoke-wheel pattern of vessels on angiograms suggest oncocytoma, not entirely specific
- Cannot confidently differentiate from RCC by PET

Hemorrhagic Renal Cyst
- > Water attenuation on CT (~ 30-70 HU)
- Should not enhance when comparing non-contrast and CE series

Transitional Cell Carcinoma (TCC)
- Renal pelvis filling defect, narrowing
- Urothelial thickening or involvement
- Rare parenchymal TCC indistinguishable from RCC

Lymphoma
- Typically more diffusely infiltrative than discrete mass

Renal Infection or Abscess
- Focal nephritis can appear mass-like
   - Short term follow-up helpful
- Clinical history and urine analysis often helpful

Metastatic Disease
- History essential
- Common primary cancers include lung, breast, colon, melanoma, pancreatic
- Typically only hypervascular metastases mistaken for RCC

RENAL CELL CARCINOMA

PATHOLOGY

General Features
- General path comments
  - Staging
    - Stage I: Solid mass ≤ 7 cm, confined to kidney
    - Stage II: > 7 cm but still organ-confined; spread to perinephric fat
    - Stage III: Invasion of renal vein or vena cava, involvement of ipsilateral adrenal gland and/or perinephric fat, or spread to one local lymph node
    - Stage IV: Invasion of adjacent organs, more than one local node or distant metastases
- Genetics: Associated with von Hippel-Lindau syndrome (autosomal dominant)
- Etiology
  - Arise from tubular epithelium
  - Bilateral lesions associated with von Hippel-Lindau syndrome, tuberous sclerosis, chronic dialysis
  - Other risk factors: Smoking, chemical exposure (diethylstilbestrol and fluoroacetamide)
- Epidemiology
  - Approximately 2% of adult malignancies (30,000/yr in US)
  - Small RCCs found at autopsy more frequently

Gross Pathologic & Surgical Features
- Solid to cystic components with necrosis, hemorrhage and rarely fat

Microscopic Features
- 70% clear cell, 13% papillary, 7% granular, 10% other

CLINICAL ISSUES

Presentation
- Most common signs/symptoms
  - Hematuria (50%), flank pain (40%), flank mass (35%)
  - Nearly half of RCCs discovered incidentally
- Other signs/symptoms
  - Fever, nausea, weight loss
  - Rarely, humoral factors such as erythropoietin, renin, parathyroid hormone, or prolactin may cause symptoms

Demographics
- Age: Generally 50-70 yrs, with wide distribution
- Gender: M > F, 2:1

Natural History & Prognosis
- 5 year survival
  - Stage I: 67%, stage II: 51%, stage III: 33.5%, stage IV: 13.5%
- Prognosis worse for larger, marginated, or necrotic tumors which tend to be ↑ grade

Treatment
- Complete surgical resection only curative treatment

DIAGNOSTIC CHECKLIST

Consider
- FDG PET for staging, evaluation of bony metastases
- Non-contrast CT followed by CECT for primary evaluation
- US to differentiate hyperdense cyst from mass if CT unclear

Image Interpretation Pearls
- RCC has variable uptake on FDG PET
- Excretory FDG in collecting system can mask small RCCs adjacent to collecting system

SELECTED REFERENCES

1. Lawrentschuk N et al: Positron emission tomography (PET), immuno-PET and radioimmunotherapy in renal cell carcinoma: a developing diagnostic and therapeutic relationship. BJU Int. 97(5):916-22, 2006
2. Ak I et al: F-18 FDG PET in detecting renal cell carcinoma. Acta Radiol. 46(8):895-9, 2005
3. Ide M et al: The detection of renal cell carcinoma with adrenal and para-aortic lymph node metastases by FDG-PET. Eur J Nucl Med Mol Imaging. 32(10):1246, 2005
4. Nguyen BD: Positron emission tomography imaging of renal vein and inferior vena cava tumor thrombus from renal cell carcinoma. Clin Nucl Med. 30(2):107-9, 2005
5. Cheow HK et al: Large renal cell carcinoma isometabolic with normal liver on F-18 FDG PET scan. Clin Nucl Med. 29(8):488-90, 2004
6. Kang DE et al: Clinical use of fluorodeoxyglucose F 18 positron emission tomography for detection of renal cell carcinoma. J Urol. 171(5):1806-9, 2004
7. Schoder H et al: Positron emission tomography for prostate, bladder, and renal cancer. Semin Nucl Med. 34(4):274-92, 2004
8. Watanabe N et al: A case of renal pelvic tumor visualized by 18F-FDG-PET imaging. Ann Nucl Med. 18(2):161-3, 2004
9. Chang CH et al: Differentiating solitary pulmonary metastases in patients with renal cell carcinomas by 18F-fluoro-2-deoxyglucose positron emission tomography--a preliminary report. Urol Int. 71(3):306-9, 2003
10. Hain SF et al: Positron emission tomography for urological tumours. BJU Int. 92(2):159-64, 2003
11. Jadvar H et al: Diagnostic role of [F-18]-FDG positron emission tomography in restaging renal cell carcinoma. Clin Nephrol. 60(6):395-400, 2003
12. Majhail NS et al: F-18 fluorodeoxyglucose positron emission tomography in the evaluation of distant metastases from renal cell carcinoma. J Clin Oncol. 21(21):3995-4000, 2003
13. Mathews D et al: Positron emission tomography in prostate and renal cell carcinoma. Curr Opin Urol. 12(5):381-5, 2002
14. Shvarts O et al: Positron emission tomography in urologic oncology. Cancer Control. 9(4):335-42, 2002
15. Bihl H et al: Metastatic Renal Cell Carcinoma (mRCC). Is There A Role of F-18-FDG-PET? Clin Positron Imaging. 2(6):340, 1999
16. Hoh CK et al: Positron emission tomography in urological oncology. J Urol. 159(2):347-56, 1998
17. Bender H et al: Possible role of FDG-PET in the evaluation of urologic malignancies. Anticancer Res. 17(3B):1655-60, 1997

RENAL CELL CARCINOMA

IMAGE GALLERY

Typical

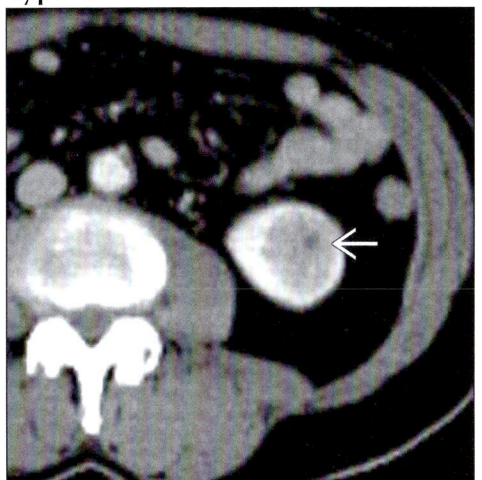

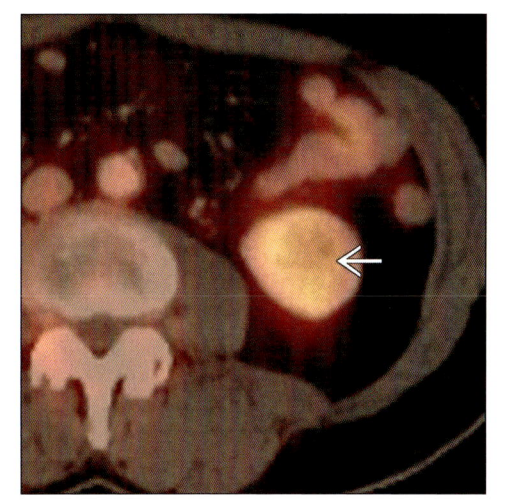

(Left) Axial CECT shows a large enhancing mass ➡ in inferior pole left kidney compatible with renal cell carcinoma. *(Right)* Axial fused PET/CT shows mild FDG uptake ➡ in the mass. FDG activity in renal cell carcinoma is variable and may show only mild uptake.

Typical

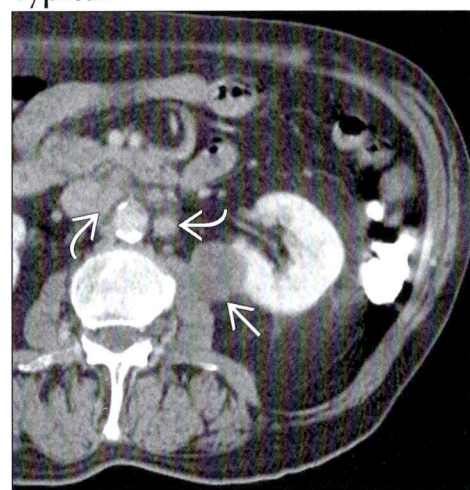

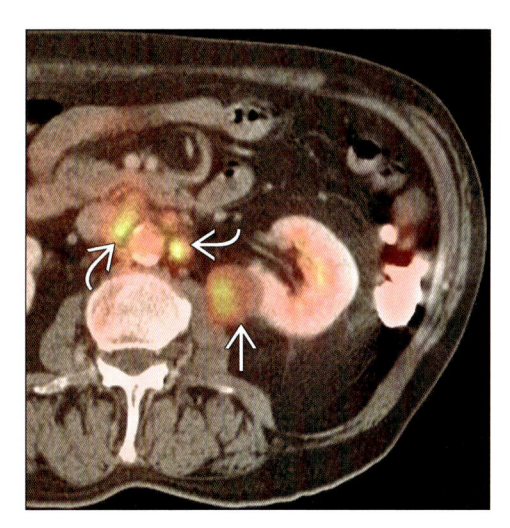

(Left) Axial CECT shows a low attenuation, solid mass ➡ in mid-pole left kidney with adjacent borderline-enlarged para-aortic lymph nodes ➡. *(Right)* Axial fused PET/CT shows moderate FDG activity within left renal mass ➡ and para-aortic lymph nodes ➡, signifying metastases.

Typical

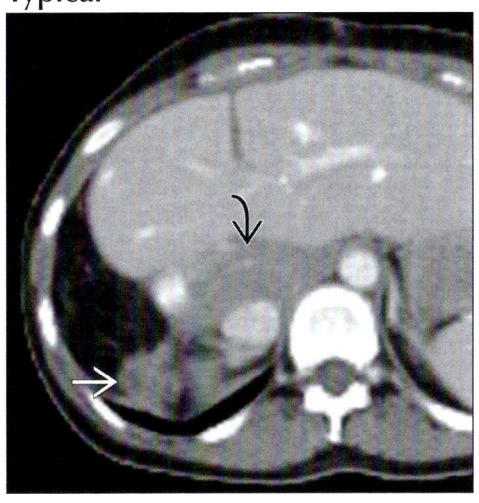

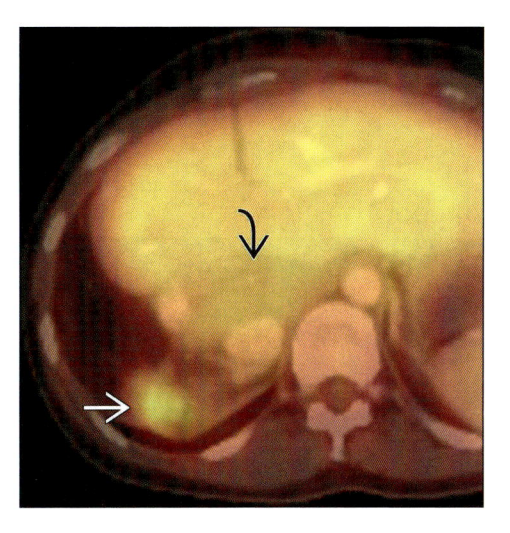

(Left) Axial CECT shows soft tissue in right nephrectomy bed ➡. The differential diagnosis includes post-operative changes and tumor. Note also mass in subhepatic region ➡. See next image. *(Right)* Axial fused PET/CT shows moderate FDG uptake in soft tissue in the renal bed ➡ and subhepatic region ➡, compatible with recurrent or residual renal cell carcinoma.

PYELONEPHRITIS

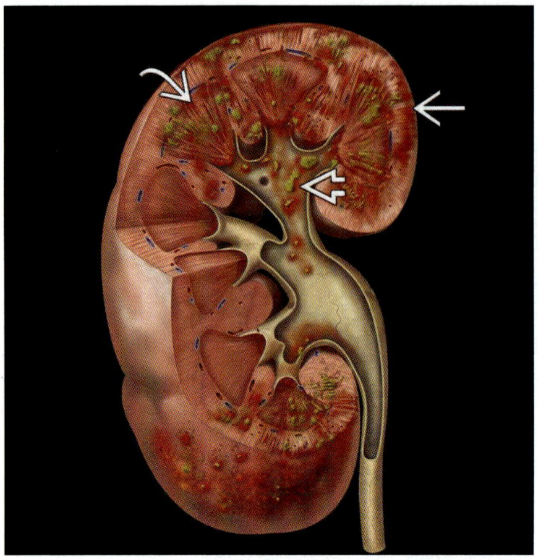

Graphic shows pattern of spread of pyelonephritis from renal pelvicaliceal system ▶ to papillae ➔, finally to renal cortical regions ➔. Extension can then progress to perirenal space.

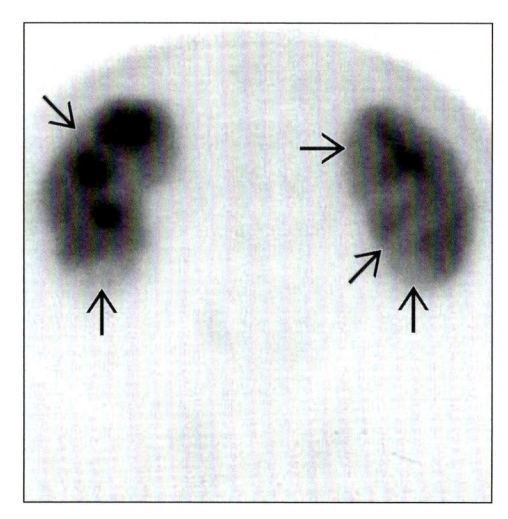

Bilateral diffuse pyelonephritis: Posterior planar Tc-99m DMSA renal cortical scan shows striated appearance ➔ due to focal decreased function from inflammation/infection.

TERMINOLOGY

Definitions
- Infection of renal pelvis, tubules & interstitium

IMAGING FINDINGS

General Features
- Best diagnostic clue
  - Renal cortical scintigraphy: Wedge-shaped regions of photopenia
  - Labeled leukocyte, Ga-67 scintigraphy: Focal or diffusely increased activity
- Location: Cortex

Nuclear Medicine Findings
- Tc-99m DMSA or glucoheptonate (GH) renal cortical scintigraphy
  - Normal scan: Homogeneous activity, ↓ activity at poles, left superior pole can show splenic indentation, fetal lobulations also seen
    - Normal split renal function: 50% ± 6%
  - Abnormal scan: ↓ Renal cortical activity in foci of inflammation/infection
    - Wedge-shaped indentation into cortex
    - Unifocal, multifocal, diffuse
  - In case of acute pyelonephritis, follow-up renal cortical scintigraphy to diagnose scar
    - Acute pyelonephritis should resolve by 3-6 months, although 12 months reported
    - If focal photopenia does not resolve on follow-up scintigraphy = renal scar
  - Tc-99m DMSA: > 90% sensitivity/specificity for acute pyelonephritis
  - Also useful for evaluation of suspected solitary, ectopic, horseshoe kidney
- Labeled leukocyte scintigraphy
  - Normal scan: No renal activity
  - Abnormal scan: ↑ Activity in kidney, portion of kidney
  - More specific than Ga-67
  - Useful for early detection of renal & perinephric infection, abscess
- Ga-67 scintigraphy
  - Normal scan: No renal activity

DDx: Mimics of Pyelonephritis

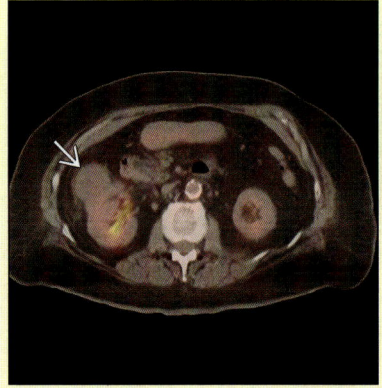

Renal Cell Carcinoma

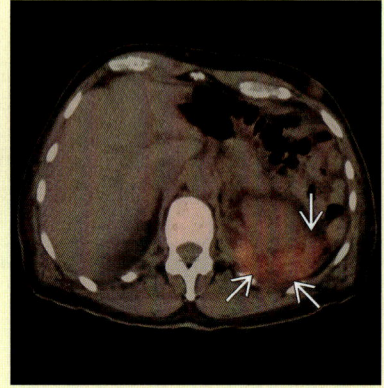

Lymphoma

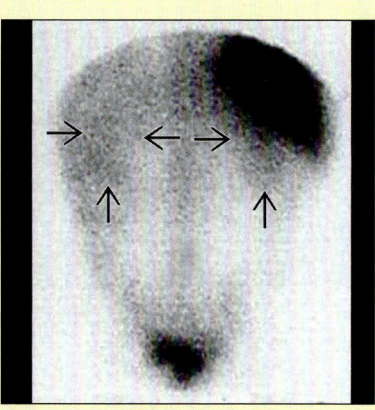

Interstitial Nephritis (Ga-67)

PYELONEPHRITIS

Key Facts

Terminology
- Infection of renal pelvis, tubules & interstitium

Imaging Findings
- Renal cortical scintigraphy: Wedge-shaped regions of photopenia
- Labeled leukocyte, Ga-67 scintigraphy: Focal or diffusely increased activity

Top Differential Diagnoses
- Renal Infarction
- Mass Lesion
- Renal Trauma
- Vasculitis
- Interstitial Nephritis

Clinical Issues
- Fever, malaise, dysuria, flank pain, tenderness
- ↑ WBC; ↑ proteinuria; + urine culture
- Age: Females < 40 yrs; males > 65 yrs; also children with risk factors

Diagnostic Checklist
- Clinical correlation important to distinguish acute pyelonephritis from renal scar (look similar on renal cortical scintigraphy)
- Serial renal cortical scans to follow for scarring
- SPECT recommended for highest quality images, low interobserver variability
- Perform anterior and posterior images if planar evaluation of pelvic, horseshoe kidneys
- SPECT: Interrenicular septum (extends from renal hilum to parenchyma) can be confused with scar

---

  ○ Abnormal scan: Unilateral or bilateral renal activity = inflammation and/or infection

Radiographic Findings
- IVP
  ○ Acute pyelonephritis
    ▪ Global or focal enlargement
    ▪ Impaired excretion: Delayed appearance, ↓ density, ↓ nephrogram
    ▪ Striated nephrogram or lucent areas (↓ filling); streaking & blushing
    ▪ Calyceal compression, pelvicaliceal or ureteral dilatation, ± calculi
  ○ Chronic pyelonephritis
    ▪ Contracted small kidney, ↓ & delayed excretion, dilated ureter
    ▪ Focal or diffuse calyceal clubbing or blunting + cortical scar
    ▪ Contralateral diffuse or focal compensatory hypertrophy

CT Findings
- Acute pyelonephritis
  ○ Renal enlargement, focal swelling, sinus obliteration
  ○ Thickening of Gerota fascia + perinephric stranding
  ○ ± Areas of ↑ HU (hemorrhagic bacterial nephritis)
  ○ Nephrographic phase: "Patchy" nephrogram
  ○ Excretory phase: Streaky linear bands, alternating ↑ + ↓ attenuation, calyceal effacement, dilated renal pelvis/ureter
  ○ Delayed phase (3-4 hrs): ↑ Enhancement in previously low density, wedge-shaped zones
- Chronic pyelonephritis
  ○ Deep cortical scarring: Focal, segmental, diffuse; unilateral or bilateral
  ○ Atrophy: Focal (> in upper pole) or diffuse
  ○ Unilateral with compensatory hypertrophy of contralateral kidney
  ○ Characteristic: Atrophy, cortical scar, dilated calices
  ○ Loss of corticomedullary differentiation
- Emphysematous pyelonephritis
  ○ Necrosis + gas with little or no pus
- Xanthogranulomatous pyelonephritis (XGPN)
  ○ Nonfunctional kidney or part of kidney with obstructing calculi
  ○ Low attenuation collections: Foot print of a bear paw (markedly dilated collecting system filled with pus, xanthoma cells + mildly dilated pelvis)
  ○ Lack of contrast excretion, rim-enhancement
  ○ Thickened Gerota fascia, perinephric stranding, abscess, extension

Ultrasonographic Findings
- Grayscale Ultrasound
  ○ Acute pyelonephritis
    ▪ Normal or swollen kidney with ↓ echogenicity; loss of sinus echoes

Imaging Recommendations
- Best imaging tool: Renal cortical scintigraphy: Follow-up and diagnosis of acute pyelonephritis, scar, split renal function
- Protocol advice
  ○ Tc-99m DMSA renal cortical scintigraphy
    ▪ Dose: 0.3-3.0 mCi (11-110 MBq) IV
    ▪ ~ 40% of dose goes to distal tubule cells
    ▪ Image 2 hrs post injection
    ▪ SPECT more sensitive than planar; ↓ interobserver variability
    ▪ With planar images, consider pinhole collimation in children
    ▪ Posterior and posterior oblique planar images, unless pelvic/horseshoe kidneys, then add anterior planar images
    ▪ Highly sensitive (> 90%) in diagnosing acute pyelonephritis
    ▪ First-line for renal cortical scintigraphy (high-quality images)
    ▪ Can get split renal function from static images
    ▪ Lower bladder, gonad exposure than with Tc-99m GH
  ○ Tc-99m GH renal cortical scintigraphy
    ▪ Dose: 0.5-8.0 mCi (20-300 MBq) IV
    ▪ ~ 10% of dose goes to proximal tubule cells
    ▪ Partially excreted in urine, therefore also shows renal excretion

PYELONEPHRITIS

- Dynamic planar images immediately post injection
- Static images ~ 30 minutes post injection, SPECT imaging more sensitive than planar
- If performing planar images, consider pinhole collimation in children
- Posterior and posterior oblique planar images, unless pelvic/horseshoe kidneys, then add anterior planar images
- Provides split renal function information
- Reports of uptake in normal uterus
- Higher bladder, gonad exposure than Tc-99m DMSA due to renal excretion
○ Labeled leukocyte scintigraphy
- Dose: 0.5-1.0 mCi (18-40 MBq) In-111 adults; 0.05-0.5 mCi (1.85-18.5 MBq) In-111 in children
- High dose to spleen; not practical for repeated use in children
- Valuable for suspected perirenal abscess
○ Ga-67 scintigraphy
- Dose: 4-6 mCi (150-220 MBq) IV adults; 0.04-0.07 mCi/kg (1.5-2.6 MBq/kg) IV children, minimum 0.25-0.5 mCi (9-18 MBq)
- Extended imaging times (24-72 hrs) not practical compared with renal cortical scintigraphy
- Positive in perirenal abscess, interstitial nephritis; no uptake in acute tubular necrosis

DIFFERENTIAL DIAGNOSIS

Renal Infarction
- Focal segmental or global photopenia

Mass Lesion
- E.g., renal cell carcinoma, lymphoma, metastases, cysts
- ↓ Activity in mass on renal cortical scintigraphy

Renal Trauma
- Wedge-shaped photopenia: Infarction
- Global photopenia: Renal artery avulsion/thrombosis
- Irregular, linear regions of ↓ activity: Laceration
- Abnormal renal contour: Mass effect from hematoma

Vasculitis
- E.g., polyarteritis nodosa, lupus, drug abuse
- Wedge-shaped or striated abnormalities

Interstitial Nephritis
- Diffusely positive on Ga-67

PATHOLOGY

General Features
- Etiology
  ○ Gram negative: E. coli, proteus, klebsiella, Enterobacter; ascending infection most common
  ○ Risk factors
    - Vesicoureteral reflux (VUR), obstruction, pregnancy, prostatic hypertrophy, urethral instrumentation, diabetes

Gross Pathologic & Surgical Features
- Acute pyelonephritis
  ○ "Polar abscesses": Microabscesses on renal surface
  ○ Narrowed calyces, enlarged kidney
- Chronic pyelonephritis
  ○ Blunted calyces + scarred shrunken kidney

Microscopic Features
- Acute pyelonephritis
  ○ Interstitial or tubular necrosis
  ○ Mononuclear cell infiltrate + fibrosis
- Chronic pyelonephritis
  ○ Chronic inflammation, atrophy, interstitial fibrosis
- XGPN
  ○ Foamy, lipid-laden histiocytes; pus & necrosis

CLINICAL ISSUES

Presentation
- Most common signs/symptoms
  ○ Acute pyelonephritis
    - Fever, malaise, dysuria, flank pain, tenderness
- Lab data
  ○ ↑ WBC; ↑ proteinuria; + urine culture

Demographics
- Age: Females < 40 yrs; males > 65 yrs; also children with risk factors

Natural History & Prognosis
- Complications
  ○ Abscess, papillary necrosis, atrophy, renal failure
  ○ Renal scarring can ⇒ hypertension (10-20% of those with scar)
- Prognosis
  ○ Acute pyelonephritis: Good
  ○ Chronic, XGPN, emphysematous types: Poor

Treatment
- Acute: Antibiotic therapy
- Chronic: Treat reflux & obstruction; nephrectomy

DIAGNOSTIC CHECKLIST

Consider
- Clinical correlation important to distinguish acute pyelonephritis from renal scar (look similar on renal cortical scintigraphy)
- Serial renal cortical scans to follow for scarring
- SPECT recommended for highest quality images, low interobserver variability
- Perform anterior and posterior images if planar evaluation of pelvic, horseshoe kidneys

Image Interpretation Pearls
- SPECT: Interrenicular septum (extends from renal hilum to parenchyma) can be confused with scar

SELECTED REFERENCES

1. Piepsz A et al: Pediatric applications of renal nuclear medicine. Semin Nucl Med. 36(1):16-35, 2006

PYELONEPHRITIS

IMAGE GALLERY

Typical

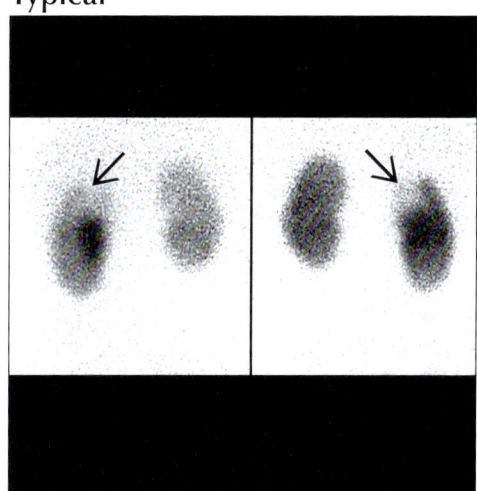

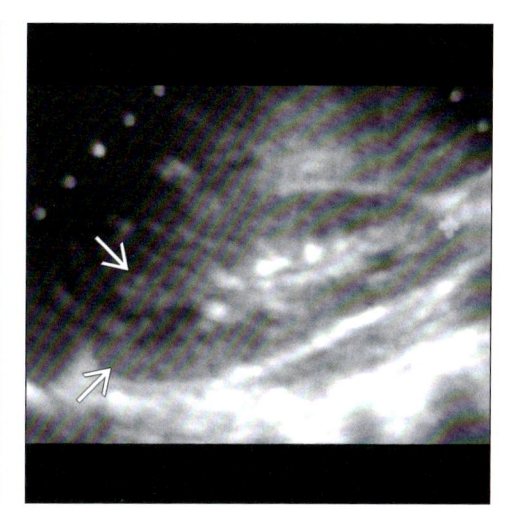

(Left) Right superior focal pyelonephritis: Anterior (left) and posterior (right) planar Tc-99m DMSA renal cortical scan shows decreased uptake ➔ in superior pole of right kidney. See next image. (Right) Longitudinal ultrasound of right kidney in same patient as previous image, shows hypoechoic superior pole ➔, consistent with focal pyelonephritis. See next image.

Typical

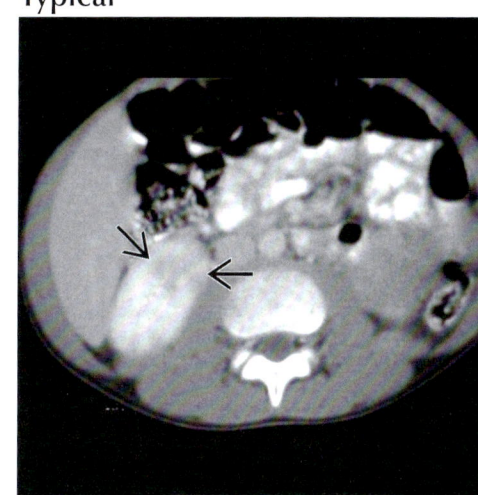

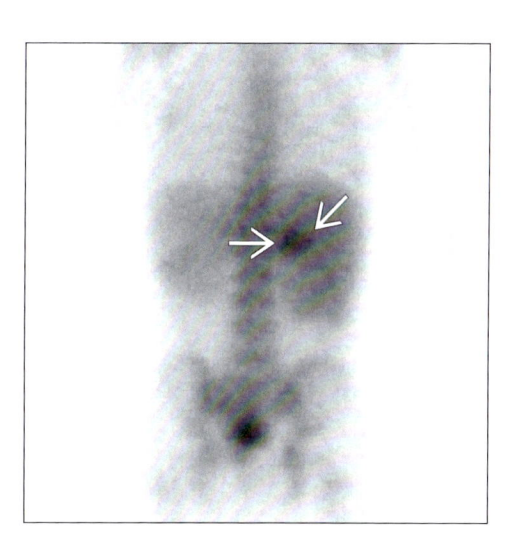

(Left) Axial CECT in same patient as previous image, shows focal decreased enhancement in superior right kidney ➔ due to focal pyelonephritis. See next image. (Right) Posterior planar Ga-67 scan in the same patient as previous image, shows increased uptake in superior pole of right kidney ➔ due to focal pyelonephritis.

Variant

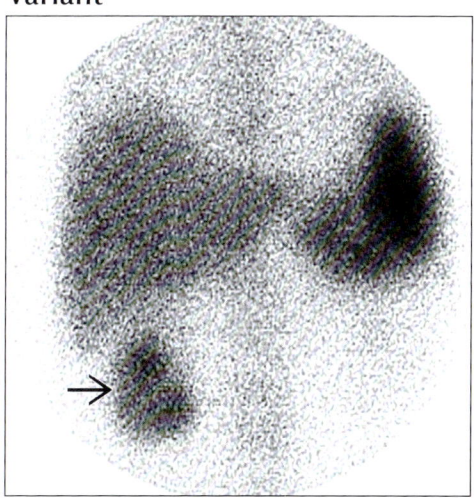

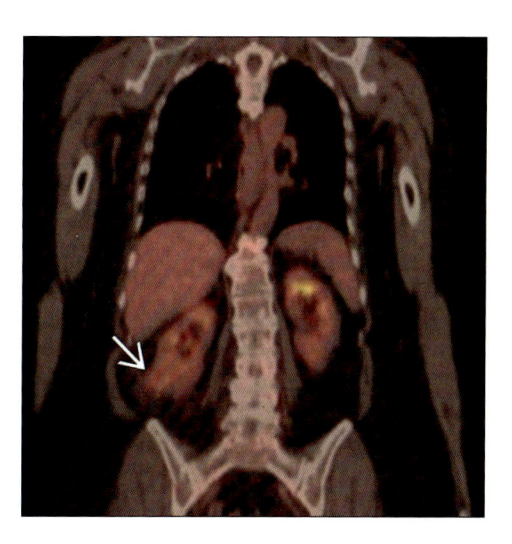

(Left) Anterior In-111 WBC scan of upper abdomen shows increased uptake in right kidney ➔ in patient with pyelonephritis. (Right) Coronal PET/CT shows increased activity in right perirenal space ➔ with surrounding hypermetabolic stranding in patient with perirenal abscess following pyelonephritis.

RENAL TRANSPLANT

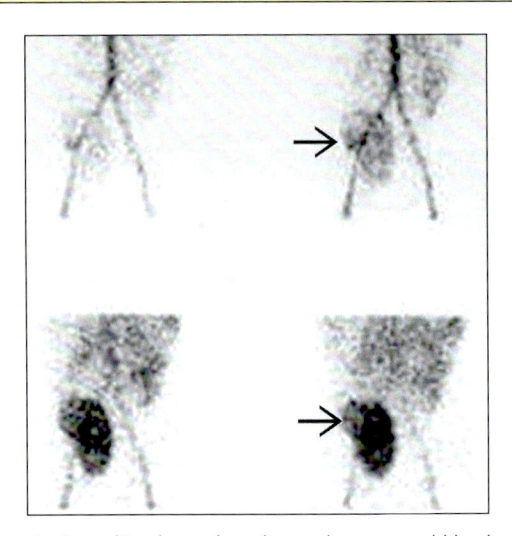

Angiographic phase of renal scan shows normal blood flow to healthy renal allograft ➡. See next image.

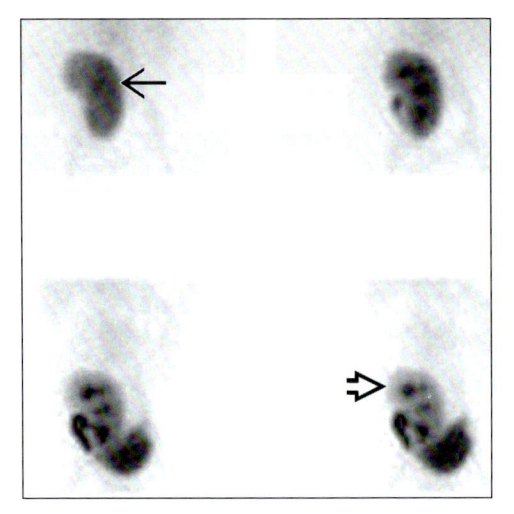

Nephrogram phase shows homogeneous early cortical concentration ➡ and good clearance ⇨ in a healthy renal allograft. 20 minute:peak cortical ratio was near-normal, at 0.32 (normal ≤ 0.3).

TERMINOLOGY

Definitions
- Acute vasomotor nephropathy (AVN)/acute transplant nephropathy: Poor function immediately post transplant from pre-operative injury to donor or kidney
  - Previously called acute tubular necrosis: May or may not be present with delayed graft function
  - More common in cadaveric allografts (up to 50%); only 5% in live donors
  - Usually resolves/improves spontaneously, severe cases which do not resolve indicate poor prognosis
- Rejection: Autoimmune response mounted against a transplanted allograft, usually T-cell mediated
  - Hyperacute: Immediate reaction leading to allograft death from preformed antibodies in major histocompatibility (HLA) or blood group mismatch
  - Accelerated: From antibodies in patients sensitized by multiple transfusions, pregnancy; usually presents 3-5 days post-transplant
  - Acute rejection (AR): Cellular or humoral antibody-mediated rejection
    - AR occurs any time: Most common ~ 5-7 d to first few months
    - AR is rare > 1st year
    - Small vessel thrombosis, arteritis, lymphocytic infiltrate
  - Chronic allograft nephropathy (CR): Untreatable delayed humoral process of fibrosis, cortical loss
    - Previously termed chronic rejection, but generally not due to underlying simmering untreated rejection
    - Development associated with prior episodes of severe AR, AVN, or effects of strong immunosuppressives
    - CR is currently most common cause of graft loss due to advances in AR therapy

IMAGING FINDINGS

Nuclear Medicine Findings
- Acute vasomotor nephropathy (AVN)
  - Also called acute transplant nephropathy [formerly, acute tubular necrosis (ATN)]

DDx: Complications of Renal Transplantation

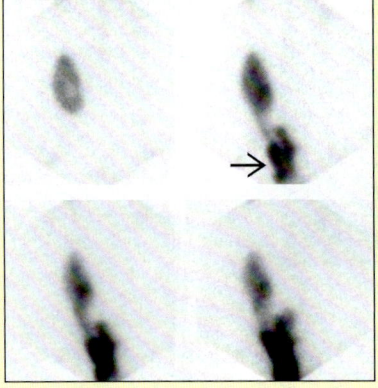

Urine Leak (Courtesy E. Dubovsky) 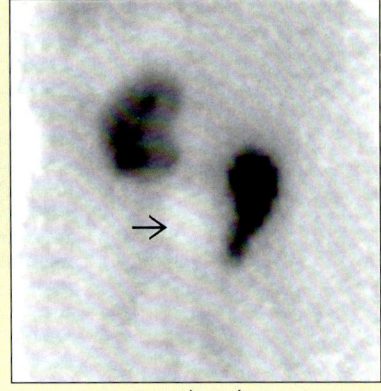 | *Lymphocele* 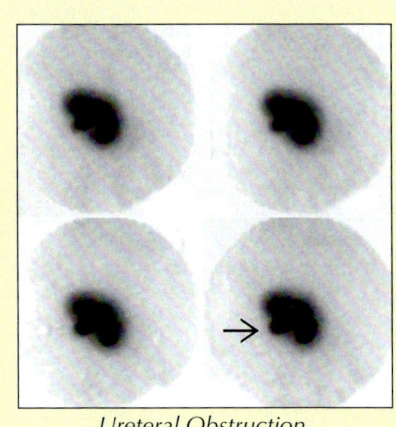 | *Ureteral Obstruction*

RENAL TRANSPLANT

Key Facts

Terminology
- Acute vasomotor nephropathy (AVN)/acute transplant nephropathy: Poor function immediately post transplant from pre-operative injury to donor or kidney
- Acute rejection (AR): Cellular or humoral antibody-mediated rejection
- AR occurs any time: Most common ~ 5-7 d to first few months
- Chronic allograft nephropathy (CR): Untreatable delayed humoral process of fibrosis, cortical loss

Imaging Findings
- Cortical retention seen in AR or AVN
- AVN: Abnormal baseline renal scan at 24 hr (AR typically occurs later)
- Perfusion in AR generally worse than function: Often technically difficult to visualize
- Late-developing AR & immunosuppressive drug toxicity appear similar
- Sensitivity and specificity lower for late AR: May be superimposed on CR (biopsy required)
- Renal artery stenosis: Typically a late complication (> 1 y post transplant)
- Activity in bladder from native kidneys may mask obstruction
- Full bladder or reflux may mimic obstruction: Empty bladder critical for renal scan
- Urinoma/urine leak: Days to weeks post-operatively; ↑ creatine due to reabsorbed urine
- Lymphocele: Typically 2-4 months post-operatively

  - AVN: Abnormal baseline renal scan at 24 hr (AR typically occurs later)
  - Relatively normal perfusion with cortical retention; function improves spontaneously over days to weeks
  - ↓ Flow, uptake & output in severe cases; differentiation from obstruction may be difficult
- Acute rejection
  - Perfusion in AR generally worse than function: Often technically difficult to visualize
  - ↑ Cortical retention compared to baseline from 1 week to < 1 year: Sensitive, fairly specific for AR
    - Hyperacute AR may occur immediately post transplant
  - Specificity of cortical retention low without baseline as scar/incomplete resolution of ATN may be present
  - Late-developing AR & immunosuppressive drug toxicity appear similar
  - Sensitivity and specificity lower for late AR: May be superimposed on CR (biopsy required)
- Chronic renal allograft nephropathy
  - Rare in transplant < 1 y unless prior episodes of severely compromised function
  - First sign: ↓ Blood flow, ERPF with relatively spared function
  - Over time, cortical thinning with worsening uptake and clearance develop, along with ↑ cortical dilation
  - Furosemide may help differentiate from obstruction
- Vascular complications
  - Fairly rare: Occlusions seen < 1% and RAS up to 10%
  - Renal vein thrombosis (RVT): Different pattern in transplant vs. native kidney RVT
    - Transplant RVT: Lack of draining collaterals, overall perfusion ↓ causing absent or photopenic transplant
    - Native kidney RVT: Large "hot" kidney as activity gets in but does not clear
  - Renal artery thrombosis: Also shows absent function
  - Renal artery stenosis: Typically a late complication (> 1 y post transplant)
    - Imaging pattern similar to that for native kidney captopril scan
- Drug toxicity
  - Cyclosporin classic cause of ↓ transplant function; rarely seen today as lower concentrations used
    - Acute cyclosporin toxicity is microvascular thrombosis: Very poor blood flow to kidney
    - Chronic cyclosporin toxicity is non-specific ↓ flow, function
  - Drug toxicity suggested if drug plasma concentration ↑ and improvement occurs when drug stopped
  - Other types of drug effects such as acute tubular necrosis can be seen with antibiotics & NSAIDs
- Surgical complications
  - Obstruction: May occur from days to years post-operatively
    - Activity in bladder from native kidneys may mask obstruction
    - Full bladder or reflux may mimic obstruction: Empty bladder critical for renal scan
  - Urinoma/urine leak: Days to weeks post-operatively; ↑ creatine due to reabsorbed urine
  - Lymphocele: Typically 2-4 months post-operatively
- Pyelonephritis: More common in allografts than general population, ↑ with vesicoureteral reflux

Ultrasonographic Findings
- Developing fluid collections (urinoma, lymphoceles, hematoma), hydronephrosis, blood flow changes
- Pulsatility and resistive indices: Nonspecific for differentiation AR from AVN

Imaging Recommendations
- Best imaging tool
  - Renal scintigraphy
    - Assess blood flow and function with Tc-99m MAG3, preferred tracer for evaluating renal transplant
    - Tc-99m MAG3 is cleared more rapidly than Tc-99m DTPA, important in cases of poor renal function
- Protocol advice
  - Perform baseline renogram at 24-48 hr to assess function & allow better differentiation of acute transplant nephropathy/AR

RENAL TRANSPLANT

- Knowing baseline uptake slope and degree of cortical retention critical in identification of deterioration in AR
- Patient preparation: 300-500 mL water po or IV hydration (7 mL/kg)
- Patient voids immediately before exam or catheterize bladder in those with incomplete emptying
- Patient position: Supine with camera anterior, centered over side of pelvis containing transplant
- Camera: Low energy collimator, windowed 15-20% around 140 keV photopeak
- Computer: Acquire study in two phases, angiogram and functional
  - Angiogram: Dynamic 1-4 sec/frame for 60 sec
  - Dynamic: 20-60 sec frames for 20-30 min followed by prevoid & postvoid images
- Radiotracer
  - Tc-99m MAG3: 3-5 mCi (111-185 MBq) IV
  - Second-line: Tc-99m DTPA, 10-15 mCi (370-555 MBq) IV
- Diuretic: Furosemide (40 mg IV adult) if obstruction suspected; administer 20 min after radiotracer injection if good function
- Processing
  - Region of interest (ROI) around kidney, avoid bladder, background ROI next to kidney
  - Background ROI preferences vary: Crescent or encircle allograft
  - Time activity curve (TAC) processing: For blood flow and dynamic function phases
  - Measures of excretion: Seen in 3rd phase of TAC and ratios of late counts to peak counts (e.g., the 20/3 ratio)
- Calculate measures of excretion/cortical retention
  - Perfusion index: Kidney to aorta (iliac artery for transplant) ratio
  - T½: Time required to go from maximal counts to half maximal counts (normal 6.6 ± 2.8 min)
  - 20/3 ratio: Ratio of counts at 20 min to counts at 3 min, may also use 20 min:peak ratio, normal ≤ 0.3
- Calculate glomerular filtration rate (GFR) or effective renal plasma flow (ERPF): May allow earliest identification chronic allograft nephropathy
- Interpretation
  - Perfusion to allograft: Normally within 4 sec of radiotracer bolus passing through iliac artery
  - Normal peak cortical activity 3-5 min post injection
  - Normal renal transit: Tracer in collecting system, bladder by 6 min
  - By end of exam, cortex should clear or be significantly less than early in exam if no cortical retention
  - Cortical retention seen in AR or AVN
  - Cortical loss & dilated pelvis helpful identifiers in CR
- Additional nuclear medicine imaging options
  - Tc-99m DMSA: Can be used to identify acute pyelonephritis (patchy areas of decreased uptake), or focal areas of infarction
  - In-111 labeled platelets: Can identify AR with high sensitivity but use not widespread, expensive
  - Labeled leukocyte scintigraphy: Patchy or focal uptake may indicate pyelonephritis (low sensitivity)
    - In-111 preferred over Tc-99m HMPAO WBCs: Tc-99m HMPAO metabolites excreted by kidneys
    - In-111 WBCs typically show diffuse uptake even in healthy transplants: Mononuclear cell residence from previous rejection
  - Tc-99m sulfur colloid scintigraphy: Diffuse uptake in transplant indicates current or previous rejection
    - Once rejection occurs, sulfur colloid uptake remains due to mononuclear cell residence
  - Ga-67 citrate: Normal transplants show uptake up to 1 year; 20% retain activity > 1 y
    - Normal uptake up to 48 h: Must image ≥ 72 h for renal disease
    - Intense or focal uptake > 48 h may indicate rejection or infection

DIFFERENTIAL DIAGNOSIS

Technical Factors (Injection Technique)
- Small IV site, poor bolus, extravasation of dose: Mimic ↓ blood flow to transplant

Hypotension
- Hypotension: Mimics ↓ blood flow to transplant

Full Bladder, Reflux
- Full bladder: May mimic obstruction

CLINICAL ISSUES

Treatment
- Complex drug regimens to prevent or treat AR
  - Steroids: The foundation of immunosuppression
  - Other medications: Calcineurin blockers (Tacrolimus), interleukin-2, antiproliferative drugs (azathioprine), monoclonal antibodies
  - Close monitoring and care to prevent toxicity-related renal failure

DIAGNOSTIC CHECKLIST

Consider
- Bladder activity from native kidneys may mask obstruction

Image Interpretation Pearls
- Bladder emptying critical to accurate interpretation

SELECTED REFERENCES
1. Russell CD et al: Prediction of renal transplant survival from early postoperative radioisotope studies. J Nucl Med. 41(8):1332-6, 2000
2. Dubovsky EV et al: Report of the Radionuclides in Nephrourology Committee for evaluation of transplanted kidney (review of techniques). Semin Nucl Med. 29(2):175-88, 1999
3. Dubovsky EV et al: Radionuclide evaluation of renal transplants. Semin Nucl Med. 25(1):49-59, 1995

RENAL TRANSPLANT

IMAGE GALLERY

Typical

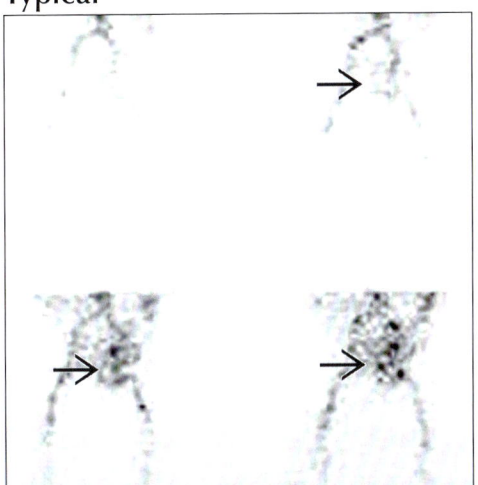

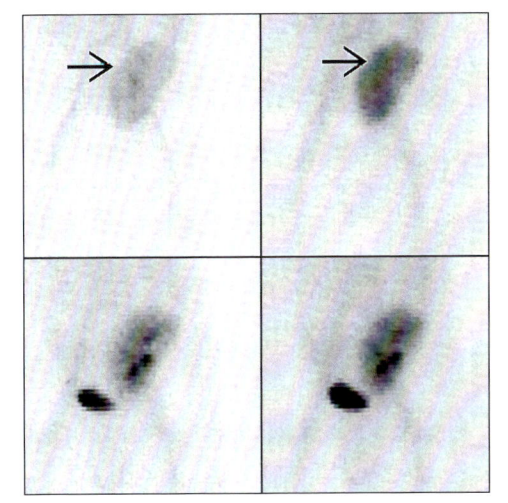

(Left) Anterior angiographic phase of renal scan shows very poor perfusion of renal allograft ➔ in a case of acute rejection. See next image. *(Right)* Nephrogram phase shows slightly heterogeneous and delayed uptake and excretion by renal allograft ➔. Blood flow is often worse than function in acute rejection.

Typical

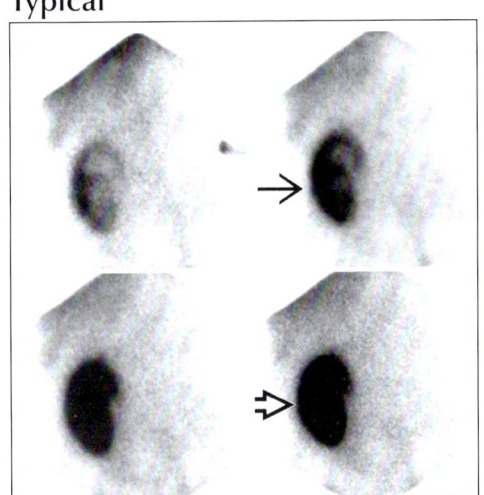

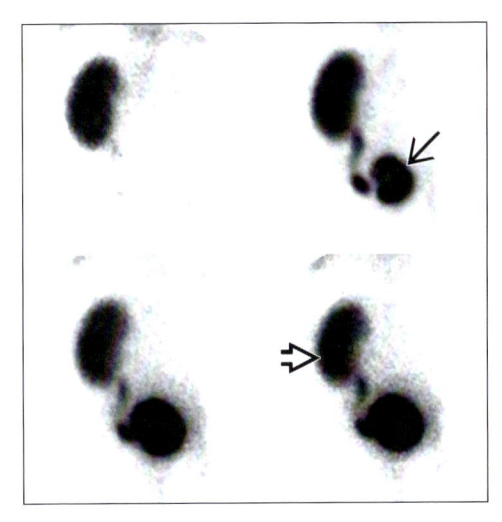

(Left) Anterior renogram two weeks after transplantation shows continual increasing activity ➔ over time without significant excretion ⇨ in a case of severe acute rejection. See next image. *(Right)* Anterior renogram in the same patient as previous image, three weeks later shows marked improvement with excretion ➔, although cortical retention ⇨ persists.

Typical

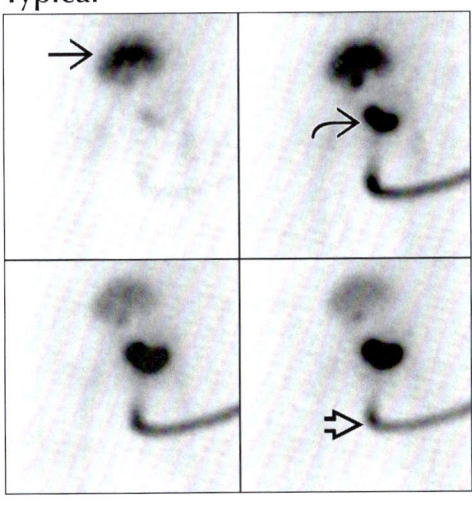

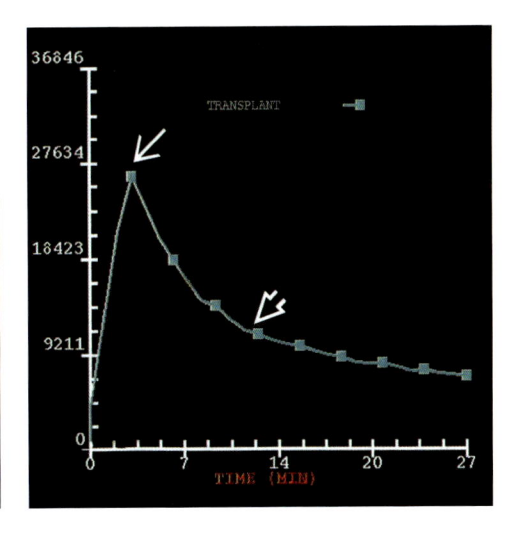

(Left) Anterior renogram shows normal renal allograft function with prompt uptake ➔ and excretion of MAG3 into the bladder ➔. A bladder catheter is in place ⇨. See next image. *(Right)* Normal time activity curve in the same patient as previous image shows rapid peak uptake ➔ and washout ⇨ of radiotracer in baseline exam of a living related donor allograft.

RENAL TRANSPLANT

(Left) Anterior renogram shows post-operative scan of a cadaveric donor allograft: Normal blood flow ➡ and typical cortical retention ⇨ of acute vascular nephropathy (formerly called ATN). (Right) Anterior renogram perfusion images show lack of flow to renal transplant (photopenia) ⇨, consistent with vascular catastrophe (arterial thrombosis in this case). (Courtesy E. Dubovsky, MD).

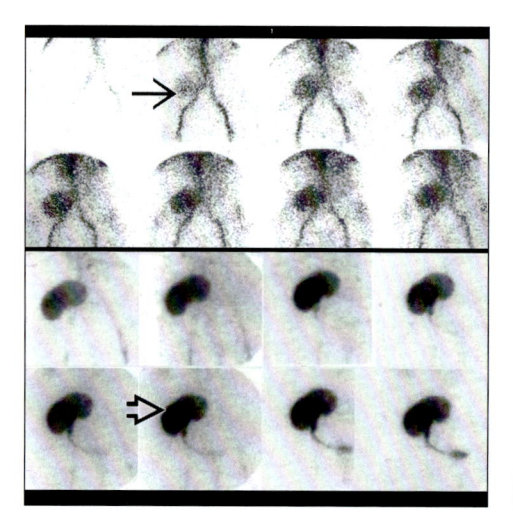

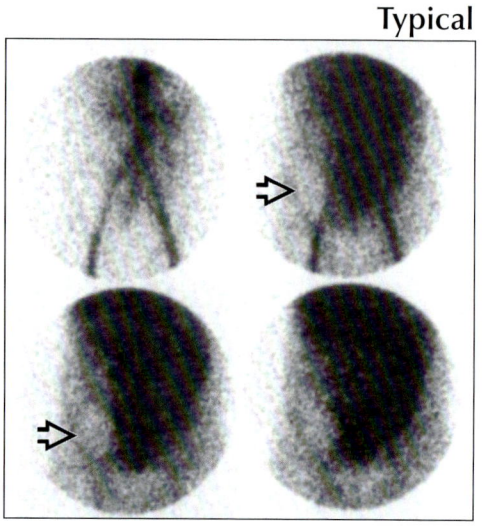

Typical

(Left) Anterior renogram shows hydronephrotic allograft ⇨ that responds to furosemide administration ➡. A bladder catheter is appropriately in place ➡. (Right) Anterior renogram of two year old allograft shows high background activity ➡ and a prominent collecting system ⇨, typical of chronic nephropathy.

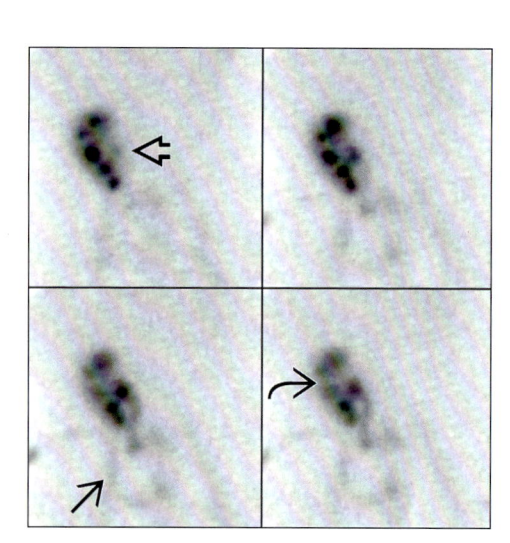

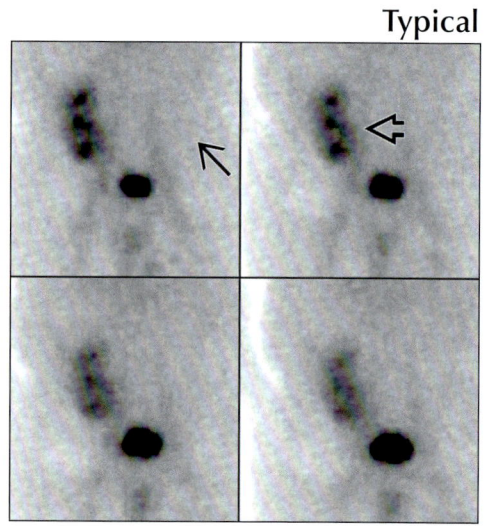

Typical

(Left) Pain and rising creatinine 3 days following transplantation of living related donor kidney prompted renal scan, which shows normal blood flow to the allograft ➡. See next image. (Right) Nephrogram phase shows progressive accumulate of labeled urine around allograft, consistent with urine leak. This will cause rising creatinine due to recycling of absorbed urine.

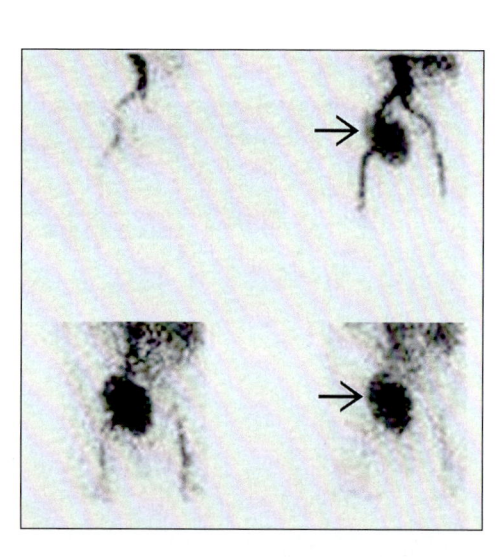

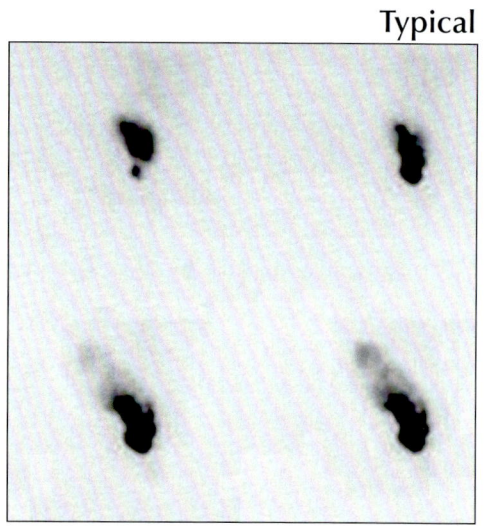

Typical

RENAL TRANSPLANT

Typical

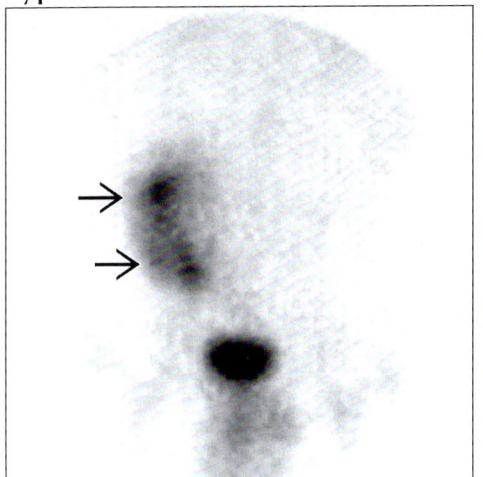

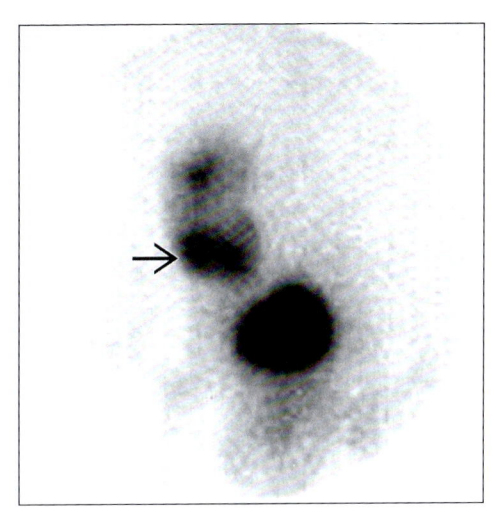

(Left) Single 20 min frame of baseline (non ACE-I) renal scan in hypertensive patient 9 years after living related donor transplant shows relatively homogeneous cortical uptake ➔. See next image. *(Right)* Repeat renal scan with ACE-I shows marked retention of tracer in cortex of inferior pole ➔ of transplanted kidney suggestive of RVHT caused by subsegmental RAS. See next image.

Typical

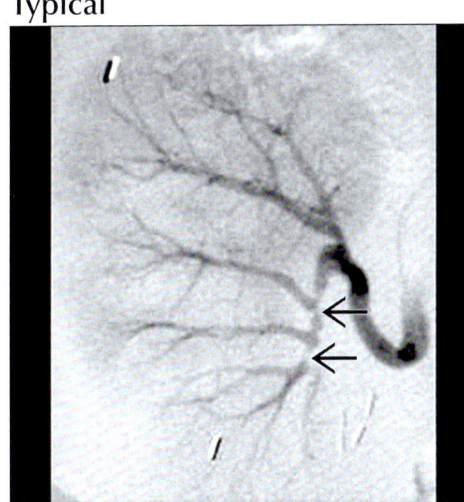

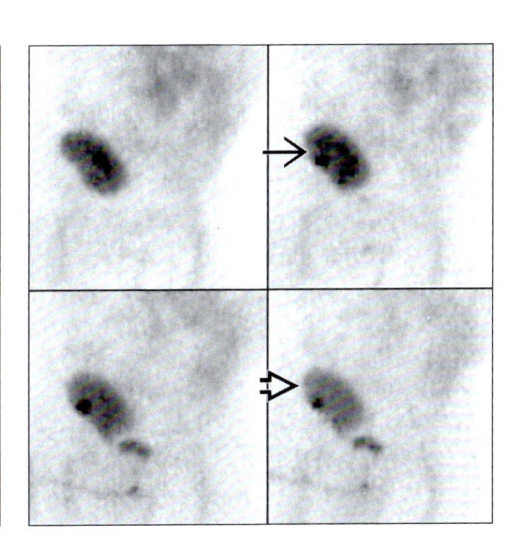

(Left) Renal transplant arteriogram shows beaded areas of stenosis in lower pole segmental renal artery branch ➔. RAS, often segmental or subsegmental, is a common late complication of renal transplantation. *(Right)* Nephrogram phase 1 day following living related donor transplant shows near normal concentration ➔ and clearance ⇨ of tracer. See next image.

Typical

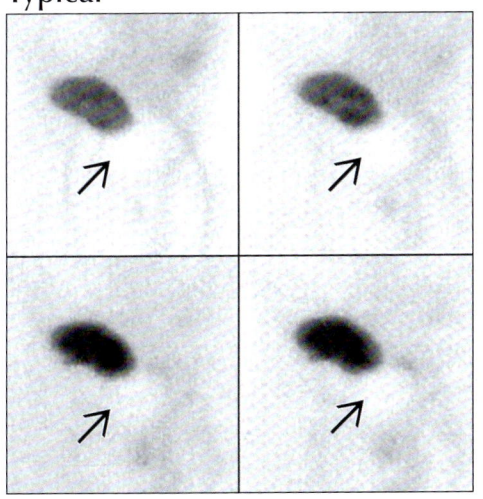

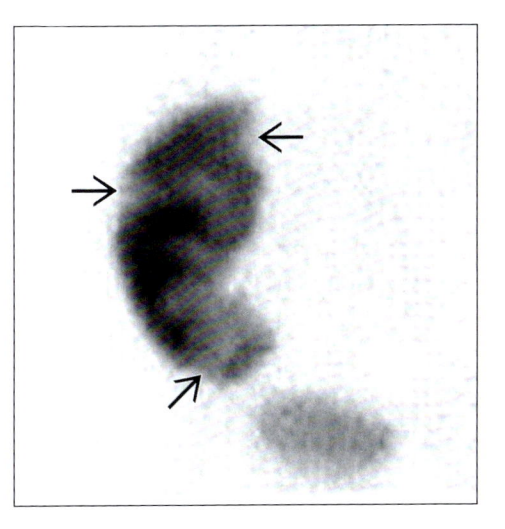

(Left) Repeat renal scan 2 months post transplant, in face of rising creatinine, shows lack of excretion of tracer, which is due to obstruction of allograft from subrenal lymphocele (photopenia) ➔. *(Right)* Single anterior frame of nephrogram phase of renal scan in a 7 year old allograft shows extensive cortical scarring ➔, typical of repeat infections, episodes of acute rejection or subsegmental renal artery disease.

RENAL FUNCTION QUANTIFICATION

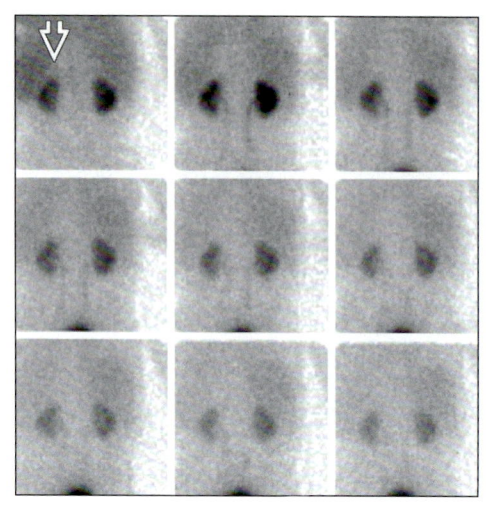

MAG3 images from a patient following aortic aneurysm surgery show subtle diminished relative function on the left ➡. While they provide valuable information, images do not measure overall function itself.

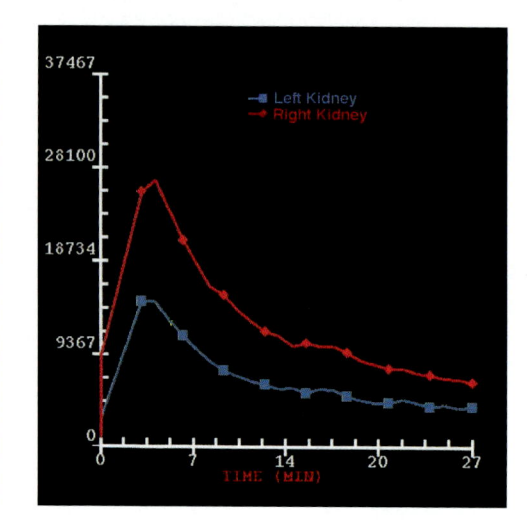

TACs from the same patient show the relative decreased left renal function. While they do not measure function, they represent the functional status of each kidney-rate of uptake, clearance, and differential contribution.

TERMINOLOGY

Background
- Renal function can be measured by determining rate a substance disappears/is cleared from plasma
  - Clearance (mL/min) = [urine concentration (mg/mL) x urine flow (mL/min)]/plasma concentration (mg/mL)
  - Maximum clearance would occur with 100% extraction, directly reflecting renal blood flow
  - Renal plasma flow (RPF) normally ~ 120 mL/min with ~ 20% blood flow filtered by glomeruli and ~ 80% passing to tubules
  - Total renal function: Sum of material filtered at glomerulus and secreted at tubules
  - Radiopharmaceuticals are available that measure tubular secretion or glomerular filtration
  - Measuring total clearance of a substance reaching kidneys reflects total RPF
  - True RPF measurement would require agent with 100% extraction
  - Because available radiopharmaceuticals attain less than 100% clearance, measurement is termed "effective" renal plasma flow (ERPF)
- ERPF: RPF measurement is approximated by highly extracted agents
  - Paraaminohippurate: Gold standard for ERPF measurement, difficult to use clinically
  - Not commercially available in US, I-131 or I-123 hippuran, cleared by tubular secretion (80%) and glomerular filtration (20%), hippuran accurately assesses ERPF
  - Tc-99m mercaptoacetyltriglycine (MAG3): Highly extracted, cleared essentially entirely by tubular secretion; currently used for ERPF
  - MAG3 clearance is ~ 60% that of hippuran; ERPF calculations with MAG3 are adjusted to reflect this difference
- Glomerular filtration rate (GFR): Measurement of substances filtered by glomerulus
  - Material freely filterable at glomerulus: Unbound by proteins and of sufficiently small size, charge; not secreted at tubules or reabsorbed
  - Inulin: Laboratory gold standard for GFR measurement
  - Creatinine clearance: Classic clinical measurement of GFR, assesses total renal function, time consuming, prone to error, insensitive to early changes
  - Radiotracers allow accurate, more rapid measurement of GFR
  - GFR may be measured with Cr-51EDTA (unavailable in US) or Tc-99m diethylenetriamine pentaacetic acid (DTPA)
  - DTPA: Cleared entirely by filtration at glomerulus, no tubular secretion, closely approximates GFR
  - Because of lower clearance of glomerular agents relative to tubular agents, tubular agents (e.g., MAG3) preferred in cases of renal failure
- Compartmental models
  - In order to measure renal clearance, simplified models have been developed outlining distribution of a substance injected intravenously
  - Slope of clearance curve reflects two phases
    - Phase 1: Initial rapid drop as activity moves out of intravascular space
    - Phase 2: Slightly slower linear second phase as material clears into urine
  - Two-compartment model: Injected material enters vascular blood pool (V1), then moves back and forth into extracellular soft tissues (V2) before being cleared into urine (V3)

RENAL FUNCTION QUANTIFICATION

Key Facts

Terminology
- Renal function can be measured by determining rate a substance disappears/is cleared from plasma
- Renal plasma flow (RPF) normally ~ 120 mL/min with ~ 20% blood flow filtered by glomeruli and ~ 80% passing to tubules
- Tc-99m mercaptoacetyltriglycine (MAG3): Highly extracted, cleared essentially entirely by tubular secretion; currently used for ERPF
- DTPA: Cleared entirely by filtration at glomerulus, no tubular secretion, closely approximates GFR
- In order to measure renal clearance, simplified models have been developed outlining distribution of a substance injected intravenously

- Single blood sample methods have been developed to measure ERPF as well as GFR following a single radiotracer injection
- Gamma camera quantitative methods are available when blood sampling methods are not practical, including lack of wet lab or scintillation detector

Procedure
- Precise technique is required for both blood sample and camera techniques
- Draw blood sample: ERPF blood single blood sample can be taken 44 min after injection while GFR sampling occurs later at 3 hr
- Camera methods measure the percentage of activity localizing in the kidneys at 1-3 min for MAG3 ERPF or 2-3 min for DTPA GFR

- By making assumptions about distribution, formulas have been developed making it possible to measure renal function without continuous infusion or urine collection
- Blood sample methods
  - Most accurate methods for measuring renal function involve blood sampling to measure plasma disappearance of a substance
    - Multiple blood samples taken during continuous radiotracer infusion are most accurate, but excellent simplified methods have been established
  - Single blood sample methods have been developed to measure ERPF as well as GFR following a single radiotracer injection
  - Highly reproducible, results utilizing single sample technique may vary ~ 10% but this represents a minimal change in rates (e.g., ≤ 10 mL/min for GFR)
- External detection (camera) methods
  - Gamma camera quantitative methods are available when blood sampling methods are not practical, including lack of wet lab or scintillation detector
  - Camera methods must correct for attenuation using renal depth measurement or assumptions
  - Results from imaging methods vary more than blood sampling methods at ~ 20%

PRE-PROCEDURE

Indications
- Follow post-procedure renal function (e.g., renal artery stent, pyeloplasty), monitor renal transplant function, assess acute renal failure

Contraindications
- None

Getting Started
- Things to Check
  - Patient preparation
    - Hydration: Hydrate well orally with ~ 500 mL water or 5-10 mL/kg IV
    - Empty bladder completely immediately prior to radiotracer injection
    - Obtain good direct venous access for injection in one arm & for blood sample (if desired) from opposite arm
    - Injection should not utilize central lines or long IV tubing as dose adhering to tube will significantly alter calculations
- Equipment List
  - Dose calibrator: Must be accurate & requires routine quality control monitoring
  - Camera: Camera method or may use image only to check injection site to confirm adequate injection
    - Low energy collimator on wide field of view camera
  - Scintillation detector for blood sample method, pipettes and dilution lab equipment
  - Syringe holder stand: To hold dose away from camera surface for preinjection counting

PROCEDURE

Procedure Steps
- Precise technique is required for both blood sample and camera techniques
- Measure patient height & weight
- Patient placed supine with camera immediately adjacent to kidneys
- Select desired radiotracer
  - GFR: 1.5 mCi (55.5 MBq) DTPA IV for camera method while 10-15 mCi (370-555 MBq) used for routine renal scintigraphy
  - ERPF: 1.5 mCi (55.5 MBq) MAG3 IV for camera method; 3-5 mCi (111-185 MBq) generally used for routine imaging
- Select desired technique
  - Blood sample technique
    - Calibrate dose and inject activity bolus in arm opposite from sample draws

RENAL FUNCTION QUANTIFICATION

- Measure syringe post-injection residual in dose calibrator
- Draw blood sample: ERPF blood single blood sample can be taken 44 min after injection while GFR sampling occurs later at 3 hr
- Dilute sample for scintillation counting
- Prepare dilute standard for comparison
○ Camera technique
- Place dose in a syringe holder 30 cm from the surface of the camera
- Count pre- and post-injection syringe activity for 1 minute
- Dead time losses are acceptable for small doses (1.5 mCi) but adjustments must be made for larger doses
- Camera methods measure the percentage of activity localizing in the kidneys at 1-3 min for MAG3 ERPF or 2-3 min for DTPA GFR
- Imaging may be completed in only a few minutes although 25 min is traditional for routine scintigraphy
- Formulas correcting for depth, body mass/surface area are used to calculate renal function

Findings and Reporting

- GFR: Normal GFR ~ 120 mL/min; sampling time varies with function
  ○ When GFR > 100 mL/min, 2 hr is a sufficient delay for sampling but when function is < 60 mL/min, closer to 4 hours is optimal

Alternative Procedures/Therapies

- Radiologic
  ○ CT quantitation of renal function is being developed using changes in contrast enhancement density (Hounsfield units) but is unproven in patients with abnormal function
  ○ MR gadolinium contrast can be used to estimate GFR but split renal function calculations vary widely and gadolinium has been implicated in the rare but severe disorder nephrogenic systemic fibrosis among patients with elevated creatinine/renal failure

POST-PROCEDURE

Image Processing

- Generate routine perfusion time activity curves (TACs): Region of interest (ROI) placement around kidneys and nearest major artery (aorta for native kidneys & iliac for transplants) as the bolus passes during 1st minute
- Function TACs: ROIs around the kidneys, background regions (either crescent or around kidney), and possible around bladder
- Calculate routine split function from the 1-3 minute nephrogram activity

PROBLEMS & COMPLICATIONS

Problems

- Inaccurate measurements occur for many reasons
  ○ Inaccurate dose delivery: Dose infiltration, inaccurate dose calibration, inaccurate post-injection residual measurement
  ○ Radiopharmaceutical issues: Impurities which can clear at different rates or radiolabel breakdown
  ○ Blood sample errors: Errors in sample dilution or standard counting
  ○ Result errors for failure to correct for patient body size as plasma volume is proportional to body surface area: Results should be normalized to 1.73 sq meters
  ○ Camera measurement errors: Incorrect dose syringe placement from camera surface, too high a dose overwhelming camera counts
  ○ Third space losses
  ○ Recent radiotracer administration with elevated background levels will alter measurements and must be corrected for
- GFR diminishes more rapidly than ERPF in cases of compromised renal function: May be limiting when function is very low
  ○ Acute tubular necrosis (ATN): Reciprocal pattern, GFR maintained at a higher level in the face of diminished ERPF

SELECTED REFERENCES

1. Piepsz A et al: Guidelines for glomerular filtration rate determination in children. Eur J Nucl Med. 28(3):BP31-6, 2001
2. Russell CD et al: Reproducibility of single-sample clearance of 99mTc-mercaptoacetyltriglycine and 131I-orthoiodohippurate. J Nucl Med. 40(7):1122-4, 1999
3. Taylor A et al: Multicenter trial validation of a camera-based method to measure Tc-99m mercaptoacetyltriglycine, or Tc-99m MAG3. Radiology. 205:47-54, 1997
4. Russell CD et al: Renal clearance of technetium-99m-MAG3: normal values. J Nucl Med. 36(4):706-8, 1995
5. Piepsz A et al: Determination of the technetium-99m mercaptoacetyltriglycine plasma clearance in children by means of a single blood sample: a multicentre study. The Paediatric Task Group of the EANM. Eur J Nucl Med. 20(3):244-8, 1993
6. Russell CD et al: Measurement of glomerular filtration rate: single injection plasma clearance method without urine collection. J Nucl Med. 26(11):1243-7, 1985
7. Dubovsky EV et al: Quantitation of renal function with glomerular and tubular agents. Semin Nucl Med. 12(4):308-29, 1982
8. Gates GF: Glomerular filtration rate: estimation from fractional renal accumulation of 99mTc-DTPA (stannous). AJR Am J Roentgenol. 138(3):565-70, 1982
9. Schlegel JU et al: Individual renal plasma flow determination in 2 minutes. J Urol. 116(3):282-5, 1976
10. Blaufox MD: Methods for measurement of the renal blood flow. Prog Nucl Med. 2:71-84, 1972
11. Blaufox MD et al: Measurement of effective renal plasma flow in man by external counting methods. J Nucl Med. 8(2):77-85, 1967
12. Sapirstein LA et al: Volumes of distribution and clearances of intravenously injected creatinine in the dog. Am J Physiol. 181:330-6, 1955

RENAL FUNCTION QUANTIFICATION

IMAGE GALLERY

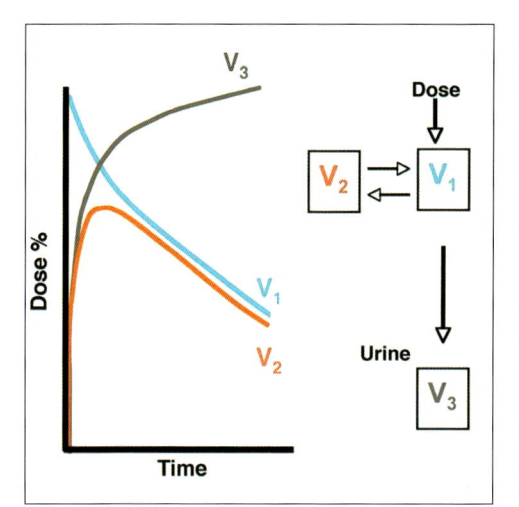

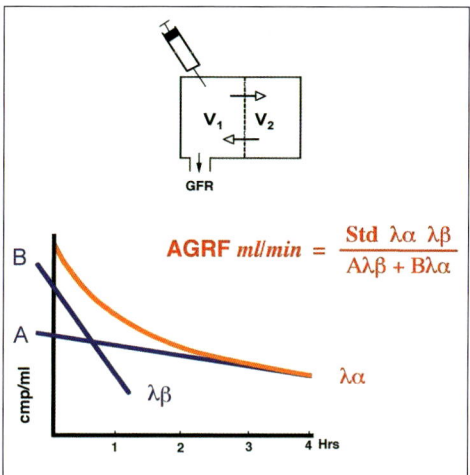

(Left) Graphical representation of a compartmental model for plasma clearance. V1 is the intravascular space, V2 is extracellular space/soft tissues, & V3 is urine output. **(Right)** Graphical representation of 2 phases of plasma clearance. Slope B = rapid movement out of intravascular space and slope A = clearance into urine. Clearance measurements depend on sampling time.

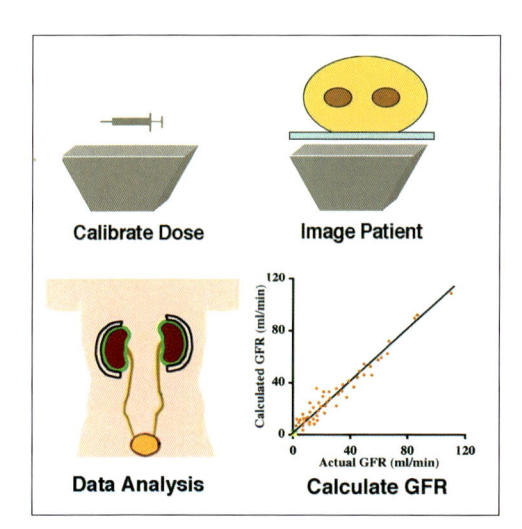

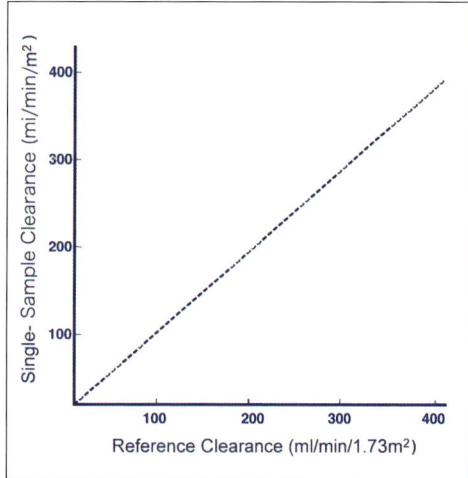

(Left) Camera method for renal function measurement (GFR here) with preinjection syringe counting, patient imaging, & processing. Such estimated measurements can closely reflect actual GFR. (Courtesy H. Liu, MD). **(Right)** Single blood sample technique accuracy for ERPF measurement using I131 hippuran. MAG3 results are proportional. Properly done, single injection/single blood sample method closely correlates with multiple sample techniques.

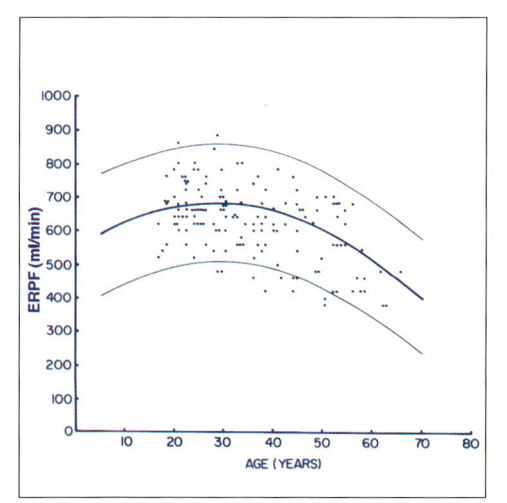

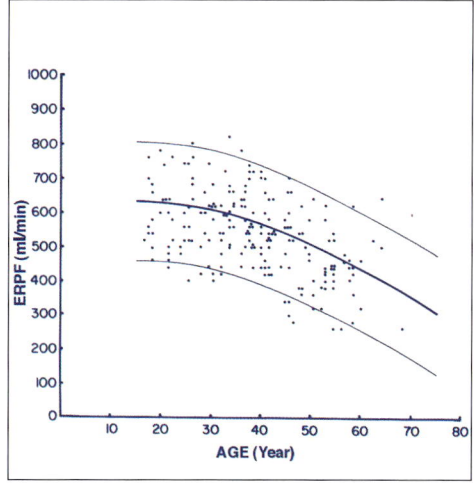

(Left) Normal renal function for men based on potential male renal donors showing expected changes in normal function (curves within 2 standard deviations from normal) with age. **(Right)** Normal ERPF function in women from female potential renal donors. Again, function normally declines with age, and normal lies within 2 standard deviations (curves). Images courtesy of Dr. Eva Dubovsky, from Nuclear Medicine in Clinical Urology by Tauxe & Dubovsky, 1985.

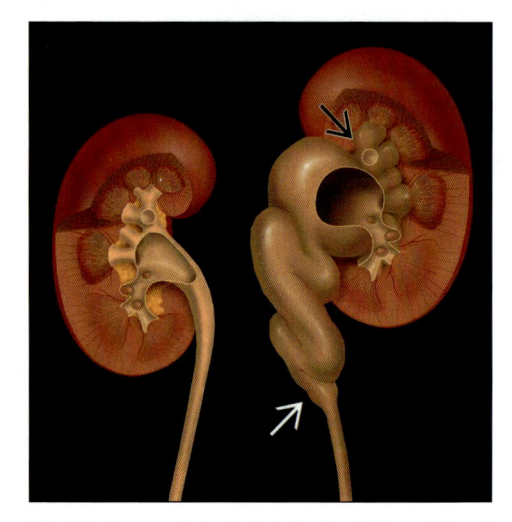

OBSTRUCTIVE UROPATHY

Graphic shows unilateral dilated calices and dilated, corkscrew renal pelvis, to the level of the ureteropelvic junction, consistent with UPJ obstruction.

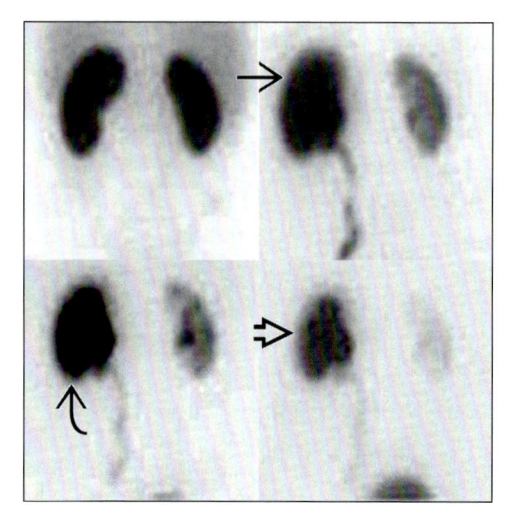

6 week old infant with left hydronephrosis. Tc-99m MAG-3 images at 5, 10, 15 and 30 min. post injection. Lasix given at 15 min. Washout T 1/2 = 24 min (high grade partial UPJ obstruction).

TERMINOLOGY

Abbreviations and Synonyms
- Ureteropelvic junction (UPJ); ureterovesical junction (UVJ)

Definitions
- Obstruction of urinary outflow producing hydronephrosis or acute or chronic renal insufficiency

IMAGING FINDINGS

General Features
- Best diagnostic clue: Lasix renography: Decreased washout from dilated collecting system
- Location: Most common sites of obstruction: UPJ, ureter, UVJ, bladder outlet
- Size
  ○ Degree of hydroureter/hydronephrosis variable
  ○ Hydronephrosis/hydroureter: May persist after obstruction relieved
  ○ Bladder outlet obstruction: May show mild or no hydronephrosis
- Morphology: Collecting system is typically dilated proximal to the level of obstruction

Nuclear Medicine Findings
- Degree of obstruction inferred by renal + collecting system washout curves: O'Reilly classification
- Normal kidney and collecting system
  ○ Type-I curve (normal): Spontaneous washout of activity from collecting system prior to Lasix (furosemide) administration (washout T 1/2 < 10 minutes)
  ○ Washout curve after Lasix often flat: Activity already eliminated from collecting system
- Very high grade or complete obstruction
  ○ Degree of hydronephrosis: Variable, dependent on acuity
  ○ ↓ Renal blood flow and differential function: Cannot predict functional potential in face of high grade obstruction
  ○ Delayed time to cortical peak and cortical clearance: "Delayed nephrogram" equivalent
  ○ Delayed or non-visualization of collecting system
  ○ Type II curve (high grade obstruction): Progressive rise in activity in collecting system, even after Lasix

DDx: Mimics of Obstruction

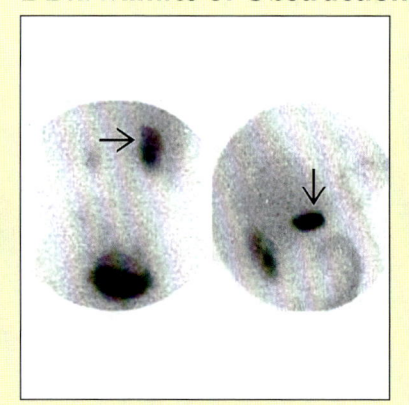

Gallbladder Activity 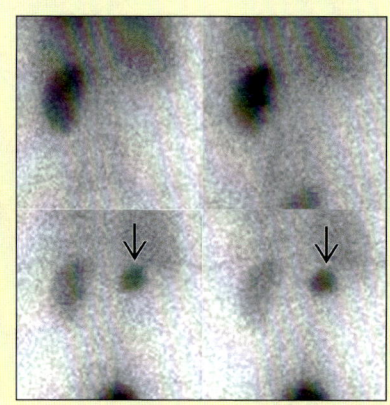   *Vesicoureteral Reflux* 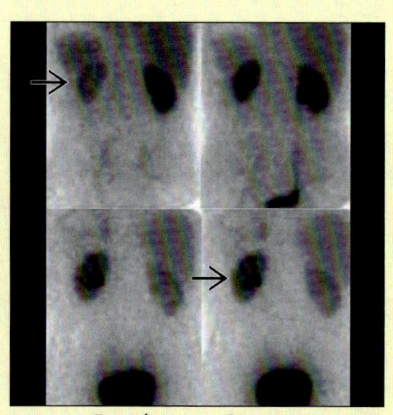   *Renal Artery Stenosis*

OBSTRUCTIVE UROPATHY

Key Facts

Imaging Findings
- Degree of obstruction inferred by renal + collecting system washout curves: O'Reilly classification
- Type-I curve (normal): Spontaneous washout of activity from collecting system prior to Lasix (furosemide) administration (washout T 1/2 < 10 minutes)
- Type II curve (high grade obstruction): Progressive rise in activity in collecting system, even after Lasix
- Type IIIa curve (dilated, non-obstructed): Activity continues to rise until Lasix given, then washes out normally (washout T 1/2 ≤ 10 min)
- Type IIIb curve (partial obstruction): Activity continues to rise until Lasix; thereafter decreases but washout T 1/2 > 10 min
- Acute obstruction: IVP or NECT
- Chronic obstruction: Tc-99m MAG-3 renography with Lasix
- Postural drainage maneuver: Greatly reduces number of false positive or indeterminate Lasix renograms
- Rationale: Many causes of false positive or indeterminate scans show normal emptying in upright position

Top Differential Diagnoses
- Dilated, Non-Obstructed Collecting System
- Renal Vein Thrombosis
- Renal Artery Stenosis
- Acute Tubular Necrosis
- Vesicoureteral Reflux
- Medical Renal Disease
- Multicystic Dysplastic Kidney

- Dilated, non-obstructed collecting system
  - Normal differential renal function (unless prior high grade obstruction)
  - Type IIIa curve (dilated, non-obstructed): Activity continues to rise until Lasix given, then washes out normally (washout T 1/2 ≤ 10 min)
- Partial obstruction
  - Renal function ↓: As function of degree, duration of obstruction
  - Type IIIb curve (partial obstruction): Activity continues to rise until Lasix; thereafter decreases but washout T 1/2 > 10 min
    - T 1/2 10-15 min: Low grade obstruction, questionable clinical significance
    - T 1/2 > 20 min: High grade obstruction
    - T 1/2 15-20 min: Partial obstruction, clinically significant
- False positive or indeterminate Lasix washout: ↓ Renal function, ↓ response to Lasix, severely dilated non-obstructed collecting system, immature kidney, dehydration

Imaging Recommendations
- Best imaging tool
  - Acute obstruction: IVP or NECT
  - Chronic obstruction: Tc-99m MAG-3 renography with Lasix
- Protocol advice
  - Patient preparation: No Lasix on day of exam, patient well-hydrated (give oral or IV fluids if dehydrated)
  - Full bladder, incomplete voiding, bladder outlet obstruction, or vesicoureteral reflux will greatly complicate results: Place Foley catheter, if necessary
  - Typical protocol
    - Adults: Inject 7-10 mCi Tc-99m MAG-3 IV, patient supine, camera posterior
    - Pediatric patients: 250 μCi/kg Tc-99m MAG-3 (minimum 2 mCi), may inject Lasix (0.5 mg/kg) and MAG-3 simultaneously
    - Immature kidneys may produce false positive or indeterminate results: Wait until 6-8 weeks of age before Lasix renography
    - Angiographic sequence 1-2 min (display in 2-4 sec/frame); dynamic acquisition x 45 min (display 2-3 min/ frame)
    - Lasix IV when collecting system well-visualized on side of obstruction; typically ~ 14-15 min post injection
    - Lasix dose: 40 mg standard adult dose; 80-150 mg required for maximum diuresis with severe azotemia
    - Inject Lasix slowly: May produce peripheral vasodilatation, hypotension
    - Regions of interest for quantitative analysis: Whole kidney for angiographic phase, differential renal function (1-2 min post injection for MAG-3); whole kidney plus dilated portions of collecting system for Lasix washout curves
- Low grade obstruction: Stability of differential renal function over time important in confirming lack of clinical significance
- Postural drainage maneuver: Greatly reduces number of false positive or indeterminate Lasix renograms
  - Rationale: Many causes of false positive or indeterminate scans show normal emptying in upright position
    - Severely dilated, non-obstructed kidney
    - Poor Lasix response: Poor renal function; already on Lasix
    - Atonic collecting system
  - At conclusion of exam, obtain supine posterior planar image x 1 min ("prevoid")
  - Patient then upright x 10 minutes (void during interval)
  - 10 minutes after prevoid image: Repeat supine posterior image x 1 min ("postvoid")
  - Determine percent retention by kidney + collecting system over 10 minutes
  - Determine upright T 1/2 for clearance of activity: T 1/2 = 0.693/(4.605-LN(%retention))
  - Percent retention (T 1/2): 95% (136 min), 90% (66 min), 85% (43 min), 80% (31 min), 75% (24 min), 70% (19 min), 65% (16 min), 60% (14 min), 55% (12 min), ≤ 50% (≤ 10 min)

OBSTRUCTIVE UROPATHY

- Interpretation: T 1/2 ≤ 10 min (no obstruction); 10 min < T 1/2 ≤ 15 min (low grade obstruction of questionable clinical significance; 15 min < T 1/2 ≤ 20 min (moderate partial obstruction), T 1/2 > 20 min (high grade obstruction)
- Correlative imaging features
  - Diuretic enhanced Doppler sonography: Elevated resistive index (RI) and pulsatile index (PI) in obstruction
  - Supine → upright decrease in size of renal pelvis on ultrasound: Lack of significant obstruction
  - Dynamic contrast-enhanced MR urography: Promising early results using renal transit times, differential renal function & time-intensity curves, crossed vessels
  - Contrast renography (intravenous pyelography, IVP): Delayed nephrogram and appearance of collecting system, dilated collecting system, dilated ureter with "standing column" of contrast to level of ureteral obstruction
  - CT: NECT (identification of stones); CECT (tumors, causes of extrinsic compression)

DIFFERENTIAL DIAGNOSIS

Dilated, Non-Obstructed Collecting System
- May show persistent hydronephrosis in absence of, or after relief of, obstruction
- May show type IIIb curve: Minimized with postural drainage maneuver

Renal Vein Thrombosis
- Similar findings to complete obstruction: Decreased renal blood flow/function, rising nephrogram, ↓ collecting system visualization

Renal Artery Stenosis
- Small kidney; +/- decreased renal blood flow; delayed nephrogram; ↓ excretion; esp. with ACE inhibitors

Acute Tubular Necrosis
- Renal blood flow normal to slightly ↓; rising ("delayed") nephrogram

Vesicoureteral Reflux
- May mimic obstruction if bladder not catheterized during Lasix renography; obstruction and reflux may coexist

Medical Renal Disease
- Impaired renal blood flow, overall decreased renal function
- Bladder outlet obstruction may mimic symmetrical medical renal disease

Multicystic Dysplastic Kidney
- Absence of functioning renal tissue

PATHOLOGY

General Features
- Etiology
  - Congenital: UPJ obstruction, neonatal hydronephrosis, crossed vessels, ectopic insertion of ureter low and medial into bladder (+/- ureterocele)
  - Acquired: Urolithiasis, post-infectious, trauma, retroperitoneal fibrosis, radiation, tumors, bladder outlet obstruction
- Epidemiology: UPJ obstruction: 1 in 500 neonates
- Associated abnormalities: VATER syndrome, cystic renal dysplasia, primary megaureter

CLINICAL ISSUES

Presentation
- Most common signs/symptoms
  - Renal colic: Adults
  - Hydronephrosis on prenatal ultrasound
- Other signs/symptoms: Impaired renal function, urinary tract infection

Demographics
- Age
  - Neonate to adult
  - 1 in 8 have stones by age 70, M:F = 3:1
- Gender: Neonatal hydronephrosis M:F = 5:1

Natural History & Prognosis
- High grade obstruction: Renal functional impairment, infection
- Low grade obstruction: Variable outcome, careful observation if no treatment

Treatment
- Mechanical relief of obstruction: Stent, nephrostomy, pyeloplasty, urinary diversion, lithotripsy

DIAGNOSTIC CHECKLIST

Image Interpretation Pearls
- Postural drainage maneuver: Increases specificity of Lasix renography

SELECTED REFERENCES

1. Hunsche A et al: Increasing the dose of furosemide in patients with azotemia and suspected obstruction. Clin Nucl Med. 29(3):149-53, 2004
2. Karam M et al: Diuretic renogram clearance half-times in the diagnosis of obstructive uropathy: effect of age and previous surgery. Nucl Med Commun. 24(7):797-807, 2003
3. O'Reilly PH; Consensus Committee of the Society of Radionuclides in Nephrourology: Standardization of the renogram technique for investigating the dilated upper urinary tract and assessing the results of surgery. BJU Int. 91(3):239-43, 2003
4. Wong DC et al: Diuretic renography with the addition of quantitative gravity-assisted drainage in infants and children. J Nucl Med. 41(6):1030-6, 2000
5. Rossleigh MA et al: Determination of the normal range of furosemide half-clearance times when using Tc-99m MAG3. Clin Nucl Med. 19(10):880-2, 1994
6. O'Reilly PH et al: The dilated non-obstructed renal pelvis. Br J Urol. 53(3):205-9, 1981
7. O'Reilly PH et al: Diuresis renography in equivocal urinary tract obstruction. Br J Urol. 50(2):76-80, 1978

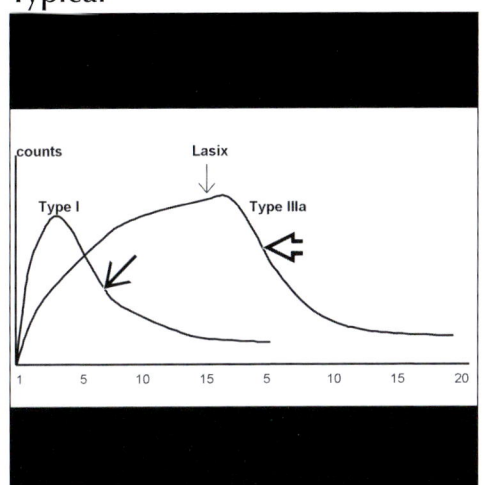

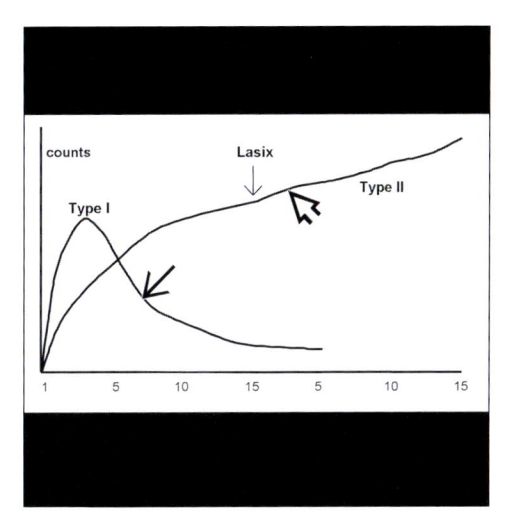

OBSTRUCTIVE UROPATHY

IMAGE GALLERY

Typical

(Left) O'Reilly type I curve (normal) ➡: Spontaneous washout without Lasix, T1/2 ≤ 10 min. O'Reilly type IIIa curve (dilated, non-obstructed collecting system) ➡: Activity rises until Lasix, then normal washout (T 1/2 ≤ 10 min). (Right) O'Reilly type II curve ➡ (very high grade or complete obstruction): Activity rises continuously, even after Lasix. Also shown is type I (normal) curve ➡ for comparison.

Typical

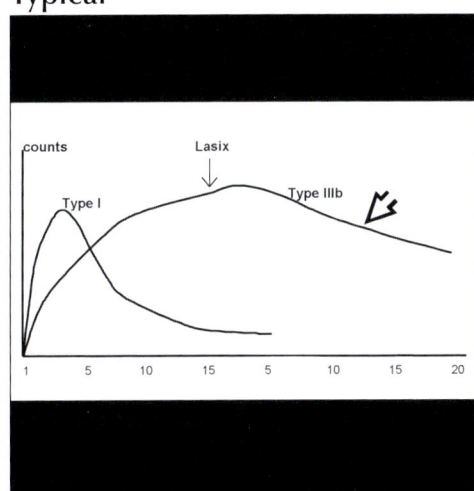

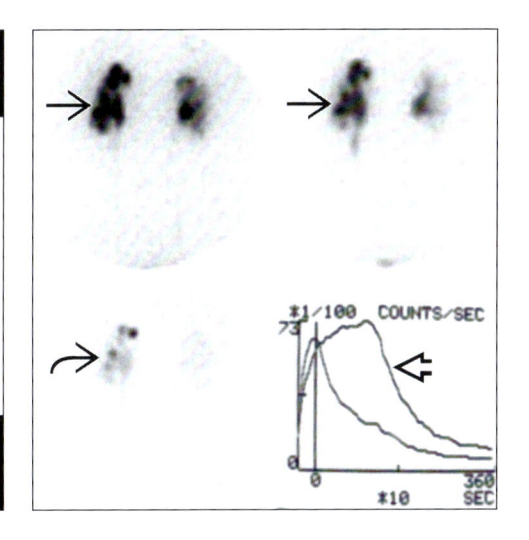

(Left) O'Reilly type IIIb curve ➡: Activity rises until Lasix, then washes out but T 1/2 10-20 min. Consistent with partial obstruction, but can also signify poor Lasix response, severe nonobstructed hydronephrosis, renal insufficiency. Postural drainage can ↑ specificity. (Right) Left hydronephrosis ➡. Normal washout ➡ after Lasix (T 1/2 6 min ➡) excludes obstruction.

Variant

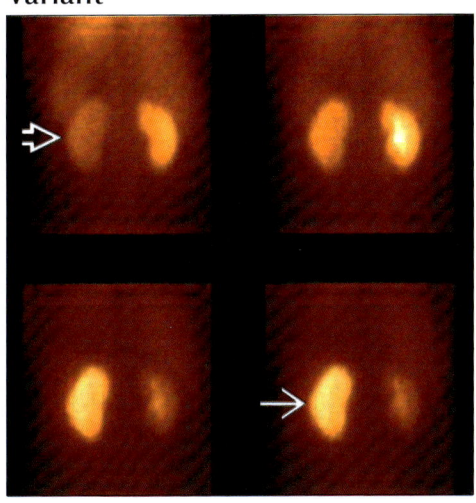

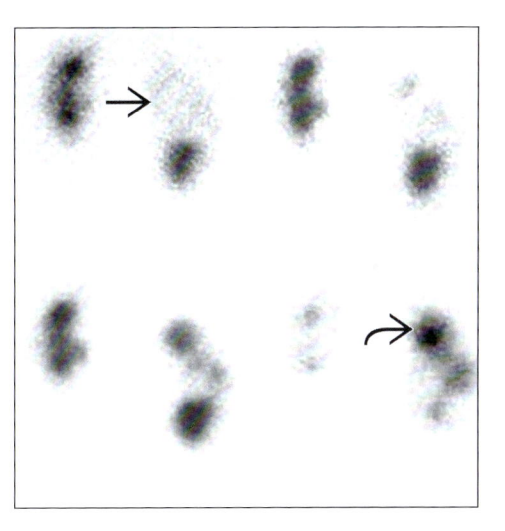

(Left) Complete left renal obstruction: Posterior Tc-99m MAG-3 images show poor uptake ➡ with delayed, rising nephrogram ➡. Collecting system never visualized, therefore Lasix not administered. (Right) Duplication of right kidney, upper pole obstruction: Posterior Tc-99m MAG-3 images show poor uptake in upper pole ➡ with rising activity, even after Lasix ➡. Lower pole refluxed, not obstructed.

REFLUX UROPATHY

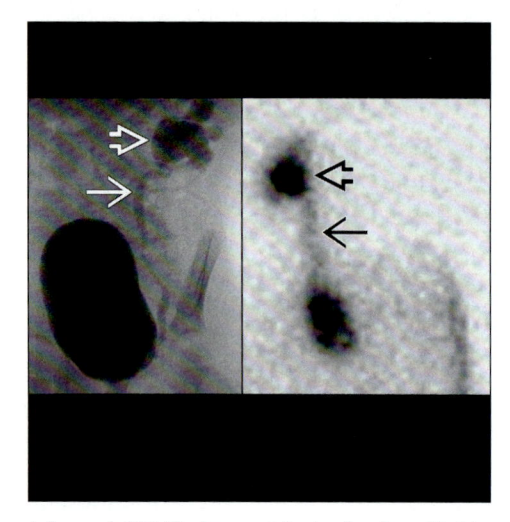

Left panel: VCUG shows grade 4 reflux from bladder into dilated left ureter ➡, intrarenal collecting system ➡. Right panel: Posterior nuclear cystogram shows reflux into ureter ➡, collecting system ➡.

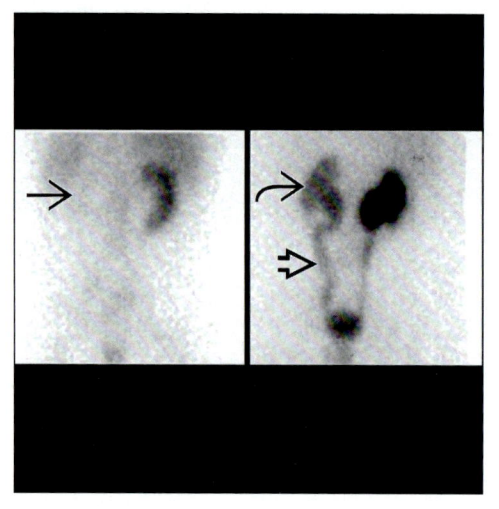

Left panel: Post Tc-99m MAG-3 3 min renogram shows virtually no functioning left kidney. Right panel: Delayed image shows VUR from bladder ➡ into dilated left ureter ➡ and intrarenal collecting system ➡.

TERMINOLOGY

Abbreviations and Synonyms
- Vesicoureteric reflux (VUR), reflux

Definitions
- Retrograde flow of urine from bladder into ureter, renal pelvis

IMAGING FINDINGS

General Features
- Best diagnostic clue
  - Nuclear cystogram: Reflux of radiotracer from bladder into ureter, intrarenal collecting system
  - Voiding cystourethrography (VCUG): Reflux of contrast from bladder into ureter, intrarenal collecting system
    - Often initial study for anatomic evaluation

Nuclear Medicine Findings
- Nuclear Cystogram
  - Performed for serial follow-up of VUR; lower radiation dose compared to VCUG
  - Radiotracer activity in ureter, renal collecting system on filling or voiding = VUR
  - Dynamic images during filling and voiding increases detection of transient VUR
  - Difficult to grade VUR due to lack of anatomic resolution: Qualitatively reported as mild, moderate, severe, or descriptive

Fluoroscopic Findings
- Voiding Cystourethrogram
  - Voiding cystourethrogram (VCUG): Anatomic information in addition to reflux evaluation
  - Early filling image of bladder best shows intraluminal abnormalities: Ureterocele, polyp, mass
  - Iodinated contrast in ureter, renal collecting system on filling or voiding = VUR
  - Oblique views of distended bladder help show periureteral diverticula and ureteric insertion into bladder in cases of VUR
  - Voiding images of urethra to exclude distal pathology: Contribute to back pressure, bladder outlet obstruction

DDx: Mimics of Neonatal Reflux Nephropathy

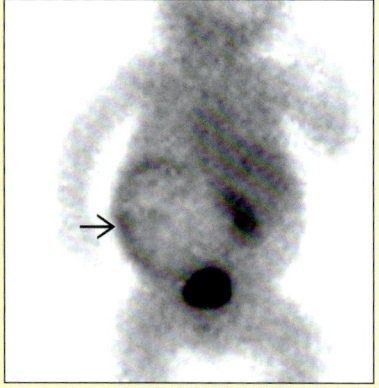

UPJ Obstruction (MAG-3)

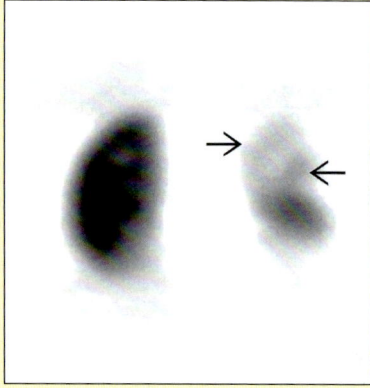

Pyelonephritis Scarring (DMSA)

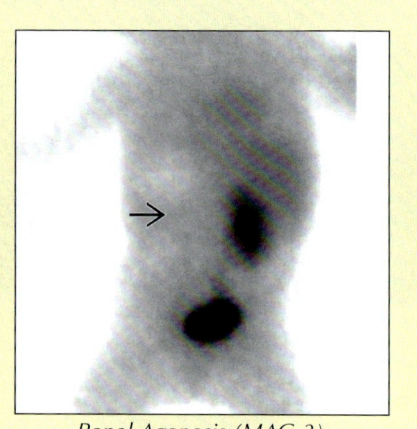

Renal Agenesis (MAG-3)

REFLUX UROPATHY

Key Facts

Imaging Findings
- Nuclear cystogram: Reflux of radiotracer from bladder into ureter, intrarenal collecting system
- Sedation of young patients during study common
- Bladder catheterization using sterile technique
- Tc-99m pertechnetate: 0.5-1 mCi (18.5-37 MBq) instilled as bolus into bladder through catheter
- Bolus administration ensures entire amount of radiotracer delivered to bladder
- Instillation of fluid volume after radiotracer bolus
- Image acquisition: Filling, voiding, post-void

Pathology
- Infancy and early childhood: Most critical period for development of reflux nephropathy
- Eighty percent of patients outgrow reflux, usually by puberty; presumably due to changes at ureterovesicle junction
- Low grade VUR more likely to resolve

Clinical Issues
- Medical management: Prophylactic antibiotics to prevent pyelonephritis
- Surgical management: Ureteral reimplantation
- Minimally invasive: Endoscopic periureteral injections of bulking agents

Diagnostic Checklist
- Nuclear cystogram: More sensitive than VCUG for VUR, but gives less anatomic detail
- DMSA most accurate method for identifying scarring

  - Grading of VUR

Ultrasonographic Findings
- Normal US
- Pelvicaliceal, ureteral, collecting system dilatation
- US not sensitive or specific for VUR

Imaging Recommendations
- Best imaging tool
  - VCUG: Preferred for anatomic detail of upper tracts and evaluation of urethral anatomy; more radiation than nuclear cystogram
  - Nuclear cystogram
    - Serial evaluation of VUR
    - Follow-up after anti-reflux procedure or after antibiotic therapy
    - Diagnosis of familial reflux
    - Initial evaluation of females with urinary tract infection (UTI)
  - Tc-99m DMSA: Best method to identify scarring secondary to reflux, infection
- Protocol advice
  - Patient voids prior to procedure
  - Sedation of young patients during study common
  - Patient position
    - Filling phase: Supine; camera head posterior
    - Voiding phase: Infant, toddler and uncooperative child supine; cooperative child sits upright on bedpan; camera head posterior
  - Bladder catheterization using sterile technique
  - Radiopharmaceutical
    - Tc-99m pertechnetate: 0.5-1 mCi (18.5-37 MBq) instilled as bolus into bladder through catheter
    - Tc-99m sulfur colloid or Tc-99m DTPA used to evaluate augmented bladders (not absorbed through bladder and bowel mucosa)
    - Bolus administration ensures entire amount of radiotracer delivered to bladder
  - Instillation of fluid volume after radiotracer bolus
    - Bladder volume goal: (Age in years + 2) x 30 cc
    - Normal saline, water
    - Gravity instill fluid 70-100 cm above patient via catheter
  - Image acquisition: Filling, voiding, post-void
    - Filling and voiding: Dynamic images at rate of 5 sec per frame, can compress for viewing
    - Post-void: Static image
- Indirect nuclear cystogram
  - Performed after conventional renogram with Tc-99m DTPA or MAG-3
  - Perform conventional dynamic renogram prior to voiding phase
  - After activity clears from kidneys and ureters, record dynamic images during voiding
  - Avoids bladder catheterization
  - Less sensitive than direct radionuclide cystography
  - Not recommended in non-toilet trained children

DIFFERENTIAL DIAGNOSIS

Fluoroscopic Mimics of VUR
- Normal bowel wall surrounded by air, contrast in bowel, or iliopectineal line can mimic contrast in ureter: Clarify with oblique views
- Ventriculoperitoneal tubing, intra-abdominal catheters can resemble contrast-filled ureter

Nuclear Cystography Mimics of VUR
- Contamination may occur with urination and activity on skin resemble reflux
- Bladder diverticula may appear as reflux

Sonographic Mimics of VUR
- Normally peristalsing ureter or renal pelvis
- Distended distal ureter in patients with very full bladders

PATHOLOGY

General Features
- General path comments
  - Shortened or abnormally angulated insertion of ureter into bladder is theorized to result in VUR

REFLUX UROPATHY

- Need adequate length of intramural ureter, adequate contraction of ureteral-trigonal muscles
- May also result from periureteral diverticulum, ureterocele, bladder outlet obstruction, voiding dysfunction, neurogenic bladder
- Infancy and early childhood: Most critical period for development of reflux nephropathy
- Eighty percent of patients outgrow reflux, usually by puberty; presumably due to changes at ureterovesicle junction
- Low grade VUR more likely to resolve
- Etiology
  - Clear association with acute pyelonephritis
  - Sterile VUR likely may be associated with scarring
- Epidemiology
  - Incidence varies, reported as low as < 1% and as high as 1-2% of general population
  - VUR: In 25-40% of children with acute pyelonephritis
  - VUR seen in 5-50% of asymptomatic siblings of children with documented VUR
- Associated abnormalities
  - Multicystic dysplastic kidney
  - Ectopic kidneys
    - Note that VUR most commonly involves contralateral orthotopic kidney
  - Repaired bladder exstrophy
  - Neurogenic bladder
  - Voiding dysfunction

Gross Pathologic & Surgical Features
- Deficiency or immaturity of longitudinal muscle in submucosal ureter
- Distortion of ureteral insertion by adjacent bladder anomaly
- Abnormal angle of ureteral insertion through bladder wall (tends to correct as ureter grows and elongates)

Staging, Grading or Classification Criteria
- International reflux study committee grading system of vesicoureteral reflux
  - I: Reflux into ureter not reaching renal pelvis
  - II: Reflux reaching pelvis but no blunting of calyces
  - III: Mild caliceal blunting
  - IV: Progressive caliceal and ureteral dilation
  - V: Very dilated and tortuous collecting system, intrarenal reflux
- Nuclear cystogram grading
  - Quantitative: Mild (reflux in ureter); moderate (reflux to nondilated pelvicaliceal system and ureter); severe (reflux in distended/redundant collecting system, dilated ureter)
  - Quantitative: Several classification systems (best to be descriptive)
    - Example of qualitative scale: Grade I (reflux in distal 1/2 of ureter); grade II (reflux to proximal 1/2 of ureter); grade III (reflux into non-dilated intrarenal collecting system); grade IV (reflux into dilated intrarenal collecting system)

CLINICAL ISSUES

Presentation
- Most common signs/symptoms
  - Most often discovered during workup of UTI
  - Higher grades of reflux may be suspected on prenatal ultrasound
  - ~ 50% of patients with UTIs have reflux
  - Prevalence of UTI's in infants, young children: 5%

Demographics
- Age: VUR most common in children < 2 yrs
- Gender: Female:male ratio = 2:1
- Ethnicity: More common in Caucasians than African-Americans (reports of 3:1 to 20:1)

Natural History & Prognosis
- 80% outgrow VUR before puberty
- Can lead to renal scar, renal insufficiency, hypertension, end-stage renal disease
- Prognosis is dependent upon: Degree and duration of VUR, presence of UTIs, scarring

Treatment
- Treat infection before performing VCUG, nuclear cystogram
- Medical management: Prophylactic antibiotics to prevent pyelonephritis
- Definitive treatment indicated with repeated infections despite antibiotic prophylaxis; evidence of renal scarring by DMSA
- Surgical management: Ureteral reimplantation
- Minimally invasive: Endoscopic periureteral injections of bulking agents

DIAGNOSTIC CHECKLIST

Consider
- Nuclear cystogram: More sensitive than VCUG for VUR, but gives less anatomic detail
- DMSA most accurate method for identifying scarring

Image Interpretation Pearls
- Reporting of nuclear cystogram
  - Number of attempted bladder fills
  - Total volume instilled into bladder
  - Bladder volume at reflux
  - Qualitative/quantitative assessment VUR magnitude
  - Whether VUR occurred at filling or voiding
  - Qualitative/quantitative residual bladder volume

SELECTED REFERENCES
1. Boubaker A et al: Radionuclide investigations of the urinary tract in the era of multimodality imaging. J Nucl Med. 47(11):1819-36, 2006
2. Piepsz A et al: Pediatric applications of renal nuclear medicine. Semin Nucl Med. 36(1):16-35, 2006
3. Unver T et al: Comparison of direct radionuclide cystography and voiding cystourethrography in detecting vesicoureteral reflux. Pediatr Int. 48(3):287-91, 2006
4. Fettich J et al: Guidelines for direct radionuclide cystography in children. Eur J Nucl Med Mol Imaging. 30(5):B39-44, 2003

REFLUX UROPATHY

IMAGE GALLERY

Typical

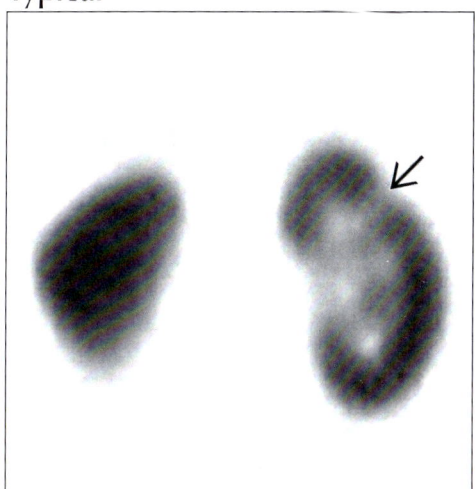

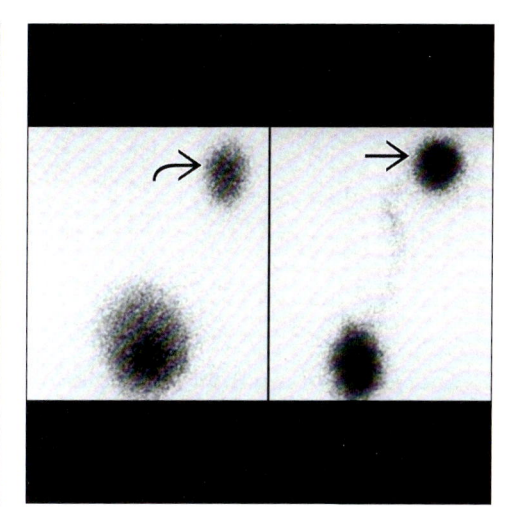

(Left) Coronal Tc-99m DMSA SPECT shows cortical scarring in superolateral upper pole of left kidney ➔, a typical pattern resulting from high grade reflux.
(Right) Left panel: Posterior filling phase of nuclear cystogram shows high grade reflux ➔ into dilated right intrarenal collecting system. Right panel: Voiding phase shows further worsening of reflux with increased bladder pressure ➔.

Typical

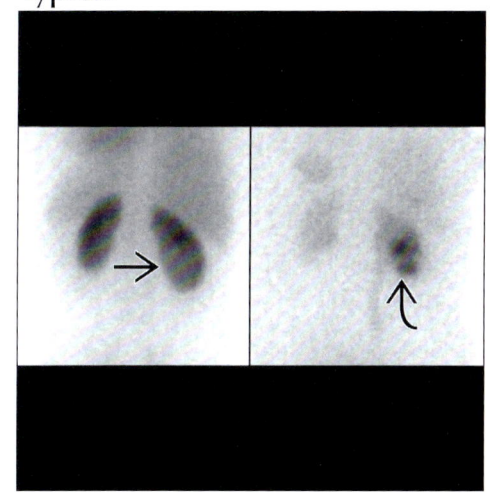

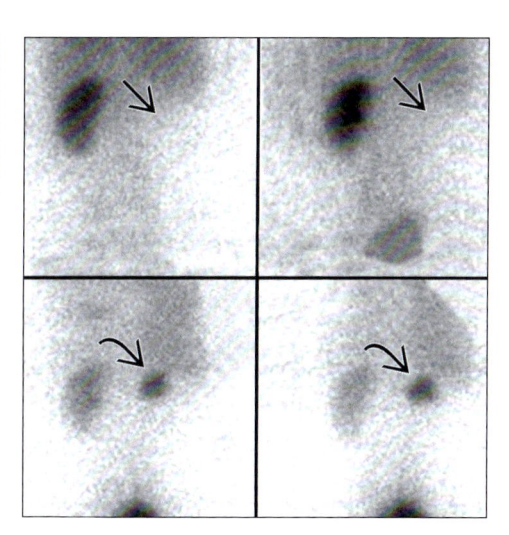

(Left) Posterior 3 min (left panel) and 20 minute Tc-99m MAG-3 renogram (right panel) frames show initial ↓ concentration ➔, subsequent apparent hydronephrosis ➔ due to reflux into lower pole of duplicated collecting system.
(Right) Serial posterior Tc-99m MAG-3 renogram images show initial absence of right renal function ➔ with delayed reflux into right kidney collecting system ➔.

Typical

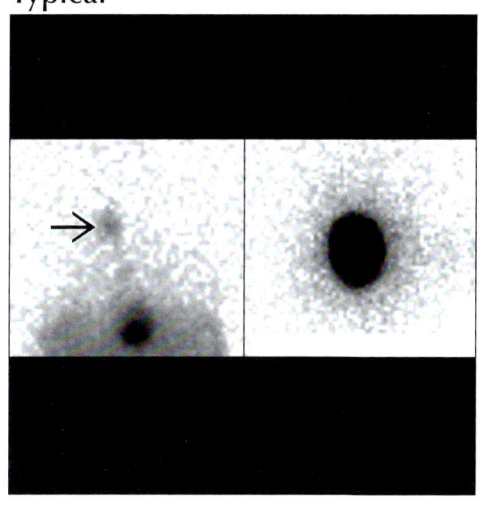

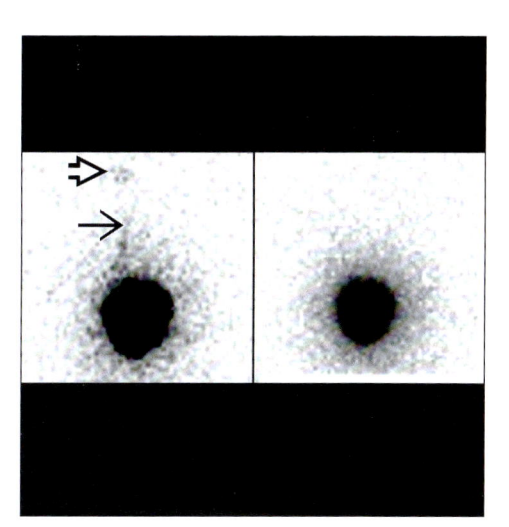

(Left) Left panel: Posterior nuclear cystogram shows moderate reflux into left renal pelvis ➔ in a 7 year old child with multiple UTIs. Right panel: Repeat exam 2 months later following Deflex injection (reflux resolved).
(Right) Left panel: Post nuclear cystogram show moderate reflux into the left ureter ➔ and intrarenal collecting system ➔ in 15 month old female treated with prophylactic antibiotics.

URINARY BLADDER & EPITHELIAL CANCER

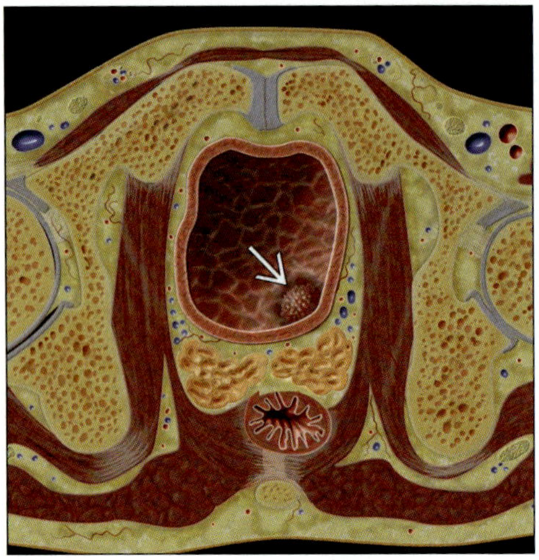

Graphic shows nodular thickening within the bladder wall ➔, typical of transitional cell carcinoma of the bladder.

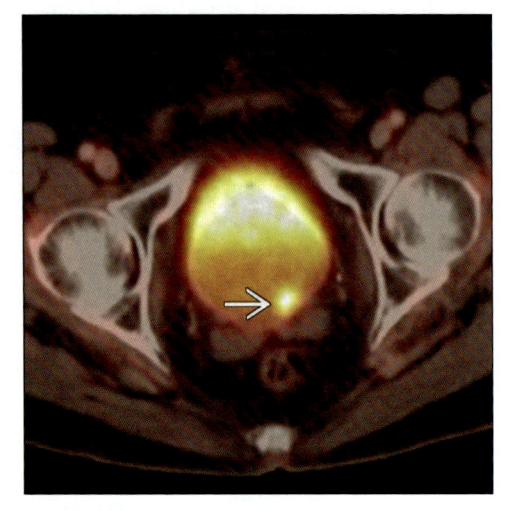

Axial fused PET/CT shows intense FDG activity in a nodular bladder lesion ➔, concerning for primary bladder malignancy.

TERMINOLOGY

Abbreviations and Synonyms
- Bladder carcinoma, urothelial carcinoma, transitional cell carcinoma

Definitions
- Malignancy of urinary bladder

IMAGING FINDINGS

General Features
- Best diagnostic clue
  - PET/CT: Focal increased FDG activity in primary tumor, regional and distant LN, lung, liver, bone
  - Bone scan: Multiple, scattered foci of increased activity in skeleton, axial > appendicular
- Location
  - Bladder wall, bladder lumen
  - Local invasion
    - Detrusor muscle, prostate, uterus, vagina
  - Lymphatic spread (30% of tumors that only involve bladder wall; 60% of those with extravesicular invasion)
    - Regional (pelvic) lymph nodes (LN)
    - Distant LN
  - Hematogenous spread
    - Lung > > liver, bone
- Morphology
  - Superficial (70-80%)
    - Confined to mucosa, lamina propria
    - Project into bladder lumen (papillary)
    - Usually low grade
  - Invasive (20-30%)
    - Within detrusor muscle
    - Solid, infiltrating
    - Usually high grade

Nuclear Medicine Findings
- PET
  - Focal increased FDG activity in primary tumor, regional and distant LN, lung, liver, bone
    - Primary tumor may be masked by excreted FDG in urine

DDx: Benign FDG Activity in Pelvis

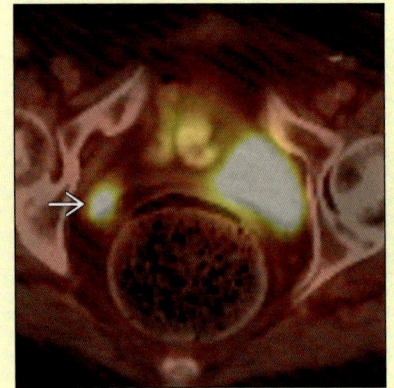

Bladder Diverticulum 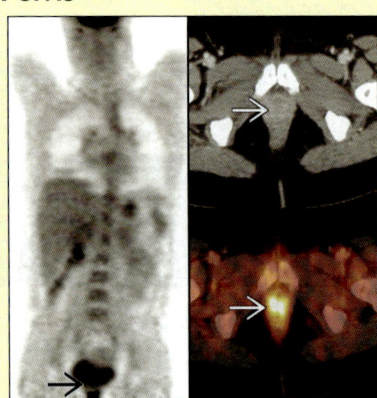   *Incontinence* 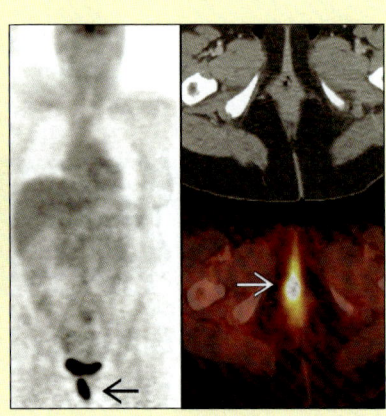   *Menstruation*

URINARY BLADDER & EPITHELIAL CANCER

Key Facts

Terminology
- Bladder carcinoma, urothelial carcinoma, transitional cell carcinoma

Imaging Findings
- Initial workup: Cystoscopy and biopsy; CT or MR for evaluation of primary tumor, LN metastases
- PET/CT: Valuable for preoperative staging, response to therapy, distinguishing post-surgical change from recurrence
- PET/CT: Minimally useful for evaluation of primary tumor
- Bone scan: Helpful if clinical suspicion of bone metastases
- PET/CT: Excreted FDG in urinary bladder can mask pelvic pathology

Top Differential Diagnoses
- Cystitis
- Hematoma
- Cystitis Cystica
- Other Neoplasm

Pathology
- ~ 90% transitional cell carcinomas (TCC); often multifocal
- 5-10% squamous cell (chronic inflammation)
- < 5% mixed TCC and squamous cell
- 2-3% adenocarcinoma (persistent urachal remnant)
- < 1% rare (e.g., leiomyomas, lymphoma, melanoma)

Diagnostic Checklist
- Bladder cancer may have variable FDG uptake; baseline PET/CT useful to confirm FDG avidity

---

- Bladder cancer may have variable uptake of FDG; baseline PET/CT useful for confirmation of FDG avidity
- Bone Scan: Bone metastases: Classically multiple, scattered foci of increased activity, axial > appendicular skeleton

Radiographic Findings
- IVP
  - Filling defect(s) in bladder
  - Hydronephrosis

CT Findings
- CT findings nonspecific, diagnosis based on biopsy
  - Focal or diffuse bladder wall thickening
  - Mass projecting into bladder ± enhancement
- Calcifications
- Hydronephrosis 2° to tumor near vesicoureteric junction
- Extravesicular extension: Nodules, irregularity of outer bladder wall, stranding of perivesicular fat
- T status of tumor most often determined by biopsy

MR Findings
- T1WI: Isointense to muscle
- T2WI: Hyperintense to muscle
- Superior to CT for assessing deep muscle involvement, invasion of adjacent organs

Imaging Recommendations
- Best imaging tool
  - Initial workup: Cystoscopy and biopsy; CT or MR for evaluation of primary tumor, LN metastases
    - CT: Reported accuracy in detecting LN involvement 70-90% with false-negative rates 25-40%
    - MR: 73-98% reported accuracy for determining nodal metastases
  - PET/CT: Valuable for preoperative staging, response to therapy, distinguishing post-surgical change from recurrence
  - PET/CT: Minimally useful for evaluation of primary tumor
  - Bone scan: Helpful if clinical suspicion of bone metastases
- Protocol advice
  - PET/CT: 10-15 mCi (370-555 MBq) F18-FDG IV, start imaging at pelvis
  - PET/CT: Excreted FDG in urinary bladder can mask pelvic pathology
    - Immediate post-void imaging, retrograde bladder irrigation with normal saline, IV Lasix administration with parenteral hydration have been recommended
    - Prone positioning may be useful
  - Bone scan: 20-30 mCi (740-1110 MBq) Tc-99m MDP, whole body scan
    - May detect hydronephrosis; upright, post-void image may exclude obstruction

DIFFERENTIAL DIAGNOSIS

Cystitis
- Infection: Chronic urinary tract infection, fungus
- Radiation or chemotherapy-induced
- Hemorrhagic cystitis

Hematoma
- Trauma
- Iatrogenic

Cystitis Cystica
- Degeneration of urothelial cells in Brunn nests

Other Neoplasm
- Endometriosis
- Metastases

PATHOLOGY

General Features
- General path comments
  - ~ 90% transitional cell carcinomas (TCC); often multifocal

URINARY BLADDER & EPITHELIAL CANCER

- 5-10% squamous cell (chronic inflammation)
- < 5% mixed TCC and squamous cell
- 2-3% adenocarcinoma (persistent urachal remnant)
- < 1% rare (e.g., leiomyomas, lymphoma, melanoma)
- Etiology
  - Risk factors
    - Cigarette smoking
    - Exposure to aniline, aromatic amines, diesel fumes
    - Phenacetin use (once used as analgesic, now often mixed with cocaine)
    - Infection: Chronic urinary tract infection, schistosomiasis
- Epidemiology
  - Most common tumor of urinary tract
  - Men: Fourth most common cancer
  - Women: Tenth most common cancer

Staging, Grading or Classification Criteria
- Preinvasive
  - TNM: To, Tis, Ta
  - Jewett-Strong-Marshall (JSM): 0
- Submucosal invasion
  - TNM: T1
  - JSM: A
- Superficial muscle invasion
  - TNM: T2a
  - JSM: B1
- Deep muscle invasion
  - TNM: T2b, T3a
  - JSM: B2
- Extravesicular spread
  - TNM: T3b
  - JSM: C
- Fixed to or invading prostate, uterus, vagina; pelvic lymph nodes
  - TNM: T4a, T4b; N1 (1 pelvic LN < 2 cm); N2 (1 pelvic LN 2-5 cm; multiple LN < 5 cm); N3 (LN > 5 cm)
  - JSM: D1
- Extrapelvic LN or distant metastases
  - TNM: M1
  - JSM: D2

CLINICAL ISSUES

Presentation
- Most common signs/symptoms
  - 80-90% have painless gross hematuria
  - Urination problems
    - Dysuria
    - Urgency
    - Frequency
- Other signs/symptoms: Hydronephrosis, renal obstruction

Demographics
- Age: Peak incidence 50-60 years
- Gender: M:F, 4:1
- Ethnicity: Caucasians:African Americans = 2:1

Natural History & Prognosis
- Most with metastatic disease die within two years

Treatment
- Surgery
  - Early stage: Transurethral resection, segmental cystectomy
  - Later stages: Radical cystectomy, pelvic LN dissection
- Chemotherapy
  - Intravesicular
  - Systemic
- Radiation
  - Early stage: Radiation implants
  - Later stages: External beam radiation
- Immunotherapy
  - Intravesicular biologic therapy (BCG)

DIAGNOSTIC CHECKLIST

Consider
- At diagnosis, 75-85% have superficial tumors and 15-25% have lymph node metastases
- As many as 50% of patients who have invasive cancer will have occult metastases that will present within five years of diagnosis
- Use PET/CT for optimal preoperative staging (N, M), evaluating response to therapy, detecting recurrence
- Bladder cancer may have variable FDG uptake; baseline PET/CT useful to confirm FDG avidity

Image Interpretation Pearls
- Primary bladder cancer often obscured by excreted FDG in urinary bladder (PET not useful for primary tumor evaluation)
- Immediate post-void imaging, retrograde bladder irrigation with normal saline, IV Lasix administration with parenteral hydration have been recommended
  - Decrease amount of FDG in urinary bladder on PET
  - Decrease rate of false negatives (small adjacent LN) in pelvis due to high FDG activity in bladder

SELECTED REFERENCES

1. Setty BN et al: State-of-the-art cross-sectional imaging in bladder cancer. Curr Probl Diagn Radiol. 36(2):83-96, 2007
2. Jana S et al: Nuclear medicine studies of the prostate, testes, and bladder. Semin Nucl Med. 36(1):51-72, 2006
3. Kamel EM et al: Forced diuresis improves the diagnostic accuracy of 18F-FDG PET in abdominopelvic malignancies. J Nucl Med. 47(11):1803-7, 2006
4. Liu IJ et al: Evaluation of fluorodeoxyglucose positron emission tomography imaging in metastatic transitional cell carcinoma with and without prior chemotherapy. Urol Int. 77(1):69-75, 2006
5. Ng CS: Radiologic diagnosis and staging of renal and bladder cancer. Semin Roentgenol. 41(2):121-38, 2006
6. Drieskens O et al: FDG-PET for preoperative staging of bladder cancer. Eur J Nucl Med Mol Imaging. 32(12):1412-7, 2005
7. Hain SF: Positron emission tomography in uro-oncology. Cancer Imaging. 5(1):1-7, 2005
8. Schoder H et al: Positron emission tomography for prostate, bladder, and renal cancer. Semin Nucl Med. 34(4):274-92, 2004

URINARY BLADDER & EPITHELIAL CANCER

IMAGE GALLERY

Typical

Typical

Typical

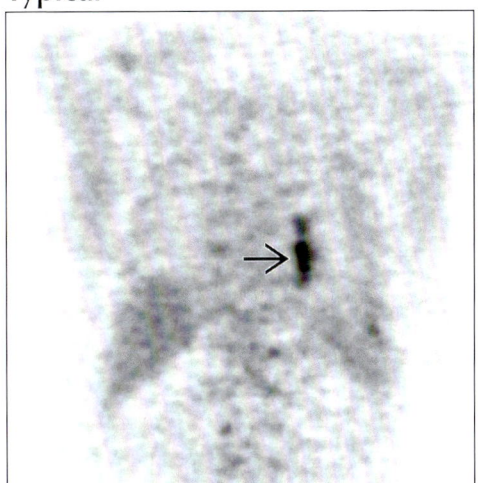

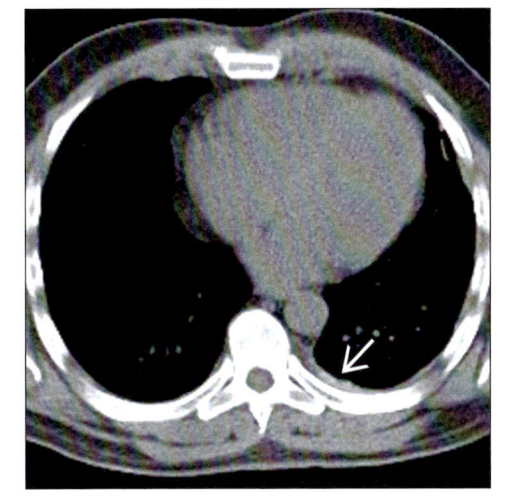

(Left) Coronal PET shows somewhat linear, intense FDG activity in left hemithorax ➡ suspicious for metastasis in patient with a history of bladder carcinoma. See next image. (Right) Axial NECT in same patient as left shows minimal, nonspecific, pleural thickening along medial posterior border of left pleural surface ➡, which prospectively was not called on CT. See next image.

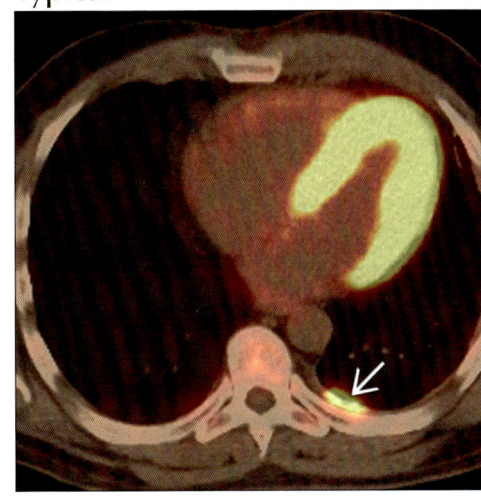

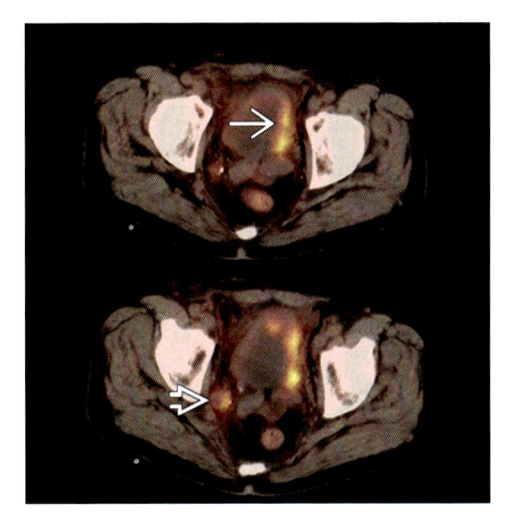

(Left) Axial fused PET/CT in same patient as previous image, shows intense FDG activity correlating to pleural thickening ➡, biopsy-proven metastatic transitional cell carcinoma. (Right) Axial fused PET/CT in patient with bladder cancer show primary cancer ➡ and pelvic lymphadenopathy ➡. See next image.

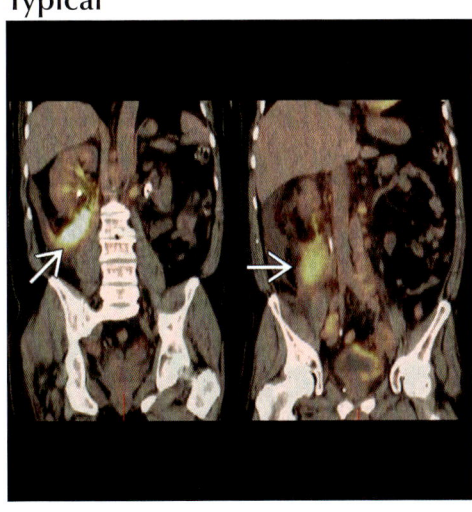

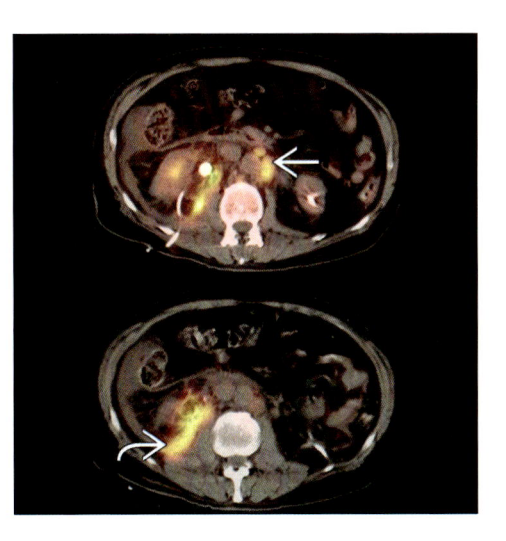

(Left) Coronal fused PET/CT in same patient as previous image shows urinoma ➡ containing renally excreted FDG, a complication of percutaneous nephrostomy for obstructed right ureter. See next image. (Right) Axial fused PET/CT in same patient as left shows periaortic lymphadenopathy ➡ and extravasated urine ➡.

TESTICULAR TORSION

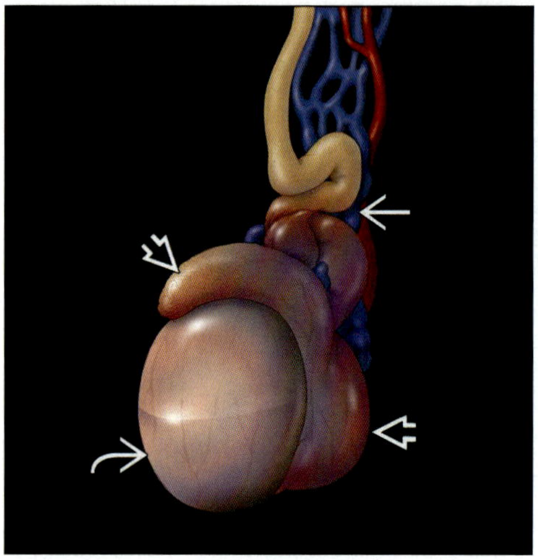

Graphic shows testicular torsion: The spermatic cord is torsed. The testis and epididymis are edematous.

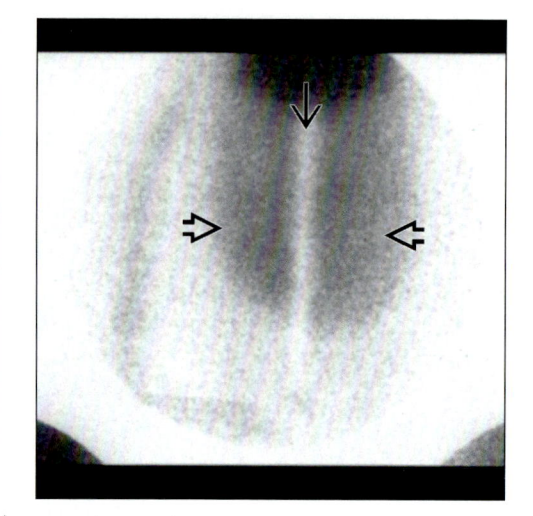

Testicular scan shows normal perfusion to both testicles in an anterior view. A lead marker is placed on the median raphe to distinguish right and left testicles on image. (Courtesy J. Ball, MD).

TERMINOLOGY

Abbreviations and Synonyms
- "Late" or "missed" torsion, acute scrotum, spermatic cord torsion

Definitions
- Spontaneous or traumatic twisting of testis & spermatic cord within scrotum, resulting in vascular occlusion/infarction
  ○ Results from inadequate fixation of testis to tunica vaginalis through gubernaculum testis (bell-clapper deformity) ⇒ testis torsing on spermatic cord
- Leads to ischemia secondary to arterial obstruction, venous outflow obstruction
- Resultant edema, congestion

IMAGING FINDINGS

General Features
- Best diagnostic clue: Decreased scintigraphic activity on painful side
- Location: Unilateral in 95% of patients

Nuclear Medicine Findings
- Tc-99m pertechnetate testicular scan: Sensitivity 80-90%
- Acute phase: 5-7 hours after onset
  ○ Blood flow: Decreased perfusion unilaterally
    ▪ During first 1-2 hours, flow may be normal
  ○ Static image: Decreased activity on affected side
- Mid phase: ~ 7-24 hours
  ○ Blood flow: Absent flow via spermatic cord
  ○ Static image: Photopenia in affected testicle when compared with normal testicle
- Late phase: > 24 hours
  ○ Blood flow: Increased (hyperemia) with testicular infarction
  ○ Static image: Halo sign = testicular infarction
    ▪ Central photopenia
    ▪ Peripheral symmetrically increased activity from pronounced scrotal hyperemia (hyperemia to dartos muscle through pudendal artery)

Ultrasonographic Findings
- Grayscale Ultrasound
  ○ May be normal, especially early after onset

DDx: Testicular Torsion

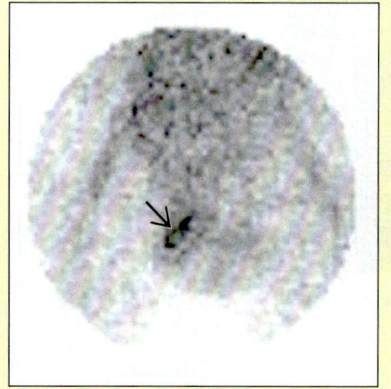

| Epididymitis | Hydrocele | Testicular Atrophy |

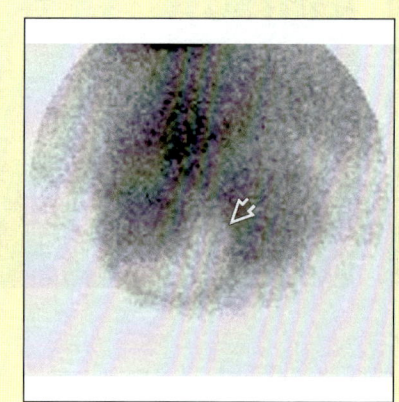

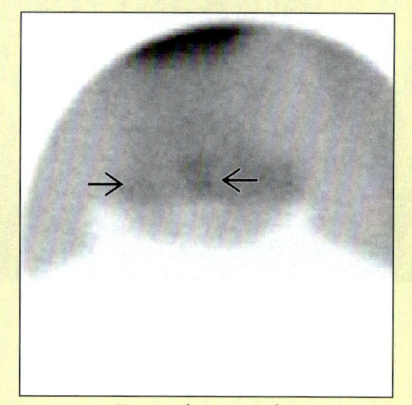

TESTICULAR TORSION

Key Facts

Terminology
- Spontaneous or traumatic twisting of testis & spermatic cord within scrotum, resulting in vascular occlusion/infarction
- Results from inadequate fixation of testis to tunica vaginalis through gubernaculum testis (bell-clapper deformity) ⇒ testis torsing on spermatic cord

Imaging Findings
- Tc-99m pertechnetate testicular scan: Sensitivity 80-90%
- During first 1-2 hours, flow may be normal
- Blood flow: Absent flow via spermatic cord
- Static image: Photopenia in affected testicle when compared with normal testicle
- Blood flow: Increased (hyperemia) with testicular infarction
- Static image: Halo sign = testicular infarction

Top Differential Diagnoses
- Epididymo-Orchitis
- Testicular Abscess
- Hydrocele
- Varicocele
- Inguinal Hernia
- Neoplasm
- Trauma

Clinical Issues
- Clinical Profile: Male child with acute scrotal pain
- Surgical emergency: Testicular infarction if torsion not treated promptly
- Spontaneous detorsion in 7%

  - Enlarged epididymis and testicle typical, with findings appearing 4-6 hours after onset
  - Inhomogeneous echotexture, most often decreased echogenicity
- Color Doppler
  - Unilateral absent or decreased flow
  - May have normal perfusion early

Imaging Recommendations
- Best imaging tool
  - First-line: US with high-frequency linear transducer & color Doppler
  - Nuclear medicine: Tc-99m pertechnetate testicular scan
    - If US equivocal, for problem-solving
- Protocol advice
  - Tc-99m pertechnetate testicular scan: Proper patient positioning critical
    - Legs abducted
    - Tape penis to pubis (point cephalad)
    - Position supine
    - Separate the testicles (left and right) with lead marker along median raphe
    - To reduce activity from thighs, place lead apron posterior to testicles
  - Blood flow images
    - Dose: 30 mCi (1.11 GBq) Tc-99m pertechnetate
    - IV bolus injection
    - 2 seconds per frame for one minute
    - Anterior planar view, converging collimator (or parallel hole collimator with magnification)
  - Static images
    - Anterior planar view, converging collimator (or parallel hole collimator with magnification)
    - Image 15 minutes after injection for 500K counts
    - May need pinhole collimator for best resolution

DIFFERENTIAL DIAGNOSIS

Epididymo-Orchitis
- Marked increased flow on angiographic phase imaging
- Increased activity on delayed images on painful side
- Common condition that may be acute, subacute, or chronic
- Infectious epididymitis
  - Chlamydia trachomatis most common organism in men < 35
  - Sexually transmitted organisms also cause epididymitis, especially gonorrhea
  - Mumps infection in adult male may result in epididymo-orchitis, with fever, scrotal swelling, severe pain; usually bilateral
- Treatment: Ice, scrotal elevation, antibiotics
- Ultrasound: Enlarged epididymis with increased flow on Doppler imaging

Testicular Abscess
- Marked increased flow
- "Donut sign" on static images (similar to "halo sign")
- May be complication of epididymitis

Testicular Atrophy/Undescended Testicle
- Unilateral decreased activity on affected side
- Non-descended testicle may be positioned anywhere along descent, may be in inguinal canal, prescrotal location, or in abdomen
- Nonpalpable or small testicle on physical exam

Torsion of Testicular Appendage
- Appendix testes: Small remnant of Müllerian duct system on anterosuperior aspect of testes
- Tc-99m pertechnetate testicular scan normal or focal mildly increased activity at appendage site
- Pedunculated morphology predisposes it to torsion
- Leading cause of acute scrotal pathology in childhood
- On physical exam may see "blue dot" sign at site of infarcted appendage
- May treat conservatively with rest, ice, anti-inflammatory medications or may have surgical excision of appendix testis

Hydrocele
- Crescent-shaped areas of decreased activity on Tc-99m pertechnetate testicular scan

TESTICULAR TORSION

- May be congenital or reactive secondary to scrotal pathology

Varicocele
- Activity in venous plexus on blood flow and static images

Inguinal Hernia
- Herniation of bowel and omentum may produce pain
- Pain may become severe with onset of incarceration

Neoplasm
- Testicular scan variable

Trauma
- Increased blood flow on Tc-99m pertechnetate testicular scan
- Variable static phase due to associated abnormalities (e.g., hematocele)

PATHOLOGY

General Features
- General path comments: Varying degrees of ischemic necrosis & fibrosis depending on duration of symptoms
- Etiology
  - Embryology-anatomy: Deficient testicular fixation related to tunica vaginalis & gubernaculum testis ("bell clapper" deformity)
  - Tunica vaginalis completely encircles epididymis, distal spermatic cord, and testis (vs. attaching to posterolateral testis)
  - Allows testicle to swing and rotate within tunica vaginalis
- Epidemiology
  - Infants and adolescent boys most often affected
  - 1:4,000 males
  - Epididymo-orchitis > > torsion of testicular appendage > testicular torsion
  - Incidence of bell-clapper deformity 12% in autopsy series, lesser incidence of torsion
  - In neonates may see extra-vaginal torsion (proximal to attachment of tunica vaginalis)
    - 5% of torsion cases
    - 20% bilateral

Gross Pathologic & Surgical Features
- Purple, edematous, ischemic testicle, may rapidly reperfuse when manually detorsed

Microscopic Features
- Hemorrhage interstitial edema, necrosis

Staging, Grading or Classification Criteria
- Previously classified acute, subacute, or delayed based on duration of symptoms

CLINICAL ISSUES

Presentation
- Most common signs/symptoms
  - Sudden onset acute scrotal/inguinal pain, onset often at night
  - Classic physical exam: Asymmetrically high-riding testicle on affected side with bell-clapper deformity, with swollen testicle
  - Absent cremasteric reflex
  - Later may have reactive hydrocele or skin erythema
  - Negative urinalysis
  - Pain not relieved by elevation of scrotum
  - Neonates: Purplish discoloration of swollen scrotum
- Other signs/symptoms: 42% have history of similar episode in same or contralateral testis
- Clinical Profile: Male child with acute scrotal pain

Demographics
- Age
  - Bimodal peak: Neonate and 14 years
  - May occur at any age
  - Increased incidence in colder weather: December, January

Natural History & Prognosis
- Surgical emergency: Testicular infarction if torsion not treated promptly
- Testicular viability depends on degree of torsion (> 540° worse), duration of symptoms & rapid surgical intervention
- Unilateral testicular loss typically does not lead to infertility problems

Treatment
- Immediate surgical exploration with detorsion
  - Orchiectomy if nonviable testicle; higher risk of subsequent torsion on contralateral side
  - Bilateral orchidopexy if viable testicle
- Higher testicular salvage rates in younger patients vs. adults
- Spontaneous detorsion in 7%

DIAGNOSTIC CHECKLIST

Image Interpretation Pearls
- Tc-99m pertechnetate testicular scan: Testicular torsion
  - Decreased or absent blood flow
    - Very early (1-2 hrs) blood flow may be normal
  - Unilateral decreased activity on static images

SELECTED REFERENCES

1. Adams BK et al: Tc-99m blood-pool imaging in torsion of an epididymal appendix. Clin Nucl Med. 28(6):526, 2003
2. Wu HC et al: Comparison of radionuclide imaging and ultrasonography in the differentiation of acute testicular torsion and inflammatory testicular disease. Clin Nucl Med. 27(7):490-3, 2002
3. Yuan Z et al: Clinical study of scrotum scintigraphy in 49 patients with acute scrotal pain: a comparison with ultrasonography. Ann Nucl Med. 15(3):225-9, 2001
4. Flores LG 2nd et al: Scintigraphic evaluation of testicular torsion and acute epididymitis. Ann Nucl Med. 10(1):89-92, 1996
5. Saxby M: Radionuclide scrotal imaging for diagnosis of testicular torsion. Br J Urol. 78(1):157-8, 1996

TESTICULAR TORSION

IMAGE GALLERY

Typical

Typical

Typical

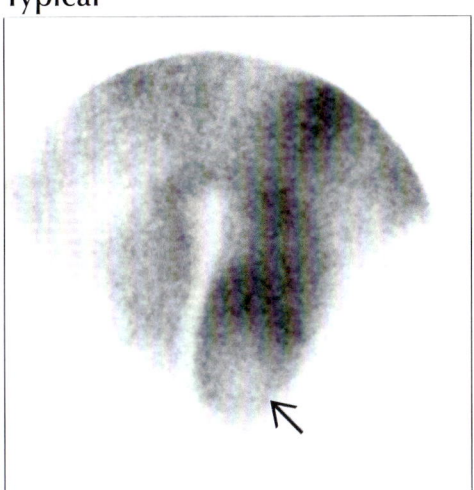

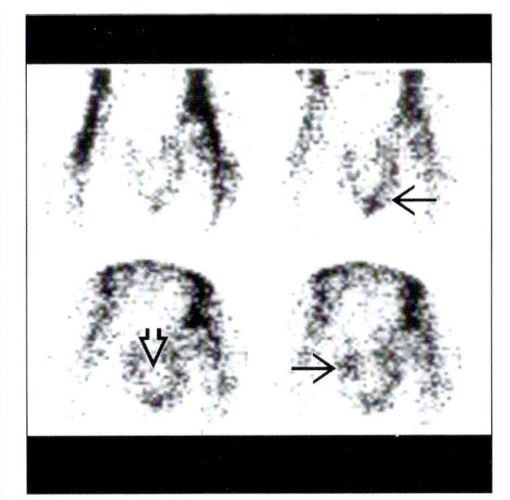

(Left) Testicular scan shows focal hypoperfusion in left testicle ➔ in a patient with mid phase testicular torsion. (Courtesy J. Ball, MD). *(Right)* Testicular scan angiographic phase images show hyperemic ring ➔ due to increased blood flow to dartos of left hemiscrotum. Central photopenia corresponds to infarcted testicle ➔ in a patient with missed torsion. (Courtesy J. Ball, MD).

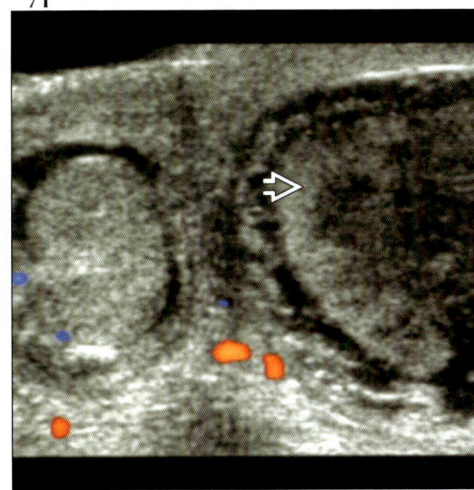

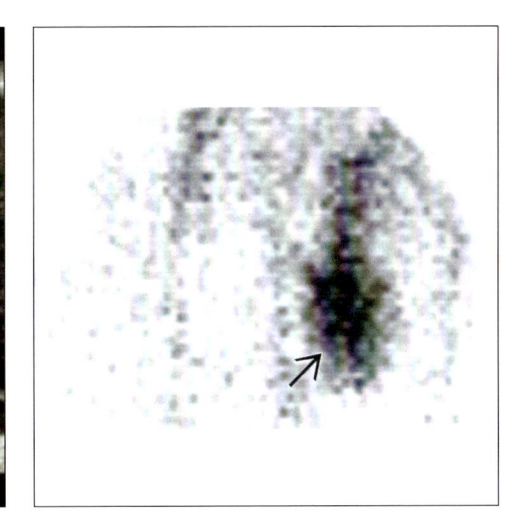

(Left) Color Doppler ultrasound shows enlarged necrotic left testicle ➔ with lack of blood flow in neonate with missed torsion. (Courtesy S. O'Hara, MD). *(Right)* Anterior testicular scan angiographic image shows marked hyperemia to left hemiscrotum ➔ in patient with epididymoorchitis. See next image. (Courtesy J. Ball, MD).

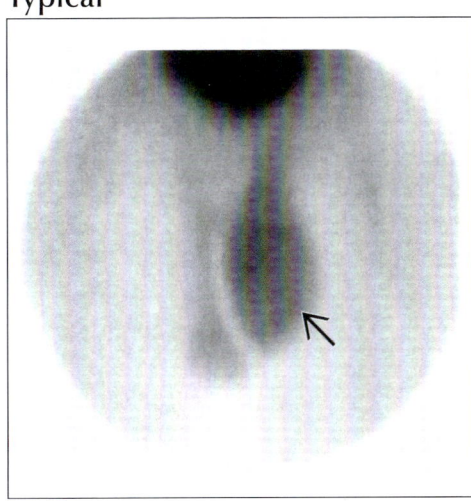

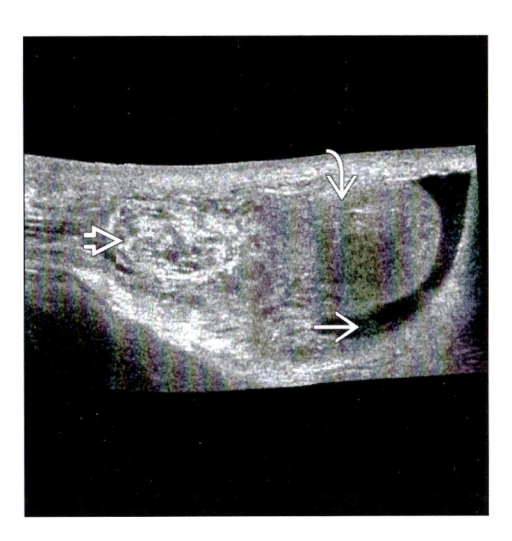

(Left) Anterior testicular scan delayed image in the same patient as previous image, shows diffusely increased uptake in left hemiscrotum ➔. (Courtesy J. Ball, MD). *(Right)* Sagittal ultrasound shows heterogeneous, mostly echogenic, enlarged epididymis ➔, enlarged testicle ➔, and small anechoic reactive hydrocele ➔ in a patient with epididymo-orchitis. (Courtesy S. O'Hara MD).

TESTICULAR CANCER

Schematic drawing of testicular carcinoma. Note heterogeneous, sold mass ➡ arising from testicular parenchyma and distending tunica albuginea.

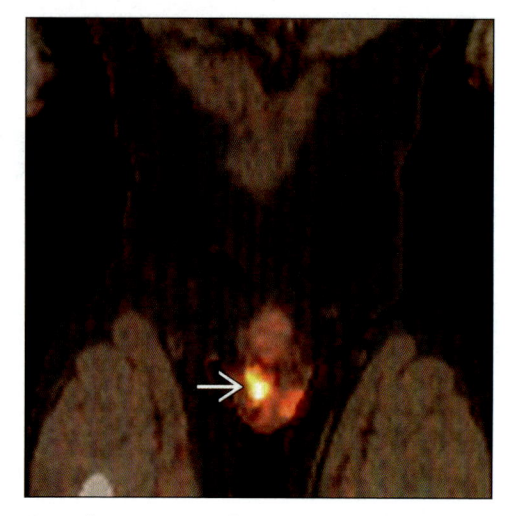

Coronal FDG PET/CT shows hypermetabolic focus in right testicle ➡. Intense uptake is more likely lymphoma (as in this case) or abscess. Primary testicular cancer is typically only moderate in metabolic activity.

TERMINOLOGY

Abbreviations and Synonyms
- Germ cell tumors = testicular carcinoma
- Non-germ cell tumors = gonadal stromal tumors = interstitial cell tumors = sex cord tumors

Definitions
- Germ cell tumors: Malignant; from germ cell elements
  - Seminomas
  - Teratoma/teratocarcinoma (embryonal cell)
  - Choriocarcinoma
- Non-germ cell tumors: Usually benign; from non-germ cell elements
  - Leydig cell tumors (LCT): From interstitial cells
  - Sertoli cell tumors (SCT): From sustentacular cells lining seminiferous tubules
  - Granulosa cell tumors: Rare benign tumors
  - Gonadoblastoma: Contains both stromal and germ cell elements

IMAGING FINDINGS

General Features
- Best diagnostic clue: Discrete hypoechoic or mixed echogenic mass on US
- Location
  - Germ cell tumors: Malignant, metastatic → lymphatic
  - Non-germ cell tumors: Bilateral in 3%; 90% benign; 10% malignant and metastatic
- Size: Non-germ cell tumors: Most benign < 3 cm; most malignant > 5 cm
- Morphology
  - Germ cell tumors: Heterogeneous solid mass
  - Non-germ cell tumors: Well-circumscribed, round-lobulated
  - Variable cystic elements, calcification, necrosis/hemorrhage

Nuclear Medicine Findings
- FDG PET
  - Initial staging of testicular germ cell tumors: FDG PET offers no statistical advantage over CT

DDx: Mimics of Testicular Cancer

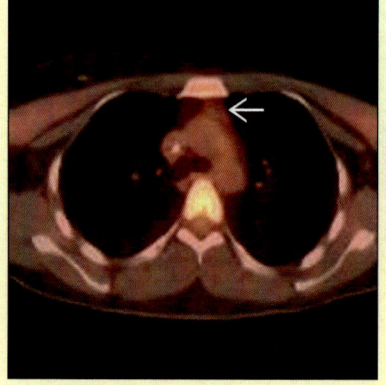

Normal Thymus

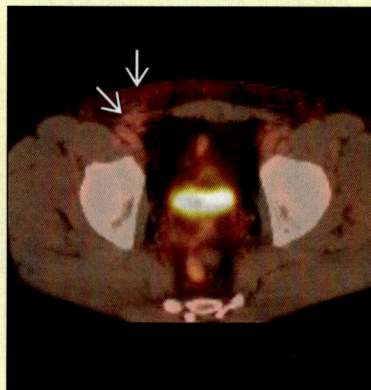

Scar Formation

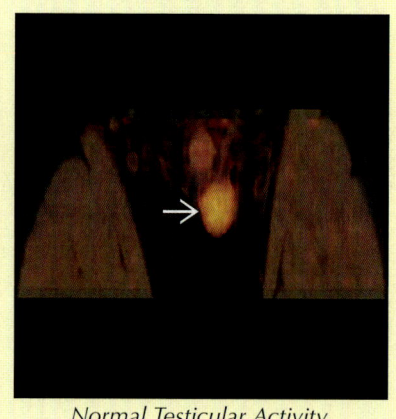

Normal Testicular Activity

TESTICULAR CANCER

Key Facts

Terminology
- Germ cell tumors: Malignant; from germ cell elements
- Non-germ cell tumors: Usually benign; from non-germ cell elements

Imaging Findings
- Therapeutic response/restaging: FDG PET is the modality of choice in malignant germ cell tumors
- For lesions > 3 cm: Negative FDG PET excludes presence of viable tumor
- For lesions < 3 cm: FDG PET sensitivity 25%, specificity 100%
- Magnitude of FDG uptake in primary testicular malignancy is often only moderate (SUV < 3), but typically > normal lymph nodes

- Raised tumor markers and negative CT: FDG PET PPV 92%, NPV 50%
- With residual mass: FDG PET PPV 96%, NPV 90%
- Late relapse: Longitudinal follow-up required despite negative FDG PET

Top Differential Diagnoses
- Epidermoid Cyst
- Lymphoma, Leukemia, Metastases
- Subacute Hematoma
- Segmental Infarct
- Focal Orchitis

Diagnostic Checklist
- US for primary diagnosis
- CT or MR for initial staging
- FDG PET/CT for therapeutic response/restaging

- ○ Therapeutic response/restaging: FDG PET is the modality of choice in malignant germ cell tumors
- ○ Limited published experience with FDG PET in evaluation of malignant non-germ cell tumors
- ○ For lesions > 3 cm: Negative FDG PET excludes presence of viable tumor
  - ▪ FDG PET sensitivity 80%, specificity 100%, positive predictive value (PPV) 100%, negative predictive value (NPV) 96% (compares to 74%, 70%, 34%, 92% for CT)
- ○ For lesions < 3 cm: FDG PET sensitivity 25%, specificity 100%
- ○ Magnitude of FDG uptake in primary testicular malignancy is often only moderate (SUV < 3), but typically > normal lymph nodes
  - ▪ Prediction of early response to chemotherapy for germ cell tumors: Non-responder mean SUV 2.7; responder mean SUV 1.8
- ○ Raised tumor markers and negative CT: FDG PET PPV 92%, NPV 50%
- ○ With residual mass: FDG PET PPV 96%, NPV 90%
- ○ Late relapse: Longitudinal follow-up required despite negative FDG PET
- Conventional testicular scintigraphy: Tagged RBCs or Tc-99m pertechnetate
  - ○ May occasionally present as acute testicular pain and mimic acute torsion
  - ○ Findings are non-specific
    - ▪ Diffuse hyperemia: Mimics orchitis, early detorsion
    - ▪ Cold defect with surrounding hyperemia: Necrosis

CT Findings
- Germ cell tumors: For staging retroperitoneum, nodal or pulmonary mets
  - ○ Low attenuation nodes: Considered positive if in typical location of left renal hilus or retrocaval on right (even if small)
  - ○ Residual low attenuation masses common after treatment in bulky disease
  - ○ Helpful in identifying retroperitoneal recurrence, "growing teratoma" syndrome

MR Findings
- Germ cell tumors: Moderate high signal intensity on T2WI, retroperitoneal lymphadenopathy
- Non-germ cell tumors: Low signal mass ± high signal capsule on T2WI; high signal central scars

Ultrasonographic Findings
- Germ cell tumors
  - ○ Seminoma: Hypoechoic, well-defined, solid mass without cystic areas or calcification
  - ○ Embryonal cell, teratocarcinoma, teratoma, choriocarcinoma: Heterogeneous, cystic areas, calcification
- Non-germ cell tumors: Similar in appearance to germ cell tumors

Imaging Recommendations
- Best imaging tool
  - ○ US to identify and characterize scrotal mass
  - ○ CT or MR for initial staging
  - ○ FDG PET/CT: Therapeutic response; restaging
- Protocol advice: US: High frequency linear array

DIFFERENTIAL DIAGNOSIS

Epidermoid Cyst
- Cystic cavity lined by stratified squamous epithelium
- "Onion skin" appearance on US, ± peripheral calcification
- No MR enhancement

Lymphoma, Leukemia, Metastases
- 50% bilateral, otherwise indistinguishable from primary testicular cancer
- Often greater FDG uptake than with primary testicular cancer
- Older age group; lymphoma most common testicular tumor > 60 yrs old
- Hypoechoic & hypervascular on US

Subacute Hematoma
- No internal color flow (US)

TESTICULAR CANCER

- Associated hematocele
- History of trauma
- FDG uptake in subacute setting (inflammatory response)

Segmental Infarct
- Acute infarct can be FDG avid (hemorrhage, inflammation)

Focal Orchitis
- Symptomatic with pain, tenderness
- FDG uptake

PATHOLOGY

General Features
- Genetics
  - Family history ↑ risk of of germ cell tumors
  - Peutz-Jeghers, Carney syndromes; Kleinfelter syndrome: Non-germ cell tumors
- Etiology: 95% of testicular tumors are malignant germ cell
- Epidemiology
  - Germ cell tumors: Most common cancer in 15-34 yr males; 1% of all cancers in men
    - Seminomas: Most common in 35-39 yrs; rare < 10 yrs
  - Non-germ cell tumors: Age 30-60 yrs; 25% before puberty; malignant LCT only in adults; SCT in all ages (1/3 < 12 yrs)
  - Lymphoma: Most common testicular tumor > 50 yrs
- Associated abnormalities
  - Germ cell tumors: Gynecomastic, pre-pubescent virilization, cryptorchidism, testicular microlithiasis, family history
  - Non-germ cell tumors: Prepubescent virilization, feminization, stigmata of Kleinfelter syndrome (LCT); Peutz-Jeghers and Carney syndromes (SCT, large calcifying type)

Gross Pathologic & Surgical Features
- Germ cell tumors: 95% of testicular tumors; multiple subtypes in 35%
  - 40-50% seminomas, 25% embryonal cell (teratocarcinoma), 5-10% teratoma
- Non-germ cell tumors: 4-5% of all testicular tumors; 10-30% in childhood; 10-13% of testicular neoplasms in children
  - LCT: 90% benign, may produce testosterone; malignant potential best dictated by metastases
  - SCT: 85-90% benign; may produce estrogen or Müllerian inhibiting factors

Microscopic Features
- Both germ cell and non-germ cell: Single or multiple cell types
- LCT: Large cells, central round nuclei, small nucleoli, eosinophilic cytoplasm, crystals of Reinke
- SCT: Sheets of uniform cells with tubule formation

Staging, Grading or Classification Criteria
- Stage I (A): Tumor confined to testis
- Stage II (B): Metastatic to nodes below diaphragm
- Stage IIA (B1): Retroperitoneal node mets < 2 cm (5 cm^3)
- Stage IIB (B2): Retroperitoneal node mets 2-5 cm (10 cm^3)
- Stage IIC (B3): Retroperitoneal node mets > 5 cm
- Stage III (C): Mets to lymph nodes above diaphragm
- Stage IIIA (C1): Mets confined to lymphatic system
- Stage IIIB (IV): Extranodal mets

CLINICAL ISSUES

Presentation
- Most common signs/symptoms: Painless testicular enlargement; Dull/acute pain < 30%
- Other signs/symptoms
  - Germ cell tumors: ↑ Tumor markers (beta-HCG, alfa-feto-protein)
  - Precocious virilization, gynecomastia, ↓ libido/impotence (adults)

Treatment
- Germ cell tumors: Radical orchiectomy; retroperitoneal nodal dissection for non-seminomatous tumor; XRT, chemotherapy for metastatic
- Non-germ cell tumors: Orchiectomy or testis-sparing surgery; same as germ cell tumors if metastatic disease

DIAGNOSTIC CHECKLIST

Consider
- US for primary diagnosis
- CT or MR for initial staging
- FDG PET/CT for therapeutic response/restaging

SELECTED REFERENCES

1. Becherer A et al: FDG PET is superior to CT in the prediction of viable tumour in post-chemotherapy seminoma residuals. Eur J Radiol. 54(2):284-8, 2005
2. De Santis M et al: 2-18fluoro-deoxy-D-glucose positron emission tomography is a reliable predictor for viable tumor in postchemotherapy seminoma: an update of the prospective multicentric SEMPET trial. J Clin Oncol. 22(6):1034-9, 2004
3. Lassen U et al: Whole-body FDG-PET in patients with stage I non-seminomatous germ cell tumours. Eur J Nucl Med Mol Imaging. 30(3):396-402, 2003
4. Sanchez D et al: 18F-fluoro-2-deoxyglucose-positron emission tomography in the evaluation of nonseminomatous germ cell tumours at relapse. BJU Int. 89(9):912-6, 2002
5. Spermon JR et al: The role of (18)fluoro-2-deoxyglucose positron emission tomography in initial staging and re-staging after chemotherapy for testicular germ cell tumours. BJU Int. 89(6):549-56, 2002
6. De Santis M et al: Predictive impact of 2-18fluoro-2-deoxy-D-glucose positron emission tomography for residual postchemotherapy masses in patients with bulky seminoma. J Clin Oncol. 19(17):3740-4, 2001
7. Hain SF et al: Fluorodeoxyglucose PET in the initial staging of germ cell tumours. Eur J Nucl Med. 27(5):590-4, 2000

TESTICULAR CANCER

IMAGE GALLERY

Typical

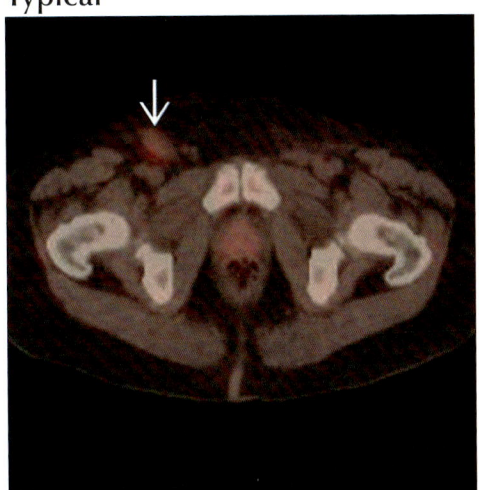

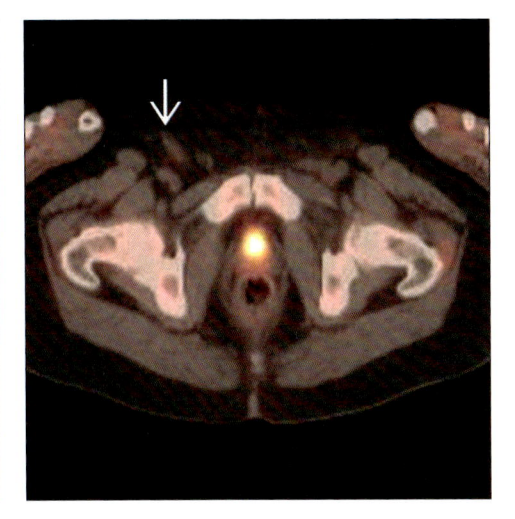

(Left) Pre-treatment axial FDG PET/CT in a patient with metastatic seminoma shows moderate metabolic activity in enlarged right inguinal node ➡, indicative of tumor involvement. SUV in this case was 2.4. See next image. *(Right)* Post-treatment axial FDG PET/CT shows interval decrease in size and metabolic activity to metastatic right inguinal lymph node ➡, indicative of good response to treatment.

Typical

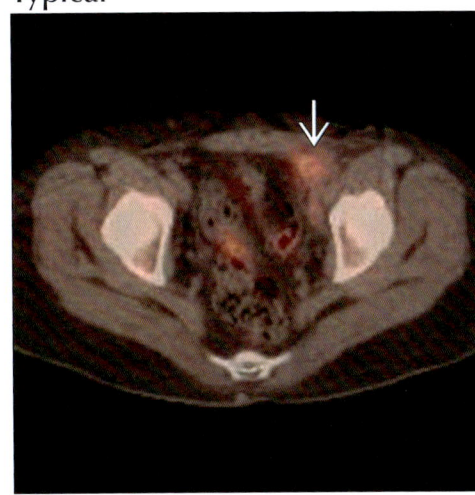

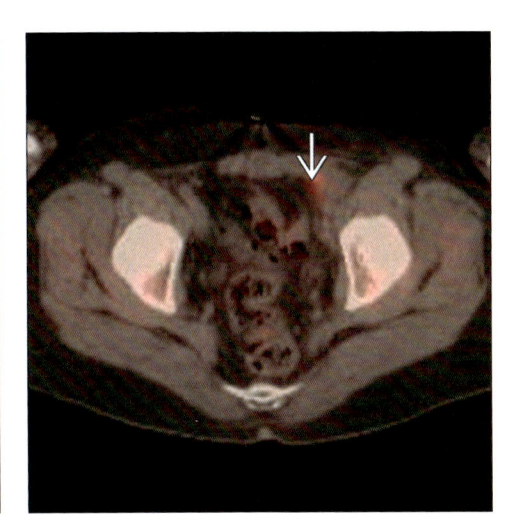

(Left) Pre-treatment axial FDG PET/CT in patient with metastatic seminoma shows increased uptake in left external iliac nodal mass ➡ consistent with tumor involvement. See next image. *(Right)* Post-treatment axial FDG PET/CT shows interval decrease in size and metabolic activity in left external iliac nodal mass. However, small metabolically active focus ➡ indicates persistent region of viable tumor.

Variant

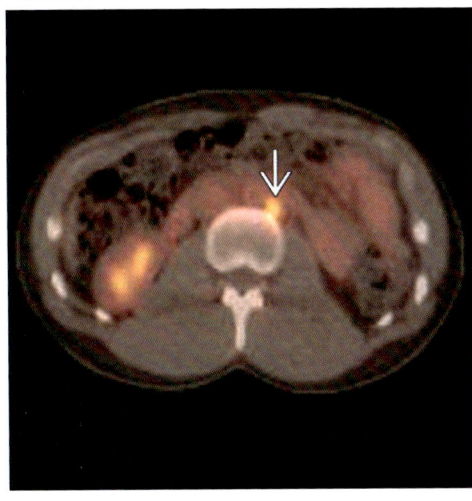

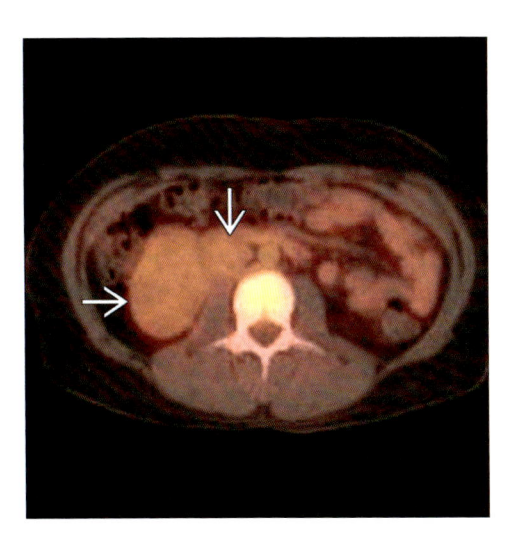

(Left) Axial FDG PET/CT in patient with metastatic mixed germ cell tumor shows small but hypermetabolic periaortic node ➡ at level of left renal vein, indicative of tumor involvement. *(Right)* Axial FDG PET/CT in patient with seminoma shows hypermetabolic, enlarged right retroperitoneal mass ➡ (SUV 2.7). Magnitude of uptake, which is only moderate in degree, is typical of seminoma.

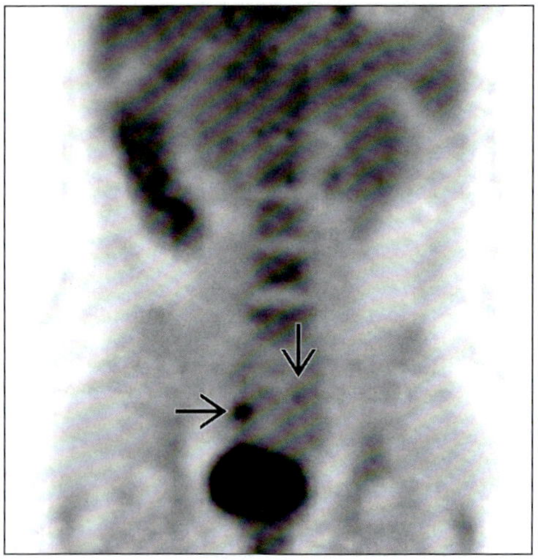

OVARIES, NORMAL & BENIGN PATHOLOGY

Coronal PET shows two focal areas of FDG activity in pelvis ➔ correlating to normal ovaries on CT, typical of physiologic ovarian activity.

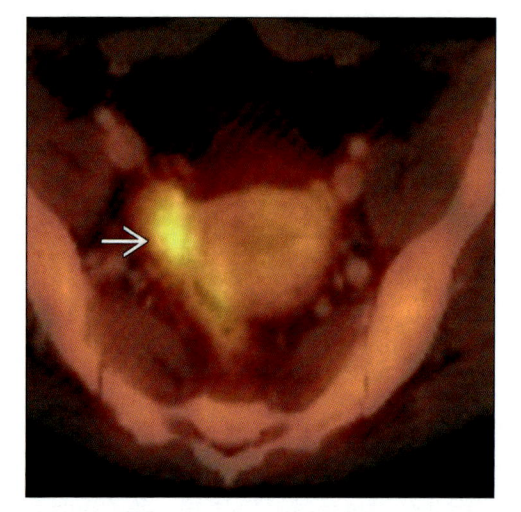

Axial fused PET/CT shows moderate FDG activity in right ovary ➔ corresponding to a normal-appearing ovary on CT, compatible with physiologic activity.

TERMINOLOGY

Definitions
- Increased activity on FDG PET due to benign or physiologic causes (e.g., reproductive cycle, infection)

IMAGING FINDINGS

General Features
- Best diagnostic clue
  - PET/CT: FDG uptake in normal and benign ovarian processes can be variable
    - Low level to intense
    - Depends on etiology
- Size: Typically 1-5 cm; < 10 cm

Nuclear Medicine Findings
- PET
  - FDG activity in ovary ranges from none to very intense, depending on etiology
  - Increased FDG activity in ovary often an incidental finding

Imaging Recommendations
- Best imaging tool
  - FDG PET/CT
    - If increased FDG activity in ovary, correlate with corresponding CT, clinical history
  - Ultrasound: First-line for suspicious ovarian masses

DIFFERENTIAL DIAGNOSIS

Physiologic or Functional Cysts
- Ovulatory follicles: Can show false + FDG uptake
  - Typically no qualitative abnormalities on CT
- Follicular, corpus luteum cysts: FDG uptake can be very high
  - Characteristic appearance of follicular cyst: Smooth, thin-walled, unilocular
  - Characteristic appearance of corpus luteum cyst: Cystic structure ± thick, enhancing rind, often complex
  - Usually < 10 cm
- Short term follow-up at two or 6 weeks with PET/CT or ultrasound may be helpful

DDx: Ovarian FDG Activity

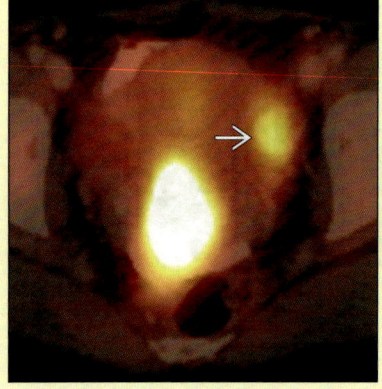

Corpus Luteum Cyst 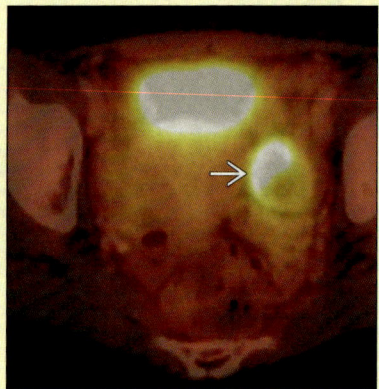 *Abscess* 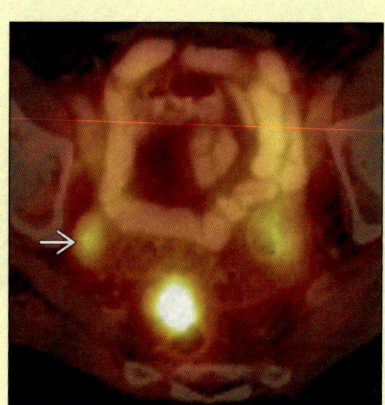 *Ovarian Metastasis*

OVARIES, NORMAL & BENIGN PATHOLOGY

Key Facts

Imaging Findings
- PET/CT: FDG uptake in normal and benign ovarian processes can be variable
- Increased FDG activity in ovary often an incidental finding
- If increased FDG activity in ovary, correlate with corresponding CT, clinical history
- Ultrasound: First-line for suspicious ovarian masses

Top Differential Diagnoses
- Physiologic or Functional Cysts
- Benign Ovarian Neoplasm
- Malignant Ovarian Neoplasm
- Tubo-Ovarian Abscess
- Ectopic Pregnancy

Diagnostic Checklist
- Short term follow-up PET/CT at 2 or 6 weeks may differentiate benign from malignant FDG uptake

Benign Ovarian Neoplasm
- Serous, mucinous cystadenoma: Classically not FDG-avid
- Endometrioma: May show increased FDG activity, would expect intrauterine endometrium to show increased FDG activity concurrently
- Mature cystic teratoma: Calcifications, complex mass on anatomic imaging; may show mild FDG activity (similar to background)

Malignant Ovarian Neoplasm
- Primary: 35% of children with ovarian mass; 6-11% of premenopausal women with ovarian mass; 30% of women > 50 yrs old with ovarian mass
- Metastatic: Breast cancer, Krukenberg tumor

Tubo-Ovarian Abscess
- Increased FDG uptake due to infectious process
- Can have similar appearance to corpus luteal cyst, usually more extensive
- Clinical: Pain, fever, vaginal discharge

Ectopic Pregnancy
- Clinical correlation with missed menstrual period, pain, vaginal bleeding

CLINICAL ISSUES

Presentation
- Most common signs/symptoms: Pelvic pain

Demographics
- Age: More common in younger women

DIAGNOSTIC CHECKLIST

Consider
- Primary and metastatic malignant etiologies if ovary shows increased FDG uptake
- Ultrasound to determine etiology of increased FDG uptake in ovary if PET/CT nondiagnostic
- Short term follow-up PET/CT at 2 or 6 weeks may differentiate benign from malignant FDG uptake

SELECTED REFERENCES
1. Ames J et al: 18F-FDG uptake in an ovary containing a hemorrhagic corpus luteal cyst: false-positive PET/CT in a patient with cervical carcinoma. AJR Am J Roentgenol. 185(4):1057-9, 2005
2. Ho KC et al: An ovary in luteal phase mimicking common iliac lymph node metastasis from a primary cutaneous peripheral primitive neuroectodermal tumour as revealed by 18-fluoro-2-deoxyglucose positron emission tomography. Br J Radiol. 78(928):343-5, 2005
3. Kim SK et al: Incidental ovarian 18F-FDG accumulation on PET: correlation with the menstrual cycle. Eur J Nucl Med Mol Imaging. 32(7):757-63, 2005
4. Lerman H et al: Normal and abnormal 18F-FDG endometrial and ovarian uptake in pre- and postmenopausal patients: assessment by PET/CT. J Nucl Med. 45(2):266-71, 2004

IMAGE GALLERY

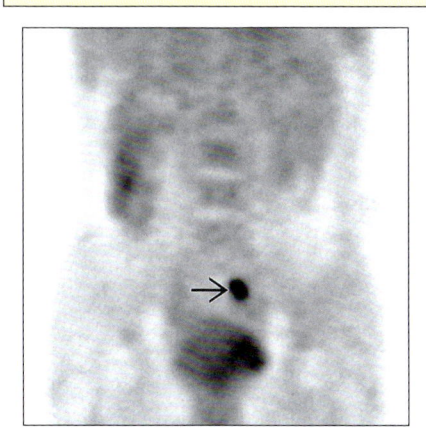

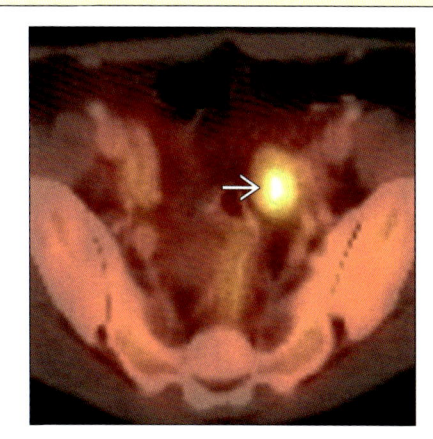

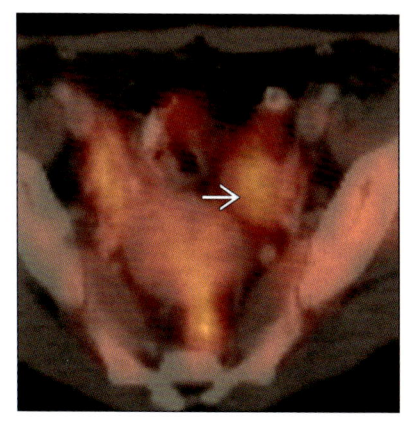

(Left) Coronal PET shows intense focal FDG activity in pelvis ➔. The differential diagnosis includes physiologic activity, functional cyst, abscess, neoplasm. (Center) Axial fused PET/CT shows intense focal FDG activity ➔ corresponding to posterior aspect of left ovary. Short term follow-up exam was recommended to help determine etiology. (Right) Axial fused PET/CT in same patient as previous image, 6 weeks later, shows complete resolution ➔ of focal intense FDG activity, suggesting benign etiology of ovarian FDG uptake.

OVARIAN CANCER

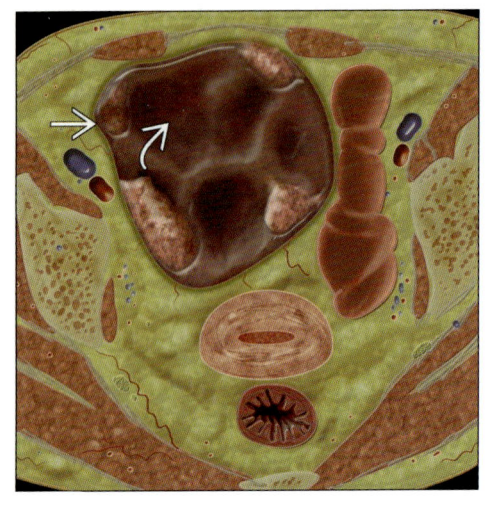

Axial graphic shows large complex ovarian mass with cystic areas centrally and mural nodularity along the periphery.

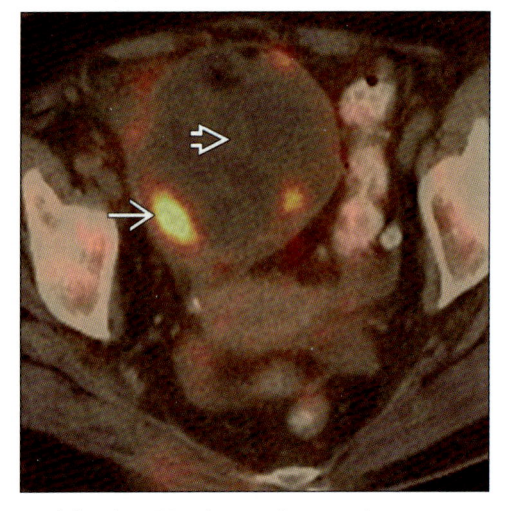

Axial fused PET/CT shows a large ovarian carcinoma with cystic and solid regions. Note intense FDG activity in solid areas of tumor.

TERMINOLOGY

Abbreviations and Synonyms
- Ovarian carcinoma

Definitions
- Primary malignancy of ovary
  - Epithelial (90%)
    - Arises from germinal epithelium on outside of ovary
  - Stromal (6%)
    - Arises from connective tissue
    - Low rate of metastasis
  - Germ cell (3%)
    - Teens/young women
    - Highly curable
- Staging of ovarian cancer
  - Stage I: Confined to one or both ovaries
  - Stage II: Spread to uterus/fallopian tube, within pelvis
  - Stage III: Lymph nodes, abdominal cavity
  - Stage IV: Outside abdomen, intrahepatic metastases

IMAGING FINDINGS

General Features
- Best diagnostic clue: Solid or complex cystic mass arising from ovary ± ascites
- Location
  - Primary generally found in ovary
  - Metastases most common to peritoneum, omentum
  - Rare intrahepatic metastases

Nuclear Medicine Findings
- PET/CT: Sensitivity > 95%, specificity 80-93% for detection of recurrence
- PET/CT: High positive predictive value of 83-94% in identifying recurrent ovarian cancer
- PET limited in detecting lymph node micrometastases
  - In one study, PET/CT failed to identify microscopic disease in 59% of pathologically positive lymph nodes
- PET limited in detecting small disseminated lesions such as peritoneal carcinosis and mesenteric or omental recurrences due to 6-8 mm limit of resolution
- Degenerative changes in pelvis, such as sacroiliac arthritis, has been mistaken for recurrence

DDx: Ovarian FDG Uptake

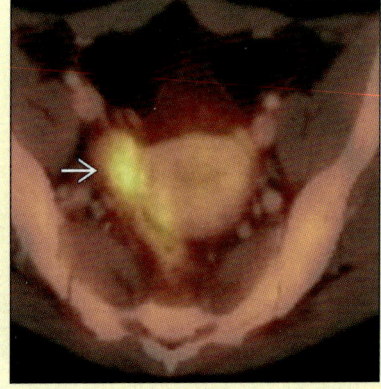

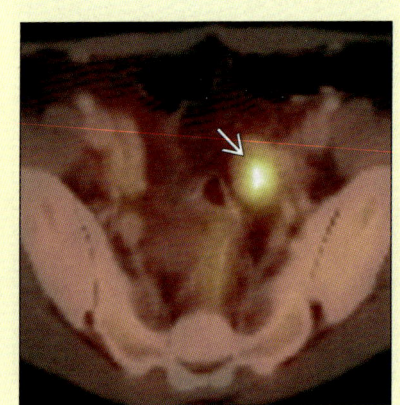

Physiologic | *Corpus Luteal Cyst* | *Metastases*

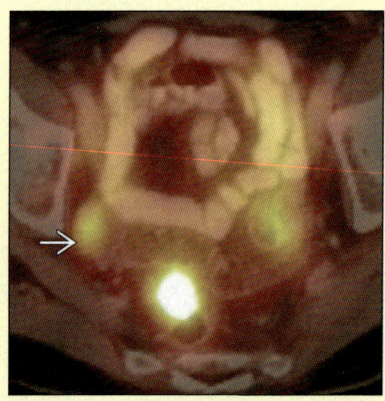

OVARIAN CANCER

Key Facts

Terminology
- Stage I: Confined to one or both ovaries
- Stage II: Spread to uterus/fallopian tube, within pelvis
- Stage III: Lymph nodes, abdominal cavity
- Stage IV: Outside abdomen, intrahepatic metastases

Imaging Findings
- PET/CT: Sensitivity > 95%, specificity 80-93% for detection of recurrence
- PET/CT: High positive predictive value of 83-94% in identifying recurrent ovarian cancer
- PET limited in detecting lymph node micrometastases
- PET limited in detecting small disseminated lesions such as peritoneal carcinosis and mesenteric or omental recurrences due to 6-8 mm limit of resolution

- PET/CT for most complete staging, suspected recurrence

Top Differential Diagnoses
- Pelvic Inflammatory Disease
- Tubo-Ovarian Abscess
- Complex Functional Cysts
- Benign Ovarian Tumors
- Borderline Ovarian Tumors

Clinical Issues
- CA-125 has accuracy of 79-95% for recurrence; increase precedes apparent recurrence by 3-6 months
- Most patients asymptomatic until disease in advanced stage
- 75-80% of patients have spread beyond ovary at time of diagnosis

---

  ○ Active degenerative change in bone can have ↑ FDG activity

CT Findings
- Primary lesion usually complex cystic mass with mural nodularity
- In general, malignancy suggested by thickness and irregularity of cavity walls, septae, enhancing nodules
- Sensitivity 92% for peritoneal metastases
- GI contrast especially helpful for distinguishing pelvic viscera from intestinal tract

MR Findings
- Sensitivity 83%, specificity 84% for discrimination of malignancy from benign lesion
- Sensitivity up to 95% for detection of peritoneal metastases
- Enhancement with gadolinium useful
  ○ Evaluate internal architecture of cystic lesions
  ○ Differentiate solid enhancing lesions from clot/debris

Ultrasonographic Findings
- Sensitivity 71-96%, specificity 23-83% for pelvic tumor
- Irregular walls, thickened septae, papillary excrescences suggest malignancy
- Tumor suspected with more solid lesions
- Intraperitoneal fluid can be sign of peritoneal spread

Imaging Recommendations
- Best imaging tool
  ○ Most common: Transvaginal ultrasound followed by MR and/or CT for evaluation of metastasis
    ▪ Risk of malignancy index (RMI) calculated using transvaginal ultrasound results, CA-125 blood level, menopausal status
  ○ PET/CT for most complete staging, suspected recurrence

DIFFERENTIAL DIAGNOSIS

Pelvic Inflammatory Disease
- CT findings nonspecific
- Disrupted fat planes
- Thickened fascial planes

Tubo-Ovarian Abscess
- Commonly depicted as a mass that is regular with debris similar to that seen with endometrioma or hemorrhagic cyst

Complex Functional Cysts
- May have intense FDG activity

Benign Ovarian Tumors
- Includes cystadenoma, dermoid tumors

Borderline Ovarian Tumors
- Pathologically difficult to differentiate between benign and malignant
- Low malignant potential

PATHOLOGY

General Features
- General path comments
  ○ Ovarian cancer spreads primarily intraperitoneally as well as to lymph nodes
    ▪ Peritoneal fluid flows upward from pelvis to paracolic gutters and subphrenic regions, carrying tumor cells that implant on abdominal viscera
  ○ Common sites of metastatic implantation
    ▪ Pelvis
    ▪ Right hemidiaphragm
    ▪ Perihepatic
    ▪ Right paracolic gutter
    ▪ Bowel
    ▪ Omentum
  ○ Distant lymph nodes are involved in approximately 7% of cases of serous ovarian adenocarcinoma
- Genetics
  ○ 10% of patients with ovarian cancer appear to have genetic predisposition
  ○ These patients may develop cancer early, between ages 30 and 50

OVARIAN CANCER

- One study suggested patients with BRCA gene have 60% risk of developing ovarian cancer
- Etiology
  - Unknown
  - Number of reproductive cycles appears to be related to risk
  - Ovulation suppression may decrease cancer incidence
- Epidemiology
  - Leading cause of death among women with gynecological malignancies
  - Third most common cancer of female reproductive organs

Microscopic Features
- Most common histologies are papillary serous adenocarcinoma and endometrioid type
- Serous adenocarcinoma comprises 40% of epithelial ovarian cancers
- Psammoma bodies may be present
  - Ovarian cancer with multiple psammoma bodies may have better prognosis

CLINICAL ISSUES

Presentation
- Most common signs/symptoms
  - Early stage: Nonspecific, pelvic pain
    - Often attributed to other causes (e.g., menstruation, irritable bowel syndrome)
  - With metastases: Abdominal/pelvic bloating, pain, pressure, early satiety, nausea/vomiting, frequent urination, feeling similar to pregnancy
- Other signs/symptoms
  - CA-125 has accuracy of 79-95% for recurrence; increase precedes apparent recurrence by 3-6 months
  - Doubling of CA-125 above normal limit has been shown to have sensitivity of 85.9% and specificity of 91.3% for detection of recurrence

Demographics
- Age: Average age at diagnosis 57 years
- Ethnicity: More common among Caucasians than African Americans

Natural History & Prognosis
- Most patients asymptomatic until disease in advanced stage
- 75-80% of patients have spread beyond ovary at time of diagnosis
- Overall survival approximately 35%

Treatment
- Surgery, chemotherapy, radiation therapy
  - Surgery for early stage: Total abdominal hysterectomy, bilateral oophorectomy, omentectomy, biopsy of lymph nodes/tissues
  - Surgery for later stage: Early stage surgery plus tumor debulking
  - Chemotherapy: Paclitaxel and/or platinum-based drugs
  - Radiation therapy: Stage II

- Exploratory laparotomy done for high suspicion of malignancy, but must perform 8-9 benign cyst operations to detect one ovarian cancer
- Benefit of optimal primary cytoreductive debulking surgery is well-established
- Stage IV patients s/p successful debulking surgery have same median survival as stage III patients
- 75% of women have complete clinical response, but the majority of these will experience recurrence

DIAGNOSTIC CHECKLIST

Consider
- Benign increased FDG uptake in ovaries can mimic ovarian primary malignancy, look for other signs of ovarian malignancy (ascites, peritoneal implants, lymphadenopathy)
- PET/CT valuable in patient with rising CA-125, negative anatomic imaging
  - Some claim PET is as valuable for detection of recurrence as second-look surgery and may be substituted as noninvasive option
- PET/CT valuable to distinguish post-surgical change from recurrence

Image Interpretation Pearls
- Serous adenocarcinoma may contain microcalcifications that can be confused with old granulomatous disease or calcifications due to treatment

SELECTED REFERENCES

1. Thrall MM et al: Clinical use of combined positron emission tomography and computed tomography (FDG-PET/CT) in recurrent ovarian cancer. Gynecol Oncol. 2007
2. Chung HH et al: Role of [(18)F]FDG PET/CT in the assessment of suspected recurrent ovarian cancer: correlation with clinical or histological findings. Eur J Nucl Med Mol Imaging. 2006
3. Kurosaki H et al: Prognostic value of FDG-PET in patients with ovarian carcinoma following surgical treatment. Ann Nucl Med. 20(3):171-4, 2006
4. Mangili G et al: Integrated PET/CT as a first-line re-staging modality in patients with suspected recurrence of ovarian cancer. Eur J Nucl Med Mol Imaging. 2006
5. Murakami M et al: Whole-body positron emission tomography and tumor marker CA125 for detection of recurrence in epithelial ovarian cancer. Int J Gynecol Cancer. 16 Suppl 1:99-107, 2006
6. Havrilesky LJ et al: FDG-PET for management of cervical and ovarian cancer. Gynecol Oncol. 97(1):183-91, 2005
7. Takekuma M et al: Positron emission tomography with 18F-fluoro-2-deoxyglucose for the detection of recurrent ovarian cancer. Int J Clin Oncol. 10(3):177-81, 2005
8. Yoshida Y et al: Incremental benefits of FDG positron emission tomography over CT alone for the preoperative staging of ovarian cancer. AJR Am J Roentgenol. 182(1):227-33, 2004

OVARIAN CANCER

IMAGE GALLERY

Typical

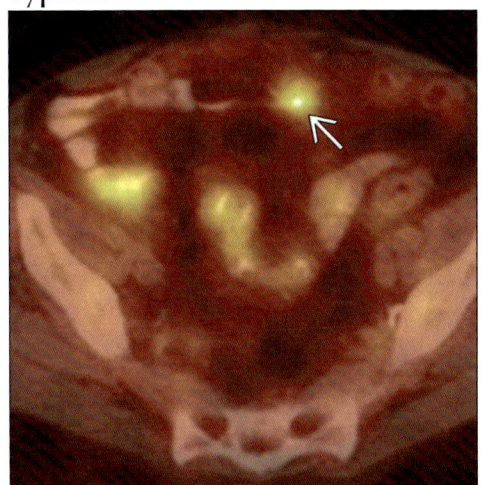

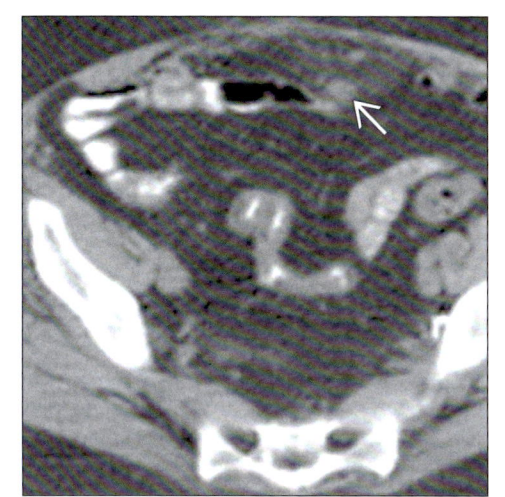

(Left) Axial fused PET/CT in patient with normal CT and elevated CA-125 shows intense FDG activity in soft tissue mass in pelvis ➡. See next image. *(Right)* Axial NECT in same patient as left shows subcentimeter nodule in mesentery adjacent to a loop of bowel ➡.

Typical

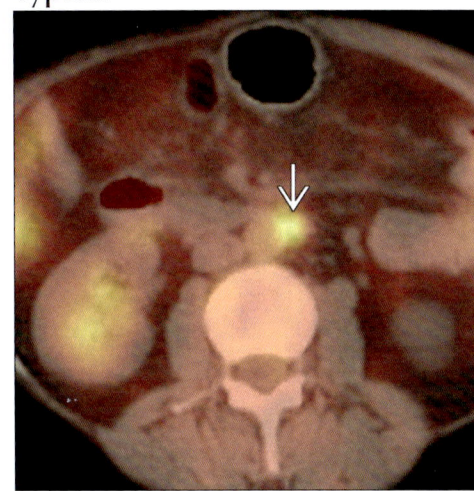

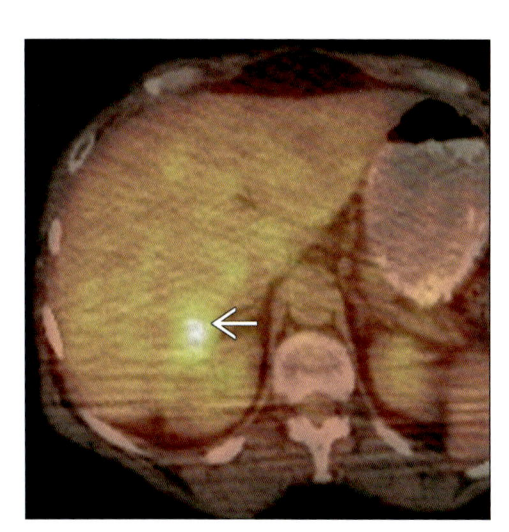

(Left) Axial fused PET/CT shows intense FDG activity in a subcentimeter left para-aortic lymph node ➡ in patient with recurrent ovarian carcinoma. *(Right)* Axial fused PET/CT shows intense FDG activity in a hepatic metastasis ➡, consistent with stage IV ovarian carcinoma.

Typical

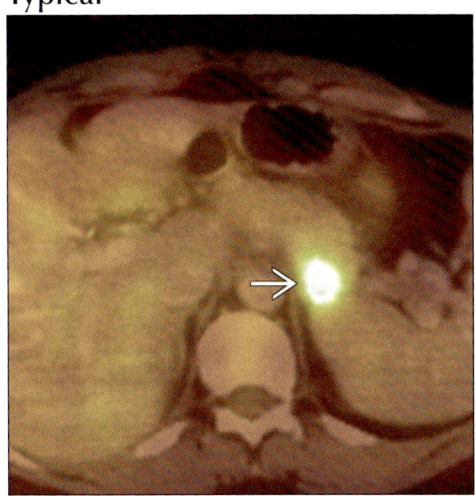

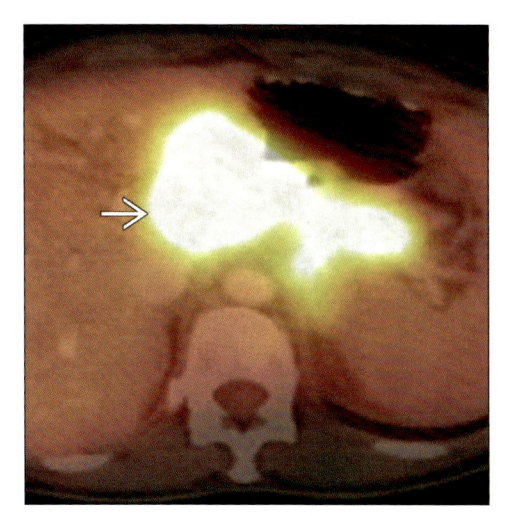

(Left) Axial fused PET/CT shows a focal area of intense FDG activity in gastrosplenic ligament region ➡. As no correlative CT abnormality could be definitively discerned, the patient was not treated. See next image. *(Right)* Axial fused PET/CT in same patient as left shows progression of disease ➡ on 9 month follow-up exam.

UTERUS, NORMAL & BENIGN PATHOLOGY

Axial fused PET/CT shows moderate FDG activity in right anterolateral border of uterus ➔ due to fibroid. Also shown is misregistered bladder activity ➔ due to difference in filling between CT & PET. See next image.

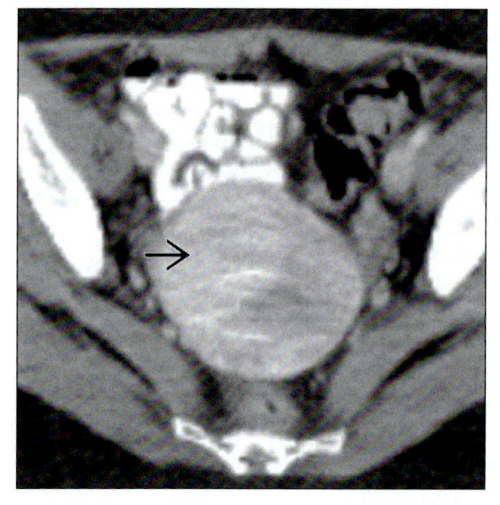

Axial CECT shows a large fibroid in the anterolateral right wall of the uterus ➔, corresponding to increased activity on PET.

TERMINOLOGY

Definitions
- Physiologic or benign activity in uterus on FDG PET

IMAGING FINDINGS

General Features
- Best diagnostic clue: Diagnosis of increased uterine FDG activity depends on clinical history, correlative CT findings, ± further imaging as necessary
- Location
  - Uterine body: Low level FDG activity can be seen throughout, focally increased with uterine fibroids
  - Endometrium: FDG activity can be seen with menstruation

Nuclear Medicine Findings
- PET
  - Low level FDG activity can be seen throughout normal uterus
  - Focal FDG activity in enlarged uterine body
    - Correlation with CT important
  - Fibroids: FDG activity ranges from minimal to intense
    - Intensity of FDG activity may correlate with fibroid degeneration, although controversial
  - Intense FDG uptake in endometrial canal
    - Young patient: Menstruation (clinical history for active menstruation should be obtained)
    - Older patient: Endometrial carcinoma (postmenopausal patient with uptake in endometrial cavity should be referred for additional workup)
  - Focal FDG activity in vagina
    - Consider cervical cancer
    - Menstruation
    - FDG-contaminated urine being wicked by tampon

Imaging Recommendations
- Best imaging tool
  - Correlation of increased FDG activity in uterus with CT portion of PET/CT
    - If etiology remains unclear, clinical examination and ultrasound/MR

DDx: Physiological Pelvic Uptake of FDG

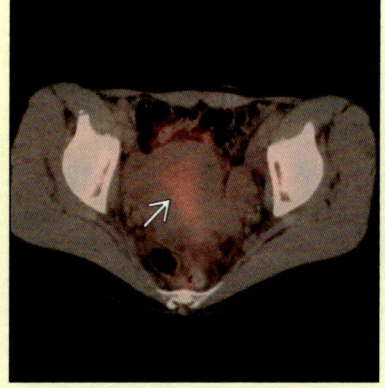

Menstruating Endometrium

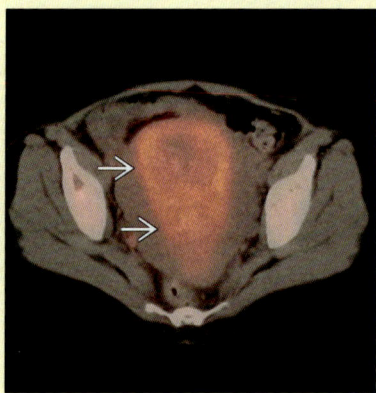

Post-Partum Uterus

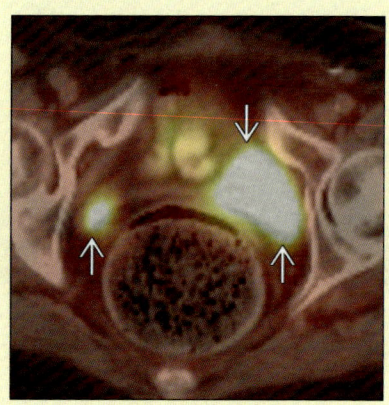

Bladder FDG Activity

UTERUS, NORMAL & BENIGN PATHOLOGY

Key Facts

Imaging Findings
- Best diagnostic clue: Diagnosis of increased uterine FDG activity depends on clinical history, correlative CT findings, ± further imaging as necessary
- Low level FDG activity can be seen throughout normal uterus
- If etiology remains unclear, clinical examination and ultrasound/MR

Top Differential Diagnoses
- Menstruation
- Fibroids
- Foreign Body
- Infection
- Endometrial Process
- Cervical Cancer
- Uterine Sarcoma

DIFFERENTIAL DIAGNOSIS

Menstruation
- Clinical history important

Fibroids
- FDG activity ranges from minimal to intense
- Unable to differentiate from early leiomyosarcoma
- CT: Variable appearance, may enhance, may have calcifications, often multiple

Foreign Body
- Increased FDG activity due to contraceptive device reported
- Tampon

Infection
- Pelvic inflammatory disease
- Myometritis, parametritis, endometritis (e.g., postpartum)

Endometrial Process
- Hyperplasia
- Polyp
- Endometrial cancer

Cervical Cancer
- Extension of primary tumor into uterus

Uterine Sarcoma
- Leiomyosarcoma
- Endometrial stromal sarcoma
- Carcinosarcoma

DIAGNOSTIC CHECKLIST

Consider
- Focal or linear FDG activity in the endometrial canal often seen with young patients
- Focal FDG activity within fibroids; can be mild or intensely FDG-avid
- Focal intense FDG activity in a postmenopausal patient: Suspect endometrial carcinoma

SELECTED REFERENCES

1. Lin E: FDG PET appearance of a postpartum uterus. Clin Nucl Med. 31(3):159-60, 2006
2. Nishizawa S et al: Physiological 18F-FDG uptake in the ovaries and uterus of healthy female volunteers. Eur J Nucl Med Mol Imaging. 32(5):549-56, 2005
3. Ak I et al: Uptake of 2-[18F]fluoro-2-deoxy-D-glucose in uterine leiomyoma: imaging of four patients by coincidence positron emission tomography. Nucl Med Commun. 25(9):941-5, 2004
4. Lerman H et al: Normal and abnormal 18F-FDG endometrial and ovarian uptake in pre- and postmenopausal patients: assessment by PET/CT. J Nucl Med. 45(2):266-71, 2004
5. Chander S et al: Physiologic uterine uptake of FDG during menstruation demonstrated with serial combined positron emission tomography and computed tomography. Clin Nucl Med. 27(1):22-4, 2002

IMAGE GALLERY

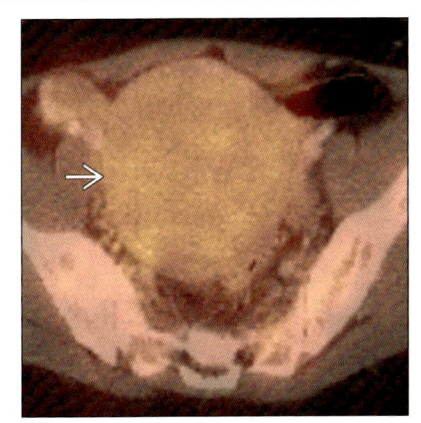

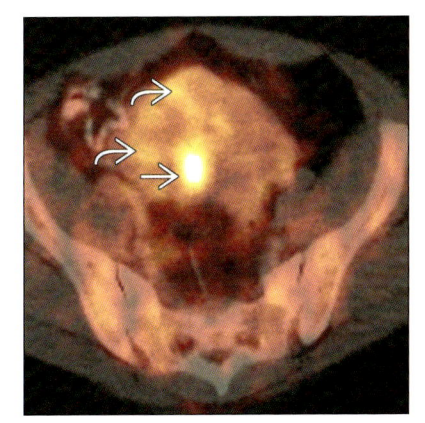

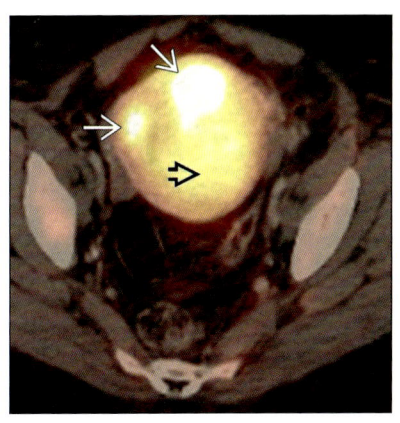

(Left) Axial fused PET/CT shows a large fibroid with no visible normal uterus. Note diffuse, low level FDG activity in the entire fibroid ➡. (Center) Axial fused PET/CT shows intense FDG uptake in an intramural uterine fibroid ➡. In addition, other fibroids with moderate FDG activity ➡ are present throughout the uterus. (Right) Axial fused PET/CT shows two fibroids with intense FDG activity ➡. A large fibroid is also present with moderate FDG activity in posterior uterus ➡.

CERVICAL CANCER

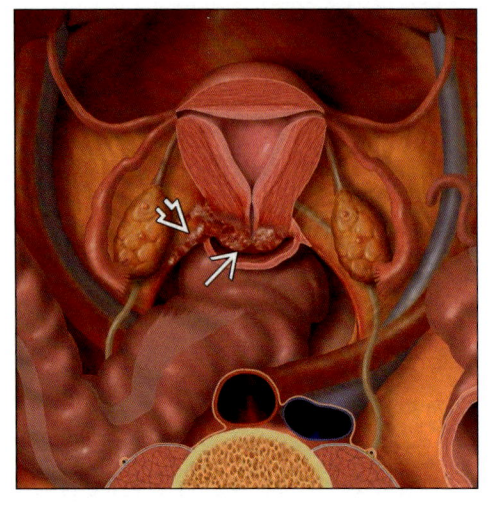

Graphic shows mass in uterine cervix with local extension. In these cases, PET/CT is used to detect lymphadenopathy and distant metastases.

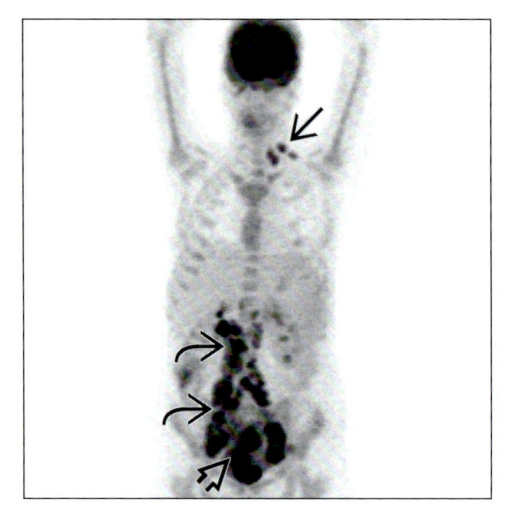

3D MIP PET/CT shows increased FDG activity in left supraclavicular, paraaortic and internal and external iliac lymph nodes in a patient with primary cervical cancer.

TERMINOLOGY

Definitions
- Primary cancer that arises from intraepithelial neoplasia of cervical cells
  - Squamous cell carcinoma (SCC): 80%
  - Adenocarcinoma: 15%
  - Adenosquamous: 3-5%
  - Rare: Lymphoma, sarcoma, rhabdomyosarcoma
- Clinical staging accurate in ~ 60% of patients
  - Undiagnosed lymphadenopathy is a major problem
- American Joint Committee on Cancer (AJCC) staging
  - 0: Carcinoma in situ
  - I: Confined to uterus
  - II: Beyond uterus, but not to pelvic side wall, lower third of vagina
  - IIIA: Extends to pelvic wall, lower third of vagina, causes hydronephrosis/nonfunctioning kidney, - lymph nodes (LN)
  - IIIB: Extends to pelvic wall, lower third of vagina, causes hydronephrosis/nonfunctioning kidney, + LN
  - IVA: Beyond true pelvis, bladder mucosa, rectal mucosa; + LN
  - IVB: Distant metastases

IMAGING FINDINGS

General Features
- Best diagnostic clue
  - PET/CT: Intense FDG activity in primary cervical mass, vagina, uterus, parametria; ± lymphadenopathy, visceral metastases
  - CT/MR: Enhancing mass in expected location of cervix; extension into vagina, uterus, parametria; ± lymphadenopathy, visceral metastases
- Location
  - Primary: Cervix
  - Local: Vaginal mucosa, extension into endometrium or myometrium, direct extension into parametrium, adjacent structures
  - Metastatic: Regional pelvic LN (any pelvic LN may be first affected), distant nodes or organs
  - Regional LN
    - Paraaortic
    - Common iliac
    - External iliac
    - Internal iliac/obturator

DDx: Benign Mimics of Cervical Cancer

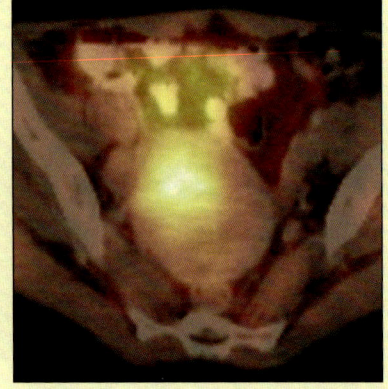

Leiomyoma

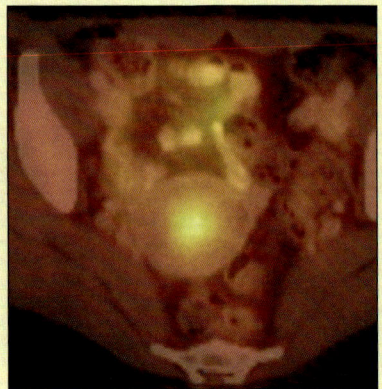

Menses: Endometrial

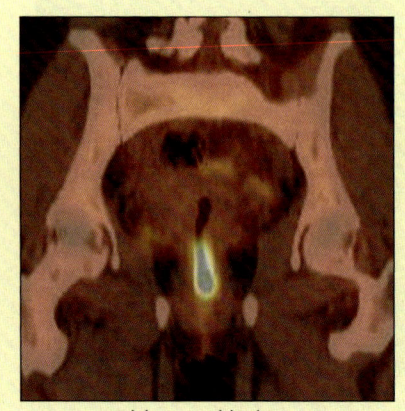

Menses: Vagina

CERVICAL CANCER

Key Facts

Terminology
- Primary cancer that arises from intraepithelial neoplasia of cervical cells
- Squamous cell carcinoma (SCC): 80%
- Adenocarcinoma: 15%
- Adenosquamous: 3-5%
- Rare: Lymphoma, sarcoma, rhabdomyosarcoma

Imaging Findings
- PET/CT: Intense FDG activity in primary cervical mass, vagina, uterus, parametria; ± lymphadenopathy, visceral metastases
- LN detection on PET: Sensitivity 75-91%, specificity 93-100%
- PET sensitivity for advanced disease 87%, specificity 100%
- Low sensitivity in LN < 1 cm
- In one study, ~ 8% of patients had distant supraclavicular lymphadenopathy detected only by PET

Top Differential Diagnoses
- Other Female Reproductive Tract Malignancy
- Leiomyoma
- Physiologic FDG Activity in Female Reproductive Organs
- Urine Contamination

Pathology
- Associated with human papillomavirus infection (strains 16, 18, 31, 33, 45)

Clinical Issues
- Surgery or radiotherapy in early stages
- Chemotherapy + radiotherapy in advanced stages

Nuclear Medicine Findings
- PET
  - Evaluation of primary cervical tumor
    - Most cervical SCC is FDG-avid ⇒ high sensitivity for sizable lesions
    - PET/CT reliable in advanced disease, may help avoid unnecessary operations, improve radiation therapy planning
    - Primary tumor SUV ≥ 10 associated with significantly lower 5-year disease-free survival than lower SUV (52% vs 71%)
    - Overall survival comparable whether SUV < or > 10
  - Evaluation of pelvic and paraaortic LN
    - LN detection on PET: Sensitivity 75-91%, specificity 93-100%
    - PET sensitivity for advanced disease 87%, specificity 100%
    - Low sensitivity in LN < 1 cm
    - Pelvic LN: Sensitivity 46%, specificity 91%.
    - Paraaortic LN: Sensitivity 40%, specificity 99%
    - Presence or absence of paraaortic LN on PET correlates most significantly with disease-free survival
  - Evaluation of distant metastases
    - In one study, ~ 8% of patients had distant supraclavicular lymphadenopathy detected only by PET

Imaging Recommendations
- Best imaging tool
  - Local and distant metastases: PET/CT (contrast-enhanced)
  - Primary tumor: CE MR
    - MR and CT: Moderate sensitivity and specificity for detecting pelvic, paraaortic lymphadenopathy, fail to identify small metastases
    - MR for detecting cervical cancer lymphadenopathy: Sensitivity 36-71%, specificity 76-100%
    - CT reveals ~ 1/3 paraaortic mets
- Protocol advice
  - FDG excretion through urinary tract and bladder can cause false +
    - Bladder voiding prior to imaging very important, although primary tumor likely well-characterized on anatomic imaging modality (MR)
    - Image from thighs toward head
    - Can repeat a bed position after voiding if unclear on initial PET scan
    - Lasix may be useful

DIFFERENTIAL DIAGNOSIS

Other Female Reproductive Tract Malignancy
- Endometrial cancer
- Ovarian cancer

Leiomyoma
- Variable FDG avidity, ranging from very minimal to intense
- Often distinguishable from cervical mass on CT portion of PET/CT

Physiologic FDG Activity in Female Reproductive Organs
- Menstruation: FDG activity in endometrial cavity, less frequently in vagina, associated with normal menstruation
  - Clinical history of current menstruation important
  - May need ultrasound, clinical correlation if patient not currently menstruating
- Ovaries: Benign and malignant etiologies
  - May need ultrasound to distinguish

Urine Contamination
- Urine containing excreted FDG can be wicked into vagina by tampon
- Incontinence can cause contamination of external genitalia

CERVICAL CANCER

PATHOLOGY

General Features
- General path comments
  - GLUT-1: Overexpressed in cervical carcinoma, may be correlated with tumor grade
    - Absence of GLUT-1 correlated with improved metastasis-free survival
  - In women with LN + cervical carcinoma, 80% of involved LN are < 1.0 cm in greatest dimension
- Etiology
  - Likely multifactorial
  - Associated with human papillomavirus infection (strains 16, 18, 31, 33, 45)
  - Other risk factors
    - Multiple sexual partners
    - Sex before age 18
    - Tobacco use
    - Diethylstilbestrol
- Epidemiology
  - In US: ~ 10,000 cases per year
    - ~ 1/3 die of disease
  - Worldwide: > 300,000 cases diagnosed per year
    - 50% mortality rate

CLINICAL ISSUES

Presentation
- Most common signs/symptoms
  - Often asymptomatic
    - Abnormal cells typically found during a cervical screening test (Pap smear)
  - Later symptoms
    - Abnormal vaginal bleeding/discharge
    - Discomfort during/after sexual intercourse

Demographics
- Age: Primarily affects younger women, although can be seen at any age

Natural History & Prognosis
- 5 year survival
  - No lymphadenopathy: 57%
  - + Pelvic lymphadenopathy: 34%
  - + Paraaortic lymphadenopathy: 12%

Treatment
- Surgery or radiotherapy in early stages
  - Single treatment modality preferred
- Chemotherapy + radiotherapy in advanced stages

DIAGNOSTIC CHECKLIST

Consider
- PET/CT for optimal staging
- Physical exam, MR for evaluation of primary tumor

SELECTED REFERENCES

1. Amit A et al: The role of hybrid PET/CT in the evaluation of patients with cervical cancer. Gynecol Oncol. 100(1):65-9, 2006
2. Chou HH et al: Low value of [18F]-fluoro-2-deoxy-D-glucose positron emission tomography in primary staging of early-stage cervical cancer before radical hysterectomy. J Clin Oncol. 24(1):123-8, 2006
3. Chung HH et al: Clinical impact of FDG-PET imaging in post-therapy surveillance of uterine cervical cancer: from diagnosis to prognosis. Gynecol Oncol. 103(1):165-70, 2006
4. Chung HH et al: Clinical impact of integrated PET/CT on the management of suspected cervical cancer recurrence. Gynecol Oncol. 2006
5. Lin CT et al: Role of [18F]fluoro-2-deoxy-D-glucose positron emission tomography in re-recurrent cervical cancer. Int J Gynecol Cancer. 16(6):1994-2003, 2006
6. Sakurai H et al: FDG-PET in the detection of recurrence of uterine cervical carcinoma following radiation therapy--tumor volume and FDG uptake value. Gynecol Oncol. 100(3):601-7, 2006
7. Sironi S et al: Lymph node metastasis in patients with clinical early-stage cervical cancer: detection with integrated FDG PET/CT. Radiology. 238(1):272-9, 2006
8. Yen TC et al: Comparative benefits and limitations of (18)F-FDG PET and CT-MRI in documented or suspected recurrent cervical cancer. Eur J Nucl Med Mol Imaging. 33(12):1399-407, 2006
9. Grosu AL et al: Positron emission tomography for radiation treatment planning. Strahlenther Onkol. 181(8):483-99, 2005
10. Park W et al: The usefulness of MRI and PET imaging for the detection of parametrial involvement and lymph node metastasis in patients with cervical cancer. Jpn J Clin Oncol. 35(5):260-4, 2005
11. Roh JW et al: Role of positron emission tomography in pretreatment lymph node staging of uterine cervical cancer: a prospective surgicopathologic correlation study. Eur J Cancer. 41(14):2086-92, 2005
12. Subhas N et al: Imaging of pelvic malignancies with in-line FDG PET-CT: case examples and common pitfalls of FDG PET. Radiographics. 25(4):1031-43, 2005
13. Belhocine TZ: 18F-FDG PET imaging in posttherapy monitoring of cervical cancers: from diagnosis to prognosis. J Nucl Med. 45(10):1602-4, 2004
14. Grigsby PW et al: Posttherapy [18F] fluorodeoxyglucose positron emission tomography in carcinoma of the cervix: response and outcome. J Clin Oncol. 22(11):2167-71, 2004
15. Lai CH et al: Restaging of recurrent cervical carcinoma with dual-phase [18F]fluoro-2-deoxy-D-glucose positron emission tomography. Cancer. 100(3):544-52, 2004
16. Wong TZ et al: Positron emission tomography with 2-deoxy-2-[(18)F]fluoro-D-glucose for evaluating local and distant disease in patients with cervical cancer. Mol Imaging Biol. 6(1):55-62, 2004
17. Lin WC et al: Usefulness of (18)F-fluorodeoxyglucose positron emission tomography to detect para-aortic lymph nodal metastasis in advanced cervical cancer with negative computed tomography findings. Gynecol Oncol. 89(1):73-6, 2003
18. Narayan K et al: Relation between FIGO stage, primary tumor volume, and presence of lymph node metastases in cervical cancer patients referred for radiotherapy. Int J Gynecol Cancer. 13(5):657-63, 2003
19. Tran BN et al: Occult supraclavicular lymph node metastasis identified by FDG-PET in patients with carcinoma of the uterine cervix. Gynecol Oncol. 90(3):572-6, 2003
20. Yen TC et al: Value of dual-phase 2-fluoro-2-deoxy-d-glucose positron emission tomography in cervical cancer. J Clin Oncol. 21(19):3651-8, 2003

CERVICAL CANCER

IMAGE GALLERY

Typical

Typical

Typical

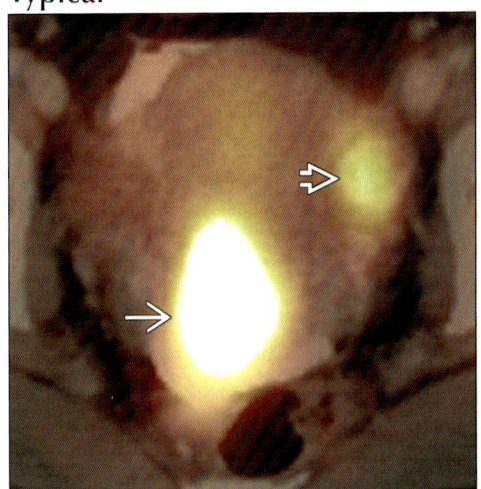

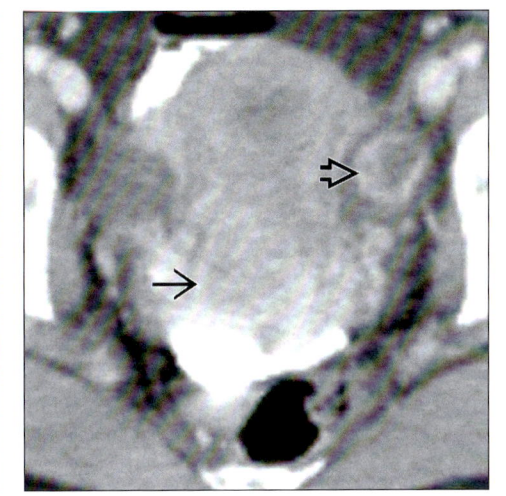

(Left) Axial fused PET/CT shows a large cervical mass ➡ with intense FDG activity in a patient with known cervical carcinoma. Note moderate FDG activity in left corpus luteum cyst ⮕. (Right) Axial CECT in same patient as left, shows large heterogeneously enhancing cervical mass ➡. Note corpus luteal cyst with thin homogeneously enhancing wall ⮕ in otherwise normal ovary.

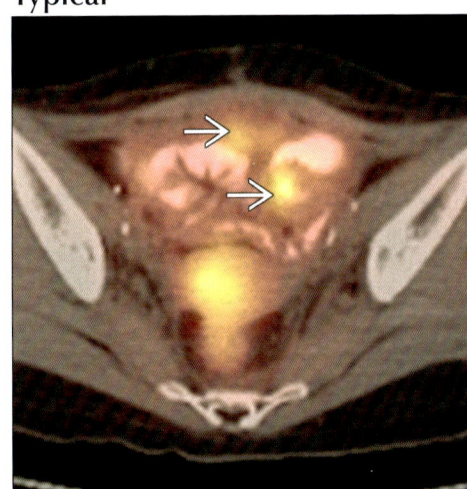

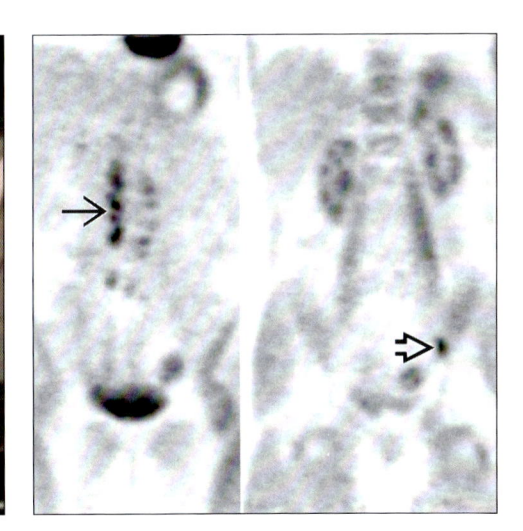

(Left) Axial fused PET/CT shows focus of moderate FDG activity in multiple soft tissue metastases ➡ in a patient with recurrent cervical carcinoma. (Right) Coronal PET shows multiple hypermetabolic paraaortic lymph nodes ➡, consistent with metastatic lymphadenopathy. Pelvic lymphadenopathy ⮕ is also evident.

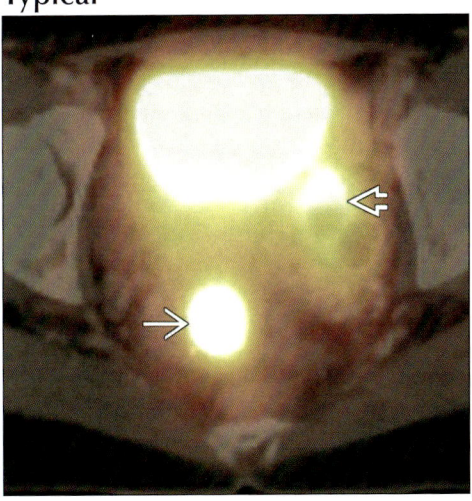

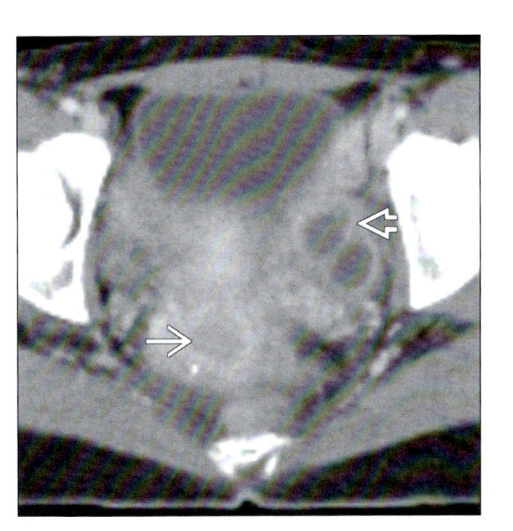

(Left) Axial fused PET/CT shows hypermetabolic activity in primary cervical mass ➡, in addition to intense activity in left ovarian cystic metastases ⮕. (Right) Axial CECT in same patient as left, shows primary cervical mass ➡. Note multiple cystic metastases in left ovary ⮕, which can also be seen in corpus luteal cysts.

ENDOMETRIAL CANCER

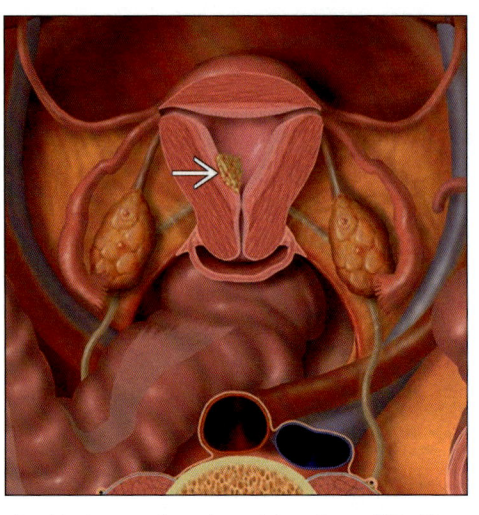

Graphic shows early endometrial carcinoma with no extension into myometrium.

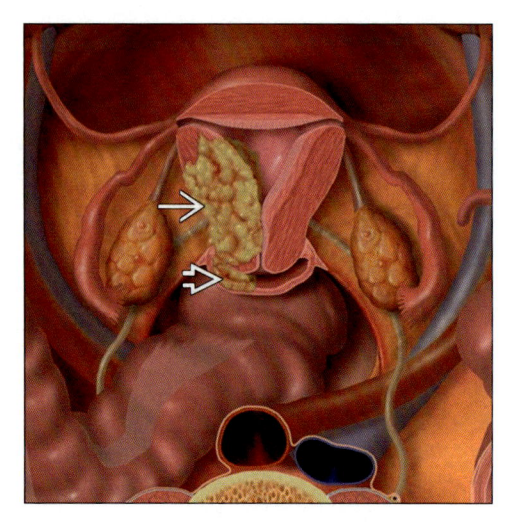

Graphic shows stage II endometrial carcinoma with invasion into cervix and myometrium.

TERMINOLOGY

Abbreviations and Synonyms
- Endometrial carcinoma

Definitions
- Malignancy of uterine endometrium, most commonly endometrioid adenocarcinoma

IMAGING FINDINGS

General Features
- Best diagnostic clue
  - Primary endometrial cancer: Thickened endometrium on CT with intense FDG activity on PET correlating to mass
  - Signs of metastatic disease on PET: Lymphadenopathy, abdominal/distant metastases
- Location
  - Usually superior endometrium, glandular component, but may spread within endo/myometrium and from fundus toward isthmus and cervix
  - May arise within an endometrial polyp

Nuclear Medicine Findings
- PET
  - Normal cycle variation of FDG activity in endometrium
  - Significant nonmalignant uptake in younger patients who are menstruating
  - Sensitivity and specificity of PET
    - Sensitivity of PET alone (87%) or plus MR or CT (91%) is higher than MR or CT alone (~ 67% in overall lesion detection)
    - PET has sensitivity/specificity 96%/78% for post-therapy surveillance
    - PET has been shown to alter treatment in 35% of patients with endometrial cancer
    - In one series, additional FDG PET had management impact in 73% of cases when performed for post-therapy surveillance
    - PET has 89% PPV and 91% NPV in patients with endometrial cancer
  - In one study, mean SUV of true-positive lesions: 13 for central pelvic lesions, 11 for metastases
  - PET most useful for detecting distant metastases

DDx: Benign Mimics of Endometrial Cancer

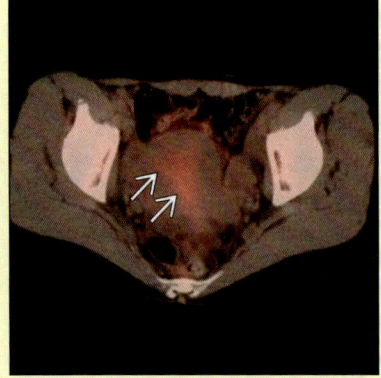

Menstruation 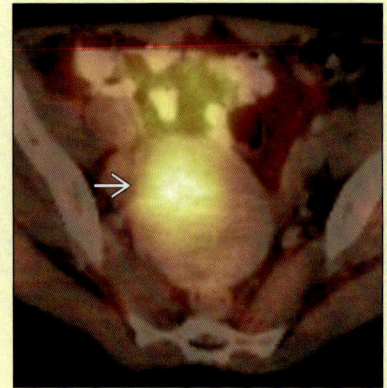   *Leiomyoma* 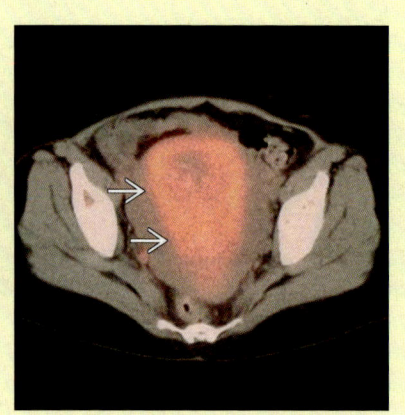   *Postpartum Uterus*

ENDOMETRIAL CANCER

Key Facts

Imaging Findings
- CT findings nonspecific for endometrial carcinoma, can be simulated by other conditions
- PET has sensitivity/specificity 96%/78% for post-therapy surveillance
- PET has been shown to alter treatment in 35% of patients with endometrial cancer
- PET has 89% PPV and 91% NPV in patients with endometrial cancer
- PET most useful for detecting distant metastases
- Accuracy of CT and MR limited by post-surgical/radiation changes for diagnosis of recurrences; PET/CT useful
- FDG PET for staging, restaging, early detection, evaluating response to therapy

Top Differential Diagnoses
- Cervical Cancer
- Uterine Leiomyoma
- Endometrial Hyperplasia
- Endometrial Polyp
- Tamoxifen-Related Endometrial Changes
- Endometrial Sarcoma

Clinical Issues
- Common gynecological cancer with good prognosis
- 75% confined to uterine corpus
- Survival rates 84% in US

Diagnostic Checklist
- MR or CT for extent of primary tumor
- PET/CT for optimal staging

CT Findings
- CT does not depict endometrium consistently
- CT not reliable for accurate evaluation of endometrial thickness
- CT appearance
  o Relatively low-attenuation mass in region of endometrial cavity which may show uniform attenuation or may be heterogeneous with or without a contrast-enhanced component
  o Polypoid mass surrounded by endometrial fluid
  o Heterogeneous soft tissue mass/masses and fluid expanding endometrial cavity
- CT findings nonspecific for endometrial carcinoma, can be simulated by other conditions

MR Findings
- T1WI: Endometrium, myometrium have similar signal intensity and cannot readily be distinguished
- T2WI: Endometrium = central zone of high signal intensity
- Myometrium depicted as zone of low signal intensity at its inner aspect and a wider zone of intermediate signal intensity at its outer aspect
- Endometrial thickness varies in menstruating women from 4 mm in early proliferative phase to 13 mm in late secretory phase

Imaging Recommendations
- Best imaging tool
  o MR/CT used to evaluate disease extension and provide information for treatment planning, ± ultrasound
  o Accuracy of CT and MR limited by post-surgical/radiation changes for diagnosis of recurrences; PET/CT useful
  o FDG PET for staging, restaging, early detection, evaluating response to therapy

DIFFERENTIAL DIAGNOSIS

Cervical Cancer
- Cervical mass on CT, although can be normal with masses up to 3 cm
- 80-90% of patients experience vaginal bleeding

Uterine Leiomyoma
- Fibroids may be indistinguishable unless calcified or necrotic
- Intramural or exophytic lesions more easy to differentiate

Endometrial Hyperplasia
- May have same findings on US as endometrial carcinoma

Endometrial Polyp
- Can mimic endometrial cancer on CT

Tamoxifen-Related Endometrial Changes
- Patients with breast cancer on prolonged tamoxifen therapy reported to have increased risk of endometrial polyps, hyperplasia, cancer

Endometrial Sarcoma
- Leiomyosarcoma tends to occur in women aged 30-50
- Carcinosarcoma, endometrial stromal sarcoma have higher incidence in women > 50 years

PATHOLOGY

General Features
- General path comments
  o Histologic subtypes
    ▪ Endometrioid carcinoma (most common)
    ▪ Adenosquamous carcinoma
    ▪ Serous papillary carcinoma
    ▪ Clear cell carcinoma
    ▪ Small cell undifferentiated carcinoma (least common)
- Etiology

ENDOMETRIAL CANCER

- Most common risk factor: Protracted exposure to endogenous or exogenous estrogen unopposed by progesterone
- Other risk factors
  - Menopause after age 52
  - Long time period between menarche and menopause
  - Estrogen replacement therapy
  - Tamoxifen use
  - Endometrial hyperplasia
  - Obesity
  - Nulliparity
- Epidemiology
  - Most common genital malignancy in US
  - Fourth most common malignancy in women after breast, lung, colorectal
  - Up to 1 in 100 women in US may develop the disease

Staging, Grading or Classification Criteria
- Staging of endometrial cancer
  - Stage I: Cancer confined to uterine corpus
    - IA: Tumor limited to endometrium and CT appearance of uterus may be normal
    - IB: Tumor extends into less than one half the width of the myometrium
    - IC: Tumor extends into one half or more of the myometrial width
  - Stage II: Cancer involving corpus and cervix, without extrauterine spread
    - IIA: Cancer extends from uterine corpus into endocervical glandular region of cervix
    - IIB: Fibromuscular stroma of cervix is involved
  - Stage III: Cancer extending outside the uterus but confined to the true pelvis
    - IIIA: Extends outside the uterus into parametria, pelvic sidewall, fallopian tube, or ovary
    - IIIB: Vaginal metastases characterize this stage
    - IIIC: Enlarged pelvic and/or para-aortic lymph nodes characterize this stage
  - Stage IV: Cancer invading the bladder or bowel mucosa and/or spreading outside the true pelvis
    - IVA: Tumor invasion spreads into urinary bladder or bowel mucosa
    - IVB: Metastases outside the true pelvis characterize this stage, including metastasis into the intra-abdominal and/or inguinal lymph nodes

CLINICAL ISSUES

Presentation
- Most common signs/symptoms
  - Postmenopausal bleeding
    - Eventually 80% present with vaginal bleeding, mostly postmenopausal
  - Early endometrial cancer usually asymptomatic
- Other signs/symptoms
  - 10% of patients present with purulent vaginal discharge, sometimes tinged with blood
  - Pelvic pain and pressure usually manifestations of advanced disease

Demographics
- Age
  - Peak incidence 55-65 years
  - 75% of patients > 50 years
  - 5% of patient < 40 years
- Ethnicity: Prevalence and survival rates higher in whites than in blacks

Natural History & Prognosis
- Common gynecological cancer with good prognosis
- 75% confined to uterine corpus
- Survival rates 84% in US

Treatment
- Complete resection includes: Total abdominal hysterectomy, bilateral salpingo-oophorectomy and pelvic/para-aortic node sampling
- Radical hysterectomy performed only for unequivocal cervical involvement
- Patients with localized recurrences are classically treated with surgery and/or radiation
- Systemic chemotherapy and/or progesterone therapy advocated for disseminated recurrent disease

DIAGNOSTIC CHECKLIST

Consider
- MR or CT for extent of primary tumor
- PET/CT for optimal staging
  - Stage IIIC: Lymphadenopathy
  - Stage IVB: Distant metastases
- Note benign causes of increased FDG activity in endometrium (e.g., menstruation)

SELECTED REFERENCES

1. Chao A et al: 18F-FDG PET in the management of endometrial cancer. Eur J Nucl Med Mol Imaging. 33(1):36-44, 2006
2. Sironi S et al: Post-therapy surveillance of patients with uterine cancers: value of integrated FDG PET/CT in the detection of recurrence. Eur J Nucl Med Mol Imaging. 2006
3. Yoshida Y et al: The positron emission tomography with F18 17beta-estradiol has the potential to benefit diagnosis and treatment of endometrial cancer. Gynecol Oncol. 2006
4. Nakamoto Y et al: Positron emission tomography application for gynecologic tumors. Int J Gynecol Cancer. 15(5):701-9, 2005
5. Pandit-Taskar N: Oncologic imaging in gynecologic malignancies. J Nucl Med. 46(11):1842-50, 2005
6. Subhas N et al: Imaging of pelvic malignancies with in-line FDG PET-CT: case examples and common pitfalls of FDG PET. Radiographics. 25(4):1031-43, 2005
7. Lerman H et al: Normal and abnormal 18F-FDG endometrial and ovarian uptake in pre- and postmenopausal patients: assessment by PET/CT. J Nucl Med. 45(2):266-71, 2004
8. Saga T et al: Clinical value of FDG-PET in the follow up of post-operative patients with endometrial cancer. Ann Nucl Med. 17(3):197-203, 2003
9. Belhocine T et al: Usefulness of (18)F-FDG PET in the post-therapy surveillance of endometrial carcinoma. Eur J Nucl Med Mol Imaging. 29(9):1132-9, 2002
10. Nakahara T et al: F-18 FDG uptake in endometrial cancer. Clin Nucl Med. 26(1):82-3, 2001

ENDOMETRIAL CANCER

IMAGE GALLERY

Typical

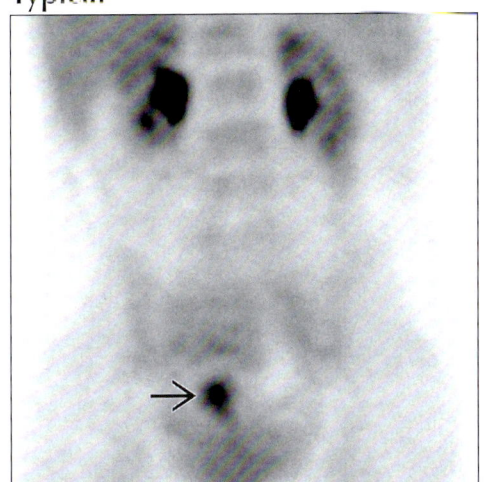

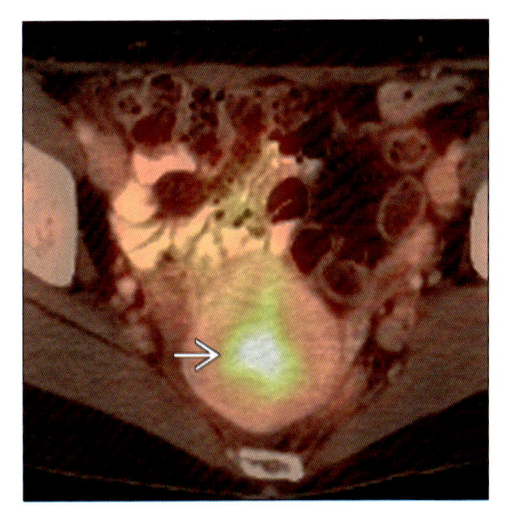

(Left) Coronal PET shows focal intense FDG uptake in pelvis ➔ in patient with endometrial carcinoma. *(Right)* Axial fused PET/CT shows intense FDG activity in endometrial cavity ➔ in patient with endometrial cancer.

Typical

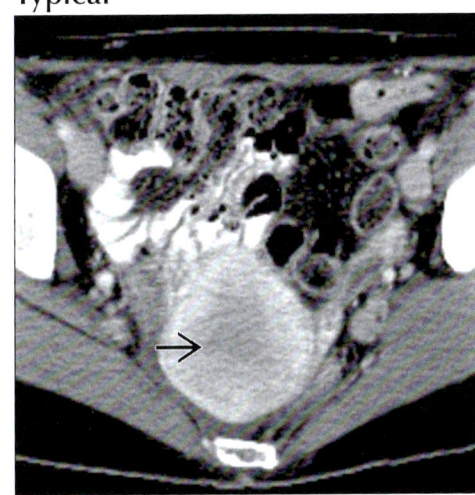

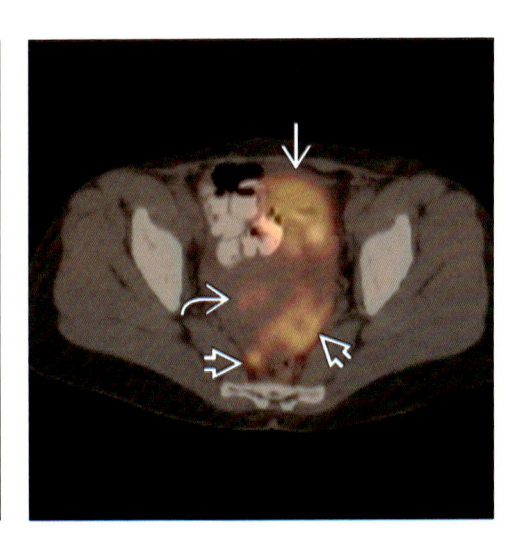

(Left) Axial CECT shows diffusely enlarged endometrial cavity ➔ with central low-attenuation compatible with fluid. There is indistinct heterogeneous enhancement of the uterine wall diffusely, difficult to appreciate much for margins of the tumor. *(Right)* Axial FDG PET/CT shows hypermetabolic endometrium ➔ in a patient with endometrial carcinoma. Tumor has spread outside uterus ➔ to left and posterior. Note normal urinary bladder activity ➔.

Typical

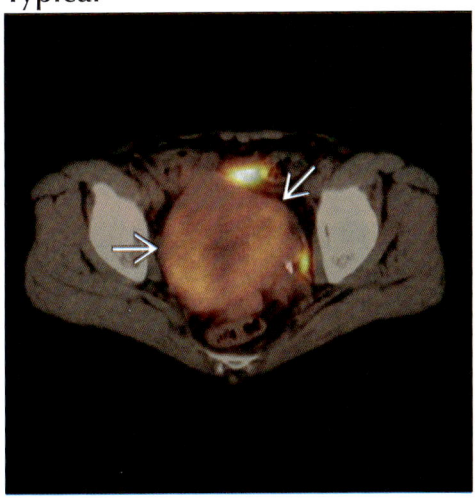

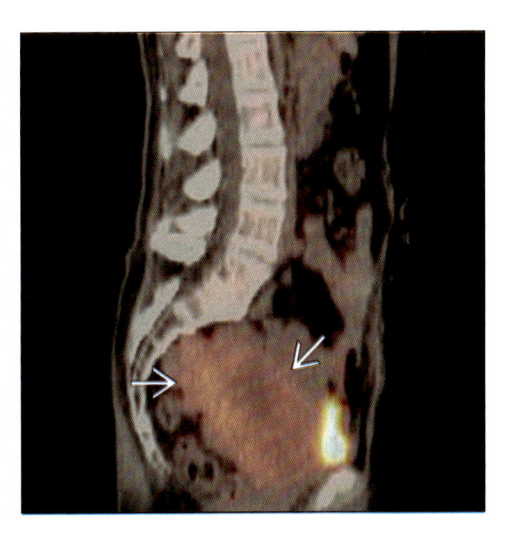

(Left) Axial FDG PET/CT shows lobular, enlarged, heterogeneously hypermetabolic uterus ➔ in a patient with endometrial carcino-sarcoma. The disease has spread to involve the entire uterus. See next image. *(Right)* Same as previous. Sagittal FDG PET/CT shows lobular, enlarged, heterogeneously hypermetabolic uterus ➔ in a patient with endometrial carcino-sarcoma.

PROSTATE CANCER, ANTIBODY SCAN

Planar In-111 capromab image shows aortocaval nodal metastases. Note normal liver and cardiac blood pool activity.

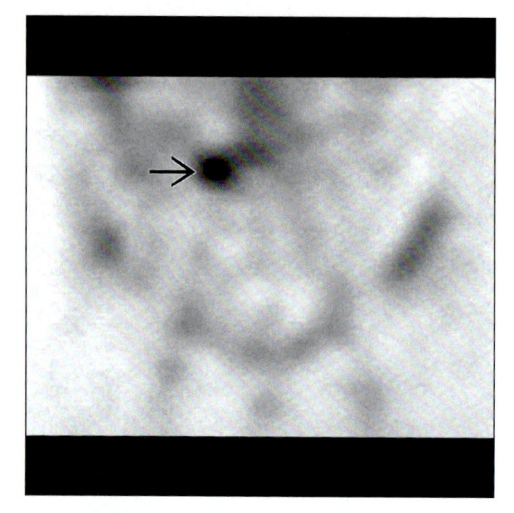

Coronal In-111 capromab SPECT image shows right proximal iliac focal uptake at site of 1.3 cm nodal metastasis.

TERMINOLOGY

Abbreviations and Synonyms
- ProstaScint: Registered trademark (Cytogen) for In-111 capromab pendetide (labeled 7E11-C5.3 murine antibody of IgG1, kappa subclass (IgG1K)

Definitions
- Prostate specific membrane antigen (PSMA): On membrane of prostate cancer cells; target for capromab

IMAGING FINDINGS

General Features
- Best diagnostic clue: Focal non-physiologic uptake of capromab: Corresponding to positive CT finding if outside prostate bed
- Indication for capromab imaging: Previous definitive treatment, then rising PSA without obvious source
  - Disease localized to prostate bed: Candidate for definitive salvage (radiation, surgery)
  - Disease spread outside prostate: Hormonal blockade, chemotherapy

Nuclear Medicine Findings
- In-111 capromab scintigraphy
  - Antibody localization in liver, marrow, urine, bowel, blood pool is normal
  - Human anti-mouse antibodies (HAMA): ↑ Liver, ↓ blood pool & bone marrow; considered non-diagnostic
  - Sens. 75%, spec. 86% in extraprostatic sites; poor specificity in prostate
  - Fusion with CT or MR may ↑ sensitivity to low 90's
- Whole body bone scan: Best applied with significant PSA elevations (> 20 ng/mL), better for bone lesions than FDG PET, capromab
  - Most common metastatic sites on bone scan: Pelvis, vertebrae via Batson plexus, generalized (late)
- Plain film: Classic sclerotic lesions, assessment of fracture risk
- CT imaging: Assessment of enlarged regional nodes
- FDG PET/CT: Poor sensitivity except with high grade, undifferentiated tumors

Imaging Recommendations
- Protocol advice
  - 222 MBq (6 mCi) In-111 capromab IV

DDx: Other Imaging Findings

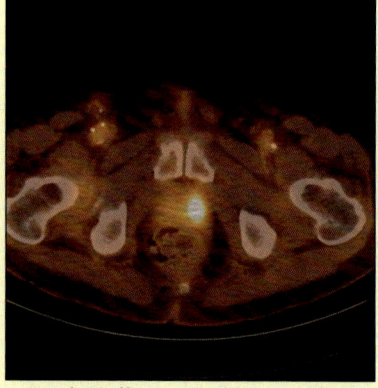

Poorly Differentiated Tumor (PET)

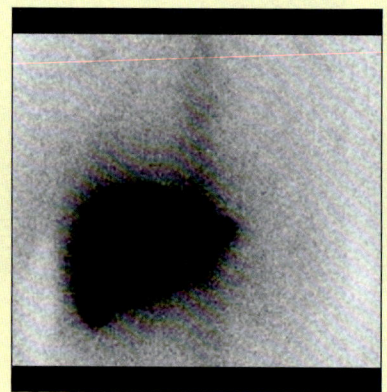

HAMA Reaction (Capromab)

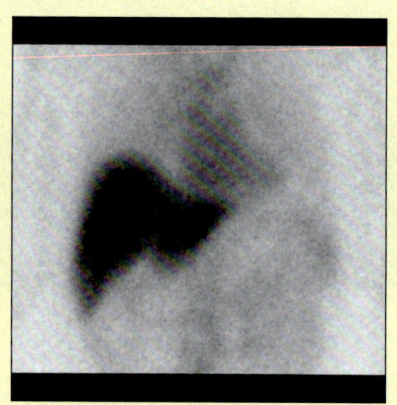

No HAMA Reaction (Capromab)

PROSTATE CANCER, ANTIBODY SCAN

Key Facts

Imaging Findings
- Best diagnostic clue: Focal non-physiologic uptake of capromab: Corresponding to positive CT finding if outside prostate bed
- Indication for capromab imaging: Previous definitive treatment, then rising PSA without obvious source
- Disease localized to prostate bed: Candidate for definitive salvage (radiation, surgery)
- Disease spread outside prostate: Hormonal blockade, chemotherapy
- Human anti-mouse antibodies (HAMA): ↑ Liver, ↓ blood pool & bone marrow; considered non-diagnostic
- Fusion with CT or MR may ↑ sensitivity to low 90's

Top Differential Diagnoses
- Inflammation, Trauma, Other Cancers
- Physiologic Uptake of Capromab

○ 4-6 days: Bowel prep, whole body planar scan, head through scrotum
○ SPECT scan of abdomen, pelvis: Fusion to CT (dedicated hybrid system or off-line)
○ If no SPECT/CT fusion options: Inject with Tc-99m-tagged RBCs, dual energy (Tc-99m and dual Indium-111 windows) SPECT of pelvis

DIFFERENTIAL DIAGNOSIS

Inflammation, Trauma, Other Cancers
- Can be positive on capromab scan

Physiologic Uptake of Capromab
- Liver, blood pool, bone marrow, GI, kidneys, bladder

CLINICAL ISSUES

Presentation
- Most common signs/symptoms: Nodular, firm prostate; elevated serum PSA, bone pain

Demographics
- Age
  ○ Age-adjusted incidence 177.8/100,000: 258.3 in African American men and 163.4 for Caucasian men
  ○ Autopsy incidence of latent prostate carcinoma: 30-39 y (3%), 50-59 y (12%), > 70 y (50+%)

Natural History & Prognosis
- 1-in-6 chance of prostate cancer in lifetime
- 200,000+ new cases diagnosed in US yearly
- 5-year survival nearly 100% (50% for stage IV)

Treatment
- Surgical: Suprapubic radical prostatectomy
- Radiation therapy: External beam, brachytherapy
- Cryotherapy: Newer method
- Complications for all methods: Impotence 80%, incontinence 60%; increases with salvage treatments

DIAGNOSTIC CHECKLIST

Consider
- PSA level: Definition of re-occurrence usually 3 successive rises, using same lab
- Rate of rise: Can be good indicator of aggressiveness

SELECTED REFERENCES
1. Jana S et al: Nuclear medicine studies of the prostate, testes, and bladder. Semin Nucl Med. 36(1):51-72, 2006
2. Ward JF et al: Biochemical recurrence after definitive prostate cancer therapy. Part I: defining and localizing biochemical recurrence of prostate cancer. Curr Opin Urol. 15(3):181-6, 2005
3. Sodee DB et al: Multicenter ProstaScint imaging findings in 2154 patients with prostate cancer. The ProstaScint Imaging Centers.

IMAGE GALLERY

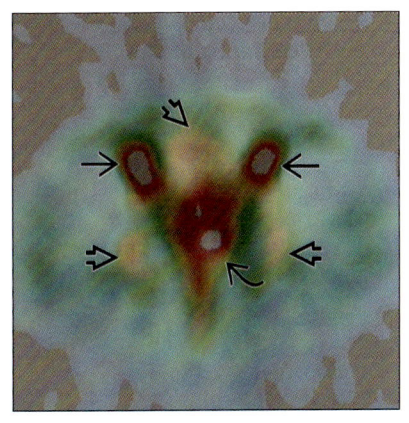

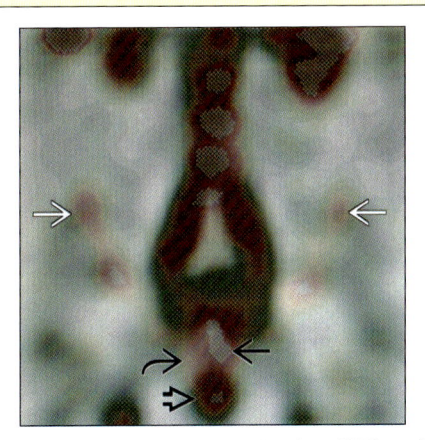

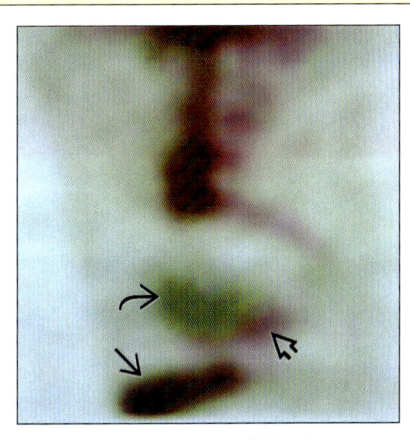

(Left) Axial dual labeled SPECT through prostate shows Tc-99m-tagged RBC blood pool ➔, and In-111 capromab in marrow ➔ and cancerous left lobe of prostate ➔. See next image. (Center) Coronal dual label SPECT in same patient shows bladder ➔, corpora cavernosa with considerable blood pool ➔, and tumor in left lobe of prostate ➔. Marrow ➔ is seen in iliac wings. (Right) Sagittal dual label fusion SPECT shows tumor ➔ involving seminal vesicles. Bladder ➔ and corpora cavernosa/penile blood pool ➔ are also shown.

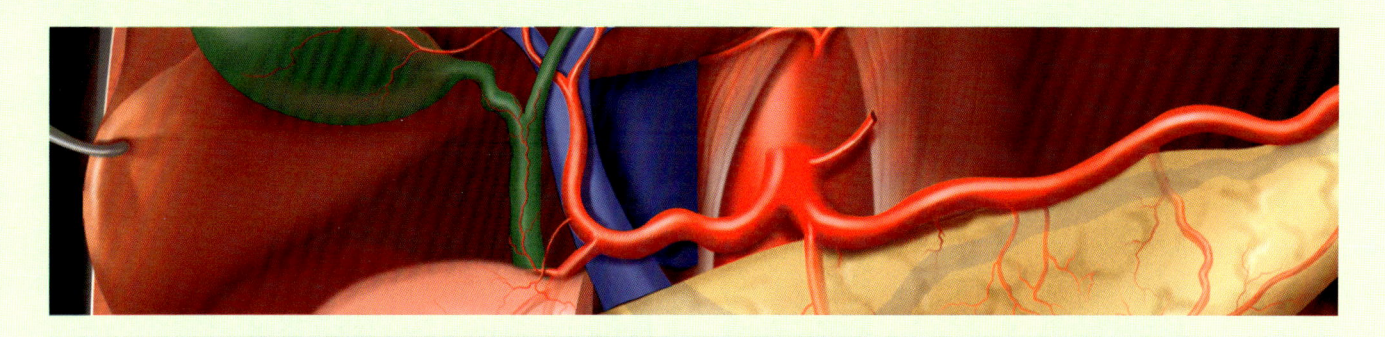

SECTION 10: HemeOnc Procedures & Therapies

Therapy - Oncology

Phosphorus-32 Therapies	10-2
Hepatic Arterial Y-90 Microspheres	10-4
Radiolabeled Antibody Therapy	10-8

Hematologic Procedures

RBC Survival & Splenic Sequestration	10-12
Red Cell Mass and Plasma Volume	10-14
Schilling Test	10-16

PHOSPHORUS-32 THERAPIES

Anterior bone scan in a patient with polycythemia vera shows increased uptake in ends of long bones, signifying marrow expansion.

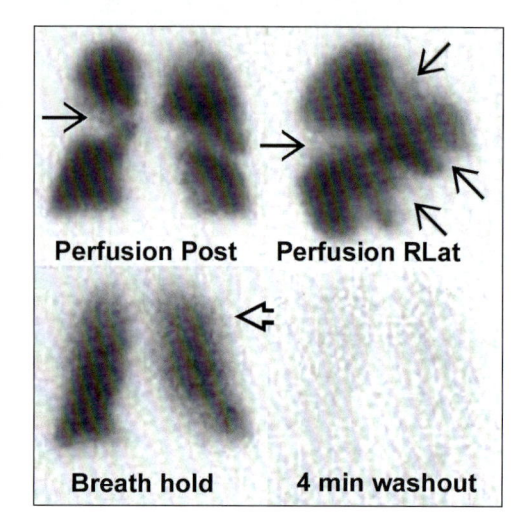

High probability lung scan shows multiple perfusion defects and normal ventilation. Pulmonary embolism is a complication of polycythemia vera and essential thrombocytosis.

TERMINOLOGY

Definitions
- Decays by pure β emission: Maximum β particle energy 1.17 MeV; mean β energy: 0.695 MeV
- Half-life: Physical 14.3 d; biological in marrow 7-9 d
- Range in soft tissue: Maximum 8 mm; therapeutic 2 mm
- Formulations: [32-P] NaH_2PO_4 (orthophosphate) or colloid chromic

PRE-PROCEDURE

Indications
- Intravenous P-32: Cytoreductive for hematoproliferative disorders (essential thrombocytosis, polycythemia vera)
  - When phlebotomy and/or conventional chemotherapy fails, not tolerated, contraindicated
  - Dosimetry: Bone 41-63 rad/mCi (11.1-17 mGy/MBq); marrow 20-40 rad/mCi (5.4-10.8 mGy/MBq); bladder 2.7 rad/mCi (0.74 mGy/MBq)
- Intracavitary P-32: Malignant fluid collections in serous cavities (peritoneum, pericardium, pleural space)
  - "Salvage" or "clean-up" therapy following successful chemotherapy in high-risk patients
  - Second-line therapy when conventional treatment not tolerated/fails
- Intraarticular P-32: For synovial proliferative/inflammatory disorders
  - Indications: When conservative treatment fails x 6 months; following surgical synovectomy; when process is monoarticular and systemic therapy is contraindicated
  - Entities amenable to intraarticular P-32 therapy: Diffuse intraarticular pigmented villonodular synovitis (PVNS), rheumatoid arthritis & other inflammatory diseases, hemophiliac joint disease
- Rarely used, experimental, historical: Intratumoral/intracystic injection of P-32 radiocolloid; P-32 orthophosphate for painful bone metastases; intraarterial tumoral embolization with P-32 glass microspheres; intralymphatic P-32 tri-n-octyl-phosphate for lymph node micrometastases

PROCEDURE

Procedure Steps
- Intravenous: P-32 orthophosphate
  - Polycythemia vera: Typical dose adult 2-3 mCi/m^2 P-32 IV (74-111 MBq/m^2), max initial dose of 5 mCi (185 MBq)
  - Essential thrombocytosis: Typical dose adult 3 mCi/m^2 P-32 IV (111 MBq/m^2), max initial dose of 5 mCi (185 MBq)
  - May repeat q 3 months: 25% dose ↑ until response, upper single dose limit 7 mCi (260MBq)
  - Inject through Angiocath (not butterfly); observe catheter site during entire injection (stop injection at first sign of extravasation or pain)
  - Inject slowly at port near catheter entry site: P-32 sticks to plastic, IV tubing
  - Allow free flowing normal saline to "carry" P-32 into vein; flush with 100-250 cc normal saline
- Intracavitary: Colloidal chromic P-32
  - Pre-procedure image of Tc-99m sulfur colloid infused in normal saline: Confirm lack of loculation
  - Dose ranges: Pericardial 1-5 mCi (37-185 MBq); peritoneal 10-110 mCi (370-4170 MBq)
  - Infuse with sufficient normal saline to allow uniform dispersion (1L peritoneal)

PHOSPHORUS-32 THERAPIES

Key Facts

Pre-procedure
- Intravenous P-32: Cytoreductive for hematoproliferative disorders (essential thrombocytosis, polycythemia vera)
- Intracavitary P-32: Malignant fluid collections in serous cavities (peritoneum, pericardium, pleural space)
- Intraarticular P-32: For synovial proliferative/inflammatory disorders

Post-procedure
- Intraperitoneal P-32: May ↑ survival or only ↓ symptoms (metastatic carcinoma)
- Essential thrombocytosis: 67% complete remission, 37% partial remission after 1st y with IV P-32
- Polycythemia vera: Average remission of disease up to 2 y
- PVNS: Reduced recurrence when intraarticular P-32 follows surgical synovectomy

---

  - Post-procedure: Patient to lie flat, rolling frequently x 12 h
- Intraarticular: Colloidal chromic P-32
  - Confirm intraarticular needle placement with contrast & fluoroscopy
  - Wide range of doses used: 1-6 mCi (37-222 MBq) in 1-4 mL normal saline with methylprednisolone, lidocaine, bupivacaine
  - Steroid injection along needle tract during withdrawal
  - Post-procedure
    - Range of motion exercise to spread throughout joint space
    - Bed rest & ACE bandage wrap x 48 h

POST-PROCEDURE

Expected Outcome
- Intraperitoneal P-32: May ↑ survival or only ↓ symptoms (metastatic carcinoma)
  - Minimal residual disease 4-year survival: 50% if P-32 plus chemotherapy; 22% chemotherapy only
  - Metastatic carcinoma: Symptomatic improvement but no survival benefit
- Essential thrombocytosis: 67% complete remission, 37% partial remission after 1st y with IV P-32
- Polycythemia vera: Average remission of disease up to 2 y
- PVNS: Reduced recurrence when intraarticular P-32 follows surgical synovectomy

PROBLEMS & COMPLICATIONS

Complications
- Most feared complication(s)
  - Intravenous P-32: Extravasation of injected dose (radiation necrosis of tissue)
  - Intravenous P-32: 2x higher incidence leukemia in polycythemia vera with P-32 Rx (no change in overall survival); secondary malignancies with P-32 + alkylating agents
  - Intracavitary P-32: Rarely peritonitis, bowel necrosis, peritoneal hemorrhage
- Other complications
  - Intrapericardial P-32 colloid: Constrictive pericarditis with repeated injections
  - Intraarticular P-32 colloid: Damage to synovial subintimal structures (bone, cartilage, ligaments); extraarticular accumulation in liver, regional lymph nodes (potential for lymphocyte chromosomal damage); periarticular erythema, skin necrosis

SELECTED REFERENCES

1. Ward WG Sr et al: Diffuse Pigmented Villonodular Synovitis: Preliminary Results with Intralesional Resection and P32 Synoviorthesis. Clin Orthop Relat Res. 454:186-191, 2007
2. Harbert JC: Phosphorous-32 Therapy in Myeloproliferative Diseases. In: Nuclear Medicine Therapy. Thieme Medical Publishers, New York. 193-205, 1986

IMAGE GALLERY

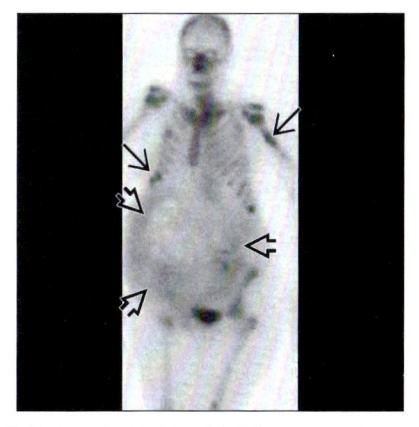

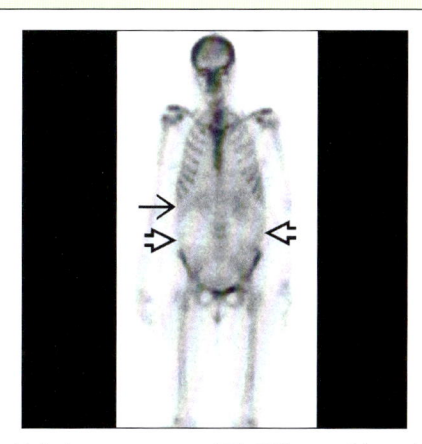

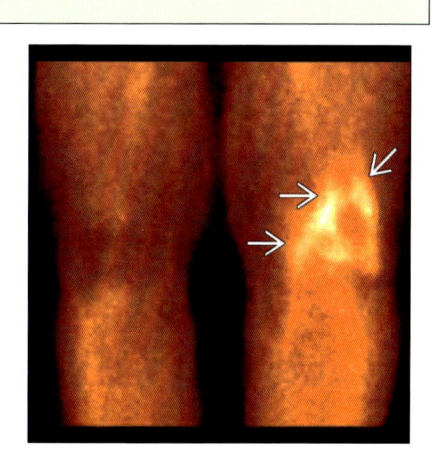

(Left) Anterior Tc-99m MDP bone scan shows multiple bone metastases ➔. Diffuse, mild uptake in ascitic fluid ➔ is often seen with malignant ascites. (Center) Anterior Tc-99m MDP bone scan shows subtle uptake in subhepatic space ➔ and pericolic gutters ➔, consistent with an exudative process in patient with peritoneal carcinomatosis/ascites. (Right) Anterior blood pool image of knees from Tc-99m MDP bone scan shows diffuse hyperemia around the left knee ➔, a finding typical for synovial inflammatory disease.

HEPATIC ARTERIAL Y-90 MICROSPHERES

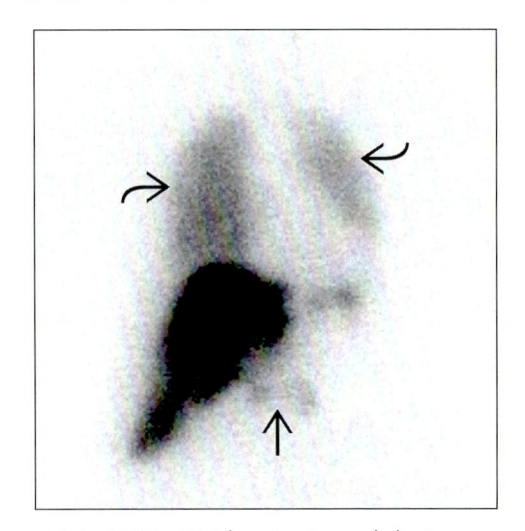

Anterior Tc-99m MAA hepatic artery embolization scan shows marked lung uptake ➔ (15% shunt), requiring Y-90 dose reduction. Extrahepatic activity ➔ evident. See next image.

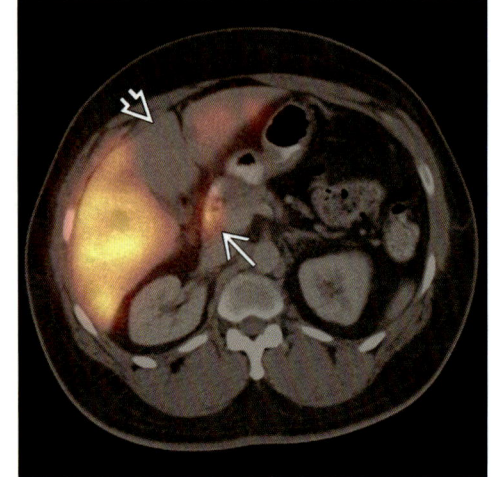

Tc-99m MAA SPECT/CT fusion of same patient at left shows minimal activity in medial left hepatic lobe ➔, supplied by replaced vessel off SMA. Note activity in duodenum ➔ due to accessory branch.

TERMINOLOGY

Abbreviations
- Yttrium-90 (Y-90): Pure beta emitter (2.28 MeV), T1/2 = 64.2 hr

Synonyms
- Sir-Sphere®: Y-90 in resin beads, 20-60 μm
- TheraSphere®: Y-90 in glass beads, 20-30 μm

Definitions
- Targeted radiotherapy of liver cancer by transhepatic arterial embolization of tumor vasculature with biocompatible Y-90 microspheres
  - Basic principal: Tumor recruits hepatic artery blood supply; normal liver spared by portal venous supply

PRE-PROCEDURE

Indications
- Indication: Inoperable liver cancer
  - Currently Sir-Sphere® FDA approved for hepatocellular carcinoma (HCC)
  - Off-label use more common for liver metastases
- Indication: Limited extrahepatic metastases

Contraindications
- Contraindication: Operable liver cancer
- Contraindication: Extensive extrahepatic metastases
- Contraindication: Liver failure
  - Bilirubin > 2.0 mg/dL; AST/ALT > 5 times upper limit normal
- Contraindication: Portal vein thrombosis
- Contraindication: > 20% Tc-99m MAA arteriovenous shunting to lungs
  - > 20% shunt to lungs: High risk of fatal radiation pneumonitis
  - May be cumulative with repeated treatments
  - Upper limit injected activity shunted to lungs: 0.61 GBq [(30 Gy), assuming lungs = 1 kg]
- Contraindication: Accessory vessels from hepatic artery to extrahepatic viscera
  - Unavoidable visceral delivery of microspheres unless detected/embolized
  - Results in radioembolization of viscera, radiation gastritis/enteritis, ulceration, perforation
- Relative contraindications
  - Bulk tumor > 70% of total liver volume
  - Infiltrative tumor
  - Tumor volume > 50% + albumin < 3 g/dL

Getting Started
- Equipment
- Authorization, training, personnel, billing issues
  - Requires appropriate institutional and authorized user approval for handling therapeutic radioactivity for medical use/brachytherapy
  - Personnel must be trained by microsphere industry representatives
  - On-site radiation safety officer/representatives required
  - Pre-authorization system in place for billing (expensive)

Decisions Prior to Treatment
- Is patient a candidate for treatment?
- Can procedure be done safely?
  - Likelihood of adequate liver function post-procedure
  - Prevention of radiation pneumonitis
  - Prevention of radiation gastritis/enteritis
- Can delivery catheter be placed via transfemoral approach?
- Concurrent/sequential systemic chemotherapy planned?
  - Many chemotherapies are radiosensitizers

HEPATIC ARTERIAL Y-90 MICROSPHERES

Key Facts

Pre-procedure
- Indication: Inoperable liver cancer
- Indication: Limited extrahepatic metastases
- Contraindication: Extensive extrahepatic metastases
- Contraindication: Liver failure
- Contraindication: Portal vein thrombosis
- Contraindication: > 20% Tc-99m MAA arteriovenous shunting to lungs
- > 20% shunt to lungs: High risk of fatal radiation pneumonitis

Procedure
- Resectability: Consider surgery for resectable liver tumor without extrahepatic metastases
- Extent of liver disease: If < 30% normal liver, ↑ likelihood of hepatic failure with Y-90 microspheres
- Accessory vessels of hepatic artery supplying extrahepatic viscera suggested by Tc-99m MAA scan
- May indicate accessory vessels not apparent on angiogram (≥ 15% of patients): Prompts "second look" angiogram
- Accessory vessels of hepatic artery ⇒ extrahepatic viscera: Must be embolized prior to procedure
- Calculate shunt fraction (F) to lungs based on MAA scan: Lungs/trunk
- Tc-99m MAA SPECT or SPECT/CT of upper abdomen: Strongly recommended

Post-procedure
- Effective duration of treatment: 92.4 hr (94% of radiation delivered in 11 days)
- PET/CT: > Accuracy than CT, MR in response assessment (prefer ≥ 50% ↓ in SUV at 1 month)

- Is intrahepatic artery chemoembolization a better initial option?
  - Currently more experience/results than with Y-90 microspheres

PROCEDURE

Patient Assessment: Clinical
- Resectability: Consider surgery for resectable liver tumor without extrahepatic metastases
- Extent of liver disease: If < 30% normal liver, ↑ likelihood of hepatic failure with Y-90 microspheres
- Assess for contraindications to therapy
- Liver function tests, including bilirubin level
- Performance status of patient: Able to tolerate?

Patient Assessment: Initial Imaging
- Pre-procedure PET/CT
  - Establish extent of metastatic disease
  - Establish baseline for assessment of therapeutic response
  - HCC typically low FDG-avidity, but PET useful in assessing response
- CECT or MR: Tumor volume, liver volume, resectability

Procedural Planning: Diagnostic Angiography
- CTA or transfemoral hepatic/visceral angiography
- Define anatomy and vascular variants
  - Replaced hepatic vessels: Suggested by reduced MAA embolization to specific lobes of liver
    - Right hepatic from SMA (20% of patients)
    - Left hepatic from left gastric (17% of patients)
    - Entire common hepatic from SMA (3% of patients)
  - Accessory vessels of hepatic artery supplying extrahepatic viscera suggested by Tc-99m MAA scan
    - May indicate accessory vessels not apparent on angiogram (≥ 15% of patients): Prompts "second look" angiogram
    - Small accessory branches to stomach, duodenum, pancreas, gallbladder, abdominal wall (from umbilical arteries) may be inapparent/insignificant by angiography

Vascular Pre-Procedure Intervention
- Accessory vessels of hepatic artery ⇒ extrahepatic viscera: Must be embolized prior to procedure
- Replaced hepatic vessels: May require surgical catheter/port if portion of liver with tumor cannot be selectively reached by transfemoral catheter
- Surgical placement of hepatic arterial port: If selective hepatic chemoembolization planned after Y-90 microspheres

Tc-99m Macroaggregated Albumin (MAA) Embolization Scan
- Last step at conclusion of angiographic procedure to assess embolization of extrahepatic structures
- Inject 3-5 mCi (111-185 MBq) Tc-99m MAA via hepatic artery catheter
  - Position catheter for MAA injection as planned for microsphere treatment
  - Slow injection to avoid reflux
  - Use freshly eluted Tc-99m to prepare Tc-99m MAA
  - Inject ≤ 30 min following preparation
    - Reduces free pertechnetate (and false positive gastric activity)
- Image soon after injection
  - Planar scan: Anterior and posterior, thorax and abdomen
    - Whole body scan mode
    - Planar spots optional: 1,000K for abdomen; same time for thorax
    - Regions of interest: Whole liver, whole lungs, background (body wall at level of diaphragm)
    - Background: Subtract anterior and posterior images separately
    - Determine geometric mean counts for trunk (liver + lung), lungs
    - Calculate shunt fraction (F) to lungs based on MAA scan: Lungs/trunk

HEPATIC ARTERIAL Y-90 MICROSPHERES

- Tc-99m MAA SPECT or SPECT/CT of upper abdomen: Strongly recommended
  - Fuse SPECT to abdominal CT/MR
  - Match inferior hepatic margins
  - Allow misregistration at superior hepatic margin (2° to respiration)
  - Visually check registration in coronal, axial, sagittal planes
- Carefully assess registered SPECT/CT(MR) images: Review with angiographer
  - Hepatic segments not embolized by MAA: May be supplied by replaced hepatic vessels
  - For foci of extrahepatic activity: Supplied by accessory visceral branches of hepatic artery

Administered Dose
- Sir-Sphere®
  - < 10% lung shunting: Full dose (2 GBq ± 10%)
  - 10-15% lung shunting: Reduce dose by 20%
  - 15-20% lung shunting: Reduce dose by 40%
  - > 20% lung shunting: Do not treat
- TheraSphere®
  - Goal: 80-150 Gy (8,000-15,000 rad) to liver
  - Activity required (GBq) = [desired dose (Gy)] [liver mass (kg)]/50
  - Liver volume/liver mass: CT or ultrasound

Post Y-90 Bremsstrahlung scan
- Planar image of chest, abdomen, pelvis to confirm delivery of dose to liver, assessment of extrahepatic embolization

POST-PROCEDURE

Expected Outcome
- Post-embolization syndrome: Fever, malaise, lethargy
  - Cytokine effect due to radiation injury of tumor, neovascularization/regeneration of normal liver
- Nausea, gastric irritation: Irritation due to radiation of adjacent liver
- Post therapy transient rise in liver function tests: Subsides in 1-2 weeks
- Therapeutic effect
  - Effective duration of treatment: 92.4 hr (94% of radiation delivered in 11 days)
  - Range of irradiation for each bead is ~ 2.5 mm

Medications
- Gastritis: Proton pump inhibitor or H2 blocker 1 week prior to 4 weeks after procedure
- Antiemetics: Commence morning of procedure
- Post-embolization syndrome: Tapering dose of oral steroids (unless contraindicated)

Assessment of Therapeutic Response
- PET/CT: > Accuracy than CT, MR in response assessment (prefer ≥ 50% ↓ in SUV at 1 month)

PROBLEMS & COMPLICATIONS

Complications
- Most feared complication(s)
  - Fatal radiation pneumonitis from arteriovenous shunting from hepatic artery → IVC → lungs
  - Embolization of extrahepatic structures via accessory branches from hepatic arteries
    - Radiation-induced gastritis, duodenitis, esophagitis: Non-healing ulceration, perforation, bleeding
    - Radiation-induced pancreatitis
    - Radiation-induced cholecystitis
- Other complications
  - Cirrhosis/liver failure with repeated treatments
  - Theoretical complication: Liver failure when chemotherapy administered during first 3-4 weeks following Y-90 microsphere treatment
    - Liver vulnerable during proliferative phase of regeneration

SELECTED REFERENCES

1. Geller DA et al: Outcome of 1000 liver cancer patients evaluated at the UPMC Liver Cancer Center. J Gastrointest Surg. 10(1):63-8, 2006
2. Gulec SA et al: Dosimetric techniques in 90Y-microsphere therapy of liver cancer: The MIRD equations for dose calculations. J Nucl Med. 47(7):1209-11, 2006
3. Kennedy AS et al: Resin 90Y-microsphere brachytherapy for unresectable colorectal liver metastases: modern USA experience. Int J Radiat Oncol Biol Phys. 65(2):412-25, 2006
4. Kim DY et al: Successful embolization of hepatocellular carcinoma with yttrium-90 glass microspheres prior to liver transplantation. J Gastrointest Surg. 10(3):413-6, 2006
5. Salem R et al: Radioembolization with 90Yttrium Microspheres: A State-of-the-Art Brachytherapy Treatment for Primary and Secondary Liver Malignancies: Part 1: Technical and Methodologic Considerations. J Vasc Interv Radiol. 17(8):1251-78, 2006
6. Sato K et al: Treatment of unresectable primary and metastatic liver cancer with yttrium-90 microspheres (TheraSphere): assessment of hepatic arterial embolization. Cardiovasc Intervent Radiol. 29(4):522-9, 2006
7. Ayav A et al: Portal hypertension secondary to 90Yttrium microspheres: an unknown complication. J Clin Oncol. 23(32):8275-6, 2005
8. Bienert M et al: 90Y microsphere treatment of unresectable liver metastases: changes in 18F-FDG uptake and tumour size on PET/CT. Eur J Nucl Med Mol Imaging. 32(7):778-87, 2005
9. Lewandowski RJ et al: 90Y microsphere (TheraSphere) treatment for unresectable colorectal cancer metastases of the liver: response to treatment at targeted doses of 135-150 Gy as measured by [18F]fluorodeoxyglucose positron emission tomography and computed tomographic imaging. J Vasc Interv Radiol. 16(12):1641-51, 2005
10. Murthy R et al: Yttrium-90 microsphere therapy for hepatic malignancy: devices, indications, technical considerations, and potential complications. Radiographics. 25 Suppl 1:S41-55, 2005
11. Salem R et al: Treatment of unresectable hepatocellular carcinoma with use of 90Y microspheres (TheraSphere): safety, tumor response, and survival. J Vasc Interv Radiol. 16(12):1627-39, 2005
12. Yip D et al: Radiation-induced ulceration of the stomach secondary to hepatic embolization with radioactive yttrium microspheres in the treatment of metastatic colon cancer. J Gastroenterol Hepatol. 19(3):347-9, 2004

HEPATIC ARTERIAL Y-90 MICROSPHERES

IMAGE GALLERY

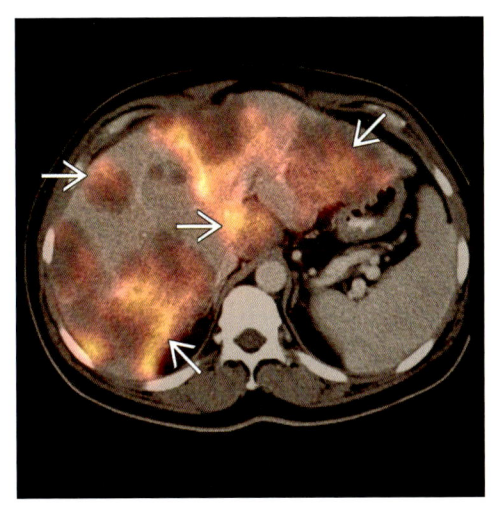

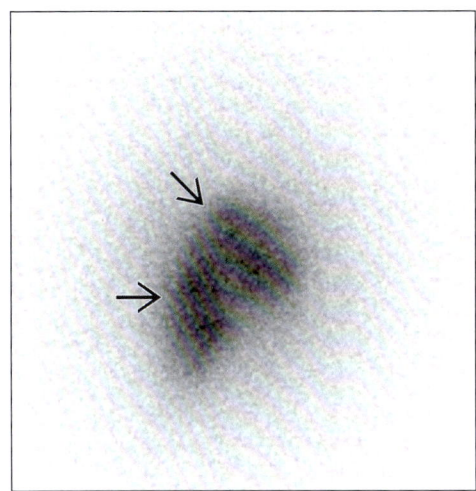

(Left) Tc-99m MAA hepatic artery embolization SPECT/CT fusion shows concentration of MAA at sites of tumor ➡, typical of hepatic artery recruitment by tumor vasculature. Necrotic regions and normal little accumulate relatively less activity. *(Right)* Bremsstrahlung scan following injection of Y-90 microspheres shows activity confined to the liver ➡. No appreciable lung activity identified.

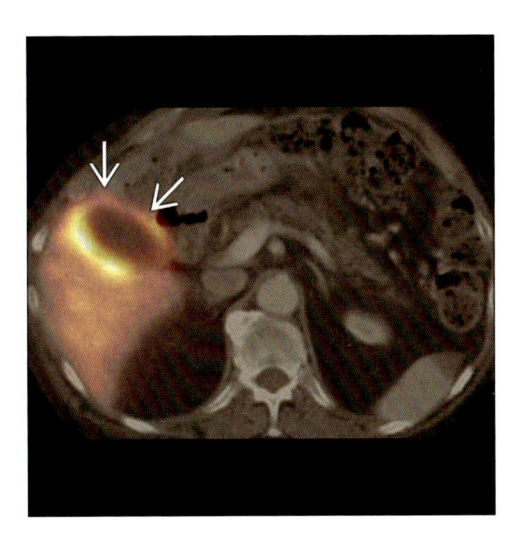

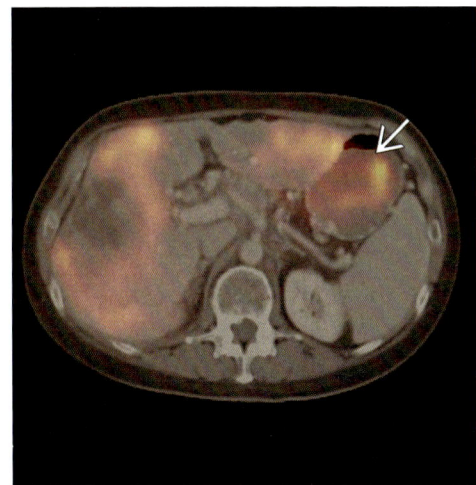

(Left) Tc-99m MAA hepatic artery embolization SPECT/CT fusion shows intense uptake in gallbladder wall ➡. Injection of Y-90 beads with similar distribution would carry risk of radiation-necrosis of gallbladder wall. *(Right)* Tc-99m MAA hepatic artery embolization SPECT/CT fusion in patient whose planar images showed marked thyroid uptake. Activity in stomach ➡ is likely due to free Tc-99m pertechnetate.

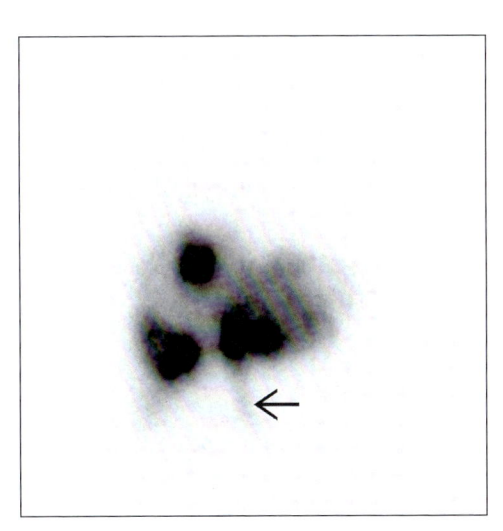

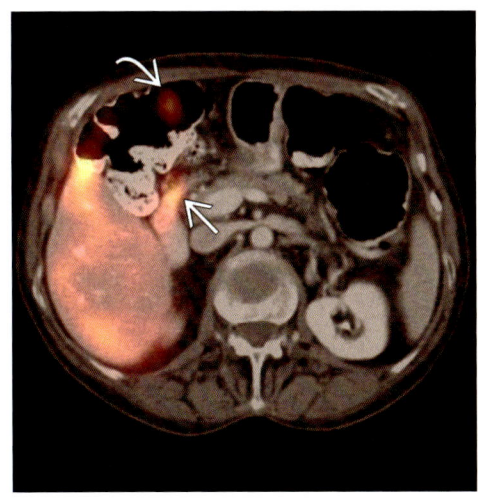

(Left) Anterior planar Tc-99m MAA hepatic artery embolization scan shows linear uptake inferior to liver ➡. See next image. *(Right)* Tc-99m MAA hepatic artery embolization SPECT/CT fusion in same patient as left shows duodenal activity ➡. Focus overlying proximal transverse colon ➡ is due to mesenteric supply from patent umbilical vessel, misregistered to colonic lumen due to different bowel distension on CT and SPECT.

RADIOLABELED ANTIBODY THERAPY

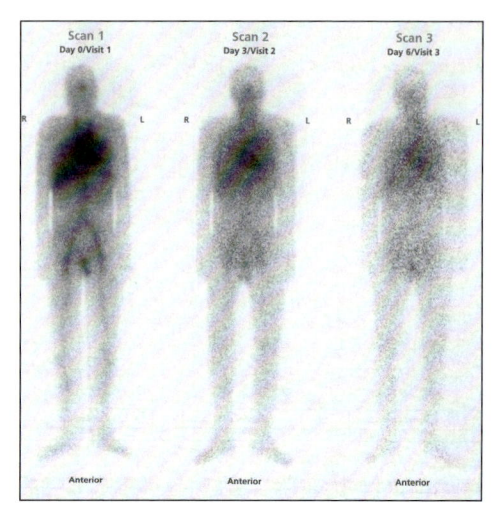

I-131 tositumomab images show expected change in biodistribution between day 0, day 3 and day 6 post injection. Note decreasing blood pool, liver, spleen activity. (Courtesy GlaxoSmithKline).

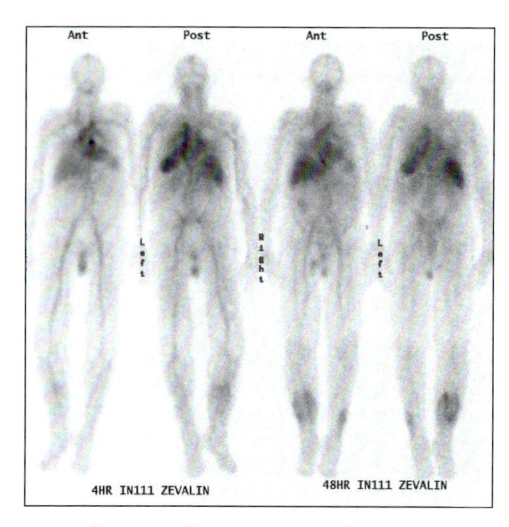

In-111 ibritumomab tiuxetan images showing expected change in biodistribution between 4 hours (image pair on left) and 48 hours (image pair on right). Note uptake in left calf lymphoma.

TERMINOLOGY

Definitions
- Radiolabeled antibody therapy
  - Monoclonal antibody-based therapy delivers radioactive treatment to CD20+ cells
  - CD20
    - Antigen expressed on pre-B and mature B-lymphocytes
    - CD20 antigen expressed on > 90% of B-cell non-Hodgkin lymphoma (NHL) cells
    - Not expressed on stem, progenitor cells
  - I-131 tositumomab (Bexxar, GlaxoSmithKline)
    - Tositumomab: Murine IgG2a λ monoclonal antibody
    - I-131 beta emission = 0.806 MeV
    - Whole-body dosimetry and biodistribution scan required prior to treatment dose
  - Yttrium-90 (Y-90) ibritumomab tiuxetan (Zevalin, Biogen Idec)
    - Ibritumomab: Murine IgG1 κ monoclonal antibody
    - Tiuxetan: Chelator provides stable linkage between antibody and radioisotope
    - Y-90 beta emission = 2.3 MeV
    - Whole-body biodistribution scan required prior to treatment dose
- Rituximab (Rituxan, Biogen Idec)
  - Nonradioactive antibody-based Rx
  - Chimeric murine/human IgG1 κ monoclonal antibody
  - Mediates B-cell lysis of NHL

PRE-PROCEDURE

Indications
- Treatment of relapsed, refractory low-grade, follicular, or transformed B-cell NHL (including rituximab refractory)
  - In rituximab-refractory patients, monoclonal antibody continues to attach to CD20 allowing for radiopharmaceutical delivery

Contraindications
- Prior myeloablative therapy, radioimmunotherapy
- Pregnancy
- > 25% marrow involvement
- Impaired bone marrow reserve
- Hypersensitivity reaction
  - Known type I hypersensitivity to murine proteins or other components of treatment regimen (including rituximab)
  - If previous exposure to murine antibodies consider human anti-mouse antibodies (HAMA) titer
- Platelets < 100,000 mm³
- Absolute neutrophil count (ANC) of < 1,500 cells/mm³
- Altered biodistribution on dosimetric imaging
- Safety and efficacy not established in children

Getting Started
- Things to Check
  - Complete blood count: ANC, platelets
  - Pregnancy test
  - ± HAMA titer
  - On thyroid-blocking agent if required
- Medications
  - No formal drug interaction studies performed
    - Use caution with any medication that affects platelet function, coagulation
  - I-131 tositumomab

RADIOLABELED ANTIBODY THERAPY

Key Facts

Terminology
- Monoclonal antibody-based therapy delivers radioactive treatment to CD20+ cells
- CD20 antigen expressed on > 90% of B-cell non-Hodgkin lymphoma (NHL) cells
- I-131 tositumomab (Bexxar, GlaxoSmithKline)
- Yttrium-90 (Y-90) ibritumomab tiuxetan (Zevalin, Biogen Idec)

Pre-procedure
- Complete blood count: ANC, platelets
- Pregnancy test
- ± HAMA titer
- On thyroid-blocking agent if required

Procedure
- Proceed with therapeutic dose if normal biodistribution
- Therapy contraindicated if altered biodistribution

Post-procedure
- Laboratory monitoring
- Avoid pregnancy
- Discontinue breastfeeding
- Radiation safety precautions

Problems & Complications
- Prolonged, severe neutropenia, thrombocytopenia
- Grade three or four neutropenia, thrombocytopenia in ~ 2/3 of patients
- Hypersensitivity reactions rare (< 1%) but can include anaphylaxis

---

- Block thyroid uptake with oral iodide 24 hrs prior to dosimetric dose, continue for 2 weeks after therapeutic dose
- Acetaminophen 650 mg and diphenhydramine 50 mg orally 30 minutes prior to antibody administration
  - No specific pre-medication for ibritumomab
- Equipment List
  - Monoclonal antibody kit
  - Dosimetric radioisotope
  - Treatment radioisotope

PROCEDURE

Equipment Preparation
- Adequate IV
  - Ensure function and rapid flow prior to radioisotope injection

Procedure Steps
- Tositumomab
  - Day -1: Begin oral iodide, continue until 14 days post therapeutic dose
  - Day 0: Premedication with acetaminophen and diphenhydramine
  - Day 0: Dosimetric dose
    - Administer unlabeled tositumomab (available binding sites on circulating B-cells and ↓ splenic targeting)
    - Unlabeled tositumomab infusion often performed in hematology/oncology clinic
    - Administer 5.0 mCi I-131 tositumomab dosimetric dose
  - Day 0: Whole body dosimetry and biodistribution images
  - Day 2, 3, or 4: Whole body dosimetry and biodistribution images
  - Day 6 or 7: Whole body dosimetry and biodistribution images
    - Evaluate biodistribution
    - If abnormal biodistribution, treatment contraindicated
  - Day 6 or 7: Calculate I-131 tositumomab treatment dose
    - 75 cGy total body dose
    - 65 cGy total body dose if platelets > 100,000 and < 150,000/mm³
  - Day 7-14: Treatment dose
    - Premedicate with acetaminophen and diphenhydramine
    - Administer unlabeled tositumomab and therapeutic I-131 tositumomab dose
- Ibritumomab tiuxetan
  - Day 1: Whole body biodistribution dose
    - IV infusion of rituximab (↓ available binding sites on circulating B-cells and ↓ splenic targeting)
    - Rituximab infusion often performed hematology/oncology clinic
    - Administer 5 mCi In-111 ibritumomab tiuxetan dosimetric dose
  - Day 3 or 4: Whole body scan
    - Evaluate biodistribution
    - If abnormal biodistribution, treatment contraindicated
  - Day 7, 8 or 9: Treatment dose
    - Dose of Y-90 based on patient weight, platelet count
    - Dosimetry not required
    - Administer unlabeled rituximab and therapeutic Y-90 ibritumomab dose

Findings and Reporting
- Normal biodistribution on whole body images
  - Tositumomab
    - On initial imaging antibody primarily in blood pool, heart, liver, spleen
    - On second and third images, blood pool, liver and spleen uptake ↓
    - Second and third images may show thyroid, kidney, bladder, and minimal lung activity
  - Ibritumomab tiuxetan
    - Blood pool generally detectable on initial scan; progressively ↓ on subsequent studies (any blood pool activity acceptable)

RADIOLABELED ANTIBODY THERAPY

- Moderate to high uptake in uninvolved liver and spleen on all images
- Low to very low uptake in uninvolved kidneys, bladder, bowel on all images
  - For both agents, sites of tumor can be seen but non-visualization not a contraindication
  - Proceed with therapeutic dose if normal biodistribution
- Altered biodistribution on whole body images
  - Tositumomab
    - Non-visualized blood pool on initial images
    - Intense liver, spleen, lung on initial images
    - Urinary obstruction or ↑ lung uptake (> blood pool) on second, third images
    - Total body residence times of < 50 or > 150 days
  - Ibritumomab tiuxetan
    - Non-visualized blood pool on initial images
    - Intense liver and spleen on initial images
    - Diffuse uptake in uninvolved lung > uninvolved liver
    - Kidneys > liver on posterior view
    - Bowel > liver
    - Prominent bone marrow uptake
  - Therapy contraindicated if altered biodistribution

POST-PROCEDURE

Expected Outcome
- Outcome data evolving
- Overall response rate (ORR) and median duration of response (MDR) in patients with rituximab-refractory disease
  - Tositumomab
    - ORR 68%
    - MDR 16 months (range 1-38 months)
  - Ibritumomab tiuxetan
    - ORR 74%
    - MDR 6.4 months (range 0.5-49.9 months)
- ORR and MDR in patients with chemotherapy-refractory disease
  - Tositumomab
    - ORR 47%
    - MDR 12 months (range 2-47 months)
  - Ibritumomab tiuxetan
    - ORR 80%
    - MDR 13.9 months (range 1-47.6 months)

Things To Do
- General post-treatment precautions
  - Laboratory monitoring
    - Monitor CBC until evidence of hematopoietic recovery (neutrophils, platelets)
    - Typically monitored by referring hematology/oncology clinic weekly
  - Avoid pregnancy
    - Contraceptive use for 12 months
  - Discontinue breastfeeding
  - Radiation safety precautions
- Tositumomab
  - Continue oral iodide for 2 weeks post-treatment
  - Standard I-131 radiation safety precautions for ↓ gamma radiation exposure to others
- Ibritumomab tiuxetan
  - Minimal radiation exposure risk to others (Y-90 = pure beta-emitter)
  - For 7 days patients must avoid body fluid transfers, clean up spilled urine, shower daily

PROBLEMS & COMPLICATIONS

Problems
- Neutropenia
  - Per patient incidence of ANC < 1000, median duration
    - Tositumomab: Incidence 63%, duration 31 days
    - Ibritumomab tiuxetan: Incidence 57%, duration 22 days
- Thrombocytopenia
  - Per patient incidence of platelet < 50,000/mm^3 and median duration
    - Tositumomab: Incidence 53%, duration 32 days
    - Ibritumomab tiuxetan: Incidence 61%, duration 24 days

Complications
- Most feared complication(s)
  - Prolonged, severe neutropenia, thrombocytopenia
    - Grade three or four neutropenia, thrombocytopenia in ~ 2/3 of patients
  - Hypersensitivity reactions rare (< 1%) but can include anaphylaxis
- Other complications
  - Tositumomab
    - Chills, fever, wheezing, nausea, fatigue, infection, nasal congestion, vomiting, pruritus, hypotension, rash
    - Hypothyroidism 2° to free I-131 (17% at 5 years)
    - Some hypersensitivity reactions fatal
  - Ibritumomab tiuxetan
    - Asthenia, nausea, infection, chills, fever, abdominal pain
    - Deaths reported with unlabeled IV rituximab

SELECTED REFERENCES

1. Fisher RI et al: Tositumomab and iodine-131 tositumomab produces durable complete remissions in a subset of heavily pretreated patients with low-grade and transformed non-Hodgkin's lymphomas. J Clin Oncol. 23(30):7565-73, 2005
2. Grillo-Lopez AJ: 90Y-ibritumomab tiuxetan: rationale for patient selection in the treatment of indolent non-Hodgkin's lymphoma. Semin Oncol. 32(1 Suppl 1):S44-9, 2005
3. Hagenbeek A et al: Report of a European consensus workshop to develop recommendations for the optimal use of (90)Y-ibritumomab tiuxetan (Zevalin) in lymphoma. Ann Oncol. 16(5):786-92, 2005
4. Horning SJ et al: Efficacy and safety of tositumomab and iodine-131 tositumomab (Bexxar) in B-cell lymphoma, progressive after rituximab. J Clin Oncol. 23(4):712-9, 2005
5. Lewington V: Development of 131I-tositumomab. Semin Oncol. 32(1 Suppl 1):S50-6, 2005
6. Marcus R: Use of 90Y-ibritumomab tiuxetan in non-Hodgkin's lymphoma. Semin Oncol. 32(1 Suppl 1):S36-43, 2005

RADIOLABELED ANTIBODY THERAPY

IMAGE GALLERY

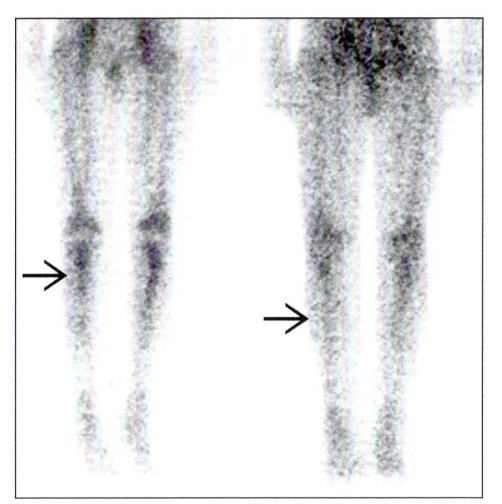

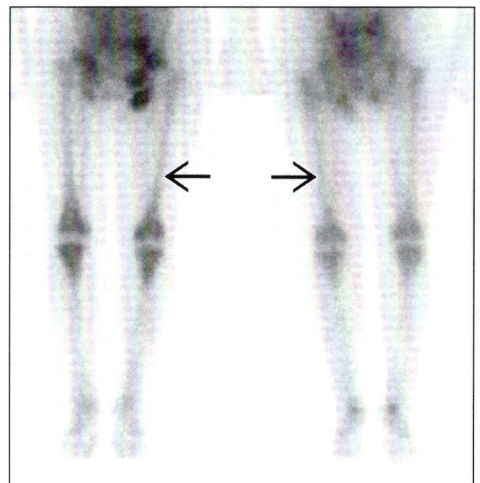

(**Left**) Anterior I-131 tositumomab image of lower extremities on day 0 (left) and day 2 (right) shows localization in areas of known tumor involvement in tibial marrow ➔ (Courtesy GlaxoSmithKline). (**Right**) Anterior and posterior In-111 ibritumomab tiuxetan image of lower extremities shows diffuse activity in the bone marrow ➔, a relative contraindication to therapy.

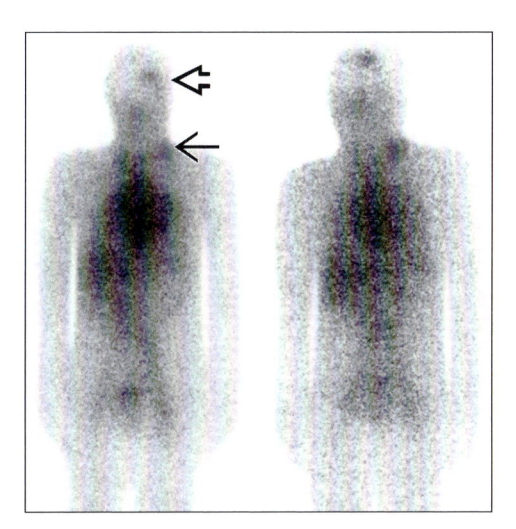

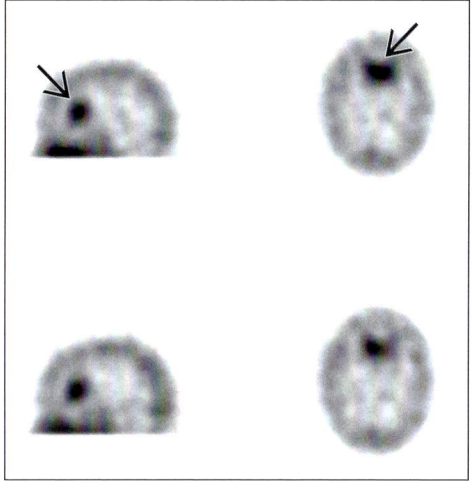

(**Left**) Anterior I-131 tositumomab images on day 3 (left) and day 6 (right) show expected biodistribution plus uptake in left supraclavicular region ➔ and head ➔. (Courtesy GlaxoSmithKline). (**Right**) Sagittal and coronal In-111 ibritumomab tiuxetan brain SPECT shows focus of CNS lymphoma ➔.

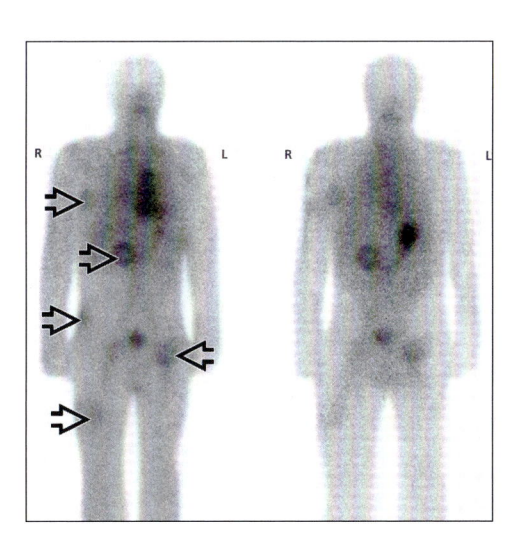

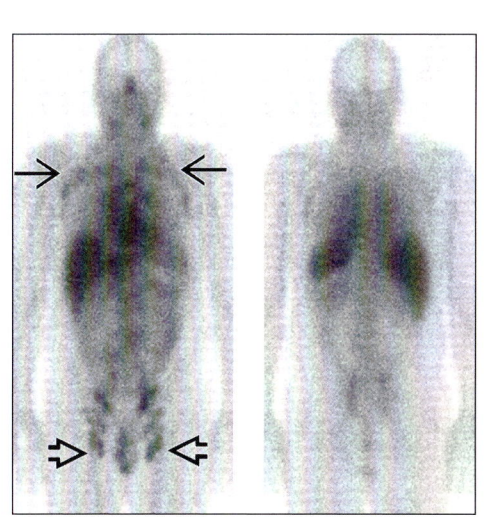

(**Left**) Anterior I-131 tositumomab imaging on day 2 (left) and day 6 (right) shows expected biodistribution and multiple cutaneous lymphoma deposits ➔ (Courtesy GlaxoSmithKline). (**Right**) Anterior and posterior In-111 ibritumomab tiuxetan image at 48 hours shows normal biodistribution plus disease in axillae ➔ and groin ➔.

RBC SURVIVAL & SPLENIC SEQUESTRATION

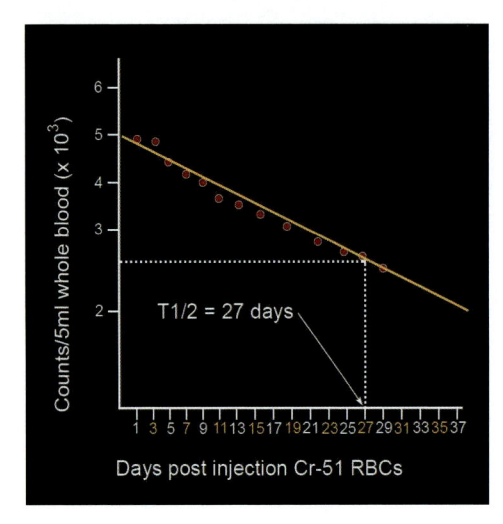

Graph shows method for calculation of T½ of RBC survival based on Cr-51 labeling method. T½ is 27 days (normal = 25-35 days).

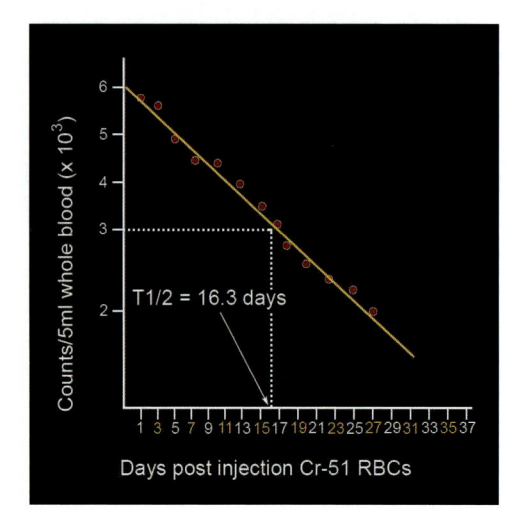

Graph shows method for calculation of T½ of RBC survival based on Cr-51 labeling method. T½ is 16.3 days, consistent with increased RBC destruction.

TERMINOLOGY

Definitions
- Determination of red blood cell (RBC) survival by measurement of disappearance of Cr-51 random-labeled RBCs from circulation
- Determination of splenic sequestration by comparison of splenic accumulation of Cr-51 RBCs over time compared to blood pool, liver levels

PRE-PROCEDURE

Indications
- Measure RBC survival time by serial measurements of dilution techniques using Cr-51 RBCs
- Determine whether RBC destruction is due to splenic sequestration of circulating RBCs

PROCEDURE

Procedure Steps
- Best procedural approach for RBC survival: Cr-51 labeled RBCs; serial blood samples x 3 weeks
- Best procedural approach for splenic sequestration: Serial precordial, liver, splenic counts
- RBC labeling
  - 10 mL venous blood withdrawn (using at least 18-g needle) into 20 mL syringe containing Strumia acid-citrate-dextrose (ACD) formula
  - Transfer to 10 mL sterile vial
  - Add 1.5 µCi/kg (55.5 kBq/kg) Cr-51 as chromate ion, very gently swirl to mix
    - Must not to exceed 2 µg chromate ion per mL packed RBCs
  - Incubate at room temperature for 16 min
  - Add 50 mg ascorbic acid
    - Stops labeling procedure, cannot cross cell membrane
  - Reinject blood into vein
- RBC survival determination
  - Draw blood sample every other day for 3 weeks
    - Obtain first sample after 24 hours: Allows removal from circulation of all cells damaged in labeling process
  - Processing of each blood sample
    - Withdraw 6 blood samples into tube containing anticoagulant (solid EDTA or concentrated heparin)
    - Invert gently 12-15 times to mix
    - Pipette exactly 5 mL well-mixed whole blood; transfer to counting tube containing tiny amount of saponin powder (lyses RBCs)
    - Take care not to allow sample to touch cap of counting tube
    - Send remaining 1 mL of blood in anticoagulant tube to lab for hematocrit determination (on day of blood withdrawal)
  - All samples counted together on last day of study
    - Gamma well counter set at 280-360 keV (Cr-51)
    - Counted to give sample error of 1% or less (approximately 10 min each)
- Splenic sequestration
  - Should do as part of any RBC survival study
  - Organ counting commences 24 hours after labeling; done every other day for 3 weeks
  - Obtain precordial, liver and spleen counts for each time point
  - Utilize counting probe with flat-field collimator, set at 280-360 keV (Cr-51)
  - Mark skin with indelible marker, cover with Tegaderm™ or similar material to allow same sampling position with each data point

RBC SURVIVAL & SPLENIC SEQUESTRATION

Key Facts

Pre-procedure
- Measure RBC survival time by serial measurements of dilution techniques using Cr-51 RBCs
- Determine whether RBC destruction is due to splenic sequestration of circulating RBCs

Procedure
- Best procedural approach for RBC survival: Cr-51 labeled RBCs; serial blood samples x 3 weeks
- Best procedural approach for splenic sequestration: Serial precordial, liver, splenic counts
- Normal T½ RBC by Cr-51 method: 25-35 days
- Increased RBC destruction (Cr-51): T½ < 25 days
- Normal spleen:precordium ratio < 2:1
- Normal spleen:liver ratio ≤ 1:1
- Active splenic sequestration: Spleen:liver ratio rises progressively to 2:1-4:1
- Large spleen, no sequestration: Initial and stable spleen:precordial ratio > 2:1 (no progressive rise)

○ Allow detector to rest on skin for each determination: Obtain sufficient counts so sample error ≤ 5%
○ Precordial counts: Patient supine, detector over left third intercostal space at sternal border
○ Liver counts: Patient supine, detector over 9th and 10th ribs, right midclavicular line
○ Spleen counts: Patient prone, detector 2/3 distance from spinous process to lateral edge of body at level of 9th and 10th ribs

Findings and Reporting
- RBC survival calculations
  ○ Net counts per min (Y-axis) plotted on semilogarithmic paper vs. time of blood withdrawal (X-axis)
  ○ Extrapolate line to time zero (Y-intercept)
  ○ Divide y-intercept by 2: At this value, draw straight line parallel to X-axis until intersects (best straight line fit through individual data points)
  ○ Drop perpendicular from this point to X-axis
  ○ Read T½ for RBC disappearance rate (survival time) off intersection with X-axis
- Interpretation: RBC survival
  ○ Normal T½ RBC by Cr-51 method: 25-35 days
  ○ True RBC survival: T½ 50-60 days (lower with Cr-51 method due to elution of Cr-51)
  ○ Increased RBC destruction (Cr-51): T½ < 25 days
- Splenic sequestration calculations
  ○ On same graph, plot organ (spleen, liver):precordial counts (Y-axis) vs. day post Cr-51 label (X-axis)
  ○ Compare spleen:liver values, trends
- Interpretation: Splenic sequestration
  ○ Normal spleen:precordium ratio < 2:1
  ○ Normal spleen:liver ratio ≤ 1:1
  ○ Active splenic sequestration: Spleen:liver ratio rises progressively to 2:1-4:1
  ○ Large spleen, no sequestration: Initial and stable spleen:precordial ratio > 2:1 (no progressive rise)

PROBLEMS & COMPLICATIONS

Problems
- RBC survival times
  ○ Not corrected for elution of Cr-51
  ○ Less critical with decreased RBC survival
  ○ Active bleeding or patient not in steady state
  ○ Blood transfusions during procedure: Results in apparent shortening of T½
- Splenic sequestration: Inaccurate or inconsistent probe position

SELECTED REFERENCES
1. Christian PE et al: Nuclear Medicine and PET: Technology and techniques. 5th Ed. St. Louis, Mosby. 525-9, 2004
2. Brecher G: Cr-51 red cell survival and corrections for hematocrit. Am J Clin Pathol. 47(1):85-7, 1967

IMAGE GALLERY

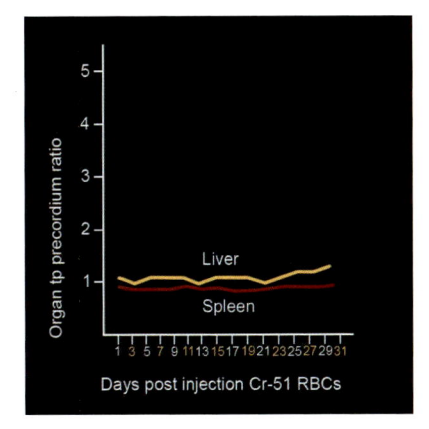

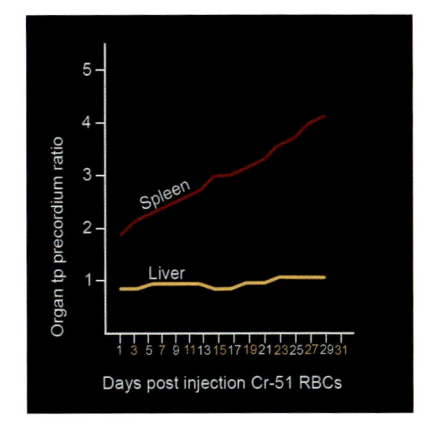

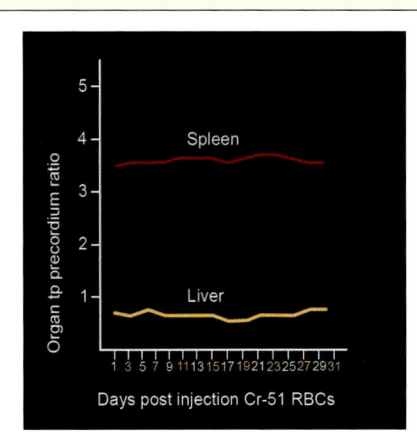

(Left) Graph of organ:precordium activity for liver & spleen in normal patient. Normal spleen:liver ratio is ≤ 1:1, normal spleen:precordium ratio is 2:1, both should be stable over study interval. *(Center)* Organ:precordium activity shows rising spleen:precordium activity (> 4:1) and spleen:liver activity (> 4:1), consistent with splenic sequestration as mechanism for RBC destruction. *(Right)* Graph shows organ:precordial activity. Stable increase in spleen:liver ratio & spleen:precordial ratio suggests hypersplenism without splenic destruction of RBCs.

RED CELL MASS AND PLASMA VOLUME

Age	Normal range
Newborn	55-68%
1 week	47-65%
1 month	37-49%
3 months	30-36%
1 year	29-41%
10 years	36-40%
Adult males	42-54%
Adult Females	38-46%

Chart shows normal hematocrit based on age and gender. Factors increasing hematocrit include polycythemia vera, high altitude, hypoxia, carboxy- and methemoglobinemia, reduced plasma volume.

Blood value compartment	Males	Females
Total blood volume (ml/kg)	55-80	50-75
Red blood cell volume (ml/kg)	25-35	20-30
Plasma volume (ml/kg)	30-45	30-45

Chart shows normal gender-based values for total blood volume, red blood cell volume, and plasma volume based on Cr-51 RBC and I-125 HSA dilutional methods.

TERMINOLOGY

Abbreviations
- Red blood cell mass (RBCM)
- Plasma volume (PV)

Definitions
- Determination of circulating RBCM and PV using radioisotopic dilutional techniques
- Used rarely if diagnosis not evident by bone marrow histology, serum erythropoietin level, other biologic markers of polycythemia vera

PRE-PROCEDURE

Indications
- To determine etiology of elevated hematocrit (Hct)
  - Polycythemia vera
  - Normal state
  - Stress polycythemia (↓ PV)

PROCEDURE

Procedure Steps
- Best procedural approach
  - RBCM: Cr-51 ascorbate labeling random red blood cells (RBC) from venous blood
    - Tc-99m Ultratag kit: Less stable label than with Cr-51, more RBC damage
  - PV: I-125 labeled human serum albumin (HSA)
    - Tc-99m albumin: Less stable label
    - PV determination can be estimated from Hct and RBCM, although less accurate than direct dilutional measurement
- RBC mass
  - 10 mL venous blood withdrawn into 20 mL syringe containing Strumia ACD formula
    - Use at least 18-g needle to avoid RBC damage
  - Transfer to 20 mL sterile vial
  - Add 30 µCi (1.1 MBq) Cr-51 as chromate ion, very gently swirl to mix
  - Incubate 15 min at room temperature
    - 80-90% of chromate ion immediately transported across cell membrane
    - Chromate ion binds to beta chain of hemoglobin
  - Add 50 mg ascorbic acid
    - Stops labeling procedure
    - Cannot cross cell membrane
  - Withdraw exactly 5 mL blood and inject into vein
    - Exercise extreme care to avoid extravasation
  - Retain remainder of labeled blood as standard
  - Wait 30 min, withdraw exactly 5 mL blood from another site into heparinized syringe
  - Remove exactly 1 mL whole blood from each sample (original labeled blood and blood withdrawn from patient)
    - Send to lab for STAT Hct or immediately measure Hct with capillary tube/centrifugation technique
    - Record Hct and plasmacrit (Plct) [Plct = (1-Hct)] as decimal values
  - Remove exactly 1 mL of whole blood (WB) from each sample, place in counting tube and label
    - WB from standard: Std WB
    - WB from patient sample: Samp WB
  - Place remainder of WB from each sample in centrifuge tube; sediment RBCs at 600-1000 x g for 5 min
  - Remove exactly 1 mL of plasma supernatant from each sample and place in counting tube and label
    - Plasma from standard: Std Plas
    - Plasma from patient sample: Samp Plas
  - Count samples centered at 320 keV photopeak of Cr-51: Long enough to ensure ≤ 1% error

RED CELL MASS AND PLASMA VOLUME

Key Facts

Terminology
- Determination of circulating RBCM and PV using radioisotopic dilutional techniques
- Used rarely if diagnosis not evident by bone marrow histology, serum erythropoietin level, other biologic markers of polycythemia vera

Procedure
- RBCM: Cr-51 ascorbate labeling random red blood cells (RBC) from venous blood

- PV: I-125 labeled human serum albumin (HSA)

Problems & Complications
- Falsely ↑ RBCM: Entire volume not injected, extravasated, RBCs damaged during labeling, white blood cells/platelets elevated
- Falsely ↓ RBCM: Contaminating radioactivity
- PV sources of error: Many factors can affect; best to report PV as "estimated"

  - Calculations
    - Formula for RBCM based on Cr-51 labeled RBC dilution method
- PV
  - Patient preparation required
    - Block thyroid with 5 drops SSKI (150 mg) 30 min before injection
    - Patient supine 10-15 min before injection
  - 10 µCi (0.37 MBq) I-125 HSA injected IV
    - Ensure complete injection, no extravasation
  - Prepare standard with separate 10 µCi (0.37 MBq) I-125 sample
    - HSA sticks to glass: Use plastic ware to prepare
  - Collect blood sample at 10 min post injection and at 10 min intervals for 3-5 samples
    - Collect blood samples at different site from injection
  - Sediment blood samples at 600-1000 x g for 5 min
  - Remove 1 mL plasma from each sample and 1 mL standard
    - Count samples in gamma counter at 20-50 keV photopeak of I-125: Long enough to ensure ≤ 1% error
  - Calculations
    - Formula for PV based on I-125 HSA dilution method

PROBLEMS & COMPLICATIONS

Problems
- Falsely ↑ RBCM: Entire volume not injected, extravasated, RBCs damaged during labeling, white blood cells/platelets elevated
- Falsely ↓ RBCM: Contaminating radioactivity
- PV sources of error: Many factors can affect; best to report PV as "estimated"
  - Edema, large 'third space", hypoproteinemia, hypoalbuminemia, obesity, recent weight loss, prolonged bed rest, body position, recent exercise

SELECTED REFERENCES

1. Lorberboym M et al: Analysis of red cell mass and plasma volume in patients with polycythemia. Arch Pathol Lab Med. 129(1):89-91, 2005
2. Sirhan S et al: Red cell mass and plasma volume measurements in polycythemia: evaluation of performance and practical utility. Cancer. 104(1):213-5, 2005
3. Christian PE et al: Nuclear medicine and PET: Technology and techniques. 5th Ed. St. Louis, Mosby, 2004
4. Pearson TC et al: The interpretation of measured red cell mass and plasma volume in patients with elevated PCV values. Clin Lab Haematol. 6(3):207-17, 1984
5. Grable E et al: Simplified method for simultaneous determinations of plasma volume and red-cell mass with 125I-labeled albumin and 51Cr-tagged red cells. J Nucl Med. 9(6):219-21, 1968

IMAGE GALLERY

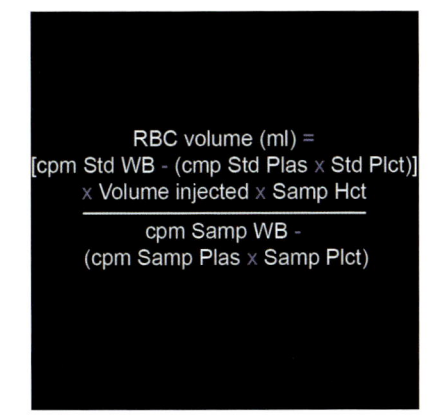

$$\text{RBC volume (ml)} = \frac{[\text{cpm Std WB} - (\text{cmp Std Plas} \times \text{Std Plct})] \times \text{Volume injected} \times \text{Samp Hct}}{\text{cpm Samp WB} - (\text{cpm Samp Plas} \times \text{Samp Plct})}$$

$$\text{Plasma volume (ml)} = \frac{\text{Volume injected} \times \text{cmp in 1ml Std} \times \text{dilution factor}}{\text{cpm of plasma obtained by back extrapolation}}$$

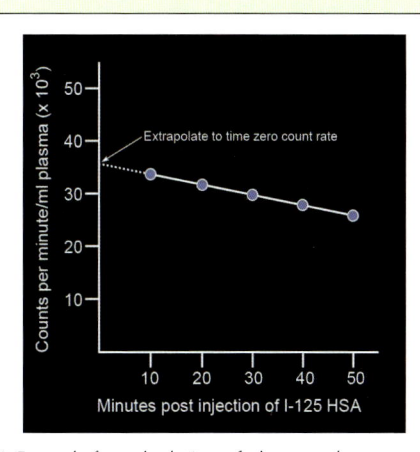

(Left) Formula for calculation of RBC mass based on Cr-51 labeled RBC dilution method. *(Center)* Formula for calculation of plasma volume based on I-125 HSA dilution method. See next image for determining cpm for plasma (denominator). *(Right)* Graph shows method for calculating cpm in plasma to be used for plasma volume formula. Cpm plasma is determined by back-extrapolation.

SCHILLING TEST

```
SCHILLING TEST

Pt name: xxxxx    MRN: xxxxx
DOB: xxxxx        Date: xxxxx

Urine vol (ml): 1512
57Co dose: 0.5
CPM: Bkgrnd: 38
57Co Std: 1237    Urine: 68

Urine cpm/ml * Urine vol (ml) * .125
           Std cpm

= % excreted: 1.2%
```

Table shows adequate urine volume → with low urinary excretion of labeled B12 → consistent with pernicious anemia or malabsorption. See next table.

```
SCHILLING TEST

Pt name: xxxxx    MRN: xxxxx
DOB: xxxxx        Date: xxxxx

Urine vol (ml): 1705
57Co dose: 0.5
CPM: Bkgrnd: 31
57Co Std: 1237    Urine: 569

Urine cpm/ml * Urine vol (ml) * .125
           Std cpm

= % excreted: 24%
```

Table shows good urine volume → and following intrinsic factor normal amount of B12 excreted in the urine → correcting the abnormality (see previous table) consistent with pernicious anemia.

TERMINOLOGY

Definitions
- Vitamin B12: Precursor of DNA synthesis, deficiency results in megaloblastic anemia, neurologic symptoms
  - Body stores of B12 last 3 to 5 years before clinical evidence of deficiency
- Intrinsic factor (IF) secreted by parietal cells of gastric fundus, required for B12 absorption in terminal ileum
- Schilling test: In vivo evaluation of B12 absorption
- Causes of B12 deficiency
  - Inadequate absorption secondary to bowel disease, bacterial overgrowth, pancreatic insufficiency, medications, inadequate intake, achlorhydria
  - Pernicious anemia: Antiparietal cell antibodies causing atrophic gastritis
  - Absence of IF secondary to gastrectomy

PRE-PROCEDURE

Indications
- Evaluation of pernicious anemia
- Low serum B12 ± hematologic, neurologic symptoms (2/3 asymptomatic)
- Determine mechanism of B12 malabsorption
- Evaluate patients at risk for B12 deficiency
  - Post gastrectomy, ileal disease, family history of pernicious anemia

Getting Started
- Things to Check
  - Serum B12, folate, peripheral blood smears, mean corpuscular volume, IF antibody, parietal cell antibody, serum methylmalonic acid
  - NPO the night prior to the study as B12 in a meal can affect absorption
  - Medications: Stop parenteral B12 supplementation at least 3 days prior to study or enterohepatic circulation will compete with B12 absorption in ileum

PROCEDURE

Procedure Steps
- Stage I
  - Oral Co-57 labeled B12 followed by a 2 hour fast
  - 24 hour urine collection starting at the time of the oral B12
  - Intramuscular administration of unlabeled B12 within two hours following oral dose
    - Saturates B12 binding sites so any absorbed B12 is excreted in urine
  - Percentage of administered dose excreted in urine over 24 hours is determined
- Stage II (optional to identify malabsorption)
  - Co-57 labeled B12-IF complex is administered orally
  - Intramuscular flushing dose of unlabeled B12 and a 24 hour urine collection as in stage I
  - Percentage of the administered dose excreted in urine over 24 hours is determined
- Stage III (optional to identify bacterial overgrowth)
  - Oral course of antibiotic (neomycin) to eliminate bacterial overgrowth, followed by repeat stage I, II Schilling test
  - Pancreatic enzyme administration x 3 days than repeat if maldigestion suspected

Findings and Reporting
- Stage I
  - Normal 24 hour urinary B12 excretion: > 9%
  - Indeterminate: 7-9%
  - Pernicious anemia or malabsorption: < 7%
- Stage II

SCHILLING TEST

Key Facts

Terminology
- Vitamin B12: Precursor of DNA synthesis, deficiency results in megaloblastic anemia, neurologic symptoms
- Schilling test: In vivo evaluation of B12 absorption

Pre-procedure
- Evaluation of pernicious anemia
- Determine mechanism of B12 malabsorption

Procedure
- Normal 24 hour urinary B12 excretion: > 9%
- Indeterminate: 7-9%
- Pernicious anemia or malabsorption: < 7%

Problems & Complications
- Falsely abnormal (up to 14% of cases)
- Incomplete urine collection is most common cause of false positive

---

  - Normalization of 24 hour urinary B12 excretion: Cause of deficiency is pernicious anemia
  - Urinary excretion of B12 remains low: Evaluate for intestinal malabsorption
    - Consider treatment with B12: Malabsorption may be due to megaloblastic changes of terminal ileum
- Stage III
  - Urinary excretion is normalized: Intestinal malabsorption due to bacterial overgrowth or pancreatic insufficiency

Alternative Procedures/Therapies
- Radiologic
  - Dual isotope Schilling test
    - Simultaneous administration of Co-58 B12 and Co-57 B12-IF complex
    - Not currently available

POST-PROCEDURE

Things To Avoid
- If repeating the study wait at least 3 days between Co-57 B12 administrations

PROBLEMS & COMPLICATIONS

Problems
- Falsely abnormal (up to 14% of cases)
  - Incomplete urine collection is most common cause of false positive

  - Old age or renal insufficiency (48 hour urine collection may be necessary)
  - Chronic B12 deficiency
    - Causes ileal mucosal atrophy
    - Results in abnormal stage II result
    - Repeat Schilling test after weeks-months B12 therapy
  - Low specific activity (> 1 microgram B12/microcurie Co-57)
- Falsely normal result
  - Normal absorption of crystalline B12 may not equal normal protein bound B12 found in food
  - Inability to absorb protein bound B12
    - Old age
    - Decreased gastric pH
    - Alcohol
  - Fecal contamination
  - Recent prior nuclear medicine study

SELECTED REFERENCES

1. Ward PC: Modern approaches to the investigation of vitamin B12 deficiency. Clin Lab Med. 22(2):435-45, 2002
2. Markle HV: Cobalamin. Crit Rev Clin Lab Sci. 33(4):247-356, 1996
3. Nickoloff E: Schilling test: physiologic basis for and use as a diagnostic test. Crit Rev Clin Lab Sci. 26(4):263-76, 1988
4. Zuckier LS et al: Schilling evaluation of pernicious anemia: current status. J Nucl Med. 25(9):1032-9, 1984

IMAGE GALLERY

SCHILLING TEST

Pt name: xxxxx   MRN: xxxxx
DOB: xxxxx   Date: xxxxx

Urine vol (ml): 475
57Co dose: 0.5
CPM: Bkgrnd: 26
57Co Std: 1197   Urine: 298

$$\frac{\text{Urine cpm/ml} * \text{Urine vol (ml)} * .125}{\text{Std cpm}}$$

= % excreted: 3.5%

SCHILLING TEST

Pt name: xxxxx   MRN: xxxxx
DOB: xxxxx   Date: xxxxx

Urine vol (ml): 1720
57Co dose: 0.5
CPM: Bkgrnd: 33
57Co Std: 1257   Urine: 261

$$\frac{\text{Urine cpm/ml} * \text{Urine vol (ml)} * .125}{\text{Std cpm}}$$

= % excreted: 10%

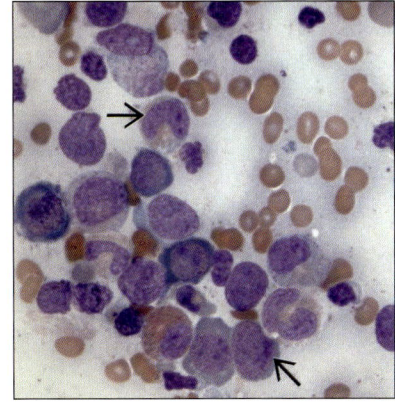

(Left) Table shows a low volume of urine collected (less than 60 cc/hour) and a low excretion of B12 which could be due to inadequate urine collection. See next table. **(Center)** Table shows (same patient as previous table) a second day collection this time with adequate volume which contains a normal excreted amount of labeled B12 consistent with a normal test. **(Right)** Bone marrow aspirate shows marked erythroid hyperplasia with megaloblastic changes in patient with severe B12 deficiency. (Courtesy K. Siechen, MD).

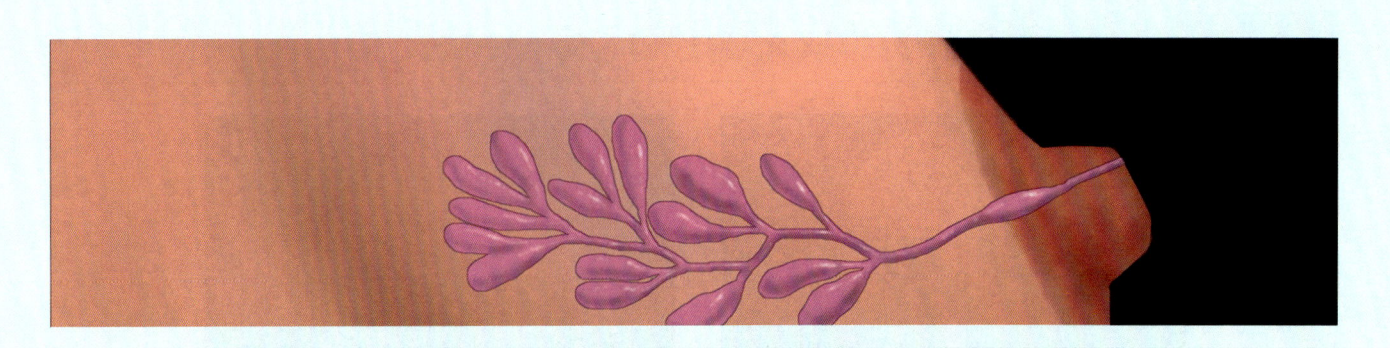

SECTION 11: Oncology, Other

Lymphoma

Lymphoma, Benign Mimics	11-2
Hodgkin Lymphoma Staging	11-6
Lymphoma Post-Therapy Evaluation	11-10
Non-Hodgkin Lymphomas, Low Grade	11-16
Non-Hodgkin Lymphoma Staging	11-20

Melanoma

Melanoma Staging	11-24
Melanoma Therapy Eval./Restaging	11-28

Breast Cancer

Breast, Benign Disease	11-32
Breast Cancer, Primary	11-34
Breast Cancer, Staging/Restaging	11-40

Miscellaneous

Adenocarcinoma of Unknown Primary	11-46
Paraneoplastic Disorders	11-48

LYMPHOMA, BENIGN MIMICS

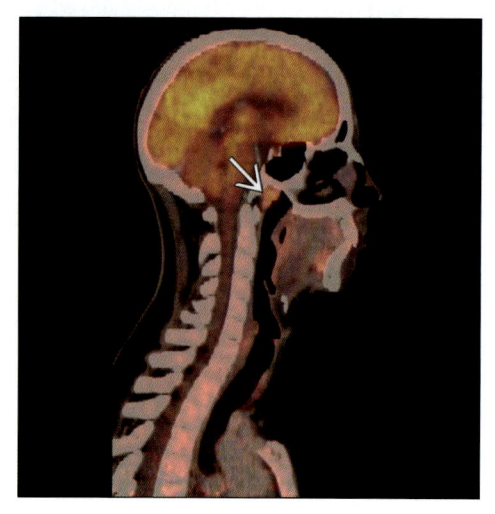

Sagittal FDG PET/CT shows increased uptake in adenoids ➡ in a patient with a recent mononucleosis-like viral illness. Finding can also be caused by interleukin, interferon treatment.

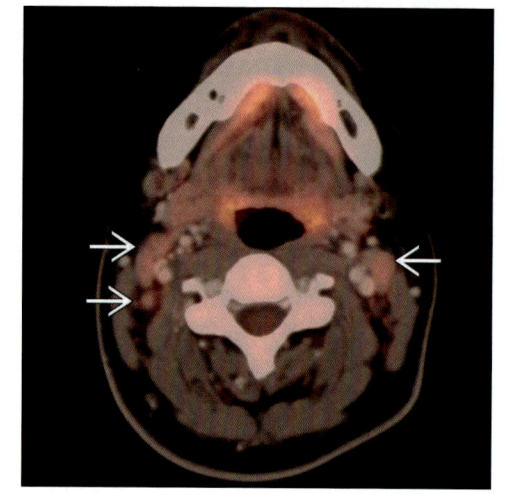

Axial FDG PET/CT, same patient as previous image, shows enlarged cervical LNs ➡ with increased FDG uptake following recent mononucleosis-like illness. Follow-up PET scan 1 month later showed resolution.

TERMINOLOGY

Definitions
- Positive FDG PET or Ga-67 findings that may mimic lymphoma

IMAGING FINDINGS

General Features
- Best diagnostic clue: Enlarged, hypermetabolic lymph nodes (LN) on FDG PET or Ga-67 scintigraphy
- Location
  ○ Lymph nodes, liver, spleen, lung nodules
  ○ Enlarged anterior mediastinal LN favors lymphoma

Nuclear Medicine Findings
- PET
  ○ Sensitivity and specificity of FDG PET: Dependent upon many factors (patient selection, endemic infectious diseases, referral bias, instrumentation, criteria for a positive or negative study)
  ○ CT based attenuation correction: Artifacts from misregistration, high attenuation structures
  ○ Prior imaging & clinical information: Best acquired through close interaction with referring clinician; helps to ensure a high level of PET accuracy
  ○ Normal physiologic FDG distribution & physiologic variants: Common mimics of lymphoma
    ▪ Normal FDG activity: Brain, myocardium, urinary tract (renal excretion), GI tract, salivary glands, liver, spleen (mild)
    ▪ Variable benign physiologic FDG uptake: Esophagus (diffuse), salivary glands, hypermetabolic brown adipose tissue (HBAT), stomach, intestine, blood pool
    ▪ Skeletal muscle FDG uptake: Focal uptake in recently exercised & myositis; diffuse uptake in ↑ insulin, hyperthyroidism (esp. psoas, rectus abdominus), ↑ dose statin therapy, hypoxia, cachexia
    ▪ Children: FDG uptake in skeletal epiphyses, thymus (thymic rebound may be seen up to 30+ y), prominent tonsillar, mild symmetrical cervical LN, diaphragm/intercostal muscles (crying)
    ▪ Diffuse fat uptake: Concurrent high dose methotrexate, cisplatinum, high dose steroids (often associated with periadrenal uptake)

DDx: Lymphoma, Benign Mimics

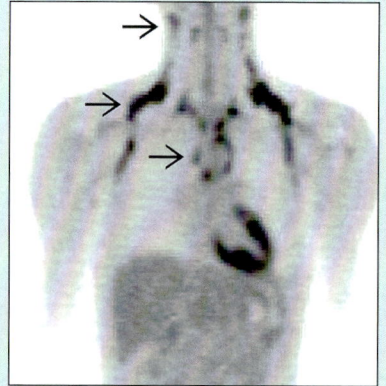

Hypermetabolic Brown Fat

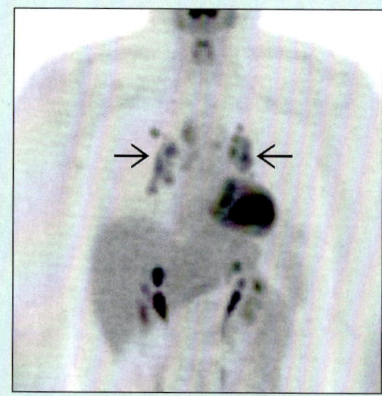

Granulomatous Disease

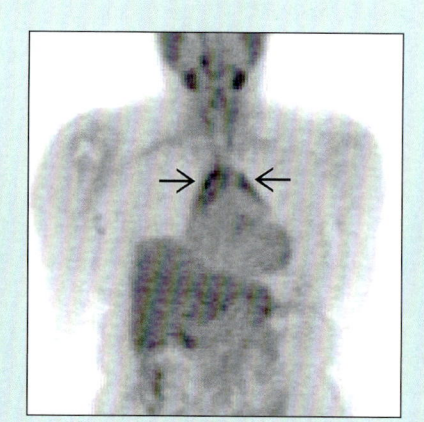

Thymic Rebound Post Chemo

LYMPHOMA, BENIGN MIMICS

Key Facts

Imaging Findings
- CT based attenuation correction: Artifacts from misregistration, high attenuation structures
- Prior imaging & clinical information: Best acquired through close interaction with referring clinician; helps to ensure a high level of PET accuracy
- Normal physiologic FDG distribution & physiologic variants: Common mimics of lymphoma
- Muscular relaxation before PET imaging recommended
- Patient warming, quiet calming environment prior to PET imaging
- Correlate with clinical history, signs & symptoms, travel history, prior imaging

Top Differential Diagnoses
- Wide Range of Infectious, Inflammatory, Granulomatous and Neoplastic Causes
- All may show uptake on FDG PET, Ga-67
- Histoplasma
- Tuberculosis (TB)
- Sarcoid
- Viral Infections; Infectious Mononucleosis
- HIV, AIDS
- Cat-Scratch Fever
- Whipple Disease
- Thoracic or Extrathoracic Malignancy
- Small Cell Lung Carcinoma
- Castleman Disease
- Immune Therapy

- False (+) PET in benign pathologic conditions
  - Infection (viral, fungal, bacterial parasitic)
  - Inflammation: Any cause
  - Granulomatous disease: Infectious, non-infectious
  - Thyroid uptake: Diffuse in thyroiditis (may be subclinical); focal in thyroid cancer, benign nodules
  - Thymic rebound in young adults
  - Diffuse marrow uptake with marrow stimulant drugs
- Ga-67 Scintigraphy
  - Normal uptake: Lacrimal glands, salivary glands, breast, epiphyses (children), bone, liver, spleen, large intestine, kidney (up to 48 h)
  - Can be seen after chemotherapy: Mild diffuse lung, marrow (stimulant drugs), diffuse stomach, thymic rebound

Imaging Recommendations
- Best imaging tool
  - PET/CT superior to CT, PET alone or Ga-67 in staging lymphoma
  - Less data on superiority of FDG PET > Ga-67 in monitoring response to treatment
- Protocol advice
  - Muscular relaxation before PET imaging recommended
  - Patient warming, quiet calming environment prior to PET imaging
  - Correlate with clinical history, signs & symptoms, travel history, prior imaging

DIFFERENTIAL DIAGNOSIS

Wide Range of Infectious, Inflammatory, Granulomatous and Neoplastic Causes
- All may show uptake on FDG PET, Ga-67
- Anatomic, clinical information may be helpful in "sorting out"

Histoplasma
- Sub-cm lung nodules that often calcify (granuloma)
- Calcified minimally or non-enlarged mildly FDG-avid mediastinal & hilar LN and calcified splenic & hepatic granulomas

Tuberculosis (TB)
- Enlarged LN ipsilateral to consolidation in primary TB
- Lung nodules which may calcify: Lung apex scarring, (+) PPD

Sarcoid
- Lung nodules: Usually sub-cm
- Sarcoid "galaxy sign": Multitude of tiny clustered lung nodules
- Garland triad (1-2-3 sign) comprises symmetrically enlarged bilateral hilar and right paratracheal LN
- Enlarged anterior mediastinal LN favors lymphoma

Viral Infections; Infectious Mononucleosis
- Variable involvement of adenoids, tonsils, anterior posterior cervical and axillary LNs, cecal-associated lymphoid tissue
- "Call back" PET scan ~ 3 weeks after resolution of symptoms: Shows improvement/regression (insurance typically won't reimburse)

HIV, AIDS
- Enlarged or non-enlarged, FDG-avid LN, liver, spleen
- Enlarged LN in HIV: Reactive follicular hyperplasia (50%), AIDS-related lymphoma (20%), mycobacterial infection (17%), Kaposi sarcoma (10%), opportunistic infection (multipathogens), metastases, drug reaction
- Diffuse uptake in HIV LNs often "blossoms" with recovery from chemotherapy

Cat-Scratch Fever
- Enlarged painful LN
- Symptoms and signs resolve over weeks

Whipple Disease
- Enlarged abdominal LN with low attenuation center

LYMPHOMA, BENIGN MIMICS

Thoracic or Extrathoracic Malignancy
- Enlarged FDG-avid LN accompanied by multiple FDG-avid lung nodules that ↑ in size & number over time
- Splenic metastases
  - Multiple (60%), solitary (31%), nodular/diffusely infiltrating (9%)
  - Breast (21%), lung (18%), ovary (8%), melanoma (6%), prostate (6%)

Small Cell Lung Carcinoma
- Markedly enlarged FDG-avid hilar & mediastinal LN

Castleman Disease
- Synonyms: Giant LN hyperplasia, angiomatous lymphoid hamartoma, angiofollicular hyperplasia
- Benign masses (lymphoid hyperplasia); unknown etiology
- 70% < 30 yr; age range 8-66 yr, M = F
- Chest: Middle & posterior mediastinum (70%), lung (rare)
- Extrathoracic: Neck, axilla, shoulder, mesentery, pelvis, retroperitoneum, within muscle
- Indistinguishable from lymphoma

Enlarged Lymph Nodes with Low-Density Center
- TB, Mycobacterium avium-intracellulare (MAI/MAC); pyogenic infection, Whipple disease, lymphoma, metastatic disease following radiation/chemotherapy

Immune Therapy
- Example: Interleukin, interferon Rx, vaccine therapies
- Stimulation of FDG uptake, diffusely, in mildly enlarged LNs, tonsils, adenoids, thymus

PATHOLOGY

Microscopic Features
- TB: Caseous necrosis; Langerhans giant cells
- Sarcoid: Noncaseating necrosis, positive Kveim reaction
- Lymphoma: FNA diagnostic in recurrent NHL; core biopsy may be required for HD
- Infections: FNA and core biopsy may aid diagnosis; more sensitive if performed prior to empiric therapy

CLINICAL ISSUES

Presentation
- Most common signs/symptoms
  - Asymptomatic, incidental finding
  - Incidentally observed lung nodules
  - Enlarged and/or calcified hilar & mediastinal LN
  - Calcified splenic & hepatic granulomas on CXR, CT
- Other signs/symptoms
  - Lymphoma
    - B-symptoms: Loss of appetite, fatigue (anemia), painless enlarged LN, abdominal fullness (enlarged liver/spleen), flu-like symptoms, night sweats
  - TB
    - Active phase: Loss of appetite, fatigue (anemia), painless LN enlargement, abdominal fullness (enlarged liver/spleen), flu-like symptoms, night sweats
    - Quiescent phase: Asymptomatic
  - Systemic malignancy
    - Loss of appetite, fatigue (anemia), painless or painful LN enlargement, abdominal fullness (enlarged liver/spleen), flu-like symptoms, symptoms referable to size/location of primary lesion and metastases
    - Malaise, anorexia, hemoptysis, pain, shortness of breath, neuropathology, paraneoplastic syndromes
  - Sarcoid: Ranges from asymptomatic in early stage to profound dyspnea in advanced stage disease
  - Infections
    - Acute: Pyrexia, cough productive of purulent sputa
    - Indolent: Asymptomatic, or, non-productive cough, shortness of breath, malaise

Treatment
- Tailored towards the diagnosed pathology

DIAGNOSTIC CHECKLIST

Image Interpretation Pearls
- Prior imaging & clinical data: Requires close contact with clinician; critical to accuracy of PET

SELECTED REFERENCES
1. Chang JM et al: False positive and false negative FDG-PET scans in various thoracic diseases. Korean J Radiol. 7(1):57-69, 2006
2. Jaruskova M et al: Role of FDG-PET and PET/CT in the diagnosis of prolonged febrile states. Eur J Nucl Med Mol Imaging. 33(8):913-8, 2006
3. Gorospe L et al: Whole-body PET/CT: spectrum of physiological variants, artifacts and interpretative pitfalls in cancer patients. Nucl Med Commun. 26(8):671-87, 2005
4. Kaste SC et al: 18F-FDG-avid sites mimicking active disease in pediatric Hodgkin's. Pediatr Radiol. 35(2):141-54, 2005
5. Manzardo C et al: Central nervous system opportunistic infections in developed countries in the highly active antiretroviral therapy era. J Neurovirol. 11 Suppl 3:72-82, 2005
6. Chen YK et al: Elevated 18F-FDG uptake in skeletal muscles and thymus: a clue for the diagnosis of Graves' disease. Nucl Med Commun. 25(2):115-21, 2004
7. Alavi A et al: Positron emission tomography imaging in nonmalignant thoracic disorders. Semin Nucl Med. 32(4):293-321, 2002
8. Montravers F et al: [(18)F]FDG in childhood lymphoma: clinical utility and impact on management. Eur J Nucl Med Mol Imaging. 29(9):1155-65, 2002
9. Brink I et al: Increased metabolic activity in the thymus gland studied with 18F-FDG PET: age dependency and frequency after chemotherapy. J Nucl Med. 42(4):591-5, 2001
10. Shreve PD et al: Pitfalls in oncologic diagnosis with FDG PET imaging: physiologic and benign variants. Radiographics. 19(1):61-77; quiz 150-1, 1999

LYMPHOMA, BENIGN MIMICS

IMAGE GALLERY

Variant

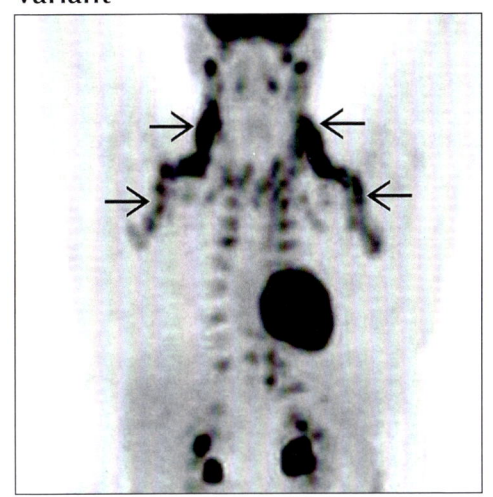

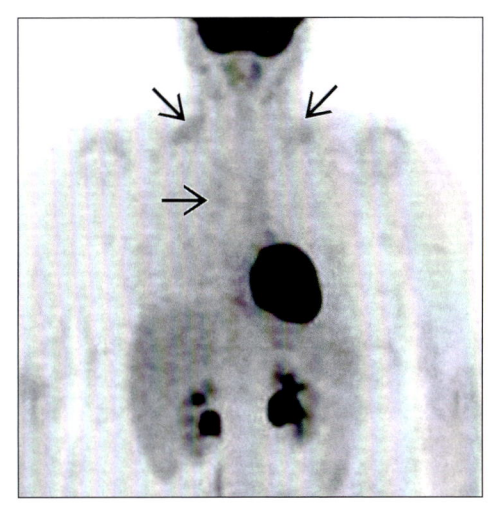

(Left) Coronal PET shows FDG uptake in sites ➔ typical for hypermetabolic brown adipose tissue (HBAT): Deep cervical, supraclavicular, axillary, intercostal paraspinous, superior mediastinal, periadrenal. See next image. *(Right)* Repeat FDG PET, same patient as previous image, following warming maneuver (environment 75° x 48 h, and during interval from injection to imaging) shows only minimal HBAT ➔.

Typical

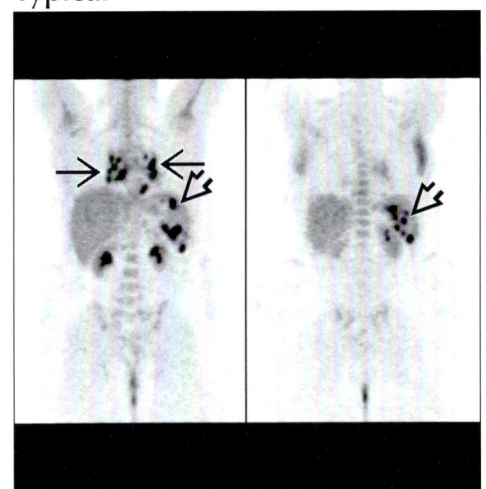

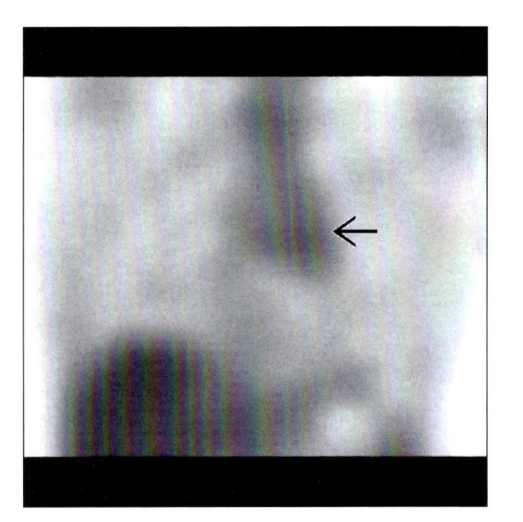

(Left) Coronal FDG PET shows balanced hypermetabolic balanced lymph nodes ➔, and multiple hypermetabolic splenic nodules ⮕ in a patient with sarcoidosis. *(Right)* Ga-67 coronal SPECT shows thymic rebound ➔ post chemotherapy for lymphoma. Chevron shape is typical for thymus, not mediastinal lymph nodes.

Variant

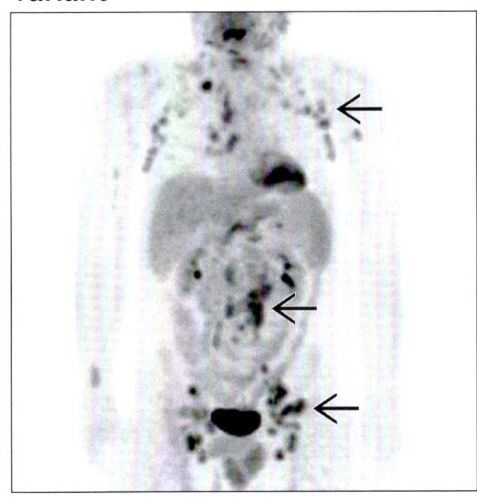

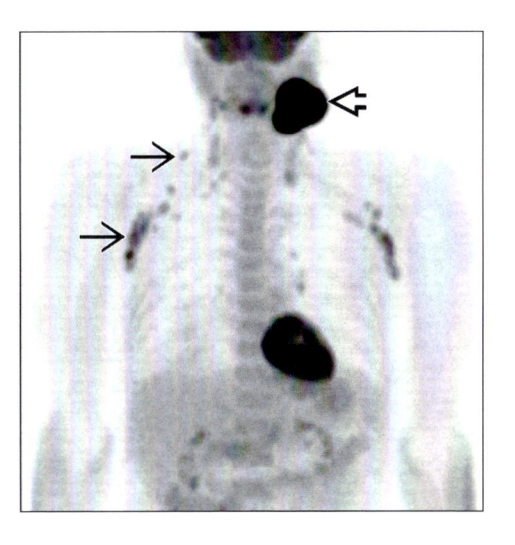

(Left) FDG PET MIP image shows widespread FDG-avid lymph nodes ➔ in a patient with AIDS and previously treated lymphoma. Multiple nodal biopsies showed no clonality/residual lymphoma. Appearance is typical for AIDS lymphadenopathy and correlates with viral burden. *(Right)* FDG PET MIP image of neck and chest shows multiple FDG-avid nodes ➔ in a HIV+ patient with left parotid NHL ⮕. Biopsies confirmed NHL only in left parotid mass.

HODGKIN LYMPHOMA STAGING

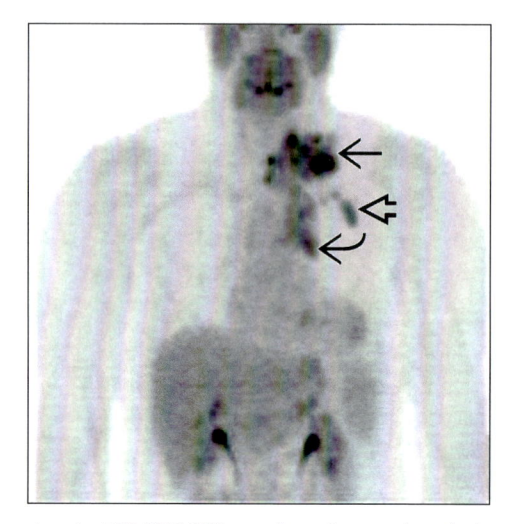

Anterior MIP FDG PET scan shows increased uptake in left neck ➡, mediastinum ➡ and high axillary ➡ regions in a patient with stage II Hodgkin lymphoma. No other sites were identified. See next image.

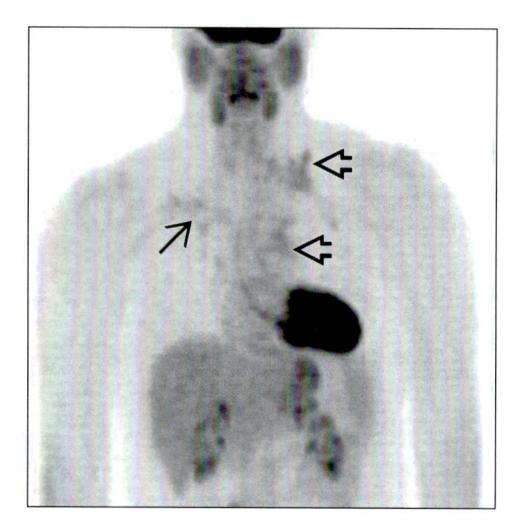

Same patient as left 4 days following placement of right sided portacath ➡ & single dose of chemo. Tumor metabolism ➡ has dropped dramatically, showing the importance of PET staging prior to any chemo.

TERMINOLOGY

Abbreviations and Synonyms
- Hodgkin lymphoma (HL); Hodgkin disease (HD)

Definitions
- Malignancy of lymphocytes, or rarely of histiocytes

IMAGING FINDINGS

General Features
- Best diagnostic clue: FDG PET/CT: Enlarged, hypermetabolic lymph nodes (LN)
- Location: Spreads in contiguous fashion to other LN and then to viscera or bone marrow

Nuclear Medicine Findings
- PET: Focal, non-physiologic ↑ uptake in nodal or extranodal tissue
- Ga-67 Scintigraphy: Focal, non-physiologic ↑ uptake in nodal, extranodal tissue
- PET and Ga-67: Abnormally ↑ uptake in spleen or liver; focal uptake more specific than diffuse

Imaging Recommendations
- Best imaging tool
  - PET/CT or PET + CT (side-by-side) is superior to contrast CT or PET alone for staging HD: PET/CT and PET + CT (side-by-side) similar
    - CT alone: Overall sensitivity (85-87%), specificity (80-91%); performance ↓ for extranodal
    - PET/CT or PET + CT (side-by-side): Overall sensitivity (94-98%), specificity (95-100%); performance similar for nodal, extranodal
  - Ga-67 inferior to FDG PET for initial staging: Sensitivity reported 71-90%
    - Pre-treatment Ga-67 scan recommended prior to treatment if used (instead of FDG PET) to evaluate response to treatment
  - Higher confidence in reading PET/CT compared to Ga-67 scintigraphy
- Protocol advice
  - FDG PET and Ga-67 should be performed prior to treatment for initial staging: One dose of chemotherapy may ↓ uptake & sensitivity
  - Knowledge of prior imaging & clinical information critical for accuracy of FDG PET & Ga-67

DDx: Hodgkin Disease

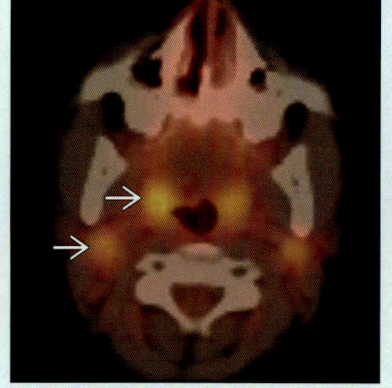

Reactive Lymph Node, Tonsils

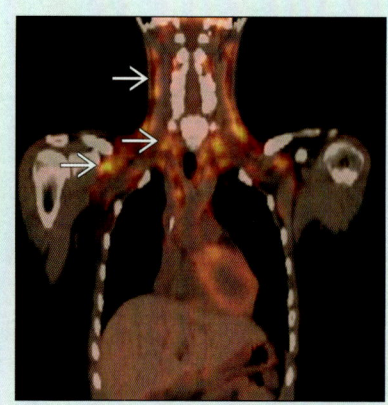

Brown Adipose Tissue

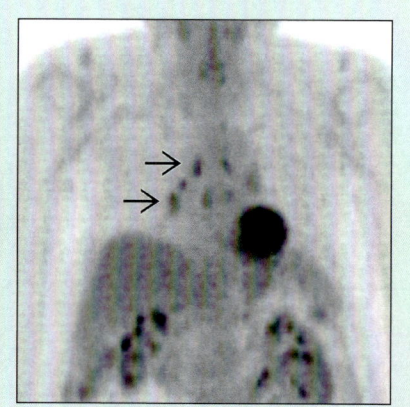

Granulomatous Disease

HODGKIN LYMPHOMA STAGING

Key Facts

Imaging Findings
- Best diagnostic clue: FDG PET/CT: Enlarged, hypermetabolic lymph nodes (LN)
- Location: Spreads in contiguous fashion to other LN and then to viscera or bone marrow
- PET: Focal, non-physiologic ↑ uptake in nodal or extranodal tissue
- Ga-67 Scintigraphy: Focal, non-physiologic ↑ uptake in nodal, extranodal tissue
- PET and Ga-67: Abnormally ↑ uptake in spleen or liver; focal uptake more specific than diffuse
- FDG PET and Ga-67 should be performed prior to treatment for initial staging: One dose of chemotherapy may ↓ uptake & sensitivity
- Knowledge of prior imaging & clinical information critical for accuracy of FDG PET & Ga-67
- FDG PET: Patient warm and relaxed/resting prior to and during uptake interval to ↓ uptake in muscle, hypermetabolic adipose tissue (HBAT)

Top Differential Diagnoses
- Granulomatous Process
- Infections
- Other Malignancy
- Normal Lymphoid Tissue

Pathology
- Staging based on history, physical examination, blood tests, imaging, biopsy

Diagnostic Checklist
- Knowledge of staging systems critical to quality of imaging report

---

- FDG PET: Patient warm and relaxed/resting prior to and during uptake interval to ↓ uptake in muscle, hypermetabolic adipose tissue (HBAT)
- Ga-67 scintigraphy: 10 mCi (adult), first imaging at 3 days, optional delayed imaging at 5-7 days, optional bowel prep, SPECT chest/abdomen recommended

DIFFERENTIAL DIAGNOSIS

Granulomatous Process
- Infectious, non-infectious
- Active disease positive on both FDG PET and Ga-67 scintigraphy

Infections
- Viral, fungal, pyogenic, parasitic, HIV-AIDS
- All positive on both FDG PET and Ga-67 scintigraphy

Other Malignancy
- More types of tumor (+) on FDG PET than Ga-67 scintigraphy

Normal Lymphoid Tissue
- Waldeyer ring, thymic tissue, mild symmetrical FDG uptake in cervical nodes

PATHOLOGY

General Features
- Etiology
  - Unknown in most
  - Reed-Sternberg cells are infected by Epstein-Barr virus (EBV) in ~ 50% of cases
  - HIV-associated HL is aggressive, often with extranodal or bone marrow involvement
  - Family history: Sibling of patient with HD has increased risk of developing HD; may be due to similar environmental, rather than genetic factors
- Epidemiology
  - 8,000 new cases occur in the US annually
  - Incidence ~ 4/100,000 per year; < 1% of all CA

Gross Pathologic & Surgical Features
- Affected LN enlarged: Shape is preserved, capsule is not invaded
- Cut surface white-grey and uniform: Nodular in nodular sclerosis subtype

Microscopic Features
- Described by Thomas Hodgkin (1832): Prominent lymphocytic infiltrate and Reed-Sternberg cells
  - Reed-Sternberg cells are large, binucleate, cells with an unusual CD15+, CD30+ immunophenotype
  - Core biopsy preferred over FNA: Tumors pleomorphic, Reed-Sternberg cells may be rare, scattered
- Core biopsy may be required to subtype HD

Staging, Grading or Classification Criteria
- Staging based on history, physical examination, blood tests, imaging, biopsy
- WHO ICD10 classification of lymphoma
  - Nature of staging is shown by: Clinical stage as obtained by exam & tests; pathological stage by exploratory laparotomy with splenectomy fallen out of favor
- Major categories of HL (preceded diagnosis by WHO classification)
  - Nodular lymphocyte predominance HL (NLPHL)
  - Classic Hodgkin lymphoma (CHL): Lymphocyte rich classic HL (LRCHL); nodular sclerosis HL (NSHL); mixed cellularity HL (MCHL); lymphocyte depletion HL (LDHL); other HD; unspecified
- Ann Arbor classification of anatomic distribution of disease
  - Stage I: Single region, usually one LN, and surrounding area (I); or a single extranodal site in absence of LN involvement (IE); usually no "B" symptoms
  - Stage II: ≥ 2 separate regions on one side of diaphragm (II); or single extralymphatic site and associated regional LN involvement on one side of diaphragm (IIE)

HODGKIN LYMPHOMA STAGING

- Stage III: Spread to both sides of diaphragm (III); may include extralymphatic extension with adjacent LN involvement (IIIE), splenic involvement (IIIS), or both (IIIE,S)
- Stage IV: Diffuse/disseminated involvement of ≥ 2 extralymphatic organs, (liver, marrow, or lung); location of stage IV disease indicated by modifier below
- Modifiers
  - A or B: Absence ("A") or presence ("B") of B-symptoms
  - E: Disease involves extralymphatic site(s) adjacent to site(s) of lymphatic involvement (± obvious direct extension)
  - X: Largest deposit is > 10 cm ("bulky disease") or mediastinum wider than 1/3 of the chest on a CXR
  - S: Splenic involvement; splenic nodule of any size, or histology proven; splenic enlargement alone insufficient to confirm involvement
  - H: Liver involvement (H) = stage IV; liver nodules of any size or histology proven; hepatomegaly alone insufficient to confirm involvement
  - M: Suspected bone marrow involvement by biopsy or imaging
  - L: Lung involvement; pulmonary nodule(s) or extension from adjacent mediastinal/hilar LN or extralymphatic extension (E lesion) = stage IV
  - Specific sites involved designated by letter subscripts: Includes "+" if biopsy proven involvement; "-" if biopsy negative
    - Spleen (S), lung (L), marrow (M), hepatic (H), pericardium (Pcard), pleura (P), Waldeyer ring (W), osseous (bone) (O), gastrointestinal (GI), skin (D), soft tissue (Softis), thyroid (Thy)
- Limitations: Staging may not predict biological behavior
  - Cotswolds modification: Introduced prognostic significance of bulky disease and other modifiers
- International Prognostic Index (IPI) risk factors
  - Age > 60 y: Ann Arbor stage III or IV, elevated LDH, reduced performance status, extranodal disease
  - Patients assigned to 5 year survival risk categories (low, low-intermediate, high-intermediate, high): Low (73%), high (26%)
  - Prognostic factors predict the success conventional Rx in patients with locally extensive or advanced stage HD: Age ≥ 45 years; stage IV disease, Hb < 10.5 mg/dl, Lymphocyte count < 600/μl or < 8%, male, Albumin < 4.0 mg/dl, WBC count ≥ 15,000/μl
  - Freedom from progression (FFP) at 5 years related to # of factors present: No factors (84%); each added factor lowers 5-year FFP by 7%, > 5 factors (42%)

CLINICAL ISSUES

Presentation
- Most common signs/symptoms
  - Asymptomatic, incidental clinical/radiologic finding
  - Enlarged non-painful LN, spleen
  - 1/3 present with systemic B-symptoms
- Other signs/symptoms
  - Enlarged LN painful for hours after alcohol consumption
  - Pel-Ebstein fever: Alternating ↑ fever for days and ↓ temperature for days to weeks
  - Pressure from enlarged mediastinal LN on airway, vessels
- Clinical Profile
  - HIV-associated HL is aggressive, often with extranodal or bone marrow involvement
    - Lower frequency of mediastinal LN involvement than non-HIV-associated HL
    - Most patients: Mixed cellularity or lymphocyte-depleted HL, B-symptoms, a CD4 count of ≤ 300/dL & express EBV-associated proteins in Reed-Sternberg cells
    - Median survival 8-20 months, < < non-HIV-HL

Demographics
- Age: Bimodal age incidence: Most common between 15-34 y and > 60 y; rare < 10 y
- Gender: M:F 3:2 except nodular sclerosis M < F

Natural History & Prognosis
- > 85% of HL is curable

Treatment
- Early stage disease (IA or IIA) now treated with abbreviated chemoRx & involved-field XRT rather than XRT alone
- Advanced disease (III, IVA, or IVB) treated with combination chemoRx alone

DIAGNOSTIC CHECKLIST

Image Interpretation Pearls
- Knowledge of staging systems critical to quality of imaging report

SELECTED REFERENCES

1. Kaste SC et al: 18F-FDG-avid sites mimicking active disease in pediatric Hodgkin's. Pediatr Radiol. 35(2):141-54, 2005
2. Hudson MM et al: PET imaging in pediatric Hodgkin's lymphoma. Pediatr Radiol. 34(3):190-8, 2004
3. AJCC Cancer Staging Handbook. 6th Ed. Springer-Verlag. 427-48, 2002
4. Jaffe ES et al: World Health Organization classification of tumors. Pathology and genetics of tumours of haematopoietic and lymphoid tissues. Lyon, IARC Press, 2001
5. Bangerter M et al: Positron emission tomography with 18-fluorodeoxyglucose in the staging and follow-up of lymphoma in the chest. Acta Oncol. 38(6):799-804, 1999
6. Devizzi L et al: Comparison of gallium scan, computed tomography, and magnetic resonance in patients with mediastinal Hodgkin's disease. Ann Oncol. 8 Suppl 1:53-6, 1997
7. Drossman SR et al: Lymphoma of the mediastinum and neck: evaluation with Ga-67 imaging and CT correlation. Radiology. 174(1):171-5, 1990
8. Front D et al: Ga-67 SPECT before and after treatment of lymphoma. Radiology. 175(2):515-9, 1990

HODGKIN LYMPHOMA STAGING

IMAGE GALLERY

Typical

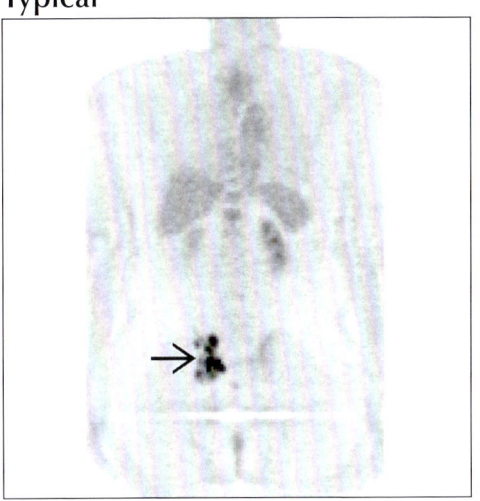

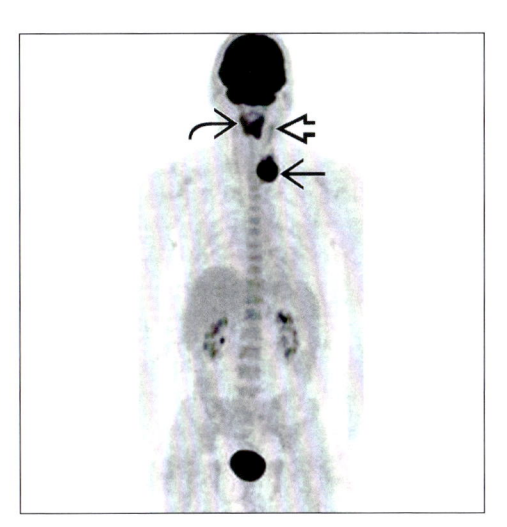

(Left) Coronal FDG PET shows increased uptake in medial right iliac bone ➔, biopsy proven Hodgkin lymphoma. No other sites identified. Involvement of a single region (LN or extralymphatic site) is stage I HD. (Right) Anterior MIP FDG PET shows tumor in left lower neck, ➔ Waldeyer tonsillar ring ➔ and left upper cervical region ➔ (all biopsy-proven Hodgkin lymphoma). ≥ 2 separate LN sites on same side of diaphragm = stage II HD.

Typical

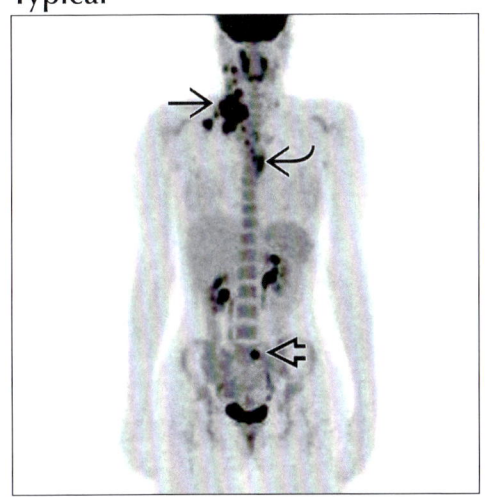

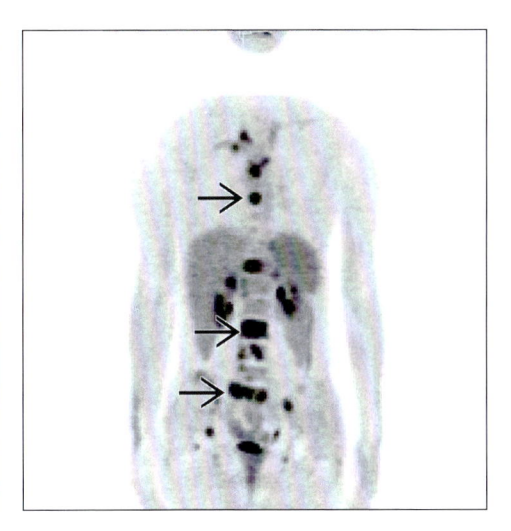

(Left) Anterior MIP FDG PET for HD staging shows increased uptake in numerous right neck ➔, and left mediastinal LNs ➔, as well as left proximal iliac node ➔. Spread to both sites of diaphragm = stage III HD. (Right) Coronal FDG PET shows diffuse tumor involvement in numerous bones ➔. Diffuse extralymphatic involvement (lung, liver, bone) = stage IV HD.

Variant

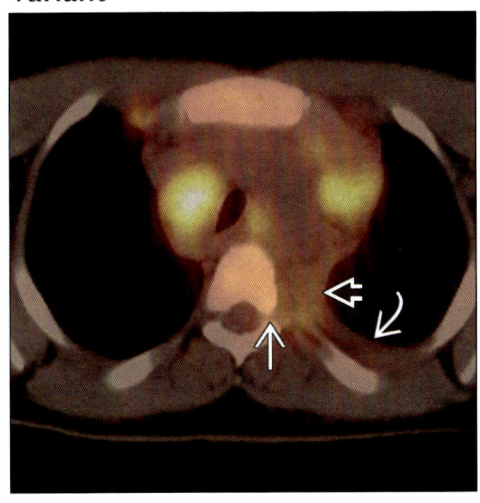

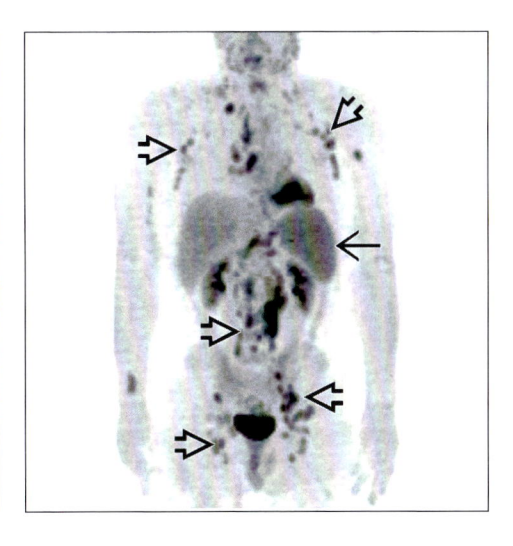

(Left) Axial FDG PET/CT of the upper chest in a patient with bulky stage IIe HD shows extranodal (e) spread of tumor to perivertebral soft tissues ➔, pleura ➔ and into bony spinal canal to involve epidural space ➔. (Right) Anterior MIP PET for HD staging shows extensive involvement of lymphatic sites ➔, plus splenic ➔ involvement. Involvement of lymph nodes on both sides of diaphragm plus splenic (s) involvement = stage IIIs HD.

LYMPHOMA POST-THERAPY EVALUATION

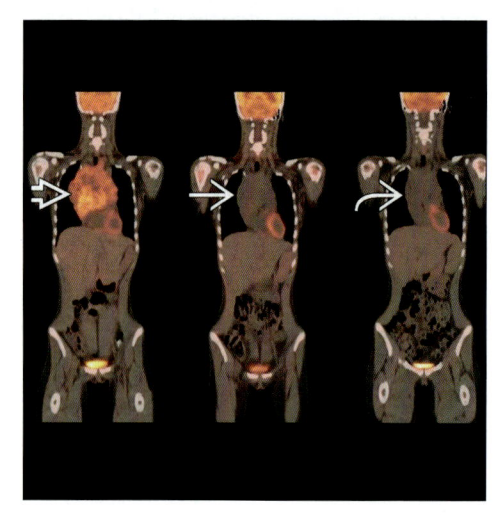

Coronal PET/CT, HL: Pre-treatment ➡, 3 weeks post-Rx ➡, 4 months post-Rx ➡. Persistent mediastinal mass without ↑ FDG uptake is consistent with fibrotic mass, not active tumor.

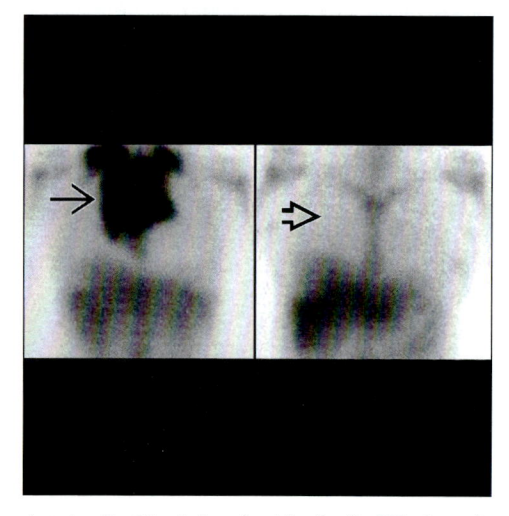

Anterior Ga-67 scintigraphy, HL: Pre-Rx ➡, 6 weeks post-Rx ➡. Resolution of metabolic activity is predictive of disease-free survival.

TERMINOLOGY

Abbreviations and Synonyms
- Hodgkin lymphoma (HL), Hodgkin disease (HD)
- Non-Hodgkin lymphoma (NHL)
- Disease free survival (DFS); overall survival (OS)

Definitions
- Malignancy of lymphocytes (rarely of histiocytes)

IMAGING FINDINGS

General Features
- Best diagnostic clue
  - Absence of metabolic activity on FDG PET following treatment: High predictive value for disease free survival
  - Persistent metabolic activity on FDG PET following treatment: Moderate predictive value for recurrence
- Rationale for FDG PET imaging mid-cycle
  - Allow change in therapy for high risk patients or those without symptomatic improvement
  - Avoid unnecessary toxicity if treatment not working
- Rational for FDG PET imaging post-Rx
  - Allow for treatment of residual/progressive disease before spreads further

Nuclear Medicine Findings
- FDG PET/CT vs. Ga-67 scintigraphy
  - Staging lymphoma: FDG PET, PET/CT clearly superior to Ga-67, CT alone
  - Assessment of response to treatment: Head-to-head comparison in small series suggest superiority of FDG PET > Ga-67
  - Confidence in interpretation: FDG PET >> Ga-67; further improved with PET/CT
- FDG PET or PET/CT
  - FDG PET in treatment (Rx) assessment
    - FDG PET in early response assessment (after 1-4 cycles): Sensitivity 79%, specificity 92%, PPV 90%, NPV 81%, accuracy 85%
    - FDG PET in post-Rx assessment (mixed population HL, NHL): Sensitivity 79%, specificity 94%, PPV 82%, NPV 93%, accuracy 91%
    - FDG PET in post-Rx assessment HL: Sensitivity 80%, specificity 91%, PPV 74%, NPV 93%, accuracy 88%

DDx: Benign Mimics of Lymphoma

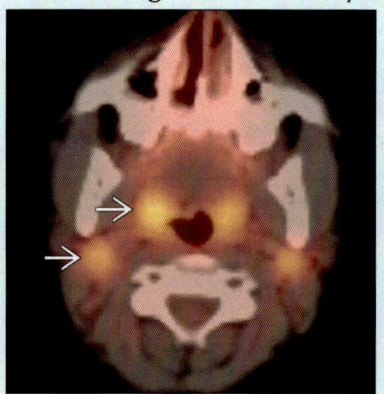

Reactive Nodes, Tonsils 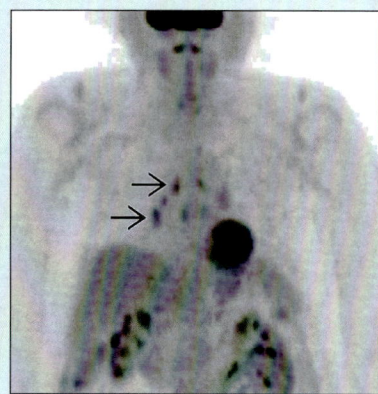 | *Granulomatous Disease* 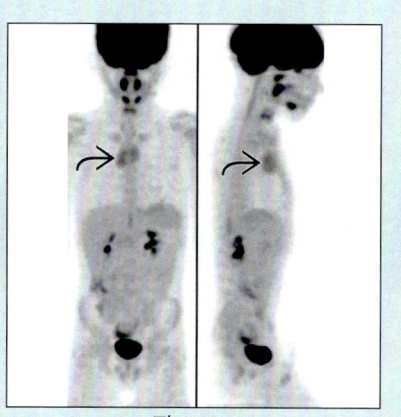 | *Thymus*

LYMPHOMA POST-THERAPY EVALUATION

Key Facts

Imaging Findings
- Staging lymphoma: FDG PET, PET/CT clearly superior to Ga-67, CT alone
- Assessment of response to treatment: Head-to-head comparison in small series suggest superiority of FDG PET > Ga-67
- FDG PET in early response assessment (after 1-4 cycles): Sensitivity 79%, specificity 92%, PPV 90%, NPV 81%, accuracy 85%
- FDG PET in post-Rx assessment (mixed population HL, NHL): Sensitivity 79%, specificity 94%, PPV 82%, NPV 93%, accuracy 91%
- FDG PET in post-Rx assessment HL: Sensitivity 80%, specificity 91%, PPV 74%, NPV 93%, accuracy 88%
- FDG PET in post-Rx assessment NHL: Sensitivity 67%, specificity 100%, PPV 100%, NPV 83%, accuracy 88%
- FDG PET in post reinduction chemo (before stem cell transplant): Sensitivity 84%, specificity 83%, PPV 84%, NPV 83%, accuracy 84%
- Low-level, patchy uptake in residual fibrotic mass, scars: Decreases over months but may persist
- Granulocyte colony stimulating factor (GCSF) or other marrow stimulant drugs: Intense red bone marrow + splenic uptake/enlargement; may persist x 2-3 months
- Following cessation of chemotherapy: Increased thymic uptake (thymic rebound); may occur in individuals up to age 40

Clinical Issues
- HL: > 85% curable
- NHL: ~ 50% curable

- FDG PET in post-Rx assessment NHL: Sensitivity 67%, specificity 100%, PPV 100%, NPV 83%, accuracy 88%
- FDG PET in post reinduction chemo (before stem cell transplant): Sensitivity 84%, specificity 83%, PPV 84%, NPV 83%, accuracy 84%
  ○ Benign patterns associated with chemotherapy: Apparent on FDG PET
    ▪ Low-level, patchy uptake in residual fibrotic mass, scars: Decreases over months but may persist
    ▪ Concurrent high dose chemotherapy: Diffuse FDG uptake in all adipose tissue (brown + yellow fat), adrenal/periadrenal regions
    ▪ Concurrent chemo + protease inhibitors (lymphoma + HIV): Skeletal muscle uptake; pattern similar to carbohydrate-insulin effect
    ▪ Granulocyte colony stimulating factor (GCSF) or other marrow stimulant drugs: Intense red bone marrow + splenic uptake/enlargement; may persist x 2-3 months
    ▪ Following cessation of chemotherapy: Increased thymic uptake (thymic rebound); may occur in individuals up to age 40
    ▪ Hypermetabolic brown adipose tissue (HBAT): Benign uptake in fat of neck, axilla, mediastinum, paraspinous, periadrenal, perirenal
- Ga-67 scintigraphy
  ○ Ga-67 in post-Rx evaluation of lymphoma for relapse with residual mass: Sensitivity 87%, PPV poor, NPV 70%
  ○ Ga-67 scintigraphy in post-Rx prediction of disease free survival (DFS) and overall survival (OS)
    ▪ Ga-67 in NHL post-Rx prediction of DFS (OS) at 24 m: 85-95% (90%) with negative scan; < 45% (35%) with positive scan
    ▪ Ga-67 in HL post-Rx prediction of DFS (OS) at 24 m: 85-95% (100%) with negative scan; < 45% (60-80%) with positive scan

Imaging Recommendations
- Best imaging tool: FDG PET/CT: Staging, evaluation of therapeutic response, restaging, post-Rx monitoring

DIFFERENTIAL DIAGNOSIS

Histoplasmosis
- Sub-cm lung nodules that often calcify (granuloma)
- Calcified unenlarged mildly FDG-avid mediastinal & hilar LN, calcified splenic & hepatic granulomas

Tuberculosis (TB)
- Enlarged LN & ipsilateral consolidation in primary TB
- Lung nodules may calcify, apical scarring, positive PPD

Sarcoid
- Lung nodules: Sarcoid "galaxy" sign; multitude of tiny clustered lung nodules
- Garland triad (1-2-3 sign): Symmetrically enlarged bilateral hilar & right paratracheal LN
- Enlarged anterior mediastinal LN favors lymphoma

Viral Infections; Infectious Mononucleosis
- Minimally enlarged LN: Possibly sub-cm lung nodules that usually resolve completely

Cat-Scratch Fever
- Enlarged painful LN: Symptoms resolve over weeks

Whipple Disease
- Enlarged abdominal LN with low-attenuation center

Cardiac Failure, Edematous State
- LN may remain minimally enlarged, usually low attenuation, for months after edema has resolved

HIV, AIDS
- Enlarged LN in HIV
  ○ Reactive follicular hyperplasia (50%)
  ○ AIDS-related lymphoma (20%)
  ○ Mycobacterial infection (17%)
  ○ Kaposi sarcoma (10%)
  ○ Opportunistic infection (multipathogen)
  ○ Metastases
  ○ Drug reaction

LYMPHOMA POST-THERAPY EVALUATION

Thoracic, Extrathoracic Malignancy
- Enlarged FDG-avid LN accompanied by multiple FDG-avid lung nodules that increase in size and number over time

Small Cell Lung Carcinoma
- Markedly enlarged, prominently FDG-avid, hilar and mediastinal LN

PATHOLOGY

General Features
- Etiology
  - Unknown in most
  - Reed-Sternberg cells (HL) are infected by Epstein-Barr virus (EBV) in ~ 50% of cases
  - Family history: Sibling of patient with HL has increased risk of developing HL
  - Gastric MALT lymphoma: Associated with H. Pylori infection, proton pump inhibitors
  - Lymphoplasmacytic lymphoma: 1/3 have evidence of Hepatitis C infection

Microscopic Features
- HL: Prominent lymphocytic infiltrate and Reed-Sternberg cells
  - Reed-Sternberg cells: Large, binucleate cells with unusual CD15+, CD30+ immunophenotype
  - Core biopsy, open biopsy often required to diagnose HL
- NHL: T- or B-cell clonality; no Reed-Sternberg cells
  - Fine needle aspirate may be sufficient for diagnosis of NHL

CLINICAL ISSUES

Presentation
- Development of B-symptoms can herald recurrence post treatment

Demographics
- Age
  - HL
    - Bimodal: 15-34 years; > 60 years
    - Rare < 10 years
  - NHL
    - > 90% in adults
    - Median age 55 years
- Gender
  - HL: M:F 3:2, except nodular sclerosing (M < F)
  - NHL: M:F 1.4:1

Natural History & Prognosis
- HL: > 85% curable
- NHL: ~ 50% curable
- High cure rates & long survival: Increased risk of second malignancies
- HIV disease and lymphoma: Reduced survival (median survival 8-10 months)

DIAGNOSTIC CHECKLIST

Consider
- FDG PET/CT mid-cycle in high risk patients

SELECTED REFERENCES

1. Brepoels L et al: PET and PET/CT for response evaluation in lymphoma: Current practice and developments. Leuk Lymphoma. 48(2):270-82, 2007
2. Alinari L et al: Discordant response to chemotherapy: an unusual pattern of fluoro-deoxy-D-glucose uptake in heavily pre-treated lymphoma patients. Leuk Lymphoma. 47(6):1048-52, 2006
3. Gallamini A et al: The predictive value of positron emission tomography scanning performed after two courses of standard therapy on treatment outcome in advanced stage Hodgkin's disease. Haematologica. 91(4):475-81, 2006
4. Kahn ST et al: Value of PET restaging after chemotherapy for non-Hodgkin's lymphoma: Implications for consolidation radiotherapy. Int J Radiat Oncol Biol Phys. 66(4):961-5, 2006
5. Kostakoglu L et al: FDG-PET after 1 cycle of therapy predicts outcome in diffuse large cell lymphoma and classic Hodgkin disease. Cancer. 107(11):2678-87, 2006
6. Meany HJ et al: Utility of PET scans to predict disease relapse in pediatric patients with hodgkin lymphoma. Pediatr Blood Cancer. 2006
7. Querellou S et al: FDG-PET/CT predicts outcome in patients with aggressive non-Hodgkin's lymphoma and Hodgkin's disease. Ann Hematol. 85(11):759-67, 2006
8. Schot BW et al: The role of serial pre-transplantation positron emission tomography in predicting progressive disease in relapsed lymphoma. Haematologica. 91(4):490-5, 2006
9. Svoboda J et al: Prognostic value of FDG-PET scan imaging in lymphoma patients undergoing autologous stem cell transplantation. Bone Marrow Transplant. 38(3):211-6, 2006
10. Zijlstra JM et al: 18F-fluoro-deoxyglucose positron emission tomography for post-treatment evaluation of malignant lymphoma: a systematic review. Haematologica. 91(4):522-9, 2006
11. Jerusalem G et al: Evaluation of therapy for lymphoma. Semin Nucl Med. 35(3):186-96, 2005
12. Reinhardt MJ et al: Computed tomography and 18F-FDG positron emission tomography for therapy control of Hodgkin's and non-Hodgkin's lymphoma patients: when do we really need FDG-PET? Ann Oncol. 16(9):1524-9, 2005
13. Rigacci L et al: 18FDG-positron emission tomography in post treatment evaluation of residual mass in Hodgkin's lymphoma: long-term results. Oncol Rep. 14(5):1209-14, 2005
14. Foo SS et al: Positron emission tomography scanning in the assessment of patients with lymphoma. Intern Med J. 34(7):388-97, 2004
15. Friedberg JW et al: FDG-PET is superior to gallium scintigraphy in staging and more sensitive in the follow-up of patients with de novo Hodgkin lymphoma: a blinded comparison. Leuk Lymphoma. 45(1):85-92, 2004
16. Jerusalem G et al: Early detection of relapse by whole-body positron emission tomography in the follow-up of patients with Hodgkin's disease. Ann Oncol. 14(1):123-30, 2003
17. Reske SN: PET and restaging of malignant lymphoma including residual masses and relapse. Eur J Nucl Med Mol Imaging. 30 Suppl 1:S89-96, 2003

LYMPHOMA POST-THERAPY EVALUATION

IMAGE GALLERY

Typical

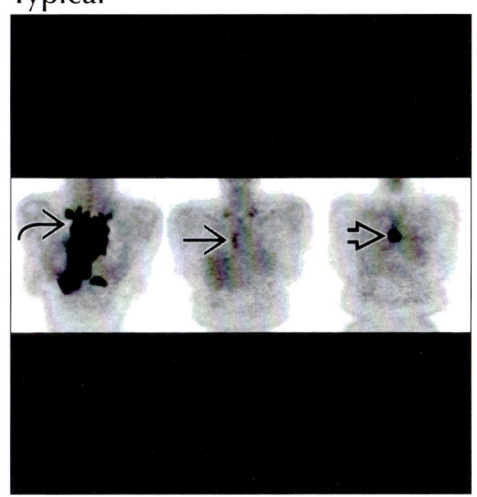

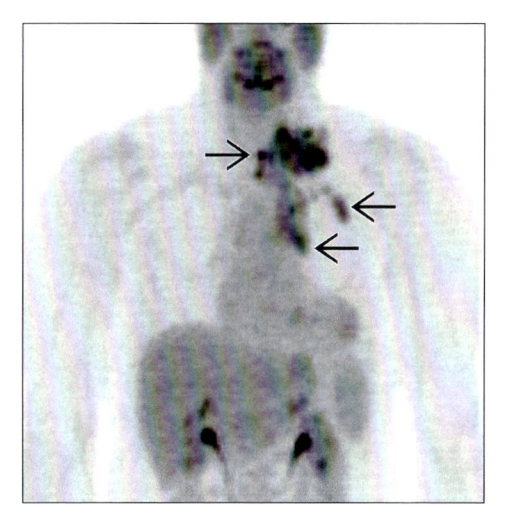

(Left) Coronal PET in patient with NHL: Pre-Rx ➔; 3 weeks post-Rx ➔; 5 months post-Rx ⇨. Immediate post-Rx scan shows faint residual activity in right mediastinum ➔, an area of subsequent recurrence ⇨. (Right) PET MIP: Pre-Rx scan shows hypermetabolic mass ➔ in left chest and neck in a patient with HL. See next.

Variant

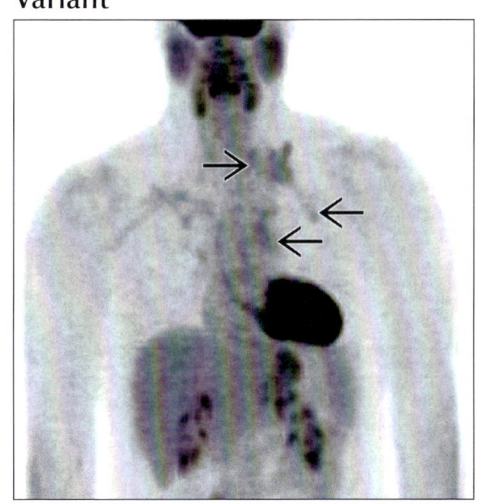

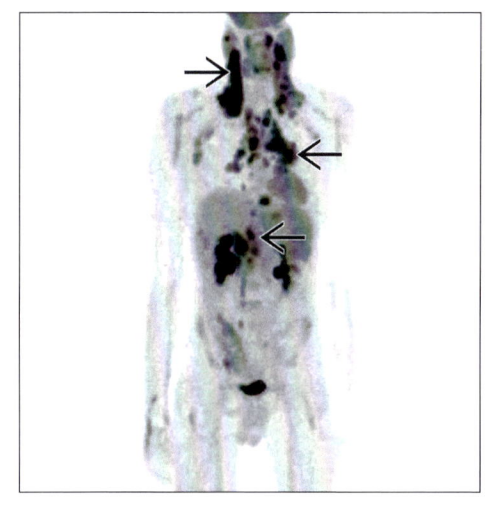

(Left) Same patient as previous. Repeat PET 4 days after 1st dose of chemo shows 70% ↓ in tumor uptake ➔, predictive of good response to chemotherapy. Also shows importance of PET staging prior to initiating chemotherapy. (Right) Anterior PET MIP image in HIV+ patient with widespread NHL shows ↑ uptake in numerous sites of tumor ➔. See next 2 images.

Variant

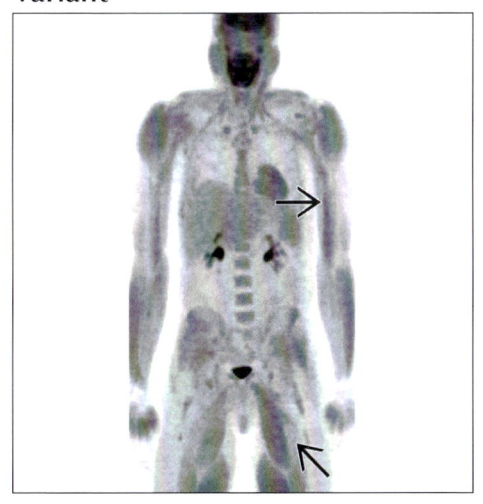

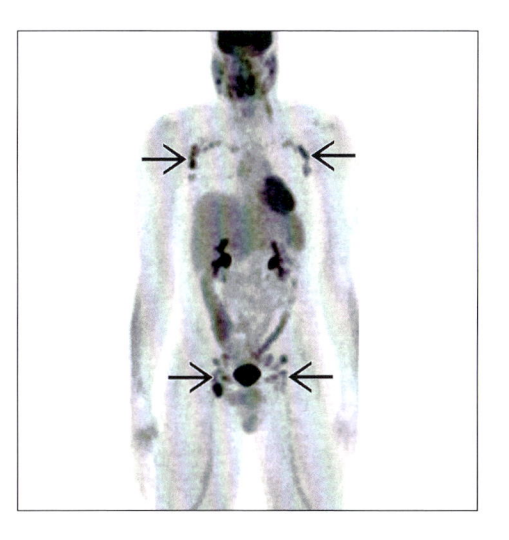

(Left) PET in same patient as previous during chemo shows resolution of activity in tumor. Diffuse skeletal muscle uptake ➔ is common with chemo + protease inhibitors, can also be seen with carbohydrate-insulin effect. See next. (Right) PET MIP in same patient as previous 3 months after chemo shows uptake in lymph nodes ➔. Biopsy: Lymphoid hyperplasia (HIV+), which commonly increases following chemo.

LYMPHOMA POST-THERAPY EVALUATION

Typical

(Left) PET MIP shows typical appearance of marrow-stimulant drugs (GCSF, etc.). Increased uptake in marrow ➔, spleen ➔ often persists for 2-3 months & can mimic marrow and splenic recurrence. (Right) Sagittal PET in patient on GCSF: Prevertebral sites of ↑ uptake ➔, associated with old compression fracture of L2 ➔, represents extramedullary hematopoiesis at site of extruded marrow, mimics recurrent tumor. (Courtesy A. Malouf, MD).

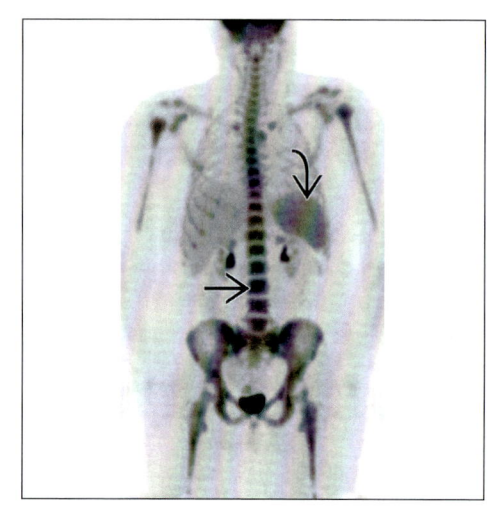

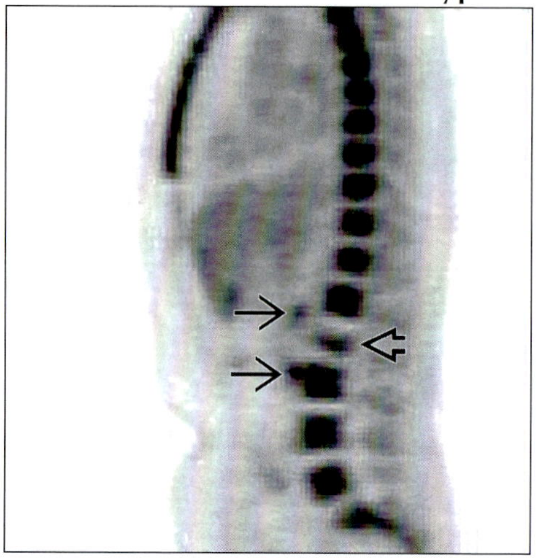

Variant

(Left) Axial CECT shows typical post-radiation change in paramediastinal regions ➔. Axial PET shows increased uptake in same regions ➔, likely chronic inflammation, which persists indefinitely. (Right) Axial PET shows diffuse increased FDG uptake in lungs ➔ with tiny pulmonary opacities on CT ➔ in patient with bleomycin-induced pulmonary toxicity, which can mimic infection or recurrent tumor.

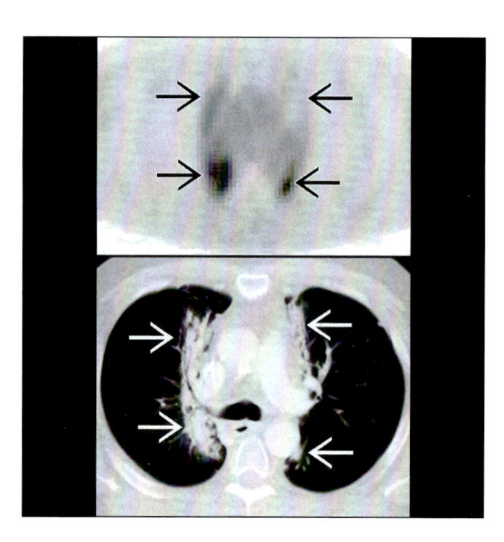

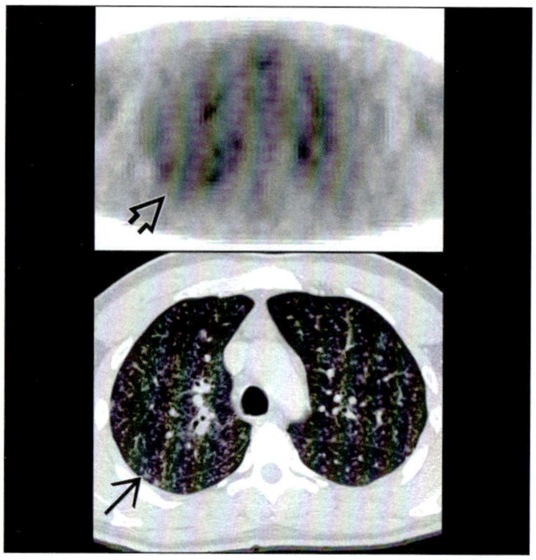

Variant

(Left) PET MIP shows diffuse uptake in adipose tissue ➔, as well as hypermetabolic brown fat ➔ and adrenal glands ➔, typical while on high dose chemo (esp. methotrexate, steroids). See next image. (Right) Axial fused PET/CT in same patient as left, confirms increased metabolism in adipose tissue ➔, called "chemo fat" pattern.

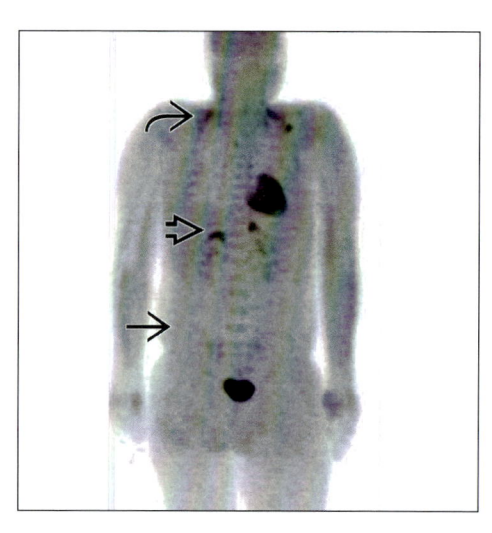

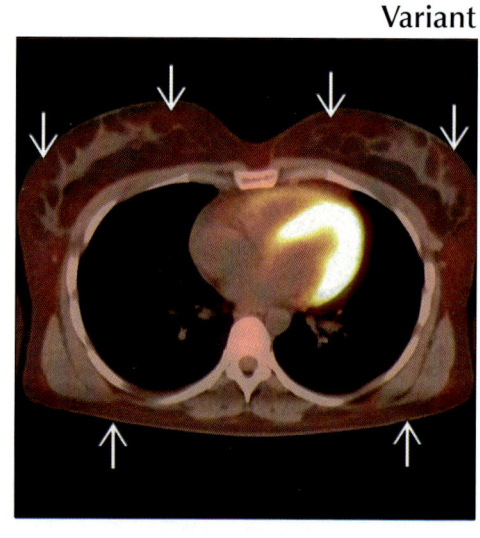

LYMPHOMA POST-THERAPY EVALUATION

Typical

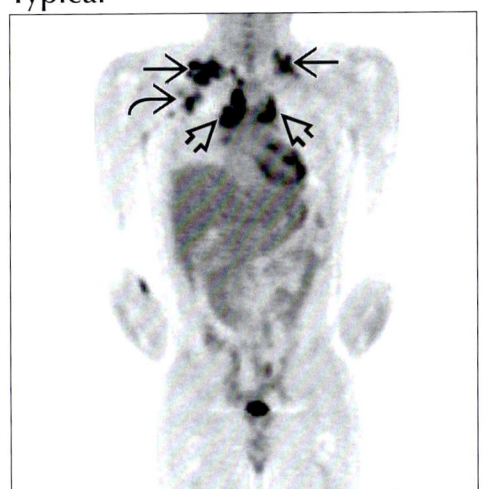

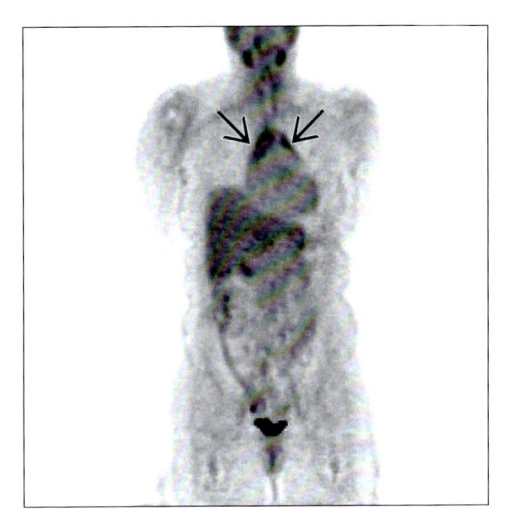

(Left) Pretreatment PET MIP in patient with HL shows ↑ uptake in supraclavicular ➡, axillary ➡ and mediastinal ➡ LNs. See next image. *(Right)* Post-treatment PET MIP in same patient as previous shows resolution of sites of tumor, development of chevron-shaped uptake in superior mediastinum ➡, typical for normal thymic rebound.

Typical

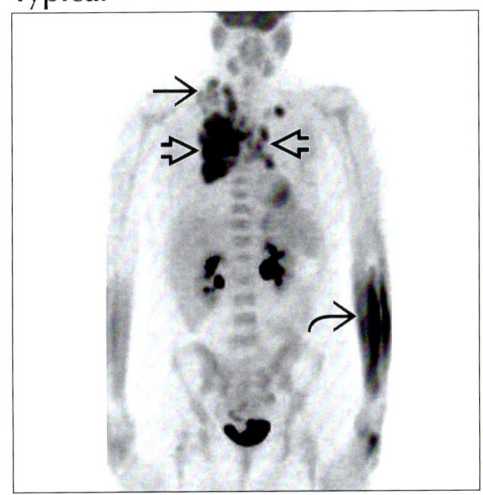

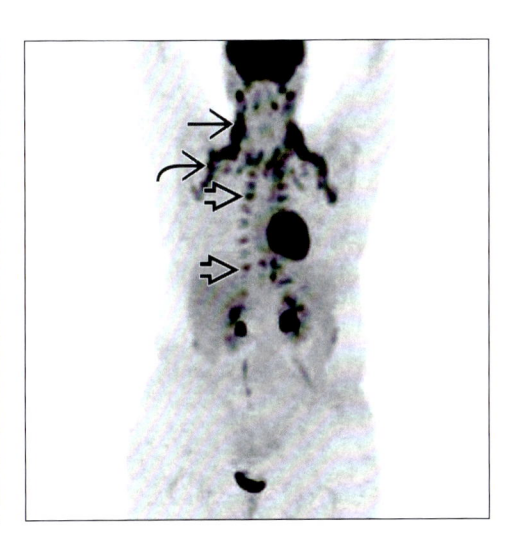

(Left) Pre-Rx PET MIP in patient with HL shows ↑ uptake in supraclavicular ➡ and mediastinal ➡ LNs. Uptake in left arm ➡ is due to recent muscle use. See next image. *(Right)* Post-Rx PET MIP in same patient at left shows resolution of sites of tumor and new uptake in neck ➡, axillary ➡, & paraspinous intercostal ➡ regions typical for hypermetabolic brown adipose tissue.

Typical

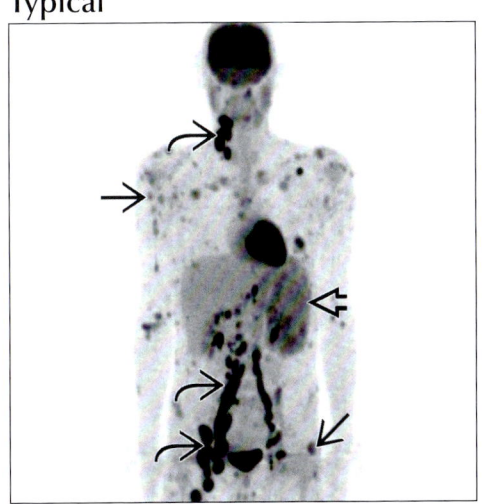

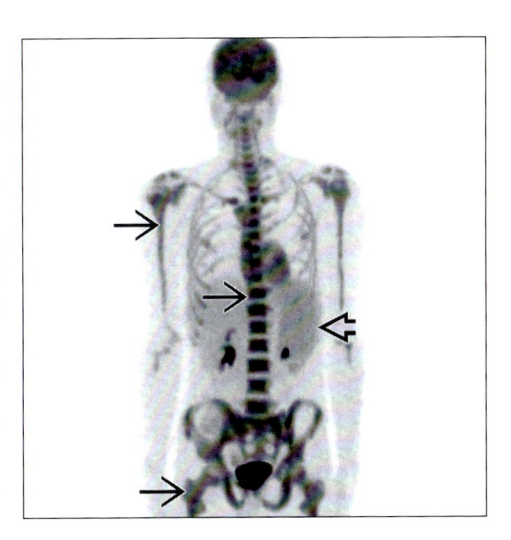

(Left) Pre-Rx PET MIP in patient with T-cell NHL shows increased uptake in numerous cutaneous ➡, splenic ➡, and ➡ nodal sites of tumor. See next image. *(Right)* Post-Rx PET MIP in same patient at left on GCSF shows resolution of sites of tumor, diffuse increased uptake in red marrow ➡ & enlarged spleen ➡, typical of hematopoietic stimulation.

NON-HODGKIN LYMPHOMAS, LOW GRADE

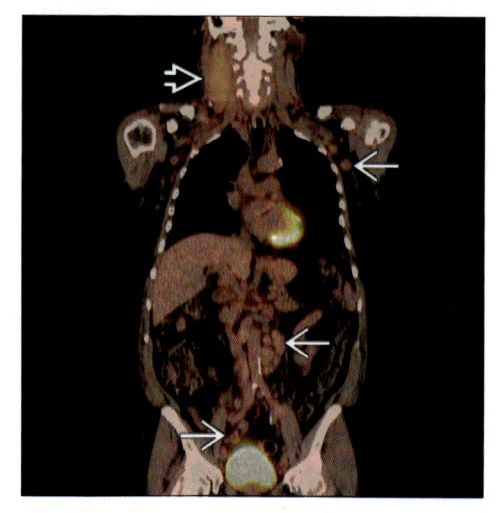

Coronal PET CT shows multiple enlarged LN's ➡ with low FDG activity in patient with CLL/SLL. Relatively higher uptake in right neck LN ➡ may indicate transformation into higher grade disease. See next.

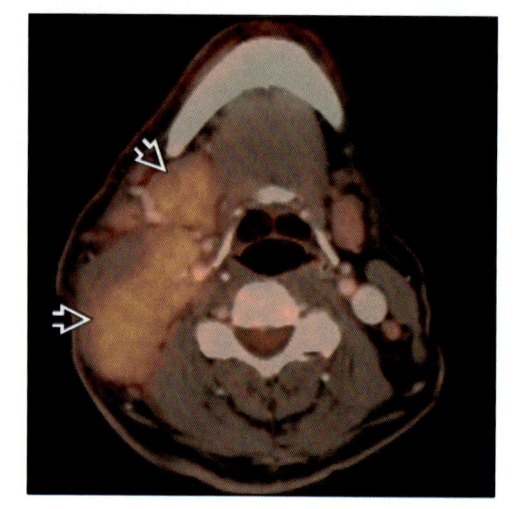

Axial PET CT in same patient as previous, shows markedly enlarged, hypermetabolic LNs ➡. PET-directed biopsy confirmed Richter transformation to higher grade large cell lymphoma.

TERMINOLOGY

Abbreviations and Synonyms
- Small lymphocytic lymphoma (SLL); chronic lymphocytic leukemia (CLL)
- Marginal zone lymphoma (MZL)
- Mucosal associated lymphoid tissue (MALT)
- Cutaneous T-cell lymphoma (CTCL)
- Low grade follicular B-cell lymphoma (FL)

Definitions
- Low grade lymphomas: Slow growing, indolent non-Hodgkin lymphoma
  - Low grade diffuse B-cell lymphomas
    - SLL: Termed CLL when 1° in blood, marrow
    - Lymphoplasmacytic lymphoma (immunocytoma)
    - MZL: MALT; nodal marginal zone; splenic marginal zone
  - FL
    - Small-cleaved cell type: < 20-25% large cells
    - Mixed small-cleaved and large cell type: Survival inversely proportionate to large cell percentage
    - Large cell type: Intermediate grade but more aggressive in nature
  - CTCL: Mycosis fungoides (MF), Sezary syndrome (leukemic variant)
    - CTCL: Rarely transforms into more aggressive large cell lymphoma
    - Not same as aggressive peripheral T-cell lymphoma (PTL) or adult T-cell lymphoma/leukemia (ATLL)

IMAGING FINDINGS

General Features
- Best diagnostic clue
  - PET/CT: Enlarged LN, extranodal mass with low to moderate FDG uptake
  - PET/CT: Marked FDG uptake = higher grade transformation

Nuclear Medicine Findings
- PET
  - CLL/SLL: PET of limited use in staging 2° ↓ FDG uptake (sens 58%)
    - SUV > 3.5 suggests Richter transformation of CLL/SLL → diffuse large B-cell lymphoma (sens 91%, spec 80%, PPV 53%, NPV 97%)

DDx: Mimics of Low Grade Lymphoma

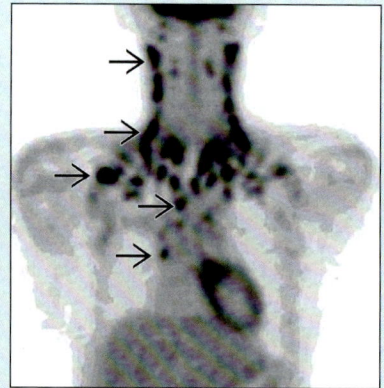

Hypermetabolic Brown Fat

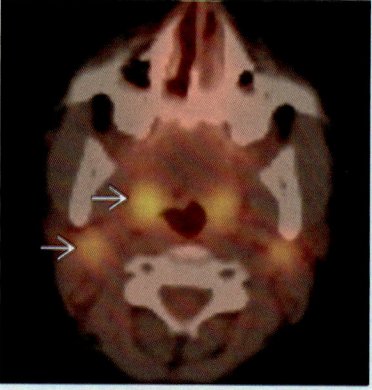

Recent Viral URI

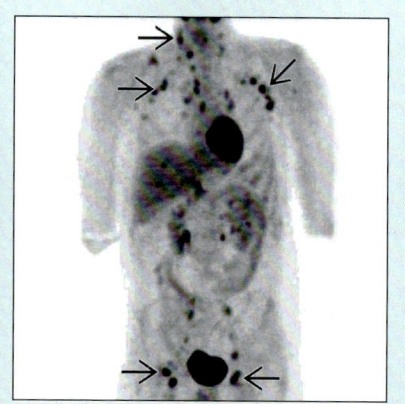

Follicular Hyperplasia (HIV)

NON-HODGKIN LYMPHOMAS, LOW GRADE

Terminology
- Small lymphocytic lymphoma (SLL); chronic lymphocytic leukemia (CLL)
- Marginal zone lymphoma (MZL)
- Mucosal associated lymphoid tissue (MALT)
- Cutaneous T-cell lymphoma (CTCL)
- Low grade follicular B-cell lymphoma (FL)
- Low grade lymphomas: Slow growing, indolent non-Hodgkin lymphoma

Imaging Findings
- PET/CT: Enlarged LN, extranodal mass with low to moderate FDG uptake
- PET/CT: Marked FDG uptake = higher grade transformation
- CLL/SLL: PET of limited use in staging 2° ↓ FDG uptake (sens 58%)

Key Facts
- MZL: FDG PET staging sens 71% (lower for extranodal)
- FL: FDG PET useful in staging all grades (sens 94%, spec 100%)

Top Differential Diagnoses
- Granulomatous Disease
- Reactive Lymph Node Hyperplasia
- Cardiac Failure, Edematous State
- Higher Grade Lymphomas on Therapy
- Other Malignancy

Diagnostic Checklist
- PET/CT useful for staging FL
- PET/CT: Intense uptake should suggest higher grade transformation, identify site to biopsy

---

- MZL: FDG PET staging sens 71% (lower for extranodal)
  - MALT lymphoma: Typically no or low FDG uptake; SUV > 3.5 suggests plasmacytic differentiation
- FL: FDG PET useful in staging all grades (sens 94%, spec 100%)
  - Wide overlap between FDG uptake by lower (SUV 2.3-13) and higher grade (SUV 3.2-43) FL
  - Emergence of sites of ↑ FDG uptake (SUV > 10): Transformation to higher grade (spec 81%)
- CTCL: FDG PET useful in staging, especially in suspected single cutaneous site
  - CTCL: Intense nodal sites suspicious for large cell transformation
- Tl-201, Tc-99m sestamibi: Superseded by PET/CT
- Ga-67
  - Poor sensitivity for low grade lymphomas; increased uptake indicative of higher grade transformation
  - Poor sensitivity in abdomen (due to colon uptake)
  - Many false positives: Granulomatous, inflammatory, infectious, normal physiologic

CT Findings
- Enlarged lymph nodes (LN), mild-moderate enhancement; low-attenuation in 20%

MR Findings
- Homogeneous, ↓ signal on T1WI, ↑ signal on T2WI, mild post-Gd enhancement

Imaging Recommendations
- Best imaging tool: FDG PET/CT: For staging FL, guiding biopsy, assess conversion to higher grade

DIFFERENTIAL DIAGNOSIS

Granulomatous Disease
- FDG uptake moderate-marked; stability over time
- Often symmetrical hilar/mediastinal LN

Reactive Lymph Node Hyperplasia
- Typically ↑ FDG uptake; numerous sites, often symmetrical, LN mild-moderately enlarged; may resolve weeks-months

Cardiac Failure, Edematous State
- LN may remain minimally enlarged, usually ↓ attenuation months after edema resolved

Higher Grade Lymphomas on Therapy
- May show ↓ FDG uptake, mimic low grade lymphoma

Other Malignancy
- FDG PET may identify best candidate site for biopsy

PATHOLOGY

General Features
- Etiology
  - MALT lymphoma (stomach) associated with H. pylori infection
  - Lymphoplasmacytic lymphoma: 1/3 associated with hepatitis C infection

Microscopic Features
- FL: Aggressiveness proportionate to percentage of large cells

CLINICAL ISSUES

Presentation
- Most common signs/symptoms: Asymptomatic, loss of appetite, fatigue, enlarged LN, flu-like symptoms
- Other signs/symptoms
  - B-symptoms: Unexplained persistent fever & chills, night sweats, fatigue, pruritus, weight loss
    - More common in aggressive (47%) than indolent lymphoma (25%)
    - Concern for progression to intermediate/high-grade lymphoma with development of B-symptoms

NON-HODGKIN LYMPHOMAS, LOW GRADE

- Enlarged LN may be painful for hours after a person consumes large amounts of alcohol
- Enlarging LN may narrow airways (cough, discomfort, stridor) or vessels (SVC syndrome)
- Lymphoplasmacytic lymphoma: Hyperviscosity syndromes 2° IgM secretion (Waldenstrom macroglobulinemia)
- Cutaneous T-cell lymphoma spectrum: Small raised red patches (MF) → plaques, bumps, ulcers → involvement of large areas of skin → entire skin red, peeling (l'homme rouge), LN, bone marrow (Sezary syndrome)

Demographics
- Age: Median age 55 years: Initial diagnosis usually > 50 years
- Gender: M:F = 1.4:1

Natural History & Prognosis
- Indolent lymphomas
  - 20-45% of all lymphomas; median survival ≥ 5 years
  - Treatment often deferred until morbidity occurs
  - Combination chemotherapy usually results in complete or partial response: Relapse rate 10-15%/year
  - Vast majority of relapses occur in first 2 years after Rx
- SLL/CLL
  - Median survival: 10 years
  - 30% progress to higher grade process: Diffuse large cell lymphoma (Richter transformation); prolymphocytic lymphoma
- MALT lymphoma: Plasmacytic differentiation to more aggressive diffuse large B-cell lymphoma
- Follicular lymphomas: Survival inversely proportionate to percentage of large cells
- Low grade lymphomas (Kiel/Lennert)
  - Follicular small cleaved cell (22.5%): Median age 54 years, 70% 5-year survival
  - Follicular mixed (7.7%): Median age 56 years, 50% 5-year survival
  - Small lymphocytic (3.6%): Median age 61 years, 59% 5-year survival

Treatment
- No standard approach to Rx of indolent lymphoma
- Watchful waiting: Indolent lymphomas may be followed with no Rx until B-symptoms develop
- Extended (regional) XRT: To cover adjacent LN prophylactically; often curative in stage I or II; adjunctive in more advanced
- Chemotherapy with XRT
- Tailored therapies: Monoclonal autoantibody therapy for FL ± chemoRx; radioimmunotherapy (e.g., Zevalin or Bexxar)
- Systemic chemoRx: Stem cell transplant allows for higher dose chemoRx
- Investigational therapies: Combinations of antibodies ± radioimmunotherapy; vaccine therapy of FL; immune modulating therapy
- Cutaneous T-cell lymphomas: Topical chemotherapy, UV light for early (limited) stage

DIAGNOSTIC CHECKLIST

Consider
- PET/CT useful for staging FL

Image Interpretation Pearls
- PET/CT: Intense uptake should suggest higher grade transformation, identify site to biopsy

SELECTED REFERENCES

1. Alinari L et al: 18F-FDG PET in mucosa-associated lymphoid tissue (MALT) lymphoma. Leuk Lymphoma. 47(10):2096-101, 2006
2. Bruzzi JF et al: Detection of Richter's transformation of chronic lymphocytic leukemia by PET/CT. J Nucl Med. 47(8):1267-73, 2006
3. Hoffmann M et al: 18F-Fluoro-deoxy-glucose positron emission tomography in lymphoma of mucosa-associated lymphoid tissue: histology makes the difference. Ann Oncol. 17(12):1761-5, 2006
4. Karam M et al: Role of fluorine-18 fluoro-deoxyglucose positron emission tomography scan in the evaluation and follow-up of patients with low-grade lymphomas. Cancer. 107(1):175-83, 2006
5. Kumar R et al: 18F-fluorodeoxyglucose-positron emission tomography in evaluation of primary cutaneous lymphoma. Br J Dermatol. 155(2):357-63, 2006
6. Tsai EY et al: Staging accuracy in mycosis fungoides and sezary syndrome using integrated positron emission tomography and computed tomography. Arch Dermatol. 142(5):577-84, 2006
7. Wohrer S et al: 18F-fluoro-deoxy-glucose positron emission tomography (18F-FDG-PET) visualizes follicular lymphoma irrespective of grading. Ann Oncol. 17(5):780-4, 2006
8. Beal KP et al: FDG-PET scanning for detection and staging of extranodal marginal zone lymphomas of the MALT type: a report of 42 cases. Ann Oncol. 16(3):473-80, 2005
9. Blum RH et al: Frequent impact of [18F]fluorodeoxyglucose positron emission tomography on the staging and management of patients with indolent non-Hodgkin's lymphoma. Clin Lymphoma. 4(1):43-9, 2003
10. Hoffmann M et al: 18F-fluorodeoxyglucose positron emission tomography (18F-FDG-PET) for staging and follow-up of marginal zone B-cell lymphoma. Oncology. 64(4):336-40, 2003
11. Jerusalem GH et al: Positron emission tomography in non-Hodgkin's lymphoma (NHL): relationship between tracer uptake and pathological findings, including preliminary experience in the staging of low-grade NHL. Clin Lymphoma. 3(1):56-61, 2002
12. Jerusalem G et al: Positron emission tomography (PET) with 18F-fluorodeoxyglucose (18F-FDG) for the staging of low-grade non-Hodgkin's lymphoma (NHL). Ann Oncol. 12(6):825-30, 2001
13. Hoffmann M et al: Positron emission tomography with fluorine-18-2-fluoro-2-deoxy-D-glucose (F18-FDG) does not visualize extranodal B-cell lymphoma of the mucosa-associated lymphoid tissue (MALT)-type. Ann Oncol. 10(10):1185-9, 1999
14. Rodriguez M et al: Predicting malignancy grade with PET in non-Hodgkin's lymphoma. J Nucl Med. 36(10):1790-6, 1995
15. Okada J et al: FDG-PET for predicting the prognosis of malignant lymphoma. Ann Nucl Med. 8(3):187-91, 1994

NON-HODGKIN LYMPHOMAS, LOW GRADE

IMAGE GALLERY

Typical

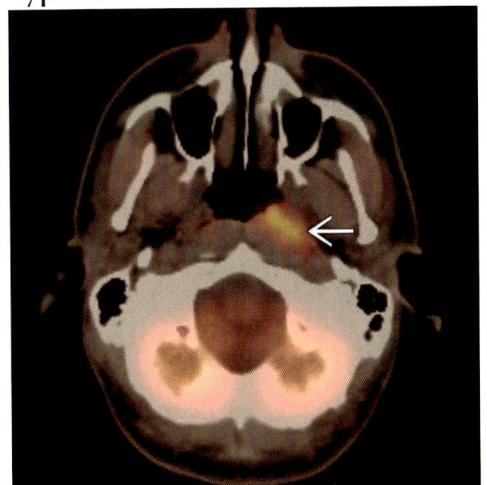

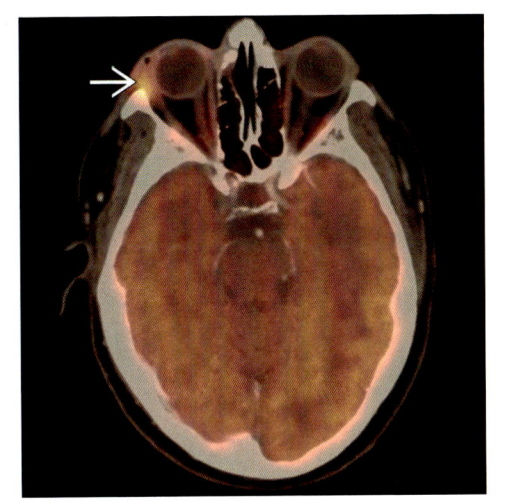

(Left) Axial PET CT shows enlarged, hypermetabolic tissue of left eustachian tube ➡. Initially thought inflammatory, biopsy subsequently showed MALT lymphoma. *(Right)* Axial PET CT shows low FDG uptake in an enlarged right lacrimal gland ➡, biopsy proven extranodal marginal zone lymphoma. Magnitude of uptake is typical for MZL.

Variant

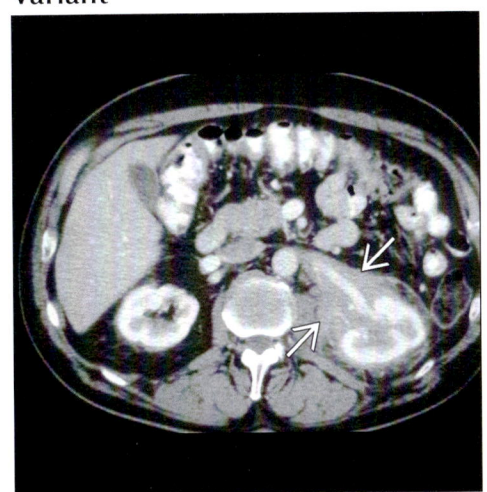

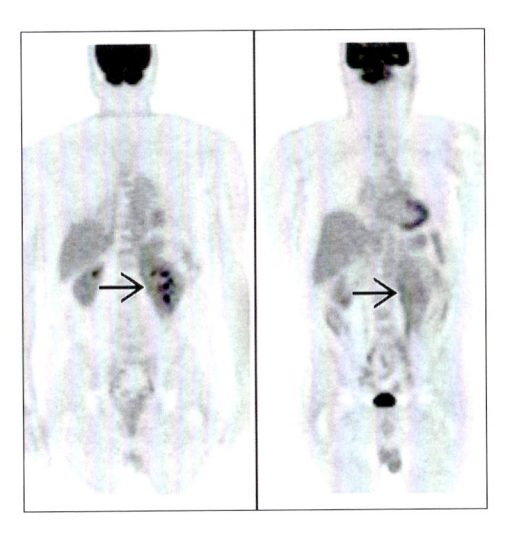

(Left) Axial CECT shows a left perirenal mass ➡ encasing (not compressing) the left renal pelvis and vessels. See next image. (Courtesy A. Malouf, MD). *(Right)* Coronal PET in same patient as left shows relatively low level FDG uptake in left perirenal mass ➡, biopsy proven low grade MALT lymphoma. Low level uptake is typical of MALT tumors. (Courtesy A. Malouf, MD).

Typical

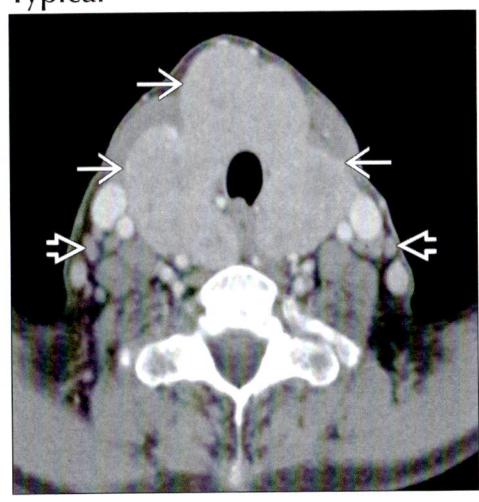

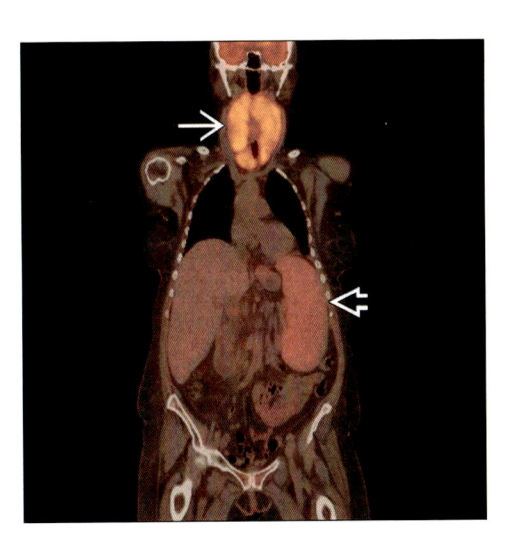

(Left) Axial CECT shows diffusely enlarged thyroid gland ➡, numerous mildly enlarged cervical LNs ➡ in patient with history of low grade MALT lymphoma of thyroid. See next image. *(Right)* Axial fused PET/CT in same patient as left shows intense metabolic activity in markedly enlarged thyroid ➡ and spleen ➡. Biopsy confirmed transformation to more aggressive tumor (diffuse large B-cell lymphoma).

NON-HODGKIN LYMPHOMA STAGING

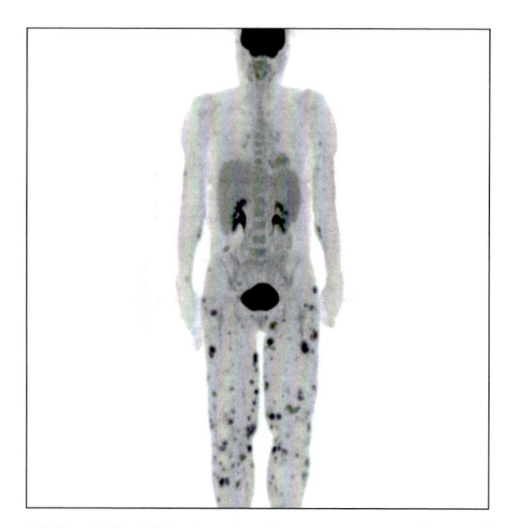

FDG PET MIP image demonstrates widespread dermal/subcutaneous tumor deposits in a patient with peripheral T-cell NHL. See next image.

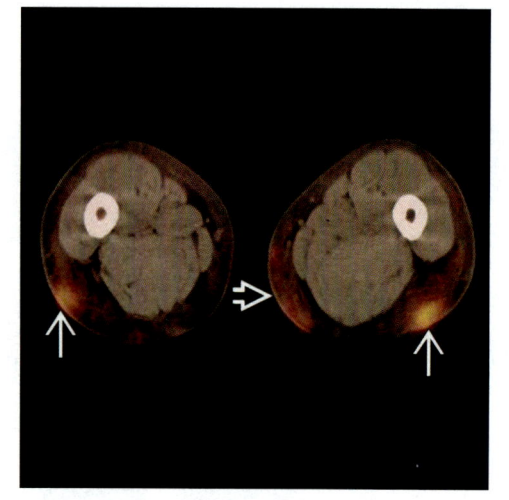

Axial FDG PET/CT in the same patient as previous, through the mid-thighs, shows multiple, subcutaneous, hypermetabolic nodules ➡ and diffuse, hazy hypermetabolism ➡ in peripheral T-cell NHL.

TERMINOLOGY

Abbreviations and Synonyms
- Non-Hodgkin lymphoma (NHL)

Definitions
- NHL: Malignancy of B or T lymphocytes

IMAGING FINDINGS

General Features
- Best diagnostic clue: Enlarged/unenlarged FDG-avid nodes, liver or spleen; "misty mesentery"
- Location
  - Superior mediastinal, paraaortic nodes common
  - NHL less predictable spread than HD
  - Spleen: Nodal in HD, extranodal in NHL

Nuclear Medicine Findings
- FDG PET or Ga-67: ↑ Uptake in nodal, extranodal tissue; ↓ sensitivity in ↓ grade NHL, MALT lymphoma

Imaging Recommendations
- Best imaging tool
  - PET/CT preferred for staging NHL over other modalities
  - Sens/spec nodal: PET/CT 91/90%, CT 88/86%
  - Sens/spec extranodal: PET/CT 88/100%, CT 50/90%
  - Ga-67: 59% sens; spec comparable to CT, PET
- Protocol advice
  - Stage with PET/CT before any therapy is administered: One dose of chemotherapy may ↓ FDG uptake
  - Ga-67: High dose (10 mCi adults); initial imaging at 3 d; imaging 5-7 d as needed (optional bowel prep); SPECT chest & abdomen
  - Clinical information regarding other imaging findings, symptoms, intercurrent or recent infection, surgery, etc. critical for both Ga-67 or FDG PET

DIFFERENTIAL DIAGNOSIS

Infection/Inflammation
- Inflammation, infection, granulomatous

Normal Structures
- Thymus, salivary glands, muscle, tonsils

DDx: Benign Mimics of NHL

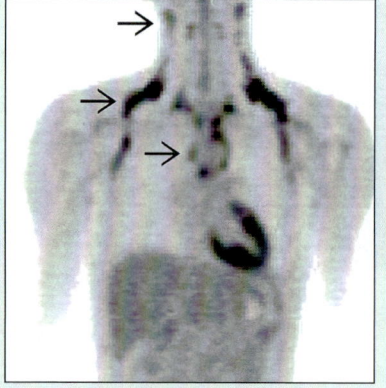

Hypermetabolic Brown Fat 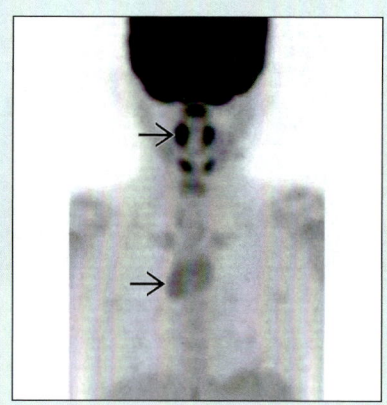 | Thymus, Tonsils 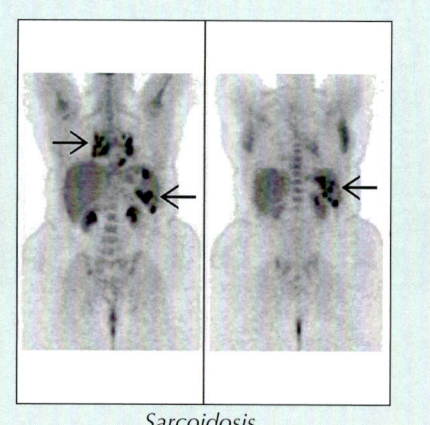 | Sarcoidosis

NON-HODGKIN LYMPHOMA STAGING

Terminology
- NHL: Malignancy of B or T lymphocytes

Imaging Findings
- NHL less predictable spread than HD
- Spleen: Nodal in HD, extranodal in NHL
- Sens/spec nodal: PET/CT 91/90%, CT 88/86%
- Sens/spec extranodal: PET/CT 88/100%, CT 50/90%
- Ga-67: 59% sens; spec comparable to CT, PET

Pathology
- Etiology: Unknown in most patients
- Epidemiology: NHL incidence ↑ 75% x 20 y; ↑ mortality
- Ann Arbor classification: Anatomic extent of disease in HD & NHL

Key Facts
- International Prognostic Index (IPI): Independent statistically significant pre-treatment risk factors

Clinical Issues
- > 90% NHL occurs in adults: Risk increases with age
- Prognosis depends on histologic type, stage and Rx
- Overall 5 y survival is ~ 50% to 60% with modern Rx
- Vast majority of relapses occur in first 2 y after Rx

Diagnostic Checklist
- Localized uptake to an unusual site may represent NHL: Infection/inflammation must be excluded
- Staging FDG PET must be done prior to initiation of any therapy: Even one dose of chemotherapy may decrease sensitivity

PATHOLOGY

General Features
- Etiology: Unknown in most patients
- Epidemiology: NHL incidence ↑ 75% x 20 y; ↑ mortality

Microscopic Features
- T- or B-cell clonality: No Reed-Sternberg cells
- FNA is diagnostic in NHL

Staging, Grading or Classification Criteria
- Clinical staging: Includes history & physical examination, imaging the chest, abdomen & pelvis, blood count, chemistry, bone marrow biopsy
- Pathologic staging: Staging laparotomy & pathologic staging are out of vogue
- REAL/WHO classification: Revised European-American Classification of Lymphoid Neoplasms (REAL), adopted by World Health Org. (WHO)
  - Distinct disease entities defined by combination of morphology, immunophenotype & genetic features, distinct clinical features
  - Relative importance of features varies by disease: There is no "gold standard"
  - Includes all lymphoid neoplasms: HD, NHL, lymphoid leukemias & plasma cell neoplasms
  - Lymphomas & lymphoid leukemias included because solid + circulating phases are present in many lymphoid neoplasms
  - Different manifestations, same neoplasm: B-cell chronic lymphocytic leukemia (CLL) & small B-cell lymphocytic lymphoma (SLL); lymphoblastic lymphomas & acute lymphoblastic leukemias (ALL)
  - HD & plasma cell myeloma are both lymphoid neoplasms of B-lineage belonging to a compilation of lymphoid neoplasms
- REAL/WHO classification of B-cell neoplasms
  - Precursor B-cell neoplasm: Precursor B-lymphoblastic leukemia/lymphoma (precursor B-cell acute lymphoblastic leukemia)
  - Mature (peripheral) B-cell neoplasms
    - B-cell CLL/small lymphocytic lymphoma (SLL); B-cell prolymphocytic leukemia
    - Lymphoplasmacytic lymphoma; splenic marginal zone B-cell lymphoma
    - Hairy cell leukemia; plasma cell myeloma/plasmacytoma
    - Marginal zone B-cell/mucosal associated lymphoid tissue (MALT) lymphoma
    - Nodal marginal zone B-cell lymphoma; follicular lymphoma; mantle cell lymphoma
    - Diffuse large B-cell lymphoma; Burkitt lymphoma/Burkitt cell leukemia
- REAL/WHO classification of T-cell and natural killer (NK)-cell neoplasms: Account for 10-15% of NHL
  - Precursor T-cell neoplasm: Precursor T-lymphoblastic lymphoma/leukemia (precursor T-cell ALL)
  - Mature (peripheral) T/NK-cell neoplasms
    - T-cell prolymphocytic leukemia; T-cell granular lymphocytic leukemia; aggressive NK-cell leukemia
    - Adult T-cell lymphoma/leukemia (HTLV1+); extranodal NK/T-cell lymphoma, nasal type
    - Enteropathy-type T-cell lymphoma; hepatosplenic T-cell lymphoma; subcutaneous panniculitis-like T-cell lymphoma
    - Mycosis fungoides/Sézary syndrome; anaplastic large cell lymphoma, T/null cell, primary cutaneous type
    - Peripheral T-cell lymphoma, not otherwise characterized; angioimmunoblastic T-cell lymphoma
    - Anaplastic large cell lymphoma, T/null cell, primary systemic type
- Ann Arbor classification: Anatomic extent of disease in HD & NHL
  - Stage 1: Single LN region (I); or localized involvement of a single extralymphatic site in the absence of LN involvement (IE) (rare in HD)

NON-HODGKIN LYMPHOMA STAGING

- Stage 2: ≥2 LN regions, same side of diaphragm (II); or single extralymphatic site with regional LN ± other LN stations, same side of diaphragm (IIE)
- Stage 3: LN regions, both sides of diaphragm (III); may have extralymphatic extension with adjacent LNs (IIIE) or + spleen (IIIS) or both (IIIE,S)
- Stage 4: Diffuse or disseminated dz. in ≥ 1 extralymphatic organ, ± LN; or isolated extralymphatic organ w/o regional LN with distant dz.; any liver, bone marrow, lung nodules
- Presence or absence of systemic symptoms; A = asymptomatic, B = B-symptoms
- Anatomic disease extent: One prognostic factor in NHL
- The NHL prognostic factors of the International Prognostic Index used for Rx decisions along with histologic cell type
- Additional factors reported to affect outcomes in preliminary studies include tumor beta-2 microglobulin & S-phase fraction
- **International Prognostic Index (IPI):** Independent statistically significant pre-treatment risk factors
  - Age (60 vs. > 60 years); Ann Arbor stage III or IV (advanced), serum LDH (normal vs. abnormal), reduced performance status (0 or 1 vs. > 2), extranodal sites of disease (1 vs. > 1)
  - Patients are assigned to 1 of 4 risk groups on the basis of presenting risk factors: Low (0 or 1); low intermediate (2); high intermediate (3); high (4, 5)
  - Outcomes: 87% complete response, 73% 5-year survival in low risk patients; 44% complete response, 26% survival rate in high risk patients

CLINICAL ISSUES

Presentation
- Most common signs/symptoms: Asymptomatic: Loss of appetite, fatigue, enlarged LN, flu-like symptoms
- Other signs/symptoms
  - Pruritus: Painful LN after drinking alcohol, cough
  - B-symptoms: Unexplained persistent fever & chills, night sweats, fatigue, pruritus, weight loss
  - B-symptoms are more common in aggressive (47%) than in indolent lymphoma (25%)

Demographics
- Age
  - Median age 55 years: Initial diagnosis usually > 50 y
  - > 90% NHL occurs in adults: Risk increases with age
- Gender: 1.4:1 (M:F)

Natural History & Prognosis
- Prognosis depends on histologic type, stage and Rx
- Two prognostic groups: Indolent and aggressive
  - Indolent NHL: Relatively good prognosis, median survival up to 10 y, but usually not curable
  - Aggressive: 30% to 60% can be cured
- Overall 5 y survival is ~ 50% to 60% with modern Rx
- Vast majority of relapses occur in first 2 y after Rx
- Risk of late relapse is > in patients with a divergent histology of both indolent and aggressive disease

Treatment
- Watchful waiting: Indolent lymphomas may be followed with no Rx until B-symptoms
- Can Rx early (stage I, II) indolent NHL with deep X-ray therapy (XRT) alone
- Extended (regional) radiation Rx to cover adjacent LN prophylactically may be curative in stage I or II, or as adjunct in more advanced
- Tailored Rx: Monoclonal autoantibodies ± radioligand (follicular lymphoma)
- Aggressive NHL has a shorter natural history, but significant number of patients can be cured with intensive combination chemoRx
- Systemic chemoRx: Stem cell transplant allows for higher dose chemoRx
- Chemotherapy + XRT

DIAGNOSTIC CHECKLIST

Consider
- Localized uptake to an unusual site may represent NHL: Infection/inflammation must be excluded

Image Interpretation Pearls
- Staging FDG PET must be done prior to initiation of any therapy: Even one dose of chemotherapy may decrease sensitivity

SELECTED REFERENCES

1. Armitage JO et al: Lymphoma 2006: classification and treatment. Oncology (Williston Park). 20(3):231-9; discussion 242, 244, 249, 2006
2. Jhanwar YS et al: The role of PET in lymphoma. J Nucl Med. 47(8):1326-34, 2006
3. Meignan M et al: Value of [18F]fluorodeoxyglucose-positron emission tomography in managing patients with aggressive non-Hodgkin's lymphoma. Clin Lymphoma Myeloma. 6(4):306-13, 2006
4. Raanani P et al: Is CT scan still necessary for staging in Hodgkin and non-Hodgkin lymphoma patients in the PET/CT era? Ann Oncol. 17(1):117-22, 2006
5. Roe RH et al: Whole-body positron emission tomography/computed tomography imaging and staging of orbital lymphoma. Ophthalmology. 113(10):1854-8, 2006
6. Isasi CR et al: A metaanalysis of 18F-2-deoxy-2-fluoro-D-glucose positron emission tomography in the staging and restaging of patients with lymphoma. Cancer. 104(5):1066-74, 2005
7. Burton C et al: The role of PET imaging in lymphoma. Br J Haematol. 126(6):772-84, 2004
8. Kumar R et al: Utility of fluorodeoxyglucose-PET imaging in the management of patients with Hodgkin's and non-Hodgkin's lymphomas. Radiol Clin North Am. 42(6):1083-100, 2004
9. Yamamoto F et al: 18F-FDG PET is superior to 67Ga SPECT in the staging of non-Hodgkin's lymphoma. Ann Nucl Med. 18(6):519-26, 2004
10. Schiepers C et al: PET for staging of Hodgkin's disease and non-Hodgkin's lymphoma. Eur J Nucl Med Mol Imaging. 30 Suppl 1:S82-8, 2003

NON-HODGKIN LYMPHOMA STAGING

IMAGE GALLERY

Variant

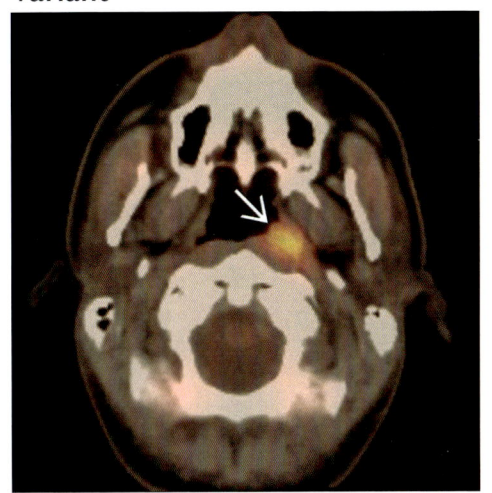

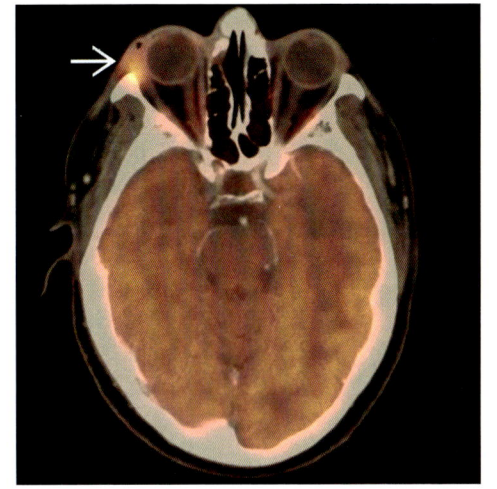

(Left) Axial FDG PET/CT shows a mass and hypermetabolism involving the left eustachian tube ➡. Biopsy proven mucosal-associated lymphoid tissue (MALT) lymphoma (stage I). (Right) Axial FDG PET/CT shows focal uptake and enlargement of right lacrimal gland ➡ in a patient with biopsy proven NHL of the lacrimal gland (stage I).

Typical

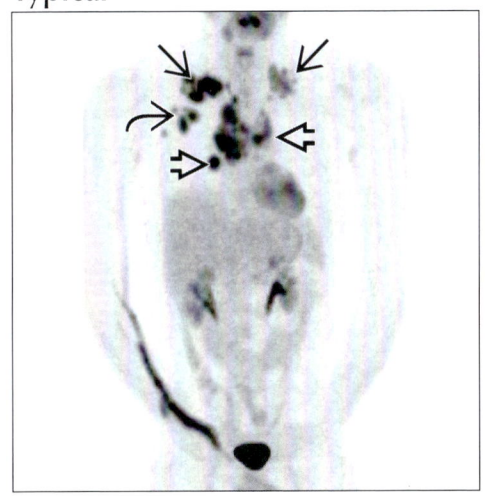

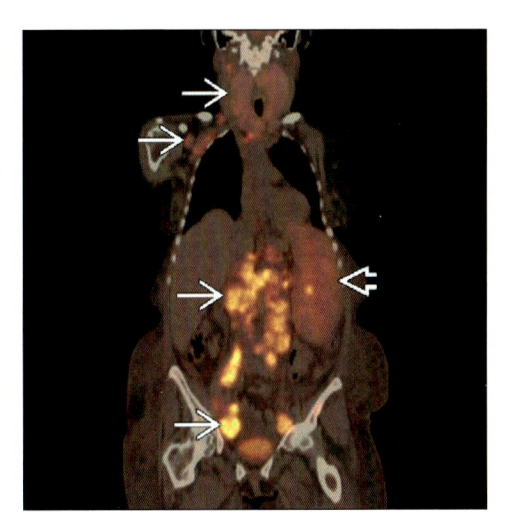

(Left) Coronal FDG PET/CT shows tumor involving supraclavicular ➡, deep axillary ➡, and hilar/mediastinal ➡ lymph nodes in a patient with stage II NHL. Linear uptake in right arm is due to extravasation of tracer at injection. (Right) Coronal FDG PET/CT shows extensive disease ➡ in the neck (including thyroid), supraclavicular region, axilla, abdomen, pelvis, spleen ➡. Represents stage IV NHL (thyroid and spleen are extranodal).

Variant

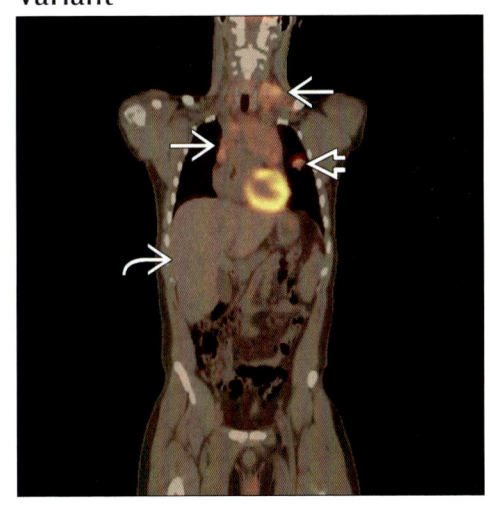

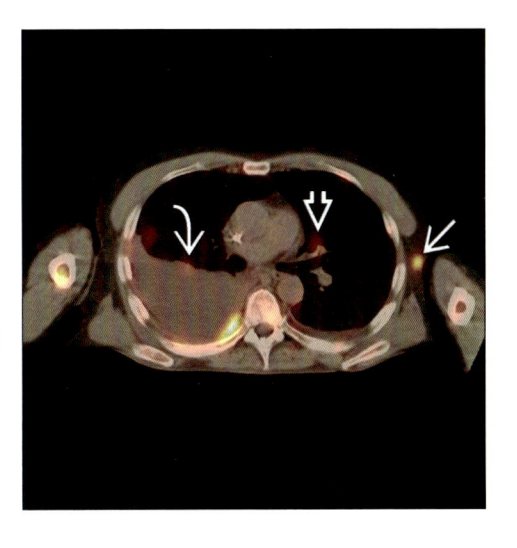

(Left) Coronal FDG PET/CT shows enlarged FDG-avid mediastinal, supraclavicular & cervical LNs ➡ & a lung lesion ➡ in a patient with NHL. Diffuse liver hypermetabolism ➡ & mild hepatomegaly suggests liver involvement (biopsy required if diffuse). Lung or liver involvement = stage IV. (Right) Axial FDG PET/CT in a patient with NHL shows a tumor involving the bone, pleura ➡, axillary ➡ & left hilar ➡ lymph nodes. Bone (> 1 site) or marrow involvement = stage IV.

MELANOMA STAGING

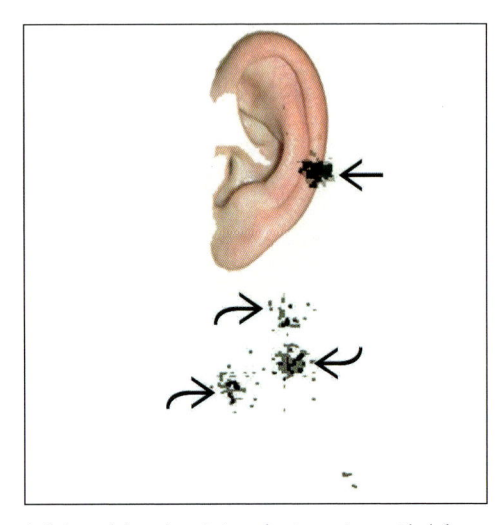

Left lateral lymphoscintigraphy in patient with left ear melanoma shows injection site ⇒ and sentinel lymph nodes ⇒ in left neck.

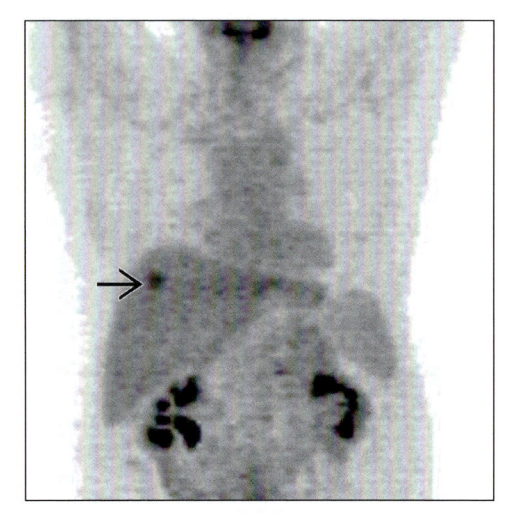

3D PET in patient with melanoma shows focus of increased activity in liver ⇒, consistent with metastasis.

TERMINOLOGY

Definitions
- Melanoma: Neoplasm of melanin-producing cells
- American Joint Committee on Cancer staging system
  - IA
    - < 1 mm thick, no ulceration/invasion
  - IB
    - < 1 mm thick, + ulceration/invasion
    - > 1 and < 2 mm thick, no ulceration/invasion
  - IIA
    - > 1 and < 2 mm thick, + ulceration/invasion
    - > 2 and < 4 mm thick, no ulceration
  - IIB
    - > 2 and < 4 mm thick, + ulceration
    - > 4 mm, no ulceration
  - IIC
    - > 4 mm, + ulceration
  - IIIA
    - 1-3 + lymph nodes (microscopic), no ulceration
  - IIIB
    - 1-3 + lymph nodes (microscopic), + ulceration
    - 1-3 + lymph nodes (macroscopic), no ulceration
  - IIIC
    - 1-3 + lymph nodes (macroscopic), + ulceration
    - ≥ 4 + lymph nodes, matted nodes, in-transit metastases with + lymph node
  - IV
    - Distant metastases
- Local staging by histologic analysis of tumor thickness, anatomic invasion
- Regional lymph node staging by surgical lymphadenectomy (sentinel lymph node)
- Distant staging by clinical exam, laboratory tests, imaging
  - Whole-body: PET, CECT
  - Brain: MR

IMAGING FINDINGS

General Features
- Best diagnostic clue
  - Lymph node metastases
    - Histopathological confirmation at sentinel lymph node biopsy
  - Extranodal metastases, large (> 1-2 cm) lymphadenopathy

DDx: Mimics of Melanoma on FDG PET

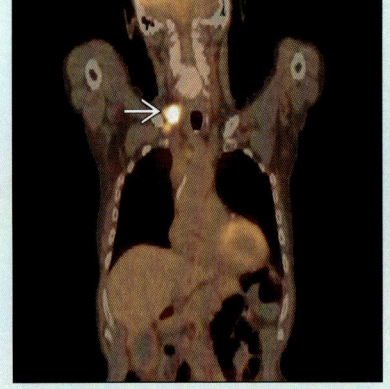

Other Malignancy (Lymphoma)

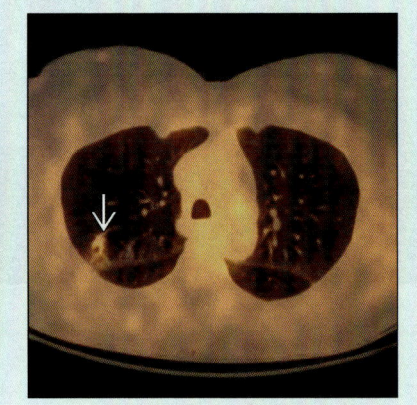

Pulmonary Infection

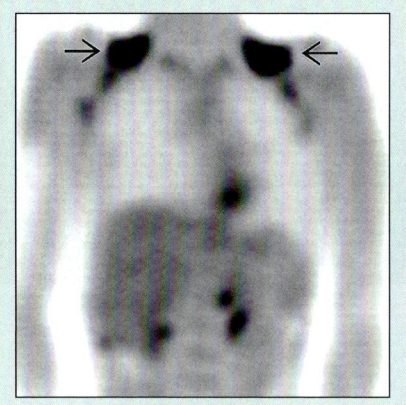

Brown Fat

MELANOMA STAGING

Key Facts

Terminology
- Local staging by histologic analysis of tumor thickness, anatomic invasion
- Regional lymph node staging by surgical lymphadenectomy (sentinel lymph node)
- Distant staging by clinical exam, laboratory tests, imaging

Imaging Findings
- Tc-99m sulfur colloid sentinel lymph node mapping and biopsy
- FDG PET for distant metastases
- CECT for small pulmonary metastases
- MR for brain metastases

Top Differential Diagnoses
- Other Neoplasms
- Inflammation/Infection
- Brown Fat

Clinical Issues
- Surgical treatment even for distant metastatic disease
- External beam radiation, interferon and vaccines are being used
- Poor response to chemotherapy

Diagnostic Checklist
- As always with FDG PET, normal physiologic and benign causes of ↑ activity must be excluded
- Both primary lesion and post-biopsy site can be positive on PET
- Attenuation correction can smooth peripheral data: Evaluate non-attenuation corrected PET images to survey skin

---

- FDG PET: Focal increased uptake in lymph node bed, soft tissue, organs
- CECT: Evident in lymph node bed, soft tissues, organs
- Location
  - Primary melanoma
    - Men: Most frequently skin of trunk
    - Women: Most frequently skin of upper extremities
    - 4-5% extracutaneous (mucous membranes of digestive, genitourinary, respiratory tracts; eyes; cerebral meninges)
  - In-transit nodal metastases
    - Between primary and regional lymph nodes
  - Lymph node metastases
    - Most commonly metastasizes to regional lymph nodes
  - Extranodal metastases to almost any organ, including unusual sites
    - Spine, lung, liver, spleen, bowel common
- Morphology
  - Metastatic lymph nodes
    - Round, no fatty hilum on CT

Imaging Recommendations
- Best imaging tool
  - Tc-99m sulfur colloid sentinel lymph node mapping and biopsy
    - Lymphoscintigraphy directs surgeon to appropriate lymph node basin for sentinel lymph node biopsy
    - Staging and detection of occult lymph node metastases
    - Recommended for tumors > 1 mm or 0.76-1 mm in presence of ulceration, reticular dermal invasion
    - FDG PET insensitive for micrometastases
  - FDG PET for distant metastases
    - Insensitive for micrometastatic disease, small lung nodules
    - Sensitivity 23% if metastases ≤ 5 mm
    - Sensitivity ≥ 90% if ≥ 1 cm
    - If stage I or II, FDG PET not sensitive for detection of lymph node metastases
    - Best indicated for ≥ stage III disease
    - Large metaanalysis: Sensitivity 83%, specificity 91% for staging
    - Changes management in ≥ 26% of patients
    - Less sensitive than MR for brain metastases
    - Reimbursable by Medicare for evaluation of extranodal metastases during initial staging
    - Not reimbursable by Medicare for evaluation of regional lymph nodes
  - CECT for small pulmonary metastases
  - MR for brain metastases
- Protocol advice
  - Tc-99m sulfur colloid sentinel lymph node mapping and biopsy
    - 1.0 mCi (37 MBq) Tc-99m sulfur colloid injected intradermally around primary melanoma
    - Imaging of all adjacent lymph node basins to determine sentinel lymph node location
    - Note: Head-and-neck and truncal melanomas may have aberrant drainage
    - Can have 2 or more sentinel lymph node basins
  - FDG PET
    - Evaluation of skin best with non-attenuation corrected emission PET
    - Incidence of multiple primary melanomas from 1.3-8%
    - Consider extending scan to include entire body (vertex to feet)
    - Clinical history crucial: False + with recent surgery, biopsy, inflammation
- Additional nuclear medicine imaging options
  - Tc-99m MDP bone scan
    - For regionally advanced disease
    - Whole body bone scan usually not helpful unless clinical suspicion of bone metastases
  - Ga-67 SPECT
    - Uncommon today
    - FDG PET superior to Ga-67 SPECT 2° resolution
- Correlative imaging features
  - Confirm positive PET with anatomic imaging
    - In retrospect, metastatic lymph node often present on CECT

MELANOMA STAGING

- Bone, liver, or spleen metastases may not be detectable on CT

DIFFERENTIAL DIAGNOSIS

Other Neoplasms
- Benign or malignant neoplasms can show ↑ activity
- Especially if low clinical suspicion of recurrence
  - Metastases from second primary
  - Other skin carcinomas including squamous or basal cell
  - Consider lymphoma if multiple enlarged lymph nodes

Inflammation/Infection
- With PET/CT scan, false positive lung nodule can be due to infection or inflammation
- Granulomatous infection can ⇒ enlarged, hypermetabolic lymph nodes
  - Mycobacterium avium intracellulare
  - Tuberculosis
  - Sarcoid
- Reactive lymph nodes
  - Look for other causes of enlarged reactive lymph nodes on CT such as colitis, pancreatitis, pneumonia

Brown Fat
- Warming maneuvers may ↓

PATHOLOGY

General Features
- Genetics
  - Family history = risk factor
    - Associated with germline mutations
    - If familial, may appear at early age
- Etiology
  - Due to proliferation of transformed melanocytes
  - UV radiation exposure causally related
- Epidemiology: ~ 100,000 cases diagnosed per year in US
- Associated abnormalities: May have bleeding or itching of primary skin lesion

Gross Pathologic & Surgical Features
- Primary melanoma
  - Asymmetric
  - Irregular border
  - Color variation
  - Diameter ≥ 6 mm
  - Changes over time

Microscopic Features
- Large atypical melanocytes

CLINICAL ISSUES

Presentation
- Most common signs/symptoms
  - Relative risk association of a changing mole with melanoma estimated at 400%
  - Metastatic lymph nodes ± palpable
- Other signs/symptoms
  - History of recurrent sunburn increases risk
  - Increased risk if previous history of skin cancer, including nonmelanoma

Demographics
- Age
  - One of more common cancers in 20-40 year olds
  - Mean age 55 years
  - In US, 1-4% of all melanomas occur in patients ≤ 20 years old
- Gender: Probably slightly more common in males
- Ethnicity: More common if fair skin

Natural History & Prognosis
- Tumor thickness = most important histologic prognostic indicator
- Number and clinically apparent metastatic lymph nodes associated with worse prognosis
- Nonvisceral metastases associated with better prognosis than visceral metastases

Treatment
- Surgical treatment even for distant metastatic disease
- External beam radiation, interferon and vaccines are being used
- Poor response to chemotherapy

DIAGNOSTIC CHECKLIST

Consider
- As always with FDG PET, normal physiologic and benign causes of ↑ activity must be excluded
- Both primary lesion and post-biopsy site can be positive on PET

Image Interpretation Pearls
- Attenuation correction can smooth peripheral data: Evaluate non-attenuation corrected PET images to survey skin

SELECTED REFERENCES

1. Belhocine TZ et al: Role of nuclear medicine in the management of cutaneous malignant melanoma. J Nucl Med. 47(6):957-67, 2006
2. Clark PB et al: Futility of fluorodeoxyglucose F 18 positron emission tomography in initial evaluation of patients with T2 to T4 melanoma. Arch Surg. 141(3):284-8, 2006
3. Wagner JD et al: Inefficacy of F-18 fluorodeoxy-D-glucose-positron emission tomography scans for initial evaluation in early-stage cutaneous melanoma. Cancer. 104(3):570-9, 2005
4. Fuster D et al: Is 18F-FDG PET more accurate than standard diagnostic procedures in the detection of suspected recurrent melanoma? J Nucl Med. 45(8):1323-7, 2004
5. Gulec SA et al: The role of fluorine-18 deoxyglucose positron emission tomography in the management of patients with metastatic melanoma: impact on surgical decision making. Clin Nucl Med. 28(12):961-5, 2003
6. Crippa F et al: Which kinds of lymph node metastases can FDG PET detect? A clinical study in melanoma. J Nucl Med. 41(9):1491-4, 2000

MELANOMA STAGING

IMAGE GALLERY

Typical

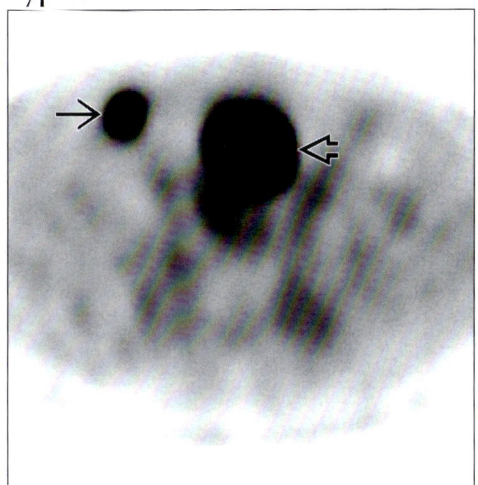

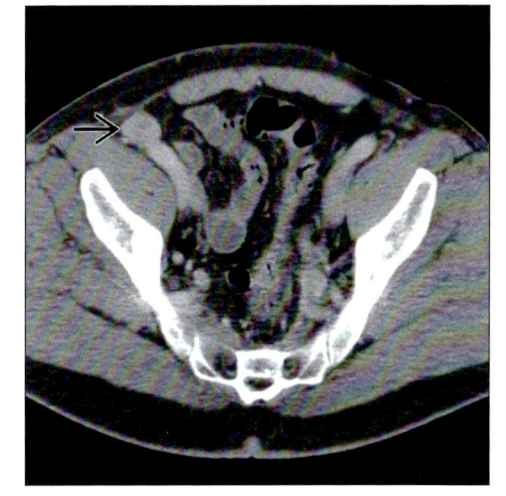

(Left) Axial PET shows lymphadenopathy ➡ in right inguinal region in patient with primary lower extremity melanoma. Normal bladder ⊳. See next image. (Right) Axial CECT shows 2 cm right inguinal lymph node ➡ which prospectively was missed on CECT, likely mistaken for adjacent small bowel.

Typical

(Left) Coronal PET shows focus of increased activity ➡ in cutaneous tissues of scalp vertex, the site of known primary melanoma. (Right) Axial fused PET/CT shows increased activity in bilateral positive neck lymph nodes ➡ in patient with primary scalp melanoma.

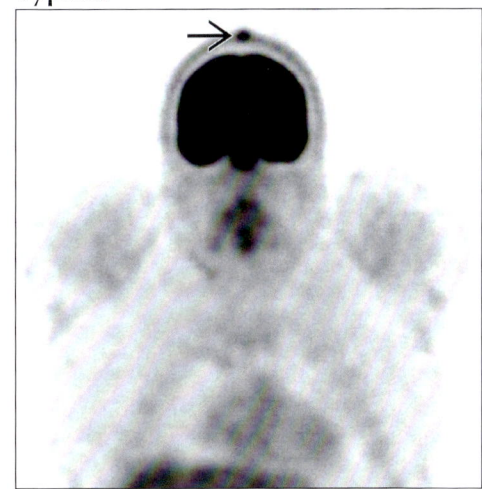

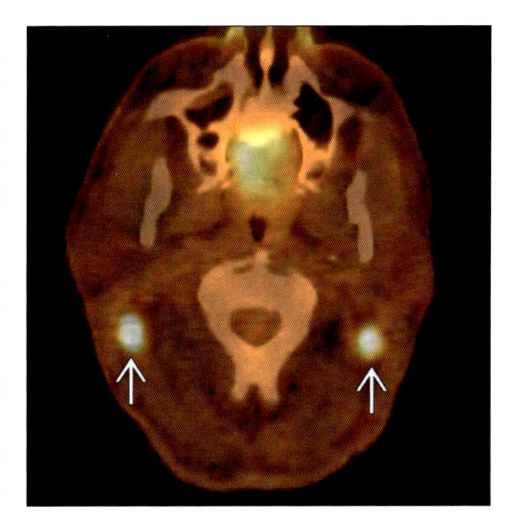

Variant

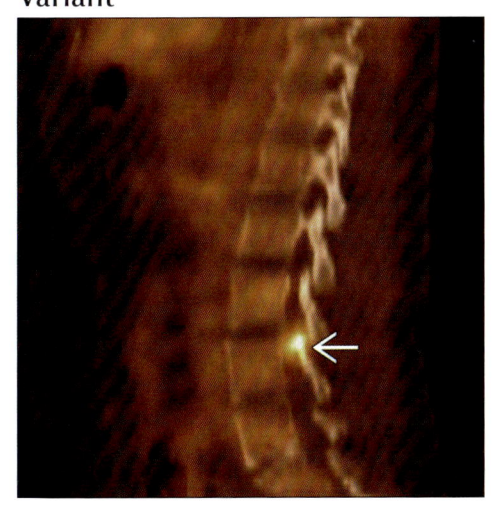

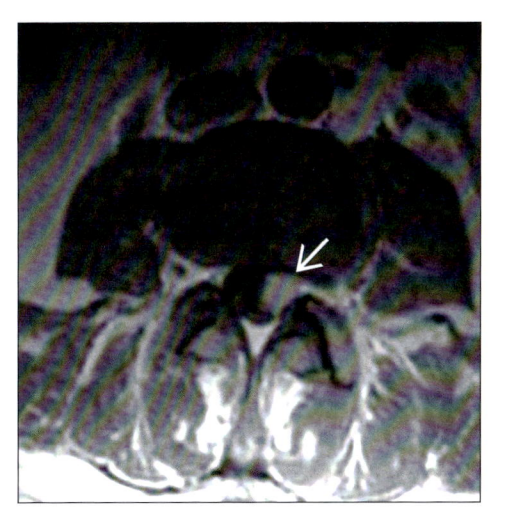

(Left) Axial fused PET/CT shows increased activity ➡ in an epidural lesion in patient with truncal melanoma and low back pain. See next image. (Right) Axial contrast-enhanced MR shows the left L4-5 epidural lesion ➡, pathologically confirmed as metastatic melanoma.

MELANOMA THERAPY EVAL./RESTAGING

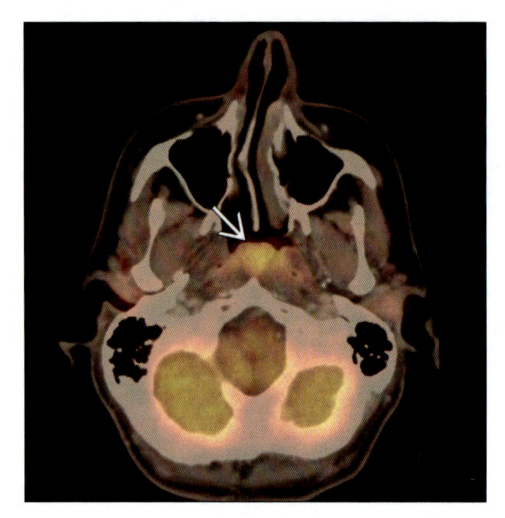

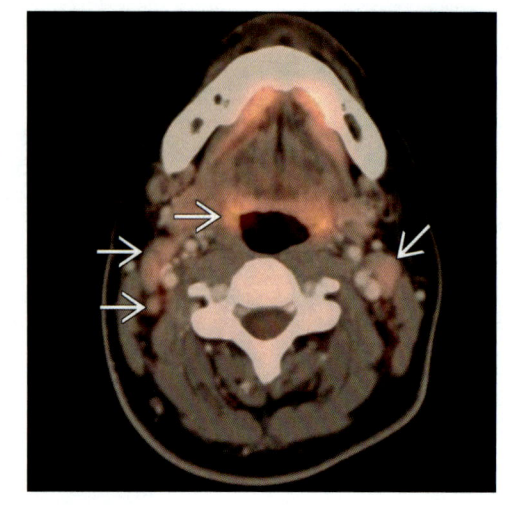

PET/CT following cytokine therapy for high risk melanoma shows increased uptake in adenoid tissue ➡. See next image.

Axial PET/CT after cytokine therapy shows increased uptake in cervical nodes ➡. Cytokine therapy (interferon, interleukin-2) results in stimulation, of lymphoid tissue which resolves over time.

TERMINOLOGY

Definitions
- Melanoma therapy evaluation: Assess response to treatment
- Melanoma restaging: Detect recurrent tumor

IMAGING FINDINGS

General Features
- Best diagnostic clue
  - Focally increased uptake on FDG PET
    - Satellite skin lesions, lymph nodes, visceral organs, bone
  - Exclude FDG uptake due to normal structure or inflammatory condition
  - Confirmation with anatomic correlation
- Location
  - Locally
    - More likely to be in patients originally with stage I or II
    - Can arise at or near previous excision site
    - Clinical history important to distinguish tumor from recent biopsy site/inflammation
    - May further stage with sentinel node resection
  - Regional lymph nodes
    - More likely in patients originally with stage I or II
  - Distant metastases
    - More likely in patients originally with stage III or IV
    - Can occur almost anywhere
    - More common sites of distant metastases: Bone, lung, liver, spleen, bowel
- Therapy evaluation
  - Few studies published regarding evaluation of response to therapy in melanoma
  - Baseline FDG PET very helpful for evaluating response to therapy
  - FDG PET pitfall: Cytokine therapy results in diffuse hypermetabolism in normal lymph nodes for months

Imaging Recommendations
- Best imaging tool
  - Combination of FDG PET and conventional imaging (CT/MR) more accurate than either one alone

DDx: Abnormal FDG Activity in Melanoma Patients

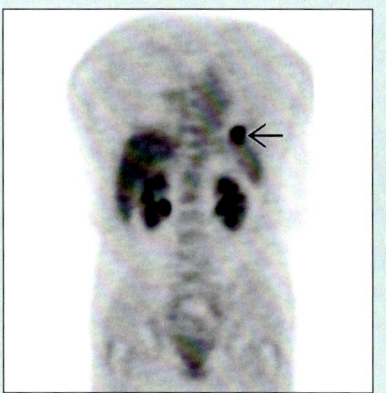

Other Malignancy: Lung

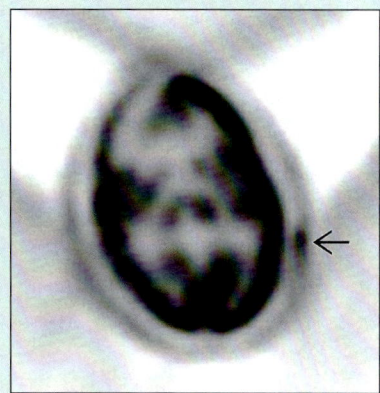

Skin Inflammation

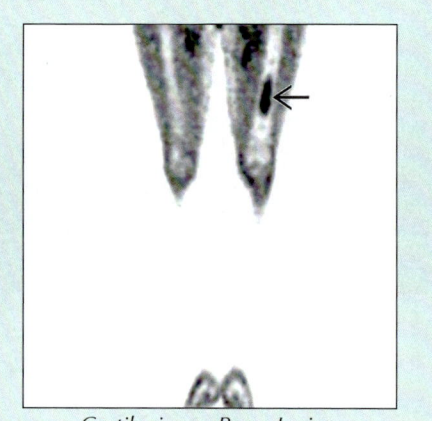

Cartilaginous Bone Lesion

MELANOMA THERAPY EVAL./RESTAGING

Key Facts

Terminology
- Melanoma therapy evaluation: Assess response to treatment
- Melanoma restaging: Detect recurrent tumor

Imaging Findings
- Focally increased uptake on FDG PET
- Exclude FDG uptake due to normal structure or inflammatory condition
- More common sites of distant metastases: Bone, lung, liver, spleen, bowel
- Baseline FDG PET very helpful for evaluating response to therapy
- FDG PET pitfall: Cytokine therapy results in diffuse hypermetabolism in normal lymph nodes for months
- Combination of FDG PET and conventional imaging (CT/MR) more accurate than either one alone
- Consider extending FDG PET to include all extremities (upper and lower)

Pathology
- Hematogenous and lymphatic spread can occur simultaneously
- Associated abnormalities: ↑ Serum lactate dehydrogenase (LDH) with recurrence

Diagnostic Checklist
- Non-attenuation corrected images best to evaluate skin
- Recent biopsy site can cause false positive
- Small (<1.5 cm) brain metastases may be missed on FDG PET
- Cytokine therapy can result in symmetrical stimulation of lymphoid tissue (tonsils, nodes)

- FDG PET
  - Reported 74% sensitive and 86% specific for recurrence
  - Indicated if clinical concern of recurrence or elevated laboratory markers
  - Important to perform prior to surgical metastasectomy as disease may be more extensive than detected on conventional imaging
  - FDG PET reimbursable by Medicare for evaluating recurrence prior to surgery (alternative to Ga-67 scan)
  - Less sensitive than MR for brain metastases (↑ ↑ FDG activity in normal brain; PET limits of resolution ~ 6-8 mm)
  - PET/CT shows anatomic and metabolic abnormality
- CT
  - Better than FDG PET scan for lung nodule detection
  - FDG PET better than CT for bone, skin, lymph node, abdominal metastases
  - May completely miss extensive bone metastases
- MR
  - Best indicated if clinical concern of brain metastases
  - FDG PET poor in distinguishing normal grey matter FDG uptake from metastases
  - Even if anatomic imaging inconclusive, FDG PET may not add additional information on brain
- Tc-99m sulfur colloid sentinel lymph node mapping and biopsy
  - Used extensively to stage primary melanoma
  - Also with local recurrence to detect locoregional lymphadenopathy
- Protocol advice
  - Consider extending FDG PET to include all extremities (upper and lower)
    - Truncal metastases not rare
  - Evaluate skin for lesions with non-attenuation corrected PET images
    - Attenuation correction can smooth data, obscuring lesions
- Additional nuclear medicine imaging options
  - Tc-99m MDP bone scan
    - Consider if signs/symptoms of bone metastases
    - FDG PET scan might be more sensitive
  - Ga-67 SPECT
    - Historically used for melanoma staging
    - Replaced by FDG PET
    - May be used for equivocal lesions on FDG PET
- Correlative imaging features
  - Confirm PET + findings with anatomic imaging

DIFFERENTIAL DIAGNOSIS

Other Neoplasms
- Benign or malignant
- Consider if distant melanoma history; low clinical suspicion of recurrence
- PET/CT reported to detect new, unexpected primaries in at least 1.2% of cancer patients
  - Most common: Lung cancer

Inflammation/Infection
- Granulomatous disease (e.g., histoplasmosis, sarcoid)
- Reactive lymph nodes
  - Clinical history important
- Lung infection
  - CT correlation, follow-up studies helpful to avoid unnecessary biopsy

Other
- Iatrogenic
  - Recent biopsy sites can ⇒ false positive
- Asymmetric muscle uptake
- Brown fat

PATHOLOGY

General Features
- Genetics: Familial melanomas behave similar to non-familial
- Etiology

MELANOMA THERAPY EVAL./RESTAGING

- Local recurrence due to two causes
  - Incomplete excision of original tumor
  - Microsatellite metastases with spread through surrounding lymphatics
- Locoregional recurrence
  - Lymphatic spread
- Distant recurrence
  - Hematogenous and lymphatic spread can occur simultaneously
- Epidemiology
  - If sentinel lymph node negative, reported 8.9% will have recurrence
  - If sentinel lymph node positive, 55% will recur by 42 months
- Associated abnormalities: ↑ Serum lactate dehydrogenase (LDH) with recurrence

Gross Pathologic & Surgical Features
- Heterogeneous pigmentation throughout lesion
- Nonpigmented lesion

Microscopic Features
- Usually highly cellular and pleomorphic
- Immunohistochemical stains
  - S-100 more sensitive
  - HMB-45 more specific

CLINICAL ISSUES

Presentation
- Most common signs/symptoms
  - May be fairly nonspecific
  - Palpable lymph nodes
  - Recurrent skin lesions
  - Increased laboratory markers (LDH, liver function tests)
- Other signs/symptoms
  - Depends on organ involved
    - Bowel obstruction
    - Neurologic changes
    - Jaundice
    - Bone pain

Demographics
- Age: Advanced age = recurrence risk factor
- Gender: Males have worse prognosis

Natural History & Prognosis
- Location of metastatic site and ↑ LDH useful prognostic factors
  - Better prognosis
    - Subcutaneous metastases, distant lymph nodes
  - Worse prognosis
    - Visceral organ, lung
- Median survival time for distant metastases ~ 7.5 months

Treatment
- Surgery
  - Satellite skin metastases
  - Metastases to regional lymph nodes
  - Metastases to limited distant sites
- External beam radiation
- Cytokines: Interferons, interleukin-2
- Vaccines
- Efficacy of systemic chemotherapy limited

DIAGNOSTIC CHECKLIST

Consider
- As always with FDG PET, normal physiologic and benign causes of increased activity must be excluded
- Image entire body (including extremities) with FDG PET

Image Interpretation Pearls
- Non-attenuation corrected images best to evaluate skin
- Recent biopsy site can cause false positive
- Small (<1.5 cm) brain metastases may be missed on FDG PET
- Cytokine therapy can result in symmetrical stimulation of lymphoid tissue (tonsils, nodes)

SELECTED REFERENCES

1. Belhocine TZ et al: Role of nuclear medicine in the management of cutaneous malignant melanoma. J Nucl Med. 47(6):957-67, 2006
2. Kettlewell S et al: Value of sentinel node status as a prognostic factor in melanoma: prospective observational study. BMJ. 332(7555):1423, 2006
3. Aydin A et al: Detection of bone marrow metastases by FDG-PET and missed by bone scintigraphy in widespread melanoma. Clin Nucl Med. 30(9):606-7, 2005
4. Florell SR et al: Population-based analysis of prognostic factors and survival in familial melanoma. J Clin Oncol. 23(28):7168-77, 2005
5. Homsi J et al: Cutaneous melanoma: prognostic factors. Cancer Control. 12(4):223-9, 2005
6. Ishimori T et al: Detection of unexpected additional primary malignancies with PET/CT. J Nucl Med. 46(5):752-7, 2005
7. Zogakis TG et al: Melanoma recurrence patterns after negative sentinel lymphadenectomy. Arch Surg. 140(9):865-71; discussion 871-2, 2005
8. Finkelstein SE et al: A prospective analysis of positron emission tomography and conventional imaging for detection of stage IV metastatic melanoma in patients undergoing metastasectomy. Ann Surg Oncol. 11(8):731-8, 2004
9. Fuster D et al: Is 18F-FDG PET more accurate than standard diagnostic procedures in the detection of suspected recurrent melanoma? J Nucl Med. 45(8):1323-7, 2004
10. MacCormack MA et al: Local melanoma recurrence: a clarification of terminology. Dermatol Surg. 30(12 Pt 2):1533-8, 2004
11. Gulec SA et al: The role of fluorine-18 deoxyglucose positron emission tomography in the management of patients with metastatic melanoma: impact on surgical decision making. Clin Nucl Med. 28(12):961-5, 2003
12. Swetter SM et al: Positron emission tomography is superior to computed tomography for metastatic detection in melanoma patients. Ann Surg Oncol. 9(7):646-53, 2002
13. Crippa F et al: Which kinds of lymph node metastases can FDG PET detect? A clinical study in melanoma. J Nucl Med. 41(9):1491-4, 2000
14. Barth A et al: Prognostic factors in 1,521 melanoma patients with distant metastases. J Am Coll Surg. 181(3):193-201, 1995

MELANOMA THERAPY EVAL./RESTAGING

IMAGE GALLERY

Typical

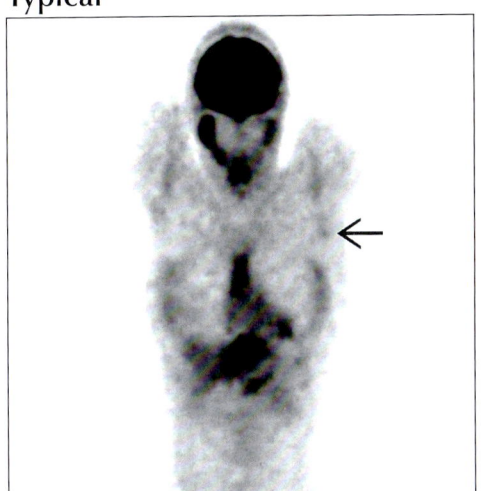

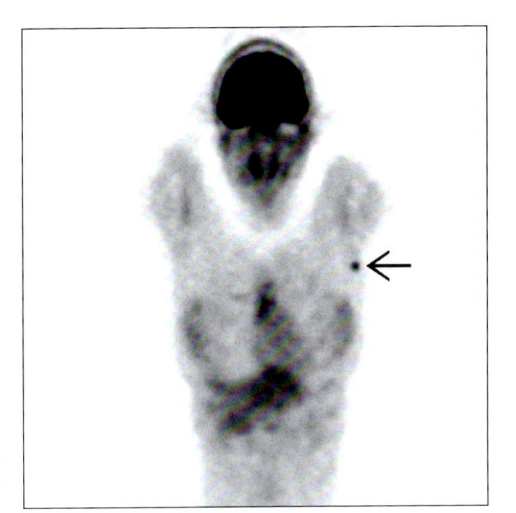

(Left) Coronal PET shows faint activity in left axilla ➔ following cytokine therapy for high risk melanoma. Follow-up was recommended for further characterization. See next 2 images. *(Right)* Coronal PET 6 months after previous image shows definite left axillary lymphadenopathy ➔. Left axillary lymphadenectomy revealed a single positive lymph node.

Typical

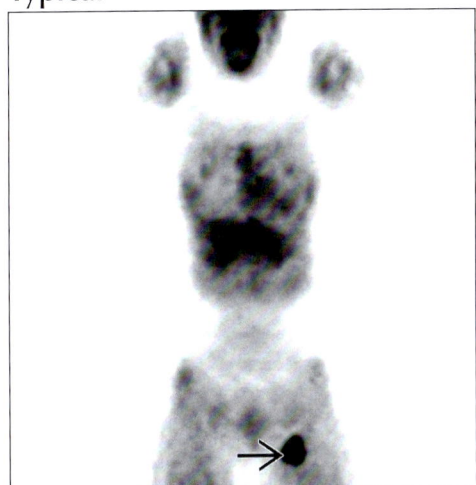

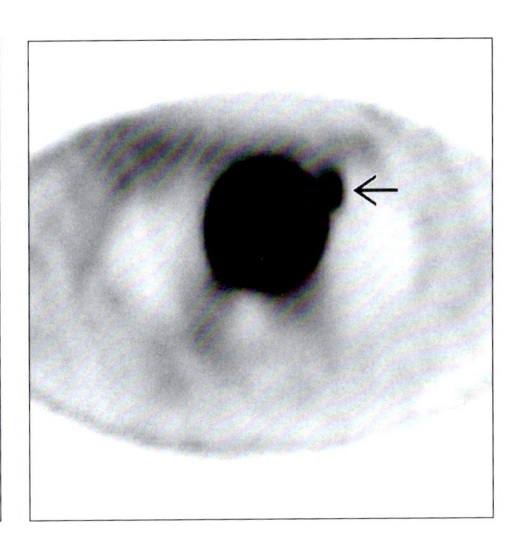

(Left) Coronal PET one year following previous study shows large left inguinal lymphadenopathy ➔. *(Right)* Axial PET shows left inguinal lymphadenopathy ➔ in patient with prior surgical resection and radiation therapy for metastatic melanoma in right groin. See next image.

Typical

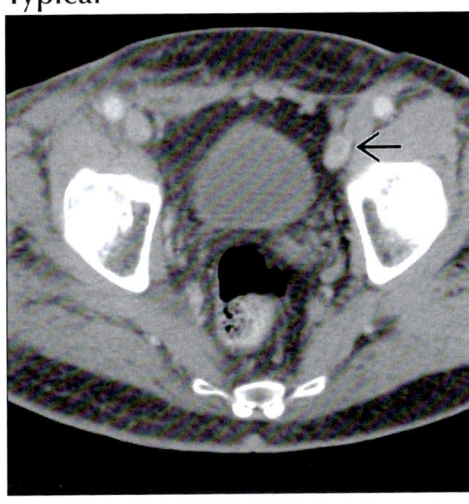

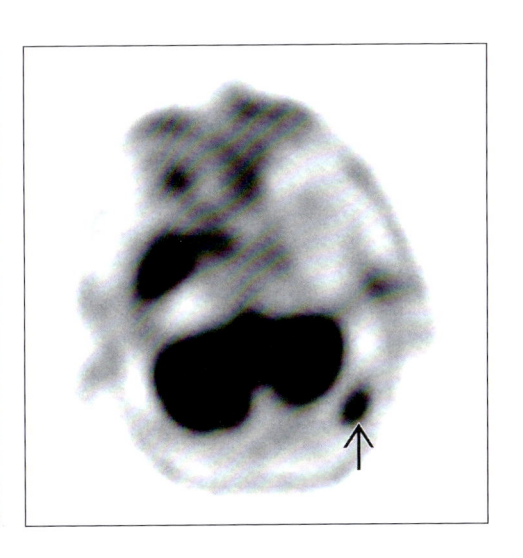

(Left) Axial CECT (same patient as previous image) shows the metastatic lymph node ➔. The node was surgically resected following ultrasound guided needle localization. *(Right)* Axial PET shows melanoma metastasis in subcutaneous left occipital lymph node ➔ in patient with previously resected left parietal scalp primary.

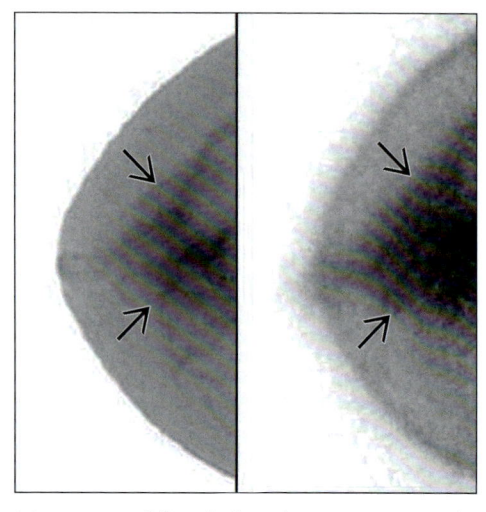

BREAST, BENIGN DISEASE

Mammogram (left) & high-resolution FDG PET (right) show concordant distribution of dense breast tissue & hypermetabolism ➔. Dense glandular tissue is more FDG avid than fat, which can obscure small cancers.

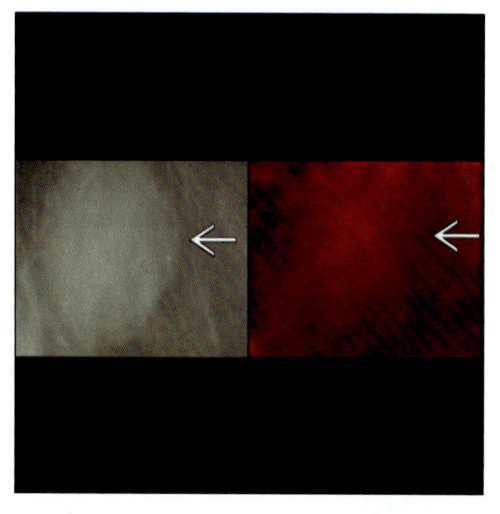

Coned down mammogram (left) and corresponding high-resolution FDG PET (right) shows minimal FDG uptake in 3 x 4 cm fibroadenoma ➔. Fibroadenomas & benign breast tumors are usually ↓ in FDG uptake.

TERMINOLOGY

Definitions
- Benign conditions of the breast that may mimic carcinoma

IMAGING FINDINGS

General Features
- Best diagnostic clue
  - Ultrasound, MR features of benign disease
  - History often important in identifying/classifying benign causes of FDG uptake on PET

Nuclear Medicine Findings
- Benign conditions with increased uptake on FDG PET
  - Normal breast tissue
    - FDG uptake is proportionate to breast density
  - Fat necrosis
    - Increased FDG uptake: May persist in fat necrosis
    - TRAM reconstruction: Typically ↑ FDG uptake along incisional margins 2° fat necrosis
  - Lactating breast
    - Lactating glandular tissue: Intense FDG uptake
    - FDG uptake returns to normal within 3-4 weeks of discontinuing breast feeding
  - Implants
    - Leaking implants: ↑ FDG uptake (silicone > saline)
    - ↑ FDG uptake at rim of calcific capsulitis
  - Infection
    - ↑ FDG uptake 2° mastitis, including overlying skin
    - Reactive intramammary, axillary, internal mammary nodes: ↑ FDG uptake
  - Trauma
    - Bruising or hematoma typically show increased uptake on FDG PET for several weeks
  - Post-surgical or biopsy
    - Focal increased FDG uptake due to core biopsy or surgery may persist for several weeks
  - Ductal, typical & atypical hyperplasia, apocrine metaplasia: Often mild FDG uptake above normal background glandular tissue
- Benign conditions without ↑ uptake on FDG PET
  - Most benign cystic lesions: ↓ FDG uptake
    - Malignant lesions with cystic, mucinous components may mimic benign cysts on FDG PET
  - Benign breast tumors: Usually ↓ FDG uptake

DDx: FDG PET: Malignant Mimics of Benign Breast Disease

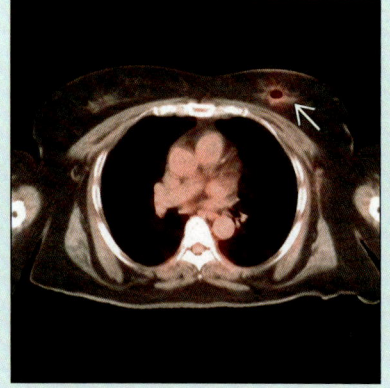

Tumor vs. Post-Bx Inflammation 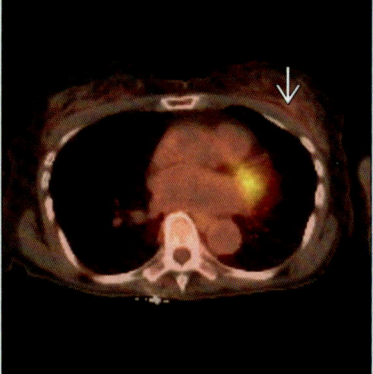 | *Lobular Cancer* 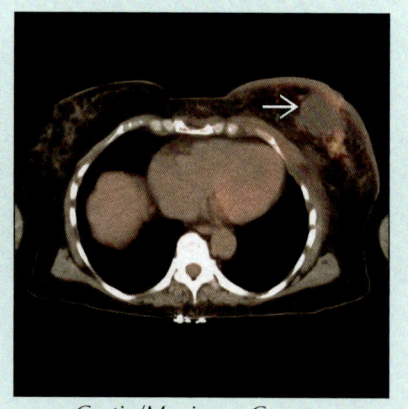 | *Cystic/Mucinous Cancer*

BREAST, BENIGN DISEASE

Key Facts

Imaging Findings
- FDG uptake is proportionate to breast density
- Increased FDG uptake: May persist in fat necrosis
- Lactating glandular tissue: Intense FDG uptake
- Leaking implants: ↑ FDG uptake (silicone > saline)
- Bruising or hematoma typically show increased uptake on FDG PET for several weeks
- Focal increased FDG uptake due to core biopsy or surgery may persist for several weeks
- Ductal, typical & atypical hyperplasia, apocrine metaplasia: Often mild FDG uptake above normal background glandular tissue
- Most benign cystic lesions: ↓ FDG uptake
- Benign breast tumors: Usually ↓ FDG uptake

Diagnostic Checklist
- Poorly FDG avid: Tiny tumors, DCIS, lobular & tubular carcinomas
- Benign disease can be FDG avid

- Non-reactive intramammary nodes: Typically ↓ FDG uptake
- Skin thickening due to post-axillary dissection lymphedema: Low FDG uptake

DIFFERENTIAL DIAGNOSIS

Poorly FDG Avid Breast Cancer
- Concurrent chemotherapy
  - May decrease uptake in still-viable tumor
  - Predictive of good response to chemotherapy
- Lobular or tubular carcinoma
  - Typically low FDG uptake
  - When exhibiting more aggressive behavior, may show greater FDG uptake
- DCIS
  - Variable linear areas of uptake
    - Greater sensitivity with high-resolution positron emission mammography units than conventional PET scanners
- Small tumors
  - Partial volume effects ↓ measured SUV in tumors < 2.5 cm diameter

CLINICAL ISSUES

Presentation
- Most common signs/symptoms: Nonspecific in breast cancer: Mimics benign disease

DIAGNOSTIC CHECKLIST

Image Interpretation Pearls
- Poorly FDG avid: Tiny tumors, DCIS, lobular & tubular carcinomas
- Benign disease can be FDG avid

SELECTED REFERENCES

1. Berg WA et al: High-resolution fluorodeoxyglucose positron emission tomography with compression ("positron emission mammography") is highly accurate in depicting primary breast cancer. Breast J. 12(4):309-23, 2006
2. Kumar R et al: Clinicopathologic factors associated with false negative FDG-PET in primary breast cancer. Breast Cancer Res Treat. 98(3):267-74, 2006
3. Abouzied MM et al: 18F-FDG imaging: pitfalls and artifacts. J Nucl Med Technol. 33(3):145-55; quiz 162-3, 2005
4. Rosen EL et al: Detection of primary breast carcinoma with a dedicated, large-field-of-view FDG PET mammography device: initial experience. Radiology. 234(2):527-34, 2005
5. Hurwitz R: F-18 FDG positron emission tomographic imaging in a case of ruptured breast implant: inflammation or recurrent tumor? Clin Nucl Med. 28(9):755-6, 2003
6. Vranjesevic D et al: Relationship between 18F-FDG uptake and breast density in women with normal breast tissue. J Nucl Med. 44(8):1238-42, 2003
7. Avril N et al: Breast imaging with positron emission tomography and fluorine-18 fluorodeoxyglucose: use and limitations. J Clin Oncol. 18(20):3495-502, 2000
8. Bakheet SM et al: F-18 FDG uptake in breast infection and inflammation. Clin Nucl Med. 25(2):100-3, 2000

IMAGE GALLERY

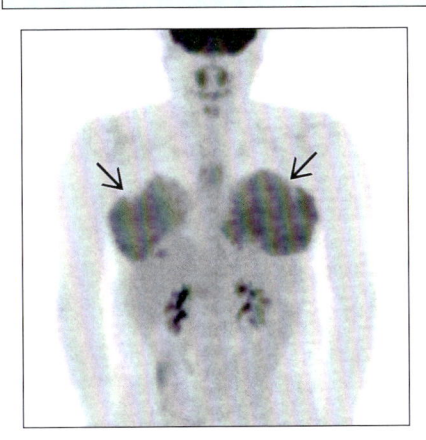

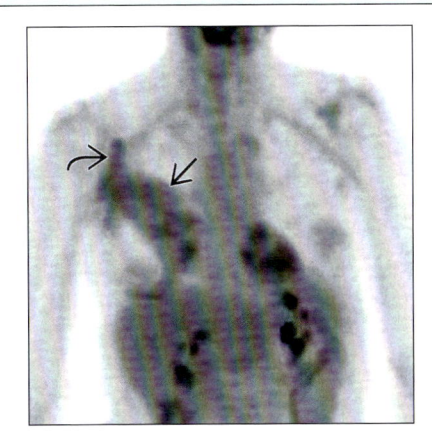

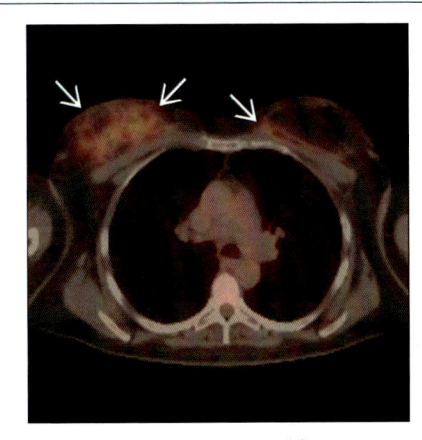

(Left) Anterior MIP FDG PET of the chest and upper abdomen shows intense uptake in both breasts ➔ due to lactation. Note mild asymmetry, which is common. *(Center)* Anterior MIP FDG PET of the chest and upper abdomen shows intense uptake around the right breast ➔, extending into the axilla ➔, due to leaking silicone implant. *(Right)* Axial FDG PET/CT shows increased uptake in regions of fat necrosis ➔ along margins of TRAM reconstruction. Fat necrosis can remain FDG avid indefinitely, obscuring detection of recurrence in mastectomy bed.

BREAST CANCER, PRIMARY

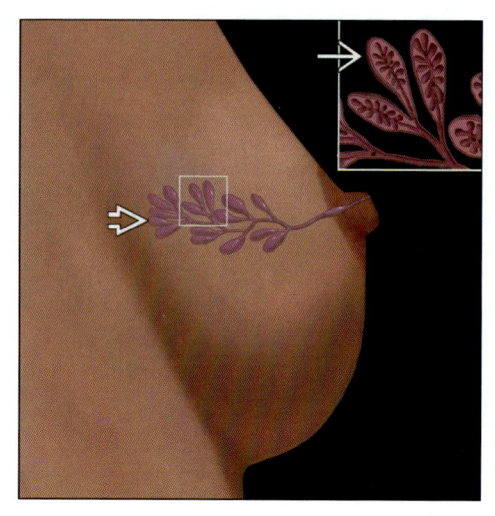

Breast tissue contains ducts and lobules in addition to fat and connective tissue. Ducts give rise to ductal cancers; lobules give rise to lobular cancers.

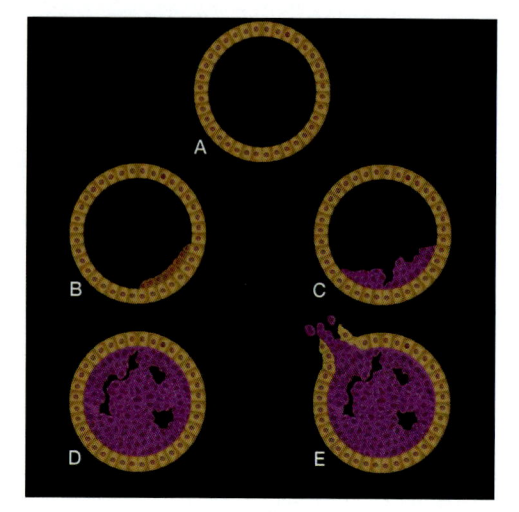

Evolution of ductal cancer. A) Normal duct with single epithelial wall. B) Ductal hyperplasia. C) Atypical ductal hyperplasia. D) Ductal carcinoma in situ. E) Invasive ductal cancer.

TERMINOLOGY

Definitions
- Primary malignant lesion of breast

IMAGING FINDINGS

General Features
- Best diagnostic clue: Focal increased activity on PET/CT or breast scintigraphy corresponding to suspicious mammographic lesion
- Location: Any site within breast tissue; contiguous skin or intramammary lymph node may also demonstrate increased activity when involved
- Size
  - Lesions < 1 cm difficult to detect on whole-body PET/CT or scintigraphy
  - Note: PET and scintigraphy performed with dedicated breast apparatus can detect 4-5 mm lesions

Nuclear Medicine Findings
- Nuclear medicine: Problem-solving technique when conventional breast imaging difficult/equivocal
  - Dense breast tissue on mammography, equivocal MR
- PET/CT
  - Performance best with dedicated high resolution positron emission mammography (PEM) scanners: Sensitivity 90%, specificity 86%
  - Conventional PET or PET/CT: Sensitivities reported in range of 79-90%
  - 5-7 mm lesions routinely detected especially if prone PET/CT used
  - Negative PET in breast lesion ≥ 10 mm likely benign (unless lobular, tubular cancer which tend to show low FDG uptake)
  - PET may detect high-grade DCIS if > 1.5-2.0 cm
  - 50% reduction in SUV on PET following 2 cycles of chemotherapy considered good response
- Tc-99m MIBI: Declining use due to inferior results compared to PET/CT
  - Tc-99m MIBI: Sensitivity reported range of 76-90%

DDx: FDG Uptake in Breast

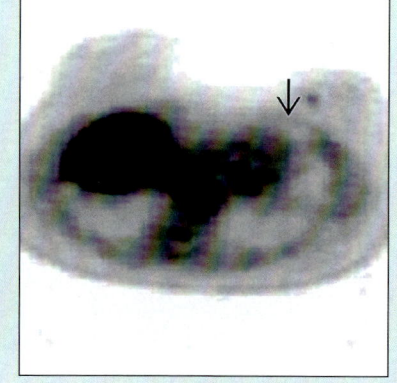

Post-Op Inflammation 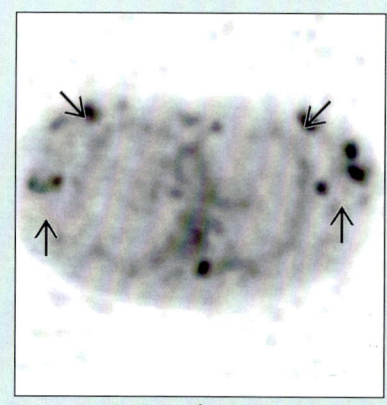 | *Lymphoma* 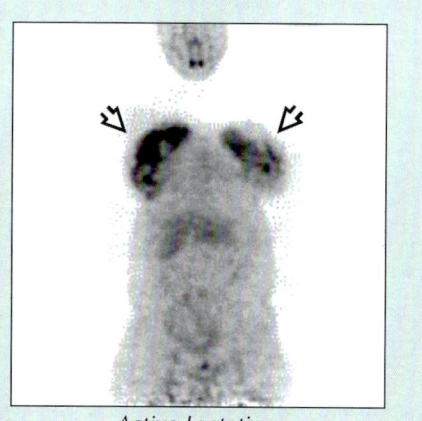 | *Active Lactation*

BREAST CANCER, PRIMARY

Key Facts

Imaging Findings
- Best diagnostic clue: Focal increased activity on PET/CT or breast scintigraphy corresponding to suspicious mammographic lesion
- Conventional PET or PET/CT: Sensitivities reported in range of 79-90%
- 50% reduction in SUV on PET following 2 cycles of chemotherapy considered good response
- Tc-99m MIBI: Sensitivity reported range of 76-90%
- Problem-solving: Prone PET/CT or PEM

Top Differential Diagnoses
- Infection/Inflammation
- Trauma and Surgery
- Nonmalignant Tumors
- Lactating Breast

Pathology
- ↑ Incidence: Close family history (mother, sister)
- BRCA-1, BRCA-2 genetics indicate a high likelihood for development of breast cancer

Diagnostic Checklist
- Detection enhanced by optimizing technique and choice of instrumentation: FDG PET with CT fusion > planar MIBI > planar Tl
- False negative PET: Small (< 10 mm) or in situ cancers
- False positive PET: Inflammation, infection, adenomas, lactation, recent trauma or surgery
- False positive PET: Low grade (lobular, tubular)
- Low or absent MIBI activity in PET positive breast cancer: Potential for poor response to chemo

---

  - Poor sensitivity for nonpalpable lesions and low grade malignancies (< 50%) including ductal cancer in situ (DCIS) or lobular cancer in situ (LCIS)
  - Special high-resolution detectors attached to mammographic devices in clinical trials (4 mm malignancies may be detected)
- Thallium (Tl)-201: Rarely used due to higher sensitivity with Tc-99m MIBI or PET/CT
  - Sensitivity for lesions < 1.5 cm poor (40-60%); sensitivity poor for low grade malignancy

Imaging Recommendations
- Best imaging tool
  - Screening: Mammography
  - Localization, tissue characterization: Ultrasound
  - Sensitivity, tissue characterization: MR
  - Problem-solving: Prone PET/CT or PEM
- Protocol advice
  - FDG PET or PET/CT
    - Supine whole-body PET/CT (arms up)
    - Prone imaging following supine study: Highest sensitivity for breast, axillary and mediastinal lesions; separates chest wall from breast
    - Patient preparation: Avoid carbohydrates x 12 hours prior to PET; NPO 6 hours prior to PET; adequate hydration
  - Tc-99m MIBI
    - Lesion uptake dependent on mitochondrial activity and concentration in tumor
    - Prone SPECT imaging desirable
    - Three serial images (each 10 minute acquisitions) beginning immediately after ~ 20 mCi (640 MBq) Tc-99m MIBI IV; prone, lateral views
    - 140 keV photopeak with 20% window
    - Special detectors available with mammographic fusion with compression imaging of breast.
  - Tl-201
    - Lesion uptake dependent on sodium/potassium pump (inactivated by ouabain) and cotransport system (inactivated by furosemide)
    - Prone imaging with single photon emission computed tomography (SPECT) has highest sensitivity
    - Anterior, and lateral views (prone) helpful for localization
    - Three serial images (each 10 minute acquisitions) beginning immediately after 3 mCi (111MBq) Tl-201 IV; prone, lateral views
    - SPECT imaging 360° rotation continuous acquisition for 30 minutes: Advantages over planar include higher contrast resolution, both breasts imaged simultaneously, 3D display
    - 80 keV photopeak with 20% window
    - Photon flux limited due to 3 mCi allowable dose

DIFFERENTIAL DIAGNOSIS

Infection/Inflammation
- Usually lower target/background ratio than tumors of comparable size

Trauma and Surgery
- Post-surgical procedure: Frequently result in FDG uptake up to 3-6 months
- Hematoma or may be FDG-avid 2° inflammation
- Low-level FDG activity may persist in scar tissue indefinitely

Fibrocystic Disease
- Multifocal low-level FDG uptake often present

Nonmalignant Tumors
- Fibroadenoma, papilloma, etc.
- Typically ↓ FDG uptake: Higher if hypercellular

Lactating Breast
- Intense FDG uptake in glandular tissue

Normal Breast
- FDG uptake proportionate to breast density

PATHOLOGY

General Features
- Genetics

BREAST CANCER, PRIMARY

- ↑ Incidence: Close family history (mother, sister)
  - \> 80-85% new breast cancer patients: No family history
- BRCA-1, BRCA-2 genetics indicate a high likelihood for development of breast cancer
- Etiology
  - Other factors: Age, radiation exposure (esp. external beam), alcohol, hormonal replacement therapy, early menarche, late menopause
  - Risk reduced with early full-term pregnancy
- Epidemiology
  - Most common women's cancer (excluding skin)
  - NCI estimates (2006): 214,640 new diagnoses; 41,430 deaths
  - Lifetime risk in women for breast cancer: 13.2%
  - Lifetime risk in women with BRCA mutation: 6-85% (3-7 x that of women without mutations)

Microscopic Features
- Ductal cancers (cancers arising from ductal cells)
  - In situ: Tumor cells contained within ducts with no stromal invasion by tumor cells
  - Invasive: Tumor has penetrated ductal epithelium, invades stroma
- Lobular cancers (cancers arising from lobule cells)
  - In situ: Tumor cells contained within lobules with no penetration of lobule walls
  - Invasive: Tumor cells invade stroma

Staging, Grading or Classification Criteria
- Tumor (T) staging for primary breast cancer
  - TX: Primary tumor cannot be assessed
  - T0: No evidence of primary tumor
  - Tis: Carcinoma in situ
    - Tis (DCIS): Intraductal carcinoma in situ
    - Tis (LCIS): Lobular carcinoma in situ
    - Tis (Paget): Paget disease of nipple with no tumor; tumor-associated Paget disease classified according to primary tumor size
  - T1: Tumor ≤ 2 cm in greatest dimension
    - T1mic: Microinvasion ≤ 0.1 cm in greatest dimension
    - T1a: Tumor > 0.1 cm but ≤ 0.5 cm in greatest dimension
    - T1b: Tumor > 0.5 cm but ≤ 1 cm in greatest dimension
    - T1c: Tumor > 1 cm but ≤ 2 cm in greatest dimension
  - T2: Tumor > 2 cm but ≤ 5 cm in greatest dimension
  - T3: Tumor > 5 cm in greatest dimension
  - T4: Tumor of any size with direct extension to (a) chest wall or (b) skin, only as described below
    - T4a: Extension to chest wall
    - T4b: Edema (including peau d'orange) or ulceration of breast skin, or satellite skin nodules confined to same breast
    - T4c: Both T4a and T4b
    - T4d: Inflammatory carcinoma

CLINICAL ISSUES

Presentation
- Most common signs/symptoms
  - Discovered by self-examination or screening mammography
  - Nipple discharge or inverted or retract nipple

DIAGNOSTIC CHECKLIST

Consider
- Detection a function of size, mitotic activity
- Detection enhanced by optimizing technique and choice of instrumentation: FDG PET with CT fusion > planar MIBI > planar Tl

Image Interpretation Pearls
- Breast cancer may be multifocal
  - Examine both breasts with any technique used
- False negative PET: Small (< 10 mm) or in situ cancers
- False positive PET: Inflammation, infection, adenomas, lactation, recent trauma or surgery
- False positive PET: Low grade (lobular, tubular)
- Low or absent MIBI activity in PET positive breast cancer: Potential for poor response to chemo
  - Multidrug resistance due to expression of a membrane P-glycoprotein

SELECTED REFERENCES

1. Berg WA et al: High-resolution fluorodeoxyglucose positron emission tomography with compression ("positron emission mammography") is highly accurate in depicting primary breast cancer. Breast J. 12(4):309-23, 2006
2. Kumar R et al: Clinicopathologic factors associated with false negative FDG-PET in primary breast cancer. Breast Cancer Res Treat. 98(3):267-74, 2006
3. Kumar R et al: Standardized uptake values of normal breast tissue with 2-deoxy-2-[F-18]fluoro-D: -glucose positron emission tomography: variations with age, breast density, and menopausal status. Mol Imaging Biol. 8(6):355-62, 2006
4. Pelosi E et al: Value of integrated PET/CT for lesion localisation in cancer patients: a comparative study. Eur J Nucl Med Mol Imaging. 31(7):932-9, 2004
5. Zangheri B et al: PET/CT and breast cancer. Eur J Nucl Med Mol Imaging. 31 Suppl 1:S135-42, 2004
6. Vranjesevic D et al: Relationship between 18F-FDG uptake and breast density in women with normal breast tissue. J Nucl Med. 44(8):1238-42, 2003
7. Bos R et al: Biologic correlates of (18)fluorodeoxyglucose uptake in human breast cancer measured by positron emission tomography. J Clin Oncol. 20(2):379-87, 2002
8. Schirrmeister H et al: Fluorine-18 2-deoxy-2-fluoro-D-glucose PET in the preoperative staging of breast cancer: comparison with the standard staging procedures. Eur J Nucl Med. 28(3):351-8, 2001
9. Palmedo H et al: Scintimammography with technetium-99m methoxyisobutylisonitrile: results of a prospective European multicentre trial. Eur J Nucl Med. 25(4):375-85, 1998
10. Waxman AD: The role of (99m)Tc methoxyisobutylisonitrile in imaging breast cancer. Semin Nucl Med. 27(1):40-54, 1997
11. Khalkhali I et al: Prone scintimammography in patients with suspicion of carcinoma of the breast. J Am Coll Surg. 178(5):491-7, 1994
12. Waxman AD et al: Thallium scintigraphy in the evaluation of mass abnormalities of the breast. J Nucl Med. 34(1):18-23, 1993

BREAST CANCER, PRIMARY

IMAGE GALLERY

Typical

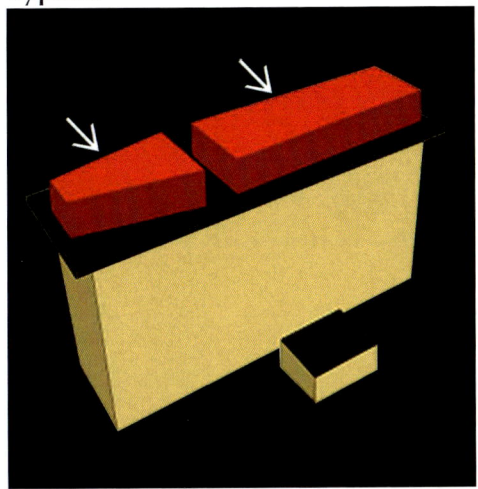

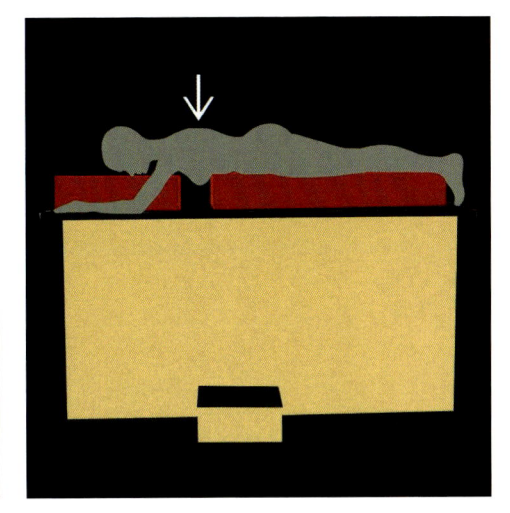

(Left) Graphic of positron emission tomography scan table with pads ⇨ configured for prone imaging. See next image. (Right) Graphic of positron emission tomography with patient positioned prone ⇨. This is ideal for a 2-3 bed position, limited study in which the axilla and breasts are imaged.

Typical

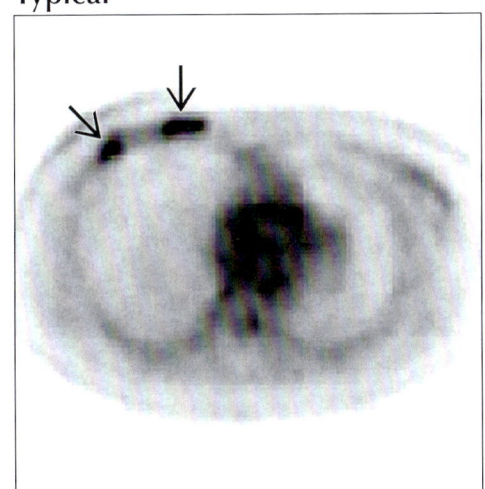

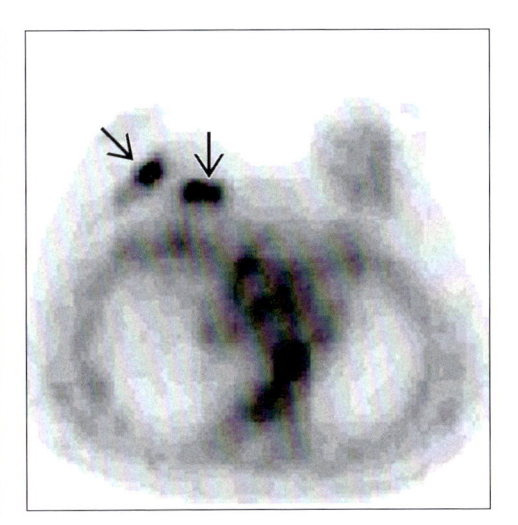

(Left) Axial supine PET image in a patient with with primary breast tumors that appear to abut the chest wall ⇨. See next image. (Right) Axial prone PET image in same patient as left, shows primary tumors do not abut the chest wall ⇨ and are more peripherally located in the breast.

Typical

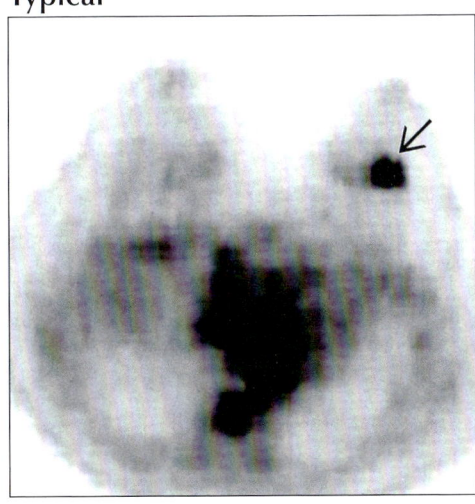

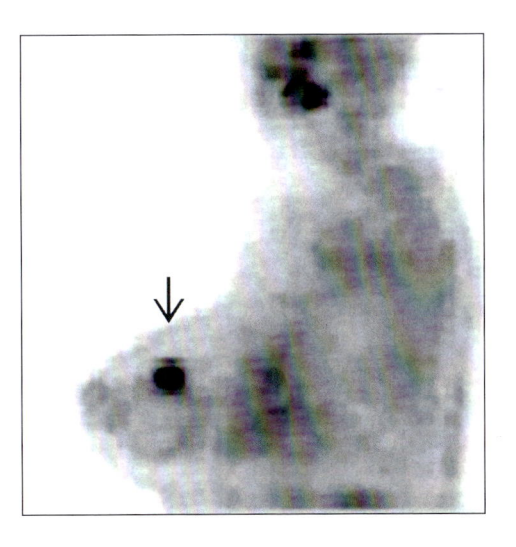

(Left) Axial prone PET shows increased FDG activity in a 16 mm invasive ductal cancer ⇨ of the left breast. See next image. (Right) Sagittal prone PET in same patient as left shows the lesion in the left upper outer quadrant ⇨.

BREAST CANCER, PRIMARY

Typical

(Left) Tl-201 LAO planar image shows increased tracer accumulation in a 16 mm invasive ductal cancer ➔. *(Right)* Tc-99m MIBI prone planar image shows focal increased activity ➔ in a patient with breast mass, at biopsy a multifocal ductal cancer.

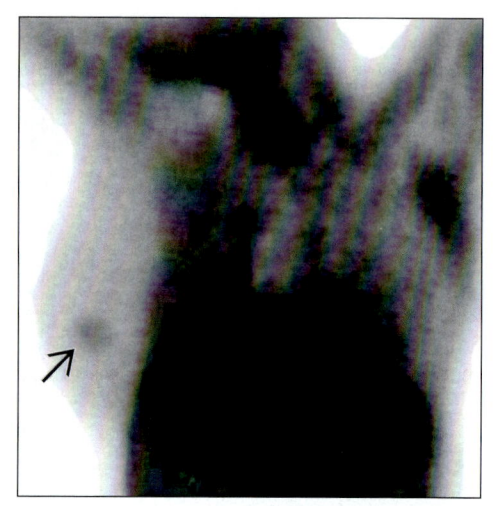

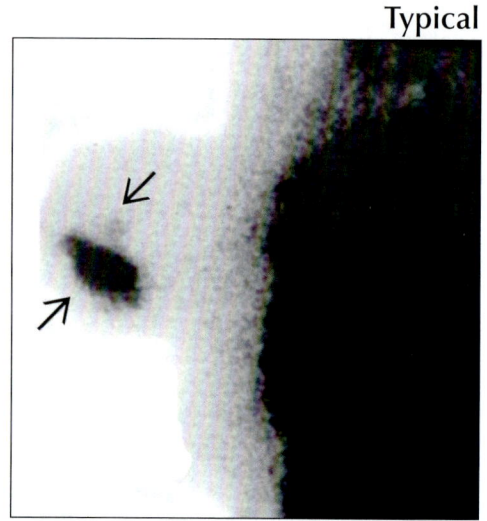

Typical

(Left) Sagittal prone PET of normal breast. Note mildly heterogeneous appearance ➔. See next image. *(Right)* Sagittal prone PET in the same patient as left with increased activity ➔ in a 14 mm invasive ductal cancer of the opposite breast.

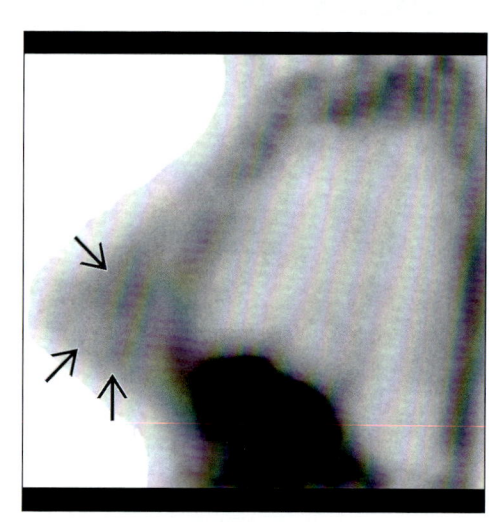

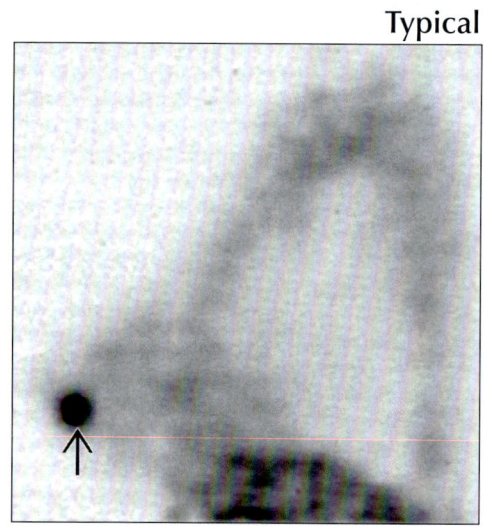

Typical

(Left) Axial CT in a patient, post bilateral mastectomy and reconstruction, shows a soft tissue nodule ➔ in the medial left breast. See next image. *(Right)* Axial PET CT in the same patient as previous, shows increased FDG activity in medial left breast lesion ➔. Biopsy showed recurrent ductal cancer.

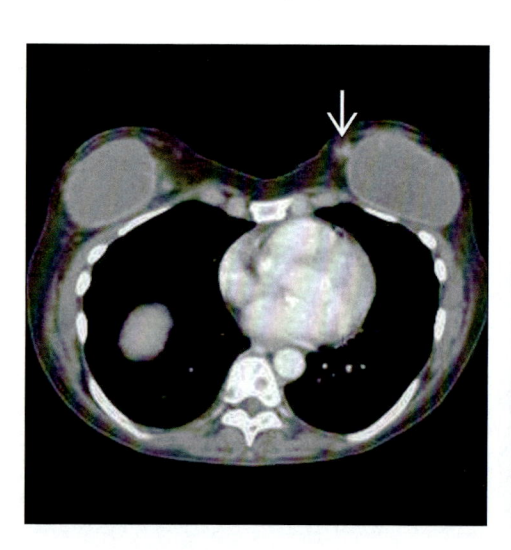

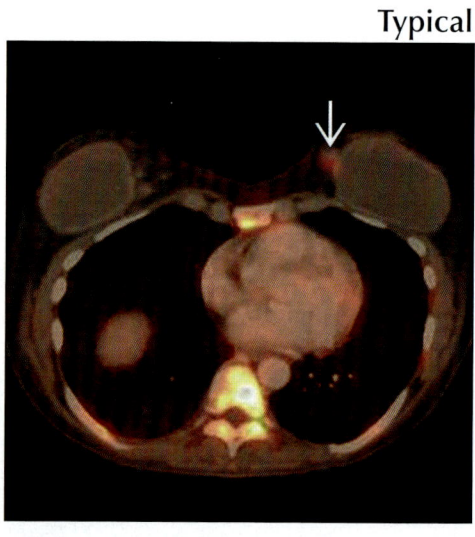

BREAST CANCER, PRIMARY

Typical

Typical

Typical

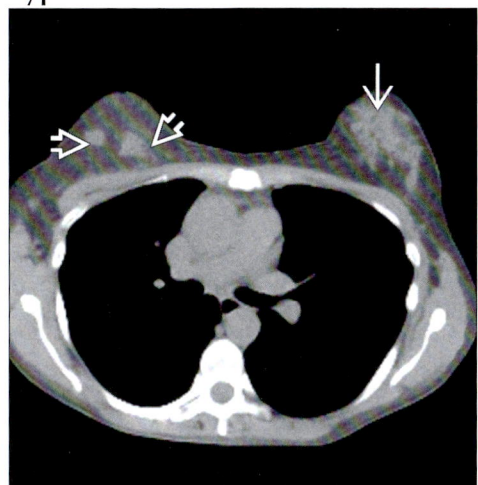

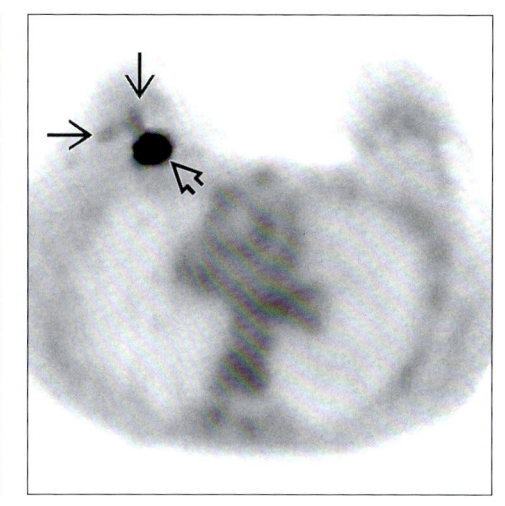

(Left) Axial CT shows hyperdense foci in the right breast ➡. Note normal high-density left breast tissue ➡. See next image. *(Right)* Axial prone PET in same patient as previous, shows increased FDG activity in dominant lesion ➡ and milder activity in surrounding lesions ➡. Biopsy showed 15 mm ductal carcinoma in dominant lesion with surrounding high grade DCIS. See next 4 images.

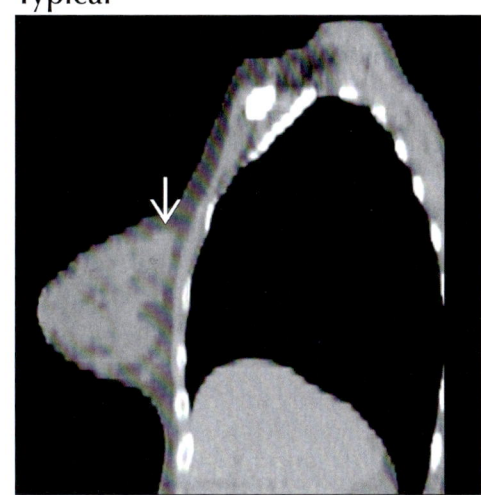

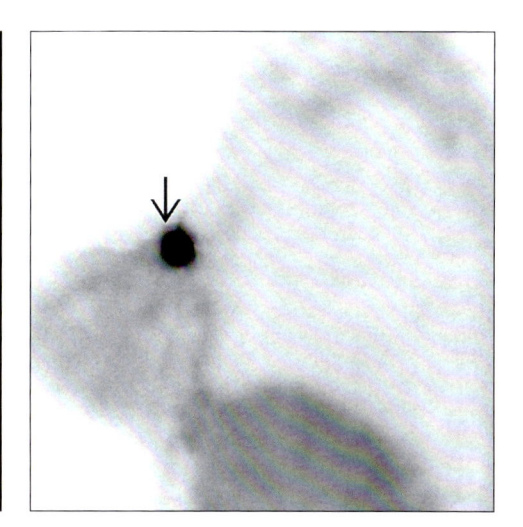

(Left) Sagittal prone CT in the same patient as previous shows dense breast tissue with slightly increased density in tumor ➡. See next image. *(Right)* Sagittal prone PET in the same patient as previous with increased activity corresponding to dominant lesion ➡.

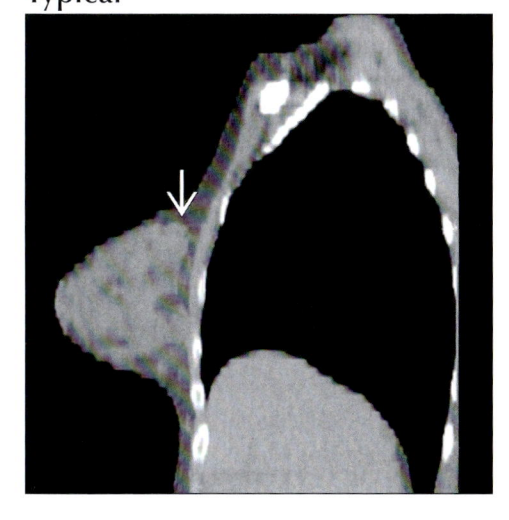

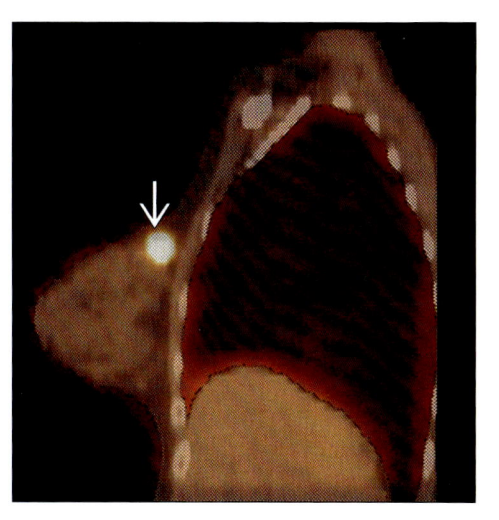

(Left) Sagittal prone CT of same patient as previous image with localizing markers shows a superior medial location ➡ of the mass. *(Right)* Sagittal prone PET/CT in the same patient as previous image, shows fused display of tumor ➡.

BREAST CANCER, STAGING/RESTAGING

Graphic shows sites of breast cancer metastases: Regional lymph nodes > bone, liver > adrenal gland, pleura/lung > brain.

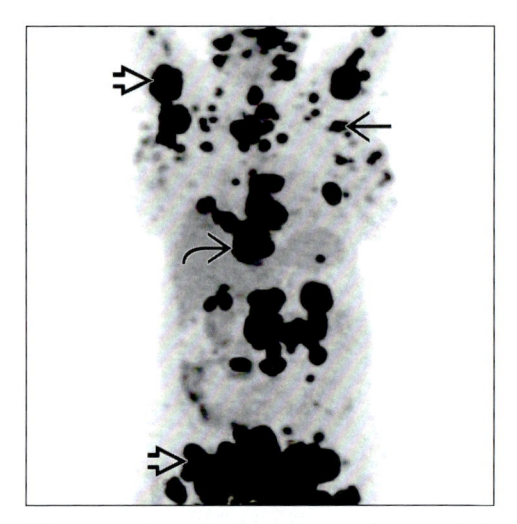

PET in a patient with breast cancer shows multiple metastatic sites in lymph nodes ⇨, liver ➔, and bones ⇾.

TERMINOLOGY

Definitions
- Primary malignancy of breast

IMAGING FINDINGS

General Features
- Best diagnostic clue
  - PET/CT: Focal increased activity in primary tumor, axillary/internal mammary and distant lymph nodes (LN), bone, liver, lung
  - Bone scan: Multiple sites of focally increased activity throughout skeleton, axial > appendicular
  - Tc-99m Sestamibi: Focal increased activity in primary tumor, axillary and distant lymph nodes (LN), lung, liver, bone
- Location: Metastasis may occur at any location but more common in axillary LN > internal mammary LN > bone > liver

Nuclear Medicine Findings
- PET/CT: Detection of distant metastases at time of initial diagnosis: 80-95% sensitivity
  - PET/CT: Negative predictive value (NPV) > 90% in the evaluation of distant metastases
  - Positive predictive value (PPV) reduced by infection, inflammation, trauma, muscle uptake, bowel activity, blood pool, ureteral urine, benign tumors
  - NPV and PPV improved with PET/CT (vs. PET alone) or fusion with MR
- Axillary metastases: Sensitivity and specificity for PET dependent on multiple factors
  - Size, number of nodes
    - PET/CT: Low sensitivity (60%) for axillary metastases: Micrometastases not detected by PET
    - Limits of resolution of PET: 6-8 mm
    - Sentinel LN biopsy procedure required for optimal axillary staging
  - Degree of nodal replacement by metastasis
  - Proliferative activity
  - Tumor type: Poor sensitivity for lobular, tubular
  - Prior lymphadenectomy
    - PET may remain positive for 3-12 months

DDx: Other Causes of Increased Activity on PET

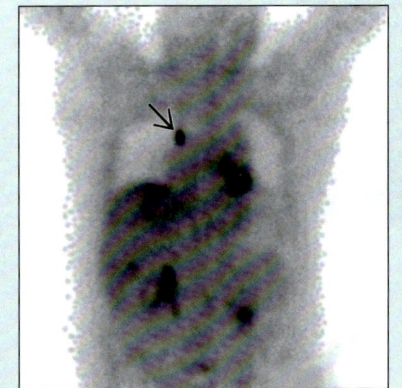

Tip of Central Line

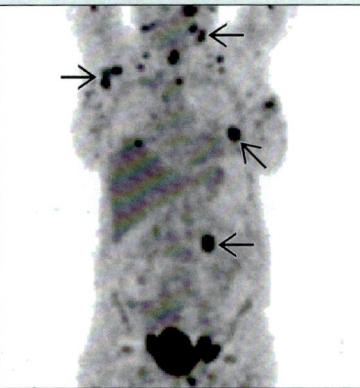

Lymphoma

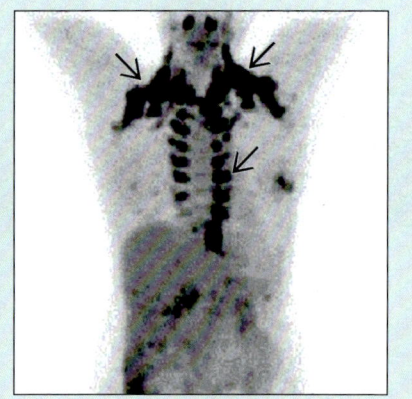

Hypermetabolic Brown Fat

BREAST CANCER, STAGING/RESTAGING

Key Facts

Imaging Findings
- PET/CT: Focal increased activity in primary tumor, axillary/internal mammary and distant lymph nodes (LN), bone, liver, lung
- PET/CT: Detection of distant metastases at time of initial diagnosis: 80-95% sensitivity
- PET/CT: Negative predictive value (NPV) > 90% in the evaluation of distant metastases
- PET/CT: Low sensitivity (60%) for axillary metastases: Micrometastases not detected by PET
- PET/CT has higher sensitivity and specificity in restaging than PET alone

Top Differential Diagnoses
- Infection/Inflammation
- Trauma
- Other Malignancy

Pathology
- Stage I: Tumor < 2 cm
- Stage II: Tumor < 2 cm, 1-3 positive axillary LN; tumor 2-5 cm, negative LN or 1-3 positive LN; tumor > 5 cm, negative LN
- Stage III: Tumor < 5 cm with 4-9 positive axillary LN or positive internal mammary LN; tumor > 5 cm, positive axillary/internal mammary LN; tumor invades chest wall, ± axillary/internal mammary LN
- Stage IV: Distant metastases

Diagnostic Checklist
- Be aware of potential pitfalls and artifacts with PET/CT including motion and misregistration
- Be aware of pertinent history, physical and other imaging findings prior to final interpretation

---

- Extensive clips or sutures: Inflammation → false positive PET scan
- If axillary LN positive on PET/CT, high PPV for malignancy
- Mediastinal and internal mammary LN evaluation
  - Best detected and localized with PET/CT
  - Important for prognosis and therapy
  - PET sensitivity > CT or MR
- Hepatic metastasis
  - Best detected with MR; PET/CT: Low-density hepatic finding on CT with ↑ FDG activity = metastasis
  - May have positive FDG PET and negative CT; MR or CECT confirmation suggested
  - False negative FDG PET: Small lesions (< 10 mm), low density CT abnormality of liver > 15 mm isometabolic on FDG PET is likely metastasis
  - False positive FDG PET
    - Infection/inflammation
    - Interposed colon
  - Bone scan may incidentally detect hepatic metastases
- Osseous metastases
  - PET: Sensitivity high for lytic or trabecular metastasis (> 90%)
    - 50-60% of patients with osseous positive FDG PET scans have no pain
  - Bone scan: High sensitivity in detection of cortical blastic metastases
    - Low sensitivity for lytic (75-80%) or trabecular metastases (< 50%)
- PET has a similar or higher diagnostic accuracy than conventional imaging for restaging
- PET/CT has higher sensitivity and specificity in restaging than PET alone
- SUV measurements helpful in determining adequate response to chemotherapy
  - Greater than 50% SUV reduction at 9 weeks accurately defined good clinical response
  - Greater than 55% response after one cycle also defined good response
- Sensitivity and specificity improved with PET/CT compared to PET alone
- Rise in SUV 7-10 days after antiestrogen therapy (metabolic flare) sign of good response
- Tc-99m Sestamibi scintigraphy
  - PET/CT has largely replaced this exam

Imaging Recommendations
- Best imaging tool
  - SLN biopsy procedure: Optimal axillary LN staging
  - PET/CT: Optimal detection of distant metastases
  - Bone scan: Osseous metastases
  - MR: Brain metastases; confirm hepatic metastases
- Protocol advice
  - Tc-99m MDP bone scan
    - 20-30 mCi (740-1110 MBq) Tc-99m MDP IV
    - Planar whole body scan 90-120 min following radiopharmaceutical administration
    - Spot views and/or SPECT of regions of interest
  - PET/CT
    - Patient preparation: No food x 6 hours, low carbohydrates x 12 hours prior to study; good hydration
    - 10-15 mCi (370-550 MBq) F18-FDG IV
    - CT: ± Oral contrast (2 hours prior to scan) and/or IV contrast
    - Prone breast study highly accurate for evaluation of breast, axilla, mediastinum
- Additional nuclear medicine imaging options
  - Positron emission mammography (PEM)
    - Investigational device
    - Used with F-18 FDG
    - May be useful for primary tumor characterization
  - F-18 Fluoride PET/CT: May ultimately replace traditional bone imaging agents (Tc-99m-MDP): Current reimbursement, FDA barriers exist
  - F-18 estradiol compounds give estrogen receptor (ER) status of primary and metastatic foci: Investigational
  - F-18 L-thymidine targets tissue with high DNA turnover: Investigational
- Correlative imaging features
  - Rapidly expanding use of PET/CT in radiation treatment planning maps

BREAST CANCER, STAGING/RESTAGING

- Impact on radiotherapy in pretreatment planning or follow-up (40-60% of patients treated in many published studies)

DIFFERENTIAL DIAGNOSIS

Infection/Inflammation
- Granulomatous disease (e.g., sarcoidosis)
- Soft tissue infection (e.g., esophagitis, abscess)
- Atherosclerosis
- Post-surgical changes, ostomy sites
- Intramuscular injection sites
- Degenerative bone disease

Trauma
- Traumatic, compression fractures
- Soft tissue trauma

Other Malignancy
- Second primary neoplasm: Thyroid, lung, colon, etc.

PATHOLOGY

General Features
- Genetics
  - \> 80% breast cancer sporadic
  - BRCA-1, BRCA-2 increase likelihood of developing breast cancer
  - BRCA-1 and BRCA-2 present in ~ 0.5% population
  - BRCA-2 may increase breast cancer risk in men
- Etiology: Risk factors: Age, estrogen exposure, dense breasts, radiation exposure, postmenopausal obesity
- Epidemiology
  - ~ 13% of women will develop breast cancer in their lifetime
  - BRCA-1, BRCA-2 confers 3-7 times risk of developing breast cancer compared to women without these mutations
  - 75% of recurrent breast cancer occurs within 5 years of initial diagnosis
  - Distant metastases ⇒ average survival of 1-2 years

Staging, Grading or Classification Criteria
- Stage I: Tumor < 2 cm
- Stage II: Tumor < 2 cm, 1-3 positive axillary LN; tumor 2-5 cm, negative LN or 1-3 positive LN; tumor > 5 cm, negative LN
- Stage III: Tumor < 5 cm with 4-9 positive axillary LN or positive internal mammary LN; tumor > 5 cm, positive axillary/internal mammary LN; tumor invades chest wall, ± axillary/internal mammary LN
- Stage IV: Distant metastases

CLINICAL ISSUES

Presentation
- Most common signs/symptoms
  - Patients with metastases often asymptomatic
  - Symptoms depend on organ involved
    - Axillary: Extremity swelling, mass
    - Brain: CNS findings
    - Bone: Most asymptomatic but pain is common; can be palliated with beta emitters (Sm-153, Sr-89)
    - Liver: Asymptomatic in most; may progress to hepatic failure or abdominal pain

Demographics
- Age: 80% of cases occur in women > 50 years
- Gender: Female breast cancer ~ 55 times more common than male

Natural History & Prognosis
- Mortality rate for African Americans > Caucasians
- Early stage: Survival rates ~ 98%
- Distant metastases: Remission ~ 10-20%, cure very rare
- In patients whose breast cancer recurs, most die of this disease

Treatment
- Surgery: Removal of primary tumor, recurrent tumor in breast
- Chemotherapy: Primary therapy, adjuvant, neoadjuvant, hormonal
- Radiation therapy: Following lumpectomy; axillary and/or mediastinal radiation dependent on lymphadenopathy; treatment/palliation of metastases

DIAGNOSTIC CHECKLIST

Consider
- PET/CT excellent for staging patients with potentially aggressive breast cancers and for monitoring response to treatment
- Precludes need for bone scan when PET/CT demonstrates osseous metastases

Image Interpretation Pearls
- Be aware of potential pitfalls and artifacts with PET/CT including motion and misregistration
- Evaluate study quality prior to interpretation
  - Insulin effect due to poor dietary preparation may produce false negative study
  - Adequate time following injection (~ 60 minutes)
  - Optimization of scan time and FDG dose for quality
- Be aware of pertinent history, physical and other imaging findings prior to final interpretation

SELECTED REFERENCES

1. Chung A et al: Preoperative FDG-PET for axillary metastases in patients with breast cancer. Arch Surg. 141(8):783-8; discussion 788-9, 2006
2. Zangheri B et al: PET/CT and breast cancer. Eur J Nucl Med Mol Imaging. 31 Suppl 1:S135-42, 2004
3. Yang SN et al: Comparing whole body (18)F-2-deoxyglucose positron emission tomography and technetium-99m methylene diphosphonate bone scan to detect bone metastases in patients with breast cancer. J Cancer Res Clin Oncol. 128(6):325-8, 2002
4. Wahl RL et al: Metabolic monitoring of breast cancer chemohormonotherapy using positron emission tomography: initial evaluation. J Clin Oncol. 11(11):2101-11, 1993

BREAST CANCER, STAGING/RESTAGING

IMAGE GALLERY

Typical

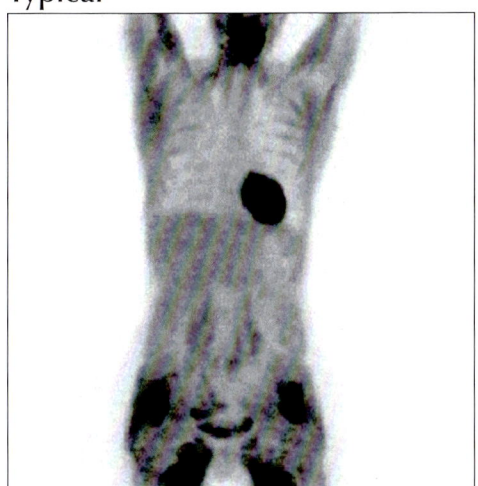

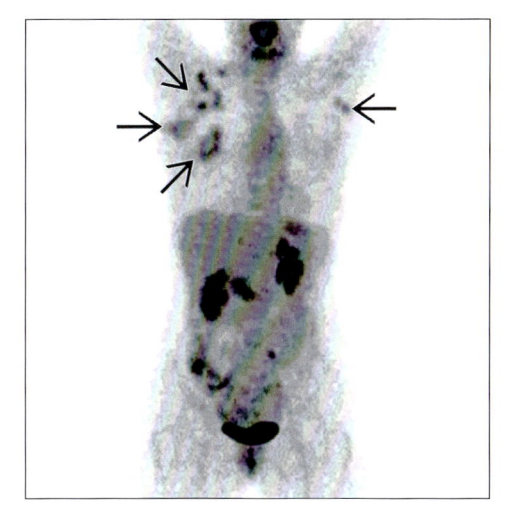

(Left) PET performed when blood glucose was 225 mg/dL in breast cancer patient with elevated tumor markers. Patient consumed high carbohydrate meal prior to study. See next image. **(Right)** PET in same patient as previous image, after appropriate preparation (no food 6 hours prior to FDG injection) shows multiple metastatic foci ➔.

Typical

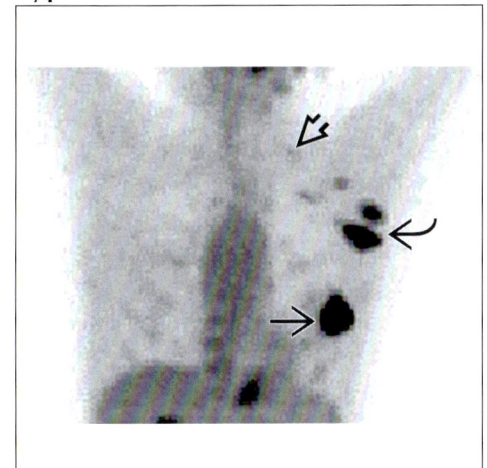

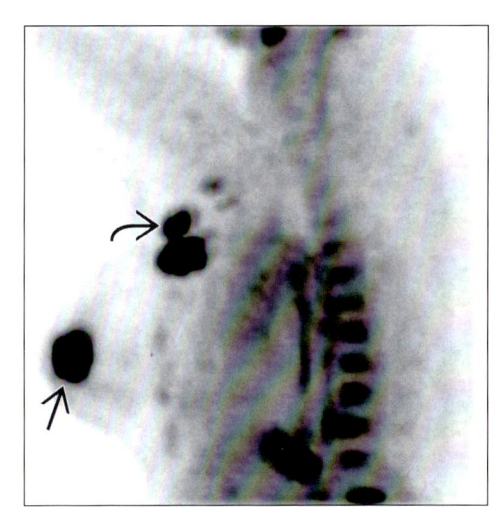

(Left) PET shows foci of abnormal activity in left breast ➔, and axillary ➔, and supraclavicular ➔ lymph nodes. See next image. **(Right)** Lateral PET in same patient as previous shows breast primary ➔ and axillary lymphadenopathy ➔.

Typical

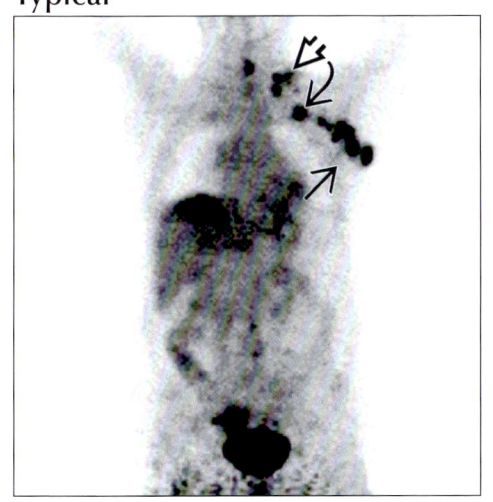

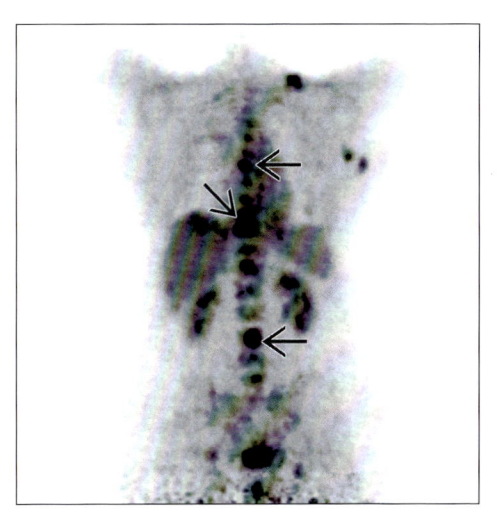

(Left) PET shows multiple axillary ➔, infraclavicular ➔, supraclavicular ➔ and cervical lymphadenopathy in patient with 4 mm primary breast cancer. See next image. **(Right)** Coronal PET in same patient as previous, shows multiple osseous metastases ➔, which were asymptomatic.

BREAST CANCER, STAGING/RESTAGING

Typical

(Left) Tc-99m MDP bone scan in asymptomatic patient with breast cancer shows subtle abnormalities in spine ➜. See next image. *(Right)* PET in same patient as previous shows extensive osseous metastases ➜. PET is superior to bone scan in detection of lytic or trabecular osseous metastases, but may underestimate sclerotic mets.

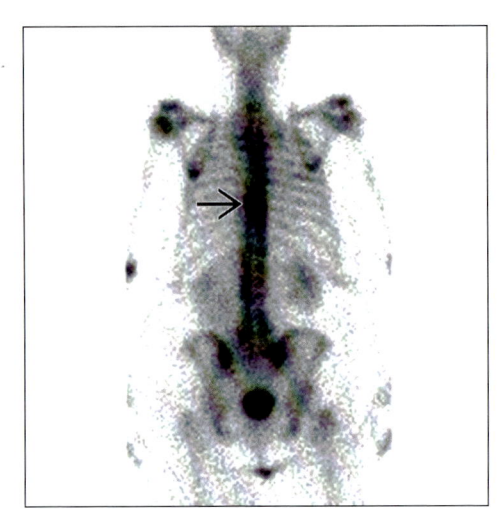

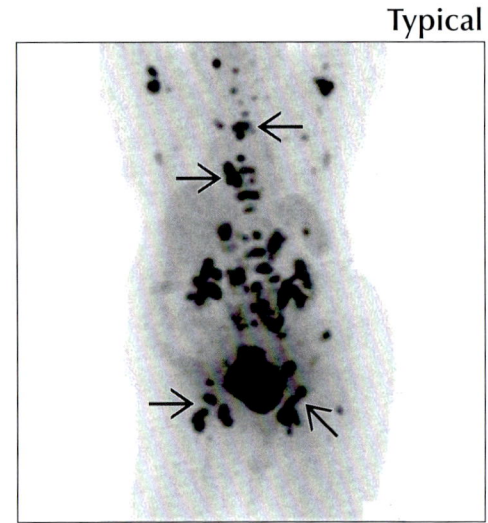

Typical

(Left) PET performed for solitary pulmonary nodule shows occult right breast cancer ➜. See next image. *(Right)* PET PET in same patient as previous, shows right axillary nodal metastasis ➜. PET cannot reliably stage the axilla (low NPV) and sentinel lymph node biopsy is required.

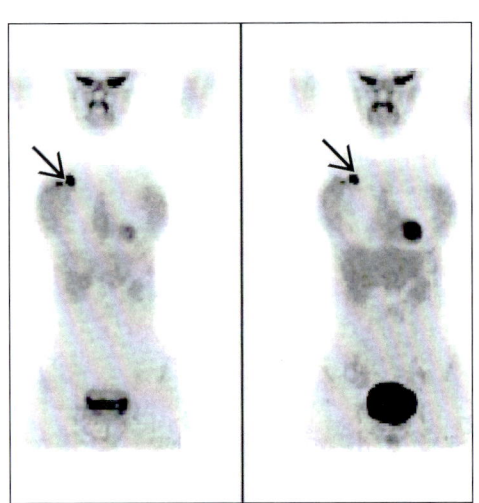

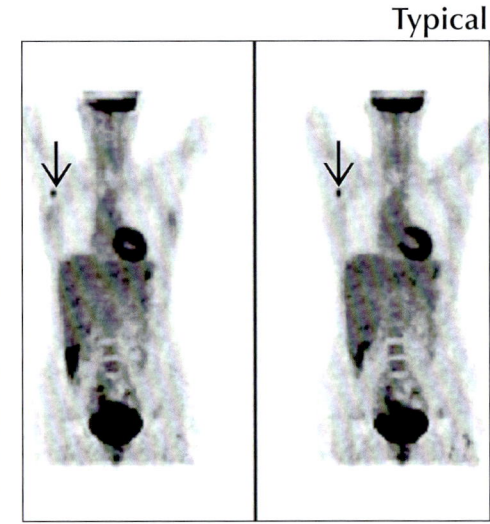

Typical

(Left) PET in patient with recurrent breast cancer shows multiple axillary ➜ and osseous metastases ➜ prior to hormonal therapy. See next image. *(Right)* PET in same patient as previous 6 months later. Note interval resolution of most abnormalities, indicating response to therapy.

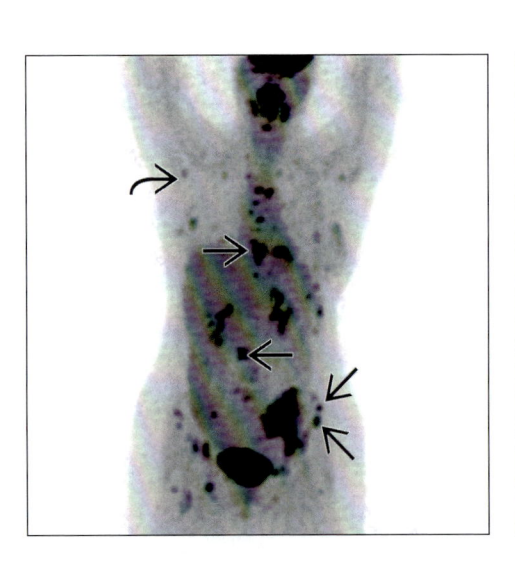

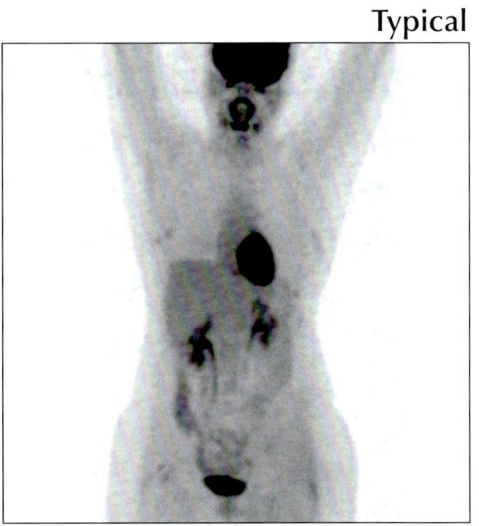

BREAST CANCER, STAGING/RESTAGING

Typical

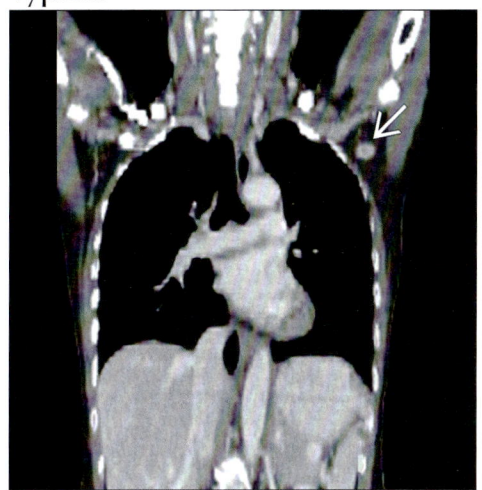

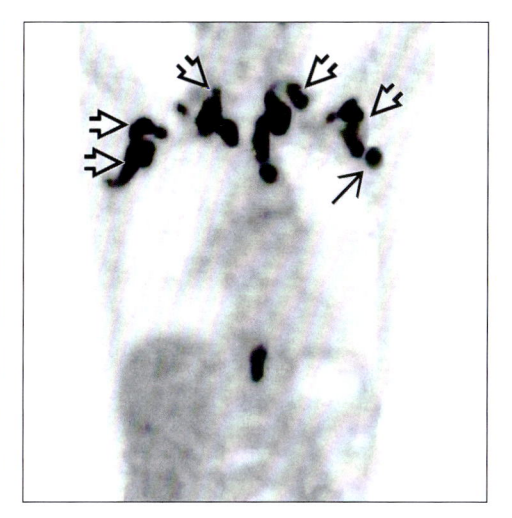

(Left) Coronal CT shows an enlarged left axillary node ➡ which contained metastatic ductal cancer. See next image. *(Right)* PET shows increased activity in corresponding LN ➡. However, symmetric hypermetabolic brown fat ➡, could easily obscure detection of metastases on PET.

Typical

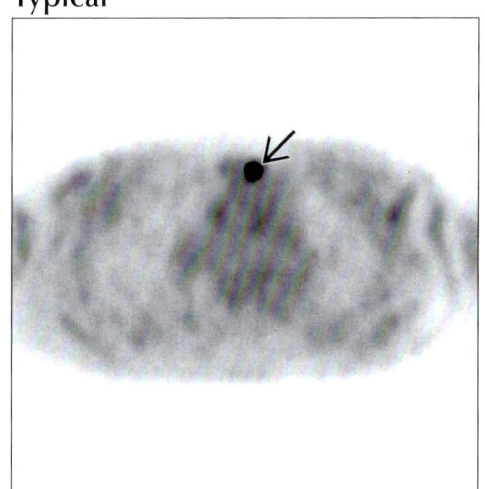

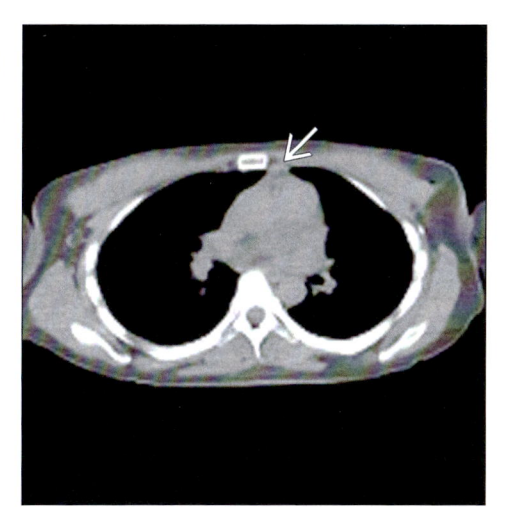

(Left) Axial PET in a patient with breast cancer demonstrates intense focus ➡ in internal mammary LN. See next image. *(Right)* Axial CT in same patient as previous shows small internal mammary LN ➡ detected only after viewing PET.

Typical

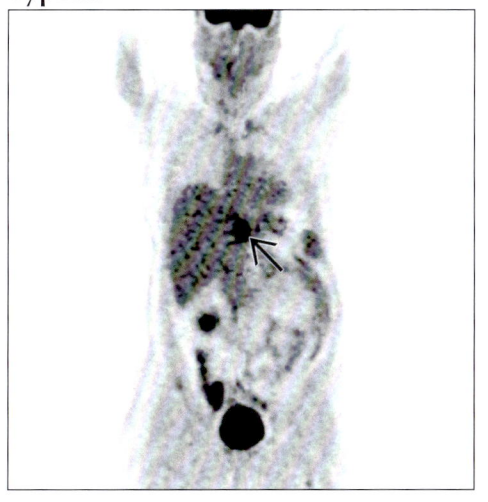

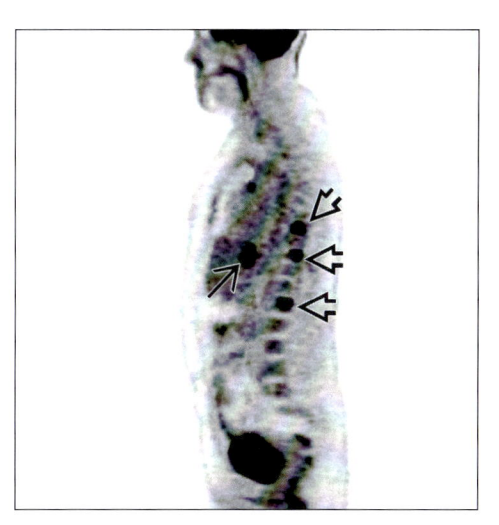

(Left) Coronal PET shows metastasis in the left hepatic lobe ➡, not evident on noncontrast CT. See next image. *(Right)* Sagittal PET in same patient as previous shows hepatic metastasis ➡ as well as multiple occult vertebral metastases ➡ that were asymptomatic.

ADENOCARCINOMA OF UNKNOWN PRIMARY

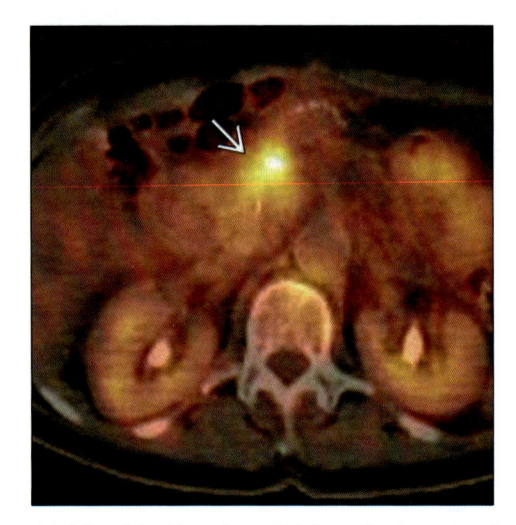

Axial fused PET/CT shows FDG activity in body of pancreas ➡ in a patient with chronic pancreatitis and hepatic CUP. Endoscopic ultrasound confirmed pancreatic adenocarcinoma.

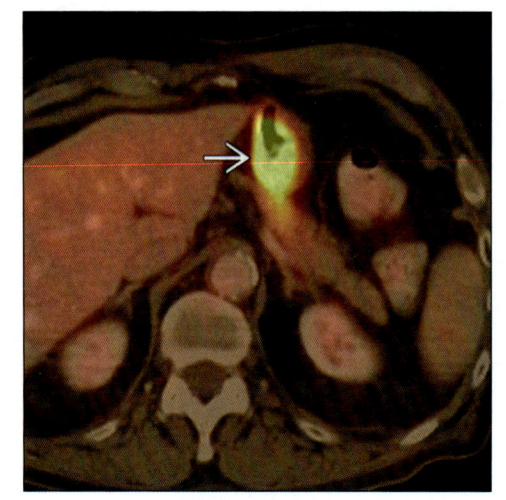

Axial fused PET/CT shows FDG activity in stomach antrum ➡ in a patient with metastatic lung disease. PET/CT suggested gastric carcinoma primary, confirmed with endoscopy.

TERMINOLOGY

Abbreviations and Synonyms
- Carcinoma of unknown primary (CUP); includes undifferentiated carcinomas in addition to adenocarcinoma

Definitions
- Metastatic cancer without known site of origin; histology inconsistent with known tumors from organ biopsied

IMAGING FINDINGS

General Features
- Location
  o Most common site: Lung; gastrointestinal and urogenital tract also common
  o Frequency of metastases by location: Lymph node (LN) 46.3%, liver 12%, brain 11%, bone 11%, lung 6%, pleura 4%, peritoneum 4%, other 10%

Nuclear Medicine Findings
- PET
  o FDG PET has been shown to identify ~ 25-40% of previously unknown primaries
  o PET may commonly reveal "missed primary" rather than unknown primary in true sense, i.e., following complete workup
  o False negative may result from low tumor uptake (e.g., carcinoid) or high background uptake (e.g., liver, high serum glucose level)
  o PET has high specificity for tumors in lung, breast, pancreas

CT Findings
- CT typically used to help identify primary, however low sensitivity (~ 25%)

Imaging Recommendations
- Best imaging tool
  o Likelihood of primary detection with PET/CT: 25-40%; CT: 25%
  o FDG PET provides whole-body survey

DDx: Benign Causes of FDG Uptake

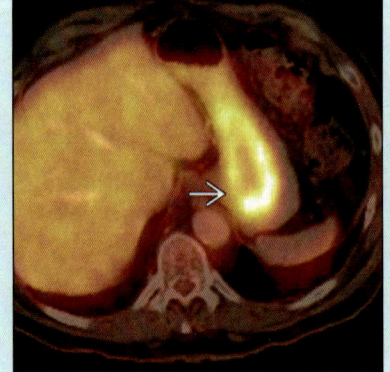

Gastritis

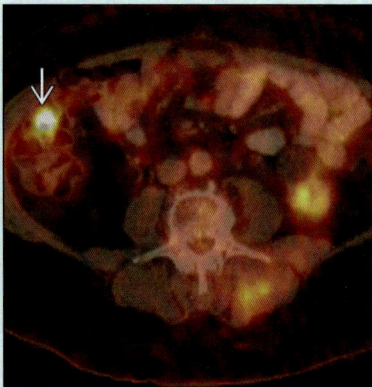

Colon Adenoma

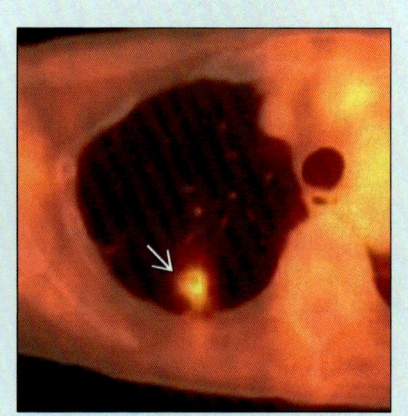

Tuberculosis

ADENOCARCINOMA OF UNKNOWN PRIMARY

Key Facts

Terminology
- Carcinoma of unknown primary (CUP); includes undifferentiated carcinomas in addition to adenocarcinoma

Imaging Findings
- Most common site: Lung; gastrointestinal and urogenital tract also common

- Frequency of metastases by location: Lymph node (LN) 46.3%, liver 12%, brain 11%, bone 11%, lung 6%, pleura 4%, peritoneum 4%, other 10%
- FDG PET has been shown to identify ~ 25-40% of previously unknown primaries
- False negative may result from low tumor uptake (e.g., carcinoid) or high background uptake (e.g., liver, high serum glucose level)
- FDG PET provides whole-body survey

DIFFERENTIAL DIAGNOSIS

Physiologic Activity
- Colon, stomach, thyroid can have short segment or occasionally focal physiologic activity that may mimic potential malignancy

Inflammation
- Several inflammatory or granulomatous conditions, such as sarcoidosis, may cause focal FDG activity and mimic malignancy

Infection
- Infectious processes such as underlying fungal infection or TB may cause focal activity

PATHOLOGY

General Features
- Epidemiology
  o High percentage of CUP patients have adenocarcinoma (60-75%)
  o CUP makes up only a small proportion of all cancer at 0.5-6%

CLINICAL ISSUES

Presentation
- Most common signs/symptoms: Variable depending on site of presenting metastasis

Demographics
- Age: Median age at presentation = 59 y

Natural History & Prognosis
- Primary will not be found in majority of cases despite full work-up
- 20% of patients still have no identifiable primary site post-mortem

Treatment
- If primary is identified, aggressive chemotherapy or hormonal therapy may be considered

DIAGNOSTIC CHECKLIST

Consider
- In patient with CUP, perform conventional laboratory work-up and combination of imaging studies, including PET/CT
- PET/CT: Image top of skull to feet to identify all possible primary sites

SELECTED REFERENCES
1. Pelosi E et al: Role of whole body positron emission tomography/computed tomography scan with 18F-fluorodeoxyglucose in patients with biopsy proven tumor metastases from unknown primary site. Q J Nucl Med Mol Imaging. 50(1):15-22, 2006

IMAGE GALLERY

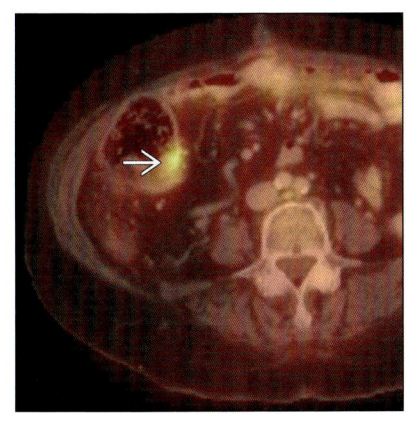

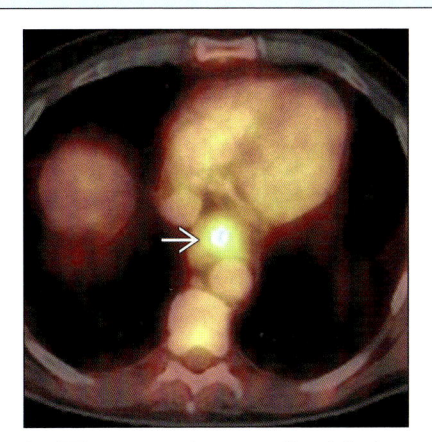

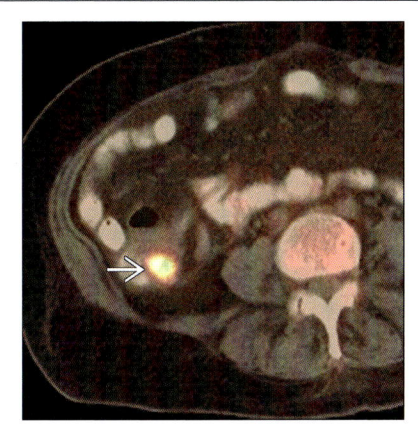

(Left) Axial fused PET/CT shows focal activity in colon ➡ corresponding to small nodular lesion in patient with single liver metastasis. Colonoscopy confirmed adenocarcinoma. *(Center)* Axial fused PET/CT shows activity in esophagus ➡ suggestive of carcinoma in patient with supraclavicular lymph node biopsy showing adenocarcinoma. *(Right)* Axial fused PET/CT shows activity in descending colon ➡. Focal bowel activity should be evaluated with colonoscopy as infection, adenoma, and adenocarcinoma can have this appearance.

PARANEOPLASTIC DISORDERS

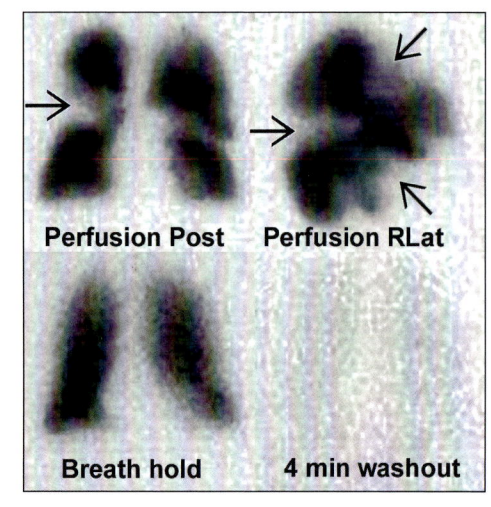

High probability VQ scan: Multiple segmental perfusion defects ➔ (upper panel) with normal ventilation (lower panel). Cancer patients have great increased risk of of venothromboembolism (VTE). See next image.

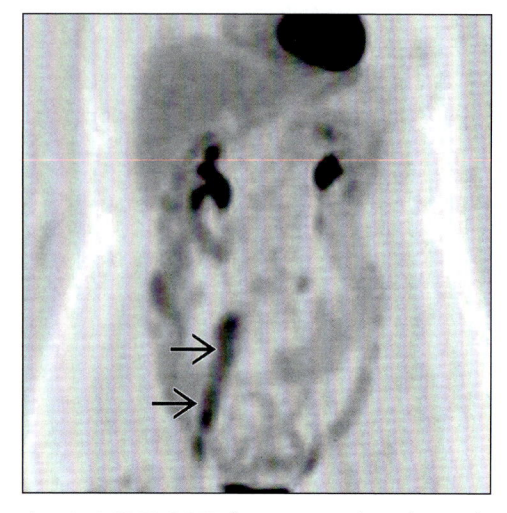

Anterior MIP FDG PET shows increased uptake in right iliac vein ➔ due to acute deep venous thrombosis. ≥ 20% of patients with unprovoked VTE have an occult malignancy.

TERMINOLOGY

Abbreviations and Synonyms
- Paraneoplastic syndrome (PNS); paraneoplastic encephalomyelitis (PEM)

Definitions
- Syndromes mediated by humoral factors produced by tumor or immune response to tumor

IMAGING FINDINGS

General Features
- Best diagnostic clue: Imaging findings in various PNS disorders: May be specific, nonspecific, or absent

Nuclear Medicine Findings
- Identification of occult cancer in patients with suspected PNS
  - FDG PET may detect occult malignancy in 23-37% of patients with suspected paraneoplastic syndromes
    - Available data from limited number of small series
  - Endocrine paraneoplastic disorders (e.g., Cushing syndrome, carcinoid-like syndrome, virilization, feminization, precocious puberty)
    - Directed anatomic imaging (CT, MR) should be performed first
    - Scintigraphy/SPECT using labeled In-111 octreotide: Where islet cell tumor, carcinoid, medullary thyroid cancer suspected
    - Scintigraphy/SPECT using labeled I-131 or -123 MIBG: Where pheochromocytoma suspected
- Diagnosis of PNS: Specific imaging findings may characterize some, but not all, PNS disorders
  - Paraneoplastic encephalomyelitis (PEM): Wide range of disorders effecting brain and central nervous system; may be degenerative
    - E.g., Lambert-Eaton myasthenic syndrome, paraneoplastic cerebellar degeneration, stiff-person syndrome, myasthenia gravis
    - Acute PEM findings: Focal uptake on FDG PET in regions of inflammation or sustained seizure activity
    - Late PEM findings: May show hypometabolism on FDG PET where neuronal damage previously occurred

DDx: Mimics of Paraneoplastic Disorders

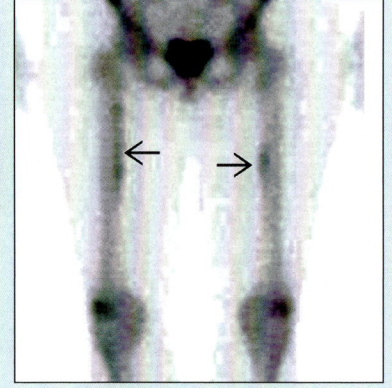

Adductor Splints

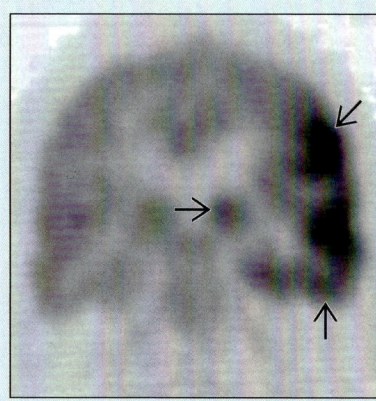

Herpes Encephalitis

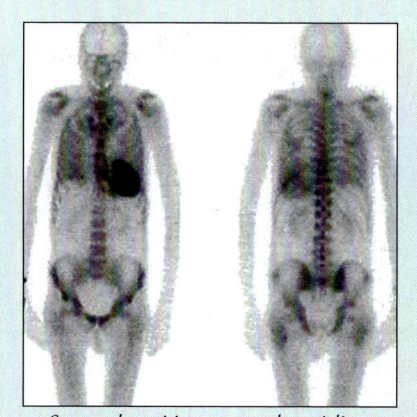

Secondary Hyperparathyroidism

PARANEOPLASTIC DISORDERS

Key Facts

Terminology
- Paraneoplastic syndrome (PNS); paraneoplastic encephalomyelitis (PEM)
- Syndromes mediated by humoral factors produced by tumor or immune response to tumor

Imaging Findings
- Best diagnostic clue: Imaging findings in various PNS disorders: May be specific, nonspecific, or absent
- FDG PET may detect occult malignancy in 23-37% of patients with suspected paraneoplastic syndromes
- Diagnosis of PNS: Specific imaging findings may characterize some, but not all, PNS disorders
- Acute PEM findings: Focal uptake on FDG PET in regions of inflammation or sustained seizure activity
- Late PEM findings: May show hypometabolism on FDG PET where neuronal damage previously occurred
- Poly/dermatomyositis: Focal FDG uptake in skeletal muscles, not attributable to recent activity
- Tc-99m diphosphonate bone scan in PTHrP syndrome: Uptake due to "metastatic calcification" in solid organs such as lungs, heart, stomach
- Secondary amyloidosis: Uptake of Tc-99m diphosphonate in involved solid organs
- HOA: Diffusely "active" Tc-99m bone scan; periosteal uptake in long bones (esp. distal femurs)
- Oncogenic osteomalacia: Fractures, increased uptake of Tc-99m diphosphonate in anterior rib ends
- Large vessel vasculitis: Diffuse FDG uptake in walls of large arteries (aorta, subclavian, iliac)
- ≥ 20% of patients with unprovoked DVT may have occult malignancy: Role of FDG PET in screening for cancer not yet established
- Acute clot shows increased uptake on FDG PET

- Paraneoplastic limbic or brainstem encephalitis: ↑ FDG activity in posterior thalamus, hippocampus, or brainstem; may be unilateral or bilateral
- Paraneoplastic cerebellar degeneration: Cerebellar foci of increased FDG uptake may occur in absence of CT or MR findings
- Polymyositis, dermatomyositis: May occur with hematologic malignancies or myelodysplastic syndromes
    - Symptoms include muscle pain, fever, elevated sed rate
    - 25% have underlying malignancy
    - Poly/dermatomyositis: Focal FDG uptake in skeletal muscles, not attributable to recent activity
- PTHrP syndrome: Hyperparathyroidism-like syndrome due to excretion of parathyroid hormone related protein (PTHrP) by tumor
    - Hypercalcemia, osteomalacia
    - Tc-99m diphosphonate bone scan in PTHrP syndrome: Uptake due to "metastatic calcification" in solid organs such as lungs, heart, stomach
    - Variable finding on Tc-99m bone scan: Prominent uptake throughout entire skeleton
- Secondary amyloidosis: Deposition of abnormal protein in solid organs due to myeloma, related disorders
    - Symptoms specific to organ involved
    - Secondary amyloidosis: Uptake of Tc-99m diphosphonate in involved solid organs
- Hypertrophic osteoarthropathy (HOA)
    - Presentation: Arthralgias (esp. peripheral), ± clubbing of digits
    - HOA: Periosteal new bone formation on CT, plain film
    - HOA: Diffusely "active" Tc-99m bone scan; periosteal uptake in long bones (esp. distal femurs)
- Oncogenic osteomalacia
    - Due to mesenchymal tumors, often benign, small & clinically inapparent
    - Plain film, CT: Poor mineralization, pathologic fractures, Looser zones
    - Oncogenic osteomalacia: Fractures, increased uptake of Tc-99m diphosphonate in anterior rib ends
    - FDG PET or In-111 octreotide: May be helpful in identifying occult primary tumor
- Large vessel vasculitis: Less common than small vessel vasculitis
    - Large vessel vasculitis: Diffuse FDG uptake in walls of large arteries (aorta, subclavian, iliac)
    - CT: Large artery vascular wall thickening, perivascular stranding
- Deep venous thrombosis (DVT)
    - ≥ 20% of patients with unprovoked DVT may have occult malignancy: Role of FDG PET in screening for cancer not yet established
    - Acute clot shows increased uptake on FDG PET

Imaging Recommendations
- Best imaging tool
    - Diagnosis of underlying occult malignancy in presence of suspected PNS: FDG PET/CT
    - Imaging findings of specific PNS disorders may mimic diseases that occur in absence of cancer
- Protocol advice: Interpretation of imaging studies in light of accurate and complete history, physical findings is critical to accuracy

DIFFERENTIAL DIAGNOSIS

Neurological
- PEM may mimic many other neurological disorders
- Infectious or post-infectious
    - Guillain-Barré syndrome, encephalitis, cerebritis
- Vascular disease
    - Stroke, vasculitis, aneurysm
- Neurodegenerative disorders
    - Myasthenia gravis, multiple sclerosis, dementia, epilepsy, toxins, poisons
- Metastatic disease to brain or spinal cord

Musculoskeletal
- Secondary HOA

PARANEOPLASTIC DISORDERS

- ○ May occur with non-malignant lung or liver disease
- ○ Also autosomal dominant primary HOA (pachydermal periostosis)
- Reflex sympathetic dystrophy, polymyalgia rheumatica, hypervitaminosis A, thyroid acropachy may mimic HOA
- Polymyositis, dermatomyositis
  - ○ Usually occurs in absence of cancer
- Oncogenic osteomalacia
  - ○ May mimic other causes of osteomalacia

Cardiovascular
- Primary amyloidosis
- Idiopathic or viral cardiomyopathy
- Hemochromatosis
- Ischemic cardiomyopathy

Vascular
- Venothromboembolism
  - ○ Many non-oncologic causes
- Giant cell or Takayasu arteritis

Endocrine
- Primary or secondary hyperparathyroidism: Clinical identical to PTHrP PNS

Hematologic
- Primary amyloidosis: May mimic PNS amyloidosis involvement of solid organs

PATHOLOGY

General Features
- Etiology
  - ○ Humoral factors evolved by tumor
    - ▪ Parathyroid hormone related proteins (PTHrP): Indistinguishable in physiologic activity from PTH
    - ▪ Neuroendocrine tumors: Produce hormones that ⇒ disease manifestations (e.g., gastrinoma, insulinoma, carcinoid, pheochromocytoma)
  - ○ Autoantibodies: Against tumor antigens; cross-react with host tissues
    - ▪ Autoantibodies to onconeural antigens in CNS: Produce multifocal inflammatory lesions in paraneoplastic encephalomyelitis (PEM)
    - ▪ PEM: Associated with serum and CSF anti Hu, Yo, Ma1, Ta, Ma2; ± association with non-neuronal antinuclear & anticytoplasmic antibodies
  - ○ T-cells: Cytotoxic cdr2-specific T-cells may play a role in paraneoplastic cerebellar degeneration
- Epidemiology: May occur in up to 10-15% of malignancies (may be underestimated)

CLINICAL ISSUES

Presentation
- Most common signs/symptoms
  - ○ Wide range of manifestations: Most nonspecific for PNS
  - ○ Nonspecific: Fever, anorexia, taste disorder, cachexia, pruritus
  - ○ Paraneoplastic encephalomyelitis: Ataxia, dizziness, nystagmus, loss of muscle tone & fine motor coordination, slurred speech, memory loss, seizure
  - ○ Musculoskeletal: Pain due to pathologic fractures, muscle pain, arthralgias
  - ○ Endocrine manifestations: Symptoms specific to humoral factors produced
  - ○ Gastrointestinal: Diarrhea, electrolyte imbalance, peptic ulcers, 2° motility & secretory humoral factors

Demographics
- Age: All ages affected
- Gender: No gender predilection

Natural History & Prognosis
- Variable: DIC associated with poor prognosis; HOA may improve prognosis

Treatment
- Treatment of underlying tumor: May result in rapid resolution of PNS
  - ○ Surgery
  - ○ Chemotherapy
  - ○ Radiation therapy
- Treatment of presumed immune mediated syndromes
  - ○ Immunosuppressive drugs, steroids, immune globulin, plasma exchange
- HOA: Ipsilateral vagus nerve resection

DIAGNOSTIC CHECKLIST

Consider
- Directed anatomic imaging with CT, MR as first-line modality
- FDG PET/CT may find occult malignancy in ~ 30-40% of suspected PNS
- Scintigraphy with In-111 octreotide, I-123/I-131 MIBG

SELECTED REFERENCES

1. Vedeler CA et al: Management of paraneoplastic neurological syndromes: report of an EFNS Task Force. Eur J Neurol. 13(7):682-90, 2006
2. Pacak K et al: The role of [(18)F]fluorodeoxyglucose positron emission tomography and [(111)In]-diethylenetriaminepentaacetate-D-Phe-pentetreotide scintigraphy in the localization of ectopic adrenocorticotropin-secreting tumors causing Cushing's syndrome. J Clin Endocrinol Metab. 89(5):2214-21, 2004
3. Scheid R et al: Serial 18F-fluoro-2-deoxy-D-glucose positron emission tomography and magnetic resonance imaging of paraneoplastic limbic encephalitis. Arch Neurol. 61(11):1785-9, 2004
4. Younes-Mhenni S et al: FDG-PET improves tumour detection in patients with paraneoplastic neurological syndromes. Brain. 127(Pt 10):2331-8, 2004
5. Berner U et al: Paraneoplastic syndromes: detection of malignant tumors using [(18)F]FDG-PET. Q J Nucl Med. 47(2):85-9, 2003
6. Kassubek J et al: Limbic encephalitis investigated by 18FDG-PET and 3D MRI. J Neuroimaging. 11(1):55-9, 2001
7. Rees JH et al: The role of [18F]fluoro-2-deoxyglucose-PET scanning in the diagnosis of paraneoplastic neurological disorders. Brain. 124(Pt 11):2223-31, 2001

PARANEOPLASTIC DISORDERS

IMAGE GALLERY

Variant

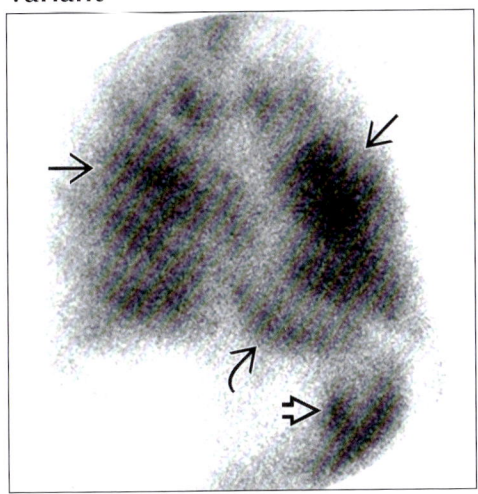

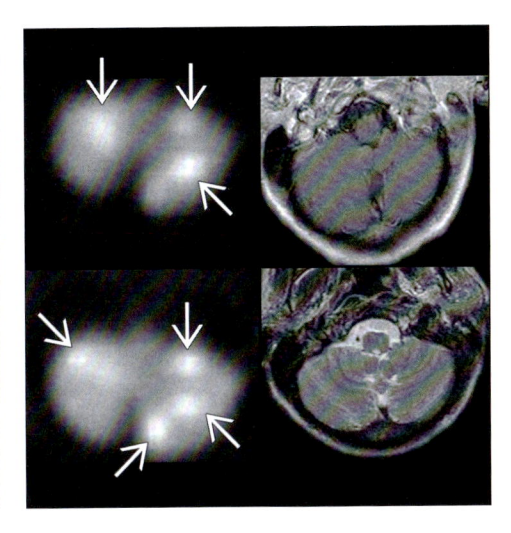

(Left) Anterior Tc-99m diphosphonate bone scan of chest shows increased uptake in lungs ➡, heart ➚, and stomach ➪ 2° hypercalcemia due to PTHrP syndrome (small cell lung cancer in this case). *(Right)* Axial FDG PET of posterior fossa (left panel) with companion MR (right panel) shows multiple foci of increased FDG uptake ➡ with normal MR (presumed paraneoplastic cerebellar degeneration). (Courtesy T. Larson, MD).

Typical

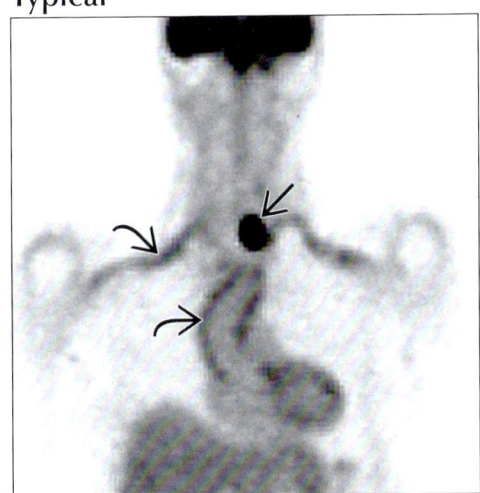

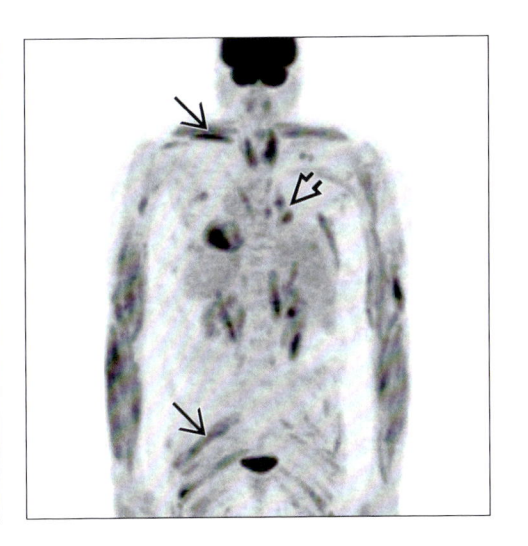

(Left) Coronal FDG PET scan in a patient with medullary thyroid cancer ➡ shows increased uptake in aortic and subclavian arteries ➚, consistent with paraneoplastic large vessel vasculitis, more common seen in hematologic/myelodysplastic malignancy. *(Right)* Posterior MIP FDG PET scan shows increased uptake in multiple muscle cords ➡ in patient with known small cell lung cancer ➪ and paraneoplastic polymyositis.

Typical

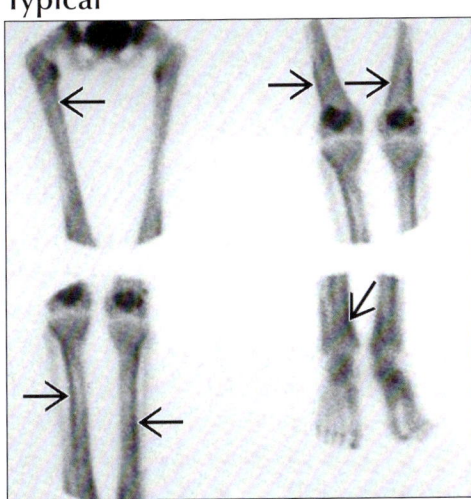

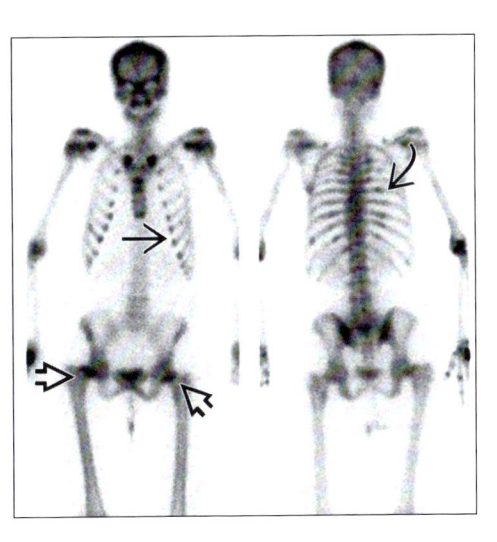

(Left) Multiple anterior planar views of the lower extremities from a Tc-99m diphosphonate bone scan shows diffuse increased activity with focal uptake along cortical surfaces ➡ in a patient with HOA 2° lung cancer. *(Right)* Anterior and posterior bone scan in patient with hemangiopericytoma of the foot shows accentuation of anterior rib ends ➡ & fractures of posterior ribs ➡ & bilateral femoral necks ➪ 2° to oncogenic osteomalacia.

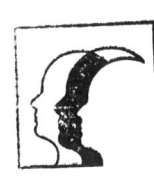

Praxis
Dr. Med. Boris Kirschsieper
Facharzt für Nuklearmedizin
Facharzt für Diagnostische Radiologie

Balger Strasse 50   Tel: (07221) 91 27 94
79832 Baden-Baden   Fax: (07221) 91 27 98

Web: www.Praxis-Kirschsieper.de
E-Mail: info@Praxis-Kirschsieper.de

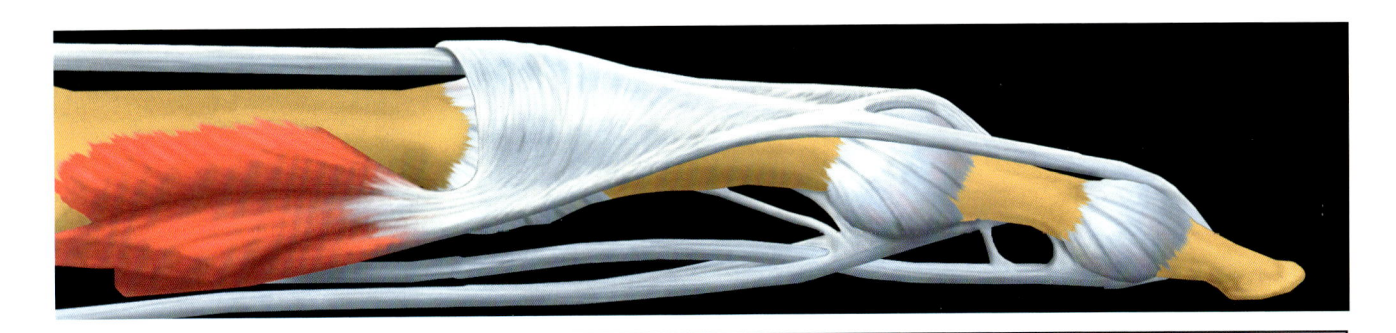

INDEX

A

Abscess
  bone, solitary (unicameral) bone cyst vs., 1–13
  central nervous system
    brain metastases vs., **5–40i**, 5–41
    gliomas and astrocytomas vs., 5–33
    primary CNS lymphoma vs., **5–36i**, 5–37
    radiation necrosis vs., 5–46
  dental, squamous cell carcinoma of head and neck vs., **6–2i**, 6–3
  gastrointestinal
    biliary leak vs., **8–20i**, 8–21
    chronic cholecystitis vs., 8–18
  hepatic, hepatic metastases vs., 8–57
  intestinal, intestinal neoplasms vs., **8–120i**, 8–121
  neck, squamous cell carcinoma of head and neck vs., **6–8i**, 6–9
  perirenal, renal mass vs., **9–20i**
  renal
    renal cell carcinoma vs., 9–23
    renal mass vs., 9–21
  testicular, testicular torsion vs., 9–53
  tubo-ovarian
    benign ovarian pathology vs., **9–60i**, 9–61
    ovarian cancer vs., 9–63
Accessory spleen. *See* Spleen, accessory and ectopic.
Acetabular labral tear, hip pain vs., 1–142
Achilles tendinitis, calcaneal pain vs., **1–150i**, 1–151
Adductor splints, paraneoplastic disorders vs., **11–48i**
Adenocarcinoma
  lung. *See* Non-small cell lung cancer.
  mucinous, hepatocellular carcinoma vs., **8–64i**
  of unknown primary, 11–46 to 11–47
  pancreatic. *See* Pancreatic neoplasms, adenocarcinoma.
Adenoids, PET studies of well-differentiated thyroid cancer and, 7–60
Adenoma
  adrenal, 8–76, 8–82
  colonic, adenocarcinoma of unknown primary vs., **11–46i**
  hepatic
    cavernous hemangioma vs., **8–70i**, 8–71 to 8–72
    focal nodular hyperplasia vs., 8–43
    intestinal neoplasms vs., **8–116i**, 8–117
  parathyroid. *See* Parathyroid adenoma.
  pleomorphic, parotid and salivary tumors vs., 6–12
  serous cystadenoma, islet cell tumors vs., 8–142
  thyroid. *See* Thyroid adenoma.
Adenomyomatosis, gallbladder cancer vs., **8–38i**, 8–40
Adipose tissue. *See also* Brown fat, hypermetabolic.
  chemotherapy-induced FDG uptake, skeletal muscle disorders vs., 1–165 to 1–166
Adrenal disorders, MIBG-positive, pheochromocytoma vs., **8–80i**, 8–81 to 8–82
Adrenal hemorrhage, 8–76
Adrenal neoplasms, 8–74 to 8–79, **8–77i** to **8–79i**
  adenoma, 8–76, 8–82
  carcinoma, 8–76, **8–80i**, 8–82
  differential diagnosis, **8–74i**, 8–76
  metastatic, **8–80i**, 8–82
  myelolipoma, 8–76, 8–82
  pheochromocytoma, 8–80 to 8–83, **8–83i**
AIDS. *See* HIV-AIDS.
Alagille syndrome, biliary atresia vs., 8–31
Alpha-1 antitrypsin deficiency, biliary atresia vs., 8–31
Alveolar proteinosis, pulmonary, pneumocystis carinii pneumonia vs., 4–17
Alzheimer disease, 5–22 to 5–25, **5–25i**
  dementia vs., 5–27
  differential diagnosis, **5–22i**, 5–23 to 5–24
  normal pressure hydrocephalus vs., 5–59
  with infarct, seizure vs., **5–16i**
Amiodarone effects
  Graves disease vs., 7–13
  Hashimoto thyroiditis vs., 7–17
  subacute thyroiditis vs., 7–29
Amyloidosis, 1–168 to 1–169
  differential diagnosis, **1–168i**, 1–169
  hyperparathyroidism vs., **1–72i**, 1–74
  paraneoplastic disorders vs., 11–50
Aneurysm
  large vessel vasculitis vs., **2–8i**, 2–9
  left ventricular, valvular heart disease vs., **3–12i**, 3–13 to 3–14
  mycotic, atherosclerosis vs., 2–12
Aneurysmal bone cyst, 1–10 to 1–11

INDEX

differential diagnosis, **1–10i**, 1–11
hip pain vs., 1–141
osteosarcoma vs., 1–29
solitary (unicameral) bone cyst vs., **1–12i**, 1–13
wrist pain vs., 1–146
Angiodysplasia, colonic, GI bleeding localization vs., 8–128
Angiomyolipoma, renal cell carcinoma vs., **9–22i**, 9–23
Anterior cruciate ligament injury, knee pain vs., 1–156
Antibody therapy, radiolabeled, 10–8 to 10–11, **10–11i**
Anxiety, 5–75
Appendicitis, chronic cholecystitis vs., 8–18
Appendicular osteomyelitis, 1–52 to 1–57, **1–55i** to **1–57i**
Arteriosclerosis. *See* Atherosclerosis.
Arteriovenous malformations, metastatic disease of lung and mediastinum vs., 4–40
Arthritis, non-infectious, 1–132 to 135, **1–135i**. *See also* Osteoarthritis.
    differential diagnosis, **1–132i**, 1–133
    foot osteomyelitis vs., 1–64
    fractures vs., **1–124i**
    hematoproliferative disorders vs., 1–172
    hip pain vs., 1–141
    insufficiency fractures vs., 1–120
    juvenile chronic, Legg-Calvé-Perthes disease vs., 1–109
    pediatric osteomyelitis vs., 1–68
    rheumatoid, hip pain vs., 1–141
    wrist pain vs., 1–145
Arthritis, septic
    non-infectious arthritis vs., **1–132i**, 1–133
    pediatric osteomyelitis vs., 1–67 to 1–68
    sickle cell osteopathy vs., 1–178
Arthrofibrosis, painful joint prosthesis vs., 1–111
Arthropathies. *See also* Osteoarthropathy.
    appendicular osteomyelitis vs., 1–54
    bone metastases vs., 1–20
    diabetic neuropathic, calcaneal pain vs., 1–151
Artifacts
    cardiomyopathy vs., 3–7
    myocardial infarction vs., **3–26i**, 3–27
    myocardial ischemia vs., **3–16i**, 3–18
Ascites, biliary leak vs., **8–20i**, 8–21
Aseptic necrosis. *See* Osteonecrosis.
Aspiration pneumonia, pneumocystis carinii pneumonia vs., **4–16i**
Asplenia/polysplenia syndromes, 8–90 to 8–93, **8–93i**
Asthma, abnormal quantitative V/Q scan due to, **4–10i**, 4–12
Astrocytomas, 5–32 to 5–35, **5–35i**
    differential diagnosis, **5–32i**, 5–33
    low-grade, seizure vs., 5–17
Asymmetrical muscle activity, squamous cell carcinoma of head and neck vs., **6–2i**, 6–3, 6–9 to 6–10
Atherosclerosis, 2–10 to 2–13, **2–13i**
    differential diagnosis, **2–10i**, 2–11 to 2–12
    large vessel vasculitis vs., **2–8i**, **2–10i**, 2–11
    vascular thrombosis vs., 2–15
Attention deficit disorder, 5–75
Avascular necrosis. *See* Osteonecrosis.
Avulsion injury
    hip pain vs., 1–141
    stress fracture vs., 1–129
Axial osteomyelitis, 1-58 to 1-59

B

Back surgery, failed. *See* Failed back surgery syndrome.
Bacterial pneumonia
    interstitial lung disease vs., **4–20i**
    pneumocystis carinii pneumonia vs., **4–16i**
Bedding contamination, sentinel lymph node vs., 2–6
Biliary tract disorders, 8–4 to 8–41
    biliary atresia, 8–30 to 8–33, **8–33i**
    biliary bypass obstruction, 8–28 to 8–29
    biliary leak, 8–20 to 8–21
        biliary bypass obstruction vs., **8–28i**, 8–29
        common bile duct obstruction vs., **8–22i**
        differential diagnosis, **8–20i**. 8–21
        peritoneal systemic shunt vs., **8–158i**, 8–159
    biloma, choledochal cyst vs., 8–25
    cholangiocarcinoma, 8–34 to 8–37, **8–37i**
    cholecystitis. *See* Cholecystitis.
    choledochal cyst, 8–24 to 8–27, **8–27i**
        biliary atresia vs., 8–31
        common bile duct obstruction vs., **8–22i**
        differential diagnosis, **8–24i**, 8–25
    common bile duct obstruction, 8–22 to 8–23
        complete, acute calculous cholecystitis vs., 8–5
        differential diagnosis, **8–22i**, 8–23
    duodenogastric reflux, chronic cholecystitis vs., **8–16i**, 8–17
    gallbladder cancer, 8–36 to 8–41, **8–41i**
    obstruction, choledochal cyst vs., **8–24i**, 8–25
    occult lithiasis, microlithiasis, chronic cholecystitis vs., 8–17
    sphincter dysfunction, chronic cholecystitis vs., **8–16i**, 8–17
Binswanger disease, normal pressure hydrocephalus vs., 5–60
Bladder. *See* Urinary bladder.
Bleeding, gastrointestinal
    inflammatory bowel disease vs., **8–130i**, 8–131

INDEX

    localization of, 8–126 to 8–129, **8–129i**
    Meckel diverticulum vs., **8–122i**, 8–123
Blood brain barrier disruption, 5–14 to 5–15
Blood pool activity
    vascular graft infection vs., **2–16i**, 2–17
    vascular thrombosis vs., **2–14i**, 2–15
Bone abscess, solitary (unicameral) bone cyst vs., 1–13
Bone cyst
    aneurysmal, 1–10 to 1–11
        differential diagnosis, **1–10i**, 1–11
        hip pain vs., 1–141
        osteosarcoma vs., 1–29
        solitary (unicameral) bone cyst vs., **1–12i**, 1–13
        wrist pain vs., 1–146
    simple, enchondroma vs., 1–7
    solitary (unicameral), 1–12 to 1–15, **1–15i**
        hip pain vs., 1–141
        wrist pain vs., 1–146
Bone disease, metabolic, 1–72 to 1–85
    bone superscan vs., 1–26
    calcaneal pain vs., 1–152
    hyperparathyroidism. *See* Hyperparathyroidism.
    hypertrophic osteoarthropathy. *See* Osteoarthropathy, hypertrophic (HOA).
    osteomalacia. *See* Osteomalacia.
    pediatric osteomyelitis vs., 1–68
Bone dysplasias. *See* Dysplasias.
Bone fractures. *See* Fractures.
Bone infarction. *See also* Osteonecrosis.
    bone metastases vs., 1–20
    chondrosarcoma vs., 1–39
    enchondroma vs., **1–6i**, 1–7
    multiple enchondromatosis vs., **1–96i**, 1–97
    non-infectious arthritis vs., 1–133
    osteosarcoma vs., 1–29
    wrist pain vs., 1–145
Bone infections, 1–48 to 1–71
    cellulitis, 1–48 to 1–51, **1–51i**
    chondrosarcoma vs., 1–39
    osteomyelitis. *See* Osteomyelitis.
    osteonecrosis vs., 1–105
    osteosarcoma vs., 1–29
    prosthetic joint vs., 1–110 to 1–111
Bone island, wrist pain vs., 1–146
Bone marrow
    disorders. *See* Hematoproliferative disorders.
    metastases, hematoproliferative disorders vs., **1–170i**
    normal activity, vascular graft infection vs., 2–17
    stimulant drugs, hypersplenism vs., 8–52
Bone metastases, 1–18 to 1–23, **1–21i** to **1–23i**
    axial osteomyelitis vs., **1–58i**, 1–59

    bone superscan vs., 1–26
    differential diagnosis, **1–18i**, 1–20
    Ewing sarcoma vs., 1–35
    failed back surgery syndrome vs., **1–112i**, 1–114
    fibrous dysplasia vs., **1–90i**
    fractures vs., **1–124i**
    hip pain vs., 1–141
    hyperparathyroidism vs., **1–72i**, 1–73
    hypertrophic osteoarthropathy vs., 1–81
    insufficiency fractures vs., **1–118i**, 1–120
    Legg-Calvé-Perthes disease vs., **1–108i**
    lytic, multiple myeloma vs., 1–181
    multiple enchondromatosis vs., **1–96i**, 1–97
    multiple myeloma vs., 1–181
    neuroblastoma, pediatric osteomyelitis vs., **1–66i**
    non-accidental trauma vs., **1–126i**, 1–127
    non-infectious arthritis vs., **1–132i**, 1–133
    osteoid osteoma vs., **1–2i**, 1–4
    osteomalacia vs., 1–77
    osteosarcoma vs., 1–29
    Paget disease vs., **1–86i**, 1–87
    palliation of bone pain, 1–44 to 1–47, **1–47i**
    prostatic, 1–42 to 1–43
    sickle cell osteopathy vs., **1–176i**
Bone neoplasms, 1–2 to 1–47
    axial osteomyelitis vs., 1–59
    benign
        chondrosarcoma vs., 1–39
        Ewing sarcoma vs., 1–35
        osteosarcoma vs., 1–29
    bone superscan for, 1–24 to 1–27, **1–27i**
    calcaneal pain vs., 1–152
    cellulitis vs., **1–48i**, 1–49
    chondrosarcoma. *See* Chondrosarcoma.
    enchondroma. *See* Enchondroma.
    Ewing sarcoma. *See* Ewing sarcoma.
    fibrous cortical defect, 1–8 to 1–9
    fibrous dysplasia vs., 1–91
    fractures vs., 1–125
    giant cell tumor. *See* Giant cell tumor.
    knee pain vs., 1–156
    lytic, sickle cell osteopathy vs., **1–176i**, 1–178
    melorheostosis vs., 1–93
    MIBG-negative/MIBG-positive, neuroblastoma vs., 8–85
    multiple myeloma vs., 1–181
    non-accidental trauma vs., **1–126i**, 1–127
    non-infectious arthritis vs., 1–133
    osteoid osteoma. *See* Osteoid osteoma.
    osteonecrosis vs., 1–105 to 1–106
    osteosarcoma. *See* Osteosarcoma.
    pediatric osteomyelitis vs., 1–68
    primary
        bone metastases vs., 1–20

INDEX

chondrosarcoma vs., 1–39
hip pain vs., **1–140i**, 1–141
osteosarcoma vs., 1–29
Paget disease vs., **1–86i**, 1–87
sclerotic, sickle cell osteopathy vs., 1–178
skeletal muscle disorders vs., 1–166
wrist pain vs., 1–146
Bone pain
metastatic, palliation of, 1–44 to 1–47, **1–47i**
sickle cell disease, 1–176 to 1–179, **1–179i**
Bone superscan, 1–24 to 1–27, **1–27i**
Bone trauma. *See also* Fractures.
bone metastases vs., 1–20
chondrosarcoma vs., 1–39
fibrous cortical defect vs., 1–9
healing, appendicular osteomyelitis vs., 1–54
multiple enchondromatosis vs., **1–96i**, 1–97
osteosarcoma vs., **1–28i**, 1–29
pediatric osteomyelitis vs., 1–67
Bowel disease
chronic cholecystitis vs., 8–18
inflammatory, 8–130 to 8–133, **8–133i**. *See also* Crohn disease.
differential diagnosis, **8–130i**, 8–131
intestinal neoplasms vs., **8–116i**, 8–117
non-infectious and ischemic colitis, intraabdominal infection vs., 8–146
ischemic, chronic cholecystitis vs., 8–18
Brachiocephalic vein/artery fistula, abnormal quantitative V/Q scan due to, **4–10i**
Bradycardia, and brain death scan, **5–4i**
Brain. *See also* Central nervous system; Cerebral vascular occlusion; Dementia; Seizures.
blood brain barrier disruption, 5–14 to 5–15
contusion, stroke vs., 5–11
heterotopic gray matter, 5–64 to 5–69, **5–69i**
imaging overview, 5–2 to 5–3
infection and inflammation, 5–70 to 5–73, **5–73i**
normal aging, normal pressure hydrocephalus vs., 5–59
normal pressure hydrocephalus. *See* Hydrocephalus, normal pressure.
psychiatric disorders, 5–74 to 5–79, **5–77i** to **5–79i**
Brain death, 5–4 to 5–9, **5–8i** to **5–9i**
Brain neoplasms
astrocytomas, 5–32 to 5–35, **5–35i**
differential diagnosis, **5–32i**, 5–33
low-grade, seizure vs., 5–17
gliomas. *See* Gliomas.
infection or inflammation vs., **5–70i**, 5–71
metastatic, 5–40 to 5–43, **5–43i**
blood brain barrier disruption vs., **5–14i**, 5–15

brain infection and inflammation vs., 5–71
differential diagnosis, **5–40i**, 5–41 to 5–42
gliomas and astrocytomas vs., 5–33
primary CNS lymphoma vs., 5–37
primary central nervous system lymphoma, 5–36 to 5–39, **5–39i**
primary tumor, brain metastases vs., 5–41
radiation necrosis vs. recurrent tumor, 5–44 to 5–49, **5–47i** to **5–49i**
stroke vs., **5–10i**, 5–11
Branchial cleft cyst, ectopic thyroid gland vs., 7–37
Breast
benign disease, 11–32 to 11–33
lactating, primary breast cancer vs., **11–34i**, 11–35
normal, primary breast cancer vs., 11–35
Breast neoplasms
benign breast disease vs., **11–32i**, 11–33
nonmalignant, primary breast cancer vs., 11–35
primary, 11–34 to 11–39, **11–37i** to **11–39i**
staging/restaging, 11–40 to 11–45, **11–43i** to **11–45i**
Bronchioalveolar carcinoma, interstitial lung disease vs., 4–22
Bronchogenic carcinoma. *See* Non-small cell lung cancer.
Brown fat, hypermetabolic
adrenal malignancy vs., **8–74i**, 8–76
benign mimics of lymphoma vs., **11–2i**
breast cancer staging/restaging vs., **11–40i**
Hodgkin lymphoma staging vs., **11–6i**
low-grade non-Hodgkin lymphoma vs., **11–16i**
medullary thyroid cancer vs., **7–62i**
melanoma staging vs., **11–24i**, 11–26
melanoma therapy evaluation/restaging vs., 11–29
non-Hodgkin lymphoma staging vs., **11–20i**
skeletal muscle disorders vs., **1–164i**, 1–165
squamous cell carcinoma of head and neck vs., **6–2i**, 6–3, 6–9 to 6–10
thymus disorder vs., **4–46i**, 4–47
Brown tumor
aneurysmal bone cyst vs., **1–10i**, 1–11
bone metastases vs., 1–20
solitary (unicameral) bone cyst vs., **1–12i**, 1–13
Budd-Chiari syndrome
focal nodular hyperplasia vs., **8–42i**, 8–44
hepatic cirrhosis vs., **8–46i**, 8–48
Bursitis
knee pain vs., 1–156
osteonecrosis vs., 1–106
painful joint prosthesis vs., 1–111
trochanteric, hip pain vs., 1–141

INDEX

C

Caffey disease, non-accidental trauma vs., 1–127
Calcaneal pain, 1–150 to 1–153, **1–153i**
Camurati-Engelmann disease, infantile cortical, hypertrophic osteoarthropathy vs., 1–81
Cancer. *See* Neoplasms.
Capromab, physiologic uptake of, prostate cancer antibody scan, 9–77
Carcinoid tumor, 8–150 to 8–153, **8–153i**
    differential diagnosis, **8–150i**, 8–151
    hepatocellular carcinoma vs., **8–64i**
    islet cell tumors vs., **8–140i**
Carcinomatosis, lymphangitic, interstitial lung disease vs., **4–20i**, 4–22
Cardiac transplantation, 3–32 to 3–35, **3–35i**
Cardiovascular disorders, 3–2 to 3–39
    cardiac transplantation, 3–32 to 3–35, **3–35i**
    cardiomyopathy, 3–6 to 3–11, **3–9i** to **3–11i**
        differential diagnosis, **3–6i**, 3–7 to 3–8
        end-stage, pre-transplant evaluation, 3–33
        heart failure
            low-grade non-Hodgkin lymphoma vs., 11–17
            post-therapy evaluation of lymphoma vs., 11–11
    imaging overview, 3–2 to 3–5, **3–5i**
    left-to-right intracardiac shunts, 3–36 to 3–39
    myocardial infarction, 3–26 to 3–31, **3–29i** to **3–31i**
        amyloidosis vs., **1–168i**, 1–169
        differential diagnosis, **3–26i**, 3–27
    myocardial ischemia, 3–16 to 3–21, **3–19i** to **3–21i**
    myocardial viability, 3–22 to 3–25, **3–25i**
    myocardial wall thickening
        pericardial disease vs., 4–51
        valvular heart disease vs., 3–13
    paraneoplastic disorders vs., 11–50
    pericardial disease
        constrictive, cardiomyopathy vs., **3–8**, 3–7
        malignant and inflammatory, 4–50 to 4–53, **4–53i**
    valvular heart disease, 3–12 to 3–15, **3–15i**
Caroli disease, biliary atresia vs., 8–31
Cartilage
    injury, chondrosarcoma vs., **1–38i**
    lesions, melanoma therapy evaluation/restaging vs., **11–28i**
Castleman disease, benign mimics of lymphoma vs., 11–4
Cat-scratch fever
    benign mimics of lymphoma vs., 11–3
    post-therapy evaluation of lymphoma vs., 11–11
Catheter tip, breast cancer staging/restaging vs., **11–40i**
Cavernous hemangioma, 8–70 to 8–73, **8–73i**
    cholangiocarcinoma vs., **8–34i**, 8–35
    differential diagnosis, **8–70i**, 8–71 to 8–72
    hepatic metastases vs., **8–56i**, 8–57
Cellulitis, 1–48 to 1–51, **1–51i**
    differential diagnosis, **1–48i**, 1–49
    foot osteomyelitis vs., **1–62i**, 1–64
    pediatric osteomyelitis vs., 1–68
Central line tip, breast cancer staging/restaging vs., **11–40i**
Central nervous system, 5–2 to 5–79. *See also* Brain entries.
    cerebrospinal fluid leak, 5–50 to 5–53, **5–53i**
    neoplasms
        astrocytomas. *See* Astrocytomas.
        gliomas. *See* Gliomas.
        primary central nervous system lymphoma, 5–36 to 5–39, **5–39i**
        primary CNS lymphoma vs., 5–37
    normal pressure hydrocephalus. *See* Hydrocephalus, normal pressure.
    psychiatric disorders, 5–74 to 5–79, **5–77i** to **5–79i**
    ventricular shunt dysfunction, 5–54 to 5–57, **5–57i**
Cerebral contusion, stroke vs., 5–11
Cerebral edema, brain death vs., 5–6
Cerebral infarction
    brain death vs., **5–4i**, 5–6
    gliomas and astrocytomas vs., 5–33
Cerebral vascular occlusion, 5–10 to 5–13, **5–13i**. *See also* Atherosclerosis.
    Alzheimer disease vs., **5–22i**, 5–23
    brain metastases vs., **5–40i**, 5–41
    differential diagnosis, **5–10i**, 5–11
    seizure vs., **5–16i**
Cerebral venous infarct, stroke vs., 5–11
Cerebritis
    radiation necrosis vs., **5–44i**
    stroke vs., 5–11
Cerebrospinal fluid, shunting of. *See* Ventricular shunt dysfunction.
Cerebrospinal fluid leak, 5–50 to 5–53, **5–53i**
Cervical neoplasms, 9–68 to 9–71, **9–71i**
    benign uterine activity vs., 9–67
    differential diagnosis, **9–68i**, 9–69
    endometrial cancer vs., 9–73
Charcot joint, foot osteomyelitis vs., 1–64
Chemotherapy-induced adipose uptake, skeletal muscle disorders vs., 1–165 to 1–166
Chest and mediastinum, 4–2 to 4–52
Children
    neuroblastoma, 8–84 to 8–89, **8–87i** to **8–89i**
    non-accidental trauma, 1–126 to 1–127

INDEX

pediatric osteomyelitis, 1–66 to 1–71, **1–69i** to **1–71i**
Cholangiocarcinoma, 8–34 to 8–37, **8–37i**
   differential diagnosis, **8–34i**, 8–35
   gallbladder cancer vs., **8–38i**, 8–40
   hepatic metastases vs., **8–56i**
   hepatocellular carcinoma vs., 8–65
   intahepatic, cavernous hemangioma vs., 8–72
Cholangitis, primary sclerosing, cholangiocarcinoma vs., 8–35
Cholecystitis
   acute acalculous, 8–10 to 8–15, **8–13i** to **8–15i**
   acute calculous, 8–4 to 8–9, **8–7i** to **8–9i**
      acute acalculous cholecystitis vs., 8–11
      differential diagnosis, **8–4i**, 8–5 to 8–6
   chronic, 8–16 to 8–19, **8–19i**
      acute calculous cholecystitis vs., 8–5
      differential diagnosis, **8–16i**, 8–17 to 8–18
      gallbladder cancer vs., **8–38i**, 8–40
Choledochal cyst, 8–24 to 8–27, **8–27i**
   biliary atresia vs., 8–31
   common bile duct obstruction vs., **8–22i**
   differential diagnosis, **8–24i**, 8–25
Choledocholithiasis, biliary atresia vs., 8–31
Cholestasis, due to total parenteral nutrition, biliary atresia vs., **8–30i**, 8–31
Chondroblastic osteosarcoma, chondrosarcoma vs., 1–39
Chondroid tumors, wrist pain vs., 1–146
Chondrosarcoma, 1–38 to 1–41, **1–41i**
   differential diagnosis, **1–38i**, 1–39
   enchondroma vs., **1–6i**, 1–7
   heterotopic ossification vs., 1–159
   hip pain vs., 1–141
   multiple hereditary exostoses vs., **1–100i**, 1–101
   multiple myeloma vs., 1–181
   Paget disease vs., 1–87
Choroid plexus, and brain death scan, **5–4i**
Choroidal fissure cyst, seizure vs., 5–17
Cirrhosis. *See* Hepatic disorders, cirrhosis.
Clot, intravascular, vascular graft infection vs., 2–17
Clothing contamination, sentinel lymph node vs., 2–6
Colitis. *See also* Inflammatory bowel disease.
   non-infectious and ischemic, intraabdominal infection vs., 8–146
Collateral ligament injury, knee pain vs., 1–156
Colon adenoma, adenocarcinoma of unknown primary vs., **11–46i**
Colonic angiodysplasia, GI bleeding localization vs., 8–128
Colorectal neoplasms. *See* Intestinal neoplasms.
Common bile duct obstruction, 8–22 to 8–23
   complete, acute calculous cholecystitis vs., 8–5
   differential diagnosis, **8–22i**, 8–23

Compartmental models, plasma clearance, 9–36
Complex regional pain syndrome, 1–136 to 1–139, **1–139i**
   differential diagnosis, **1–136i**, 1–137 to 1–138
   wrist pain vs., 1–145
Compression fractures
   axial osteomyelitis vs., **1–58i**, 1–59
   spinal, in elderly, prostatic bone metastases vs., **1–42i**
Congenital hypothyroidism. *See* Hypothyroidism, congenital.
Contracture, complex regional pain syndrome vs., **1–136i**
Coronary artery disease. *See* Atherosclerosis.
Corpus luteum cysts
   benign ovarian pathology vs., **9–60i**
   ovarian cancer vs., **9–62i**
Cortical dysplasia, seizure vs., 5–17
Corticobasal degeneration, Alzheimer disease vs., 5–23
Creutzfeldt-Jakob disease, Alzheimer disease vs., 5–23
Cricoarytenoid muscles, PET studies of well-differentiated thyroid cancer and, 7–60
Criminal and antisocial behavior, 5–75
Crohn disease
   gastric carcinoma vs., 8–114
   gastritis vs., 8–107
   intestinal neoplasms vs., 8–117
   intraabdominal infection vs., **8–144i**
Cruciate ligament injury, knee pain vs., 1–156
CSF fluid, shunting of. *See* Ventricular shunt dysfunction.
Cushing disease, bone metastases vs., 1–20
Cutaneous lymphoma, neuroendocrine tumors of head and neck vs., **6–14i**, 6–15
Cystic fibrosis, biliary atresia vs., 8–31
Cystitis, bladder epithelial cancer vs., 9–49
Cystitis cystica, bladder epithelial cancer vs., 9–49
Cysts
   bone. *See* Bone cyst.
   choledochal. *See* Choledochal cyst.
   choroidal fissure, seizure vs., 5–17
   complex functional, ovarian cancer vs., 9–63
   corpus luteum
      benign ovarian pathology vs., **9–60i**
      ovarian cancer vs., **9–62i**
   dermoid/epidermoid, tongue, ectopic thyroid gland vs., 7–37
   epidermoid, testicular cancer vs., 9–57
   ganglion, wrist pain vs., 1–146
   hemorrhagic renal, renal cell carcinoma vs., **9–22i**, 9–23
   hepatic, choledochal cyst vs., 8–25
   mesenteric or omental, choledochal cyst vs., 8–25

INDEX

ovarian, benign ovarian pathology vs., **9–60i**
pancreatic pseudocyst, choledochal cyst vs., **8–24i**, 8–25
popliteal, knee pain vs., **1–154i**, 1–156
renal
    hemorrhagic, renal cell carcinoma vs., **9–22i**, 9–23
    renal cortical scar vs., **9–2i**, 9–4
thyroglossal duct, ectopic thyroid gland vs., **7–36i**, 7–37
Cytomegalovirus infection, heterotopic gray matter vs., 5–65
Cytomegalovirus pneumonitis, pneumocystis carinii pneumonia vs., 4–17

D

Deep venous thrombosis
    heterotopic ossification vs., 1–159
    lymphedema vs., **2–2i**
Degenerative process(es). *See also* Arthritis, non-infectious; Osteoarthritis.
    bone metastases vs., **1–18i**, 1–20
    fractures vs., **1–124i**
    sickle cell osteopathy vs., **1–176i**
Dehydration, renovascular hypertension vs., **9–10i**
Delayed imaging, bone superscan vs., 1–26
Dementia, 5–26 to 5–31, **5–29i** to **5–31i**. *See also* Alzheimer disease.
    autoimmune, 5–28
    differential diagnosis, **5–26i**, 5–27 to 5–28
    drug-related, 5–28
    frontotemporal, Alzheimer disease vs., 5–23
    multi-infarct, normal pressure hydrocephalus vs., 5–60
    post-traumatic, **5–26i**, 5–27 to 5–28
    reversible, Alzheimer disease vs., **5–22i**, 5–23
    vascular
        Alzheimer disease vs., **5–22i**, 5–23
        radiation necrosis vs., 5–46
Demyelination disorder, primary CNS lymphoma vs., 5–37
Dental abscess, squamous cell carcinoma of head and neck vs., **6–2i**, 6–3
Depression, 5–75
Dermatomyositis, paraneoplastic disorders vs., 11–50
Dermoid/epidermoid cyst, tongue, ectopic thyroid gland vs., 7–37
Diabetic neuropathic arthropathy, calcaneal pain vs., 1–151
Diaphragmatic patency determination, 8–162 to 8–163
Discitis
    axial osteomyelitis vs., 1–59
    fractures vs., **1–124i**
    insufficiency fractures vs., **1–118i**, 1–119

Discogenic sclerosis
    axial osteomyelitis vs., 1–59
    fractures vs., **1–124i**
Disuse, complex regional pain syndrome vs., **1–136i**, 1–137
Diverticulosis, GI bleeding localization vs., 8–128
Drug addiction, 5–74 to 5–79, **5–77i** to **5–79i**
Drug effects. *See* Medication effects.
Drug-related dementia, 5–28
Duodenal bulb, acute calculous cholecystitis vs., **8–4i**
Duodenal neoplasm, adrenal malignancy vs., **8–74i**
Duodenal pooling, choledochal cyst vs., **8–24i**
Duodenogastric reflux, chronic cholecystitis vs., **8–16i**, 8–17
Dysplasias, 1–86 to 1–103
    fibrous. *See* Fibrous dysplasia.
    melorheostosis, 1–92 to 1–95, **1–95i**
    metaphyseal (Rickets mimic), osteomalacia vs., 1–77
    mixed sclerosing, melorheostosis vs., 1–94
    multiple enchondromatoses. *See* Enchondromatoses, multiple.
    multiple hereditary exostoses. *See* Multiple hereditary exostoses.
    Paget disease. *See* Paget disease.
    progressive diaphyseal, melorheostosis vs., **1–92i**

E

Ectopic and accessory spleen, 8–94 to 8–97, **8–97i**
    asplenia/polysplenia syndromes vs., **8–90i**, 8–91
    differential diagnosis, **8–94i**, **8–95**
Ectopic parathyroid adenoma, 7–10 to 7–11
Ectopic pregnancy, benign ovarian pathology vs., **9–60i**, 9–61
Ectopic thyroid, 7–36 to 7–39, **7–39i**
    congenital hypothyroidism vs., **7–40i**, 7–41
    differential diagnosis, **7–36i**, 7–37 to 7–38
    ectopic parathyroid adenoma vs., **7–10i**
Ectopy, renal, 9–6 to 9–9, **9–9i**
    acute renal failure vs., **9–14i**, 9–16
    differential diagnosis, **9–6i**, 9–7
Ectropion, lacrimal complex dysfunction vs., **6–18i**, 6–19
Edema
    cardiac
        low-grade non-Hodgkin lymphoma vs., 11–17
        post-therapy evaluation of lymphoma vs., 11–11
    cerebral, brain death vs., 5–6
    nonlymphatic, lymphedema vs., **2–2i**
    pulmonary
        interstitial lung disease vs., 4–22
        pneumocystis carinii pneumonia vs., 4–17

INDEX

Effective renal plasma flow, 9–36
Embolism
    cerebral, stroke vs., 5–11
    pulmonary. *See* Pulmonary embolism.
Embolus, septic, pulmonary embolism vs., 4–8
Encephalitis
    brain infection and inflammation, 5–70 to 5–73, **5–73i**
    herpes, paraneoplastic disorders vs., **11–48i**
    limbic, brain infection and inflammation vs., 5–71
    paraneoplastic disorders vs., **11–48i**, 11–49
Encephalopathy, subcortical arteriosclerotic, normal pressure hydrocephalus vs., 5–60
Enchondroma, 1–6 to 1–7
    aneurysmal bone cyst vs., **1–10i**, 1–11
    chondrosarcoma vs., **1–38i**, 1–39
    differential diagnosis, with or without calcification, **1–6i**, 1–7
    osteoid osteoma vs., **1–2i**
    osteosarcoma vs., 1–29
    solitary (unicameral) bone cyst vs., 1–13
Enchondromatoses, multiple, 1–96 to 1–99, **1–99i**
    differential diagnosis, **1–96i**, 1–97
    enchondroma vs., 1–7
    multiple hereditary exostoses vs., **1–100i**, 1–101
Endobronchial carcinoma, metastatic disease of lung and mediastinum vs., 4–40
Endometrium
    carcinoma, 9–72 to 9–75, **9–75i**
    hyperplasia
        benign uterine activity vs., 9–67
        endometrial cancer vs., 9–73
    polyp
        benign uterine activity vs., 9–67
        endometrial cancer vs., 9–73
    tamoxifen-related changes, endometrial cancer vs., 9–73
Enthesopathy, hip pain vs., 1–142
Eosinophilic granuloma
    enchondroma vs., 1–7
    Ewing sarcoma vs., 1–35
    osteoid osteoma vs., 1–4
    osteosarcoma vs., 1–29
Epidermoid cyst, testicular cancer vs., 9–57
Epididymo-orchitis, testicular torsion vs., **9–52i**, 9–53
Epilepsy. *See* Seizures; Status epilepticus.
Epiphysis, slipped capital femoral
    hip pain vs., 1–142
    Legg-Calvé-Perthes disease vs., 1–109
Epistaxis
    inflammatory bowel disease vs., 8–131
    intraabdominal infection vs., **8–144i**
Esophageal neoplasms, 8–98 to 8–101, **8–101i**
    differential diagnosis, **8–98i**, 8–99 to 8–100
    esophageal dysmotility vs., **8–102i**, 8–104
Esophagitis
    inflammatory, esophageal neoplasms vs., 8–99
    with stricture, esophageal dysmotility vs., **8–102i**, 8–104
Esophagus
    diverticulum, gastric emptying disorders vs., **8–108i**
    dysmotility, 8–102 to 8–105, **8–105i**
    normal variants, esophageal neoplasms vs., 8–100
    varices, GI bleeding localization vs., 8–128
Ewing sarcoma, 1–34 to 1–37, **1–37i**
    appendicular osteomyelitis vs., **1–52i**, 1–54
    differential diagnosis, **1–34i**, 1–35 to 1–36
    hip pain vs., 1–141
    skeletal metastases vs., **1–18i**
Exostoses, multiple hereditary. *See* Multiple hereditary exostoses.
External radiation (XRT) changes. *See* Radiation necrosis.
Extramedullary hematopoiesis, renal mass vs., **9–20i**, 9–21

F

Facet joint, degenerative, PET studies of well-differentiated thyroid cancer and, **7–58i**
Failed back surgery syndrome
    differential diagnosis, **1–112i**, 1–114
    surgical assessment, 1–112 to 1–117, **1–115i** to **1–117i**
False-negative scan, myocardial viability vs., **3–22i**, 3–23
False-positive scan
    adrenal malignancy vs., **8–74i**, 8–76
    myocardial viability vs., **3–22i**, 3–23
Fasciitis, necrotizing, cellulitis vs., 1–49
Femoral fracture, proximal, insufficiency fractures vs., 1–120
Fetal lobulation, persistent, renal cortical scar vs., **9–2i**, 9–4
Fibrocystic breast disease, primary breast cancer vs., 11–35
Fibroid tumors, benign uterine activity vs., 9–67
Fibroma, nonossifying, 1–8 to 1–9
    differential diagnosis, **1–8i** to 1–9
    enchondroma vs., 1–7
Fibrosarcoma
    chondrosarcoma vs., 1–39
    hip pain vs., 1–141
Fibrothorax, pleural disease vs., 4–43
Fibrous cortical defect, 1–8 to 1–9
Fibrous dysplasia, 1–90 to 1–91
    axial osteomyelitis vs., **1–58i**

INDEX

chondrosarcoma vs., 1–39
differential diagnosis, **1–90i**, 1–91
enchondroma vs., 1–7
fibrous cortical defect vs., **1–8i**, 1–9
hip pain vs., 1–142
osteosarcoma vs., 1–29
Paget disease vs., **1–86i**, 1–87 to 1–88
solitary (unicameral) bone cyst vs., 1–13
temporal bone osteomyelitis vs., **1–60i**
wrist pain vs., 1–146
Fibroxanthoma, solitary (unicameral) bone cyst vs., 1–13
Focal fat, hepatic metastases vs., 8–58
Focal nodular hyperplasia, 8–42 to 8–45, **8–45i**
    cavernous hemangioma vs., 8–71
    cholangiocarcinoma vs., 8–35
    differential diagnosis, **8–42i**, 8–43 to 8–44
    hepatic metastases vs., 8–57
    hepatocellular carcinoma vs., 8–66
Foot, osteomyelitis, 1–62 to 1–65, **1–65i**
Foreign body
    benign uterine activity vs., 9–67
    lung, pulmonary embolism vs., 4–8
Foreign body reaction, radiation necrosis vs., 5–46
Forensics, 5–74 to 5–79, **5–77i** to **5–79i**
Fractures, 1–124 to 1–125
    calcaneal pain vs., 1–151
    cellulitis vs., **1–48i**, 1–49
    compression
        axial osteomyelitis vs., **1–58i**, 1–59
        spinal, in elderly, prostatic bone metastases vs., **1–42i**
    differential diagnosis, **1–124i**, 1–125
    Ewing sarcoma vs., **1–34i**, 1–36
    giant cell tumor vs., 1–17
    healing, bone metastases vs., 1–20
    hip pain vs., **1–140i** to 1–141
    insufficiency, 1–118 to 1–123, **1–121i** to **1–123i**
        differential diagnosis, **1–118i**, 1–119 to 1–120
        hip pain vs., 1–140 to 1–141
        osteonecrosis vs., **1–104i**, 1–105
    knee pain vs., 1–156
    non-accidental, neuroblastoma vs., **8–84i**
    occult
        failed back surgery syndrome vs., 1–114
        in elderly, prostatic bone metastases vs., **1–42i**
        wrist pain vs., 1–145
    osteogenesis imperfecta, neuroblastoma vs., **8–84i**
    osteonecrosis vs., **1–104i**, 1–105
    osteosarcoma vs., **1–28i**, 1–29
    patellar
        knee pain vs., **1–154i**
        painful joint prosthesis vs., **1–110i**
    pathologic
        fibrous cortical defect vs., **1–8i**
        stress fractures vs., **1–128i**, 1–130
    pediatric osteomyelitis vs., **1–66i**, 1–67
    periprosthetic, painful joint prosthesis vs., 1–111
    sesamoid, foot osteomyelitis vs., **1–62i**, 1–64
    spinal compression, in elderly, prostatic bone metastases vs., **1–42i**
    stress. *See* Stress fractures.
    trampoline, non-accidental trauma vs., **1–126i**
Frontotemporal dementia, Alzheimer disease vs., 5–23
Fungal infection, pulmonary, interstitial lung disease vs., 4–22

G

Gallbladder
    cancer, 8–36 to 8–41, **8–41i**
    mass, acute acalculous cholecystitis vs., **8–10i**
    non-fasting normal, acute calculous cholecystitis vs., 8–5
    nonvisualizing, rare causes of, 8–5
    polyp, gallbladder cancer vs., 8–40
    postcholecystectomy, acute calculous cholecystitis vs., 8–5
    prolonged fasting, acute calculous cholecystitis vs., 8–5
Gallstones. *See* Cholecystitis.
Ganglion cyst, wrist pain vs., 1–146
Gastric emptying disorders, 8–108 to 8–111, **8–111i**
Gastric obstruction, gastric emptying disorders vs., 8–110
Gastric ulcer
    gastric carcinoma vs., 8–113
    gastritis vs., 8–107
Gastritis, 8–106 to 8–107
    adenocarcinoma of unknown primary vs., **11–46i**
    differential diagnosis, **8–106i**, 8–106 to 8–107
    erosive, GI bleeding localization vs., 8–128
    gastric carcinoma vs., **8–112i**, 8–113
Gastroesophageal reflux disease, gastric emptying disorders vs., **8–108i**, 8–110
Gastrointestinal neoplasms
    adrenal neoplasms, 8–74 to 8–79, **8–77i** to **8–79i**
        differential diagnosis, **8–74i**, 8–76
        pheochromocytoma, 8–80 to 8–83, **8–83i**
    carcinoid tumor, 8–150 to 8–153, **8–153i**
    esophageal neoplasms, 8–98 to 8–101, **8–101i**
    gastric carcinoma, 8–112 to 8–115, **8–115i**
        differential diagnosis, **8–112i**, 8–113 to 8–114
        gastritis vs., **8–106i**
        gastric emptying disorders vs., 8–110
        gastric wall tumors, gastrointestinal stromal tumors vs., 8–155

INDEX

gastrointestinal stromal tumors, 8–154 to 8–157, **8–157i**
    differential diagnosis, **8–154i**, 8–155
    gastric carcinoma vs., **8–112i**, 8–113
    intestinal neoplasms
        primary and staging, 8–116 to 8–119, **8–119i**
        therapy evaluation/restaging, 8–120 to 8–121
    lymphoma
        gastric carcinoma vs., **8–112i**, 8–113
        gastritis vs., **8–106i**
Gastrointestinal system, 8–2 to 8–165
    anatomy and imaging issues, 8–2 to 8–3
    biliary tract disorders. *See* Biliary tract disorders.
    bleeding
        inflammatory bowel disease vs., **8–130i**, 8–131
        localization of, 8–126 to 8–129, **8–129i**
        Meckel diverticulum vs., **8–122i**, 8–123
    diaphragmatic patency determination, 8–162 to 8–163
    duplications containing gastric mucosa, Meckel diverticulum vs., **8–122i**, 8–123
    esophageal disorders
        dysmotility, 8–102 to 8–105, **8–105i**
        neoplasms, 8–98 to 8–101, **8–101i**
    gastric disorders. *See Gastric* entries.
    hepatic disorders. *See* Hepatic disorders.
    intraabdominal infection, 8–144 to 8–149, **8–147i** to **8–149i**
    Meckel diverticulum, 8–122 to 8–125, **8–125i**
    pancreatic disorders. *See Pancreatic* entries.
    peritoneal systemic shunt evaluation, 8–158 to 8–161, **8–161i**
    physiologic activity, adenocarcinoma of unknown primary vs., 11–47
    splenic
        asplenia/polysplenia syndromes, 8–90 to 8–93, **8–93i**
        hypersplenism, 8–52 to 8–55, **8–55i**
Genitourinary system, 9–2 to 9–77. *See also Renal* entries.
    cervical cancer, 9–68 to 9–71, **9–71i**
        benign uterine activity vs., 9–67
        differential diagnosis, **9–68i**, 9–69
        endometrial cancer vs., 9–73
    endometrial cancer, 9–72 to 9–75, **9–75i**
    obstructive uropathy, 9–40 to 9–43, **9–43i**
    ovarian cancer. *See* Ovarian neoplasms.
    ovaries, normal and benign pathology, 9–60 to 9–61
    prostate cancer
        antibody scan, 9–76 to 9–77
        metastatic to bone, 1–42 to 1–43
    reflux uropathy, 9–44 to 9–47, **9–47i**
    testicular cancer, 9–56 to 9–59, **9–59i**
    testicular torsion, 9–52 to 9–55, **9–55i**
    urinary bladder and epithelial cancer, 9–48 to 9–51, **9–51i**
    uterine cancer
        endometrial, 9–72 to 9–75, **9–75i**
        leiomyoma, endometrial cancer vs., **9–72i**, 9–73
        sarcoma, benign uterine activity vs., 9–67
    uterus, normal and benign pathology, 9–66 to 9–67
Germ cell tumors, thymus disorder vs., 4–48
Giant cell arteritis. *See* Large vessel vasculitis.
Giant cell tumor, 1–16 to 1–17
    aneurysmal bone cyst vs., **1–10i**, 1–11
    differential diagnosis, **1–16i**, 1–17
    Ewing sarcoma vs., 1–35
    hip pain vs., 1–141
    Paget disease vs., **1–86i**, 1–87
    solitary (unicameral) bone cyst vs., 1–13
    wrist pain vs., 1–146
Glioblastoma multiforme, primary CNS lymphoma vs., 5–37
Gliomas, 5–32 to 5–35, **5–35i**
    differential diagnosis, **5–32i**, 5–33
    high-grade
        brain infection and inflammation vs., **5–70i**, 5–71
        primary CNS lymphoma vs., **5–36i**
        radiation necrosis vs., **5–44i**
    low-grade, **5–32i**
        brain infection and inflammation vs., 5–71
        stroke vs., **5–10i**
Glomerular filtration rate, 9–36
Goiter
    diffuse nontoxic or endemic
        congenital hypothyroidism vs., **7–40i**
        Hashimoto thyroiditis vs., **7–16i**, 7–17
    Graves disease, 7–12 to 7–15, **7–15i**
    multinodular, 7–20 to 7–23, **7–23i**
        differential diagnosis, **7–20i**, 7–21 to 7–22
        ectopic parathyroid adenoma vs., 7–11
        Graves disease vs., **7–12i**, 7–13
        Hashimoto thyroiditis vs., **7–16i**, 7–17
        medullary thyroid cancer vs., 7–63
    toxic
        hyperfunctioning thyroid adenoma vs., **7–24i**, 7–25
        subacute thyroiditis vs., **7–28i**, 7–29
Gout, sickle cell osteopathy vs., 1–178
Graft vs. host disease
    inflammatory bowel disease vs., 8–131
    intraabdominal infection vs., **8–144i**
Granuloma, eosinophilic. *See* Eosinophilic granuloma.
Granulomatosis, Wegener. *See* Wegener granulomatosis.
Granulomatous disease

INDEX

adenocarcinoma of unknown primary vs., 11–47
benign mimics of lymphoma vs., **11–2i**, 11–3
gastrointestinal
    hepatic metastases vs., 8–58
    hypersplenism vs., 8–54
Hodgkin lymphoma staging vs., **11–6i**, 11–7
low-grade non-Hodgkin lymphoma vs., 11–17
lung, 4–24 to 4–27, **4–27i**
melanoma staging vs., 11–26
pheochromocytoma vs.
post-therapy evaluation of lymphoma vs., **11–10i**, 11–11
thoracic
    metastatic disease of lung and mediastinum vs., 4–40
    non-small cell lung cancer vs., **4–32i**, 4–33 to 4–34
Granulomatous pneumonia, pneumocystis carinii pneumonia vs., **4–16i**
Graves disease, 7–12 to 7–15, **7–15i**
    differential diagnosis, **7–12i**, 7–13
    multinodular goiter vs., **7–20i**, 7–21
    subacute thyroiditis vs., **7–28i**, 7–29
    with cystic nodule, hyperfunctioning thyroid adenoma vs., **7–24i**, 7–25
Gray matter
    heterotopic, 5–64 to 5–69, **5–69i**
        differential diagnosis, **5–64i**, 5–65
        syndromes including, 5–65
    normal, heterotopic gray matter vs., **5–64i**, 5–65
Growth plates, wrist pain vs., **1–144i**

H

Hamartoma
    mesenchymal, hepatoblastoma vs., 8–62
    non-small cell lung cancer vs., 4–34
    solitary pulmonary nodule vs., **4–28i**, 4–30
Hashimoto thyroiditis, 7–16 to 7–19, **7–19i**
    congenital hypothyroidism vs., 7–42
    differential diagnosis, **7–16i**, 7–17
    hyperfunctioning thyroid adenoma vs., **7–24i**, 7–25
    multinodular goiter vs., **7–20i**, 7–21
    subacute thyroiditis vs., 7–29
Head and neck, 6–2 to 6–19. *See also Thyroid* entries.
    lacrimal complex dysfunction, 6–18 to 6–19
    physiologic activity, squamous cell carcinoma vs., **6–6i**
Head and neck neoplasms
    ectopic parathyroid adenoma vs., 7–10
    neuroendocrine tumors, 6–14 to 6–17, **6–17i**
    parathyroid adenoma vs., 7–7
    parotid and salivary tumors, 6–12 to 6–13
    squamous cell carcinoma. *See* Squamous cell carcinoma.
    well-differentiated thyroid cancer vs., 7–59
Head injury, brain imaging and, 5–74
Heart disorders. *See* Cardiovascular disorders; *Myocardial* entries.
Heart transplantation, 3–32 to 3–35, **3–35i**
Heel (calcaneal) pain, 1–150 to 1–153, **1–153i**
Hemangioendothelioma, hepatoblastoma vs., 8–61
Hemangioma
    atypical, hepatic metastases vs., 8–57
    cavernous. *See* Cavernous hemangioma.
    focal nodular hyperplasia vs., 8–43
    hepatic, hepatocellular carcinoma vs., 8–66
Hematologic oncology, therapies
    hepatic arterial Y-90 microspheres, 10–4 to 10–7, **10–7i**
    phosphorus-32 therapies, 10–2 to 10–3
    radiolabeled antibody therapy, 10–8 to 10–11, **10–11i**
Hematologic procedures
    RBC survival and splenic sequestration, 10–12 to 10–13
    red cell mass and plasma volume, 10–14 to 10–15
    Schilling test, 10–16 to 10–17
Hematoma
    bladder epithelial cancer vs., 9–49
    heterotopic ossification vs., 1–160
    intraabdominal infection vs., 8–146
    retroperitoneal, renal ectopy vs., **9–6i**
    subacute, testicular cancer vs., 9–57 to 9–58
Hematopoiesis, extramedullary, renal mass vs., **9–20i**, 9–21
Hematoproliferative disorders, 1–170 to 1–175, **1–173i** to **1–175i**. *See also* Sickle cell disease.
    differential diagnosis, **1–170i**, 1–172
    multiple myeloma, 1–180 to 1–183, **1–183i**
        differential diagnosis, **1–180i**, 1–181 to 1–182
        osteomalacia vs., 1–77
Hepatic disorders. *See also* Hepatic neoplasms; Hepatitis.
    abscess, hepatic metastases vs., 8–57
    cirrhosis, 8–46 to 8–51, **8–49i** to **8–51i**
        differential diagnosis, **8–46i**, 8–48
        hepatic metastases vs., 8–48, **8–56i**
    cyst, choledochal cyst vs., 8–25
    hydatid, hepatic metastases vs., 8–58
    infarct, intraabdominal infection vs., 8–146
    severe hepatocellular disease, acute calculous cholecystitis vs., 8–5
    venous occlusive disease, focal nodular hyperplasia vs., 8–44
Hepatic neoplasms
    adenoma
        cavernous hemangioma vs., **8–70i**, 8–71 to 8–72
        focal nodular hyperplasia vs., 8–43

INDEX

cavernous hemangioma, 8–70 to 8–73, **8–73i**
   cholangiocarcinoma vs., **8–34i**, 8–35
     differential diagnosis, **8–70i**, 8–71 to 8–72
     hepatic metastases vs., **8–56i**, 8–57
  focal nodular hyperplasia. *See* Focal nodular hyperplasia.
  hepatic arterial Y-90 microsphere therapy, 10–4 to 10–7, **10–7i**
  hepatoblastoma, 8–60 to 8–63, **8–63i**
  hepatocellular carcinoma. *See* Hepatocellular carcinoma.
  intraarterial hepatic pump evaluation, 8–164 to 8–165
  metastatic, 8–56 to 8–59, **8–59i**
    differential diagnosis, **8–56i**, 8–57 to 8–58
    focal nodular hyperplasia vs., **8–42i**, 8–43
    hypervascular
      cavernous hemangioma vs., 8–71
        hepatocellular carcinoma vs., 8–66
      treated
        cavernous hemangioma vs., **8–70i**, 8–71
        cirrhosis vs., 8–48
    primary, cavernous hemangioma vs., 8–71
    sarcoidosis, cirrhosis vs., 8–48
Hepatic pump, intraarterial, evaluation, 8–164 to 8–165
Hepatitis
  alcoholic, common bile duct obstruction vs., **8–22i**
  chronic cholecystitis vs., **8–16i**, 8–17
  cirrhosis vs., **8–46i**, 8–48
  neonatal, biliary atresia vs., 8–31
Hepatobiliary disease, gastric emptying disorders vs., 8–110
Hepatoblastoma, 8–60 to 8–63, **8–63i**
Hepatocellular carcinoma, 8–64 to 8–69, **8–67i** to **8–69i**
  cholangiocarcinoma vs., **8–34i**, 8–35
  differential diagnosis, **8–64i**, 8–65 to 8–66
  focal nodular hyperplasia vs., **8–42i**, 8–43
  hepatic metastases vs., 8–58
  hepatoblastoma vs., 8–62
Hereditary exostoses, multiple. *See* Multiple hereditary exostoses.
Herpes encephalitis, paraneoplastic disorders vs., **11–48i**
Heterotopic gray matter, 5–64 to 5–69, **5–69i**
  differential diagnosis, **5–64i**, 5–65
  syndromes including, 5–65
Heterotopic ossification, 1–158 to 1–163, **1–161i** to **1–163i**
  cellulitis vs., **1–48i**
  differential diagnosis, **1–158i**, 1–159 to 1–160
  multiple hereditary exostoses vs., **1–100i**
  osteosarcoma vs., **1–28i**
  painful joint prosthesis vs., **1–110i**, 1–111

Hiatal hernia, gastric emptying disorders vs., **8–108i**
Hip pain, 1–140 to 1–143, **1–143i**
Hip prosthesis, hip pain vs., 1–142
Hippocampal sulcus remnant, seizure vs., 5–17 to 5–18
Histoplasmosis
  benign mimics of lymphoma vs., 11–3
  post-therapy evaluation of lymphoma vs., 11–11
HIV-AIDS
  benign mimics of lymphoma vs., 11–3
  post-therapy evaluation of lymphoma vs., 11–11
Hodgkin lymphoma
  post-therapy evaluation, 11–10 to 11–15, **11–13i** to **11–15i**
  staging, 11–6 to 11–9, **11–9i**
Horseshoe kidney. *See* Renal ectopy.
Human anti-mouse antibody (HAMA) reaction, prostate cancer antibody scan, **9–76i**
Huntington disease. *See also* Dementia.
  dementia vs., 5–27
Hydatid liver disease, hepatic metastases vs., 8–58
Hydrocele, testicular torsion vs., **9–52i**, 9–53 to 9–54
Hydrocephalus, normal pressure, 5–58 to 5–63, **5–61i** to **5–63i**. *See also* Dementia.
  Alzheimer disease vs., **5–22i**, 5–23
  dementia vs., **5–26i**, 5–27
  differential diagnosis, **5–58i**, 5–59 to 5–60
Hypermetabolic brown fat. *See* Brown fat, hypermetabolic.
Hyperostosis, infantile cortical, hypertrophic osteoarthropathy vs., 1–81
Hyperparathyroidism, 1–72 to 1–75, **1–75i**
  amyloidosis vs., **1–168i**, 1–169
  aneurysmal bone cyst vs., 1–11
  bone superscan vs., 1–26
  differential diagnosis, **1–72i**, 1–73 to 1–74
  hematoproliferative disorders vs., 1–172
  osteomalacia vs., **1–76i**, 1–77
  paraneoplastic disorders vs., **11–48i**, 11–50
Hyperplasia
  endometrial
    benign uterine activity vs., 9–67
    endometrial cancer vs., 9–73
  focal nodular. *See* Focal nodular hyperplasia.
  reactive lymph node, low-grade non-Hodgkin lymphoma vs., **11–16i**, 11–17
Hypersensitivity pneumonitis, pneumocystis carinii pneumonia vs., 4–17
Hypersplenism, 8–52 to 8–55, **8–55i**
Hypertension, renovascular, 9–10 to 9–13, **9–13i**
Hyperthyroid autoimmune thyroiditis, Graves disease vs., 7–13
hypertrophic osteoarthropathy (HOA). *See* Osteoarthropathy, hypertrophic (HOA).

INDEX

Hypervitaminosis A
    hypertrophic osteoarthropathy vs., 1–81
    paraneoplastic disorders vs., 11–50
Hypophosphatasia, (Rickets mimic), osteomalacia vs., 1–77
Hypotension, renal transplant complication vs., 9–32
Hypothyroidism
    central
        congenital hypothyroidism vs., 7–42
        ectopic thyroid gland vs., 7–37 to 7–38
    congenital, 7–40 to 7–43, **7–43i**
        differential diagnosis, **7–40i**, 7–41 to 7–42
        ectopic thyroid gland vs., 7–37

I

I-131 hyperthyroid therapy, 7–32 to 7–35, **7–35i**
    congenital hypothyroidism vs., 7–42
    overview, 7–3
    post-procedure steps, 7–34
    pre-procedure steps, 7–32 to 7–33
    problems and complications, 7–34
    procedure steps, 7–33 to 7–34
I-131 thyroid cancer therapy, 7–54 to 7–57, **7–57i**
Iliotibial band syndrome, knee pain vs., 1–156
Immune therapy, benign mimics of lymphoma vs., 11–4
Infantile cortical hyperostosis, hypertrophic osteoarthropathy vs., 1–81
Infarction
    bone. *See* Bone infarction.
    myocardial. *See* Myocardial infarction.
    pulmonary, non-small cell lung cancer vs., **4–32i**, 4–33
Infections. *See also* Abscess; Bone infections; Septic arthritis.
    adenocarcinoma of unknown primary vs., 11–47
    benign mimics of lymphoma vs., 11–3
    benign uterine activity vs., 9–67
    brain, 5–70 to 5–73, **5–73i**
    breast cancer staging/restaging vs., 11–42
    ectopic parathyroid adenoma vs., 7–11
    fungal, interstitial lung disease vs., 4–22
    Hodgkin lymphoma staging vs., 11–7
    intraabdominal, 8–144 to 8–149, **8–147i** to **8–149i**
    knee pain vs., 1–156
    low-grade non-Hodgkin lymphoma vs., **11–16i**
    lungs
        melanoma staging vs., **11–24i**
        non-small cell lung cancer vs., 4–34
    melanoma staging vs., 11–26
    melanoma therapy evaluation/restaging vs., 11–29
    non-Hodgkin lymphoma staging vs., 11–20
    parathyroid adenoma vs., 7–7
    post-therapy evaluation of lymphoma vs., 11–11
    primary breast cancer vs., 11–35
    renal
        renal cell carcinoma vs., 9–23
        renal mass vs., 9–21
    splenic, hypersplenism vs., 8–54
    vascular grafts, 2–16 to 2–21, **2–19i** to **2–21i**
        atherosclerosis vs., 2–12
        differential diagnosis, **2–16i**, 2–17
        vascular thrombosis vs., **2–14i**, 2–15
    viral
        benign mimics of lymphoma vs., 11–3
        low-grade non-Hodgkin lymphoma vs., **11–16i**
        post-therapy evaluation of lymphoma vs., 11–11
Infectious colitides, inflammatory bowel disease vs., 8–131
Inflammation
    adenocarcinoma of unknown primary vs., 11–47
    amyloidosis vs., **1–168i**, 1–169
    benign mimics of lymphoma vs., 11–3
    brain, 5–70 to 5–73, **5–73i**
    breast cancer staging/restaging vs., 11–42
    chronic, sickle cell osteopathy vs., 1–178
    ectopic parathyroid adenoma vs., 7–11
    melanoma staging vs., 11–26
    melanoma therapy evaluation/restaging vs., **11–28i**, 11–29
    non-Hodgkin lymphoma staging vs., 11–20
    parathyroid adenoma vs., 7–7
    postoperative, primary breast cancer vs., **11–34i**, 11–35
    primary breast cancer vs., **11–34i**, 11–35
    prostate cancer antibody scan vs., 9–77
    radiation-induced, squamous cell carcinoma of head and neck vs., **6–8i**, 6–9
    skin, melanoma therapy evaluation/restaging vs., **11–28i**
Inflammatory bowel disease, 8–130 to 8–133, **8–133i**. *See also* Crohn disease.
    differential diagnosis, **8–130i**, 8–131
    intestinal neoplasms vs., **8–116i**, 8–117
    non-infectious and ischemic colitis, intraabdominal infection vs., 8–146
Inflammatory disorders
    esophagitis, esophageal neoplasms vs., 8–99
    pelvic inflammatory disease, ovarian cancer vs., 9–63
    pericardial, malignant and inflammatory, 4–50 to 4–53, **4–53i**
    pleural, malignant and inflammatory, 4–42 to 4–45, **4–45i**
Inguinal hernia, testicular torsion vs., 9–54

INDEX

Inspissated bile syndrome/cystic fibrosis, biliary atresia vs., 8–31
Insufficiency fractures, 1–118 to 1–123, **1–121i** to **1–123i**. *See also* Stress fractures.
   differential diagnosis, **1–118i**, 1–119 to 1–120
   hip pain vs., 1–140 to 1–141
   osteonecrosis vs., **1–104i**, 1–105
Interferon effects
   Hashimoto thyroiditis vs., 7–17
   subacute thyroiditis vs., 7–30
Interstitial lung disease, 4–20 to 4–23, **4–23**
   differential diagnosis, **4–20i**, 4–22
   granulomatous disease vs., **4–24i**
   metastatic disease of lung and mediastinum vs., 4–40
Interstitial nephritis
   pyelonephritis vs., **9–26i**, 9–28
   renal cortical scar vs., 9–4
Intestinal malrotation. *See* Midgut malrotation.
Intestinal neoplasms
   primary and staging, 8–116 to 8–119, **8–119i**
   therapy evaluation/restaging, 8–120 to 8–121
Intra-arterial injection, wrist pain vs., **1–144i**
Intraabdominal infection, 8–144 to 8–149, **8–147i** to **8–149i**
Intraarterial hepatic pump evaluation, 8–164 to 8–165
Intracardiac shunts
   left-to-right, 3–36 to 3–39
   right-to-left, 3–38 to 3–39
Iodine contrast effects
   congenital hypothyroidism vs., **7–40i**
   Graves disease vs., 7–13
   subacute thyroiditis vs., 7–29
Iodine deficiency, congenital hypothyroidism vs., 7–42
Ischemia
   balanced, myocardial ischemia vs., 3–18
   bowel, chronic cholecystitis vs., 8–18
   brain infection and inflammation vs., 5–72
   mesenteric, inflammatory bowel disease vs., **8–130i**, 8–131
   myocardial, 3–16 to 3–21, **3–19i** to **3–21i**
Islet cell tumors, 8–140 to 8–143, **8–143i**
   differential diagnosis, **8–140i**, 8–142
   pancreatic adenocarcinoma vs., 8–138
   pancreatitis vs., 8–135

J

Jod-Basedow phenomenon, Graves disease vs., 7–13
Joint derangement
   pediatric osteomyelitis vs., 1–67
   stress fractures vs., 1–130
Joint prosthesis, painful
   differential diagnosis, **1–110i** to **1–111**
   hip pain vs., 1–142
   surgical assessment, 1–110 to 1–111
Juvenile chronic arthritis, Legg-Calvé-Perthes disease vs., 1–109
Juvenile osteonecrosis, Legg-Calvé-Perthes disease vs., 1–109

K

Kidney. *See also Renal* entries.
   displaced by space-occupying lesion, renal ectopy vs., 9–7
   function quantification, 9–36 to 9–39
   horseshoe. *See* Renal ectopy.
   infarction, pyelonephritis vs., 9–28
   infection/abscess
      renal cell carcinoma vs., 9–23
      renal mass vs., 9–21
   interstitial nephritis
      pyelonephritis vs., **9–26i**, 9–28
      renal cortical scar vs., 9–4
   masses, 9–20 to 9–21
   medical disease, obstructive uropathy vs., 9–42
   multicystic dysplastic, obstructive uropathy vs., 9–42
   obstructive uropathy. *See* Uropathy, obstructive.
   polycystic, acute renal failure vs., **9–14i**
   ptotic
      acute renal failure vs., 9–16
      renal ectopy vs., **9–6i**, 9–7
   pyelonephritis. *See* Pyelonephritis.
   transplantation. *See* Renal transplant.
   trauma, pyelonephritis vs., 9–28
Kidney failure. *See* Renal failure.
Knee effusion, knee pain vs., 1–156
Knee pain, 1–154 to 1–157, **1–157i**

L

Lacrimal complex dysfunction, 6–18 to 6–19
Lacrimal mucoceles, lacrimal complex dysfunction vs., **6–18i**
Lactation, primary breast cancer vs., **11–34i**, 11–35
Langerhans cell histiocytosis, solitary (unicameral) bone cyst vs., 1–13
Large cell carcinoma of lung. *See* Non-small cell lung cancer.
Large vessel vasculitis, 2–8 to 2–9
   atherosclerosis vs., **2–8i**, **2–10i**, 2–11
   differential diagnosis, **2–8i**, 2–8 to 2–9
Lateral collateral ligament injury, knee pain vs., 1–156
Left bundle branch block, myocardial ischemia vs., **3–16i**, 3–18
Left-to-right shunts
   extracardiac, **3–36i**, 3–37

INDEX

intracardiac, 3–36 to 3–39
Legg-Calvé-Perthes disease, 1–108 to 1–109
    differential diagnosis, **1–108i**, 1–109
    hip pain vs., 1–142
Leiomyoma
    cervical cancer vs., **9–68i**, 9–69
    uterine, endometrial cancer vs., **9–72i**, 9–73
Leiomyosarcoma
    gastrointestinal stromal tumors vs., **8–154i**, 8–155
    metastatic, solitary pulmonary nodule vs., **4–28i**
Leukemia
    acute, Ewing sarcoma vs., 1–35
    lymphocytic, hypersplenism vs., **8–52**
    neuroblastoma vs., 8–85
    testicular cancer vs., 9–57
Leukoencephalopathy, progressive multifocal
    primary CNS lymphoma vs., 5–37
    radiation necrosis vs., 5–46
Lewy body disease
    Alzheimer disease vs., **5–22i**, 5–23
    seizure vs., **5–16i**
Ligamentous injury, knee pain vs., 1–156
Limbic encephalitis, brain infection and inflammation vs., 5–71
Lithium-induced hypothyroidism, Hashimoto thyroiditis vs., 7–17
Liver. *See also* Hepatic disorders; Hepatic neoplasms.
    abscess, hepatic metastases vs., 8–57
    regenerative nodules
        cavernous hemangioma vs., 8–71
        focal nodular hyperplasia vs., **8–42i**, 8–43
        hepatoblastoma vs., **8–60i**, 8–62
        hepatocellular carcinoma vs., 8–65
Lumbar spine, CSF leak, **5–50i**
Lung(s). *See also* V/Q scan.
    chronic consolidation vs. post-obstructive pneumonitis, metastatic disease of lung and mediastinum vs., 4–40
    diffuse hemorrhage syndromes, pneumocystis carinii pneumonia vs., 4–17
    embolism. *See* Pulmonary embolism.
    infarct, non-small cell lung cancer vs., **4–32i**, 4–33
    infection
        melanoma staging vs., **11–24i**
        non-small cell lung cancer vs., 4–34
    non-thromboembolic intraluminal occlusions, pulmonary embolism vs., **4–6i**, 4–8
    vascular abnormalities, pulmonary embolism vs., **4–6i**, 4–8
Lung disorders
    granulomatous disease, 4–24 to 4–27, **4–27i**
    interstitial lung disease, 4–20 to 4–23, **4–23**
        differential diagnosis, **4–20i**, 4–22
        granulomatous disease vs., **4–24i**
    metastatic disease of lung and mediastinum vs., 4–40
    pleural disease, malignant and inflammatory, 4–42 to 4–45, **4–45i**
    pneumonia. *See* Pneumonia.
    pulmonary embolism. *See* Pulmonary embolism.
Lung neoplasms
    central, abnormal quantitative V/Q scan due to, 4–12
    ectopic parathyroid adenoma vs., 7–11
    granulomatous disease vs., 4–25
    melanoma therapy evaluation/restaging vs., **11–28i**
    metastatic, 4–38 to 4–41, **4–41i**
        differential diagnosis, **4–38i**, 4–40
        small cell carcinoma, neuroendocrine tumors of head and neck vs., 6–15
    non-small cell, 4–32 to 4–37, **4–35i** to **4–37i**
    parathyroid adenoma vs., 7–7
    pulmonary embolism vs., **4–6i**, 4–8
    small cell carcinoma
        benign mimics of lymphoma vs., 11–4
        post-therapy evaluation of lymphoma vs., 11–12
    solitary pulmonary nodule, 4–28 to 4–31, **4–31i**
Lymph nodes
    enlarged, benign mimics of lymphoma vs., 11–4
    metastatic, benign thyroid conditions vs., 7–45
    reactive
        benign thyroid conditions vs., 7–45
        melanoma staging vs., 11–26
        PET studies of well-differentiated thyroid cancer and, 7–60
        squamous cell carcinoma of head and neck vs., 6–3
    tonsils
        Hodgkin lymphoma staging vs., **11–6i**
        post-therapy evaluation of lymphoma vs., **11–10i**
    reactive hyperplasia, low-grade non-Hodgkin lymphoma vs., **11–16i**, 11–17
    sentinel lymph node mapping, 2–4 to 2–7, **2–7i**
Lymphangioma, ectopic thyroid gland vs., **7–36i**, 7–37
Lymphangitic carcinomatosis, interstitial lung disease vs., **4–20i**, 4–22
Lymphangitis, metastatic disease of lung and mediastinum vs., 4–40
Lymphatic and vascular systems, 2–2 to 2–21
Lymphatic valves or channels, sentinel lymph node vs., 2–6
Lymphatic vessels, peritoneal, diaphragmatic patency determination, 8–163
Lymphedema, 2–2 to 2–3
Lymphocele, renal transplant complication vs., **9–30i**
Lymphocytic leukemia, hypersplenism vs., **8–52**

INDEX

Lymphoid tissue, normal, Hodgkin lymphoma
  staging vs., 11–7
Lymphoma
  adrenal, pheochromocytoma vs., 8–82
  benign mimics, 112 to 115, **11–5i**
  benign thyroid conditions vs., **7–44i**, 7–45
  breast cancer vs.
    primary, **11–34i**
    staging/restaging, **11–40i**
  carcinoid tumor vs., 8–151
  central nervous system, primary, 5–36 to 5–39,
    5–39i
    brain infection and inflammation vs., **5–70i**,
      5–71
    differential diagnosis, **5–36i**, 5–37
  cutaneous, neuroendocrine tumors of head and
    neck vs., **6–14i**, 6–15
  ectopic parathyroid adenoma vs., **7–10i**, 7–11
  gastric, gastric carcinoma vs., **8–112i**, 8–113
  gastritis vs., **8–106i**
  gastrointestinal stromal tumors vs., **8–154i**,
    8–155
  granulomatous disease vs., 4–25
  high grade on therapy, post-therapy evaluation
    of lymphoma vs., 11–11
  Hodgkin, staging, 11–6 to 11–9, **11–9i**
  hypersplenism vs., **8–52**, 8–54
  melanoma staging vs., **11–24i**
  multiple myeloma vs., 1–181
  non-Hodgkin. *See* Non-Hodgkin lymphoma.
  non-small cell lung cancer vs., **4–32i**, 4–34
  pancreatic, pancreatic adenocarcinoma vs.,
    8–136i, 8–138
  parathyroid adenoma vs., 7–7
  post-therapy evaluation, 11–10 to 11–15, **11–13i**
    to **11–15i**
  primary bone, Ewing sarcoma vs., 1–35
  pyelonephritis vs., **9–26i**, 9–28
  renal cell carcinoma vs., **9–22i**, 9–23
  squamous cell carcinoma of head and neck vs.,
    6–3
  temporal bone osteomyelitis vs., 1–60
  testicular cancer vs., 9–57
  thymus disorder vs., **4–46i**, 4–48

M

Maffucci syndrome. *See* Enchondromatoses,
  multiple.
Malignant fibrous histiocytoma
  Ewing sarcoma vs., 1–35
  hip pain vs., 1–141
Marijuana, acute exposure effect, **5–74i**
Mastoiditis, temporal bone osteomyelitis vs., 1–60
Meckel diverticulum, 8–122 to 8–125, **8–125i**
Medial collateral ligament injury, knee pain vs.,
  1–156
Mediastinum
  mass, non-small cell lung cancer vs., **4–32i**, 4–34
  metastatic disease, 4–38 to 4–41, **4–41i**
Medication effects
  acute acalculous cholecystitis vs., 8–11
  congenital hypothyroidism vs., 7–42
  gastric emptying disorders vs., 8–110
  Graves disease vs., 7–13
  Hashimoto thyroiditis vs., 7–17
  subacute thyroiditis vs., 7–29
  Tamoxifen-related endometrial changes,
    endometrial cancer vs., 9–73
Medullary thyroid cancer, 7–62 to 7–65, **7–65i**
Melanoma
  metastatic, squamous cell carcinoma of head
    and neck vs., 6–3
  neuroendocrine tumors of head and neck vs.,
    6–14i, 6–15
  staging, 11–24 to 11–27, **11–27i**
  temporal bone osteomyelitis vs., 1–60
  therapy evaluation/restaging, 11–28 to 11–31,
    11–31i
Melorheostosis, 1–92 to 1–95, **1–95i**
Meningioma, brain metastases vs., 5–41
Meniscal tear, knee pain vs., **1–154i**, 1–156
Menstruation
  benign uterine activity vs., **9–66i**, 9–67
  bladder epithelial cancer vs., **9–48i**
  cervical cancer vs., **9–68i**, 9–69
  endometrial cancer vs., **9–72i**
Mesenteric cyst, choledochal cyst vs., 8–25
Mesenteric ischemia, inflammatory bowel disease
  vs., **8–130i**, 8–131
Metabolic bone disease. *See* Bone disease,
  metabolic.
Metachondromatosis. *See* Enchondromatoses,
  multiple.
Metastatic disease
  adenocarcinoma of unknown primary, 11–46 to
    11–47
  adrenal, **8–80i**, 8–82
  bone. *See* Bone metastases.
  bone marrow metastases, hematoproliferative
    disorders vs., **1–170i**
  brain/central nervous system, 5–40 to 5–43,
    5–43i
    blood brain barrier disruption vs., **5–14i**,
      5–15
    brain infection and inflammation vs., 5–71
    differential diagnosis, **5–40i**, 5–41 to 5–42
    gliomas and astrocytomas vs., 5–33
    primary CNS lymphoma vs., 5–37
  breast, ectopic parathyroid adenoma vs., **7–10i**
  gastrointestinal

INDEX

gallbladder cancer vs., 8–40
gastrointestinal stromal tumors vs., **8–154i**, 8–155
mucinous, cholangiocarcinoma vs., **8–34i**
pancreatic adenocarcinoma vs., **8–136i**, 8–138
peritoneal systemic shunt vs., **8–158i**, 8–159
granulomatous disease vs., **4–24i**, 4–25 to 4–26
hepatic. *See* Hepatic neoplasms, metastatic.
leiomyosarcoma, solitary pulmonary nodule vs., **4–28i**
lung and mediastinum, 4–38 to 4–41, **4–41i**
  differential diagnosis, **4–38i**, 4–40
  small cell carcinoma, neuroendocrine tumors of head and neck vs., 6–15
lymphoma, hypersplenism vs., **8–52**, 8–54
melanoma, squamous cell carcinoma of head and neck vs., 6–3
mucinous neoplasms, cholangiocarcinoma vs., **8–34i**
neuroblastoma
  hematoproliferative disorders vs., **1–170i**
  hepatoblastoma vs., 8–62
ovarian
  benign ovarian pathology vs., **9–60i**
  ovarian cancer vs., **9–62i**
pancreatic
  islet cell tumors vs., 8–142
  pancreatic adenocarcinoma vs., **8–136i**, 8–138
parotid gland, **6–12i**, 6–13
peritoneal, peritoneal systemic shunt vs., **8–158i**, 8–159
pleural, pleural disease vs., 4–43
renal cell carcinoma vs., 9–23
solitary pulmonary nodule vs., **4–28i**, 4–30
splenic, benign mimics of lymphoma vs., 11–4
testicular cancer vs., 9–57
thymus disorder vs., 4–47
thyroid
  benign thyroid conditions vs., 7–45
  squamous cell carcinoma of head and neck vs., 6–3
Microvascular coronary disease, myocardial ischemia vs., 3–18
Midgut malrotation
  biliary leak vs., 8–21
  Meckel diverticulum vs., 8–123
Miliary tuberculosis, interstitial lung disease vs., 4–22
Mixed sclerosing osteodystrophy, melorheostosis vs., 1–93 to 1–94
Monoclonal antibody therapy, radiolabeled, 10–8 to 10–11, **10–11i**
Mononucleosis
  benign mimics of lymphoma vs., 11–3
  post-therapy evaluation of lymphoma vs., 11–11
Mouth floor masses, ectopic thyroid gland vs., **7–36i**, 7–37
Mucinous neoplasms
  adenocarcinoma, hepatocellular carcinoma vs., **8–64i**
  cystic
    islet cell tumors vs., 8–142
    pancreatitis vs., **8–134i**, 8–135
  metastatic, cholangiocarcinoma vs., **8–34i**
Mucoceles, lacrimal, lacrimal complex dysfunction vs., **6–18i**
Mucosal neoplasm, squamous cell carcinoma of head and neck vs., 6–7
Multi-infarct dementia, normal pressure hydrocephalus vs., 5–60
Multicystic dysplastic kidney, obstructive uropathy vs., 9–42
Multinodular goiter. *See* Goiter, multinodular.
Multiple enchondromatoses. *See* Enchondromatoses, multiple.
Multiple hereditary exostoses, 1–100 to 1–103, **1–103i**
  chondrosarcoma vs., **1–38i**, 1–39
  differential diagnosis, **1–100i**, 1–101
  multiple enchondromatosis vs., **1–96i**, 1–97
  osteosarcoma vs., 1–29
Multiple myeloma, 1–180 to 1–183, **1–183i**
  differential diagnosis, **1–180i**, 1–181 to 1–182
  osteomalacia vs., 1–77
Multiple sclerosis
  gliomas and astrocytomas vs., 5–33
  radiation necrosis vs., 5–46
Multiple system atrophy. *See* Dementia.
Muscle activity, asymmetrical, squamous cell carcinoma of head and neck vs., **6–2i**, 6–3, 6–9 to 6–10
Musculoskeletal disorders, 1–2 to 1–183. *See also* Bone entries.
  amyloidosis, 1–168 to 1–169
  paraneoplastic disorders vs., 11–49 to 11–50
  skeletal muscle disorders, 1–164 to 1–167, **1–167i**
  soft tissue pathology, stress fractures vs., 1–130
Myelitis, primary CNS lymphoma vs., **5–36i**, 5–37
Myelodysplastic disease. *See* Hematoproliferative disorders.
Myelolipoma, adrenal, 8–76, 8–82
Myocardial hibernation/stunning. *See* Myocardial viability.
Myocardial infarction, 3–26 to 3–31, **3–29i** to **3–31i**
Myocardial ischemia, 3–16 to 3–21, **3–19i** to **3–21i**
Myocardial perfusion scintigraphy, 3–2 to 3–5, **3–5i**
Myocardial viability, 3–22 to 3–25, **3–25i**
  differential diagnosis, **3–22i**, 3–23
  myocardial infarction vs., 3–27

INDEX

Myocardial wall thickening
    pericardial disease vs., 4–51
    valvular heart disease vs., 3–13
Myositis (skeletal muscle disorders), 1–164 to 1–167, **1–167i**
    heterotopic ossification vs., **1–158i**
    stress fractures vs., **1–128i**, 1–130
    wrist pain vs., 1–145

N

Nasolacrimal fracture, lacrimal complex dysfunction vs., **6–18i**
Nasopharynx, CSF leak and, **5–50i**
Necrotizing fasciitis, cellulitis vs., 1–49
Neoplasms, 11–2 to 11–51
    adenocarcinoma
        lung. *See* Non-small cell lung cancer.
        mucinous, hepatocellular carcinoma vs., **8–64i**
        of unknown primary, 11–46 to 11–47
        pancreatic. *See* Pancreatic neoplasms, adenocarcinoma.
    adenoma. *See* Adenoma.
    adrenal. *See* Adrenal neoplasms.
    amyloidosis vs., 1–169
    astrocytomas, 5–32 to 5–35, **5–35i**
        differential diagnosis, **5–32i**, 5–33
        low-grade, seizure vs., 5–17
    benign mimics of lymphoma vs., 11–3
    bladder epithelial cancer vs., 9–49
    bone. *See* Bone neoplasms.
    brain. *See* Brain neoplasms.
    breast
        benign breast disease vs., **11–32i**, 11–33
        nonmalignant, primary breast cancer vs., 11–35
        primary, 11–34 to 11–39, **11–37i** to **11–39i**
        staging/restaging, 11–40 to 11–45, **11–43i** to **11–45i**
    breast cancer staging/restaging vs., 11–42
    carcinoid tumor. *See* Carcinoid tumor.
    cavernous hemangioma, 8–70 to 8–73, **8–73i**
        cholangiocarcinoma vs., **8–34i**, 8–35
        differential diagnosis, **8–70i**, 8–71 to 8–72
        hepatic metastases vs., **8–56i**, 8–57
    central nervous system. *See* Brain neoplasms.
    cervical, 9–68 to 9–71, **9–71i**
        benign uterine activity vs., 9–67
        differential diagnosis, **9–68i**, 9–69
        endometrial cancer vs., 9–73
    cholangiocarcinoma. *See* Cholangiocarcinoma.
    chondrosarcoma. *See* Chondrosarcoma.
    enchondroma. *See* Enchondroma.
    endobronchial carcinoma, metastatic disease of lung and mediastinum vs., 4–40
    endometrial, 9–72 to 9–75, **9–75i**
    esophageal, 8–98 to 8–101, **8–101i**
        differential diagnosis, **8–98i**, 8–99 to 8–100
        esophageal dysmotility vs., **8–102i**, 8–104
    Ewing sarcoma. *See* Ewing sarcoma.
    focal nodular hyperplasia. *See* Focal nodular hyperplasia.
    gallbladder, 8–36 to 8–41, **8–41i**
    gastrointestinal. *See* Gastrointestinal neoplasms.
    germ cell tumors, thymus disorder vs., 4–48
    giant cell tumor. *See* Giant cell tumor.
    gliomas. *See* Gliomas.
    head and neck. *See* Head and neck neoplasms.
    hemangioma
        atypical, hepatic metastases vs., 8–57
        focal nodular hyperplasia vs., 8–43
        hepatic, hepatocellular carcinoma vs., 8–66
    hematologic oncology, therapies
        hepatic arterial Y-90 microspheres, 10–4 to 10–7, **10–7i**
        phosphorus-32 therapies, 10–2 to 10–3
        radiolabeled antibody therapy, 10–8 to 10–11, **10–11i**
    hepatic. *See* Hepatic neoplasms.
    Hodgkin lymphoma staging vs., 11–7
    islet cell tumors, 8–140 to 8–143, **8–143i**
        differential diagnosis, **8–140i**, 8–142
        pancreatic adenocarcinoma vs., 8–138
        pancreatitis vs., 8–135
    lung. *See* Lung neoplasms.
    lymphoma. *See* Lymphoma.
    melanoma. *See* Melanoma.
    metastatic. *See* Metastatic disease.
    mucinous. *See* Mucinous neoplasms.
    multiple myeloma, 1–180 to 1–183, **1–183i**
        differential diagnosis, **1–180i**, 1–181 to 1–182
        osteomalacia vs., 1–77
    neuroblastoma, 8–84 to 8–89, **8–87i** to **8–89i**
        differential diagnosis, **8–84i**, 8–85
        metastatic
            hematoproliferative disorders vs., **1–170i**
            hepatoblastoma vs., 8–62
        pediatric osteomyelitis vs., **1–66i**
    neuroendocrine, 6–14 to 6–17, **6–17i**
        carcinoid tumor vs., 8–151
    non-Hodgkin lymphoma. *See* Non-Hodgkin lymphoma.
    osteoid osteoma. *See* Osteoid osteoma.
    osteosarcoma. *See* Osteosarcoma.
    ovarian. *See* Ovarian neoplasms.
    pancreatic. *See* Pancreatic neoplasms.
    paraneoplastic disorders, 11–48 to 11–51, **11–51i**
    parotid gland, 6–12 to 6–13
    pheochromocytoma, 8–80 to 8–83, **8–83i**
        differential diagnosis, **8–80i**, 8–81 to 8–82
        islet cell tumors vs., **8–140i**

INDEX

post-therapy evaluation of lymphoma vs., 11–11
prostatic
    antibody scan, 9–76 to 9–77
    metastatic to bone, 1–42 to 1–43
renal cell carcinoma, 9–22 to 9–25, **9–25i**
    differential diagnosis, **9–22i**, 9–23
    pyelonephritis vs., **9–26i**, 9–28
renal masses, 9–20 to 9–21
    pyelonephritis vs., **9–26i**, 9–28
    renal cortical scar vs., 9–4
rhabdomyosarcoma, wrist pain vs., 1–146
salivary glands, 6–12 to 6–13
sarcoma. *See* Sarcoma.
splenic, primary, hypersplenism vs., 8–54
squamous cell carcinoma. *See* Squamous cell carcinoma.
testicular, 9–56 to 9–59, **9–59i**
thoracic/extrathoracic malignancy
    benign mimics of lymphoma vs., 11–4
    post-therapy evaluation of lymphoma vs., 11–12
thymolipoma, thymus disorder vs., 4–47
thymoma, ectopic parathyroid adenoma vs., 7–11
urinary bladder epithelial, 9–48 to 9–51, **9–51i**
uterine
    endometrial, 9–72 to 9–75, **9–75i**
    leiomyoma, endometrial cancer vs., **9–72i**, 9–73
    sarcoma, benign uterine activity vs., 9–67
Nephritis, interstitial
    pyelonephritis vs., **9–26i**, 9–28
    renal cortical scar vs., 9–4
Nephroptosis, renal ectopy vs., **9–6i**, 9–7
Neuroblastoma, 8–84 to 8–89, **8–87i** to **8–89i**
    differential diagnosis, **8–84i**, 8–85
    metastatic
        hematoproliferative disorders vs., **1–170i**
        hepatoblastoma vs., 8–62
    pediatric osteomyelitis vs., **1–66i**
Neuroendocrine tumors
    carcinoid tumor vs., 8–151
    head and neck, 6–14 to 6–17, **6–17i**
Neurofibromatosis, fibrous dysplasia vs., 1–91
Neurologic disorders, paraneoplastic disorders vs., **11–48i**, 11–49
Neuropathic osteoarthropathy (Charcot joint), foot osteomyelitis vs., 1–64
Non-Hodgkin lymphoma
    low-grade, 11–16 to 11–19, **11–19i**
    parotid and salivary tumors vs., 6–13
    post-therapy evaluation, 11–10 to 11–15, **11–13i** to **11–15i**
    squamous cell carcinoma of head and neck vs., 6–7
    staging, 11–20 to 11–23, **11–23i**

thyroid gland, medullary thyroid cancer vs., 7–63
Non-small cell lung cancer, 4–32 to 4–37, **4–35i** to **4–37i**
Nonossifying fibroma. *See* Fibroma, nonossifying.
Normal pressure hydrocephalus. *See* Hydrocephalus, normal pressure.

O

Obsessive-compulsive disorder, 5–74
Obstructive uropathy. *See* Uropathy, obstructive.
Ollier disease. *See* Enchondromatoses, multiple.
Omental cyst, choledochal cyst vs., 8–25
Oncology. *See* Neoplasms.
Orchitis
    focal, testicular cancer vs., 9–58
    testicular torsion vs., **9–52i**, 9–53
Orthopedic hardware complications, bone metastases vs., 1–20
Ossification, heterotopic. *See* Heterotopic ossification.
Osteitis deformans, appendicular osteomyelitis vs., 1–54
Osteoarthritis. *See also* Arthritis, non-infectious.
    bone metastases vs., **1–18i**, 1–20
    hip pain vs., 1–141
    knee pain vs., 1–156
    osteonecrosis vs., **1–104i**, 1–106
    prostatic bone metastases vs., **1–42i**, 1–43
    wrist pain vs., 1–145
Osteoarthropathy
    hypertrophic (HOA), 1–80 to 1–85, **1–83i** to **1–85i**
        bone superscan vs., 1–26
        differential diagnosis, **1–80i**, 1–81
        hematoproliferative disorders vs., **1–170i**, 1–172
        paraneoplastic disorders vs., 11–49 to 11–50
    hypertrophic pulmonary (HPOA), hyperparathyroidism vs., 1–73
    neuropathic (Charcot joint), foot osteomyelitis vs., 1–64
Osteoblastoma
    aneurysmal bone cyst vs., 1–11
    osteoid osteoma vs., 1–4
    wrist pain vs., 1–146
Osteochondroma
    chondrosarcoma vs., 1–39
    osteosarcoma vs., 1–29
    skeletal muscle disorders vs., 1–166
    solitary, multiple hereditary exostoses vs., 1–101
Osteodystrophy, mixed sclerosing, melorheostosis vs., 1–93 to 1–94
Osteogenesis imperfecta
    fibrous dysplasia vs., 1–91

INDEX

fractures, neuroblastoma vs., **8–84i**
non-accidental trauma vs., **1–126i**, 1–127
Osteoid osteoma, 1–2 to 1–5, **1–5i**
    appendicular osteomyelitis vs., **1–52i**, 1–54
    differential diagnosis, **1–2i**, 1–3 to 1–4
    fibrous cortical defect vs., 1–9
    hip pain vs., **1–140i**, 1–141
    Legg-Calvé-Perthes disease vs., 1–109
    osteosarcoma vs., 1–29
    wrist pain vs., 1–146
Osteoma, osteoid osteoma vs., 1–4
Osteomalacia, 1–76 to 1–79, **1–79i**
    bone superscan vs., 1–26
    differential diagnosis, **1–76i**, 1–77
    hyperparathyroidism vs., **1–72i**, 1–73
    oncogenic, paraneoplastic disorders vs., 11–50
Osteomyelitis
    appendicular, 1–52 to 1–57, **1–55i** to **1–57i**
    axial, 1–58 to 1–59
    calcaneal pain vs., 1–151 to 1–152
    chronic
        osteoid osteoma vs., **1–2i**, 1–3 to 1–4
        osteosarcoma vs., 1–29
    chronic recurrent multifocal, pediatric
        osteomyelitis vs., 1–68
    Ewing sarcoma vs., **1–34i**, 1–35
    foot, 1–62 to 1–65, **1–65i**
    fractures vs., 1–125
    giant cell tumor vs., 1–17
    hip pain vs., 1–142
    Legg-Calvé-Perthes disease vs., **1–108i**
    multiple myeloma vs., **1–180i**
    non-infectious arthritis vs., 1–133
    pediatric, 1–66 to 1–71, **1–69i** to **1–71i**
    temporal bone, 1–60 to 1–61
    wrist pain vs., 1–145
Osteonecrosis, 1–104 to 1–107, **1–107i**. *See also*
    Bone infarction.
    bone metastases vs., **1–18i**, 1–20
    differential diagnosis, **1–104i**, 1–105 to 1–106
    foot osteomyelitis vs., 1–64
    hip pain vs., **1–140i**, 1–141
    juvenile
        hip pain vs., 1–142
        Legg-Calvé-Perthes disease vs., 1–109
    Legg-Calvé-Perthes disease, 1–108 to 1–109
    non-infectious arthritis vs., 1–133
    pediatric osteomyelitis vs., **1–66i**, 1–68
Osteopathia stria, melorheostosis vs., 1–94
Osteopenia, multiple myeloma vs., 1–181
Osteopoikilosis, melorheostosis vs., 1–93 to 1–94
Osteoporosis
    calcaneal pain vs., 1–152
    hyperparathyroidism vs., 1–74
    multiple myeloma vs., 1–181
    non-accidental trauma vs., 1–127
    osteomalacia vs., **1–76i**, 1–77
    transient
        hip pain vs., 1–142
        osteonecrosis vs., 1–105
Osteosarcoma, 1–28 to 1–23, **1–31i** to **1–33i**
    aneurysmal bone cyst vs., 1–11
    chondroblastic, chondrosarcoma vs., 1–39
    differential diagnosis, **1–28i**, 1–29
    Ewing sarcoma vs., **1–34i**, 1–35
    hip pain vs., 1–141
    melorheostosis vs., **1–92i**, 1–93
    multiple myeloma vs., 1–181
    Paget disease vs., 1–87
    parosteal
        heterotopic ossification vs., **1–158i**, 1–159
        skeletal muscle disorders vs., **1–164i**, 1–166
    skeletal muscle disorders vs., 1–166
Ostomy sites
    carcinoid tumor vs., **8–150i**
    intraabdominal infection vs., 8–146
Ovarian cysts, benign ovarian pathology vs., **9–60i**
Ovarian neoplasms, 9–62 to 9–65, **9–65i**
    benign
        benign ovarian pathology vs., 9–61
        ovarian cancer vs., 9–63
    borderline, ovarian cancer vs., 9–63
    differential diagnosis, **9–62i**, 9–63
    malignant, benign ovarian pathology vs., 9–61
    metastatic, benign ovarian pathology vs., **9–60i**
Ovaries, normal and benign pathology, 9–60 to
    9–61
    cervical cancer vs., 9–69
    differential diagnosis, **9–60i** to 9–61

P

Paget disease, 1–86 to 1–89, **1–89i**
    appendicular osteomyelitis vs., **1–52i**, 1–54
    bone metastases vs., 1–20
    bone superscan vs., 1–26
    calcaneal pain vs., 1–152
    differential diagnosis, **1–86i**, 1–87 to 1–88
    failed back surgery syndrome vs., **1–112i**, 1–114
    fibrous dysplasia vs., **1–90i**
    hematoproliferative disorders vs., 1–172
    hip pain vs., 1–141 to 1–142
    hypertrophic osteoarthropathy vs., 1–81
    insufficiency fracture vs., **1–118i**
    melorheostosis vs., 1–93
    multiple myeloma vs., **1–180i**
    osteosarcoma vs., **1–28i**, 1–29
    prostatic bone metastases vs., **1–42i**, 1–43
    temporal bone osteomyelitis vs., **1–60i**
Pain evaluation, 1–136 to 1–157
    calcaneal pain, 1–150 to 1–153, **1–153i**

INDEX

complex regional pain syndrome, 1–136 to
1–139, **1–139i**
hip pain, 1–140 to 1–143, **1–143i**
knee pain, 1–154 to 1–157, **1–157i**
wrist pain, 1–144 to 1–149, **1–147i** to **1–149i**
Pain insensitivity, congenital, non-accidental
trauma vs., 1–127
Painful joint prosthesis
differential diagnosis, **1–110i** to 1–111
surgical assessment, 1–110 to 1–111
Palate, squamous cell carcinoma of head and neck
vs., **6–6i**
Palliation of metastatic bone pain, 1–44 to 1–47,
1–47i
Palsy, progressive supranuclear, Alzheimer disease
vs., 5–23
Pancreatic disorders. *See also* Pancreatitis.
pseudocyst, choledochal cyst vs., **8–24i**, 8–25
sphincter dysfunction, chronic cholecystitis vs.,
8–16i, 8–17
Pancreatic neoplasms. *See also* Islet cell tumors.
adenocarcinoma, 8–136 to 8–139, **8–139i**
differential diagnosis, **8–136i**, 8–138
pancreatitis vs., **8–134i**
cholangiocarcinoma vs., 8–35
cystic, pancreatic adenocarcinoma vs., 8–138
ductal, islet cell tumors vs., 8–142
lymphoma, pancreatic adenocarcinoma vs.,
8–136i, 8–138
metastatic
islet cell tumors vs., 8–142
pancreatic adenocarcinoma vs., **8–136i**,
8–138
nonepithelial, pancreatic adenocarcinoma vs.,
8–138
periampullary, pancreatic adenocarcinoma vs.,
8–138
serous cystadenoma, islet cell tumors vs., 8–142
Pancreatitis, 8–134 to 8–135
biliary leak vs., 8–21
choledochal cyst vs., **8–24i**
chronic or autoimmune, chronic cholecystitis
vs., 8–17
differential diagnosis, **8–134i**, 8–134 to 8–135
inflammatory bowel disease vs., **8–130i**, 8–131
intraabdominal infection vs., 8–146
pancreatic adenocarcinoma vs., **8–136i**, 8–138
Panic disorder, 5–75
Paraganglioma, islet cell tumors vs., **8–140i**
Paraneoplastic disorders, 11–48 to 11–51, **11–51i**
differential diagnosis, **11–48i**, 11–49 to 11–50
hyperparathyroidism vs., 1–73
Parathyroid adenoma
benign thyroid conditions vs., 7–45 to 7–46
ectopic, 7–10 to 7–11
medullary thyroid cancer vs., **7–62i**, 7–63
typical, 7–6 to 7–9, **7–9i**
Parathyroid carcinoma, parathyroid adenoma vs.,
7–6i, 7–7
Parietal infarct, bilateral, dementia vs., **5–26i**
Parosteal osteosarcoma. *See* Osteosarcoma.
Parotid tumors, 6–12 to 6–13
metastatic, **6–12i**, 6–13
primary carcinoma, 6–13
Patellar fracture
knee pain vs., **1–154i**
painful joint prosthesis vs., **1–110i**
Patellofemoral pain syndrome, knee pain vs., 1–156
Pediatric osteomyelitis, 1–66 to 1–71, **1–69i** to
1–71i
Pelvic inflammatory disease, ovarian cancer vs.,
9–63
Penile activity, GI bleeding localization vs., **8–126i**
Peptic ulcer disease
chronic cholecystitis vs., 8–17
gastric emptying disorders vs., 8–110
GI bleeding localization vs., 8–128
Pericardial disease
constrictive, cardiomyopathy vs., **3–8**, 3–7
malignant and inflammatory, 4–50 to 4–53,
4–53i
Pericardial thickening/mass, pericardial disease vs.,
4–51
Periodontal disease, bone metastases vs., 1–20
Periosteal contusion, calcaneal pain vs., 1–152
Perirenal abscess, renal mass vs., **9–20i**
Peritoneal systemic shunt evaluation, 8–158 to
8–161, **8–161i**
Peritoneum
adhesions, chronic cholecystitis vs., 8–18
dispersion of radiotracer, ventricular shunt
dysfunction and, **5–54i**, 5–56
metastases, peritoneal systemic shunt vs.,
8–158i, 8–159
Peroxisomal disorder, heterotopic gray matter vs.,
5–65
Persistent fetal lobulation, renal cortical scar vs.,
9–2i, 9–4
Pheochromocytoma, 8–80 to 8–83, **8–83i**
differential diagnosis, **8–80i**, 8–81 to 8–82
islet cell tumors vs., **8–140i**
Phosphorus-32 therapies, 10–2 to 10–3
Physiologic activity, bone metastases vs., 1–20
Pick disease, Alzheimer disease vs., 5–23
PIOPED (prospective investigation of pulmonary
embolism diagnosis), modified, interpretation,
4–4
Pituitary neoplasms, carcinoid tumor vs., **8–150i**
Plantar fasciitis
calcaneal pain vs., **1–150i**, 1–151
foot osteomyelitis vs., **1–62i**
Plasma cell neoplasms, multiple myeloma vs., 1–182

INDEX

Plasma clearance, compartmental models, 9–36
Plasma volume and red cell mass, 10–14 to 10–15
Plasmacytoma, hip pain vs., 1–141
Pleomorphic adenoma, parotid and salivary tumors vs., 6–12
Pleural disease
  benign asbestos-related, malignant and inflammatory pleural disease vs., 4–43
  malignant and inflammatory, 4–42 to 4–45, **4–45i**
Pleural effusion/thickening
  diaphragmatic patency determination, 8–163
  medial, pericardial disease vs., 4–51
  post pneumonectomy, pleural disease vs., 4–43
Pleurodesis, malignant and inflammatory pleural disease vs., 4–43
Plummer disease (hyperfunctioning thyroid adenoma), 7–24 to 7–27, **7–27i**
Pneumocystis carinii pneumonia, 4–16 to 4–19, **4–19i**
  differential diagnosis, **4–16i**, 4–17
  interstitial lung disease vs., **4–20i**
Pneumonia
  abnormal quantitative V/Q scan due to, 4–12
  aspiration, pneumocystis carinii pneumonia vs., **4–16i**
  bacterial
    interstitial lung disease vs., **4–20i**
    pneumocystis carinii pneumonia vs., **4–16i**
  granulomatous, pneumocystis carinii pneumonia vs., **4–16i**
  pneumocystis carinii, 4–16 to 4–19, **4–19i**
    differential diagnosis, **4–16i**, 4–17
    interstitial lung disease vs., **4–20i**
Pneumonitis
  cytomegalovirus, pneumocystis carinii pneumonia vs., 4–17
  hypersensitivity, pneumocystis carinii pneumonia vs., 4–17
  post-obstructive vs. chronic consolidation, metastatic disease of lung and mediastinum vs., 4–40
Polyarteritis nodosa, renal cortical scar vs., 9–4
Polycystic kidney, acute renal failure vs., **9–14i**
Polymyalgia rheumatica, paraneoplastic disorders vs., 11–50
Polymyositis, paraneoplastic disorders vs., 11–50
Polysplenia/asplenia syndrome, 8–90 to 8–93, **8–93i**
  accessory and ectopic spleen vs., 8–95
  differential diagnosis, **8–90i**, 8–91
Popliteal cyst, knee pain vs., **1–154i**, 1–156
Post-treatment effects, brain metastases vs., **5–40i**, 5–41
Posterior cruciate ligament injury, knee pain vs., 1–156

Pregnancy, ectopic, benign ovarian pathology vs., **9–60i**, 9–61
Progressive multifocal leukoencephalopathy
  primary CNS lymphoma vs., 5–37
  radiation necrosis vs., 5–46
Progressive supranuclear palsy, Alzheimer disease vs., 5–23
Prospective investigation of pulmonary embolism diagnosis (PIOPED), modified, interpretation, 4–4
Prostate neoplasms
  antibody scan, 9–76 to 9–77
  metastatic to bone, 1–42 to 1–43
Prosthetic joint. *See* Joint prosthesis, painful.
Psychiatric disorders, 5–74 to 5–79, **5–77i** to **5–79i**
Pterygoid muscle, squamous cell carcinoma of head and neck vs., **6–6i**
Ptotic kidney. *See* Kidney, ptotic.
Pulmonary alveolar proteinosis, pneumocystis carinii pneumonia vs., 4–17
Pulmonary artery hypertension, valvular heart disease vs., 3–14
Pulmonary edema
  interstitial lung disease vs., 4–22
  pneumocystis carinii pneumonia vs., 4–17
Pulmonary embolism
  abnormal quantitative V/Q scan due to, **4–10i**, 4–12
  chronic or unresolved pulmonary embolism vs., **4–6i**, 4–8
  differential diagnosis, **4–6i**, 4–8
  metastatic disease of lung and mediastinum vs., 4–40
  V/Q scan, 4–6 to 4–9, **4–9i**
Pulmonary hemorrhage syndromes, diffuse, pneumocystis carinii pneumonia vs., 4–17
Pulmonary nodule
  multiple benign, metastatic disease of lung and mediastinum vs., 4–40
  solitary, 4–28 to 4–31, **4–31i**
Pulmonary vascular abnormalities, pulmonary embolism vs., **4–6i**, 4–8
Pyelonephritis, 9–26 to 9–29, **9–29i**
  differential diagnosis, **9–26i**, 9–28
  reflux uropathy vs., **9–44i**
  renal cortical scar vs., 9–4

Q

Quantitative V/Q scan, 4–10 to 4–15, **4–13i** to **4–15i**

R

Radial/ulnar artery thrombosis, wrist pain vs., 1–146

INDEX

Radiation effects
    brain, stroke vs., **5–10i**
    intestinal neoplasms vs., 8–121
Radiation-induced inflammation, squamous cell carcinoma of head and neck vs., **6–8i**, 6–9
Radiation necrosis
    differential diagnosis, **5–44i**, 5–46
    gliomas and astrocytomas vs., **5–32i**, 5–33
    recurrent tumor vs., 5–44 to 5–49, **5–47i** to **5–49i**
Radiation therapy, blood brain barrier disruption vs., 5–15
Radioiodine therapy. *See* I-131 hyperthyroid therapy.
Radiolabeled antibody therapy, 10–8 to 10–11, **10–11i**
Radiopharmaceuticals
    brain imaging, 5–2
    cardiovascular imaging, 3–4
    thyroid scan, 7–2 to 7–3
    V/Q scan, 4–2
Ranula, salivary, ectopic thyroid gland vs., **7–36i**, 7–37
Raynaud syndrome, complex regional pain syndrome vs., **1–136i**, 1–137 to 1–138
RBC survival and splenic sequestration, 10–12 to 10–13
Reactive hyperemia, wrist pain vs., **1–144i**
Reactive lymph nodes. *See* Lymph nodes, reactive.
Red blood cells
    RBC survival and splenic sequestration, 10–12 to 10–13
    red cell mass and plasma volume, 10–14 to 10–15
Reflex Sympathetic Dystrophy (RSD). *See also* Complex regional pain syndrome.
    paraneoplastic disorders vs., 11–50
    wrist pain vs., 1–145
Reflux uropathy, 9–44 to 9–47, **9–47i**
    fluoroscopic mimics, 9–45
    nuclear cystography mimics, 9–45
    obstructive uropathy vs., **9–40i**, 9–42
    sonographic mimics, 9–45
Regional pain evaluation. *See* Complex regional pain syndrome; Pain evaluation.
Renal. See also Kidney.
Renal agenesis, reflux uropathy vs., **9–44i**
Renal artery stenosis, obstructive uropathy vs., **9–40i**, 9–42
Renal calculi, obstructing, acute renal failure vs., **9–14i**
Renal cell carcinoma, 9–22 to 9–25, **9–25i**
    differential diagnosis, **9–22i**, 9–23
    pyelonephritis vs., **9–26i**, 9–28
Renal collecting system
    adrenal malignancy vs., **8–74i**, 8–76
    dilated, non-obstructed, obstructive uropathy vs., 9–42
    GI bleeding localization vs., **8–126i**
Renal cortical scar, 9–2 to 9–5, **9–5i**
Renal cyst
    hemorrhagic, renal cell carcinoma vs., **9–22i**, 9–23
    renal cortical scar vs., **9–2i**, 9–4
Renal ectopy, 9–6 to 9–9, **9–9i**
    acute renal failure vs., **9–14i**, 9–16
    differential diagnosis, **9–6i**, 9–7
Renal failure
    acute, 9–14 to 9–19, **9–17i** to **9–19i**
        differential diagnosis, **9–14i**, 9–16
        renovascular hypertension vs., 9–12
    chronic
        acute renal failure vs., 9–16
        renovascular hypertension vs., 9–12
Renal function quantification, 9–36 to 9–39
Renal masses, 9–20 to 9–21
    pyelonephritis vs., **9–26i**, 9–28
    renal cortical scar vs., 9–4
Renal oncocytoma, renal cell carcinoma vs., 9–23
Renal pelvis, Meckel diverticulum vs., **8–122i**
Renal plasma flow, effective, 9–36
Renal transplant, 9–30 to 9–35, **9–33i** to **9–35i**
    complications, differential diagnosis, **9–30i**, 9–32
    intraabdominal infection vs., 8–146
    renal ectopy vs., 9–7
Renal vein thrombosis, obstructive uropathy vs., 9–42
Renovascular hypertension, 9–10 to 9–13, **9–13i**
Reproductive System. *See* Genitourinary system.
Retroperitoneal hematoma, renal ectopy vs., **9–6i**
Rhabdomyolysis, hip pain vs., 1–142
Rhabdomyosarcoma, wrist pain vs., 1–146
Rheumatoid arthritis, hip pain vs., 1–141
Rheumatologic disease. *See* Arthritis, non-infectious.
Rickets, mimics of, osteomalacia vs., 1–77
Riedel struma (thyroiditis)
    Hashimoto thyroiditis vs., **7–16i**, 7–17
    multinodular goiter vs., 7–22
Right-to-left intracardiac shunts, 3–38 to 3–39

S

Sacral insufficiency fracture, 1–119
Salivary glands
    PET studies of well-differentiated thyroid cancer and, 7–60
    tumors, 6–12 to 6–13
Salivary ranula, ectopic thyroid gland vs., **7–36i**, 7–37
Sarcoidosis

INDEX

benign mimics of lymphoma vs., 11–3
hepatic, cirrhosis vs., 8–48
interstitial lung disease vs., 4–22
metastatic disease of lung and mediastinum vs., **4–38i**, 4–40
non-Hodgkin lymphoma staging vs., **11–20i**
post-therapy evaluation of lymphoma vs., 11–11
Sarcoma
    endometrial, benign uterine activity vs., 9–67
    fibrosarcoma
        chondrosarcoma vs., 1–39
        hip pain vs., 1–141
    osseous, wrist pain vs., 1–146
    soft tissue
        heterotopic ossification vs., **1–158i**
        wrist pain vs., 1–146
    synovial, heterotopic ossification vs., 1–159
    uterine, benign uterine activity vs., 9–67
SCCHN. *See* Squamous cell carcinoma.
Schilling test, 10–16 to 10–17
Schizophrenia, 5–74 to 5–75
Sclerosing osteodystrophy, mixed, melorheostosis vs., 1–93 to 1–94
Secondary hypertrophic osteoarthropathy (HOA). *See* Osteoarthropathy, hypertrophic (HOA).
Seizures
    brain metastases vs., 5–41
    differential diagnosis, **5–16i**, 5–17 to 5–18
    evaluation, 5–16 to 5–21, **5–19i** to **5–21i**
    interictal, stroke vs., **5–10i**
    radiation necrosis vs., **5–44i**
Sentinel lymph node
    false negative, 2–6
    mapping, 2–4 to 2–7, **2–7i**
Septic arthritis
    non-infectious arthritis vs., **1–132i**, 1–133
    pediatric osteomyelitis vs., 1–67 to 1–68
    sickle cell osteopathy vs., 1–178
Septic hip, Legg-Calvé-Perthes disease vs., **1–108i**, 1–109
Seroma, intestinal neoplasms vs., **8–120i**, 8–121
Sesamoid fracture, foot osteomyelitis vs., **1–62i**
Shin splints
    melorheostosis vs., **1–92i**
    stress fractures vs., **1–128i**, 1–129
Shunts
    left-to-right shunts
        extracardiac, **3–36i**, 3–37
        intracardiac, 3–36 to 3–39
    peritoneal systemic shunt evaluation, 8–158 to 8–161, **8–161i**
    right-to-left intracardiac shunts, 3–38 to 3–39
    ventricular shunt dysfunction, 5–54 to 5–57, **5–57i**
Sickle cell disease
    amyloidosis vs., **1–168i**, 1–169
    bone pain due to, 1–176 to 1–179, **1–179i**
    with bone infarcts, neuroblastoma vs., **8–84i**, 8–85
Skeletal metastases. *See* Bone metastases.
Skeletal muscle disorders, 1–164 to 1–167, **1–167i**
Skeletally immature patient, normal, hematoproliferative disorders vs., 1–172
Skin
    contamination, sentinel lymph node vs., 2–6
    inflammation, melanoma therapy evaluation/restaging vs., **11–28i**
Slipped capital femoral epiphysis
    hip pain vs., 1–142
    Legg-Calvé-Perthes disease vs., 1–109
Small cell carcinoma of lung
    benign mimics of lymphoma vs., 11–4
    metastatic, neuroendocrine tumors of head and neck vs., 6–15
    post-therapy evaluation of lymphoma vs., 11–12
Soft tissue pathology
    stress fractures vs., 1–130
    vascular mass, wrist pain vs., 1–146
Soft tissue sarcoma. *See* Sarcoma.
Solitary (unicameral) bone cyst, 1–12 to 1–15, **1–15i**
    hip pain vs., 1–141
    wrist pain vs., 1–146
Solitary pulmonary nodule, 4–28 to 4–31, **4–31i**
Spine
    compression fractures, in elderly, prostatic bone metastases vs., **1–42i**
    insufficiency fractures, 1–118 to 1–123, **1–121** to **1–123i**
Spleen
    accessory and ectopic, 8–94 to 8–97, **8–97i**
        asplenia/polysplenia syndromes vs., **8–90i**, 8–91
        differential diagnosis, **8–94i**, 8–95
    metastatic disease, benign mimics of lymphoma vs., 11–4
    wandering, 8–91
Splenectomy, asplenia/polysplenia syndromes vs., **8–90i**, 8–91
Splenic disorders
    asplenia/polysplenia syndromes, 8–90 to 8–93, **8–93i**
    granulomatous, hypersplenism vs., 8–54
    hypersplenism, 8–52 to 8–55, **8–55i**
    infarct, intraabdominal infection vs., 8–146
    infection, hypersplenism vs., 8–54
    splenosis
        accessory and ectopic spleen vs., 8–95
        asplenia/polysplenia syndromes vs., **8–90i**, 8–91
Splenic impression, renal cortical scar vs., **9–2i**, 9–4

INDEX

Splenic neoplasms, primary, hypersplenism vs., 8–54
Splenic sequestration and RBC survival, 10–12 to 10–13
Squamous cell carcinoma
  head and neck
    neuroendocrine tumors of head and neck vs., **6–14i**, 6–15
    primary unknown, 6–6 to 6–7
    staging, 6–2 to 6–5, **6–5i**
    therapeutic assessment/restaging, 6–8 to 6–11, **6–11i**
  lung. *See* Non-small cell lung cancer.
Status epilepticus
  brain infection and inflammation vs., **5–70i**, 5–71
  seizure vs., 5–17
Stomach disorders. *See Gastric* entries.
Stress fractures, 1–128 to 1–131, **1–131i**. *See also* Insufficiency fractures.
  calcaneal pain vs., 1–151
  differential diagnosis, **1–128i**, 1–129 to 1–130
  Ewing sarcoma vs., **1–34i**, 1–36
  fibrous cortical defect vs., **1–8i**
  fibrous dysplasia vs., **1–90i**
  hip pain vs., **1–140i**
  hypertrophic osteoarthropathy vs., **1–80i**, 1–81
  knee pain vs., 1–156
  melorheostosis vs., 1–93
  osteoid osteoma vs., 1–3
  osteomalacia vs., **1–76i**, 1–77
  osteonecrosis vs., **1–104i**, 1–105
  periprosthetic, painful joint prosthesis vs., 1–111
Stroke. *See* Cerebral vascular occlusion.
Subacute thyroiditis. *See* Thyroiditis, subacute.
Subcortical arteriosclerotic encephalopathy, normal pressure hydrocephalus vs., 5–60
Subependymal tumors, heterotopic gray matter vs., **5–64i**, 5–65
Substance abuse, 5–75
Subtalar synovitis, calcaneal pain vs., 1–152
Superior vena cava syndrome, focal nodular hyperplasia vs., 8–44
Superscan, bone, 1–24 to 1–27, **1–27i**
Surgery, postoperative inflammation, primary breast cancer vs., **11–34i**, 11–35
Surgical assessment, 1–110 to 1–117
  failed back surgery syndrome, 1–112 to 1–117, **1–115i** to **1–117i**
  painful joint prosthesis, 1–110 to 1–111
Surgical incision
  carcinoid tumor vs., **8–150i**
  uninfected, intraabdominal infection vs., 8–146
Synovial sarcoma, heterotopic ossification vs., 1–159
Synovitis
  hip pain vs., 1–141
  painful joint prosthesis vs., 1–111
  subtalar, calcaneal pain vs., 1–152
  toxic
    Legg-Calvé-Perthes disease vs., 1–109
    pediatric osteomyelitis vs., 1–68
  wrist pain vs., 1–145

T

Takayasu arteritis. *See* Large vessel vasculitis.
Tamoxifen-related endometrial changes, endometrial cancer vs., 9–73
Tarsal coalition, calcaneal pain vs., 1–152
Tears, overproduction, lacrimal complex dysfunction vs., 6–19
Temporal arteritis. *See* Large vessel vasculitis.
Temporal bone osteomyelitis, 1–60 to 1–61
Temporal lobe epilepsy. *See* Seizures.
Tendinitis, wrist pain vs., 1–145
Testicular appendage, torsion of, testicular torsion vs., 9–53
Testicular neoplasms, 9–56 to 9–59, **9–59i**
  differential diagnosis, **9–56i**, 9–57 to 9–58
  testicular torsion vs., 9–54
Testicular torsion, 9–52 to 9–55, **9–55i**
Testis
  abscess, testicular torsion vs., 9–53
  atrophy, testicular torsion vs., **9–52i**, 9–53
  normal activity, testicular cancer vs., **9–56i**
  scar formation, testicular cancer vs., **9–56i**
  segmental infarct, testicular cancer vs., 9–58
  testicular torsion vs., **9–52i**, 9–53
  trauma, testicular torsion vs., 9–54
  undescended, testicular torsion vs., 9–53
Thoracic/extrathoracic malignancy
  benign mimics of lymphoma vs., 11–4
  post-therapy evaluation of lymphoma vs., 11–12
Thoracolumbar tube, ventricular shunt dysfunction and, **5–54i**, 5–56
Thrombophlebitis, pediatric osteomyelitis vs., 1–68
Thrombosis, 2–14 to 2–15
  deep venous
    heterotopic ossification vs., 1–159
    lymphedema vs., **2–2i**
  differential diagnosis, **2–14i**, 2–15
  large vessel vasculitis vs., **2–8i**, **2–14i**, 2–15
  radial/ulnar artery, wrist pain vs., 1–146
  renal vein, obstructive uropathy vs., 9–42
  vascular graft infection vs., **2–16i**, 2–17
Thymolipoma, thymus disorder vs., 4–47
Thymoma, ectopic parathyroid adenoma vs., 7–11
Thymus
  cystic, thymus disorder vs., 4–47
  disorders
    differential diagnosis, **4–46i**, 4–47 to 4–48
    evaluation of, 4–46 to 4–49, **4–49i**

INDEX

non-Hodgkin lymphoma staging vs., **11–20i**
normal
    granulomatous disease vs., **4–24i**
    testicular cancer vs., **9–56i**
post-chemotherapy rebound, benign mimics of lymphoma vs., **11–2i**
post-therapy evaluation of lymphoma vs., **11–10i**
primary neoplasms, thymus disorder vs., 4–47
well-differentiated thyroid cancer vs., **7–48i**, 7–50
Thyroglossal duct cyst, ectopic thyroid gland vs., **7–36i**, 7–37
Thyroid acropachy
    hypertrophic osteoarthropathy vs., 1–81
    paraneoplastic disorders vs., 11–50
Thyroid adenoma. *See also* Parathyroid adenoma; Thyroid neoplasms.
    follicular, medullary thyroid cancer vs., 7–63
    hyperfunctioning, 7–24 to 7–27, **7–27i**
    parathyroid adenoma vs., **7–6i**, 7–7
    toxic
        Graves disease vs., **7–12i**, 7–13
        subacute thyroiditis vs., **7–28i**, 7–29
    toxic or autonomous, multinodular goiter vs., **7–20i**, 7–21
Thyroid disorders, 7–2 to 7–65
    benign
        parathyroid adenoma vs., 7–7
        PET studies, 7–44 to 7–47, **7–47i**
        PET studies of well-differentiated thyroid cancer vs., 7–59
    goiter. *See* Goiter.
    hypothyroidism. *See* Hypothyroidism.
    I-131 hyperthyroid therapy, 7–32 to 7–35, **7–35i**
    infiltrative, subacute thyroiditis vs., 7–29
    neoplasms. *See* Thyroid neoplasms.
    thyroiditis. *See* Thyroiditis.
Thyroid gland
    agenesis or hypoplasia, congenital hypothyroidism vs., 7–41
    dysgenesis, congenital hypothyroidism vs., 7–41
    ectopic, 7–36 to 7–39, **7–39i**
        congenital hypothyroidism vs., **7–40i**, 7–41
        differential diagnosis, **7–36i**, 7–37 to 7–38
        ectopic parathyroid adenoma vs., **7–10i**
    extrathyroidal structures, PET studies of well-differentiated thyroid cancer and, 7–59 to 7–60
    normal extrathyroidal, benign thyroid conditions vs., 7–45
    normal physiologic uptake, well-differentiated thyroid cancer vs., 7–49
    substernal, thymus disorder vs., 4–47
    trauma, subacute thyroiditis vs., 7–30
    unilobar agenesis, hyperfunctioning thyroid adenoma vs., 7–25
Thyroid hormone
    dyshormogenesis, congenital hypothyroidism vs., 7–41 to 7–42
    endogenous sources, Graves disease vs., 7–13
    exogenous sources, Graves disease vs., 7–13
Thyroid neoplasms. *See also* Parathyroid adenoma; Thyroid adenoma.
    anaplastic, benign thyroid conditions vs., **7–44i**, 7–45
    carcinoid tumor vs., **8–150i**
    ectopic parathyroid adenoma vs., 7–11
    hyperfunctioning thyroid adenoma vs., 7–25
    I-131 therapy, 7–54 to 7–57, **7–57i**
    invasive/infiltrative, Hashimoto thyroiditis vs., 7–17
    medullary, 7–62 to 7–65, **7–65i**
    metastatic
        benign thyroid conditions vs., 7–45
        squamous cell carcinoma of head and neck vs., 6–3
    multinodular goiter vs., 7–22
    well-differentiated, 7–48 to 7–53, **7–51i** to **7–53i**
        benign thyroid conditions vs., **7–44i**, 7–45
        differential diagnosis, **7–48i**, 7–49 to 7–50
        medullary thyroid cancer vs., **7–62i**, 7–63
        PET studies, 7–58 to 7–61, **7–61i**
            differential diagnosis, **7–58i**, 7–59 to 7–60
Thyroid scan
    Nuclear Regulatory Agency requirements, 7–3 to 7–4
    overview, 7–2 to 7–5, **7–5i**
Thyroiditis
    acute
        benign thyroid conditions vs., 7–45
        subacute thyroiditis vs., 7–29
    autoimmune, congenital hypothyroidism vs., 7–42
    Hashimoto. *See* Hashimoto thyroiditis.

INDEX

hyperthyroid autoimmune, Graves disease vs., 7–13
  subacute, 7–28 to 7–31, **7–31i**
    benign thyroid conditions vs., 7–45
    congenital hypothyroidism vs., **7–40i**
    differential diagnosis, **7–28i**, 7–29 to 7–30
    Graves disease vs., **7–12i**, 7–13
    hyperfunctioning thyroid adenoma vs., 7–25
    post-viral, multinodular goiter vs., 7–21
    recovering, Hashimoto thyroiditis vs., 7–17
Thyroiditis facticia
  Graves disease vs., 7–13
  subacute thyroiditis vs., 7–29
Tibial periostitis, stress fractures vs., 1–129
Tibialis posterior tendinitis, calcaneal pain vs., **1–150i**, 1–151
Tonsils
  non-Hodgkin lymphoma staging vs., **11–20i**
  PET studies of well-differentiated thyroid cancer and, 7–60
  reactive lymph nodes
    Hodgkin lymphoma staging vs., **11–6i**
    post-therapy evaluation of lymphoma vs., **11–10i**
Total parenteral nutrition, cholestasis due to, biliary atresia vs., **8–30i**, 8–31
Toxic exposure and multiple chemical sensitivity, 5–75
Toxic synovitis
  Legg-Calvé-Perthes disease vs., 1–109
  pediatric osteomyelitis vs., 1–68
Toxoplasmosis, primary CNS lymphoma vs., 5–37
Tracheostomy site
  benign thyroid conditions vs., 7–46
  PET studies of well-differentiated thyroid cancer and, **7–58i**
Transitional cell carcinoma, renal cell carcinoma vs., 9–23
Transplant rejection, cardiac, differential diagnosis, **3–32i**, 3–33
Trauma
  amyloidosis vs., **1–168i**, 1–169
  blood brain barrier disruption vs., **5–14i**, 5–15
  bone. *See* Bone trauma.
  breast cancer staging/restaging vs., 11–42
  multiple myeloma vs., **1–180i**
  non-accidental, 1–126 to 1–127
  non-infectious arthritis vs., 1–133
  primary breast cancer vs., 11–35
  prostate cancer antibody scan vs., 9–77
  renal, pyelonephritis vs., 9–28
  testicular, testicular torsion vs., 9–54
Trochanteric bursitis, hip pain vs., 1–141
Tuberculosis
  adenocarcinoma of unknown primary vs., **11–46i**
  benign mimics of lymphoma vs., 11–3
  miliary, interstitial lung disease vs., 4–22
  post-therapy evaluation of lymphoma vs., 11–11
Tuberous sclerosis, heterotopic gray matter vs., 5–65
Tubo-ovarian abscess
  benign ovarian pathology vs., **9–60i**, 9–61
  ovarian cancer vs., 9–63
Tubular necrosis, acute
  obstructive uropathy vs., 9–42
  renovascular hypertension vs., **9–10i**
Tumoral calcinosis, heterotopic ossification vs., 1–160

U

Ulcerative colitis, intestinal neoplasms vs., **8–116i**, 8–117
Unicameral bone cyst. *See* Solitary (unicameral) bone cyst.
Ureter
  obstruction, renal transplant complication vs., **9–30i**
  visualization of, Meckel diverticulum vs., **8–122i**, 8–123
Ureteropelvic junction obstruction. *See* Uropathy, obstructive.
Urinary bladder
  epithelial cancer, 9–48 to 9–51, **9–51i**
  FDG activity, benign uterine activity vs., **9–66i**
  full, renal transplant complication vs., 9–32
  incontinence, bladder epithelial cancer vs., **9–48i**
  reflux, renal transplant complication vs., 9–32
  ventricular shunt dysfunction and, **5–54i**, 5–56
Urinary system. *See* Genitourinary system.
Urine contamination, cervical cancer vs., 9–69
Urine leak
  acute renal failure vs., 9–16
  renal mass vs., **9–20i**, 9–21
  renal transplant complication vs., **9–30i**
Uropathy
  obstructive, 9–40 to 9–43, **9–43i**
    differential diagnosis, **9–40i**, 9–42
    reflux uropathy vs., **9–44i**

INDEX

renovascular hypertension vs., **9–10i**
reflux, 9–44 to 9–47, **9–47i**
    fluoroscopic mimics, 9–45
    nuclear cystography mimics, 9–45
    obstructive uropathy vs., **9–40i**, 9–42
    sonographic mimics, 9–45
Uterine neoplasms
    endometrial cancer, 9–72 to 9–75, **9–75i**
    leiomyoma, endometrial cancer vs., **9–72i**, 9–73
    sarcoma, benign uterine activity vs., 9–67
Uterus
    normal and benign pathology, 9–66 to 9–67
    postpartum, endometrial cancer vs., **9–72i**

V

V/Q scan
    interpretation: modified PIOPED, 4–4
    overview, 4–2 to 4–5, **4–5i**
    pulmonary embolism, 4–6 to 4–9, **4–9i**
    quantitative, 4–10 to 4–15, **4–13i to 4–15i**
    radiopharmaceuticals, 4–2
    technique, 4–2 to 4–3
Valvular heart disease, 3–12 to 3–15, **3–15i**
Varicocele, testicular torsion vs., 9–54
Vascular and lymphatic systems, 2–2 to 2–21
Vascular dementia
    Alzheimer disease vs., **5–22i**, 5–23
    radiation necrosis vs., 5–46
Vascular disorders
    paraneoplastic disorders vs., 11–49, 11–50
    thrombosis. *See* Thrombosis.
Vascular grafts
    infected, 2–16 to 2–21, **2–19i to 2–21i**
        atherosclerosis vs., 2–12
        differential diagnosis, **2–16i**, 2–17
        vascular thrombosis vs., **2–14i**, 2–15
    large vessel vasculitis vs., **2–8i**
    normal
        atherosclerosis vs., **2–10i**, 2–12
        vascular graft infection vs., 2–17
Vasculitis
    complex regional pain syndrome vs., **1–136i**, 1–137
    inflammatory bowel disease vs., 8–131
    large vessel, 2–8 to 2–9
        atherosclerosis vs., **2–8i**, **2–10i**, 2–11
        differential diagnosis, **2–8i**, 2–8 to 2–9
    pulmonary embolism vs., **4–6i**, 4–8
    pyelonephritis vs., 9–28
    radiation necrosis vs., 5–46
Venous insufficiency, hypertrophic osteoarthropathy vs., **1–80i**, 1–81
Venous vascular malformations, ectopic thyroid gland vs., 7–37

Ventilation/Perfusion scan. *See* V/Q scan.
Ventricle (cardiac)
    aneurysm, valvular heart disease vs., **3–12i**, 3–13 to 3–14
    radionuclide ventriculography, 5–54 to 5–57, **5–57i**
    ventricular failure, valvular heart disease vs., 3–14
Ventricular shunt dysfunction, 5–54 to 5–57, **5–57i**
Ventriculoperitoneal shunt, peritoneal systemic shunt vs., **8–158i**, 8–159
Vertebrae
    discitis. *See* Discitis.
    discogenic sclerosis, axial osteomyelitis vs., 1–59
    insufficiency fracture, **1–118i**, 1–119
Vesicoureteral reflux. *See* Reflux uropathy.
Violence, 5–75
Viral infections
    benign mimics of lymphoma vs., 11–3
    low-grade non-Hodgkin lymphoma vs., **11–16i**
    post-therapy evaluation of lymphoma vs., 11–11
Vocal cord paralysis, PET studies of well-differentiated thyroid cancer and, **7–58i**, 7–60

W

Wandering spleen, 8–91
Warthin tumor, parotid and salivary tumors vs., 6–13
Wegener granulomatosis
    metastatic disease of lung and mediastinum vs., 4–40
    pneumocystis carinii pneumonia vs., 4–17
    solitary pulmonary nodule vs., **4–28i**, 4–30
Well-differentiated thyroid cancer. *See* Thyroid neoplasms, well-differentiated.
Whipple disease
    benign mimics of lymphoma vs., 11–3
    post-therapy evaluation of lymphoma vs., 11–11
Wrist pain, 1–144 to 1–149, **1–147i to 1–149i**

Y

Yttrium-90 microspheres, hepatic arterial, 10–4 to 10–7, **10–7i**

Z

Zellweger syndrome, heterotopic gray matter vs., 5–65